Water-Soluble Vitamins							Minerals						
Vitamin C (mg)	Thiamin (mg)	kibo-flavin (mg)	Niacin (mg NE)[#]	Vitamin B_6 (mg)	Folate (µg)	Vitamin B_{12} (µg)	Calcium (mg)	Phos-phorus (mg)	Mag-nesium (mg)	Iron (mg)	Zinc (mg)	Iodine (µg)	Sele-nium (µg)
30	0.3	0.4	5	0.3	25	0.3	400	300	40	6	5	40	10
35	0.4	0.5	6	0.6	35	0.5	600	500	60	10	5	50	15
40	0.7	0.8	9	1.0	50	0.7	800	800	80	10	10	70	20
45	0.9	1.1	12	1.1	75	1.0	800	800	120	10	10	90	20
45	1.0	1.2	13	1.4	100	1.4	800	800	170	10	10	120	30
50	1.3	1.5	17	1.7	150	2.0	1,200	1,200	270	12	15	150	40
60	1.5	1.8	20	2.0	200	2.0	1,200	1,200	400	12	15	150	50
60	1.5	1.7	19	2.0	200	2.0	1,200	1,200	350	10	15	150	70
60	1.5	1.7	19	2.0	200	2.0	800	800	350	10	15	150	70
60	1.2	1.4	15	2.0	200	2.0	800	800	350	10	15	150	70
50	1.1	1.3	15	1.4	150	2.0	1,200	1,200	280	15	12	150	45
60	1.1	1.3	15	1.5	180	2.0	1,200	1,200	300	15	12	150	50
60	1.1	1.3	15	1.6	180	2.0	1,200	1,200	280	15	12	150	55
60	1.1	1.3	15	1.6	180	2.0	800	800	280	15	12	150	55
60	1.0	1.2	13	1.6	180	2.0	800	800	280	10	12	150	55
70	1.5	1.6	17	2.2	400	2.2	1,200	1,200	320	30	15	175	65
95	1.6	1.8	20	2.1	280	2.6	1,200	1,200	355	15	19	200	75
90	1.6	1.7	20	2.1	260	2.6	1,200	1,200	340	15	16	200	75

[‡]Retinol equivalents. 1 retinol equivalent = 1 µg retinol or 6 µg β-carotene. See text for calculation of vitamin A activity of diets as retinol equivalents.

[§]As cholecalciferol. 10 µg cholecalciferol = 400 IU of vitamin D.

[‖] α-Tocopherol equivalents. 1mg d-α tocopherol = 1 α-TE. See text for variation in allowances and calculation of vitamin E activity of the diet as α-tocopheral equivalents.

[#]1 NE (niacin equivalent) is equal to 1 mg of niacin or 60 mg of dietary tryptophan.

Elements[†]			Electrolytes		
Chromium (mg)	Selenium (mg)	Molybdenum (mg)	Sodium (mg)	Potassium (mg)	Chloride (mg)
0.01–0.04	0.01–0.04	0.03–0.06	115–350	350–925	275–700
0.02–0.06	0.02–0.06	0.04–0.08	250–750	425–1275	400–1200
0.02–0.08	0.02–0.08	0.05–0.1	325–975	550–1650	500–1500
0.03–0.12	0.03–0.12	0.06–0.15	450–1350	775–2325	700–2100
0.05–0.2	0.05–0.2	0.1–0.3	600–1800	1000–3000	925–2775
0.05–0.2	0.05–0.2	0.15–0.5	900–2700	1525–4275	1400–4200
0.05–0.2	0.05–0.2	0.15–0.5	1100–3300	1875–5625	1700–5100

[†] Since the toxic levels for many trace elements may be only several times usual intakes, the upper levels for the trace elements in this table should not be habitually exceeded.

Source: Food and Nutrition Board, National Academy of Sciences—National Research Council, Washington, D.C., 1980.

NORMAL and
THERAPEUTIC NUTRITION

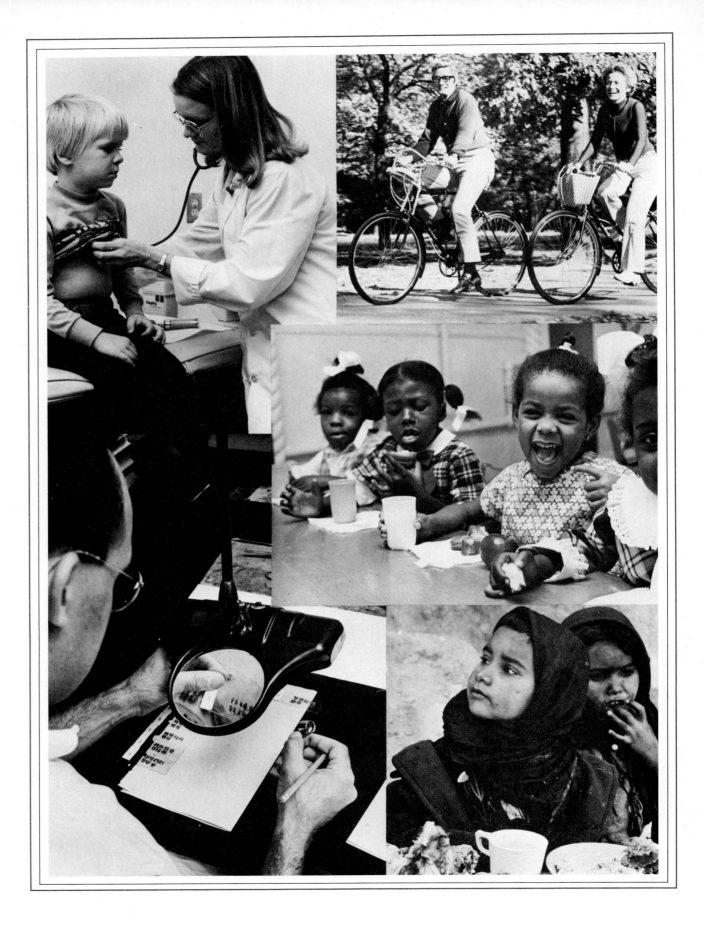

NORMAL and THERAPEUTIC NUTRITION

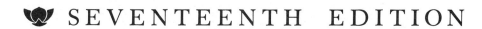 SEVENTEENTH EDITION

Corinne H. Robinson, M.S., D.Sc. (Hon.), R.D.

Professor of Nutrition Emeritus
Formerly Head, Department of Nutrition and Food
Drexel University
Philadelphia, Pennsylvania

Marilyn R. Lawler, M.S., Ph.D., R.D.

Director of Clinical Nutrition Services
Lecturer, Department of Medicine
University of Chicago Medical Center
Chicago, Illinois

Wanda L. Chenoweth, M.S., Ph.D., R.D.

Professor
Department of Food Science and Human Nutrition and
Department of Pediatrics
Michigan State University
East Lansing, Michigan

Ann E. Garwick, M.S., R.N.

Assistant Professor
Department of Nursing
Gustavus Adolphus College
St. Peter, Minnesota

Macmillan Publishing Company
NEW YORK

Collier Macmillan Canada
TORONTO

Maxwell Macmillan International
NEW YORK   OXFORD   SINGAPORE   SYDNEY

Earlier edition(s), entitled *Dietetics for Nurses* by Fairfax T. Proudfit copyright 1918, 1922, 1924, 1927 by Macmillan Publishing Co.,
Inc., copyright renewed 1946, 1950, 1952, 1955 by Fairfax T. Proudfit; *Nutrition and Diet Therapy* by Fairfax T. Proudfit copyright
1930, 1934, 1938, 1942 by Macmillan Publishing Co., Inc., copy-
right renewed 1958 by Fairfax T. Proudfit, 1962, 1966 by The First
National Bank of Memphis; *Nutrition and Diet Therapy* by Fair-
fax T. Proudfit and Corinne H. Robinson © 1961 by Macmillan
Publishing Co., Inc.; *Proudfit-Robinson's Normal and Therapeutic
Nutrition* by Corinne H. Robinson © copyright 1967 by Macmillan
Publishing Co., Inc.; *Normal and Therapeutic Nutrition* by Corinne
H. Robinson copyright © 1972 by Macmillan Publishing Co., Inc.;
Case Studies in Clinical Nutrition by Corinne H. Robinson, Mari-
lyn R. Lawler, and Ann E. Garwick, copyright © 1977 and 1982 by
Macmillan Publishing Co., Inc.; *Normal and Therapeutic Nutrition*
by Corinne H. Robinson and Marilyn R. Lawler © 1977 and 1982
by Macmillan Publishing Co., Inc.

Revised 1990 Printing with 1989 Recommended Daily Allowances.

MACMILLAN PUBLISHING COMPANY
866 Third Avenue • New York, N.Y. 10022

COLLIER MACMILLAN CANADA, INC.
1200 Eglinton Avenue, E.
Don Mills, Ontario M3C 3N1

Library of Congress Cataloging in Publication Data

Normal and therapeutic nutrition.

Rev. ed. of: Normal and therapeutic nutrition /
Corinne H. Robinson, Marilyn R. Lawler. 16th ed. c1982.
   Includes bibliographies and index.
   1. Diet therapy.   2. Nutrition.   3. Food—Composition
—Tables.   I. Robinson, Corinne H. (Corinne Hogden)
[DNLM: 1. Diet Therapy.   2. Nutrition. WB 400 N842]
RM216.N76   1986   613.2   86–157
ISBN 0-02–402605-0

Printing: 1 2 3 4 5 6 7   Year: 1 2 3 4 5 6 7

PREFACE

This revised 1980 printing includes the 1989 Recommended Dietary Allowances throughout.

Public interest in nutrition is more evident today than ever before. This presents health care professionals with unprecedented opportunities to provide nutrition services, nutrition education, and dietary counseling. The 17th edition extends the tradition of excellence established in previous editions to meet the needs of today's students in nursing, dietetics, and other health professions. It is also a useful reference for the practicing nurse, dietitian, dental hygienist, physician, and dentist. As in earlier editions, the objectives for this book are

to provide a background in the science of nutrition that individuals can use as the basis for making decisions for dietary planning for themselves or for others in any age group in health or in illness;

to show how the principles of nutrition may be integrated with the physiologic, cultural, and socioeconomic factors in the daily selection of meals:

to furnish guidelines for nutrition education, dietary counseling, and community nutrition services.

The concept of dietary balance to maintain or restore the best possible level of health is emphasized; that is, the diet must furnish sufficient energy and nutrients to meet the metabolic needs at all stages of the life cycle. On the other hand, the excesses that are believed to be risk factors in chronic disease ranging from dental caries to cardiovascular diseases are to be avoided. The issues and unresolved controversies that concern so many are highlighted in many of the chapters, and the reader is provided with information that can help him or her take a responsible position based upon current research.

New Content and Organization

Four new chapters are the result of expanding and reorganizing content:

Food Composition and Dietary Evaluation: Tools for Dietary Planning (Chapter 4)

Physical Fitness, Exercise, and Weight Control (Chapter 25)

Food, Nutrient, and Drug Interactions (Chapter 27)

Computer Applications in Clinical Nutrition (Chapter 44)

Reflecting our completely revised framework, the book is now divided into three parts. Part I, "Fundamentals of Nutrition Science," includes four chapters that provide an introduction to nutrition study and nine chapters on individual nutrients. Chapter 2 presents an overview of the processes of digestion and absorption together with an expanded discussion of gastrointestinal hormones and peptides. The Recommended Dietary Allowances and the Daily Food Guide are presented in Chapter 3. Also, four guidelines aimed to reduce the risks of cardiovascular diseases and cancer are compared. The new Chapter 4 brings together a discussion of food compostion, a calculation of a basic dietary pattern that is referred to throughout the text, the procedure for calculations using the Exchange Lists, and a discussion of the concept of nutrient density.

Newer findings related to digestion and absorption are described for protein (Chapter 5), fat (Chapter 7), zinc (Chapter 9), and vitamin B-12 (Chapter 13). The possible roles of fat (Chapter 7), selenium (Chapter 9), vitamin A (Chapter 11), and ascorbic acid (Chapter 12) in the etiology of cancer are discussed.

Other additions for Part I include protein supplements (Chapter 5); brown adipose tissue (Chapter 7), the possible role of calcium in hypertension (Chapter 9); neurologic disturbances associated with vitamin E deficiency (Chapter 12); possible toxicity of vitamin B-6 (Chapter 13); and carnitine (Chapter 13).

Part II, "Practical Applications of the Principles for Normal Nutrition," includes 12 chapters that pertain to dietary planning, food habits and cultural food patterns, food safety, meeting nutritional needs throughout the life cycle, nutritional assessment and dietary counseling, and prevailing nutrition problems in the United States and throughout the world.

Among the revisions in this part are the following: 1983 low-cost food plan (Chapter 14); revised discussion of mechanisms of hunger and appetite (Chapter 15); calculations for a lacto-ovo-vegetarian diet (Chapter 16); "fast foods," "junk foods," "organic/natural/health foods" (Chapter 16), herbal teas, food irradiation, ethylene dibromide (Chapter 17), and recently adopted standards for sodium and low-calorie labeling (Chapter 18).

In Chapters 19 through 22 increased emphasis is placed on nutritional assessment and nutritional status. Several topics such as anemia, obesity, underweight, and growth failure, formerly covered in the section on therapeutic nutrition, are now covered in the study of the life cycle. Alcoholism, smoking, and pica are identified as serious problems in pregnancy (Chapter 19); discussions of breast feeding, infant feeding problems, and feeding of low-birth-weight infants have been expanded (Chapter 20). Hyperactivity in children is included in Chapter 21 and osteoporosis in Chapter 22.

Methods of nutritional assessment and practical guidelines for dietary counseling are described in Chapter 23. The concepts for nutrition education recently developed by the Society for Nutrition Education are included in Chapter 24. A new chapter, "Physical Fitness, Exercise, and Weight Control," concludes Part II. This chapter presents guidelines for exercise programs to improve physical fitness and to aid in weight control, a critique of current height-weight tables, and discussion of several dietary approaches to weight control. The problem of underweight and the eating disorders anorexia nervosa and bulimia are discussed as well.

Part III, "Therapeutic Nutrition," includes 18 chapters in which the principles described in Parts I and II are applied in a variety of clinical situations. Chapter 26 presents an overview of the nutritional care process including assessment, intervention, documentation, and evaluation of nutritional care in the acute-care setting. Also included in this chapter are nutritional considerations for the physically handicapped and for those receiving care in the home, in nursing homes, or in mental hospitals.

Chapter 27, "Food, Nutrient, and Drug Interactions," describes specific ways in which selected prescription drugs or alcohol interfere with nutrient utilization and, conversely, ways in which foods or nutrients may interfere with the effectiveness of drug therapy. This new chapter lays the foundation for discussion in subsequent chapters on the nutritional effects of drugs in specific conditions.

Expanded coverage of the characteristics, composition, and use of enteral feeding formulas and paren-

teral nutrition is presented in Chapter 28. Chapters 29 through 32 describe dietary modifications used in the management of diseases involving the gastrointestinal tract, pancreas, and liver.

Chapters 33 and 34 are concerned with immunity and stress. New in this edition are a discussion of levels of stress, metabolic and nutritional considerations in stress, and nutritional management of the trauma patient and the critically ill.

Also new in Part III are a discussion of dietary factors implicated in the etiology of cancer and hospice care (Chapter 35) and of glycosylated hemoglobin, insulin pump therapy, and glycemic index (Chapter 36). Other additions include the American Heart Association Three-Phase approach to fat-modified diets and the Pritikin diet (Chapter 38); the role of various dietary factors in hypertension and nutrition following heart transplant (Chapter 39); nutritional considerations in chronic ambulatory peritoneal dialysis (Chapter 40); types of allergic reactions (Chapter 41); management of variant forms of phenylketonuria and homocystinuria (Chapter 42); and inflammatory bowel disease in children (Chapter 43).

Part III concludes with the new Chapter, 44, "Computer Applications in Clinical Nutrition." This chapter describes the use of computers in nutritional assessment, dietary counseling, and computer-assisted instruction.

The Appendix includes six tables on nutritive values in foods, twenty tables of standards for nutritional assessment, two tables of normal blood and urine constituents, and 1983 revisions of the Recommended Nutrient Intake for Canadians. New to this edition are Table A–6, a compilation of the nutritive values of fast foods, and Tables A–11 to A–14 providing additional NCHS measures of physical growth of children. Other tables include 1983 Metropolital Life standards for height and weight for adults, NHanes percentiles for triceps, arm circumference, and arm muscle circumference.

Contemporary Design and Format

We have enlarged the book in this edition for several reasons. Today's health care professionals are required to have more and more information at their command. Also, students and clinicians need the information arranged so that it can be easily found and understood, and so that learning will be reinforced. The seventeenth edition has been designed to use space economically while maximizing quick access to the multiple features offered. Color, illustrations, shading and other design features have been carefully planned to offer students an engaging learning experience, facilitating mastery of the content.

Learning Aids Within the Text

In response to faculty recommendations, new learning aids have been included and all learning aids are more highly emphasized in this edition.

Twenty-eight case studies have been added. Nine case studies pertain to normal nutrition throughout the life cycle and 19 case studies apply to a variety of pathologic conditions. Questions on pathophysiologic conditions, nutritional assessment, meal planning, and dietary counseling combine a review of text material, journal references, and the application of problem-solving techniques.

Current issues and controversies appear in shaded boxes. Background information is provided to help the student arrive at a responsible position.

Dietary counseling guidelines have been shaded within the text to foster application of nutrition education principles.

Meal plans for normal and therapeutic diets are boxed for a quick reference.

Review questions and problems conclude many chapters.

References indicate sources for further study.

Food, nutrient, and drug interactions are summarized in Appendix B.

A form for a dietary history and nutritional assessment appears in Appendix C.

An expanded glossary is provided to facilitate mastery of important terms introduced in the text. The correct pronunciation is indicated for each term.

Numerous tables and illustrations are located throughout the chapters and the appendix to emphasize key concepts and support clinical application.

Our Approach to the Teaching/ Learning Experience

Each of the four coauthors of this edition currently holds, or previously held, a teaching position in a college or university. In addition to extensive experience with basic students in nursing, dietetics, allied health and medicine, we have taught graduate students in those fields as well as non-majors with a general interest in nutrition.

To our teaching of future clinicians, and to the writing of this text, we bring years of practical wisdom acquired in our own clinical work. We have all experienced daily responsibility for nutritional services to patients in hospitals, including assessment, planning, implementation, and evaluation. We have all faced the challenges of teaching and counseling individual patients.

Our combined experiences encompass community settings as well as hospital-based practice. This text reflects our clinical work in home health services, programs for the elderly, and education for the lay public.

In addition to extensive classroom and clinical experience, all of us have conducted basic and applied research, publishing the results in numerous journal articles. This research orientation has helped us to evaluate objectively the many issues and controversies that persist in nutrition today.

As each page of this text was developed, we drew upon our experiences with students, our own clinical practice, and the latest scientific findings in the field. Our primary goals have been to provide students and instructors with a textbook that is a dynamic teaching/learning tool, to share what we have learned in an accessible and engaging style, and to provide a sound basis for practice and continued study in normal and therapeutic nutrition.

Acknowledgments

The authors express appreciation to the many faculty in dietetic and nursing schools who participated in a survey conducted by our publisher. The suggestions of the faculty were most helpful in planning for the seventeenth edition of this book. We are grateful to those who gave permission to use illustrations and quoted materials. These sources are cited at the points of use throughout the book.

We thank Dr. Darla E. Danford for her authoritative and timely chapter on "Computer Applications in Clinical Nutrition." Dr. Danford is staff officer, Committee on the Inter-American Conference on Food Protection, Food and Nutrition Board, National Research Council, National Academy of Sciences, Washington, D.C. Appreciation is also extended to Edna Kendall-Doss and Mary Schneider for their secretarial assistance.

Our editor, Carol Wolfe, has given many valuable suggestions for the format of the book, has been supportive throughout the preparation of the manuscript, and has skillfully guided the book throughout the various stages of production.

Corinne H. Robinson
Marilyn R. Lawler
Wanda L. Chenoweth
Ann E. Garwick

CONTENTS IN BRIEF

CONTENTS IN DETAIL

❧ PART II
Practical Applications of the Principles for Normal Nutrition   203

CASE STUDIES

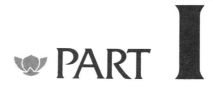

PART I

Fundamentals of Nutrition Science

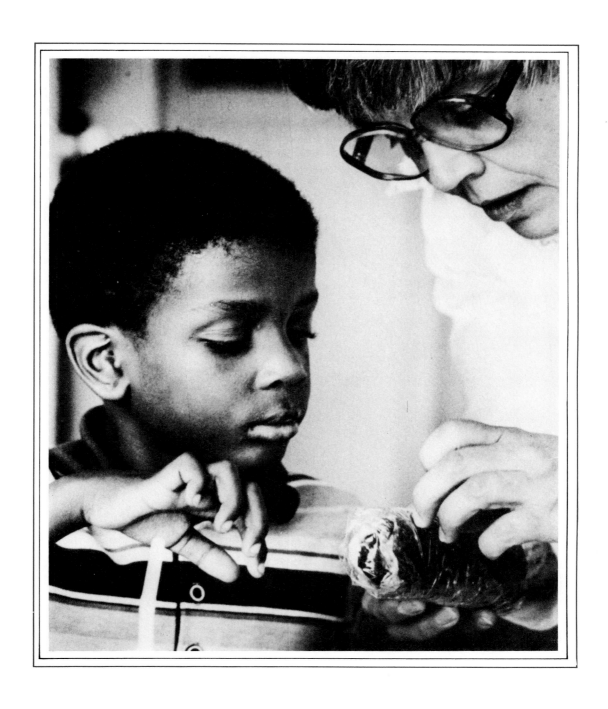

In Part I you will find the fundamentals of nutrition science. The facts and concepts presented here will become the basis of your future clinical decisions and interventions.

You are becoming a health care professional at a time when advances in nutrition represent one of the greatest achievements in public health in the 20th century. Classic nutritional deficiency diseases have been almost completely eliminated in the developed countries of the world and their incidence has been considerably reduced in the developing countries. Through applications of the science of nutrition the quality and years of life continue to improve for the worlds' people. Such progress has been possible because of knowledge gained through basic and applied research on animal models and human beings.

Continually expanding knowledge gained through research has established the need for some 50 or more nutrients. We know more than ever before about the roles that these nutrients play in growth, maintenance and regulation of the myriad activities occurring within the body, and reproduction; the ways in which these nutrients interact with one another; and the body's quantitative needs at various stages of the life cycle in widely different circumstances.

Parallel research in food science has led to knowledge about the nutrient composition of foods and the stability of nutrients under conditions of processing, storage, and preparation in the home and institution. Through agricultural sciences and food technology an unsurpassed abundance and variety of foods is available to the consumer.

During the last quarter century much public health emphasis in nutrition has been directed toward the role that diet plays as a risk factor in chronic diseases such as cancer and heart disease. Epidemiologic and clinical research have established a strong case for the relationships, and major public health organizations have promoted specific dietary guidelines for reducing the risks of disease. Controversies exist among health professionals as well as the public, and definitive answers may not be available for many years.

To the health professional is given the responsibility to translate the science of nutrition into food selection to meet the needs of clients at various stages of the life cycle in health and in illness. Health professionals are also expected to take positions on current issues and controversies that are based on a knowledge of nutrition science, and to adjust these positions as current issues are clarified through research.

1

Food, Nutrition, and Health

An Introduction

NUTRITION is "the science of foods, the nutrients and other substances therein; their action, interaction, and balance in relationship to health and disease; the processes by which the organism ingests, digests, absorbs, transports, and utilizes nutrients and disposes of their end products. In addition, nutrition must be concerned with social, economic, cultural, and psychological implications of food and eating."*

The Meanings of Food, Nutrition, and Nutritional Care

What Does Food Mean to You? Food—menu—diet—hunger—nutrition—malnutrition. What images do these words bring to your mind? Are they oriented to your physical senses? To your social enjoyment? To your concerns about your own well-being? To your emotions? Do they raise questions about the quality of life for your fellow human beings?

When you sit down to your next meal you will have definite ideas—positive or negative—about that meal and the specific foods that are served to you. Through your eyes you will delight in the texture variations and color combinations of the food, the artistic touch of a garnish, and the beautiful table appointments; or perhaps your interest will be diminished because the food lacks color and is carelessly served. Through your nose you will enjoy the tantalizing odors of meat or of freshly baked rolls, or the fragrance of fully ripened fruit; or possibly you will be repelled because of the odor of grease which is too hot or of vegetables which have been cooked too long. Through your sense of taste you will experience countless flavors—the salty,

sweet, bitter, and sour and their variations; you will feel the textures of smooth or fibrous, crisp or soft, creamy or oily, moist or dry foods.

But the experiences of your senses alone do not determine what your next meal, or any meal, means to you. Is the meal merely a way of staying alive and keeping in health? Is it an opportunity for fellowship with your family and friends; a way to celebrate an event; an occasion for stimulating conversation; a means of satisfying your feelings when you are hurt and depressed; a display of prestige by which you show that you can afford certain foods others cannot; a token of security and love; a concern because some foods might make you ill? Will you leisurely enjoy the meal; take it for granted as your right; consider it as a precious gift from God for which you are thankful? What other feelings are evoked by the food you eat?

Next to the air you breathe and the water you drink, food has been basic to your existence. In fact, food has been the primary concern of humankind in its physical environment throughout all recorded history. By food, or the lack of it, the destinies of individuals are greatly influenced. People must eat to live, and what they eat will affect in a high degree their ability to keep well, to work, to be happy, and to live long.

Some Important Definitions HEALTH is defined by the World Health Organization of the United Nations as the "state of complete physical, mental and social well-being and not merely the absence of disease or infirmity."*

NUTRIENTS are the constituents in food that must be supplied to the body in suitable amounts. These include water, proteins and the amino acids of which

---

* Robinson, W.D.: "Nutrition in Medical Education," in *Proceedings Western Hemisphere Nutrition Congress—1965*, American Medical Association, Chicago, 1966, p. 206.

* *World Health Organization—What It Is, What It Does, How It Works.* Leaflet, Geneva, Switzerland, 1956.

they are composed, fats and fatty acids, carbohydrates, minerals, and vitamins.

NUTRITIONAL STATUS is the condition of health of the individual as influenced by the utilization of the nutrients. It can be determined only by the correlation of information obtained through a careful medical and dietary history, a thorough physical examination, and appropriate laboratory investigations.

NUTRITIONAL CARE is "the application of the science and art of human nutrition in helping people select and obtain food for the primary purpose of nourishing their bodies in health or in disease throughout the life cycle. This participation may be in single or combined functions: in feeding groups involving food selection and management; in extending knowledge of food and nutrition principles; in teaching these principles for application according to particular situations; and in dietary counseling."*

MALNUTRITION is an impairment of health resulting from a deficiency, excess, or imbalance of nutrients. It includes UNDERNUTRITION, which refers to a deficiency of calories and/or one or more essential nutrients, and OVERNUTRITION, which is an excess of one or more nutrients and usually of calories.

The Science of Nutrition Observations concerning the relationship of food to health have been made throughout recorded history. Occasionally these observations have withstood scientific scrutiny. Others have persisted to this day although their validity has never been established. Knowledge concerning nutrition has its origin in research conducted by chemists, biochemists, microbiologists, molecular biologists, physiologists, pathologists, nutritionists, and others over approximately two centuries.

The science of nutrition had its beginnings during the late eighteenth century with the discovery of the respiratory gases and especially the studies on the nature and the quantification of energy metabolism by Lavoisier, a Frenchman often referred to as the Father of the Science of Nutrition. During the nineteenth century many chemists and physiologists added important information on the need for protein and some minerals such as calcium, phosphorus, and iron. Knowledge of vitamins has been gained in the twentieth century. Indeed, more knowledge concerning nutrition has been gained during this century than in all the preceding centuries combined.

The facts of nutrition are gained by applying the scientific method, that is, setting up an hypothesis,

* Committee on Goals of Education for Dietetics, Dietetic Internship Council: "Goals of the Lifetime Education of the Dietitian," *J. Am. Diet. Assoc.,* **54:**92, *1969.*

testing the hypothesis under carefully controlled conditions, observing the results, and interpreting them. The research may take place within the borders of a community or within the walls of a laboratory. Epidemiologic studies, surveys, and laboratory investigations are cited frequently in this book. A brief description of each of these will help the reader to understand the several ways by which knowledge of nutrition is obtained.

EPIDEMIOLOGY is the science of epidemic disease. Epidemiologic studies are based on observing the associations that exist between given environmental conditions and the incidence of disease conditions. For example, recent studies have shown that rural Africans who consume a large amount of fiber have a low incidence of gastrointestinal diseases such as diverticulitis and colon cancer. But in western European countries and the United States the incidence of these diseases is high and the fiber intake is low. These studies establish association, not cause! For example, one might also find that the low incidence of these diseases among rural Africans is associated with the presence of few automobiles, and their consequent pollution, or the scarcity of television sets, or the high rate of physical activity of these Africans! Although the epidemiologic study does not establish cause, it is valuable because it suggests hypotheses to be tested. Indeed, much research is now taking place under controlled conditions to determine whether fiber intake is related to gastrointestinal diseases.

Experimental Studies. Colleges, universities, the food industry, and government agencies such as the U.S. Department of Agriculture, the Food and Drug Administration, the National Institutes of Health, and others are engaged in a wide spectrum of research projects in nutrition. Much research is conducted directly on human beings with their informed consent. For example, under controlled conditions of diet, exercise, and weight maintenance the investigator might study the changes in the blood cholesterol of persons of a given age group when they consume high- or low-fiber diets. Or a carefully selected group of volunteers, often college or medical students, might participate in very exacting balance studies. In a balance study the diets consumed are rigidly controlled in kinds and amounts of foods, analyses are made of the diet for nutrient composition, fecal and urine excretions are collected and analyzed, and changes in blood composition are determined. Such balance studies require weeks or months of participation. Through such studies the requirements for specific nutrients have been determined.

For obvious reasons many types of studies preclude the use of human beings, so the researcher uses animal models. Rats are widely used because their life span is relatively short and they can be studied over the entire life cycle, they are omnivorous as are humans, they can be handled with relative ease, and the costs of studies with them are realistic. The results obtained from animal studies cannot always be directly applied to human beings, but they indicate the direction for further studies that will be appropriate on human beings.

Nutrition Surveys. The nutritive quality of diets consumed by a given population and the nutritional status of the people in the sample can be ascertained by using survey techniques. This approach also is used to evaluate the nutrition knowledge of a specific group or to determine factors such as attitudes and beliefs that may influence food selection. To illustrate, students in a nutrition course might conduct a survey to compare the breakfast habits of students living in a dormitory with those of students commuting to classes. Or they might survey the snacking habits of normal-weight and overweight students.

Nationwide surveys referred to frequently in this book include the Ten-State Nutrition Survey, 1968–70; the Survey of Preschool Children, 1968–70; the Health and Nutrition Examination Survey (HANES), 1971–72; and the National Food Consumption Survey, 1977–78.[1–4]

Good Nutrition: A Multidisciplinary Effort To meet the nutritional needs of the population of a nation requires a complex system involving many disciplines. Each step in the food chain must provide conditions that ensure retention of maximum nutritive values, safety, and quality. These requirements are met by (1) application of agricultural science and technology to produce sufficient amounts of animal and plant foods; (2) harvesting and transporting of foods to processors; (3) processing and packaging of foods; (4) adequate storage, transportation, and marketing facilities to make foods available at times and places where needed; (5) appropriate governmental controls to ensure wholesomeness and nutritive quality of the food supply; (6) economic conditions that make it possible to procure the necessary foods at a cost within the reach of all; (7) educational programs in nutrition within the schools and at the community level; and (8) efficient use of food within the home, public eating place, and institution.

The perspectives of nutrition held by each of the specialists who help ensure an adequate food supply obviously would be quite different. Thus, the disciplines of the life sciences, human behavior, economics, government, and communications are intertwined in nutrition study. The benefits of good nutrition—health, happiness, efficiency, and longevity—are sought by people all over the world. The achievement of these benefits is like a utopian dream to most of the world's people. (See Figure 1-1.)

Dietary Trends in the United States

Changes in Patterns of Living Since the beginning of this century the population of the United States has shifted from rural to urban areas. Most people must purchase all their foods, and even on the farm most families purchase a substantial proportion of the foods that they consume. Americans have the benefit of many labor-saving devices both in their occupations and in their homes. They work fewer hours per week, so that the way in which they spend their leisure may be decisive in determining their food needs. Leisure, to many people, means little activity—riding rather than walking, watching television rather than leading an active outdoor life, and so on.

Greater numbers of married women are working away from home than ever before, which means that less time is available for food preparation, more expensive prepared foods are used, and shopping is less frequent. Husbands, as well as wives, are shopping for and preparing foods; sometimes children, especially teenagers, are given too much freedom in their food choices. Increased numbers of women seeking to establish careers are postponing pregnancy and often are older than 30 years of age when their first child is born. At the same time, significant numbers of teenage girls, often unmarried, are experiencing the stresses of pregnancy before their own growth and development are complete.

The average American family of today has a higher income and is spending more of it for food. With this higher income, more meals are eaten in restaurants. The growth of the fast-food industry during the past decade has been phenomenal. These restaurants appeal not only to teenagers but to many families who can no longer afford to eat in traditional restaurants. More workers are eating in cafeterias at their place of work rather than carrying lunches, and more children are participating in school breakfast and lunch programs. The family eats fewer meals together, and in far too many families some meals may be skipped by one or more persons. In a recent consumer survey nearly three quarters admitted skipping meals. Of

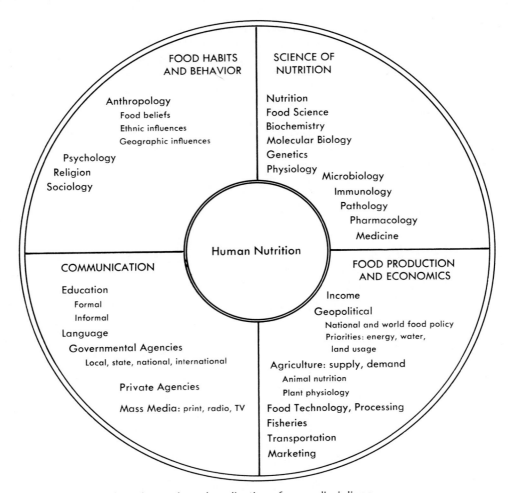

Figure 1-1. Human nutrition involves the study and application of many disciplines.

these, approximately 62 percent were women; 24 percent, men; and 16 percent, children. Breakfast was skipped by 62 percent, lunch by 26 percent and dinner by 7 percent.[5]

The scientific and technologic advances reach into every aspect of daily life, including the quantity, quality, variety, and attractiveness of the foods we eat. Fewer foods are produced in the home from basic ingredients. Frozen foods including complete meals, baked foods of all kinds, mixes, and snacks are commonplace among the 10,000 or so items in a supermarket. An increasing number of fabricated foods are replacing conventional foods. The number of brands and the variety are so great that the shopper finds it difficult indeed to make wise selections.

Social changes often have an adverse effect on nutrition: the large number of young as well as elderly persons living alone; the increasing proportion of older people; long periods of unemployment; the breakup of families by divorce or death with the at-

tendant emotional turmoil and also the dual role that must be assumed in maintenance of the home and the supply of the income; and the high incidence of alcoholism and drug addiction.

The Changing American Diet Major changes have taken place in the American diet during the present century. One way to review these changes is to look at the nutrient values of the food supply available for consumption each year. The U.S. Department of Agriculture keeps such records annually. (See Figures 1-2, 1-3, and 1-4.)

Since the beginning of this century, protein in the available food supply has varied within a range of about 15 g. By contrast, the source of protein has changed considerably, with animal foods supplying about one half the total available protein in 1909 compared with about two thirds of the total protein today.[6] The increasing consumption of meat, especially beef and poultry, together with a substantial decrease

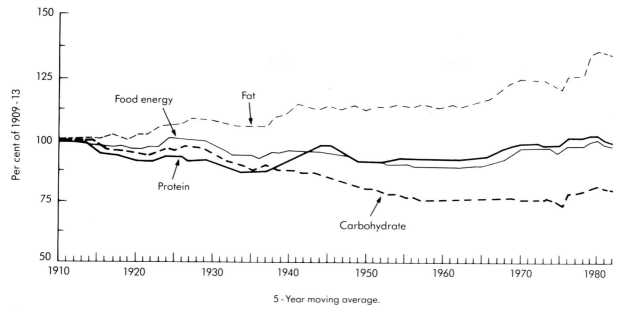

5 - Year moving average.

Figure 1-2. Since the beginning of the century, there has been a decrease in the consumption of carbohydrate by about one fourth and an increase in fat consumption by about one fourth. (Courtesy, U.S. Department of Agriculture.)

in the consumption of grain foods accounts for this shift in the proportion of animal to plant foods. With increasing affluence Americans and people of other countries consume more animal protein foods and less plant protein foods.

In 1909 carbohydrates represented 56 percent of the total available calories and now account for about 46 percent of the food energy.[7] The consumption of grain foods is about half as high as it was at beginning of the century, while the amount of available sweeteners, primarily sucrose and corn syrups, has increased by approximately one half. In 1980 sweeteners accounted for about 17 percent of total available calories.

Figure 1-3. Per-capita consumption of selected livestock products since 1967. Note the marked increase in poultry consumption and the decline in egg consumption. (Courtesy, U.S. Department of Agriculture.)

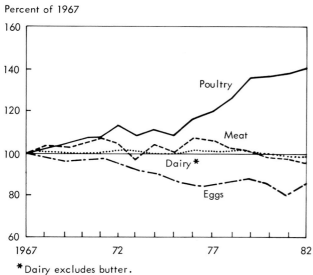

Percent of 1967

*Dairy excludes butter.

Figure 1-4. Per-capita consumption of selected crop products. More fruits, vegetables, and sugars and sweeteners has resulted from the greater use of corn sugars and syrups. (Courtesy, U.S. Department of Agriculture.)

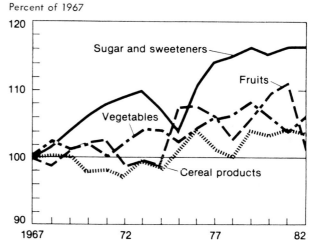

Percent of 1967

Vegetables exclude potatoes, peas, beans, and melons.

The level of total fat in the food supply increased about 30 percent since 1909. It is now at 162 g per capita.[6] Fats and oils, including butter, supply about one fifth of total available calories. Margarine and butter supply some vitamin A, and most vegetable oils are good sources of linoleic acid and vitamin E. Except for these nutrient contributions, fats are poor contributors to the nutritive value of the diet. Thus, sugars and fats and oils together account for more than one third of the available calories in the food supply.

National Food Consumption Survey   Since 1936 the U.S. Department of Agriculture has conducted surveys of food consumption at approximately 10-year intervals. The most recent nationwide survey was conducted in 1977–78. It included a survey of foods brought into the home and also the food intake by individuals in the various age–sex categories. Among the preliminary findings are these [4,8–11]:

1. Of the people questioned in this survey, 3 percent of the entire population but 9 percent of the lowest income group said they "sometimes or often did not have enough to eat." Translated in terms of the U.S. population this represents several million people.[4]
2. About 24 percent of the food dollar was spent away from home, compared with 17 percent in 1965. This increase is attributed to more women working away from home, higher income, and greater access to fast-food restaurants. People with higher incomes ate more meals away from home than did those with the lowest income.[4]
3. Diets of people in the lowest income group had improved the most. There was less difference in adequacy of the diet between persons in the several income categories than in 1965. The food assistance programs probably were significant factors in this improvement.[4,9]
4. When compared with 1965, there was an increased intake of meat, poultry, and fish; fruits; soft drinks; and alcoholic beverages. The intake declined for milk, cream, and cheese; grain products; vegetables; eggs, legumes, and nuts; and sugar, syrup, jelly, and candy.[4]
5. Although the energy value of the available food supply is about 3,500 kcal, the caloric value of food actually brought into the household was 2,900 kcal, and the actual intake was 1,800 to 1,900 kcal. Hegsted[8] raises these questions: Where does all the extra food go? Is it wasted?

6. For all age categories, the average protein intake exceeded the recommended allowances. (See Table inside front cover.) Although the average intake of all vegetables declined, the consumption of dark green vegetables increased, thus improving the vitamin A intake. The consumption of grain products had decreased, but more universal enrichment of all grain foods together with higher fortification levels resulted in improvement of the intake of B-complex vitamins. Ascorbic acid intake was 35 percent higher than in 1965 owing to increased consumption of citrus fruits and fortified fruit drinks and ades.[9,10] The calcium intake declined by 4 percent. The average intake for females over 12 years was about 25 percent below the recommended allowances. Iron intakes of women aged 12 to 50 years were 35 to 40 percent below recommended allowances, and magnesium intakes of this group were about 30 percent below allowances.[9,10]
7. According to Hegsted, the intakes of vitamin B-6, magnesium, iron, and zinc should be watched more closely. He also indicated that the survey shows that the major problem is one of overconsumption—of calories, fat, cholesterol, sugars, salt, and alcohol.[8]

Nutritional Problems in the United States

Public Concerns about Nutrition   In recent years the American public has shown increasing interest and concern about food supplies and nutritional needs. This has come about through dramatic, often exaggerated presentations of newscasts, documentaries, and advertising on radio and television and in the print media. Nutritional terms such as protein, saturated and polyunsaturated fats, cholesterol, minerals, and vitamins are familiar, although there are many misconceptions concerning them. This interest provides an excellent opportunity for nutrition education. It also places a responsibility on the professional person in nutrition to provide a sound informational basis for judging the safety of the food supply and for meeting community and world food needs.

What are some of these concerns? For some people the major issues center around possible disruptions in the ecologic balance. They believe that there is excessive use of pesticides that may harm plant and animal life and of additives in food processing. They respond to this concern by selecting foods grown on soils fertilized by manures and without use of pesticides or chemical fertilizers; they also avoid foods to which additives have been included in food processing. These concerns are often exaggerated, as later discussions in the text will show. (See Chapter 17.)

In developing countries people consume an average of 400 pounds of grains per capita annually. In the United States, Canada, and western Europe about 1,500 to 2,000 pounds of grains are consumed per capita, but most of this is fed to animals that are in turn used for food. Most of the world's people consume diets that contain very little animal protein and manage to maintain health when the plant food supply is varied and abundant. Various forms of vegetarianism have been adopted by significant numbers of Americans in the belief that such diets are more healthful and that they represent a more efficient use of world resources, since the food is eaten directly rather than consumed by animals first. Some forms of vegetarianism are nutritionally satisfactory; others are not. (See Chapter 16.)

As people approach middle age they are more likely to question whether the present American diet poses health risks. They are constantly reminded through advertising that some products may reduce one's blood cholesterol and thus lower the risk of cardiovascular disease. More recently the role of diet in prevention of cancer has been emphasized through communications media.

Nutritional Problems   An analysis of recent surveys of nutritional status has identified the following problems[1-3,11-13]:

1. Some people at all socioeconomic levels fail to obtain a nutritionally satisfactory diet. People at the lowest income level spend as much as 40 percent of their income for food—yet they remain the most vulnerable. They often have limited access to food, as on Indian reservations, in Appalachia, or in ghetto sections of large cities. Lack of knowledge is a further contributing factor.
2. Infant mortality has decreased since the beginning of the century to the present rate of 10.5 per 1,000 live births for whites, which is comparable to the rate found in western European countries. The rate for blacks, however, is twice as high—20.0 per 1,000 live births. Two thirds of all babies who die have low birth weights. The rate is higher for infants born to young women in their teens who are also poor.
3. Anemia occurs frequently in all age categories and

is especially prevalent in children under 6 years. The incidence is twice as high in persons below the poverty level.
4. Dental problems affect about nine of every ten persons. These include decayed teeth, missing teeth, and periodontal disease. One in five persons has severe periodontal disease, and one of every six persons over 10 years has trouble in biting or chewing.
5. Retarded growth and retarded bone development have been observed in some children 1 to 3 years of age. Protein-energy malnutrition has occasionally been found.
6. Chronic illness is a fact of life for the elderly; about 80 percent have some chronic condition. Low income, poor nutrition and social isolation are contributing factors.

Problems of Nutrient Excesses   Many Americans consume diets that are excessively high in calories, saturated fat, cholesterol, and sugars, and that are also excessively refined. All these excesses are believed to increase the risk of chronic diseases. It must be remembered, however, that other factors relate to the incidence of chronic diseases as well:

1. Excessive caloric intake leads to obesity, which is highly prevalent in the American population, and which is associated with chronic diseases such as diabetes mellitus, gallbladder disease, gout, cardiovascular diseases and cancer.
2. Excessive intake of fats and sugars that are practically devoid of minerals, vitamins, and proteins may result in suboptimal intakes of these essential nutrients. This imbalance may lead to some of the deficiencies described previously.
3. Excessive intakes of saturated fats and cholesterol are believed by many clinicians to be among the important risk factors in the incidence of cardiovascular and cerebrovascular diseases. (See Chapter 38.)
4. Excessive and frequent intake of sugars contributes to an increase in dental caries.
5. Excessive intake of salt has been associated with hypertension.
6. Excessive use of refined foods low in dietary fiber, on the basis of epidemiologic studies, is believed to increase the incidence of gastrointestinal disorders such as diverticulosis, irritable colon, and possibly colon cancer. (See Chapter 30.)
7. Excessive intakes of vitamins A and D are known to be toxic. (See Chapter 11.)

Global Problems in Nutrition

Scope of Malnutrition   Throughout history most of the world's people have been engaged in a struggle for food. The magnitude of the hunger problem, however, has never been greater than now. There are no completely reliable statistics on hunger, but according to one estimate approximately 12.5 percent of the world population, or one half billion people, do not receive close to an adequate quantity of food.[14] Furthermore, possibly one half the world's people are marginally fed, being caught up in a relentless sequence of ignorance, poverty, malnutrition, disease, and early death. It has been stated that one of every four children dies before age 5, most as the result of malnutrition.[15]

A major social factor contributing to world hunger is growth in population. Although new methods of contraception and family planning have been promoted, populations continue to increase except in a select group of countries.[14,16] Serious impediments to success include the need for children who will sustain their parents when they are old, the need for child labor in the fields, and religious beliefs.

The lack of success in population control has been partially offset by a rather dramatic increase in world food production since 1950, so that the overall per-capita food production has improved. However, food conditions vary widely among countries and even within countries. Whereas a greatly improved food situation may be true for some people, others may be much worse off. In contrast to the improvements occurring in Latin American and East Asia, per-capita food production in Africa has actually decreased. This decrease in combination with persistent and widespread drought have led to extreme conditions of hunger, starvation, and death in certain areas—a situation with no immediate or easy solution.

The energy crisis experienced throughout the world also directly affects the food supply. Energy is required for the production of fertilizers, to run farm machinery, to transport foods, and to process foods. Short supplies of energy together with high costs of energy have affected the poor countries most severely.

The first need is for sufficient food to meet the energy requirements of the population. Qualitatively, the next need is for sufficient protein to supply the amino acids used to build and maintain body structures.

Protein-energy malnutrition is the single greatest world problem in nutrition. In its severe forms, kwashiorkor and marasmus, it affects millions of preschool children. Those children who survive may be physically and mentally retarded—perhaps irreversibly. (See Chapter 24.)

Anemia (especially in mothers and young children), blindness resulting from vitamin A deficiency, and riboflavin deficiency are especially frequent. Rickets, scurvy, pellagra, beriberi, and endemic goiter occur in severe forms in some parts of the world. The characteristics of these deficiencies will be described in the chapters related to the specific nutrients involved.

Responsibility for World Nutrition   No thinking man or woman can afford to avoid the fact that so many of the world's people simply do not have enough to eat, nor can he or she, even in self-interest, evade the responsibility for alleviating hunger. In chronic starvation lie the frustration, tension, and envy of masses of people who will ultimately resort to violence.

World peace cannot be guaranteed by supplying adequate food alone, but one road to world peace is surely through a better-fed world population. Beyond this, charity and brotherhood are at the root of the Judeo-Christian religions and indeed of all ethical systems, and to practice them should be on the conscience of mankind.

A number of groups under the United Nations are directly concerned with global problems of nutrition, namely the Food and Agriculture Organization (FAO); World Health Organization (WHO); United Nations Children's Fund (UNICEF); and United Nations Educational, Scientific and Cultural Organization (UNESCO). (See Chapter 24.) Efforts of the United States to alleviate world hunger have been in the form of food aid, help to developing countries to improve their economic condition, and promotion of sound world agricultural policies.[15]

Achieving Nutritional Balance

Nutritional Balance   From the preceding discussion it becomes evident that the concept of nutritional balance is important. A good diet must fulfill these criteria: (1) it must furnish the appropriate levels of all nutrients to meet the physiologic and biochemical needs of the body at all stages of the life cycle; and (2) it must avoid the excesses of calories, fat, sugar, salt, and alcohol associated with increased risk of diet-related diseases. Giving more attention to avoiding excesses does not mean that one gives less attention to dietary adequacy. The key words in achieving the two criteria are *moderation* and *prudence*. (See Figure 1-5.)

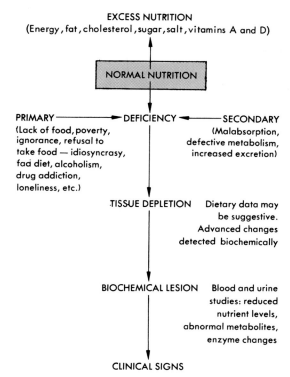

EXCESS NUTRITION
(Energy, fat, cholesterol, sugar, salt, vitamins A and D)

NORMAL NUTRITION

PRIMARY ─────────→ DEFICIENCY ◄─────── SECONDARY
(Lack of food, poverty,   (Malabsorption,
ignorance, refusal to   defective metabolism,
take food — idiosyncrasy,   increased excretion)
fad diet, alcoholism,
drug addiction,
loneliness, etc.)

TISSUE DEPLETION   Dietary data may
be suggestive.
Advanced changes
detected biochemically

BIOCHEMICAL LESION   Blood and urine
studies: reduced
nutrient levels,
abnormal metabolites,
enzyme changes

CLINICAL SIGNS

Figure 1-5.   Normal nutrition implies a balance that avoids deficiency of intake, on one hand, and excessive intake, on the other.

Nutrition and Disease Prevention   Traditionally, health care has been concerned primarily with healing the sick and helping them maintain health. Today prevention is described as a "unifying theme" among public health professionals, consumers, employers, workers, physicians, nurses, nutritionists, legislators, and policy makers.[12] Of 10 health problems that have been given high priority for prevention research, five are related in some degree to nutrition: alcohol-related problems; cancers of medium and high prevalence; cardiovascular disease; dental disease; and infant mortality.[17]

The preventive measures described in this book are related to nutrition. However, it must be emphasized that the etiology of chronic disease is complex and that there are many other risk factors such as cigarette smoking, alcohol and drug abuse, stress, lack of exercise, heredity, poverty, age, sex, and occupation. One cannot change one's heredity, age, or sex, but one can control most of the environmental factors.

In assessing the value of preventive measures one must differentiate between that which has been proven and that for which final proof is not yet available. To illustrate, the following measures are of

proven value: the adequate intake of specific vitamins to prevent scurvy, pellagra, beriberi, rickets, and other deficiency diseases; adequate prenatal diets to reduce infant mortality; iodinization of salt to prevent endemic goiter; fluoridation of water supplies to reduce dental decay; and many others.

There is much evidence to support some widely recommended measures, but final proof is not yet forthcoming. Thus, lowering the intake of saturated fat and cholesterol is associated with a lower serum cholesterol, but not everyone agrees that there is proof of less frequent premature heart attacks. High salt intake is associated with hypertension, but it has not been proven that reducing salt intake over the life span will reduce the occurrence of hypertension.

Since moderation of fat, cholesterol, and salt intake carries no health risks, and since a reduced intake of fats and sugars is likely to improve the nutrient quality of the diet, it seems prudent to adopt such measures even though final proof is not yet available. Indeed, it seems irresponsible to wait for final proofs or to wait for disease signs to appear before making any modifications in diet.

The case for prevention of breast and colon cancer by changes in diet is on much more tenuous grounds. Epidemiologic studies have shown an association between lack of dietary fiber and colon cancer and between a high fat intake and breast cancer. Much research will be required before these relationships can be proven. Although an increase in fiber intake and a reduction in fat intake is prudent, the health professional should be cautious about making firm claims when evidence is still lacking.

Nutrition Issues and Research Priorities   At every level of government, food and nutrition are important issues. Legislation imposes controls on food production, marketing, distribution, safety, and assistance to the needy of this nation and to food-deficit countries. Nutritional guidelines have been developed by governmental and voluntary agencies. (See Chapter 3.) Many chapters in this book identify important issues that concern the consumer and the health professional.

Research workers throughout the world are continually adding to nutrition knowledge. But there is urgent need to extend knowledge by basic and applied research. The Joint Subcommittee on Human Nutrition Research, representing federal agencies responsible for human nutrition research, identified the following goals for human nutrition research in the 1980s:

1. Determine the food and nutritional needs for maintaining health throughout the life cycle and for preventing and treating diseases, particularly chronic degenerative diseases.
2. Improve the assessment of dietary intake and nutritional status, as well as monitoring of populations.
3. Elucidate the interactions of nutrients with each other and with other ingested substances (including drugs and alcohol), and improve the methods for determination of nutrient toxicity.
4. Improve our understanding of the safety, quality, and nutritional value of foods, diets, and the national food supply.
5. Expand research training and research manpower development in the biomedical and behavioral aspects of nutrition and in food sciences.
6. Develop programs in nutrition education for professionals and expand the programs in nutrition education research and nutrition education and information for the public.
7. Expand international collaborative research efforts with both developed and less developed countries. *

Some Objectives in the Study of Nutrition

You bring to the study of nutrition your lifetime experience with food that may serve you well in further improving your nutritional status and the nutritional health of others. But you also may have misconceptions and strong feelings about food that will require much effort and perseverance on your part in order to change your attitudes and motivations. As you enter upon this study it is a good idea for you to examine carefully your present feelings about food, as well as your current knowledge of nutrition, so that you can build on what is good in your dietary pattern and correct that which is undesirable.

Personal and Family Nutrition Regardless of one's future career plans, the study of nutrition should first be directed to oneself. Many young men and women today live alone and are solely responsible for their own nutritional well-being. Physical and mental health are essential assets to meet the exciting and sometimes arduous requirements of one's life work. Those who expect to help other people to achieve better health through nutrition must themselves be enthusiastic living examples of the benefits of the application of nutrition knowledge.

* *Joint Subcommittee on Human Nutrition Research, Federal Coordination Council on Science, Engineering, and Technology: "Federally-Supported Human Nutrition Research, Training, and Education: Update for the 1980s," Am. J. Clin. Nutr., (Suppl.) 34:981–1030, 1981.*

Nutrition education applied to the individual also reaches the family. This is especially important for young men and women as they establish their own families. In most families the wife and mother is still the principal decision maker concerning the family's food. She plans the menus, purchases the food, and prepares the meals. In some families men are assuming more responsibility for meal planning, food purchasing, and preparation. Thus, the prevailing attitudes and practices of both parents are significant in helping children form good food habits.

Professional Opportunities in Nutrition Professional people in any discipline related to health are engaged in activities related to education, prevention, and therapy.

Nutrition Education in Schools. Education of the population holds promise of long-range benefits to the greatest numbers. Teachers, nurses, nutritionists, dietitians, home economists, dentists, and physicians assume varying responsibilities for individual and group education. Preschool, elementary, and secondary schools afford the single best opportunity for helping the child to establish attitudes and practices concerning food selection that will lead to a more healthful, productive live. Nutrition education can be successfully initiated even in preschool and should continue as a planned curriculum until the twelfth grade if maximum effectiveness is to be achieved. It is the responsibility of elementary teachers as well as teachers of home economics, health, and physical education.

The school nurse, physician, and dentist have many opportunities to note defects in health that suggest the need for improved nutrition; they can influence children in changing their food habits, provide experiences in the classroom, and lend their support to school food service and nutrition education programs.

The school breakfasts and lunches demonstrate that good nutrition and good food are, in fact, partners. School dietitians serve as teachers and also as consultants to teachers.

Nutrition Programs for the Public. Voluntary and governmental agencies together with industry are accepting responsibility for nutrition programs. The focus of nutrition programs is on maintaining *wellness* by avoiding excesses as well as protecting against deficiencies. The researcher in nutrition and food sciences is equally at home in the laboratories of a food company, a university, a hospital, or in the public health field. Nutritionists, dietitians, and home economists, depending on their education and particular interests, are the experts who interpret a product for a company; develop new uses for a food; advise mothers and children concerning their diets in a clinic; serve as consultants to a public health team; supervise food service in a college dormitory, industrial cafeteria, or hospital; assist individuals and groups in dietary selection; and teach in nursing schools, colleges, and universities.

Nutrition and Health Care.   The concern of today's health worker is for the maintenance as well as the restoration of health. Traditionally, health care has been directed to the hospitalized patient. Today, health care includes the concept of continuity of care. Earlier discharge from hospitals is occurring because of government-mandated changes in rates for care of Medicare patients. Ambulatory services have also increased. The health worker soon learns that there must be concern for the patient who makes the transition from the hospital to the home. Home-based services during convalescence may need to increase because of earlier discharge. To implement continuity of care with respect to nutritional needs, the patient may require counseling in the proper choice of foods in the market, assistance in planning for the best use of food money, and practical suggestions for food preparation with meager facilities or in the face of physical handicaps. Some of the assistance required by the patient may be provided by the nurse, but more often a team effort—nurse, dietitian, social worker—is needed. (See also Chapter 26.)

In the community the nurse is often the coordinator of services. The nurse encounters a legion of problems and needs related to nutrition; perhaps a mother needs to know how to prepare an infant formula; another person would like some help in budgeting her limited income so that she can feed her family adequately; another needs instruction in preparing food for an ill member of the family; and another needs counseling so that the diet conforms to religious beliefs. In some of these situations the nurse can use nutrition knowledge to assist the client. For more complex problems she or he may need to either consult a nutritionist or refer the client to the nutritionist.

Some Guidelines for Nutrition Study   It is often said that one can judge a worker by the way in which he or she uses tools. This is also true of the use a student makes of the study tools available. First, one must become acquainted with a tool and gain some practice in using it before it becomes comfortable to use. With your text, for example, look through the table of contents to learn something of the topics that are covered and the sequence of their presentation. Then browse through the book to become aware of the kinds of study aids that are provided.

Terminology in any study is basic to understanding, and the time used in developing the ability to use nutrition terms with accuracy and ease is well spent. Terms with which you should be familiar are set in small capital letters and are defined at the point of their first use. Terms that are used frequently throughout the text have also been listed in the Glossary in the Appendix.

Many tables, diagrams, charts, and photographs emphasize and summarize important points made in the discussion. If you study these, you will find that they reinforce the reading of the text itself. The tables of food composition in the Appendix contain a gold mine of information. Perhaps half of all the questions people will pose to you are concerned with nutritive values, and in these tables you can find the answers. But to use them with confidence means that you must consult them often.

Review questions at the end of each chapter will help you to focus on the important points that have been made. The suggested problems are examples of situations that may be encountered in making applications of the principles of nutrition. You will soon learn to find answers to problems that come within your own daily experiences.

Any student of nutrition should be aware of the current issues before the public. You will find that your interest will be deeper if you try to relate your course of study to some of the reporting in newspapers and magazines, for example. Try to evaluate what you read in the popular publications with what you learn in your study.

The references for each chapter will enable you to read more extensively on selected topics, to familiarize you with reliable publications in nutrition, to foster the habit of consulting the literature, and perhaps even to provide the starting point for a paper you may wish to develop.

In your reading you need to begin to become critical of the contents. Has there been scientific testing of the issue? Are the authors recognized practitioners in the field about which they are writing? Are there explanations for contradictory findings? Is there bias in the article in favor of a product, device, or belief? Has the information been gained through repeated research, or is it based on a single study? The ability to identify reliable sources of nutrition information and to distinguish between fact and fallacy should be a major goal in your study of nutrition.

Problems and Review

1. What is your understanding of the following terms: nutrition, malnutrition, nutrient, health, food, nutritional care?
2. Industrial and economic developments have been a powerful factor in the changing of our food habits. List several of these which have had an influence on our dietary habits within your lifetime.
3. Within your experience give an example of a situation in which the community has fostered better nutrition.
4. Select an article related to food from the daily newspaper or a popular magazine and discuss its merits.
5. In what ways is a knowledge of the following sciences helpful in the study of nutrition: bacteriology, chemistry, sociology, psychology, anthropology?
6. What is the difference between a dietary survey and a nutritional status study?
7. *Problem.* Start a list of resources for the study of nutrition and dietetics. Add to this list as you continue in your study. Include only those books and journals that you have examined. Include the names of official and voluntary agencies in your own community and at state, federal, and international levels as you become familiar with the work they do in the area of nutrition.
8. *Problem.* Compile a list of characteristics that describe a person who is in good nutritional status. How do you measure up with this?
9. *Problem.* Review the suggested objectives for study in this chapter. Then prepare a statement in your own words that best describes the goals that are most important to you. Limit your statement to 300 words; be concise but specific.

References

1. U.S. Department of Health, Education and Welfare: *Ten State Nutrition Survey, 1968–70.* Pub. No. (HSM) 72–813–8134, Government Printing Office, Washington, D.C., 1972.
2. Owen, G., et al.: "A Study of Nutritional Status of Preschool Children in the United States, 1968–70," *Pediatrics* (Suppl.), **53:**597–646, 1974.
3. U.S. Department of Health, Education and Welfare: *Preliminary Findings of the First Health and Nutrition Examination Survey, 1971–72.* Pub. No. (HRA) 74–1219–1, Government Printing Office, Washington, D.C., 1974.
4. Hama, M. Y.: "Household Food Consumption, 1977 and 1965," *Family Econ. Rev.,* 4–9, Winter 1980.
5. Sloan, A. E., et al.: "Changing Consumer Lifestyles," *Food Technol.,* 38:99–103, 1984.
6. Marston, R. M., and Welsh, S. O.: "Nutrient Content of the U.S. Food Supply, 1982," *Nat. Food Rev.,* 7–13, Winter 1984.
7. Woteki, C., et al.: "Recent Trends and Levels of Dietary Sugars and Other Calorie Sweeteners," in Reiser, S., ed.: *Metabolic Effects of Utilizable Dietary Carbohydrates.* M. Dekker, New York, 1982, pp. 1–27.
8. Hegsted, D. M.: "Nationwide Food Consumption Survey—Implications," *Family Econ. Rev.,* 20–22, Winter 1980.
9. Cronin, F. J.: "Nutrient Levels and Food Used by Households, 1977 and 1965," *Family Econ. Rev.,* 10–15, Winter 1980.
10. Pao, E. M.: "Nutrient Consumption Patterns of Individuals, 1977 and 1965," *Family Econ. Rev., 16–20, Winter 1980.*
11. Pao, E. M., and Mickle, S. J.: "Problem Nutrients in the United States," *Food Technol.,* 35:58–69, 1981.
12. U.S. Public Health Service: *Healthy People. The Surgeon General's Report on Health Promotion and Disease Prevention.* DHEW (PHS) Pub. No. 79–55071A, Government Printing Office, Washington, D.C., 1979.
13. Boehm, W. T., et al.: *Progress Toward Eliminating Hunger in America.* Ag. Econ. Rep. No. 446, U.S. Department of Agriculture, Washington, D.C., 1980.
14. Kahn, S. G.: "World Hunger: An Overview," *Food Technol.,* 35:93–98, 1981.
15. Block, J. R. Hearings before the Committee on Agriculture, House of Representatives, 98th Congress, Oct. 25, 1983, p. 96.
16. Coole, A. J.: "Recent Trends in Fertility in Less Developed Countries," *Science,* 221:828–32, 1983.
17. Ruby, G.: "Increasing the Knowledge Base for Prevention," in *Healthy People,* U.S. Department of Health, Education and Welfare, Washington, D.C., 1979, pp. 459–70.

2

Introduction to the Study of Nutritional Processes
Digestion, Absorption, and Metabolism

Many complex and interrelated processes are involved in the utilization of food by the body. These include physical and chemical activities that take place within the cells as well as the relationships that exist between the cells and their surrounding environment. In this chapter basic concepts from the sciences of physiology and biochemistry will be reviewed that describe these processes and that are necessary for an understanding of nutrition. The discussions in the chapters pertaining to each nutrient will provide further details.

Body Structures

Composition of the Body   Approximately 96 percent of body weight is composed of the chemical elements carbon, hydrogen, oxygen, and nitrogen in the form of protein, fat, water, and a small amount of carbohydrate. The remaining 4 percent of body weight is made up of mineral elements, with calcium and phosphorus accounting for three fourths of the total.

Water is present in all body tissues and accounts for 55 to 70 percent of body weight. The water content varies inversely with the amount of fat in the body. Infant bodies have a low fat content and a high water content. Lean adults have a higher body water content than obese adults.

About three fourths of the body water is in the IN-TRACELLULAR compartment (fluid within the cells), and one fourth is in the EXTRACELLULAR compartment, which includes the blood plasma, the lymph, and the interstitial fluids that bathe all cells. Tissues vary considerably in their water content, with bones, teeth,

and adipose tissue, for example, containing appreciably less water than muscle and nervous tissue.

Proteins account for about 16 percent of body weight. The normal body fat content is 15 to 18 percent for men and is 20 to 25 percent for women.[1] Body fat content in excess of 25 percent for men and 30 percent for women is generally regarded as obesity. A gradual increase in body fat content occurs in both sexes with aging.

Only about 300 gm carbohydrate in the form of glycogen is present in the body, with very small additional amounts involved in the structure of various tissues. Many of the most important body constituents such as vitamins, hormones, and enzymes are present in such small amounts that they have no significant effect on total body weight.

Body components except fat may be referred to as LEAN BODY MASS or, more accurately, as FAT-FREE BODY. Various methods can be used to estimate lean body mass. (See Chapter 23.) Body fat then can be computed by subtracting the value for lean body mass from the total body weight.

Cells as Functioning Units   The simplest living organism consists of a single cell such as a bacterium or yeast cell that is capable of respiration, ingestion, digestion, absorption, circulation, synthesis of new materials, breakdown of materials for energy, response to the environment, excretion, and reproduction. Survival of the cell is dependent on a favorable external environment. The cells of complex organisms such as those in the human being carry out these multiple activities but cannot exist independently; they function through intricate coordination with other cells. Cells are so tiny that they can be seen only with a light microscope. Many structures within cells have been identified by means of the electron microscope that permits magnification of 100,000 times or more. Cells are of infinite variety in size, shape, and specialized functions. They also possess some structures and functions in common so that it is possible to diagram and describe a so-called typical cell. (See Figure 2-1.)

The CELL MEMBRANE surrounds the protoplasm, maintains the constancy of the internal environment, and establishes dynamic equilibrium with the external environment by its highly selective ability to regulate the kinds and amounts of materials that enter and leave the cell.

The NUCLEUS of the cell is the storehouse for deoxyribonucleic acid (DNA), the genetic plan for the construction of proteins that enable new cells to have the characteristics of the parent cell.

The CYTOPLASMIC MATRIX is the continuous phase extending from the cell membrane throughout the cell and surrounding the ORGANELLES, or living structures,

as well as certain lifeless materials known as INCLUSIONS. The organelles include the mitochondria, lysosomes, and endoplasmic reticulum.

MITOCHONDRIA are rod-shaped or round structures that vary in size and shape depending upon their activity. Within the mitochondria are hundreds to thousands of oxidative enzymes that are responsible for carrying on the reactions that yield the high-energy compound adenosine triphosphate (ATP). ATP supplies the energy needed by the cell to carry on its activities.

LYSOSOMES are small, spherical, or oval bodies that contain digestive enzymes. Lysosomes function to break down various intracellular constituents such as other organelles that have been damaged, bacteria that have been engulfed by the cell, or other cellular debris.

The ENDOPLASMIC RETICULUM is a system of membranes scattered throughout the cytoplasm that form

Figure 2-1.   Diagram of a cell as it would appear under an electron microscope.

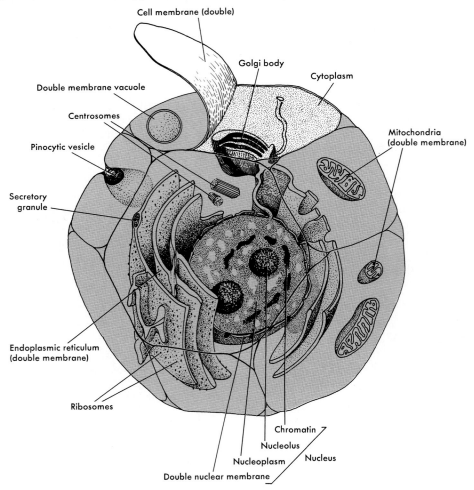

a series of flat sheets which interconnect with each other, facilitating the flow of materials within the cell. RIBOSOMES attached to the rough endoplasmic reticulum are the site of protein synthesis. The proteins then enter the channels of the endoplasmic reticulum and are transported to other parts of the cell. Another type of endoplasmic reticulum, the smooth endoplasmic reticulum, is involved in the synthesis of steroids and other lipids.[2]

The GOLGI APPARATUS appears as a series of flattened membranous sacs and vesicles. It stores and concentrates cellular secretions and releases them on demand.

Utilization of Food

Functions of Food "You are what you eat" is, in a sense, true inasmuch as the nutrients derived from food supply the *energy* for the activity of the body, the *structural materials* for every cell of the body, and the thousands of *regulatory substances* essential for all body processes.

Energy is supplied by carbohydrates, fats, and proteins. Minerals and vitamins are not sources of energy, but they are required in many steps of the release of energy.

Amino acids and mineral elements are constantly required for the growth and maintenance of body tissues. Carbohydrates and lipids enter into specialized tissues—often at very low but vital concentrations. All the structural elements contain water.

Regulatory activities of the body require innumerable substances composed of water, amino acids, fatty acids, sugars, mineral elements, and vitamins.

Processes in Food Utilization A series of processes are involved in providing the nutrients needed for cellular function:

1. Ingestion: the intake of food
2. Digestion: the breakdown of foods into their constituent nutrients
3. Absorption: transfer of nutrients from the gastrointestinal tract into the circulation
4. Transportation of nutrients: movement of nutrients through the circulatory system to sites for their use
5. Respiration: provision of oxygen to the tissues for the oxidation of food and removal of waste carbon dioxide, with the circulatory system responsible for transport of these gases
6. Metabolism of nutrients: oxidation to create heat and energy, as well as incorporation into new cells and tissues

7. Excretion of wastes: undigested food wastes and certain body wastes from the bowel; carbon dioxide from the lungs; nitrogenous, mineral and other wastes from metabolism by the kidneys and by the skin

The pathway involved in utilization of a single nutrient may be traced. For example, the digestion, absorption, and metabolism of a specific carbohydrate or mineral can be traced. This oversimplifies the complex manner by which the body uses nutrients, since processes involving individual nutrients never occur in isolation but are always interlinked with a multitude of other nutritional processes. Each of these processes is affected by others that preceded it or that occur at the same moment.

Numerous physical and chemical methods have been developed for measuring the changes that occur during the utilization of food. Analyses of blood, of urine, and, somewhat less frequently, of feces for various constituents are utilized in nutrition research. Part of the study of nutrition is concerned with a knowledge of such changes and an interpretation of their significance in assessing the quality of nutrition.

Role of Enzymes Many steps in the utilization of nutrients cannot take place without the participation of enzymes. ENZYMES are proteins that act as catalysts in chemical reactions in the body. They greatly accelerate the rate of reactions but do not undergo any net change in their own structure. A small amount of enzyme will accomplish a chemical change on a great deal of substance, sometimes as much as 4 million times its own weight. As some wastage of enzymes occurs, they must be continuously synthesized by the living cell.

Some enzymes are simple proteins, whereas others consist of a protein and another grouping loosely or firmly bound to the protein molecule. In an enzyme system the protein molecule is called the APOENZYME; its attached grouping is called the PROSTHETIC GROUP. For many enzyme systems the prosthetic group is made up of COENZYMES, which are organic compounds, including several of the vitamins. The same coenzyme, it should be noted, may be used in different enzyme systems; it is the protein molecule that gives an enzyme its particular specificity. Some enzymes may require the presence of a COFACTOR for their proper functioning. Several minerals provided by foods serve as important cofactors in enzymatic reactions.

Some enzymes are produced in an inactive form known as PROENZYME or ZYMOGEN and require some other substance to activate them. For example:

$$\text{Trypsinogen} \xrightarrow[\text{(activator)}]{\text{enterokinase}} \text{Trypsin}$$
(proenzyme or   (active enzyme)
zymogen)

Most enzymes participate in only one chemical reaction on a single substance, although some act on a class of compounds. They are named for the substances upon which they act, for example, *proteases* for proteins, *lipases* for fats, and so on. Thus a single cell contains hundreds to thousands of enzymes that are responsible for as many different actions. The enzyme lactase, for example, will split only the sugar lactose; it exerts no action on the sugar sucrose or on any other sugar, protein, or fat.

Enzymes are classified broadly by the functions they perform. Among the many important functions are hydrolysis, oxidation, dehydrogenation, and transfer of chemical groupings—thus, hydrolases, oxidases, dehydrogenases, and transferases.

Each enzyme has optimum activity at a specific acidity or alkalinity. Pepsin, which digests proteins in the stomach, is one of the few enzymes active in the very acid reaction of the stomach, whereas the enzymes found in the small intestine are active in a slightly alkaline medium.

Enzyme activity is also affected by temperature. Heat causes denaturation of proteins and leads to loss of enzyme activity in foods or in isolated body tissues such as plasma. Enzymes are inactivated but not necessarily destroyed at freezing temperatures. When a frozen food or other substance is thawed, the enzyme activity may proceed normally.

Digestion

Purposes Only a few substances contained in foods are suitable for use by the body without change, namely, water, simple sugars, and some mineral salts and vitamins. DIGESTION includes the mechanical and chemical processes whereby complex food materials are hydrolyzed to forms that are suitable in size and composition for absorption into the mucosal wall and for utilization by the body. The nutrients that are absorbed include amino acids, small peptides, fatty acids, monoglycerides, glycerol, simple sugars, minerals, and vitamins.

In addition to its hydrolytic activities the gastrointestinal tract controls the amounts of certain substances that will be absorbed, for example, calcium and iron; prevents the absorption of unwanted molecules; synthesizes enzymes and hormones required for the digestive process; eliminates the wastes remaining

from the digestion of food as well as certain endogenous wastes; and renews its own structure every 24 to 48 hours.

The Digestive Organs The gastrointestinal tract is a tube about 7.5 to 9 meters (25 to 30 feet) long in the adult and includes the mouth, esophagus, stomach, small intestine (duodenum, jejunum, and ileum), and large intestine (cecum, colon, rectum, and anal canal). The liver and pancreas, although situated apart from the tract itself, are important for the secretions that they contribute to the digestive process. (See Figure 2-2.)

The layers of the intestinal wall have the following general characteristics[3]:

Figure 2-2. The digestive system. (Courtesy, Ben Pansky: *Dynamic Anatomy and Physiology,* Macmillan Publishing Company, Inc., 1975, p. 412.)

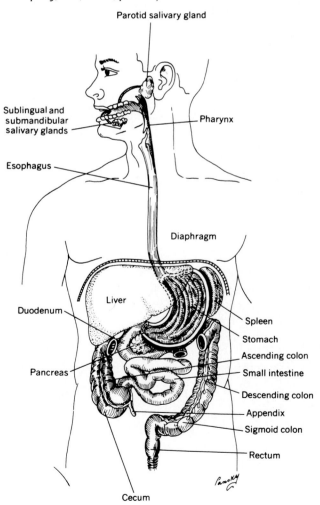

1. The mucosal lining has a layer of surface epithelium and glands lying in loose connective tissue known as the LAMINA PROPRIA. It is richly supplied with blood and lymph vessels. A thin layer of muscle facilitates the constant increase and decrease of the mucosal folds. The mucosal layer secretes hormones and enzymes, brings about absorption, and is the first line of defense against infection.
2. The submucosa is a dense layer of connective tissue with blood and lymph vessels.
3. The muscular layer includes muscle fibers arranged in circular and longitudinal bands and also supplied with blood and lymph vessels. This layer regulates the size of the intestinal lumen and the movements of the intestinal wall.
4. The serosa is the outer covering of the wall, which is supplied with blood and lymph vessels and nerve branches.

Muscular controls are in effect at several points along the tract to permit the influx of food to the next site for digestion and, under normal conditions, to prevent the backward flow of food (regurgitation). These are the cardiac opening from the esophagus to the stomach; the pyloric sphincter at the gastric–duodenal juncture; and the ileocecal valve, which regulates the passage of material from the ileum into the large intestine.

Controls for Activity of the Digestive Tract The secretion of digestive juices and the motor activity of the tract, and hence the speed and completeness of digestion, are regulated by nervous, chemical, and physical factors.

Everyone is familiar with the fact that the thought, sight, or smell of foods creates the desire for food and increases the flow of saliva and gastric juices. On the other hand, an unpleasant environment or worry and fear are likely to depress the secretion of digestive juices and thus delay digestion. Strong emotions such as anger often increase gastric secretion but sometimes depress it.

Of the many digestive processes, the only activities under voluntary control are mastication and defecation. The central nervous system and local nerve circuits exercise control over the secretory and motor activity throughout the entire tract. One example of the feedback mechanism pertains to the regulation of stomach acid. Release of the hormone gastrin from the stomach is stimulated by specific substances such as alcohol or caffeine and by distention of the antral portion of the stomach in response to the presence of food. Gastrin in turn stimulates the flow of gastric acid. Once there is a sufficient amount of acid in the stomach, the secretion of gastrin is turned off and no more acid is produced.

Hormones and Regulatory Peptides Secretory and motor activities involved in digestion are affected by a number of peptides synthesized in the gastrointestinal tract and pancreas. Some of these peptides satisfy the traditional definition of hormones in that they act as chemical messengers that travel in the bloodstream to reach their target cells. Gastrin, which is described above, in addition to secretin and cholecystokinin are familiar examples of peptides that function in this manner. Other peptides act as chemical messengers as well but reach their target cells by different pathways. In a paracrine system the peptide is secreted by the regulator cell into the interstitial fluid in the immediate vicinity of the target cell. Thus, a rise in the blood concentration of the peptide usually cannot be detected, although increased concentrations occur in local tissues. In a neurocrine system the messenger is released from neural tissue in the immediate vicinity of its target. In spite of many advances in our understanding of these regulatory peptides, the physiologic functions of several are still poorly understood. Evidence exists indicating that important interactions occur among them and that the mode of function of individual peptides may vary. Table 2-1 summarizes the characteristics of some of the major gastrointestinal regulatory peptides.

Mechanical Digestion Rhythmic coordinated muscle activity causes foods to be reduced to minute particles and intimately mixed with digestive juices so as to facilitate movement throughout the tract and to provide for maximum exposure to the hydrolyzing enzymes and contact with the absorbing surfaces of the mucosal wall.

By mastication solid foods are cut, ground, mixed with saliva, and prepared for swallowing. Within seconds rhythmic contractions of the muscles of the esophagus force the food particles into the fundus of the stomach, which serves as a reservoir. Each addition of food expands the stomach walls just enough to hold the contents and pushes the mass preceding it forward toward the central part of the organ. Because little motor or secretory activity takes place in the fundus, food may remain there for an hour or more. Small, regular contractions in the middle region of the stomach gradually increase in rate and intensity. The food is mixed with gastric juice, broken up further, and finally reduced to a thin, souplike consistency called CHYME.

Table 2-1. **Characteristics of Major Gastrointestinal Hormones and Regulatory Peptides**

Peptide	Origin	Stimulus to Secretion	Action
Gastrin	Antral and duodenal mucosa	Food in the stomach, especially proteins, caffeine, alcohol	Stimulates secretion of HCl; stimulates antral contraction
Cholecystokinin	Small intestine	Fatty acids in duodenum; peptides and amino acids	Stimulates pancreatic enzyme production, gallbladder contraction
Secretin	Duodenal and jejunal mucosa	Acid chyme in duodenum	Secretion of bicarbonate in pancreatic juice; inhibits gastric motility
Gastric inhibitory peptide (GIP)	Small intestine	Emulsified fat, glucose, amino acids	Inhibits gastric secretion; stimulates intestinal secretion and pancreatic insulin release
Vasoactive intestinal peptide (VIP)	Neurons in intestine	Acid chyme in duodenum; fat, alcohol	Increases intestinal secretions; inhibits gastric acid; smooth muscle relaxant
Motilin	Upper small intestine	Acid chyme; fat	Stimulates upper gastrointestinal motor effects
Pancreatic polypeptide	Pancreas	Protein; neural stimulation	Inhibits pancreatic enzymes and gallbladder contraction

The principal digestive activity is in the small intestine. Because the stomach has considerable storage capacity and because of the controls exerted by the pyloric valve, only small amounts of chyme enter the duodenum at a given time. The rhythmic movements of the intestine are known as PERISTALSIS. In the small intestine the circular muscle fibers have a constricting and squeezing action; thus the chyme is constantly mixed with the digestive enzymes and given maximum exposure to the absorbing surfaces. This motion of the circular muscles is referred to as a segmentation. As the longitudinal muscle fibers contract, a wavelike motion is produced that gradually moves the food mass forward. The muscular activity of the tract also serves as a stimulus to the secretion of the digestive juices and increases the blood supply to the digestive organs.

Motility Through the Tract. The rate at which foods move through the digestive tract depends on the consistency, composition, and amount of food eaten. Liquids begin to leave the stomach from 15 minutes to ½ hour after ingestion, a fact that explains why liquid diets do not have great satiety value. Water and dilute fluids such as fruit juices empty more rapidly than do fluid meals of high nutrient content such as cream soups and milk shakes. In liquid meals carbohydrates, fats, and amino acids all slow gastric emptying, with their effect being proportional to their concentration.[4] In mixed meals the inclusion of large amounts of fat has a strong inhibitory effect on gastric motility, which is initiated when the partially digested fats be-

gin to enter the duodenum. Solid particles of food, particularly nondigestible solids, remain in the stomach longer than other components. As would be expected on the basis of their greater nutrient load, larger meals are emptied more slowly than small meals. Normally the stomach empties within 2 to 6 hours.

The unabsorbed food residue from the small intestine begins to pass through the ileocecal valve into the large intestine in from 2 to 5½ hours, but 9 hours or more from the time of eating may be required for the last of a large meal to pass this point. The length of time required to eliminate food residues as feces varies widely; a range of 20 to 36 hours after the consumption of the meal is typical.

Chemical Digestion A complex mixture of substances is presented to the various sites of the tract for hydrolysis. Depending on the location, these substances include food materials in various stages of hydrolysis, secretions of digestive fluids containing enzymes and hormones, cellular materials from the desquamating mucosa, bile, bacteria, and various products of metabolism within the body that have entered the tract.

About 8 to 9 liters of digestive juices are produced daily by the secretory cells of the digestive tract and by the pancreas and liver. (See Figure 2-3.) These juices are 98 to 99 percent water and contain varying proportions of inorganic and organic compounds. One of the organic compounds of importance is MUCIN, a glycoprotein that lends the slippery quality to

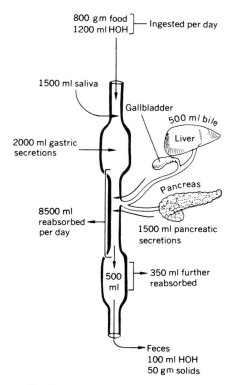

800 gm food ⎤
1200 ml HOH ⎦ — Ingested per day

1500 ml saliva

Gallbladder

500 ml *bile*

Liver

2000 ml gastric
secretions

Pancreas

8500 ml
reabsorbed
per day

1500 ml pancreatic
secretions

500
ml → 350 ml further
reabsorbed

Feces
100 ml HOH
50 gm solids

Figure 2-3. The large volumes of fluid and secretions entering the digestive tract are nearly completely absorbed in the intestines and colon. (Courtesy, B. Pansky: *Dynamic Anatomy and Physiology,* Macmillan Publishing Co., Inc., 1975, p. 427.)

mucus and thus facilitates the smooth movement of food throughout the tract. Mucus also furnishes a protective coating to the gastric and duodenal mucosa against the corrosive action of hydrochloric acid. Except for bile, the digestive juices contain enzymes that are appropriate for a particular stage of hydrolysis. The final stages of hydrolysis for some nutrients, for example, the disaccharides, occurs within the mucosal cell itself and not in the lumen. Table 2-2 presents a summary of the digestive juices, their components, and the results of enzyme activity. See Chapters 5 to 7 for details of digestion of proteins, fats, and carbohydrates.

Functions of the Large Intestine By the time chyme reaches the large intestine practically all the nutrients and water have been absorbed and the volume has been reduced to about 500 ml. The cecum fills slowly, and the peristaltic waves forcing the residues forward together with antiperistaltic waves forcing them back enable additional amounts of water to be absorbed. The large intestine secretes alkaline juices with a large amount of mucus but no hydrolytic

enzymes, so that there is practically no hydrolysis or absorption of nutrients at this point. The activity of the large intestine is greatest after meals and after exercise.

The daily excretion of feces is about 100 to 200 g. The fecal material consists of small amounts of food residues, especially indigestible fiber, billions of microflora, wastes from desquamated cells, bile pigments, cholesterol and unabsorbed minerals such as calcium and iron.

The microflora present in the large intestine have an important role in maintaining normal intestinal structure and function. Although minor alterations in numbers and types of microorganisms can be achieved by dietary manipulation, they tend to be remarkably resistant to dietary changes.

The predominant bacteria in the large intestine are *Escherichia coli*. Bacteria that are fermentative are favored by a high carbohydrate intake and those that are putrefactive by a high protein intake. Bacterial action in the large intestine releases (1) gases including ammonia, methane, carbon dioxide, and hydrogen; (2) lactic and acetic acids; and (3) certain substances such as indole and phenol that may have toxic properties. Various vitamins also are synthesized by intestinal bacteria. Although absorption of some of these may be limited, microbial synthesis of vitamin K in the colon is a major source of the vitamin.

Physicians and clinicians are reemphasizing the importance of ample amounts of fiber in the diet in order to reduce the time fecal residues remain in the large intestine.[5] The reasons for this emphasis are (1) diverticula, present in large proportions of the population by middle age, are less likely to form if the intraluminal pressure in the colon is reduced by the presence of bulk, and (2) a more rapid elimination reduces the length of time a potentially toxic substance has contact with the mucosa. (See also pages 76–77.)

Absorption

The Nature of Absorption The process whereby nutrients are moved from the intestinal lumen into the blood or lymph circulation is known as ABSORPTION and results in a net gain of nutrients to the body. It is an *active process* in that substances are moved into the body against forces that would normally cause a flow in the opposite direction. It is also a *selective process* by which some materials, such as glucose, are transported in their entirety across the cell. Others, for example, calcium and iron, are absorbed

Table 2-2.   **Digestive Juices and Their Actions**

Site of Secretion	Stimuli to Secretion	Daily Volume and pH	Important Constituents	Action
Mouth: saliva Salivary glands	Psychic: thought, sight, smell, taste Mechanical: Presence of food in mouth Chemical: contact of sugar, salt, spices, etc., on taste buds	1,000–1,500 ml pH 5.9–6.8	Mucin *Amylase** (ptyalin)	Lubrication Cooked starch→dextrins, maltose Enzyme activity in the mouth is not extensive
Serous glands	? Fats		*Lipase*	In stomach, fat→mono-, diglycerides
Stomach: gastric juice Parietal cells	Psychic: as above Mechanical: contact with mucosa; distension Hormonal: gastrin increases flow	1,500–2,500 ml pH 2.0–2.5	HCl	Pepsinogen→pepsin Bactericidal Reduces ferric iron to ferrous iron
			Intrinsic factor	Required for vitamin B-12 absorption
Chief cells			*Pepsinogen* *Pepsin*	Inactive form of pepsin Proteins→polypeptides
Columnar epithelium			Mucin	Lubrication; protects gastric and duodenal lining
			?Lipase	Fats→fatty acids + glycerol (action is negligible)
			?Rennin (infants only)	Casein→paracasein
Liver: bile	Cholecystokinin contracts gallbladder and releases bile to duodenum	500–1,100 ml pH 6.9–8.6	Bile salts	Neutralizes acid chyme Emulsifies fats for action of lipase Facilitates lipid absorption
			Bile acids Bile pigments Cholesterol	
Pancreas: pancreatic juice	Secretin	600–800 ml pH 7–8	Thin, watery, alkaline, enzyme-poor juice	Neutralizes acid chyme
			Amylase *Chymotrypsinogen* *Chymotrypsin* *Trypsinogen* *Trypsin* *Lipase*	Starch→dextrins, maltose Inactive form of enzyme Proteins→polypeptides Inactive enzyme Proteins→polypeptides Fats→monoglycerides, fatty acids, glycerol
			Carboxypeptidases	Splits off amino acid with free COOH group
			Nucleases	Nucleic acid→nucleotides
Small intestine: Intestinal juice In microvilli of mucosal cells	Presence of food in small intestine	2,000–3,000 ml pH 7–8	*Enterokinase* *Sucrase* (invertase) *Maltase* *Lactase* *Aminopeptidase*	Trypsinogen→trypsin Sucrose→glucose + fructose Maltose→glucose + glucose Lactose→glucose + galactose Splits off amino acid having free amino group
			Dipeptidase *Nuclease* *Nucleotidase*	Dipeptides→amino acids Nucleic acid→nucleotides Nucleotides→nucleosides + phosphoric acid
			Nucleosidase	Nucleosides→purine or pyrimidine base + pentose
			Lecithinase	Lecithin→diglycerides + choline phosphate

* Constituents in italics are enzymes.

only according to body need, and still others, such as intact proteins, are held back.

Absorption requires that the nutrient penetrate the cell membrane, cross the cell, exit from the cell into the lamina propria, and cross the epithelium of the blood or lymph vessels. In some instances absorption includes a metabolic change within the cell before it is transferred to the circulation. The absorption of specific nutrients will be discussed in Chapters 5 to 13.

Sites and Rates of Absorption Absorption appears to take place primarily from the duodenum and jejunum. A notable exception is vitamin B-12, which has a specific absorption site in the lower ileum. Bile is reabsorbed from the distal part of the intestine. Most, if not all, substances that are proximally absorbed can also be absorbed by the ileum; thus, those substances that escaped absorption proximally are absorbed distally.

Normally, 98 percent of the carbohydrate, 95 percent of the fat, and 92 percent of the protein in the diet is hydrolyzed, and the end products are absorbed. These percentages are sometimes referred to as COEFFICIENTS OF DIGESTIBILITY.

Malabsorption can occur under a variety of circumstances: a reduction in the number of functioning villi; an increase in motility so that the time of exposure to absorptive surfaces is inadequate; a lack of specific enzymes or of bile; an interference by insoluble compounds or of an excess of one nutrient over another; and removal of part of the intestine by surgery.

The Absorptive Surface The small intestine provides an absorbing surface that is probably 600 times as great as its external surface area.[6] This is possible because of the arrangement of the mucosal wall in numerous folds, the 4 to 5 million villi that constitute the mucosal lining, and the 500 to 600 MICROVILLI that form the "brush border" of each epithelial cell of the villus.

VILLI are visible under a light microscope. These tiny fingerlike projections of the mucosa consist of a single layer of epithelial cells resting on the lamina propria, which is a bed of supporting connective tissue supplied by arterial and venous blood vessels and lacteals or lymph channels. (See Figure 2-4.)

At the base of each villus is the *crypt of Lieberkühn*. This is where the epithelial cells are formed. As new cells are formed they migrate up the sides of the villus. When they reach the tip of the villus, about 1 to 3 days later, they are extruded into the intestinal lumen and are constantly replaced by newly functioning cells.

Microvilli can be seen only by means of an electron microscope. They elaborate some of the hydrolytic enzymes, and the final stages of hydrolysis of some substances such as disaccharides are completed here and not in the lumen of the intestine.

Figure 2-4. Intestinal villus. (*A*) Lining of the small intestine; villi with cores of the lamina propria that extend into the lumen. Note that crypts (of Lieberkuhn) are glands that dip down into the lamina propria. (*B*) An enlarged view of a typical villus. (Courtesy, Ben Pansky: *Dynamic Anatomy and Physiology,* Macmillan Publishing Co., Inc., 1975, p. 427.)

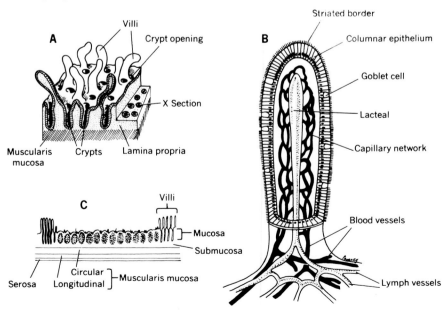

Mechanisms of Absorption   Various mechanisms are involved in the transfer of nutrients across the membrane of intestinal cells for absorption.[2,7]

1. SIMPLE DIFFUSION. The movement of molecules from an area having a high concentration to a lower one involves simple diffusion. Most of the molecules that move easily across membranes by diffusion are characterized by their ability to become dissolved in the lipid layers of the membrane. In addition, substances of very low molecular weight, such as water and some electrolytes, can enter the intestinal cell by diffusion. It is postulated that the cell membrane contains very small holes or pores through which these substances can pass. The molecular size of most nutrients is too great for diffusion by pores.

2. CARRIER-FACILITATED PASSIVE DIFFUSION. Water-soluble nutrients cannot penetrate the lipid-rich membrane of the cell. Therefore, they are attached to "carriers" or "ferries" that facilitate crossing the cell membrane. This is known as *facilitated diffusion.* The carriers are believed to be specific protein-binding sites in the membrane that combine with the nutrient. In facilitated diffusion the nutrients move downhill, that is, from an area of higher concentration to one of lower concentration; no energy is required for this mechanism. When the concentration of nutrients in the circulation is equal to or exceeds that in the lumen, nutrients can no longer passively diffuse. They remain in the intestinal tract until excreted in the feces.

3. ACTIVE TRANSPORT. The absorption of most nutrients is accounted for by active transport. As in passive diffusion, carriers are necessary for the penetration of the cell membrane. Active transport involves the uphill pumping of nutrients from the lumen into the circulation; that is, the nutrient is moved from a site of lower concentration to one of higher concentration. Energy is required for active transport and is supplied by ATP from the metabolism of glucose within the cell. Sodium plays an essential role in the active transport of water, sugars, and amino acids. The metabolic energy required for the operation of the sodium pump also serves for the transport of these other nutrients, and is thus an energy-saving device.

4. PINOCYTOSIS. In some instances the cell appears to "drink up" or surround a substance and to extrude it into the interior of the cell. Occasionally, intact proteins may be absorbed in this fashion, which helps explain the incidence of allergy. Pinocytosis is probably of little importance in the normal absorption the nutrients.

Metabolism

The Nature of Metabolism   METABOLISM can be defined as all the chemical reactions that occur in cells or living organisms. In the study of nutrition it may be used as a broad term to encompass all the processes a nutrient in food undergoes, including digestion, absorption, transport, and cellular oxidation. Often, however, the term is used primarily to indicate those physical and chemical changes that take place in cells.

Metabolism is the composite of two concurrent processes: anabolism and catabolism.

ANABOLISM refers to those processes by which new substances are synthesized from simpler compounds, for example, enzymes, hormones, and tissue proteins from amino acids; glycogen from glucose; and cholesterol from two-carbon units. CATABOLISM refers to the breakdown of complex substances to simpler compounds, for example, the oxidation of glucose to yield energy, carbon dioxide, and water; and the hydrolysis of fats to yield glycerol and fatty acids.

The enzyme systems of a given cell determine the specific functioning of that cell. A compound—for example, glucose—that is to be utilized by the cell is acted on by one enzyme after another in assembly-line fashion until the desired end product has been achieved. If only one of the necessary enzymes is missing, there is a breakdown in the assembly line. All sorts of problems then may arise because of accumulation of metabolites in the pathway prior to the step involving the missing enzyme or because of insufficient formation of essential products. During the past 30 years a better understanding of enzyme activities has led to the identification, and in some cases effective treatment, of the so-called inborn errors of metabolism seen in far too many infants. The condition *galactosemia* results from the lack of a specific enzyme needed for using galactose; *phenylketonuria* likewise results from an enzyme defect that leads to failure to utilize the amino acid phenylalanine. (See Chapter 42.)

The Metabolic Pool   The term METABOLIC POOL is often used to refer to the total supply of a given nutrient that is momentarily available for metabolic purposes. It represents the environment surrounding and within the cells and tissues from which nutrients are drawn. For example, the metabolic pool of amino acids at any given moment would include those available from absorption into the circulation from the digestive tract as well as those available from cellular breakdown. From this mixture of amino acids the cells withdraw those needed for the synthesis of a specific protein.

Common Pathways Carbohydrate, fat, and protein are metabolized in an interdependent fashion. Glucose, fatty acids, glycerol, and amino acids can enter a common pathway that yields energy. (See Figure 2-5.) Glucose can also be metabolized to fatty acids and cholesterol, and some oxidative products of glucose can combine with amino groups to form amino acids. Amino acids are potential sources of both glucose and fatty acids, and so on. Not only are these major nutrients intertwined in their utilization, but they are dependent on the correct concentrations of electrolytes and vitamins for making these changes take place. Further details of the metabolic pathways will be presented in Chapters 5, 6, and 7.

Homeostasis Cellular materials are constantly being broken down and equally rapidly synthesized. The rate of cellular turnover is exceedingly high, especially in the most active organs such as the intestinal wall. In spite of the remarkable rate of turnover, the body tends to maintain a state of equilibrium, often referred to as DYNAMIC EQUILIBRIUM or HOMEOSTASIS, that is, the removal of cells is accompanied by an equal replacement. Likewise, there are checks and balances for the biochemical reactions that take place at each level. The maintenance of equilibrium is governed by an adequate supply of nutrients, a balance between the nutrients, a normal complement of enzyme systems, the secretion of hormones that regulate metabolic rates, and controls by the nervous system.

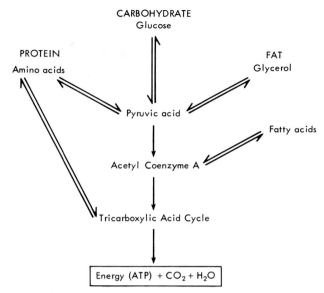

Figure 2-5. Glucose, amino acids, glycerol, and fatty acids enter a common pathway to yield energy. Details of these pathways are shown in Figures 5-5, 6-4, and 7-5.

Problems and Review

1. *Key terms*: absorption; active transport; anabolism; catabolism; coefficient of digestibility; coenzyme; diffusion; digestion; enzyme; homeostasis; metabolic pool; metabolism; prosthetic group; selective absorption; villus.
2. List five characteristics of enzymes.
3. In what way does the chewing of food facilitate digestion?
4. What is the influence of attractive service of food on digestion?
5. Differentiate between pepsin and pepsinogen. What is the substrate on which pepsin acts?
6. A meal consisted of 25 g protein, 35 g fat, and 50 g carbohydrate. Using coefficients of digestibility of typical American diets, calculate the amounts that would actually be absorbed.
7. What is meant by a feedback mechanism?
8. Explain the differences between active transport and facilitated diffusion.

References

1. Bray, G. A.: "Definition, Measurement, and Classification of the Syndromes of Obesity," in Bray, G. A., ed.: *Obesity: Comparative Methods of Weight Control.* Technomic Publishing Company, Inc., Westport, Conn., 1980, pp. 1–14.
2. Luciano, D. S., et al: *Human Anatomy and Physiology,* 2nd ed. McGraw-Hill Book Company, New York, 1983.
3. Pansky, B.: *Dynamic Anatomy and Physiology.* Macmillan Publishing Co., Inc., New York, 1975.
4. Malagelada, J. R.: "Gastric, Pancreatic, and Biliary Responses to a Meal," in Johnson, L. R., et al., eds.: *Physiology of the Gastrointestinal Tract,* Raven Press, New York, 1981, pp. 893–924.
5. Eastwood, M. A., and Passmore, R.: "Dietary Fibre," *Lancet,* 2:202–206, 1983.
6. Ingelfinger, I. J.: "Gastrointestinal Absorption," *Nutr. Today,* 2:2–10, 1967.
7. Pike, R. L., and Brown, M. L.: *Nutrition—An Integrated Approach,* 3rd ed. John Wiley & Sons, New York, 1984.

3

Dietary Guides and Their Uses

Health professionals sometimes become so concerned about diet modifications used in the treatment of various diseases that they forget the basics of what constitutes a "normal," nutritionally adequate diet. The average consumer, however, is more likely to seek answers to such questions as: How can I be sure I am getting all the nutrients I need? Am I eating enough protein? Do I need more vitamins? Should I reduce my intake of fat and salt? The Recommended Dietary Allowances represent an important standard used to plan diets that supply an adequate intake of nutrients. Translation of these allowances into practical food guides makes it possible for the consumer to select the amounts and types of foods needed to achieve the recommended intakes without being concerned about individual nutrients. Growing appreciation of the role of diet in the etiology of various chronic diseases has led to the development of dietary guidelines designed to prevent these conditions.

Recommended Dietary Allowances

Development of Dietary Allowances Humans have always been concerned about the kinds and amounts of foods that would keep them physically fit. Nevertheless, significant progress in identifying the nutrients needed by the body and the amounts required under varying circumstances has come about principally in this century as a result of thousands of investigations in research laboratories. Periodically, summaries of such research have been made in order to recommend the levels of intake desirable for various categories of the population. The first national effort in the United States came about late in 1940 when the Food and Nutrition Board of the National Research Council was organized to guide the government in its wartime nutrition program. One of the first activities of this board was the careful review of research on human requirements for the various nu-

trients. This led to the publication of the *Recommended Dietary Allowances* (RDAs) in 1943. Since that time the board has evaluated new research and has published revisions of the standards every 4 to 6 years.

The 1989 RDAs, listed in the inside front cover of this book, include 17 age–sex categories. Each category is described in terms of height and weight. For example, the "reference" man weighs 79 kg (174 lb) and is 176 cm (70 in) tall; the "reference" woman weighs 63 kg (138 lb) and is 163 cm (64 in) tall. Adjustments for variations in body size within a given category are sometimes indicated.

In the current revision the requirements for energy are listed separately. (See Table 8–3.) Unlike the nutrient allowances that are intended to meet the needs of most of the population, the energy levels are average requirements that will maintain health and normal weight in adults and support growth in children. The requirements for energy vary widely from one individual to another.

An important addition to the 1989 revision is the inclusion of a table of estimated allowances for seven nutrients for which data, as yet, are limited. (See inside front cover of this book.) Because some trace elements can be toxic, safe ranges of intake are listed. Habitual intakes that exceed the maximum level could lead to signs of toxicity.

In addition to the tables of allowances, the Food and Nutrition Board has described the basis for establishing each nutrient allowance.[1] It also provides some recommendations for water, fat, essential fatty acids, carbohydrate, and fiber in the diet. The allowances for specific nutrients and the factors that influence their needs are covered in more detail in Chapters 5 through 13.

Interpretation of the RDA The Food and Nutrition Board defines the RDA thus:

CONTROVERSIAL ISSUES

Although tremendous progress has been made in defining the nutritional needs of people, full agreement on the answers to questions such as the following has not yet been reached.

1. What are the best guidelines for dietary planning for a healthy population? A discussion of the recommended dietary allowances and of several practical guidelines will provide a background of information upon which to base one's choices.

2. What types of diet recommendations should be made that might be important in prevention of chronic diseases? Should these recommendations apply to everyone or only to high-risk segments of the population? Several recent guidelines will be presented that illustrate the major dietary factors of concern and the issues that arise when recommendations are proposed for changes in the diet of the general public.

Recommended Dietary Allowances (RDAs) are the levels of intake of essential nutrients that, on the basis of scientific knowledge, are judged by the Food and Nutrition Board to be adequate to meet the known nutrient needs of practically all healthy persons.*

The word "allowance" should not be confused with the word "requirement." An individual's requirement for nutrients is influenced by numerous interdependent physical, environmental, social, and dietary characteristics. Thus, people vary widely in their needs. Since it is not practical to determine each individual's exact needs, the allowances have been set high enough to take care of almost all healthy people. (See Figure 3-1.)

The allowances are the amounts of nutrients to be actually consumed. The food supply brought into the kitchen for a given group must be sufficient to allow for waste in preparation, losses of nutrients in cooking, and plate waste.

In the practice of dietetics the allowances are frequently used to determine the adequacy of the food intake of an individual. When the nutrient intake of a healthy individual equals or exceeds the recommended allowances, it is highly likely that the diet is meeting the needs of that person to achieve his or her full potential for growth or productivity. An intake below the recommended allowances for a prolonged period of time increases the possibility of nutritional deficiency.

Uses for the RDA   The dietary allowances are a professional tool that is appropriately used in the following ways:

*Food and Nutrition Board, *Recommended Dietary Allowances*, 10th ed. National Research Council–National Academy of Sciences, Washington, D.C., 1989, p. 10.

Evaluating the adequacy of the national food supply; setting goals for food production.

Setting standards for menu planning for publicly funded nutrition programs such as school food services, day-care centers, programs for the elderly, and others.

Establishing nutrition policy for public assistance, nursing homes, and institutions such as children's homes, mental institutions, and prisons.

Interpreting the adequacy of diets in food consumption studies. The Household Food Consumption Survey, the Health and Nutrition Examination Survey, and the Ten-State Survey have evaluated diets on the basis of the RDA or some modification of it.

Developing materials for nutrition education. The

Figure 3-1.   Normal distribution curve of the variation of requirements among individuals. Relatively small numbers of people have either low or high requirements. Most people have needs that are near the average. The RDAs are set high enough so that most people with high needs are also protected. Conversely, a given allowance will be higher than most people actually need.

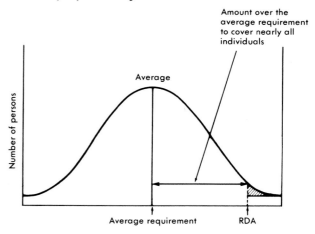

RDA are used to develop food guides and other educational materials for the public.

Setting the pattern for the normal diet used in hospitals. Although modified diets may require increased or decreased amounts of nutrients, the normal diet is the reference point for making these modifications.

Establishing labeling regulations. The USRDA labeling standard is an adaptation of the RDA.

Setting guidelines for the formulation of new food products or the fortification of specific foods.

Limitations and Misuse of the RDA   Those who use the RDAs should also understand their limitations.[1,2]

They are too complex for direct use by consumers.

They do not state *ideal* or *optimal* levels of intake. These are concepts that cannot be realized.

The allowances for some age categories such as adolescents and the elderly are based on limited data.

Data on the food content of some nutrients such as trace minerals are limited. Therefore, reliable evaluation of diets against the RDAs cannot always be achieved.

The RDAs do not evaluate nutritional status. Because the allowances are higher than the requirements of most people, failure to achieve the recommended allowance for one or more nutrients does not mean that nutritional deficiency is present. However, the risk of nutritional deficiency increases the further below the RDA a given nutrient intake habitually falls. Nutritional status can be determined only by physical, clinical, and biochemical examination of the individual. (See Chapter 23.)

The RDAs do not apply to people who are ill and who require increased or decreased levels of nutrients because of pathology or because of the use of medications.

Other Standards

Canadian Dietary Standard   Since 1938 the Canadian Council on Nutrition has published recommendations for nutrient levels for age and sex categories. The most recent revision was published in 1983.[3] (See Table A-30 in the Appendix.)

The purpose of the Canadian standard is essentially the same as that of the Food and Nutrition Board, namely, to recommend nutrient intakes at levels adequate for good health for most Canadians. The standards are above minimum levels and take individual variations into account. The data are derived from essentially the same base lines. The standards are to be used for "planning diets and processing food supplies for individuals and groups" and are not to be used as a measure of nutritional status.

An examination of the two tables shows that there are some differences in the recommended levels for nutrients, for example, iron, zinc, ascorbic acid, and folic acid, among others. These differences emphasize that there still exists a good deal of ignorance regarding the criteria for optimum health, the desirable margin of safety, and so on. The assigned levels for each nutrient represent the best judgment of the committees that set up each table.

Dietary Guides in Other Countries   Dietary allowances have been established for populations of many countries. In addition, the Food and Agriculture Organization and the World Health Organization have adopted recommendations for allowances for many nutrients. The aim of the various standards is essentially to provide a level of nutrition that maintains good health for substantially all of the population.[4] The allowances are not minimum requirements, nor are they average needs.

The allowances in various countries differ because they are intended for the population of a given environment—for example, climate, occupation and activity, dietary practices—and therefore they are not interchangeable. For example, more calories would be allowed for men and women in a country where considerable physical activity is involved in daily work than in a country where work is mechanized and activity is sedentary. The increased calorie allowances in turn necessitate increased allowances for some of the B-complex vitamins such as thiamin. The allowances in the various countries also differ because of varying interpretations of data by committees who set up the allowances.[4] As research becomes more extensive these differences are narrowing somewhat. A comparison of allowances set up for men and women for several groups is shown in Table 3-1.

Labeling   The U.S. Recommended Daily Allowances (USRDA) was established by the Food and Drug Administration as a standard for labeling the numerous packaged foods in the marketplace. (See page 260.) This standard should not be used in place of the RDAs for planning diets.

A Daily Food Guide

Development of a Food Guide   The RDAs should be translated into diets consisting of a wide variety of foods. On a given day a diet may not always furnish

Table 3-1. Dietary Allowances for Adults by Four Standards

	United States 1989		Canada 1983*		Food and Agriculture Organization†		United Kingdom 1979‡	
	M	F	M	F	M	F	M	F
Body weight, kg	79	63	74	59	65	55	65	55
Energy, kcal	2,900	2,200	3,000	1,900	3,000	2,200	2,900#	2,150
Protein	63	50	57	41	37	29	72	54
Calcium, mg	800	800	800	700	400–500§		500	500
Iron, mg	10	15	8	14	5–9	14–28	10	12
Vitamin A, RE	1,000	800	1,000	800	750	750	750	750
Thiamin, mg	1.5	1.1	1.2	0.8	1.2	0.9	1.2	0.9
Riboflavin, mg	1.7	1.3	1.5	1.0	1.8	1.3	1.6	1.3
Niacin, mg	19	15	22	14	19.8	14.5	18	15
Ascorbic acid, mg	60	60	60	45	30	30	30	30

* Bureau of Nutritional Sciences: *Recommended Nutrient Intakes for Canadians.* Department of National Health and Welfare, Canada, 1983.

† FAO/WHO: *Handbook of Human Nutritional Requirements.* FAO Nutritional Studies No. 28, Rome, 1974.

‡ Committee on Medical Aspects of Food Policy: *Recommended Daily Amounts of Food Energy and Nutrients for Groups of People in the United Kingdom.* Her Majesty's Stationery Office, London, 1979.

§ This allowance for calcium represents a range for men and women.

Allowances for moderately active men aged 18–34 years.

all nutrients at recommended levels. However, the body has sufficient adaptability that an average intake over a 5- to 8-day period that meets the allowance is satisfactory.

The RDAs have been translated into food guides such as the "Basic Seven" and later the "Basic Four," also known as the "Four Food Groups."[5] Recently the U.S. Department of Agriculture issued a revision of the Daily Food Guide.[6] The revised guide retains the four food groups but adds a fifth group—fats, sweets, and alcohol. (See Table 3-2.) Daily selections from these groups can be adjusted to comply with the dietary guidelines described below.

Limitations of the Daily Food Guide The Daily Food Guide is intended primarily for consumers. Its limitations should also be recognized.

1. A food guide appropriate for one group of people is not necessarily applicable to another group; for example, guides based on the food supplies in the United States would not be suitable for nations in Africa or the Far East.
2. Some new foods, mixtures of foods, and many convenience foods are not easily classified according to the food groups.
3. Foods within a group vary widely in caloric content. There are also wide variations of nutrient levels within each group. Some fruits and vegetables are outstanding for their content of ascorbic acid

and vitamin A, whereas others supply only small amounts. Thus, the user must become acquainted with these variations.

4. Adherence to a food guide does not guarantee nutritive adequacy. The nutrient needs are more likely to be met when a wide variety of foods is selected from each group.

A Basic Diet A diet that includes the minimum number of servings for the adult from each of the four food groups is used in this text as a basis for dietary planning. (See Tables 4-1 and 4-2 for calculations of the basic diet.) The plan substantially furnishes the recommended nutrient levels and approximately 1,300 kcal. Additional selections from the four food groups that make up the diet will significantly increase the nutrient intake. If additional calories are selected from the fats, sweets, and alcohol group there will be little increase in nutrient intake.

Dietary Guidelines

With the ever-increasing costs of health care and the high incidence of chronic diseases such as coronary heart disease, stroke, and cancer, professional and public interest has increased rapidly concerning the possible role that diet may play in preventing these diseases. For many years the American Heart Association has recommended that the general public modify food intake to maintain desirable weight and to con-

Table 3-2.   A Daily Food Guide*

Vegetable–Fruit Group: 4 basic servings daily.
  One serving is ½ cup or a typical portion such as one orange, half a medium grapefruit, a medium potato, or a bowl of salad.
  Include one good vitamin C source daily.
  Include deep yellow or dark green vegetables frequently.
  Include unpeeled fruits and vegetables and those with edible seeds for fiber.

Bread–Cereal Group: 4 basic servings whole-grain and enriched or fortified products.
  One serving is 1 slice bread or ½ to ¾ cup cooked cereal, cornmeal, grits, macaroni, noodles, rice, or spaghetti; or 1 ounce ready-to-eat cereal.
  Include some whole-grain breads and cereals for fiber.

Milk–Cheese Group: children under 9—2–3 servings
                 children, 9 to 12—3 servings
                 teenagers—4 servings
                 adults—2 servings
                 pregnant women—3 servings
                 nursing mothers—4 servings
One serving is one 8-ounce cup of milk: whole, skim, low fat, evaporated, buttermilk, or nonfat dry milk
Equivalents for calcium are

1 cup plain yogurt	= 1 cup milk
1 ounce Cheddar or Swiss cheese	= ¾ cup milk
1-inch cube Cheddar or Swiss cheese (natural or processed)	= ½ cup milk
1 ounce processed cheese food	= ½ cup milk
½ cup ice cream or ice milk	= ⅓ cup milk
1 tablespoon or ½ ounce processed cheese spread; or 1 tablespoon grated Parmesan cheese	= ¼ cup milk
½ cup cottage cheese	= ¼ cup milk

Meat, Fish, Poultry, and Beans Group: 2 basic servings daily.
  One serving is 2 to 3 ounces of lean, cooked meat, poultry, or fish without bone.
  Count as 1 ounce of meat, poultry, or fish:
   1 egg
   ½ to ¾ cup cooked dry beans, dry peas, soybeans, or lentils
   2 tablespoons peanut butter
   ¼ to ½ cup nuts, sesame seeds, sunflower seeds

Fats, Sweets, Alcohol Group: no basic servings suggested.
  Includes butter, margarine, salad dressings, mayonnaise, fats, oils; candy, sugar, jams, jellies, syrups, sweet toppings; soft drinks and other highly sugared beverages; wine, beer, and liquor; also unenriched breads, pastries, and flour products.

* *Food.* HG228. U.S. Department of Agriculture, Washington, D.C. 1980.

sume less saturated fat, cholesterol, sugar, and salt. With much fanfare by the media, various guidelines have been published in recent years. Each has been subjected to much criticism by nutrition scientists, clinicians, politicians, the food industry, and advocates for the public. None of the guidelines is considered a substitute for the Daily Food Guide, but each of them can be adapted to use with the guide.

Dietary Goals for the United States   In February 1977 the Senate Select Committee on Nutrition and Human Needs published a report on the Dietary Goals.[7] After revisions suggested by nutrition and medical scientists, the revised form of the report issued in December 1977 recommended the goals shown in Table 3-3. To implement the Goals the fol-

lowing changes in food selection and preparation were suggested:

1. Increase consumption of fruits and vegetables and whole grains.
2. Decrease consumption of foods high in total fat and partially substitute polyunsaturated fat for saturated fat.
3. Decrease consumption of animal fats. Choose meat, poultry, and fish that are low in saturated fat.
4. Except for young children, substitute low-fat or nonfat milk for whole milk, and low-fat dairy products for high-fat dairy products.
5. Decrease consumption of butterfat, eggs, and other high-cholesterol sources.

Table 3-3. A Comparison of Three Dietary Guides*

Dietary Goals for the United States 1977†	Dietary Guidelines for Americans 1985‡	Toward Healthful Diets 1980§
		Select a nutritionally adequate diet from the foods available by consuming each day appropriate servings of dairy products, meats or legumes, vegetables and fruits, and cereals and breads.
	Eat a variety of foods	Select as wide a variety of foods in each of the major food groups as is practicable in order to ensure a high probability of consuming adequate quantities of all essential nutrients
To avoid overweight, consume only as much energy (calories) as is expended; if overweight, decrease energy intake and increase energy expenditure	Maintain reasonable weight	Adjust dietary intake and energy expenditure so as to maintain appropriate weight for height; if overweight, achieve appropriate weight reduction by decreasing total food and fat intake and by increasing physical activity
Increase the consumption of complex carbohydrates and naturally occurring sugars from about 28 percent of energy intake to about 48 percent of energy intake	Eat foods with adequate starch and fiber	
Reduce the consumption of refined and processed sugars by about 45 percent to account for about 10 percent of total energy intake	Avoid too much sugar	If the requirement for energy is low (e.g., reducing diet), reduce consumption of foods such as alcohol, sugars, fats, and oils, which provide calories but few essential nutrients
Reduce overall fat consumption from approximately 40 percent to about 30 percent of energy intake	Avoid too much fat, saturated fat, cholesterol	See preceding statement
Reduce saturated fat consumption to account for about 10 percent of total energy intake; and balance that with polyunsaturated and monounsaturated fats, which should account for about 10 percent of energy intake each	See above statement	
Reduce cholesterol consumption to about 300 mg per day	See above statement	
Limit the intake of sodium by reducing the intake of salt to about 5 g per day	Avoid too much sodium	Use salt in moderation; adequate but safe intakes are considered to range between 3 and 8 g of sodium chloride per day
	If you drink alcohol, do so in moderation	

*Robinson, C. H., and Weigley, E. S.: *Basic Nutrition and Diet Therapy*, 5th ed. Macmillan Publishing Company, Inc., 1984, pp. 42–43.

†U.S. Senate Select Committee on Nutrition and Human Needs: *Dietary Goals for the United States*, rev. Washington, D.C. Government Printing Office, 1977.

‡*Nutrition and Your Health: Dietary Guidelines for Americans*. Washington, D.C.: U.S. Department of Agriculture and U.S. Department of Health and Human Services, 1985.

§Food and Nutrition Board: *Toward Healthful Diets*. Washington, D.C.: National Research Council–National Academy of Sciences, 1980.

6. Decrease consumption of sugar and foods high in sugar content.
7. Decrease consumption of salt and foods high in salt content.

No issue in nutrition in recent years has provoked as much controversy as these Goals. Those who support the Goals believe that the scientific evidence supports the hypothesis that present eating habits are contributing to disease. They agree that the overall adoption of the Goals will improve public health, although not everyone will necessarily benefit because of genetic and individual variability. They view the Goals as applicable to the general population, and not modifications intended only for persons who are at risk or who are ill. They maintain that there is no evidence that consuming the diet lower in saturated fat, cholesterol, sugar, and salt will cause harm to the population. Finally, they regard the Goals as a first step in a national nutrition policy, which are subject to revision with new research findings.

Those who oppose the Goals state that the evidence supporting them is limited and often confusing. The Goals do not provide guidelines for a nutritionally adequate diet, but place emphasis on the prevention of disease. It is maintained that the Goals promise too much and that this can only lead to disillusionment of the public. By themselves, the Goals are too simplistic an approach to the prevention of diseases that are known to have multiple risk factors. Finally, the present American diet is believed to be a good one that should not be tampered with until more research has been accomplished.

Dietary Guidelines for Americans In 1980 a joint publication by the U.S. Department of Agriculture and the U.S. Department of Health and Human Services identified seven guidelines designed to promote good eating habits that will help keep Americans healthy and possibly even improve health. As shown in Table 3-3, these guidelines slightly revised in 1985 resemble the Dietary Goals in the overall recommendations, but no quantitative levels of restriction for fat, cholesterol, sugar, and sodium are indicated.[8] Although the consumer is cautioned to "avoid too much . . ." there is no indication what is meant by "too much." However, the bulletin that accompanies these Guidelines describes food selections that should be avoided.

Toward Healthful Diets Recommendations made by the Food and Nutrition Board in response to the Goals and Dietary Guidelines were presented in the document, *Toward Healthful Diets*.[9] In developing their recommendations, the Food and Nutrition Board has stated:

> A fundamental element of any national nutrition policy, inherent in the recommendations of the Board, is to ensure the provision of a supply of diverse, safe, and attractive foods that will meet nutritional requirements of the population at reasonable cost.[9]

The Board has expressed concern about excessive hopes and fears resulting from some present claims for food and nutrition. Nutritionists will recognize the recommendations of the Board summarized in Table 3-3 as important concepts that have governed their efforts in nutrition education for many years.

Diet, Nutrition, and Cancer: Interim Dietary Guidelines The Dietary Goals and Dietary Guidelines focus primarily on diet changes believed to reduce the risk of coronary heart disease. The role of diet in cancer, another leading cause of death in the United States, was reviewed by a special committee appointed by the National Research Council. Their report issued in 1982 listed several interim guidelines that they believe would be beneficial in reducing the incidence of cancer (Table 3-4).[10] Like the previous guidelines, these recommendations also created considerable controversy. Most critics contend that there are insufficient experimental or even epidemiologic data to show that these changes would have any significant impact in preventing cancer and that it is unwise to make any recommendation until more research has been completed.

Discussion in the media of these diet–cancer guidelines as well as the Dietary Goals and Guidelines has often tended to emphasize differences and conflicting opinions among various scientific groups. Nevertheless, it is apparent from Tables 3-3 and 3-4 that despite differences in the specific details of the recommendations, many of the major areas of concern are similar. Control of energy intake to maintain appropriate body weight, reduction of total fat and salt intake, moderate use of alcohol, and consumption of a variety of foods with an emphasis on generous intakes of fruits, vegetables, and whole grains are recommendations agreed upon by most authorities as important in promoting general well-being, with a possible bonus of prevention of certain diseases. No set of guidelines should be considered irrefutable; guidelines should be reexamined and revised regularly on the basis of new knowledge.

Problems and Review

1. *Key terms*: Recommended Dietary Allowances; Safe and Adequate Intakes; USRDAs; Daily Food Guide; Dietary Goals; Dietary Guidelines; Toward Healthful Diets; Food and Nutrition Board.
2. List the Recommended Allowances for yourself. If a dietary calculation indicates that you were getting less than this allowance in one or more nutrients, how should you interpret this?
3. Identify the similarities and the differences between the dietary guidelines of the Senate Select Committee on Nutrition, the USDA/USHHS, and the Food and Nutrition Board.
4. Which of the diet recommendations listed in the Goals and the Dietary Guidelines may also be beneficial in the prevention of cancer?
5. Knowing that we cannot guarantee that adherence to the diet recommendations given in the Dietary Goals or

Table 3-4. Interim Dietary Guidelines to Prevent Cancer*

Reduce the intake of fat from 40% to 30% of total calories in the diet

Emphasize the consumption of whole-grain cereals, fruits (especially citrus), and vegetables (especially carotene-rich and cruciferous)

Minimize the consumption of foods preserved by salt curing, salt pickling, or smoking

Minimize contamination of the food supply with carcinogens from any source and continue efforts to monitor the food safety

Avoid excessive consumption of alcoholic beverages, especially by cigarette smokers

* Committee on Diet, Nutrition, and Cancer: *Diet, Nutrition and Cancer,* Washington D.C.: National Research Council–National Academy of Sciences, 1982.

diet–cancer interim guidelines will prevent heart disease or cancer, do you believe that the general public should be encouraged to follow the recommendations? Defend your answer. Are you convinced enough of their importance to change your own diet to conform to the recommendations?
6. Which of the recommendations listed in the various dietary guidelines would you find most difficult to follow? Why?

References

1. Food and Nutrition Board: *Recommended Dietary Allowances,* 10th ed. National Research Council–National Academy of Sciences, Washington, D.C., 1989.
2. Report by the Comptroller General of the United States: *Recommended Dietary Allowances: More Research and Better Food Guides Needed.* U.S. General Accounting Office, Washington, D.C., 1978.
3. Bureau of Nutritional Sciences: *Recommended Nutrient Intakes for Canadians.* Department of National Health and Welfare, Canada, 1983.
4. Patwardhan, V. A.: "Dietary Allowances—An International Point of View," *J. Am. Diet. Assoc.,* **56:**191–94, 1970.
5. Hertzler, A. A., and Anderson, H. L.: "Food Guides in the United States," *J. Am. Diet. Assoc.,* **64:**19–28, 1974.
6. Science and Education Administration: *Food.* HG 228. U.S. Department of Agriculture, Washington, D.C., 1980.
7. U.S. Senate Select Committee on Nutrition and Human Needs: *Dietary Goals for the United States,* rev. ed. Government Printing Office, Washington, D.C., December 1977.
8. *Nutrition and Your Health: Dietary Guidelines for Americans.* U.S. Department of Agriculture and U.S. Department of Health, Education and Welfare, Washington, D.C., 1985.
9. Food and Nutrition Board: *Toward Healthful Diets.* National Research Council–National Academy of Sciences, Washington, D.C., 1980.
10. Committee on Diet, Nutrition, and Cancer: *Diet, Nutrition and Cancer.* National Research Council–National Academy of Sciences, Washington, D.C., 1982.

4

Food Composition and Dietary Evaluation
Tools for Dietary Planning

The Nutritive Value of Foods

Factors Affecting Food Composition Foods are complex substances that contain many chemical compounds, more than 50 of which are required to nourish the body. Both genetic and environmental factors determine the composition of foods.

1. The variety of plants and the climate are important determinants of nutritive value. Although climate cannot be controlled, much progress has been made in developing plant varieties that have superior nutritive qualities as well as taste acceptance. For example, new strains of corn and wheat are helping to improve the food supply in many developing countries.
2. The nutritive value of animal foods varies from one animal to another and also from one species to another. Within a given species some nutrients such as fat may vary according to the diet fed to the animal—grass-fed or grain-fed. From one species to another the fatty acid content of the fat in beef, pork, lamb, poultry, and fish varies widely.

3. The compositon of the soil influences some of the nutritive values of foods grown on it. It has long been known that a low iodine content of the soil produces foods with a low iodine content. More recently it has been shown that some soils are depleted of other trace minerals, resulting in mineral-deficient foods. For example, livestock suffer severe disease when they eat food containing either a deficiency or an excess of selenium because of a soil deficiency or excess.
4. The conditions of storage—length of time, temperature, light—are known to modify the nutritive value of foods. Some nutrients such as vitamin C are rapidly lost when the temperature is high or when foods are bruised. Other nutrients may be lost to a varying degree but not quite as rapidly as ascorbic acid.
5. Processing techniques enhance or interfere with the nutritive values of foods. Dehydration, canning, and freezing yield foods of high nutritive value, but in certain ways each process modifies somewhat the nutrient contribution of a given food.

Dietitians and nurses are frequently asked questions such as these: "Are potatoes more fattening than rice and spaghetti?" "What foods should I avoid to cut down on my sodium intake?" "How does the amount of calcium in a slice of cheese compare with that in a cup of milk?" "I am allergic to citrus fruits. What foods can I use to get enough vitamin C?" "Can you help me to plan a good low-calorie diet, since I need to lose 15 pounds?" All these questions and hundreds of others can be easily answered if you have a knowledge of the composition of foods and know how to translate this knowledge with the help of tables of food composition.

This chapter will include a discussion of food composition and tables of nutritive values, the calculation of a basic dietary pattern using the Daily Food Guide, and a rapid method for planning normal and modified diets using the Exchange Lists.

6. Divergent procedures in food preparation are major factors that affect the nutritive value of a food as it is consumed. Losses in food preparation may be brought about because the nutrient is soluble in water, which is later discarded. Overcooking of a product can reduce the amount of some nutrients. The amount of peelings removed, the size of pieces exposed to the air, and the length of time food is held before it is served—for example, on a steam table—may result in wide differences in nutritive value.

Tables of Food Composition The first table of food composition in the United States was published in 1896 by Dr. W. O. Atwater and C. D. Woods, who compiled data for the United States Department of Agriculture for the now classic *Bulletin 28. The Chemical Composition of American Food Materials.* This table included the percentages for inedible waste, water, ash, energy, protein, fat, and carbohydrate in foods.

Since that first publication, research on food composition by the USDA, colleges and universities, and the food industry have provided data for the publication of numerous tables of food composition. The discovery of vitamins, one by one, led to studies on the vitamin content of foods during the 1930s and thereafter. In recent years the determination of the fatty acid, sodium, potassium, trace minerals such as zinc and copper, and fiber contents of foods has been a response to the need for data in planning diets to conform to new developments in laboratory and clinical research.

Handbook No. 8. Composition of Foods: Raw, Processed, Prepared has been the reference used to develop the shorter tables of food composition that appear in textbooks on nutrition as well as numerous books written especially for the lay person. The USDA is extensively revising this handbook and issuing the tables in looseleaf form by food categories. An invaluable reference for the dietitian and the researcher in nutrition, the scope of this table is beyond the limits of books such as this.

College and university laboratories and the food industry report data on food analysis to the Nutrient Data Research Center of the USDA. The data are stored in the computerized Nutrient Data Bank and can be retrieved for a variety of purposes.

In the Appendix of this book you will find six tables of food composition (A-1 through A-6). To use these tables effectively you should become familiar with (1) the arrangement of foods in each table; (2) the amount of food in each listing—household measure, weight of household measure, 100 g; (3) the nutrients listed in each table; and (4) the units of measure for each nutrient—grams, milligrams, micrograms, international units.

Uses for Tables of Food Composition As a health professional, you will find a variety of uses for a table of food composition:

1. To provide answers to the many questions that clients ask about foods
2. To develop lists of foods that can provide a client with alternate choices, for example, a list of foods high in zinc, low in sodium, or comparable in protein, and so on
3. To calculate the nutritive value of the daily diet record provided by a client and to compare it with the RDA (see table inside front cover)
4. To plan and calculate a dietary pattern that meets the nutritional needs for a group of people such as schoolchildren or clients in a nursing home
5. To plan diets that meet specific requirements such as 100 g protein or 500 mg sodium

Limitations in Tables of Food Composition The tables of food composition provide values that are representative for each given food as it is used in the United States on a year-round basis. The apple you ate today may be higher or lower in one or more nutrients than the values given in the table. However, for all practical purposes, the stated nutrient values are a reliable estimate of the nutrients you actually received from the apple.

The reliability of any calculation that you make also depends on the care you have used in describing the actual intake. Is the portion size carefully described? How was the food prepared—stewed, broiled, baked, or fried? Was the food fresh, canned, frozen, or dried? Were breads plain, whole-grain, or enriched? Were fats, sauces and gravies, or sweetenings added to the product?

Only limited data are available for some nutrients such as trace minerals and amino acids, as well as for fiber. In addition, the methods for the determination in some laboratories differ from those used in others, resulting in variation in the results obtained. Usually each table that is published provides information on the uses and limitations of that table.

Tables of food composition give no indication of the bioavailability of a nutrient. BIOAVAILABILITY refers to the amount of a nutrient absorbed and available for body use. In healthy persons the absorption of protein, fat, and carbohydrate exceeds 90 percent. But for some minerals such as calcium, iron, and zinc the percentage absorbed is relatively low. For iron, the absorption by healthy individuals may vary from about 5 to 25 percent or so, depending on the food source and also on the other foods that were eaten in the same meal. Thus, if you eat a food that is a good source of vitamin C, such as grapefruit, in the same meal with breakfast cereal, you will absorb more iron from the cereal than if you did not include the vitamin C-rich food. Also, a meal that contains meat will increase the amount of iron that the body can use from a vegetable such as sweet potato. On the other hand, some compounds such as phytic acid or excessive amounts of fiber can reduce the amount of nutrients absorbed, hence a lower bioavailability. Much research remains to be done on the bioavailability of various nutrients, most especially minerals. The chapters on the nutrients will present further discussion on nutrient availability.

What Is Meant by a "Nutritious" Food?   All foods are nourishing, depending on the circumstances. Even fats and sugars are important when the primary need is energy, although it is generally agreed that these foods have a low concentration (low density) of nutrients.

The nutritive quality of foods may be expressed in a variety of ways. A common method is to consult a table of food values and to arrange foods in groups, classifying them as "excellent," "good," "fair," or "poor." But this is subject to confusion, since it is difficult to decide where to draw the boundary for each category.

To compare the nutritive values of foods, one might consult a table of nutritive values and prepare lists for each given nutrient, arranging these lists from highest to lowest values. Thus, for a list of foods providing vitamin C one could readily see that strawberries and cantaloupe in typical serving portions are far better sources of vitamin C than are serving portions of peaches and bananas.

Many people in our society lead sedentary lifestyles—the office worker with no pattern of exercise away from work, the elderly person who is now less mobile, and others. For them it is important each 100 kcal supplied by the food eaten also "carry its weight" in terms of nutrients. Many years ago Dr. Mary Schwartz Rose, one of the pioneers in nutrition education, devised a "share system" that showed the nutritive contribution in relationship to its caloric content.[1] More recently this method has been modified by the National Dairy Council to show graphically the nutritive values of foods compared with the United States Recommended Daily Allowances

(USRDA).[2] The USRDA is a labeling standard that will be discussed further in Chapter 18. It should not be confused with the RDA.

Nutrient Density   The relationship of the nutrient content of a food to its caloric contribution is known as NUTRIENT DENSITY. This relationship can be expressed by the following equation[3]:

$$\text{INDEX OF NUTRITIONAL QUALITY (INQ)} = \frac{\text{percentage of nutrient allowance}}{\text{percentage of energy requirement}}$$

If the index is 1.0, the food is supplying the nutrient need in the same proportion as the caloric need. If the index is above 1.0, the food is providing the nutrient in greater proportion than the caloric need. Conversely, an index below 1.0 indicates that the food fails to provide a proportionate amount of the nutrient.

Before these calculations can be made, one must agree on the standards to be used. The RDA might seem a logical choice. One could determine the nutrient density for a given category—for example, the teenage girl. But somewhat different values would be obtained if the calculations were made for another category—for example, an elderly woman. Using the RDA to determine nutrient density is useful for health professionals who are planning diets for specific age–sex groups.

For purposes of comparing nutrient density of one food with that of another, without regard to age–sex categories, the USRDA (see page 262) is a practical standard. Although this standard does not specify a caloric level, an appropriate energy level of 2,300 kcal has been suggested.[3] A sample calculation follows:

2 tablespoons peanut butter contain 190 kcal and 8 g protein (Table A-1):

$$\frac{190 \text{ kcal}}{2,300 \text{ kcal}} \times 100 = 8.3\% \text{ of standard caloric allowance}$$

The USRDA for protein is 65 g (Table 18–1):

$$\frac{8 \text{ g}}{65 \text{ g}} \times 100 = 12.3\% \text{ of USRDA for protein}$$

$$\text{INQ} = \frac{12.3\%}{8.3\%} = 1.5$$

Figure 4-1 illustrates the profile for 2 tablespoons of peanut butter. With computers nutritionists are able to arrive at indexes for numerous foods and to obtain printouts of these nutrient profiles.

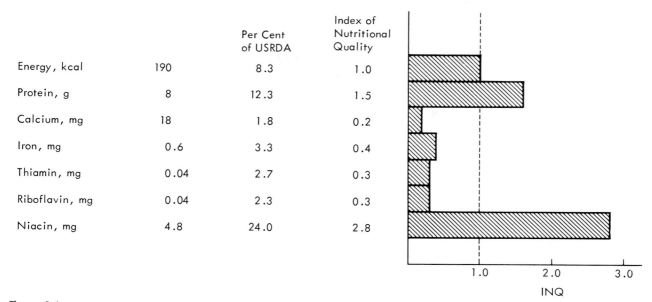

		Per Cent of USRDA	Index of Nutritional Quality
Energy, kcal	190	8.3	1.0
Protein, g	8	12.3	1.5
Calcium, mg	18	1.8	0.2
Iron, mg	0.6	3.3	0.4
Thiamin, mg	0.04	2.7	0.3
Riboflavin, mg	0.04	2.3	0.3
Niacin, mg	4.8	24.0	2.8

Figure 4-1. Index of nutritional quality (INQ) for peanut butter. Protein and niacin indexes above 1.0 indicate that peanut butter is a good source of these nutrients in relationship to the caloric content. Note that 2 tablespoons peanut butter is listed in the Daily Food Guide as equivalent to 1 ounce meat.

A Basic Dietary Pattern

Evaluation of the Daily Food Guide Tables 4-1 and 4-2 summarize the nutritive values that may be expected when one selects the recommended amounts of food from each of the groups of the Daily Food Guide. The contributions that the Basic Diet makes to each of the nutrient needs will be discussed fully in the chapters on nutrients that follow.

From the calculations in Table 4-1 and from Figure 4-2 it becomes evident that the Basic Diet provides about one-half the caloric requirement for adults. The only serious shortcoming for women is that the iron level is about one-half the recommended 18 mg. If women were to meet their caloric needs by emphasis on iron-rich foods such as liver, dried fruits, molasses, additional meat, and iron-enriched breads and cereals, they might achieve the recommended level. On a day-to-day basis this becomes difficult. (See Chapter 9.)

For men, the basic pattern is somewhat below the recommended level for thiamin. When a modest part of the additional calories is selected from the bread–cereal group and or from the meat group, this deficiency can be overcome. Although the niacin level appears to be low, additional niacin is also available through the conversion of tryptophan, an amino acid, to niacin. (See Figure 4-2 and page 188.)

Other Minerals and Vitamins Table 4-2 shows a calculation of the Basic Diet for certain minerals and vitamins for which data on food composition are less complete and reliable. Moreover, for some of these nutrients the Food and Nutrition Board has pointed out that more research needs to be done on which to base the allowances and that changes will be made as more information becomes available. It may be that some of the allowances have been set too high.

From Table 4-2 it becomes evident that the Basic Diet does not supply the daily allowances for magnesium, zinc, folacin, vitamin B-6, and vitamin E. If one observes the following guidelines, these deficiencies will be substantially corrected:

1. To complete the caloric requirement, select most of the additional foods from the four food groups, with minimum choices from the sweets, alcohol, and fat groups.
2. From day to day vary the choice of foods from each group rather than depending on a few favorite items. A variety of dark green leafy vegetables are excellent sources of magnesium and folacin. Whole-grain breads and cereals are far superior to enriched white breads and refined cereals for magnesium, zinc, folacin, vitamin B-6, and vitamin E.
3. One to two tablespoons of vegetable oils—corn, soybean, cottonseed, safflower—used in cooking and in salad dressings will furnish generous amounts of vitamin E.

Table 4-1. Nutritive Value of a Basic Diet Pattern for the Adult in Health*

Food	Measure	Weight (g)	Energy (kcal)	Protein (g)	Fat Total (g)	Fat Saturated (g)	Fat Linoleic (g)	Carbohydrate (g)	Ca (mg)	P (mg)	Fe (mg)	K (mg)	A (IU)	Thiamin (mg)	Riboflavin (mg)	Niacin (mg)	Ascorbic Acid (mg)
Vegetable–fruit group																	
Dark leafy green or deep yellow†	¼–⅓ cup	50	15	1	tr			3	14	16	0.4	112	3,810	0.03	0.04	0.3	15
Other vegetable‡	¼–⅓ cup	50	20	2	tr			4	11	18	0.4	97	270	0.03	0.03	0.4	7
Potato	1 medium	135	90	3	tr			20	8	57	0.7	385	tr	0.12	0.05	1.6	22
Vitamin C-rich fruit§	½ cup	125	55	1	tr			14	22	22	0.4	226	266	0.11	0.03	0.4	52
Other fruit‖	1 serving	100	60	tr	tr			15	8	15	0.4	180	340	0.03	0.03	0.4	5
Bread–cereal group																	
Cereal, whole-grain or enriched#	¾ cup	30 (dry)	96	3	1	0.1	0.1	21	11	60	1.4	66	433	0.17	0.15	1.6	3
Bread, whole-grain or enriched#	3 slices	75	195	8	3	0.4	0.9	38	70	121	2.1	141	tr	0.24	0.14	2.3	
Milk group																	
Milk (2 percent fat)	2 cups	488	240	16	10	5.8	0.2	24	594	464	0.2	754	1,000	0.20	0.80	0.4	4
Meat group																	
Meat, fish, poultry, eggs, legumes**	5 ounces (cooked)	140	335	39	18	5.2	2.5	5	41	370	4.3	568	186	0.42	0.36	8.7	
Total			1,106	73	32	11.5	3.7	144	779	1,143	10.3	2,529	6,305	1.35	1.63	16.1	†† 108
Fats																	
Margarine—soft	1 tablespoon	14	100	tr	12	2.0	4.1		3	3	tr	4	470	tr	tr	tr	0
Oil (corn)	1 tablespoon	14	120	0	14	1.7	7.8	0	0	0	0	0	0	0	0	0	
			1,306	73	58	15.2	15.6	144	782	1,146	10.3	2,533	6,775	1.35	1.63	16.1	108
Recommended dietary allowances																	
Woman (25–50 years)				50					800	800	15		4,000	1.1	1.3	15	60
Man (25–50 years)				63					800	800	10		5,000	1.5	1.7	19	60

* Values for foods in the vegetable–fruit, bread–cereal, and meat groups are weighted averages based on the approximate consumption in the United States.

† Includes broccoli, carrots, escarole, kale, green peppers, pumpkin, and spinach. Assumes 1 serving (½–⅔ cup) every other day.

‡ Includes snap beans, lima beans, cabbage, cauliflower, celery, corn, cucumbers, lettuce, onions, peas, tomatoes. Assumes ½–⅔ cup every other day.

§ Includes oranges, grapefruit, canned and frozen orange, and grapefruit juices.

‖ Includes fresh, canned, and frozen fruits: apples, apricots, bananas, cherries, grapes, peaches, pears, pineapple, plums.

Includes oatmeal, shredded wheat, cornflakes, wheat flakes with added iron, enriched rice, enriched macaroni; whole wheat and white bread.

** Includes per week: 4 eggs; 2 ounces peanut butter, 1 ounce dry beans; 2 ounces tuna fish; 3 ounces flounder; 7 ounces pork; 9 ounces chicken; 7 ounces beef—based on edible, cooked portion weights for meats.

†† The protein in this diet contains about 730 mg tryptophan, equivalent to 12 mg niacin; thus, the niacin equivalent is 28 mg.

Table 4-2.   Additional Mineral and Vitamin Values for the Basic Diet Pattern*

Food	Measure	Weight (g)	Minerals				Vitamins				
			Sodium† (mg)	Magne-sium (mg)	Copper (mg)	Zinc (mg)	Folacin (µg)	Pantothenic Acid (µg)	Vitamin B-6 (µg)	Vitamin B-12 (µg)	Vitamin E§ (mg)
Vegetable–fruit group											
Dark green leafy or deep yellow	¼–⅓ cup	50	18	13	0.06	0.2	23	139	80	0	0.3
Other vegetable	¼–⅓ cup	50	7	9	0.07	0.2	13	120	56	0	0.2
Potato	1 medium	135	6	24	0.2	0.6	11	540	211	0	0.05
Citrus fruit	½ cup	125	1	13	0.03	0.09	47	245	43	0	0.2
Other fruit	1 serving	100	2	13	0.01	0.1	11	139	127	0	0.4
Bread-cereal group‡											
Cereal, whole-grain or enriched	¾ cup	30 (dry)	1	19	0.05	0.4	11	166	47	0	0.1
Bread, whole-grain or enriched	3 slices	75	15	37	0.2	0.9	37	446	83	tr	0.08
Milk group											
Milk (2 percent fat)	2 cups	488	244	66	2.0	1.9	24	1,562	210	1.8	0.2
Meat group											
Meat, fish, poultry eggs, legumes	5 ounces (cooked)	140	112	48	0.2	4.0	34	1,386	376	1.6	1.1
Fats											
Margarine—soft (corn)	1 tablespoon	14	1	tr	0.01	0.03	tr	0	0	0	1.8
Oil (corn)	1 tablespoon	14	0	0	0	0	0	0	0	0	2.0
Total			407	242	2.9	8.4	211	4,743	1,233	3.4	6.4
Recommended dietary allowances											
Woman (25–50 years)				280		12	180		1,600	2.0	8
Man (25–50 years)				350		15	200		2,000	2.0	10

* Values calculated on basis of same foods used for Table 4–1. (See footnote descriptions.) Table A-2 used for calculations. Values are to be regarded as approximations because of limited availability of data.

† Sodium values are based on foods processed and prepared without the addition of salt or other sodium compounds. As consumed in the ordinary diet, the sodium intake would range widely—about 2,500 to 5,000 mg.

‡ Average of whole-grain and enriched breads and cereals.

§ Values for vitamin E are for alpha-tocopherol only; this slightly underestimates the total vitamin E activity of the diet.

Exchange Lists for Meal Planning

Nurses and dietitians are frequently expected to make quick yet reasonably accurate estimations of the nutritive values of diets or to calculate diets that must be controlled for one or more nutrients. The exchange lists widely used in the United States were first published in 1950 by a joint committee of The American Dietetic Association, the American Diabetes Association, and the U.S. Public Health Service.[4] They were revised in 1976 and again in 1986.[5] (See Appendix Table A-4). The Food Group System developed by the Canadian Diabetes Association differs in a number of ways from the exchange lists used in the United States.[6]

SIX EXCHANGE LISTS

An EXCHANGE LIST is a grouping of foods in which specified amounts of all the foods listed are of approximately equal carbohydrate, protein, and fat value. (See Table 4-3.) Specific foods within the lists may differ slightly in nutritive value from the averages stated in the group. These differences in

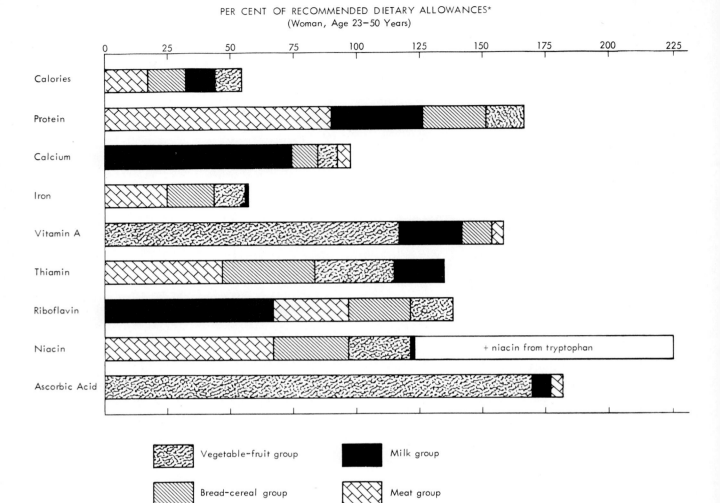

PER CENT OF RECOMMENDED DIETARY ALLOWANCES*
(Woman, Age 23–50 Years)

Legend:
- Vegetable-fruit group
- Bread-cereal group
- Milk group
- Meat group

Niacin: + niacin from tryptophan

Figure 4-2. The four essential food groups of the Basic Diet meet or nearly meet the recommended allowances for nutrients except calories and iron for the woman of 23 to 50 years. See Table 4-1 for calculations.

composition tend to cancel out because of the variety of foods selected from day to day. Thus, any food within a given list can be substituted or exchanged for any other food in that list. In the fruit list, for example, 1 2-in. apple, or 1/2 banana, or 3 prunes, or 1/2 cup orange juice would contain 15 g carbohydrate.

Starch/Bread List One slice of bread is the basis for the exchange in this list. Each exchange supplies 15 g carbohydrate 3 g protein and a trace of fat. Included are *breads*, such as bagels, English muffins, rolls; *cereals*, which include dry and cooked breakfast cereals, grits, rice, pastas; *crackers*; *dried beans, peas, and lentils*; *starchy vegetables*, such as corn, lima beans, potatoes;

and *prepared foods*, such as biscuits, muffins, pancakes.

Meat List One ounce of cooked meat, fish, or poultry supplying 7 g protein is the basis for this exchange list. Luncheon meats, canned fish, shellfish, Cheddar, American, Swiss, and cottage cheese, eggs, and peanut butter in the amounts specified are exchanges for meat. The meat exchanges are subdivided into three groups: lean, medium, and high fat, with fat contents being 3, 5, and 8 g, respectively. In some modified diets, such as a low-calorie diet or low-fat diet, the client's choices might be restricted to those in the low-fat category.

Vegetable List An exchange of most vegetables in this list is 1/2 cup and provides 5 g carbohydrate and 2 g protein. Vegetables high in carbohydrate are included in the bread list. A few salad greens may be used as desired. (See Free List)

Fruit List Each fruit in the amount stated supplies 15 g carbohydrate. Many of the fruits are in average-size servings, but some are not. For example, 1 1/2 figs or 1/2 banana would be smaller-than-average servings. It is therefore important not to use the terms "exchange" and "serving" interchangeably.

Milk List One cup of skim milk is the basis for an exchange in this list. But if 2 percent milk or whole milk is used, the calculation for the fat level is adjusted.

Note that cheeses are listed with meat exchanges and that cream, butter, and cream cheese are included with the fat exchanges.

Fat List This list is based on 1 teaspoon margarine. It includes two groups: fats that are low in saturated fat and high in polyunsaturated fat, and fats that are high in saturated fat.

Free Foods Included in this list are foods that contain less than 20 kcal per serving. They include sugar-free beverages; some vegetables; sugar-free candies, jellies, sugar substitutes, and condiments.

Supplementary Lists. The *Exchange Lists for Meal Planning* booklet also includes the exchange equivalents for some frequently used combination foods such as casseroles, soups. "Foods for Occasional Use" such as cake, cookies, ice cream, and snacks are also included.

Assuring Mineral and Vitamin Adequacy Some discretion in dietary planning with exchange lists is necessary to ensure adequate levels of minerals and vitamins. Generally, if diets are planned to include, as a minimum, the amounts of foods recommended in the Daily Food Guide, the mineral and vitamin levels will be satisfactory. Good sources of vitamin A and ascorbic acid are identified in the vegetable and fruit lists. Some of each day's vegetable and fruit selection should come from these identified sources.

Procedure for Calculation

Let us suppose that a 1,200-calorie diet is to be planned with the following levels: carbohydrate, 120 g; protein, 70 g; and fat, 50 g. The data from

Table 4-3. Composition of Exchange Lists for Meal Planning*

Exchange List	Carbohydrate (grams)	Protein (grams)	Fat (grams)	Calories
Starch/Bread	15	3	trace	80
Meat				
Lean	—	7	3	55
Medium-Fat	—	7	5	75
High-Fat	—	7	8	100
Vegetable	5	2	—	25
Fruit	15	—	—	60
Milk				
Skim	12	8	trace	90
Low-fat	12	8	5	120
Whole	12	8	8	150
Fat	—	—	5	45

*Used by permission from The American Dietetic Association and The American Diabetes Association. See Table A-4 for food selections.

Table 4-3 can be used to calculate the dietary plan shown in Table 4-4. The following steps in calculation are taken:

1. Estimate the amounts of starch/bread, vegetables, fruits, and milk to be included. The following are minimum levels that should ordinarily be included:
   Starch/bread—2 to 4 or more exchanges
   Vegetables—2 exchanges
   Fruits—2 exchanges
   Milk—2 cups for adults; 3 to 4 cups for children and pregnant and lactating women.
2. Fill in the tentative carbohydrate, protein, and fat values.
3. Add up the carbohydrate value of the four food groups. Subtract this total from the total amount of carbohydrate prescribed. Select foods from one or more of the four lists to provide the difference. For example, in the calculation in Table 4-4, the 26 g carbohydrate could be provided as follows:
   2 exchanges fruit (30 g), or
   2 exchanges bread (30 g), or
   1 exchange milk + 1 exchange fruit (27 g)
4. Total the carbohydrate column. If the total deviates more than 3 or 4 g from the prescribed amount, adjust the amounts of vegetable, fruit, and bread. No diet should be planned with fractions of an exchange, since awkward measures of food would sometimes be encountered.
5. Determine the number of meat exchanges. Add up the protein value of all foods so far cal-

Table 4-4. **Calculation of Diet Using Exchange Lists**

Food	Exchanges	Carbohydrate (g)	Protein (g)	Fat (g)	Energy (kcal)
Starch/Bread	2	30	6	—	160
Vegetables	2	10	4	—	50
Fruits	2	30	—	—	120
Milk, 2 percent	2	24	16	10	240
		94			
Fruit	2	30	—	—	120
		124	26		
Meat, lean	6	—	42	18	330
				28	
Fat	4	—	—	20	180
		124	68	48	1200

120 g carbohydrate prescribed total
− 94 g carbohydrate from four groups
  26 g carbohydrate to be added
          26 ÷ 15 = 2 fruit exchanges. Note: total fruit exchanges = 4

  70 g protein prescribed total
− 26 g protein from first four groups
  44 g protein to be supplied by meat exchanges
          44 ÷ 7 = 6 meat exchanges

  50 g fat prescribed total
− 28 g fat from other food groups
  22 g fat to be supplied from fat exchanges
          22 ÷ 5 = 4 fat exchanges

culated. Subtract this total from the amount of protein prescribed. Divide the remainder by 7 (the protein value of one meat exchange). Use the nearest whole number of meat exchanges. Fill in the protein and fat values.

6. Determine the number of fat exchanges. Add up the fat values from the milk and meat. Subtract this total from the amount of fat prescribed. Divide the remainder by 5 (the fat content of one fat exchange). Fill in the fat value.

7. Check the entire diet for the accuracy of the computations. Divide the day's food allowance into a meal pattern suitable for the client.

Problems and Review

1. *Key terms*: basic diet; bioavailability; index of nutritional quality; nutrient density; exchange list.
2. List five reasons that might account for the differences in ascorbic acid content in two oranges.
3. *Problem*. Consulting the tables in the Appendix, list the values for each of the following:
   a. The protein value of one exchange of meat (A-4)
   b. The cholesterol content of one whole egg (A-5)
   c. The total dietary fiber in one shredded wheat biscuit (A-3)
   d. The copper and zinc in 100 g peanut butter (A-2)
   e. The calcium, iron, and vitamin C in 1 cup mashed potatoes with milk and butter added (A-1)
4. *Problem*. Using Table A-1, list five fresh fruits that are the most outstanding sources of vitamin A. Of vitamin C.
5. *Problem*. Keep a careful record of your own food intake for three days. Indicate on your record the time of day when you ate the foods and snacks.
   a. Score your diet according to the Daily Food Guide. What food group, if any, requires more emphasis in order to improve your diet?
   b. Select one day that is most typical of your usual food intake. Calculate the nutritive values using Table A-1. Compare the day's totals with the recommended allowances.
   c. Using the exchange lists calculate the carbohydrate, protein, fat, and energy values for the same diet used for the calculation in (b) above. For foods that are not covered in the exchange lists, use values from Table A-1.
   d. Keep these calculations for reference as you study the nutrients in the chapters that follow.
6. *Problem*. Plan a menu for a lunch that permits the following exchanges: one milk; two vegetables; one fruit; three bread; two meat; three fat.
7. *Problem*. Write three breakfast menus based on the following exchange requirements: one milk; one fruit; two bread; two meat; and two fat.

References

1. Rose, M. S.: *A Laboratory Handbook for Dietetics.* Macmillan Publishing Company, New York, 1929.

2. *USRDA Comparison Charts.* National Dairy Council, Chicago, 1974.

3. Sorenson, A. W., et al.: "An Index of Nutritional Quality for a Balanced Diet," *J. Am. Diet. Assoc.*, **68**:236–42, 1976.

4. Case, E.: "Calculation of Diabetic Diets," *J. Am. Diet. Assoc.*, **26**:575–83, 1950.

5. American Diabetes Association, Inc., and The American Dietetic Association: *Exchange Lists for Meal Planning.* The American Dietetic Association, Chicago, 1986.

6. Canadian Diabetes Association: *Good Health Eating Guide.* Toronto, Ont., 1982.

5

Proteins and Amino Acids

In 1838 a Dutch chemist, Mulder, described certain organic material that is "unquestionably the most important of all known substances in the organic kingdom. Without it no life appears possible on our planet. Through its means the chief phenomena of life are produced."* Berzelius, a contemporary of Mulder, suggested that this complex nitrogen-bearing substance be called *protein* from the Greek word meaning to "take the first place."[1]

Composition, Structure, and Classification

PROTEIN is now retained as a group name to designate the principal nitrogenous constituents of the protoplasm of all plant and animal tissues; proteins are necessary for the synthesis of all body tissues and for innumerable regulatory functions. To say that proteins are more important than other nutrients is not appropriate, however, for we shall see in the study of nutrition that an inadequate dietary supply or an interference with the utilization of any nutrient can have serious consequences.

Composition Proteins are extremely complex nitrogenous organic compounds in which amino acids are the basic units of structure. They contain the elements carbon, hydrogen, oxygen, nitrogen, and, with few exceptions, sulfur. Most proteins also contain phosphorus, and some specialized proteins contain very small amounts of iron, copper, and other inorganic elements.

The presence of nitrogen distinguishes protein from carbohydrate and fat. Proteins contain an average of 16 percent nitrogen and have a molecular weight that varies from 13,000 or less to many millions. Thus, the protein molecule is much larger than those of carbo-

hydrates and lipids. The large protein molecules form colloidal solutions that do not readily diffuse through membranes.

Structure AMINO ACIDS are organic compounds possessing an amino (NH_2) group and an acid or carboxyl (COOH) group. All the amino acids obtained by hydrolysis from native proteins are alpha-amino acids; that is, the amino group is attached to the carbon adjacent to the acid group. The structure of an amino acid may be represented thus:

$$\begin{array}{c} NH_2 \\ | \\ R-C-COOH \\ | \\ H \end{array}$$

By varying the grouping (R) that is attached to the carbon containing the amino group, many different amino acids are possible. The R grouping might contain a straight or a branched chain; an aromatic or heterocyclic ring structure; or a sulfur grouping.

Most amino acids are neutral in reaction; that is, they have one amino and one carboxyl group. Amino acids with two carboxyl groups and one amino group are acid in reaction, whereas those with two amino and one carboxyl group are basic in reaction. (See Table 5-1 and Figure 5-1.)

Twenty-two amino acids are widely distributed in proteins, and small amounts of four or five additional amino acids have been isolated from one or more proteins. Some amino acids—ornithine and citrulline—are important intermediates in metabolism but are not constituents of intact proteins. (See page 53.)

Proteins consist of chains of amino acids joined to each other by the PEPTIDE LINKAGE; that is, the amino group of one amino acid is linked to the carboxyl group of another amino acid by the removal of water. (See Figure 5-2.) Thus, two amino acids form a dipeptide, three amino acids form a tripeptide, and so on. Proteins consist of hundreds of such linkages.

The PRIMARY STRUCTURE of the protein molecule is determined by the chain of amino acids. Chains vary

---

* Mulder, G. J.: *The Chemistry of Animal and Vegetable Physiology.* Quoted in Mendel, L. B.; *Nutrition: The Chemistry of Life.* Yale University Press, New Haven, Conn., 1923, p. 16.

IMPORTANT ISSUES

Proteins are abundantly supplied in the diets of most people living in the western world, but protein shortages are second only to energy deficits for people living in the developing nations. The plight of hungry, malnourished children is especially sad. The contrast between the diets of the affluent and the economically deprived is indeed great. On one hand is the abundance of high-quality protein available from animal foods, and on the other a food supply consisting chiefly of plant foods that furnish inadequate amounts as well as quality of protein. That the protein content of the diet has attracted the attention of the public is not surprising. This has led to a number of ambiguous, misleading, or even erroneous ideas.

People have been encouraged to consume more and more animal foods. To be sure, these foods are excellent sources of high-quality proteins and of other nutrients as well. But how much protein do we really need? What factors influence the need for protein? Are there any dangers attached to the overconsumption of protein-rich foods?

In the United States vegetarianism is applauded by many and criticized by others. Since most of the world's population consumes diets that are largely, if not completely, made up of plant foods, what are some ways by which the quality of the protein in the diet can be ensured?

Protein supplements are advertised as aids to increased vitality and well-being. Athletes have been led to believe that their performance will improve if they use such products. Others are convinced that these supplements are needed to replace worn-out tissues. Although patients with some disease states may require protein supplementation of their diets, do healthy people really need them? Do athletes and laborers engaged in vigorous physical activity have an increased need for protein?

Some advocates of "health foods" proclaim the exceptional nutritional attributes of specific foods: for example, foods rich in nucleoproteins such as organ meats, "red meats," seeds and sprouts, and so on. Based upon the body's metabolism of protein, are such claims valid?

Table 5-1. **Classification of Amino Acids**

Classification	Essential Amino Acids	Nonessential Amino Acids
Aliphatic amino acids		
Neutral reaction	Threonine	Glycine
	Valine*	Alanine
	Leucine*	
	Isoleucine*	Serine
Sulfur-containing	Methionine	Cysteine
		Cystine
Acid reaction		Aspartic acid
		Asparagine
		Glutamic acid
		Glutamine
Basic reaction	Lysine	Arginine
		Hydroxylysine
Aromatic amino acids		
Neutral reaction	Phenylalanine	Tyrosine
Heterocyclic amino acids		
Neutral reaction	Tryptophan	Proline
	Histidine (slightly basic)	Hydroxyproline

* Also referred to as branched-chain amino acids; sometimes classified as semiessential. See page 47.

from one another according to (1) the number and kinds of amino acids, (2) the number of times and sequence in which each amino acid might appear in the chain, and (3) the length of the chain. A tripeptide consisting of only three amino acids could vary in six ways. With 20 or more amino acids occurring in protein molecules, it becomes evident that almost innumerable combinations are possible.

The SECONDARY STRUCTURE of the protein pertains to bonds such as hydrogen and sulfur that occur between amino acids in the chain that are near each other. The TERTIARY STRUCTURE of the protein refers to the way in which the amino acid chains are bound together to give the shape and characteristics of performance needed by the protein. In certain proteins made up of protein subunits the QUATERNARY STRUCTURE represents the manner of association or binding between the units.

Some estimates place the number of functioning proteins in the human body at more than 100,000. Each protein is synthesized to perform a specific function, and that function generally cannot be assumed by another. Hemoglobin, insulin, albumin, myosin,

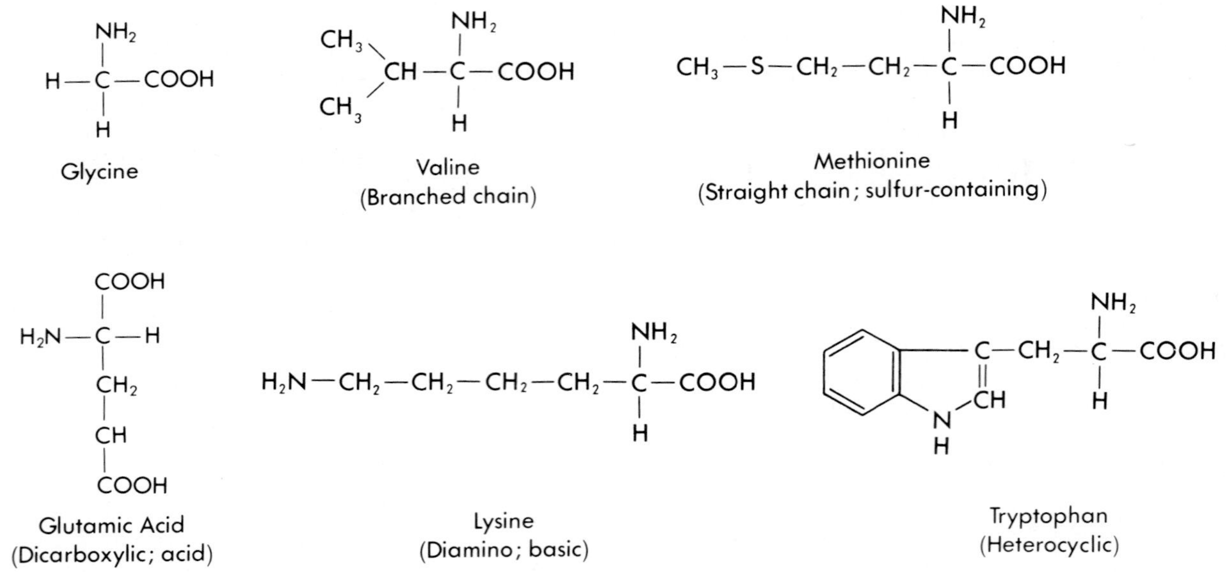

Figure 5-1. Amino acids with different groupings attached to the carbon that holds the amino group.

keratin, collagen, retinene, and carboxylase are only a few examples of proteins that differ widely in their structure, properties, and functions. Moreover, specific proteins of one species differ from those of another. For example, insulins from pig, horse, and sheep are distinct because of differences in one or two amino acids in the peptide chains.

Classification   Proteins may be classified in a number of ways, including physical and chemical properties, physical shape, and nutritional properties.

Physicochemical properties.   Each of the three groups within this classification may be subdivided into a number of classes according to solubility.

1. SIMPLE PROTEINS upon hydrolysis by acids, alkalies, or enzymes yield only amino acids or their derivatives. Examples of this group are albumin in blood plasma and lactalbumin in milk; keratin, collagen, and elastin in supportive tissues of the body and in hair and nails; globin in hemoglobin and myoglobin; zein in corn; gliadin and glutenin in wheat.

2. CONJUGATED PROTEINS are composed of simple proteins combined with a nonprotein substance. This group includes *lipoproteins*, the vehicles for the transport of fats in the blood; *nucleoproteins*, the proteins of the cell nuclei; *phosphoproteins*, such as casein in milk and ovovitellin in eggs; *metalloproteins*, such as the enzymes that contain mineral elements; *mucoproteins*, found in connective tissues, mucin, and gonadotropic hormones; *chromoproteins*, such as hemoglobin and visual purple; and *flavoproteins*, which are enzymes that contain the vitamin riboflavin.

3. DERIVED PROTEINS are substances resulting from the decomposition of simple and conjugated proteins. These include rearrangements within the molecule

Figure 5-2. Peptide linkage (CONH). The carboxyl group of one amino acid is linked to the amino group of another amino acid by the removal of water. This reaction is reversed by hydrolysis, as in the digestion of proteins.

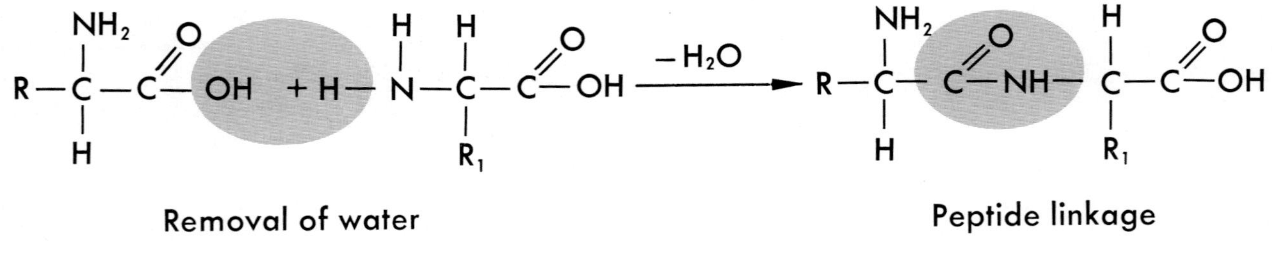

without breaking the peptide bond, such as that occurring with coagulation, and also substances formed by hydrolysis of the protein to smaller fragments.

Physical Shape. FIBROUS PROTEINS consist of long polypeptide chains bound together in more or less parallel fashion to form a linear shape. They are generally insoluble in body fluids and give strength to tissues in which they appear. Keratin in hair and nails, collagen in tendons and bone matrices, and elastin in the blood vessel walls are a few examples.

GLOBULAR PROTEINS are chains of amino acids that are coiled and tightly packed together in a round or ellipsoidal shape. They are generally soluble in body fluids and include such proteins as hemoglobin, insulin, enzymes, albumin, and others.

Nutritional Properties. The body requires 20 or so amino acids for the synthesis of its proteins. In 1915 Osborne and Mendel observed that rats failed to grow or even survive if some amino acids were omitted from the diet but that the elimination of other amino acids had no such harmful effects. Later work by others, especially Dr. William C. Rose,[2] established that this was also true for humans. Thus, amino acids came to be classified as *essential* or *indispensable* and *nonessential* or *dispensable*. (See Table 5-1.)

ESSENTIAL AMINO ACIDS are those that cannot be synthesized in the body at a rate sufficient to meet body needs. Histidine, for which the requirement by adults has long been uncertain, is now believed to be essential.[3] Thus, humans require nine essential amino acids.

Methionine, an essential amino acid, can be converted to cystine, but cystine cannot be converted to methionine. Likewise, phenylalanine can be converted to tyrosine, but tyrosine cannot be converted to phenylalanine. When cystine and tyrosine are present in the diet, the requirements for methionine and phenylalanine are reduced. Thus, cystine and tyrosine are sometimes classified as *semiessential*.

NONESSENTIAL or DISPENSABLE AMINO ACIDS are those that the body can synthesize from an available source of nitrogen and a carbon skeleton. Typical mixed diets contain ample amounts of both essential and nonessential amino acids.

Based on their content of amino acids, foods are often classified as sources of *complete*, *partially complete*, or *incomplete proteins*. A COMPLETE PROTEIN contains enough of the essential amino acids to maintain body tissues and to promote a normal rate of growth and is sometimes referred to as having a HIGH-BIOLOGIC VALUE. Egg, milk, and meat (including poultry and fish) proteins are all complete but are not necessarily identical in quality. Wheat germ and dried yeast have a biologic value approaching that of animal sources.

PARTIALLY COMPLETE PROTEINS will maintain life, but they lack sufficient amounts of some of the amino acids necessary for growth. Gliadin, which is one of a number of proteins found in wheat, is a notable example of proteins of this class. Adults under no physiologic stress can maintain satisfactory nutrition for indefinite periods when consuming sufficient amounts of protein from certain cereals or legumes.

Totally INCOMPLETE PROTEINS are incapable of replacing or building new tissue, hence cannot support life, let alone promote growth. Zein, one of the proteins found in corn, and gelatin are classic examples of proteins that are incapable of even permitting life to continue. This is an inexact and sometimes misleading classification since single foods are rarely eaten alone. We shall see in the discussion that follows that one food can effectively make up for the lack in another.

Functions

Maintenance and Growth Proteins constitute the chief solid matter of muscles, organs, and endocrine glands. They are major constituents of the matrix of bones and teeth; skin, nails, and hair; and blood cells and serum. In fact, every living cell and all body fluids, except bile and urine, contain protein. The first need for amino acids, then, is to supply the materials for the building and the continuous replacement of the cell proteins throughout life.

Regulation of Body Processes Body proteins have highly specialized functions in the regulation of body processes. Some of these can be classified as follows:

Nucleoproteins contain the blueprint for the synthesis of all body proteins.

Catalytic proteins, that is, the enzymes, number in the thousands to facilitate each step of digestion, absorption, anabolism, and catabolism.

Hormonal proteins set or release the brakes that control metabolic processes.

Immune proteins maintain the body's resistance to disease.

Contractile proteins (myosin, actin) regulate muscle contraction.

Blood proteins are involved in a wide variety of functions. The *transport* proteins ferry nutrients to the tissues; for example, hemoglobin, lipoproteins, transferrin (iron transport), retinol-binding protein (vitamin A transport), and others. Hemoglobin is involved not only in the transport of oxygen and carbon dioxide but contributes to acid–base balance. The plasma proteins, especially albumin, are of fundamental importance in the regulation of osmotic pressure and in the maintenance of fluid balance.

Individual amino acids also have specific functions in metabolism. Tryptophan serves as a precursor for niacin and also for serotonin, a vasoconstrictor; methionine supplies labile methyl groups for the synthesis of choline, a compound needed for the formation of acetylcholine, a neurotransmitter; glycine contributes to the formation of the porphyrin ring in the hemoglobin molecule and is also an important constituent of the purines and pyrimidines in nucleic acid.

Energy Proteins are a potential source of energy, each gram of protein yielding on the average 4 kcal. The energy needs of the body take priority over other needs, and if the diet does not furnish sufficient calories from carbohydrate and fat, the protein of the diet as well as tissue proteins will be catabolized for energy. When amino acids are used for energy, they are then lost for synthetic purposes. Conversely, when amino acids are incorporated into the protein molecule, they are not furnishing energy until such time as the tissue proteins are again being catabolized.

Digestion and Absorption

Digestion The purposes of digestion are to hydrolyze proteins to small peptides and amino acids so that they can be absorbed. (See also Chapter 2.) The protein to be digested in the intestinal tract includes that provided by food (exogenous source) and also that available from worn-out cells of the mucosa and of the digestive enzymes (endogenous source). The total protein requiring digestion could be as much as 160 g or so (90 to 100 g from food and 70 g from endogenous sources).[4] Within the digestive tract the endogenous and exogenous sources are indistinguishable.

Saliva contains no proteolytic enzyme, and thus the only action in the mouth is an increase in the surface area of the food mass as a result of the chewing of food. Most of the hydrolysis of protein occurs in the stomach, duodenum, and jejunum. The protein molecule is split into smaller fragments by the proteases with final cleavage by the peptidases. Several of the enzymes are secreted in their inactive form and are

activated when they are needed for protein hydrolysis. Some enzymes are highly specific and are capable of splitting only one type of peptide linkage. For example, trypsin attacks only those peptide linkages involving the carboxyl groups of arginine and lysine.

For many years proteins were believed to be completely hydrolyzed in the intestinal lumen to free amino acids. It is now generally accepted that small peptides are the major products, and these are subsequently acted on by enzymes in the brush border and cytoplasm of intestinal cells to form amino acids. Table 5-2 summarizes important gastrointestinal enzymes involved in protein hydrolysis as well as the linkages with which they react.

Effect of Protein Denaturation. Proteolytic enzymes not only bring about the splitting of the peptide linkages but they also split the crosslinks that connect the peptide chains. During moderate heating of proteins some of the crosslinkages are split, thereby facilitating digestion. On the other hand, excessive heating results in the formation of linkages that are resistant to the digestive enzymes.

One resistant linkage known as the *Maillard* or *browning reaction* is that formed between lysine and carbohydrate as a result of high, usually prolonged heat. Some breakfast cereals processed at high temperatures are subject to such losses. These changes may assume some importance when the diet supplies limited amounts of low-quality proteins.

Effect of Enzyme Inhibitors. Some foods such as navy beans and soybeans contain substances that inhibit the activity of enzymes such as trypsin. Heating inactivates these inhibitors, thereby improving the digestibility of the protein.

Coefficient of Digestibility. The digestibility of a protein is the percentage of protein intake available for absorption. Determination of digestibility requires nitrogen analyses of foods and feces. Because part of the fecal nitrogen comes from endogenous sources and occurs even when no protein is eaten, a correction must be made to determine the true digestibility of a protein. The calculation is as follows:

$$CD = \frac{\text{N intake} - (\text{fecal N} - \text{fecal N on protein-free diet})}{\text{N intake}} \times 100$$

Milk and eggs have a coefficient of digestibility of about 97; meat, fish, and poultry slightly less than that; and plant proteins about 75 to 85. Thus, diets containing substantial amounts of animal foods will

Table 5-2.   Enzyme Activity in Protein Digestion

Enzyme and Its Location	Action
Stomach	
Pepsinogen	Activated to pepsin by hydrochloric acid
Pepsin	Splits peptide bonds where aromatic amino acids or leucine furnishes amino group
Small intestine	
Trypsin*	Splits peptide chain where lysine or arginine furnishes carboxyl group
Chymotrypsin*	Splits peptide chain where carboxyl group is furnished by tryptophan, tyrosine, phenylalanine
Carboxypeptidases*	Splits peptide linkages next to terminal carboxyl group
Intestinal cell	
Brush border	
Aminooligopeptidases	Splits short peptides at amino terminal end
Dipeptidases	Splits dipeptides to amino acids
Cytoplasm	
Di- and tripeptidases	Splits di- and tripeptides to amino acids

* Precursor forms of these enzymes are secreted by the pancreas. Trypsinogen is converted to active form in intestine by enterokinase; chymotrypsinogen and procarboxypeptidases by trypsin.

have a higher digestibility than those consisting primarily of plant foods. Typical mixed American diets have a protein digestibility of about 92 percent.

Absorption   The small peptides and amino acids present in the intestinal lumen after digestion are taken up by the intestinal cell by independent processes. Rates of absorption frequently are faster for amino acids in peptides than for free amino acids. This relationship has useful practical application in providing nutritional therapy for persons with digestive and absorptive disorders. In contrast to amino acids, which are absorbed more rapidly in the proximal jejunum, peptides appear to be absorbed equally well in both the proximal and distal intestine.[5]

Intestinal uptake of peptides is limited to di- and tripeptides and is mediated by a specific carrier system. Longer peptides appear to be cleaved by brush-border enzymes on the surface of the cell: the products, including both dipeptides and amino acids, are absorbed by their respective transport mechanisms. Relatively little is known about the factors affecting peptide absorption.

Amino acids are absorbed by active transport, but some diffusion of amino acids also occurs. Separate carriers exist for the transport of four specific groups of amino acids, and competition occurs among the groups of amino acids for the shared carrier. Because of this competition, the absorption of a protein having an excess amount of a rapidly absorbed amino acid may be less effective than that of a more balanced protein, inasmuch as carriers would be less available for the amino acids with the lower rates of absorption. The absorption of amino acids is energy dependent and is coupled with sodium absorption.

The rates of absorption of amino acids are regulated by complex mechanisms not fully understood. These rates are dependent on (1) the total load of amino acids released through digestion, (2) the proportions of the various amino acids present in the mixture to be absorbed, (3) the availability of carriers to transport the amino acids into the mucosal cells, and (4) the uptake of amino acids by tissues. Amino acids are transported from the mucosal cell into the portal circulation and are rapidly removed from the blood as it circulates. The concentration of amino acids in the blood at any given time is relatively low.

Metabolism

Strictly speaking, the metabolism of proteins is the metabolism of the amino acids. Each cell within the body utilizes the available amino acids to synthesize all the numerous proteins required for its own functions and also makes use of amino acids to furnish energy. In addition, some specialized cells, such as those of the liver, also synthesize proteins and nonprotein nitrogenous substances that are required for the functioning of the body as a whole. Whether the fate of an amino acid, at any given moment, is that of anabolism or catabolism is determined by a number of interrelated factors.

Methods for Study of Protein Metabolism   The biochemist and the nutrition scientist use many techniques for the study of protein metabolism. The nitrogen balance technique described in more detail on page 54 is a classic method for determining the amino acid and protein requirements of humans under varying conditions. The quality of food proteins has been assayed by animal growth studies, by nitrogen balance studies on animals, and by analyses for amino acid content (see page 57).

Biochemical methods are available for evaluating nutritional status with respect to protein and also for tracing metabolic pathways of amino acids. The determination of hemoglobin, total serum protein, serum albumin, and gamma globulins provides information on the ability to fulfill such diverse functions as supplying oxygen to the tissues, maintaining water balance, and resisting infections. Measurement of the nonprotein nitrogenous constituents of the blood—total nonprotein nitrogen, urea, creatinine, and uric acid—gives clues to renal function. (See Tables A-27 and A-28.) The researcher in cellular nutrition uses highly sophisticated procedures for tracing the pathways of metabolism of individual acids. Many of these studies are possible today because of automated techniques, availability of stable and radioactive isotopes and the application of computer science.

Dynamic Equilibrium   The liver is the key organ in the metabolism of protein. As amino acids are absorbed, the concentration in the portal circulation rises considerably. The liver rapidly removes the amino acids from the portal circulation for the synthesis of its own proteins and for many of the specialized proteins such as lipoproteins, plasma albumins, globulins, and fibrinogen as well as nonprotein nitrogenous substances such as creatine. The liver is also the principal organ for the synthesis of urea.

Amino acids are transported throughout the body by the systemic circulation and are rapidly taken up by the various tissue cells. Likewise, amino acids and products of amino acid metabolism are constantly added to the circulation by the tissues. The AMINO ACID POOL available to any given tissue at any given moment thus includes dietary sources (exogenous) and tissue breakdown (endogenous sources). These sources are indistinguishable. Body proteins are not static structures, but there is a continuous turnover, taking up and release of amino acids. In the adult the gains and losses are about equal, and the state is known as *dynamic equilibrium*, (See Figure 5-3.)

The rate of turnover varies widely in body tissues. The intestinal mucosa, for example, renews itself every 1 to 3 days—a fantastic rate of repletion! The liver also has a high rate of turnover. Muscle proteins have a much slower rate of turnover, but the size of the muscle mass in the body is so great that the turnover of muscle protein alone has been estimated to be about 75 g per day.[4] The turnover rate of collagen is very slow, and that of the brain cells is negligible.

Protein Reserves.   Although the body does not store protein in the sense that it stores fat, or glycogen, or vitamin A, certain "reserves" are available from practically all body tissues for use in an emergency. Based on animal studies, about one fourth of the body protein can be depleted and repleted.[6] Thus, the vital functions of the organism may be protected for 30 to 50 days of total starvation or for much longer periods of partial starvation. It should be apparent that the use of these reserves eventually requires restoration of tissue to their normal protein composition.

Anabolism or Catabolism   Whether an amino acid is utilized for the synthesis of new proteins or is deaminized and used for energy depends on a number of factors.

1. *The "all-or-none" law*. All the amino acids needed for the synthesis of a given protein must be simultaneously present in sufficient amounts. If a single amino acid is missing, the protein cannot be constructed. If a given amino acid is present only to a limited extent, the protein can be formed only as long as the supply of that amino acid lasts. The amino acid in short supply is known as the LIMITING AMINO ACID. If one or more amino acids are missing from the pool, the remaining amino acids are unavailable for later synthesis and will be catabolized for energy.
2. *Adequacy of calorie intake*. For protein synthesis to proceed at an optimum rate, the calorie intake must be sufficient to supply the energy needs. A deficiency of calories necessitates the use of some dietary and tissue proteins for energy.
3. *The nutritional and physiologic state of the individual*. The rate of synthesis is high during growth and in tissue repletion following illness or injury. In the adult synthesis just balances tissue depletion when the calorie intake is adequate. Protein catabolism is greatly increased immediately following an injury, burns, and immobilization because of illness. It is also increased as a result of fear, anxiety, or anger. For example, unmarried pregnant girls who are worried about their future often have a negative nitrogen balance in spite of diets that appear to be adequate.

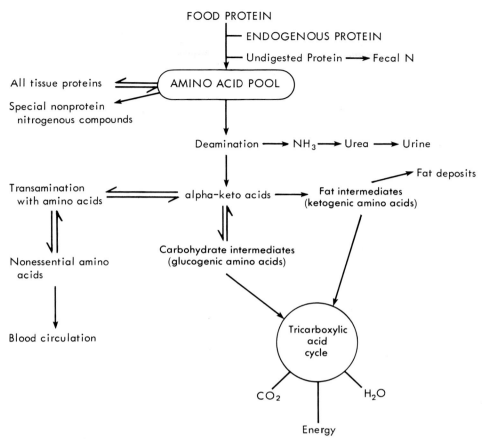

Figure 5-3.   Amino acids may be synthesized to body proteins or may be deaminized to yield carbon skeletons that lead to formation of carbohydrates or fats or to the production of energy. By transamination these carbon skeletons can also be used to form nonessential amino acids.

4. *Development of specific tissues.* Some tissues may be synthesized even though the overall nitrogen balance might be negative. Thus, the fetus and maternal tissues may be developed at the expense of the mother when her diet is inadequate. Another example of specific tissue development is that of rapidly growing tumors that use amino acids at the expense of normal tissues.

5. *Hormonal controls.* The pituitary growth hormone has an anabolic effect during infancy and childhood, and the estrogens and androgens exert an anabolic effect during preadolescent and adolescent years. By bringing about normal carbohydrate metabolism insulin has an indirect anabolic effect by reducing the breakdown of proteins to supply glucose. Insulin facilitates the transport of amino acids into the cell. In normal amounts thyroid hormone also stimulates growth.

Among the hormones that increase the catabolism of body tissues are adrenocortical hormones which stimulate the breakdown of tissue proteins to yield glucose. An excessive production of thyroxine also increases the breakdown of proteins.

Synthesis of Proteins   Each cell is capable of synthesizing an enormous number of proteins. Some of these proteins remain within the cell to carry out cellular functions. Other proteins, for example, pancreatic enzymes and insulin, leave the cell to carry out specialized functions.

The synthesis of each protein requires (1) a source of information or a pattern, (2) a "transcription" of that pattern to the site of synthesis, and (3) a "translation" of that pattern into a new protein. (See Figure 5-4.)

The Source of Information.   The pattern for each protein exists within the nucleus of the cell in giant molecules known as DEOXYRIBONUCLEIC ACID (DNA). These molecules consist of a large number of subunits called nucleotides, which are joined together to form two intertwining chains having a double helical struc-

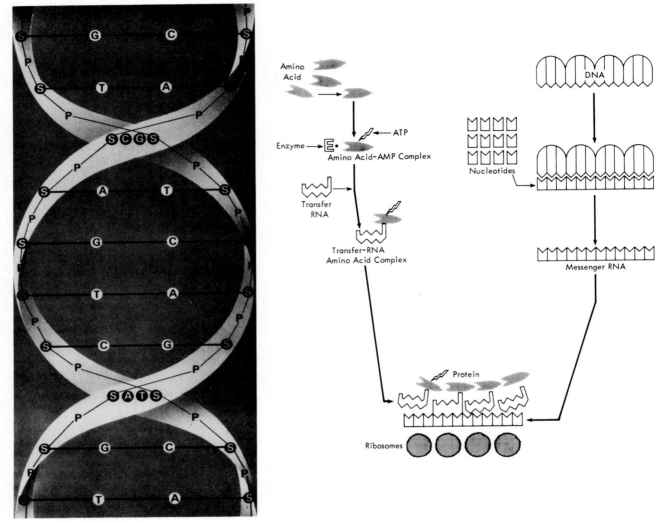

Figure 5-4. (*Left*) The Watson-Crick DNA model. Shown here are only a few of the thousands of turns in the double-helic structure of the molecule. The two outer ribbons are the backbone of the molecule, consisting of the sugar (S) deoxyribose and phosphate (P). Crosslinks between the two ribbons are pairs of bases: adenine (A) with thymine (T) and guanine (G) with cytosine (C). (Courtesy, World Health Organization.) (*Right*) Schematic representation of protein synthesis. The transfer of amino acids by transfer RNA causes the two halves to line up according to the pattern brought from the nucleus by messenger RNA. (Courtesy, Dr. J. Paul Burnett and Eli Lilly and Company.)

ture. The five-carbon sugar, deoxyribose, and the phosphate groups of the nucleotides form the backbone for the chains. The four nitrogen-containing purine and pyrimidine bases in the nucleotides of adjacent chains are joined in pairs by hydrogen bonding to give a firm structure resembling a spiral staircase. Adenine forms bonds only with thymine; guanine forms bonds only with cytosine.

The sequence of the nucleotides in the DNA is the code for the synthesis of new proteins. The coding

unit (codon) consists of a combination of three nucleotides.

Transcription. Since the DNA is within the nucleus and protein synthesis takes place in the cytoplasm, how is the code transferred to the site of synthesis? A special type of ribonucleic acid (RNA) called *messenger RNA (mRNA)* brings this about. RNA is very similar to DNA in its structure except that (1) it contains the sugar ribose instead of deoxyribose, (2) the pyrimidine base uracil replaces thymine, and (3) RNA consists of one strand instead of two. The information from DNA is copied in the nucleus by mRNA which then moves into the cytoplasm to the ribosomes that are the site of protein synthesis.

Translation. Some of the amino acids in the cytoplasm have entered the cell from the amino acid pool, and other nonessential amino acids may have been synthesized within the cell. Before these amino acids can be used in the synthesis of proteins they must be activated by a reaction that requires a specific activating enzyme and a source of energy, ATP. Each activated amino acid then becomes attached to another kind of RNA, known as *transfer RNA (tRNA)*. The amino acid–tRNA complex moves to the ribosomal-mRNA site and is positioned into the peptide linkage in exactly the sequence of the mRNA pattern. When the peptide bond has been formed the tRNA is released so that it can again combine with another activated amino acid to repeat its function. When the new protein molecule is complete, it is released from the template.

The daily protein synthesis in the body has been estimated to be about 300 g by the adult, an amount that is three to four times the daily intake of protein.[4]

Synthesis of Nonessential Amino Acids The materials for the formation of the nonessential amino acids come from carbohydrates, fats, and other amino acids. In a process known as TRANSAMINATION the amino group of one amino acid can be transferred to a ketoacid, usually those formed in the metabolism of carbohydrates. (See Figure 6-4.) This process is catalyzed by enzymes known as *transaminases*. These require the vitamin B-6 coenzyme, pyridoxal phosphate, for their activity. By this mechanism a new amino acid is formed. The general reaction is as follows:

$$R_1CHNH_2COOH + R_2COCOOH \rightleftharpoons$$
Amino acid$_1$ · · · · · Ketoacid$_2$

$$R_2CHNH_2COOH + R_1COCOOH$$
Amino acid$_2$ · · · · · Ketoacid$_1$

Catabolism When amino acids are used for energy, the amino group is removed first leaving a ketoacid. Removal of the amino group can be accomplished by transamination, as described above. The reaction frequently involves alpha-ketoglutaric acid, with subsequent formation of glutamic acid. Removal of the amino group from glutamic acid can then occur by oxidative deamination to form ammonia (ammonium ion, NH_4^+, at body pH). Deamination occurs primarily in the liver, but it occurs to some extent in

the kidney as well. Ketoacids and ammonia formed during these processes are disposed of in the following ways:

Ketoacids. The ketoacid fractions enter the common pathway for energy metabolism at various points of the cycle depending on the amino acids from which they were derived. There they may be completely oxidized to yield energy, carbon dioxide, and water. The common pathway for the release of energy is described in Chapter 6 (page 72). (See also Figure 5-5.)

Some of the amino acids, accounting for about 58 percent of the protein by weight, are said to be GLUCOGENIC; that is, after deamination they can be synthesized to glucose. Other amino acids, slightly less than half of the protein, are potentially KETOGENIC; that is, they can be synthesized to fat. These distinctions are not fully valid. For example, in Figure 5-5 it may be noted that a number of amino acids are converted to pyruvic acid, which, in turn, can form glucose or can combine with coenzyme A and proceed to form fatty acids.

Disposal of Ammonia. Most of the ammonia released through deamination is synthesized to urea. A small amount of ammonia may be used in the formation of new amino acids or purines, pyrimidines, creatine, and other important nonprotein nitrogenous substances.

The liver is the primary organ for the synthesis of urea. This is an essential mechanism for the disposal of ammonia, which is highly toxic if it enters the systemic circulation. When the function of the liver is seriously impaired, ammonia enters the circulation and produces harmful effects on the central nervous system.

The KREBS–HENSELEIT CYCLE is a mechanism that explains the formation of urea. (See Figure 5-6.) This is an energy-requiring process. The ammonia combines with carbon dioxide (available from oxidation in the Krebs cycle) and ATP to form a carbamyl phosphate. This compound combines with ornithine—an amino acid—to initiate the urea cycle. A second molecule of ammonia is contributed to the cycle from aspartic acid. In the presence of arginase, an enzyme, and magnesium, arginine yields one molecule of urea and of ornithine. Thus, one turn of the cycle has effected the release of ammonia in the form of urea and is able to recycle again.

The excretion of urea and other nitrogenous products in the urine entails an obligatory excretion of fluid as well. In the absence of sufficient fluid the work of the kidney will be increased.

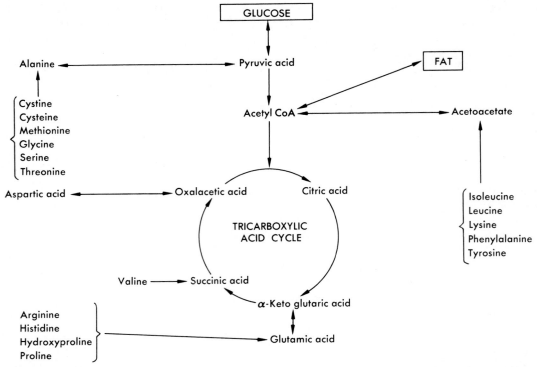

Figure 5-5. Amino acids enter the pathways common to carbohydrate and fat metabolism. Most amino acids are glucogenic; some are ketogenic; and a few are either ketogenic or glucogenic.

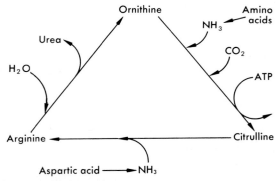

Figure 5-6. The Krebs-Henseleit cycle. A mechanism for disposing of ammonia by urea synthesis.

Dietary Protein Requirements and Allowances

Nitrogen Balance The protein requirement of individuals of varying ages has been determined primarily by the nitrogen balance technique. Nitrogen balance studies utilize the fact that protein, on the average, contains 16 percent nitrogen; thus, 1 g nitrogen is equivalent to 6.25 g protein. The balance may be expressed thus:

$$\text{Nitrogen balance} = \text{nitrogen intake} - \text{nitrogen excretion (urine} + \text{feces} + \text{skin)}$$

Nitrogen Excretion. The fecal nitrogen includes that from unabsorbed dietary protein and also nitrogen from undigested endogenous sources. The latter are composed of the undigested protein fractions of desquamated cells of the intestinal mucosa, the used-up enzymes from the digestive juices, and bacterial cells. The daily fecal excretion of nitrogen by the adult is approximately 1 g, but this varies with the quality of the protein fed, the gastrointestinal motility, and so on. The amount of nitrogen absorbed and available for tissue use is calculated as the difference between the amount of nitrogen in the diet and the fecal nitrogen. This value is referred to as *apparent* absorption because it does not take into consideration the amount of protein entering the intestines from endogenous sources.

More than 90 percent of the urinary nitrogen results from the deamination of the amino acids in the body and is excreted chiefly as urea with small amounts of ammonia. Nonprotein nitrogenous end products include creatinine, uric acid, and a number of others. When the calorie intake is fully adequate and the protein intake is just sufficient to cover the repletion of body tissues, the urinary nitrogen is at its lowest level. As the protein intake increases above the tissue maintenance requirement, the excess amino acids are not stored but are deaminized and used for energy or stored as fat, thereby increasing the amount of urinary nitrogen. Therefore, in studies of the minimum protein requirement by the nitrogen balance technique it is always necessary to determine the balance at gradually decreasing levels of intake until the point of negative balance is reached. That level just above negative balance that is just sufficient for tissue replacement represents the *minimum* protein requirement under the conditions of the experiment.

Nitrogen is also lost through perspiration and from the desquamated cells of the skin surfaces, the hair, and the nails. Such losses are extremely difficult to measure. Reported daily sweat losses have varied from 0.36 to 1.74 g per day with protein intakes of 85 to 100 g. Increased physical activity and high environmental temperatures augment sweat nitrogen losses and losses of 16 to 18 g protein per day have been reported.[7]

States of Balance. Nitrogen equilibrium is that state of balance when the intake of nitrogen is equal to that which is excreted. A state of equilibrium is normal for the healthy adult. It is established at any level of protein intake that exceeds the minimum requirement, provided that the calorie intake is also adequate.

Positive nitrogen balance is that state in which the intake of nitrogen exceeds the excretion. It indicates that new protein tissues are being synthesized, as in growing children or during pregnancy. Positive nitrogen balance also occurs when tissues depleted of protein during illness or injury are being replenished, or when muscles are being developed, as in athletic training. Positive nitrogen balance should not be interpreted as storage in the usual sense of the word. There is no further addition of protein to already well-nourished cells.

Negative nitrogen balance is that condition in which the excretion of nitrogen exceeds the intake. An individual with a negative nitrogen balance is losing nitrogen from tissues more rapidly than it is being replaced—an undesirable state of affairs. It may occur because (1) the calorie content of the diet is inadequate and therefore tissues are being broken down to supply energy; (2) the quality of the protein is poor and/or the amount fed is inadequate for tissue replacement; or (3) injury, immobilization, or disease are causing excessive breakdown of tissues.

Factors Affecting the Protein Requirement The following list summarizes the factors that determine the protein requirement of a given individual:

1. Sufficient protein for adults is needed to cover daily nitrogen losses in the urine, feces, desquamated skin, hair, nails, perspiration, and other secretions.
2. Essential amino acids must be present in sufficient amounts to meet needs for tissue regeneration.
3. Sufficient calories must be furnished to meet energy needs so that protein is not preferentially used for energy. Thus, carbohydrate and fat "spare" protein for its synthetic functions.
4. Growth needs of infants and children increase the protein requirements per kilogram of body weight.
5. Development of maternal tissues and the fetus during pregnancy increases the protein need.
6. Milk production by the mother increases the protein need.
7. A poor state of nutrition necessitates additional protein for repletion.
8. Infections, immobilization, surgery, burns, and other injuries increase protein catabolism and hence the protein requirement.
9. Emotional stress increases protein catabolism.
10. Diseases of malabsorption can seriously interfere with digestion and absorption, thus increasing the amount of protein needed or the manner of its feeding or both.

Essential Amino Acid Requirements Dr. Rose[8] has determined the quantitative requirements of the essential amino acids for healthy young men by feeding a controlled diet that included a mixture of pure amino acids flavored with lemon juice and sugar, as well as wafers made of cornstarch, sucrose, centrifuged butterfat, corn oil, and vitamins. Similar studies have been reported for young women and for infants.[9,10] The requirements on the basis of these studies are summarized in Table 5-3; they suffice only when the diet provides enough nitrogen for the synthesis of the nonessential amino acids so that the essential amino acids will not be used for this purpose. On a weight basis, it will be noted that the infant requirements are several times higher—a fact that one would expect in view of the high rate of tissue synthesis during infancy. For adults, only 20 percent of the total nitrogen requirement need be supplied by essential amino acids. For infants, essential amino acids should furnish about 35 percent of the total nitrogen requirement.[11]

Table 5-3. **Estimates of Amino Acid Requirements**[*]

| Amino Acid | Requirements, mg/kg per day, by age group | | | |
	Infants, Age 3–4 mo[†]	Children, Age ~2 yr[‡]	Children, Age 10–12 yr[§]	Adults[‖]
Histidine	28	?	?	8–12
Isoleucine	70	31	28	10
Leucine	161	73	42	14
Lysine	103	64	44	12
Methionine plus cystine	58	27	22	13
Phenylalanine plus tyrosine	125	69	22	14
Threonine	87	37	28	7
Tryptophan	17	12.5	3.3	3.5
Valine	93	38	25	10
Total without histidine	714	352	214	84

[*]From WHO (1985).

[†]Based on amounts of amino acids in human milk or cow's milk formulas fed at levels that supported good growth. Data from Fomon and Filer (1967).

[‡]Based on achievement of nitrogen balance sufficient to support adequate lean tissue gain (16 mg N/kg per day). Data from Pineda et al. (1981).

[§]Based on upper range of requirement for positive nitrogen balance. Recalculated by Williams et al. (1974) from data of Nakagawa et al. (1964).

[‖]Based on highest estimate of requirement to achieve nitrogen balance. Data from several investigators (reviewed in FAO/WHO, 1973).

Recommended Dietary Allowances On an experimental basis when a protein-free diet adequate in calories is fed to healthy adults the body becomes very efficient in conserving its tissue proteins. Although tissue breakdown continues, most of the amino acids released are used again to resynthesize new tissue. However, small losses of amino acids do occur, and their nitrogen is excreted in the urine. These losses are referred to as the *obligatory nitrogen loss*. Many studies on adults have shown that the daily nitrogen losses on the protein-free diet average 53 mg per kg. The protein equivalent of this loss is 331 mg per kg (53 × 6.25) or 0.33 g per kg. For a 50 kg individual this loss is equivalent to 16.5 g protein.

Several factors must be taken into account to assure adequate protein intake under normal living situations. Although a protein such as egg is almost perfectly utilized at submaintenance levels, there is a loss of efficiency as the maintenance level is approached. Based upon the reference protein, the requirement for adult males was found to be 0.61 g per kg daily.

Allowances must also be made for the variability of protein efficiency in typical mixed diets. Some proteins may be more completely digested than others. The proteins in mixed diets differ in their amino acid composition. Finally, variability also occurs from one individual to another. Based on these considerations, the recommended allowance for adults has been set at 0.75 g per kg per day—rounded off to 0.8 g per kg.

An allowance of 60 g protein per day during pregnancy will take care of the growth of the fetus and of the maternal tissues. During lactation an increase in the protein allowance of 15 g is satisfactory for the production of milk during the first 6 months, and an increase of 12 g daily thereafter.

Some studies suggest that the elderly require more protein than younger adults; others indicate a lesser requirement; and still others no difference. At present the adult allowance of 0.8 g per kg appears to be satisfactory for the older adult.

Allowances for growth. The allowance for infants is based on human milk as the source of protein. The allowance decreases from 2.2 g per kg during the first 6 months to 1.6 g per kg by the second half year. For children 1 to 10 years the daily allowances range from 16 to 28 g. On the basis of body weight, these are equivalent to 1.2 to 1.0 g per kg, the higher level being given during the second and third years and gradually decreasing with age. Protein allowance for teenage boys ranges from 45 to 59 g daily, and for teenage girls from 44 to 46 g.

Quality of Food Proteins

Measurement of Protein Quality The *protein efficiency ratio* (*PER*) is one of the simplest techniques for determining protein quality. The growth of young rats is observed over 28 days while they are fed an adequate diet that contains the test protein. The ratio is calculated thus:

$$PER = \frac{\text{grams weight gain}}{\text{grams protein consumed}}$$

Animal foods, except gelatin, yield high ratios, and plant foods have lower, widely varying ratios.

The PER is used in determining the amount of protein for the USRDA labeling standard. (See page 260.) The standard is 45 g protein for foods that have a PER equal to or greater than that of casein (PER = 2.5). The USRDA for protein is 65 g for foods having a PER less than that of casein.

Amino Acid Score (Chemical Score). The protein quality of a food can be determined by comparing its amino acid composition with the amino acid pattern of a reference protein such as the high-quality protein listed in the right column of Table 5-3. The calculation of the score for each amino acid is as follows:

$$AA\ score = \frac{\begin{array}{c}\text{milligrams of amino acid}\\\text{in 1 g test protein}\end{array}}{\begin{array}{c}\text{milligrams of amino acid}\\\text{in 1 g high-quality}\\\text{protein}\end{array}} \times 100$$

The amino acid that has the lowest score for any of the nine essential amino acids is the limiting amino acid for that protein and determines its chemical score. Amino acid scores do not take the absorption of amino acids into account, and thus the actual utilization from a given food might differ.

Table 5-4 shows a comparison of the scores for the three limiting amino acids in beans and rice. Note that methionine plus cystine is most limiting in beans, while lysine is most limiting in rice. But when beans and rice are eaten together, the two foods are *complementary*, or each may be said to *supplement* the other.

Biologic Value (BV). The biologic value is the percentage of absorbed nitrogen that is retained by the body. This determination requires measurement of the nitrogen content of food ingested and of the urinary and fecal excretions by the test animal under controlled conditions with the protein intake set below the requirement level.[11] In order to arrive at the

Table 5-4. **Comparison of the Content of Three Limiting Amino Acids in Beans and Rice with a High-Quality Protein**

	Lysine	Methionine + Cystine	Tryptophan
Amino acid pattern for high-quality protein* Milligrams per gram protein	51	26	11
Beans Milligrams per gram protein	74	20	9
Amino acid score	145	77†	82
Rice Milligrams per gram protein	39	32	11
Amino acid score	77†	123	100
Average, rice and beans Milligrams per gram protein	57	26	10
Amino acid score	112	100	90†

* See Table 5–3 for pattern for high-quality protein.
† Limiting amino acid.

true biologic value it is also necessary to take into account the urinary and fecal nitrogen excretion (N_0) that would occur when a protein-free diet is fed. The following equation shows the calculation:

$$BV = \frac{\text{food N} - [(\text{urine N} - N_0) + (\text{fecal N} - N_0)]}{\text{food N} - (\text{fecal N} - N_0)} \times 100$$

A protein that has a biologic value of 70 or more is capable of supporting growth provided that sufficient calories are also ingested. Biologic values of typical protein sources are as follows: egg, 100; milk, 93; rice, 86; casein, fish, and beef, 75; corn, 72; peanut flour, 56; and wheat gluten, 44.

Net Protein Utilization (NPU). This is the proportion of nitrogen consumed that is retained by the body under standard conditions. It takes into account the digestibility of food proteins. When food proteins are completely digested, the NPU and BV would be the same. When foods contain much fiber and have a lower digestibility, the NPU would be lower than the BV.

Like the biologic value, the intake of nitrogen and the urinary and fecal nitrogen must be determined. A correction must also be made for the nitrogen excretion on a protein-free diet.

$$NPU = \frac{\text{food N} - [(\text{urine N} - N_0) + (\text{fecal N} - N_0)]}{\text{Food N}} \times 100$$

Improving Protein Quality of Foods Most of the world's people consume diets in which the protein is derived principally or solely from plant foods. When foods are combined so that they supply sufficient amounts of all essential amino acids satisfactory protein nutrition is possible. This state is more readily achieved for adults than for infants and children. The principle of complementarity provides several possibilities for improving the protein quality of foods.

The Vegetarian Way. In the United States millions of people have adopted vegetarian diets for religious, ecologic, or economic reasons. (See pages 230–233 for fuller description.)

Lactovegetarians consume milk and cheese along with a variety of plant foods. Lacto-ovo-vegetarians eat eggs as well as milk and cheese. When appreciable amounts of plant proteins are fed with a small amount of animal protein foods, the quality of the mixture is as effective as if only animal proteins had been fed. For example, small amounts of milk, cheese, or egg will supply the lysine that is limiting in cereal foods. Thus, macaroni and cheese, cereal and milk, and bread and milk are complementary.

Legumes, whole grains, nuts, and vegetables provide a satisfactory combination of amino acids for strict vegetarians who eliminate all animal food.[12] However, in order for plant foods to supply all essential amino acids simultaneously, food combinations must be consumed at the same meal. The amino acid composition of foods within each category varies considerably; thus, selections should be made from a variety within each category.

Legumes (low in methionine plus cystine; good sources of lysine): peas, chickpeas (garbanzos), black-eyed peas, white beans, red beans, lima beans, soybeans, peanuts, lentils

Cereal grains, nuts, seeds (low in lysine; good sources of methionine plus cystine): whole wheat, cracked wheat, bulgur, oatmeal, millet, rye, barley, cornmeal; almonds, Brazil nuts, cashews, filberts, pecans, walnuts; pumpkin, sesame, and sunflower seeds

The adequacy of vegetarian diets depends not only on the combination of foods that are used but on the total amount of food as well. In a recent longitudinal study comparing growth of children up to 6 years of age, weights and lengths of vegetarian children were less than those of nonvegetarian children, although the differences were small. Interestingly, analysis of food records suggested that energy intakes were below recommended levels but protein intakes did not appear to be limiting.[13]

Vegetarian diets that offer little variety can be extremely dangerous. One example is the Zen macrobiotic diet, in which the final stage consists principally of brown rice.[14] It is true that rice can meet the protein needs of the healthy adult when sufficient amounts are consumed to meet caloric requirements as well. But rice alone cannot meet the protein needs of infants, children, pregnant women, and protein-depleted persons. Moreover, a diet consisting principally of rice fails to supply essential minerals and vitamins, and metabolic derangements occur, including interference with protein metabolism.

Amino Acid Supplementation. Lysine and methionine can be produced at costs sufficiently low to make it practical to add them to foods in which they are limiting. Thus, the addition of lysine to white bread improves the biologic value of the bread. Amino acid supplementation is not yet employed in food processing because the possibility exists that the addition of one or more amino acids could create an imbalance of amino acids in low-protein diets, which would actually retard growth.

Plant Food Mixtures. In many developing countries animal protein sources are scarce and expensive. For children a protein supply of satisfactory quality is particularly critical. A number of mixtures using locally available plant foods have been developed that are comparable to milk in biologic value.

Food Sources of Protein

Protein Content of Foods The average protein composition of common foods is shown in Table 5-5. The protein concentration is high in dry milk, meat, poultry, fish, cheese, and nuts; intermediate in eggs, legumes, flours, cereals, and liquid milk; and low in most fruits and vegetables. One pint of liquid milk furnishes one fourth to one third of the recommended allowance for most age categories. Breads and cereals supply an appreciable amount of protein by virtue of the amounts consumed in a day.

The protein contribution made by the recommended number of servings from each food group in the Basic Diet is shown in Figure 5-7. About three fourths of this protein is supplied by high-quality protein from animal sources. Inasmuch as some of the foods added to this Basic Diet would contain some protein, the daily intake would be more than sufficient to meet the needs of healthy people of all ages.

Table 5-5. Average Protein Content of Foods in Four Food Groups*

Food	Average Serving	Protein (g)	Protein Quality Limiting Amino Acids
Milk group			
Milk, whole or skim	1 cup	8	Complete
Nonfat dry milk	0.8 ounce (3–5 tablespoons)	8	Complete
Cottage cheese	2 ounces	8	Complete
American cheese	1 ounce	7	Complete
Ice cream	⅛ quart	3	Complete
Meat group			
Meat, fish, poultry	3 ounces, cooked	15–25	Complete
Egg	1 whole	6	Complete
Dried beans or peas	½ cup cooked	7–8	Incomplete; methionine
Peanut butter	1 tablespoon	4	Incomplete; several amino acids borderline
Seeds (sunflower; sesame)	¼ cup	9	Incomplete; lysine
Vegetable–fruit group			
Vegetables	½ cup	1–3	Incomplete
Fruits	½ cup	1–2	Incomplete
Bread–cereals group			
Breakfast cereals, wheat	½ cup cooked	2–3	Incomplete; lysine
	¾ cup dry	2–3	Incomplete; lysine
Bread, wheat	1 slice	2–3	Incomplete; lysine
Macroni, noodles, spaghetti	½ cup cooked	2–3	Incomplete; lysine
Rice	½ cup cooked	2	Incomplete; lysine and threonine
Cornmeal and cereals	½ cup cooked	2	Incomplete; lysine and tryptophan

* These values represent approximate group averages. For specific food items, consult Table A-1, in the Appendix.

Total protein content of this diet pattern calculated with the average values of the Exchange Lists (see Table A-4) is shown below and likewise exceeds recommended intakes.

Exchanges	Protein (g)
5 meat	35
2 milk	16
4 bread	12
2 vegetable	4
2 fruit	—
	67

The generous amount of protein-rich foods in the Basic Diet pattern and typical American diet often supplies much of the requirement for minerals such as iron and zinc as well as many of the B-complex vitamins. Indeed, if the protein intake were to be kept at recommended levels, diet planning to achieve recommended intakes of these nutrients would be more difficult.

Protein in the United States Food Supply Since 1910 the available food supply has furnished 88 to 103 g protein per capita daily. This corresponds to approximately 12 percent of the calories available in the food supply. Although the total protein available in the food supply has not varied greatly from year to year, the sources of this protein have changed significantly. In 1910 just over half of the protein was derived from animal sources and more than one third was obtained from flour and cereal foods. Gradually the consumption of animal foods has increased and that of flour–cereal foods decreased until presently more than two thirds of the protein is derived from animal sources and about one sixth from flour–cereal foods. (See Table 5-6.)

Protein Supplements Supplements of protein or amino acids have been promoted for various purposes. In spite of evidence showing that most Americans consume far more protein than is recommended, some people are led to believe that their health would be improved by taking more protein or specific types of protein. The amount of protein or amino acids supplied by some of the products represents a negligible percentage of the total recommended intake. No evidence exists that increased protein intake will enhance physical performance or endurance. Likewise,

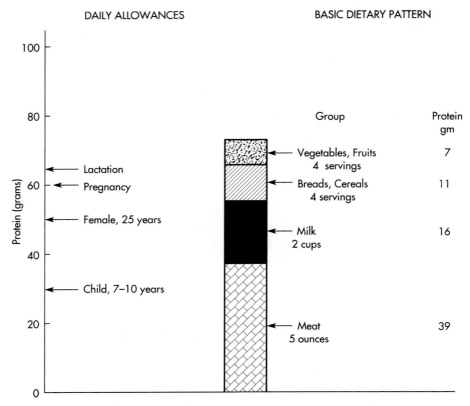

Figure 5-7.   The Basic Diet furnishes sufficient protein to meet the recommended dietary allowances for most categories of the population. The addition of 1 cup of milk or 1 ounce of meat will fulfill the increased needs of the pregnant woman. Note that the milk and meat groups supply about three fourths of the total protein in this pattern. See Table 4-1 for calculations.

Table 5-6.   Sources of Protein in the American Food Supply*†

Food Group	Percentage Contribution to the Total Protein Supply		
	1909–1913	1957–1959	1982
Meat, poultry, fish	29.9	35.7	42.4
Dairy, excluding butter	16.4	24.5	21.3
Eggs	5.2	6.8	4.8
Total–animal sources	51.5	67.0	68.5
Flour, cereals	35.8	19.9	18.9
Dry beans, peas, nuts	4.5	5.2	5.0
Potatoes, sweet	4.2	2.4	2.4
Other vegetables, and fruits	3.7	5.0	4.8
Total—plant sources	48.2	32.5	31.1

* *U.S. Food Consumption: Sources of Data and Trends, 1909–63.* Statistical Bulletin No. 364, U.S. Department of Agriculture, Washington, D.C., 1965.
† Marston, R. M., and Welsh, S. O.: "Nutrient Content of The U.S. Food Supply, 1982," *National Food Review*, U.S. Department of Agriculture, Washington, D.C., Winter 1984, pp. 7–13.

many of the claims for specific proteins, such as gelatin for treatment of brittle nails, are not based on scientific data. Although some evidence exists that tryptophan may have some value in treating insomnia, use of megadose supplements of tryptophan without medical supervision is unwise. Its long-term safety is unknown, and imbalances in amino acids may arise.[15]

Effects of Protein Excess or Deficiency

Liberal Protein Intakes   Although protein intakes by most people in the United States far exceed the recommended allowances, there is little evidence that such intakes by healthy persons are harmful. Arctic explorers who consumed diets consisting mainly of meats for several years showed no pathologic effects. Consumption of a high-protein diet is wasteful, however. Since the body does not store protein in the sense that it stores other nutrients, the excess amino acids are deaminized and then enter the common pathway of metabolism for fat and carbohydrate. Protein foods thus entail more work for the liver and kidney and also cost more in the marketplace.

High-protein diets are undesirable in some circumstances. As the protein intakes increases, the urinary losses of calcium also increase. (See Chapter 9.) With an increase in nitrogenous wastes there also is an increased need for water to excrete them. Premature and very young infants do not have the ability to excrete the additional nitrogenous wastes incurred from high-protein formulas. Persons who have chronic renal failure also have less ability to excrete nitrogenous wastes, and blood urea levels are elevated when protein is fed in excess of synthetic needs.

Diets that provide a high proportion of protein from animal sources also furnish considerable amounts of saturated fats and cholesterol, two factors that may lead to elevation of serum cholesterol and low-density lipoproteins. The intake of saturated fats and cholesterol from protein foods can be effectively reduced in the following ways:

1. Substitute low-fat or skim milk for whole milk and low-fat cheeses for whole-milk cheeses.
2. Select only lean cuts of meat; trim off visible fat.
3. Use more poultry, fish, and legumes, and less beef.
4. Restrict the size of portions of meat, poultry, and fish to the recommended 4 to 5 ounces daily.

Protein Deficiency   Results in both the Nationwide Food Consumption Survey and the first Health and Nutrition Examination Survey (HANES) showed that the mean intakes of protein for each age–sex category exceeded the recommended allowances.[16,17] In the Nationwide Food Consumption Survey, 3 percent of the population had protein intakes less than 70 percent of their respective recommended intakes. The HANES data showed that protein intakes were below standard for 12 percent of children aged 1 to 5 years, for 32 percent of women aged 18 to 44 years, and for 27 percent of persons over 60 years of age. The protein intake per 1,000 kcal was 38 to 40 g and varied little regardless of income. Thus, the failure to ingest the recommended amount of protein appeared to be related to the inadequate quantity of food. The lower intakes of protein were not correlated with lower blood protein levels. In fact, not a single case of severe protein deficiency showing clinical signs and a serum albumin below 2.5 g was found in the HANES survey.

Clinicians sometimes do encounter persons with protein deficiency. Among these are young children who have had diets grossly deficient in protein and calories because of parental abuse or ignorance. Some elderly people show signs of protein deficiency be-

cause their incomes are too small to purchase enough food, they have insufficient understanding of their nutritional needs, they lack the incentive to cook and eat, and they have little appetite because of poor health.

A protein intake that fails to meet the individual requirements leads first to depletion of tissue reserves and then to a lowering of the blood protein levels. Nutritional edema is a clinical sign, but it does not appear until substantial depletion of tissue reserves has taken place and the serum albumin level is decreased. It must be differentiated from the edema that is caused by fluid–electrolyte imbalance in cardiac failure. Protein deficiency sometimes becomes abruptly evident when an infection, injury, or surgery occurs.

Protein-Calorie Malnutrition (PCM)   On a worldwide basis the shortage of protein is second only to the shortage of calories. Protein-calorie malnutrition, also known as protein-energy malnutrition (PEM), is a broad term that encompasses kwashiorkor and marasmus together with milder stages of these diseases. Literally millions of infants and young children are victims of these diseases in Asia, Africa, Central America, the West Indies, and South America. Many of the children who survive are unable to achieve their full physical growth and development. Even more serious is the threat that the most severely malnourished may be retarded in their mental development, and that this retardation may be irreversible.

Kwashiorkor (meaning "the displaced child") occurs in children shortly after weaning, usually between the ages 1 and 4 years, and is characterized by growth failure, skin lesions, edema, and changes in hair color. The liver is extensively infiltrated with fat. The principal dietary defect is a lack of good quality protein in the foods available to the child when he or she is weaned. (See Figure 5-8.)

Marasmus (from a Greek word meaning "withering") is usually seen at a somewhat earlier age than kwashiorkor and is caused by a deficiency of both protein and calories. Growth failure is even more severe than in kwashiorkor, but edema is usually absent. Not infrequently the deficiency has resulted because the mother has substituted inadequate quantities of a formula for breast milk (See also Chapter 24.)

SOME POINTS FOR EMPHASIS IN NUTRITION EDUCATION

1. Proteins are made up of building units called amino acids. They are required by people of all ages to replace the tissues that are constantly being broken down. Children and pregnant

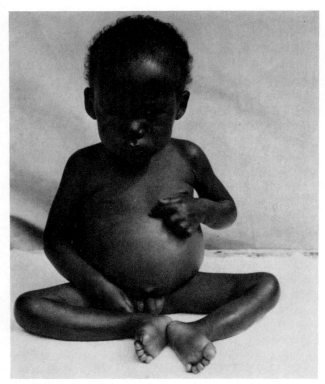

Figure 5-8. Child suffering from kwashiorkor—Africa. (Courtesy, M. Autret and the Food and Agriculture Organization.)

and lactating women need additional protein for synthesis of new proteins.

2. Proteins, like carbohydrates and fats, contribute calories to the diet. If too few calories are included in the diet, protein will be used for energy. Then it cannot also be used for building tissues.

3. Muscular work does not increase the requirement for protein.

4. Nine amino acids, called essential, must be supplied in the diet because the body cannot make them.

5. Animal protein foods, except gelatin, are complete because they contain balanced proportions of the essential amino acids. Include some good-quality protein at each meal.

6. About one seventh to one sixth of the day's allowance for protein for the adult will be supplied by 1 ounce meat, fish, or poultry, or 1 cup milk, or 1 egg, or 1 ounce cheese.

7. Proteins from plant foods are incomplete but they are useful in reducing the amount of expensive animal protein that is needed. Breads, cereals, dry beans and peas, and peanut butter when combined with small amounts of eggs, cheese, meat, fish, and poultry give just as good an assortment of amino acids as a large amount of animal foods.

8. In vegetarian diets a variety of plant proteins can provide the amounts and kinds of essential amino acids required. Thus, cereal grains and legumes when consumed together provide satisfactory biologic value. Since the protein concentration in plant foods is lower than that in flesh foods, the bulk of the diet is greater.

Problems and Review

1. *Key terms*: amino acid; amino acid pool; biologic value; browning reaction; coefficient of digestibility; complete protein; deoxyribonucleic acid; essential amino acid; glucogenic acid; incomplete protein; ketogenic acid; kwashiorkor; marasmus; net protein utilization; nitrogen balance; nonessential amino acid; peptide linkage; protein complementarity; protein efficiency ratio; ribonucleic acid; urea cycle.

2. Describe the synthesis of tissue proteins. Under what circumstances would synthesis be accelerated?

3. List four ways in which proteins are used in the regulation of body functions.

4. Explain why proteins are considered a wasteful source of energy.

5. *Problem.* Prepare an outline or diagram that shows the steps in the digestion of protein.

6. Under what circumstances does positive nitrogen balance occur? Negative nitrogen balance?

7. How can you explain the fact that a person on a low-protein, high-calorie diet is less likely to go into negative nitrogen balance than one who is on a low-calorie diet of the same protein level?

8. How can you explain the fact that some vegetarians maintain good protein nutrition while others do not?

9. *Problem.* Plan a diet for a woman that provides 44 g protein, of which not more than one third is in the form of animal protein. What foods are especially important in such a diet plan?

10. What happens to protein that is eaten in excess of body requirements? Why is it important to provide a margin of safety in planning for the daily protein allowance?

11. What foods would you include in your own diet to ensure an adequate protein intake? How would you modify this plan for a growing child?

12. *Problem.* A diet contains 3,000 kcal and 150 g protein. What percentage of the calories is supplied by protein?

13. *Problem.* One pint of milk supplies 16 g protein. What amounts of these foods would be required to replace the protein of the milk: nonfat dry milk; ice cream; Cheddar cheese; eggs; halibut; beef liver; sirloin steak; peanut butter; dry navy beans; oatmeal? How does the quality of protein in the various foods listed compare?

14. *Problem.* On the basis of current market prices, calculate the cost for the amounts of foods that were needed to replace the protein of 1 pint milk (problem 13). What conclusions can you draw from this calculation?

15. A friend asks you whether she should buy lysine-enriched bread in preference to the usual enriched loaf of bread. How would you reply?

16. What are the consequences of insufficient protein in the diet?

References

1. Vickery, H. B.: "The Origin of the Word Protein," *Yale J. Biol. Med.*, **22**:387–93, 1950.
2. Rose, W. C., et al.: "Further Experiments on the Role of Amino Acids in Human Nutrition," *J. Biol. Chem.*, **148**:457–58, 1943.
3. Kopple, J. D., and Swendseid, M. E.: "Evidence That Histidine is an Essential Amino Acid in Normal and Chronically Uremic Man," *J. Clin. Invest.*, **55**:881–91, 1975.
4. Munro, H. N., and Crim, M. C.: "The Proteins and Amino Acids," in Goodhart, R. S., and Shils, M. E., ed.: *Modern Nutrition in Health and Disease*. Lea & Febiger, Philadelphia, 1980, pp. 51–98.
5. Freeman, H. J., and Kim, Y. S.: "Digestion and Absorption of Protein," *Annu. Rev. Med.*, **29**:99–116, 1978.
6. Allison, J. B., and Wannamacher, R. N., Jr.: "The Concept and Significance of Labile and Over-all Protein Reserves of the Body," *Am. J. Clin. Nutr.*, **16**:445–52, 1965.
7. Consolazio, C. F.: "Nutrition and Performance. Sweat Losses," *Prog. Food Nutr. Sci.*, **7**:113–128, 1983.
8. Rose, W. C., et al.: "The Amino Acid Requirements of Man. XV. The Valine Requirements: Summary and Final Observations," *J. Biol. Chem.*, **217**:987–95, 1955.
9. Leverton, R. M., et al.: "The Quantitative Amino Acid Requirements of Young Women," *J. Nutr.*, **58**:59, 83, 219, 341, 355, 1956.
10. Holt, L. E., and Snyderman, S. E.: "The Amino Acid Requirements of Children," in Cole, W. H., ed.: *Some Aspects of Amino Acid Supplementation*. Rutgers University Press, New Brunswick, N.J., 1956, pp. 60–68.
11. Food and Nutrition Board: *Recommended Dietary Allowances*, 10th ed. National Research Council–National Academy of Sciences, Washington D.C., 1989.
12. American Dietetic Association: "Position Paper on the Vegetarian Approach to Eating." *J. Am. Diet. Assoc.*, **77**:61–69, 1980.
13. Dwyer, J. T., et al.: "Growth in 'New' Vegetarian Preschool Children Using the Jenss-Bayley Curve Fitting Technique." *Am. J. Clin. Nutr.*, **37**:815–827, 1983.
14. Council of Foods and Nutrition: "Zen Macrobiotic Diets," *JAMA*, **218**:397, 1971.
15. Dubick, M. A.: "Dietary Supplements and Health Aids—A Critical Evaluation. Part 2. Macronutrients and Fiber," *J. Nutr. Ed.*, **15**:88–93, 1983.
16. Chopra, J. G., et al.: "Protein in the U.S. Diet," *J. Am. Diet. Assoc.*, **72**:253–58, 1978.
17. Pao, E. M., and Mickle, S. J.: "Problem Nutrients in the United States." *Food Technol.*, **35**:58–69, 1981.

6

Carbohydrates

In our culture "starchy foods" and "sugar" are regarded by some as undesirable or unnecessary dietary components, that must be eliminated or avoided if a person wishes to lose weight or practice good nutrition. For most people in the world, however, high-starch cereal grains not only provide most of the energy in the diet but supply an appreciable portion of the protein as well. From 45 to 80 percent of the energy requirement of people throughout the world is met by consumption of starches and sugars stored in the leaves, stems, fruits, seeds, and roots of plants. The ability of plants to harness solar energy in the form of usable carbohydrates is basic to the continuance of life by all species.

Composition and Synthesis

Composition Carbohydrates are simple sugars or polymers of sugars such as starch that can be hydrolyzed to simple sugars by the action of digestive enzymes or by heating with dilute acids. Like thousands of organic compounds, they contain carbon, hydrogen, and oxygen. Generally, but not always, the hydrogen and oxygen are in the proportions to form water, hence the term *carbohydrate*.

Photosynthesis An exceedingly complex process known as PHOTOSYNTHESIS is used by plants to synthesize the carbohydrate that is unique for each plant. Sunlight is absorbed by several pigments in the plant, the most important of which is the green pigment, CHLOROPHYLL. The absorbed solar energy is used by the plant to bring about a complicated sequence of chemical reactions that essentially transfer two atoms of hydrogen from a molecule of water to a molecule of carbon dioxide. The result is the release of oxygen to the air and the fixation of carbon as carbohydrate.

$$6 \, CO_2 + 6 \, H_2O + \text{light energy} \xrightarrow[\substack{\text{plant} \\ \text{enzymes}}]{\text{chlorophyll}}$$

$$\underset{\substack{\text{chemical} \\ \text{energy}}}{C_6H_{12}O_6 + 6 \, O_2}$$

The plant uses some of the carbohydrate to meet its own metabolic needs such as the synthesis of the amino acids that make up its proteins. The rest is

CURRENT ISSUES

Several aspects of carbohydrate nutrition are of particular concern to the public at the present time.

1. Sugars account for 24 percent of the caloric composition of the American diet. According to the Dietary Goals (see page 31) an intake of 10 percent of calories as refined sugar is preferable. What are the effects of a high sugar intake on nutritive adequacy? What advantages would be gained by substituting starchy foods for part of the sugar? What evidence exists that a high sugar intake contributes to disease or affects behavior? What dietary adjustments can be made to reduce sugar intake?

2. High-fiber diets currently are popular with many consumers and health professionals alike. Are the claims that a liberal intake of fiber will reduce the risks of gastrointestinal disorders, cancer of the colon, coronary heart disease, and many other disease conditions justified? What are the characteristics of dietary fiber? How does fiber react within the intestinal environment? We shall see that there are some answers for these concerns, but there are also theories that remain to be proven.

stored in the form of polysaccharides. Carbohydrates are the most abundant compounds in the universe. Cellulose, which makes up the structural parts of plants, accounts for about half the carbon in vegetation. Plants are valued as food for their large stores of starches and sugars.

Classification, Distribution, and Characteristics

Monosaccharides The simplest form of carbohydrates are the MONOSACCHARIDES, or simple sugars. Although naturally occurring simple sugars may contain three to seven carbon atoms, only the hexoses (6-carbon atoms) are of dietary importance.

Glucose, galactose, fructose, and mannose have the same empiric formula, $C_6H_{12}O_6$. They differ in the arrangement of the groupings about the carbon atoms (see Figure 6-1) and are distinctive in their physical properties, such as solubility and sweetness. Glucose, galactose, and mannose possess an aldehyde grouping (CHO) and are known as aldohexoses. Fructose possesses a ketone grouping (CO) and is known as a keto-hexose.

Glucose, also known as dextrose, grape sugar, or corn sugar, is somewhat less sweet than cane sugar and is soluble in hot or cold water. It is found in sweet fruits such as grapes, berries, and oranges and in some vegetables such as sweet corn and carrots. It is prepared commercially as corn syrup or in its crystalline form by the hydrolysis of starch with acids. Glucose is the chief end product of the digestion of the oligo- and polysaccharides, is the form of carbohydrate circulating in the blood, and is the primary carbohydrate utilized by the cell for energy.

Fructose (levulose or fruit sugar) is a highly soluble sugar that does not readily crystallize. It is much sweeter than cane sugar and is found in honey, ripe fruits, and some vegetables. It is also a product of the hydrolysis of sucrose.

Galactose is not found free in nature, its only source being from the hydrolysis of lactose. *Mannose* is of limited distribution in foods, is poorly absorbed, and is of little consequence in nutrition.

Ribose, *xylose*, and *arabinose* are three pentoses (5-carbon sugars) of little dietary significance. Xylose and arabinose are widely distributed in many root vegetables and fruits. Ribose is of great physiologic importance as a constituent of riboflavin, a B-complex vitamin, and of ribonucleic acid (RNA) and deoxyribonucleic acid (DNA). It is rapidly synthesized by the body and is not a dietary essential.

Oligosaccharides This group of carbohydrates is composed of 2 to 10 monosaccharides joined together. The most common oligosaccharides are sucrose, lactose, and maltose. These substances are DISACCHARIDES, or double sugars, formed from the combination of two hexoses with loss of one molecule of water. They are water soluble, diffusible, and crystallizable and vary widely in their sweetness. They are split to simple sugars by acid hydrolysis or by digestive enzymes.

Sucrose is the table sugar with which we are familiar and is found in cane or beet sugar, brown sugar, sorghum, molasses, and maple sugar. Many fruits and some vegetables contain small amounts of sucrose.

Lactose, or milk sugar, is produced by mammals and is the only carbohydrate of animal origin of significance in the diet. It is about one sixth as sweet as sucrose and dissolves poorly in cold water. The con-

Figure 6-1. These hexoses differ in the arrangement of the groupings about the carbon atoms. The encircled grouping shows how the sugar differs from glucose in its structure. Fructose is a ketose; the others are aldoses.

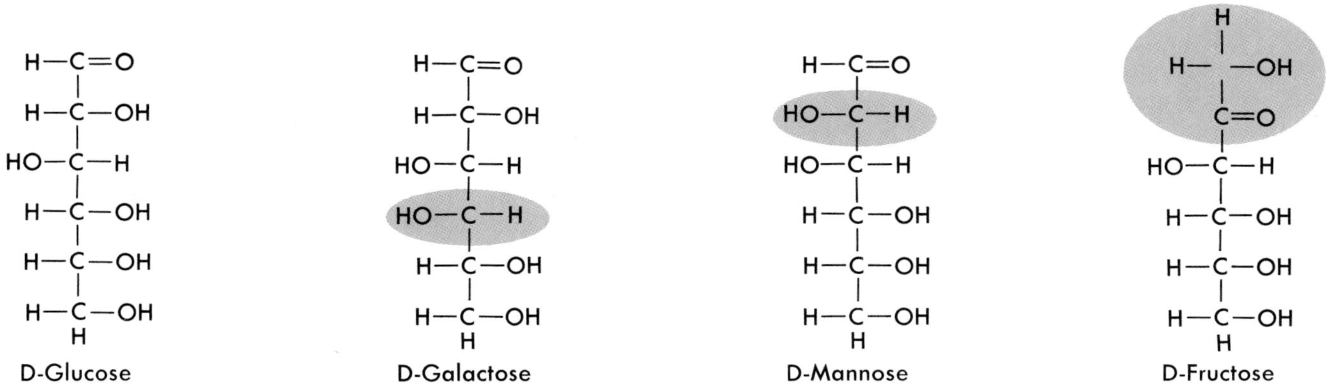

D-Glucose   D-Galactose   D-Mannose   D-Fructose

centration of lactose in milk varies from 2 to 8 percent, depending on the species of animal.

Maltose, or malt sugar, does not occur to any appreciable extent in foods. It is an intermediate product in the hydrolysis of starch. Maltose is produced in the malting and fermentation of grains and is present in beer and malted breakfast cereals. It is also used with dextrins as the source of carbohydrate for some infant formulas.

Small amounts of other oligosaccharides are found in foods. Raffinose, a trisaccharide, and stachyose, a tetrasaccharide, are nondigestible carbohydrates found primarily in legumes. Fermentation of these oligosaccharides by intestinal microorganisms is largely responsible for the flatulence associated with consumption of legumes.

Polysaccharides These carbohydrates are complex compounds composed of many molecules of simple sugars. They have a relatively high molecular weight, are amorphous rather than crystalline, are not sweet, are insoluble in water, and are digested with varying degrees of completeness. Starches, dextrins, glycogen, and several indigestible carbohydrates are of nutritional interest.

Starch is the storage form of carbohydrate in the plant and a valuable contributor to the energy content of the diet. The starch granules are encased in a cellulose-type wall and are distinctive in size and shape for each source. The characteristics of the starch molecule depend upon the way in which the 2,000 or so glucose units that make up the molecule are linked. Two types of glucose chains are present: (1) *amylose*, consisting of long straight chains of glucose, accounts for 10 to 20 percent of the molecule; and (2) *amylopectin*, consisting of short branched chains of glucose units, accounts for the major part of the molecule.

When starch is cooked in moist heat, the granules absorb water and swell, and the walls of the cell are ruptured, thus permitting more ready access to the digestive enzymes. Amylopectin has colloidal properties so that thickening of a starch–water mixture occurs when heat is applied.

Dextrins are intermediate products in the hydrolysis of starch and consist of shorter chains of glucose units. Some dextrins are produced when flour is browned or bread is toasted.

Glycogen, the so-called "animal starch," is similar in structure to the amylopectin of starch but contains many more branched chains of glucose. It is rapidly synthesized from glucose in the liver and muscle.

Indigestible polysaccharides include cellulose, hemicellulose, pectins, gums, and mucilages. They will be discussed fully under the heading Dietary Fiber in this chapter. (See page 76.)

Carbohydrate Derivatives Sugars react chemically to form sugar alcohols, amino sugars, glycosides, uronic acids, and many complex compounds with lipids and proteins. *Glycerol* is the 3-carbon alcohol that is a component of glycerides. *Sorbitol, mannitol,* and *xylitol* are sugar alcohols that contain 4 kcal per g, the same as sucrose. They occur naturally in fruits but are commercially produced from sources such as sucrose. Xylitol is equal in sweetness to sucrose, whereas sorbitol and mannitol are only half as sweet. All are absorbed more slowly and less efficiently than glucose and sucrose and consequently cause lower blood glucose and insulin responses. Ingestion of excessive amounts may produce an osmotic diarrhea. Sorbitol is a common sweetener in "sugar-free" candies and gums. *Inositol* is an alcohol related to the hexoses. It occurs in the bran of cereal grains. When combined with phosphate it forms phytic acid, a compound that interferes with the absorption of minerals such as calcium, iron, and zinc.

Ascorbic acid, one of the water-soluble vitamins, is a hexose derivative that can by synthesized by plants and by some animals but not by the human being. Numerous carbohydrate derivatives are constituents of connective, nervous, and other tissues and are involved in many metabolic functions.

Functions

Body Distribution The amount of carbohydrate in the adult body is about 300 to 350 g. Of this, 100 g is stored as glycogen in the liver, another 200 to 250 g is present as glycogen in cardiac, smooth, and skeletal muscles, and about 15 g makes up the glucose in the blood and extracellular fluid. Carbohydrates provide the carbon skeletons for the synthesis of the nonessential amino acids by the body (See page 53.) Very small amounts of carbohydrate are constituents of numerous essential body compounds such as the following:

Glucuronic acid, which occurs in the liver and is also a constituent of a number of mucopolysaccharides. Glucuronic acid in the liver combines with toxic chemicals and bacterial byproducts and is thus a detoxifying agent.

Hyaluronic acid, a viscous substance that forms the matrix of connective tissue.

Heparin, a mucopolysaccharide, a substance that prevents the clotting of blood.

Chondroitin sulfates found in skin, tendons, cartilage, bone, and heart values.

Immunopolysaccharides as part of the body's mechanism to resist infections.

Deoxyribonucleic acid (DNA) and ribonucleic acid (RNA), the compounds that possess and transfer the genetic characteristics of the cell.

Galactolipins as constituents of nervous tissue.

Glycosides as components of steroid and adrenal hormones.

Energy Carbohydrates are the least expensive source of energy to the body. Each gram of carbohydrate when oxidized yields, on the average, 4 kcal. Glucose is the primary source of energy for the nervous system and the lungs. After absorption from the intestinal tract, the carbohydrate meets the following principal fates: (1) immediate use to meet energy needs of tissue cells; (2) conversion to glycogen and storage in the liver or muscle for later release to meet energy needs; and (3) conversion to fat as a larger reserve for energy. The total glycogen reserves in the body would meet about half of one day's energy needs of the adult. Glycogen stored in the liver can be converted to glucose to maintain the sugar level of the blood. Glycogen in muscle can be used to supply energy needs of muscle cells but is not available for regulation of the blood sugar level. The amount of energy stored as fat can be large and is a ready and continuing supply to meet energy needs when glycogen stores are depleted.

Protein-Sparing Action. The body will use carbohydrate preferentially as a source of energy when it is adequately supplied in the diet, thus sparing protein for tissue building. Since meeting energy needs of the body takes priority over other functions, any deficiency of calories in the diet will be made up by using adipose and protein tissues.

Regulation of Fat Metabolism Some carbohydrate is necessary in the diet so that the oxidation of fats can proceed normally. When carbohydrate is severely restricted in the diet, fats will be metabolized faster than the body can take care of the intermediate products. The accumulation of these incompletely oxidized products leads to dehydration, loss of body sodium, and ketosis. As little as 50 g carbohydrate in the diet will prevent ketosis under normal conditions. In uncontrolled diabetes mellitus, ketosis is often present.

Role in Gastrointestinal Function Lactose has several functions in the gastrointestinal tract. It promotes the growth of desirable bacteria, some of which are useful in the synthesis of B-complex vitamins. Lactose also enhances the absorption of calcium. It is undoubtedly no accident of nature that milk, which is the outstanding source of calcium, is also the only source of lactose.

Dietary fiber is a negligible source of energy to the body. It does aid, however, in the stimulation of peristaltic movements in the gastrointestinal tract, gives bulk to the intestinal contents, and reduces the length of time that food wastes remain in the colon (see page 77).

Digestion and Absorption

Digestion The purpose of carbohydrate digestion is to hydrolyze the di- and polysaccharides of the diet to their constituent simple sugars. This process is accomplished by enzymes of the digestive juices and yields several end products:

$$\text{Starch} \xrightarrow{\text{amylase}} \text{Maltose} + \text{glucose}$$

$$\text{Sucrose} \xrightarrow{\text{sucrase}} \text{Glucose} + \text{fructose}$$

$$\text{Maltose} \xrightarrow{\text{maltase}} \text{Glucose} + \text{glucose}$$

$$\text{Lactose} \xrightarrow{\text{lactase}} \text{Glucose} + \text{galactose}$$

Although some hydrolysis of starch to maltose occurs in the mouth by the action of salivary amylase and continues in the stomach until the food mass is acidified, the principal site of digestion of carbohydrate is in the small intestine. Salivary amylase does not act upon raw starch, but pancreatic amylase hydrolyzes both raw and cooked starch to dextrins and, in turn, to maltose. Cooked starch is more rapidly hydrolyzed because the cell walls have been ruptured and the enzymes have more ready access to the starch granules.

Disaccharidases are produced within the mucosal cell and are not secreted into the lumen of the intestine. Sucrose, lactose, and maltose are hydrolyzed within the brush border of the epithelial cell.

Dietary fiber is resistant to hydrolysis by human digestive enzymes. Degradation of some types of dietary fiber may occur in the lower intestine and colon through the action of bacterial enzymes. Some of the products formed are potential sources of energy but usually are of minor importance.

Absorption The process by which the monosaccharides are absorbed is by no means simple. The single sugars must enter the epithelial cell, be transported across the cell, enter the interstitial fluid, and then pass through the walls of the blood capillaries for transport to the portal circulation and the liver, and be dispensed according to need to the systemic circulation.

When the concentration in the circulation exceeds that at the luminal surfaces of the intestine, an energy-requiring process called active transport is needed. Active transport accounts for most of the absorption of glucose and galactose. It is effected by the sodium pump and a mobile carrier system. The same energy that is required to pump sodium out of the cell also serves to transport glucose and galactose. The energy required to operate the sodium pump is provided by ATP that has been generated from a supply of glucose within the cell.

Glucose and galactose also can be absorbed by passive diffusion when intraluminal concentrations of the sugars are high. Passive diffusion accounts for only a small amount of the total glucose absorbed. Fructose apparently is not absorbed by active transport. Its absorption occurs by facilitated diffusion, which utilizes a carrier but is not energy dependent. This process occurs only when concentrations in the intestinal lumen exceed those in the circulation.[1]

Most absorption of sugars occurs in the jejunum, although some absorption occurs along the length of the small intestine. The rate of absorption is about equal for galactose and glucose, whereas fructose is absorbed about half as rapidly. Mannose and xylose are poorly absorbed, indicating a high level of selectivity at the absorption sites.

About 97 to 98 percent of the carbohydrate in diversified American diets is digested and absorbed. The fuel factor of 4 kcal (17 kJ) per g is based on this level of absorption. In countries where plant foods comprise most of the diet, the percentage of carbohydrate absorbed is lower, and the energy value per gram of dietary carbohydrate is somewhat lower.

Metabolism

Glucose is quantitatively the most important carbohydrate available to the body whether it be by absorption from the diet or by synthesis within the body. Galactose from the diet or from endogenous sources is rapidly converted to glucose in the liver. Similarly, fructose is converted to products identical to those formed in the initial steps in the breakdown of

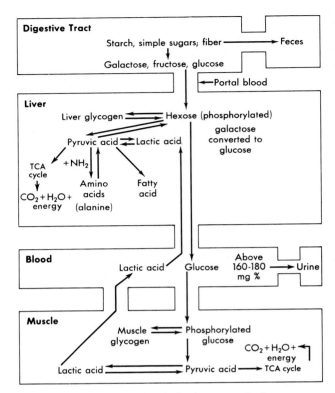

Figure 6-2. Pathways of carbohydrate metabolism.

glucose. Therefore, any discussion of carbohydrate metabolism is essentially that of glucose. (See Figure 6-2.)

Interrelation with Other Nutrients Glucose metabolism consists of an interrelated series of biochemical reactions facilitated by enzymatic activity. Glucose metabolism cannot be completely separated from the metabolism of fats and proteins. On the one hand, proteins are potential sources of glucose, and on the other, glucose can be converted to fatty acids, glycerol, and certain amino acids. A number of points in the sequence of glucose metabolism are also the crossroads for amino acid and fatty acid metabolism, and in some respects one nutrient can substitute for another. For example, a decrease in carbohydrate metabolism is accompanied by an increase in fatty acid oxidation.

Trace amounts of magnesium, iron, and other mineral elements and several of the B-complex vitamins are essential for enzyme activity. Thus, the metabolism of the nutrients is interdependent, and the lack of any one of them affects the total metabolism of the organism. For example, a deficiency of any one of the vitamins results in a failure of the reaction to take place at the point where that vitamin is essential. Any reactions subsequent to this point, therefore, cannot occur.

The details of these elegant metabolic mechanisms are beyond the scope of this text, but they are well described in a number of texts on biochemistry. Nevertheless, the nurse and nutritionist frequently encounter patients with some defect in carbohydrate metabolism. The following paragraphs will furnish a general understanding of the mechanisms for the regulation of the blood glucose and a broad outline of the anaerobic and aerobic phases of glucose metabolism.

The Liver in Carbohydrate Metabolism Following absorption from the small intestine, the monosaccharides are carried by the portal vein to the liver. Just as the control tower in an airport regulates the flow of traffic in the air, so the liver exercises the principal control of the pathways that glucose (and other nutrients) shall take. The liver converts galactose and fructose to intermediates in glucose metabolism. It synthesizes glycogen (GLYCOGENESIS) from glucose, stores it, and reconverts it to glucose (GLYCOGENOLYSIS) according to need. It deaminizes amino acids so that the carbon skeletons can be used for the synthesis of glucose (GLUCONEOGENESIS) if the glycogen stores are depleted. It can transform excess glucose into fatty acids (LIPOGENESIS) and can also use the glycerol fraction of lipids to form glucose. Many carbohydrate compounds that have a regulatory function throughout the body are synthesized by the liver. (See page 66.) From carbon skeletons donated by carbohydrate, the liver can also synthesize nonessential amino acids.

These many chemical transformations are facilitated by enzymes that are specific for each reaction and that are under the influence of hormones secreted by the pancreas and the adrenal, pituitary, and thyroid glands.

The Blood Glucose By means of the blood circulation glucose is made continuously available to each and every cell of the body as a source of energy and for the synthesis of a variety of substances. The glucose taken from the circulation by the cells is constantly replaced by the liver so that the blood glucose level is maintained within relatively narrow limits.

In the fasting state the blood glucose concentration is normally 60 to 85 mg per deciliter (dl). Shortly after a meal it rises to about 140 to 150 mg per dl, but within a few hours the concentration will have returned to the fasting level. Should the blood sugar level reach 160 to 180 mg per dl, some glucose will be

excreted in the urine (GLUCOSURIA). This level, varying somewhat from one individual to another, is known as the RENAL THRESHOLD FOR GLUCOSE. The regulation of the blood sugar level by the liver is so efficient that glucosuria does not normally occur. Occasionally, an individual who has a lower renal threshold for glucose but who has no other abnormalities will excrete some glucose after meals that are especially rich in carbohydrate.

A blood sugar concentration in excess of normal levels is known as HYPERGLYCEMIA; this is characteristic of diabetes mellitus. A glucose concentration below normal levels is known as HYPOGLYCEMIA and may occur in certain abnormalities of liver function or when insulin is produced in excessive amounts by the pancreas.

Regulation of the Blood Sugar Level The liver is the only organ able to supply glucose to the circulation, and it also participates in the removal of glucose not immediately needed. The sources of glucose to the blood and the avenues of its removal are shown in Figure 6-3. Glucose is made available to the circulation by (1) the absorbed sugars from the diet, (2) glycogenolysis, (3) gluconeogenesis, and, (4) to a lesser extent, the reconversion of pyruvic and lactic acids formed in the glycolytic pathway.

Several hormones bring about an increased supply of glucose to the blood. *Thyroid hormone* increases the rate of absorption from the gastrointestinal tract. *Glucagon*, a hormone secreted by the cells of the pancreas, is believed to activate glycogenolysis. *Epinephrine*, produced by the adrenal gland under conditions of stress, increases the rate of glycogen breakdown. *Steroid hormones* accelerate the catabolism of proteins, thus bringing about gluconeogenesis. *Adrenocorticotropic hormone* is antagonistic to the action of insulin and thus prevents the blood sugar level from dropping.

Removal of Glucose from the Blood. Six pathways are available for the removal of glucose from the blood: (1) the continuous uptake of glucose by every cell in the body and its oxidation for energy; (2) the conversion of glucose to glycogen by the liver (GLYCOGENESIS); (3) the synthesis of fats from glucose (LIPOGENESIS); (4) the synthesis of numerous carbohydrate derivatives (see page 66); (5) glycolysis in the red blood cells; and (6) elimination of glucose in the urine when the renal threshold is exceeded.

The amount of glycogen that can be formed is limited, but there is no limit to the amount of fat that is

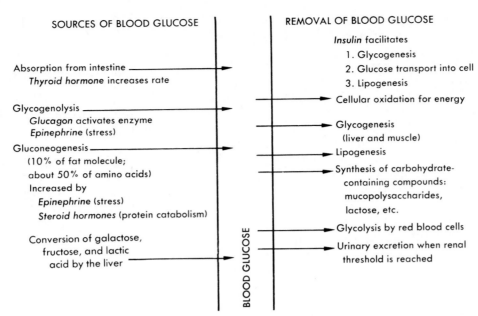

SOURCES OF BLOOD GLUCOSE

Absorption from intestine
Thyroid hormone increases rate

Glycogenolysis
    Glucagon activates enzyme
    Epinephrine (stress)
Gluconeogenesis
    (10% of fat molecule;
    about 50% of amino acids)
    Increased by
      Epinephrine (stress)
      Steroid hormones (protein catabolism)

Conversion of galactose,
    fructose, and lactic
    acid by the liver

REMOVAL OF BLOOD GLUCOSE

Insulin facilitates
    1. Glycogenesis
    2. Glucose transport into cell
    3. Lipogenesis
Cellular oxidation for energy

Glycogenesis
(liver and muscle)
Lipogenesis
Synthesis of carbohydrate-
    containing compounds:
    mucopolysaccharides,
    lactose, etc.
Glycolysis by red blood cells
Urinary excretion when renal
    threshold is reached

BLOOD GLUCOSE

Figure 6-3. The blood glucose is maintained within physiologic limits by replacement as rapidly as it is removed to meet metabolic needs. Glycogenesis and lipogenesis are mechanisms that prevent hyperglycemia in the normal individual. The renal threshold is rarely exceeded in the healthy person.

formed. Glycogen reserves are maintained at their maximum level by diets high in carbohydrate. A diet high in protein and relatively low in carbohydrate will result in moderate glycogen reserves, but a diet high in fat and low in carbohydrate and protein will result in poor glycogen reserves.

Insulin. Only one hormone is known to lower the blood sugar. An increase in the concentration of blood glucose stimulates the release of INSULIN, the hormone produced by the beta cells of the islands of Langerhans. Insulin lowers the blood glucose by several actions: (1) facilitation of the synthesis of glycogen in the liver; (2) the active transport of glucose across cell membranes; and (3) the conversion of glucose to fatty acids.

Oxidation of Glucose Within each of the billions of cells of the body the oxidation of glucose is continuously taking place. The end products of this oxidation are carbon dioxide, water, and energy. If the potential energy of glucose, fatty acids, and amino acids were released in an explosive reaction, much of it would be lost and wasted as heat. The cell utilizes energy efficiently by releasing a small amount of it at a time in a series of steps that occur in the mitochondria of the cell. The energy liberated in these steps is trapped in the form of ADENOSINE TRIPHOSPHATE (ATP). This is

the compound consisting of adenine (a nitrogenous base), ribose, and three phosphate groupings, two of which are high-energy phosphate bonds, designated thus ~ . One of these bonds is broken to release energy whenever required for the innumerable transactions of the cell (ATP→ADP). As energy is liberated in the catabolism of glucose, fatty acids, or amino acids, ATP is again formed (ADP→ATP). ATP is sometimes called the "currency" or the "legal tender" for energy of the living organism, because, like coins of money, it is the convenient form for small bursts of energy.

The first step in glucose catabolism is GLYCOLYSIS, principally an anaerobic phase that results in the formation of two molecules of pyruvic acid from each molecule of glucose. The second phase of glucose catabolism is an aerobic phase that includes the decarboxylation of pyruvic acid to acetic acid, the condensation of acetic acid with coenzyme A, and the transfers through the TRICARBOXYLIC ACID CYCLE (TCA) to yield hydrogen and electrons, carbon dioxide, and water. This is the common pathway for the oxidation of deaminized amino acids and fatty acids as well as for glucose. The final step in the release of energy is the immediate trapping of the energy in ATP through the ELECTRON TRANSPORT SYSTEM. Each of these phases involves many reactions, a broad outline of which is described in the paragraphs that follow. (See Figure 6-4.)

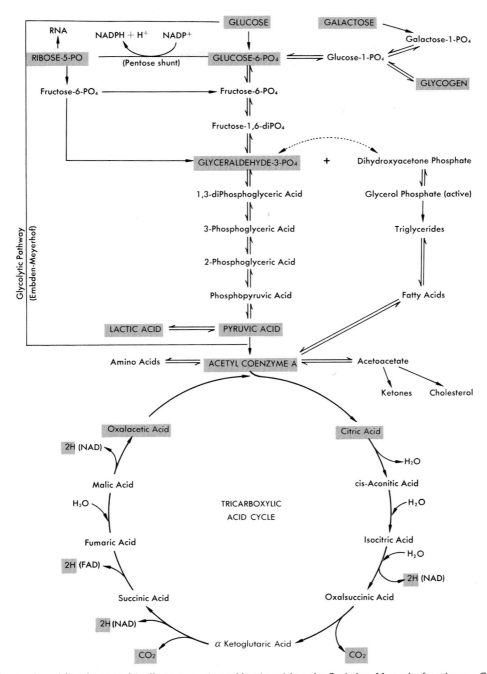

Figure 6-4. Glucose is oxidized anaerobically to pyruvic and lactic acids—the Embden-Meyerhof pathway. Glucose may also be oxidized through the pentose shunt. Pyruvic acid is decarboxylated to form acetyl CoA. This condenses with oxalacetic acid, and each turn of the TCA cycle releases two molecules of CO_2 and eight hydrogen ions and uses up two molecules of water.

Glycolysis The chemical reactions that constitute glycolysis, also known as the *Embden-Meyerhof pathway* for the men who first described them, take place in the cytoplasmic matrix of the cell. These reactions degrade glucose to pyruvic acid in preparation for entrance into the mitochondria. They are catalyzed by a specific enzyme in each case, some of which require the presence of inorganic phosphate, inorganic ions, nicotinamide adenine dinucleotide (NAD), and nicotinamide adenine dinucleotide phosphate (NADP).

The reactions do not require oxygen. Most of the glucose catabolized in the body undergoes breakdown through these steps.

The entrance of glucose into the cell is facilitated by insulin. Within the cell the first step in glycolysis is the phosphorylation of glucose with ATP in the presence of glucokinase and magnesium to form glucose 6-phosphate and ADP. The phosphorylated glucose then proceeds through the glycolytic pathway to pyruvic acid and lactic acid, or to the synthesis of glycogen, or, to a lesser extent, through an alternative oxidative pathway known as the *pentose shunt*.

Conversion to Trioses. The hexose molecule is split into trioses, which undergo a series of changes until pyruvic acid ($CH_3COCOOH$) is formed. One of the trioses—glyceraldehyde 3-phosphate—instead of proceeding to pyruvic acid may be sidetracked to form alpha-glycerophosphate, which furnishes the glycerol molecule for the synthesis of neutral fats. (See page 92.)

Lactic Acid. Pyruvic acid can proceed anaerobically to form lactic acid, which is utilized for muscle contraction under conditions when the energy need exceeds the supply of oxygen. Thus, the runner in a race can continue beyond his or her capacity to supply oxygen to muscles. Under normal conditions only a small amount of lactic acid is formed. About one fifth of the lactic acid produced in the muscle is further oxidized through the citric acid cycle; the rest enters the blood circulation and is synthesized to glycogen by the liver.

The Pentose Shunt An aerobic bypass for glycolysis may be utilized especially by the liver and adipose tissue. This is also known as the *hexose monophosphate shunt* or the *oxidative shunt*. Through the reactions occurring in this pathway, ribose, which is a constituent of RNA, is synthesized. Also, NADPH is produced, which is essential for the synthesis of fatty acids and for the utilization of lactic acid in muscular work.

Aerobic Metabolism Most of the pyruvic acid formed in the glycolytic pathway enters the mitochondria of the cells where it is oxidized. By a complex series of steps pyruvic acid is decarboxylated to a 2-carbon fragment (acetate), which reacts with coenzyme A to form ACETYL COENZYME A also known as ACTIVE ACETATE. These reactions require NAD, flavin adenine dinucleotide (FAD), thiamin pyrophosphate, lipoic acid, magnesium, coenzyme A, and a series of enzymes. As a consequence of this reaction, 3 molecules of ATP eventually can be formed, or 6 molecules for each glucose molecule.

COENZYME A (CoA) is a complex molecule of which pantothenic acid, a B-complex vitamin, is a constituent. It plays an important role in numerous cellular reactions. Acetyl CoA is derived not only from pyruvic acid but also from the oxidation of fatty acids (see page 92) and from certain amino acids (see page 53). Acetyl CoA is something like the hub of a wheel in that it can proceed in a number of directions, namely, through the TCA cycle to yield energy or to form a number of new compounds.

Tricarboxylic Acid Cycle. The TCA cycle is also known as the *citric acid cycle* or the *Krebs cycle* (for the man who first formulated the sequence). Through this cycle about 90 percent of the energy of the body is produced.

The TCA cycle is initiated by the condensation of acetyl CoA with oxaloacetic acid to form citric acid. In one turn of the cycle two molecules of carbon dioxide and four pairs of hydrogens and electrons are produced. The overall reaction is as follows:

$$CH_3COOH + 2\,H_2O \rightarrow 2\,CO_2 + 8\,H^+$$

One molecule of carbon dioxide is released in the formation of alpha-ketoglutaric acid and one in the formation of succinyl CoA. (See Figure 6-4.) A full turn of the cycle again yields one molecule of oxaloacetic acid, which then combines with a new molecule of acetyl CoA for another cycle.

Electron Transport System The hydrogens released in the catabolism of glucose are never in the free state but are accepted by enzymes complexes containing NAD or FAD. These important coenzymes contain the vitamins niacin (NAD) and riboflavin (FAD) as part of their structure. Their function depends on their ability to be oxidized and reduced ($NAD \leftrightarrow NADH_2$ and $FAD \leftrightarrow FADH_2$). The hydrogen transferred to these enzyme complexes is subsequently transported through the cytochrome system, also known as the *respiratory chain* or the *electron transport system*. In this transport the oxidation of hydrogen to water and phosphorylation are coupled; hence, this is referred to as OXIDATIVE PHOSPHORYLATION.

The CYTOCHROMES are a series of iron-containing enzymes. They accept hydrogens and transfer them step by step from one cytochrome to another until they react with oxygen to form water. The transfer of each pair of electrons from NAD-dehydrogenases

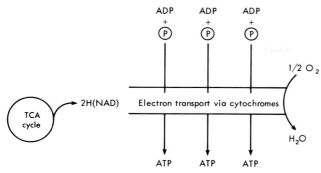

Figure 6-5. Each pair of hydrogens generated in glucose catabolism is carried by niacin- or riboflavin-containing enzymes and transferred step by step through a series of cytochromes in the electron transport system. The oxidation of hydrogen is coupled with the phosphorylation of ADP to ATP. Each pair of hydrogens yields three ATP molecules.

along the respiratory chain yields three molecules of ATP. (See Figure 6-5.)

The amount of energy converted to ATP from glucose and fat is, at a maximum, 38 to 40 percent of the potential energy. The remainder is dissipated as heat. Theoretically each molecule of glucose can yield 38 molecules of ATP: 8 through the glycolytic pathway, 6 in the conversion of pyruvic acid to acetyl coenzyme A, and 24 in the TCA cycle. A variety of factors may contribute to failure in generating a complete yield of 38 molecules of ATP.

Carbohydrate in the Diet

Dietary Allowance The low-carbohydrate diet of the Eskimos and the high-carbohydrate diet of many people in Far Eastern countries indicate that humans can be healthy with wide variations in carbohydrate intake. This wide variation is compatible with health because of the interrelations with fatty acids and amino acids in meeting the energy needs of the body.

The minimum requirement for carbohydrate is not known, but at least 50 to 100 g carbohydrate daily is desirable to prevent ketosis.[2] Intakes considerably above this level are customary and desirable.

The revised Dietary Goals recommend that complex carbohydrates and naturally occurring sugars provide about 48 percent of the total caloric intake and that refined sugars provide no more than 10 percent of the energy requirement.[3]

Dietary Sources The carbohydrate composition of typical foods is shown in Table 6-1. Pure sugars are 100 percent carbohydrate, and syrups, jellies, and

jams contain 69 to 80 percent. Cereal foods, flours, and crackers contain 65 to 85 percent carbohydrate on a dry weight basis, chiefly in the form of starch.

Fruits and vegetables vary widely in their carbohydrate concentration. Those with a high water content such as spinach, cabbage, other leafy vegetables, and melons contain 6 percent or less of carbohydrate and are correspondingly low in calories. Potatoes, sweet potatoes, lima beans, corn, and bananas are somewhat lower in water content and furnish approximately 20 percent carbohydrate or more. Dried beans and peas and dried fruits have a carbohydrate content in excess of 60 percent.

For convenience in dietary planning, the Exchange Lists for Meal Planing group vegetables with a high water content together as the Vegetable Exchange with a serving of 1/2 cup supplying an average of 5 g carbohydrate. (See page 40 and Table A-4.) Vegetables with a higher carbohydrate content, such as potatoes, corn, peas, and Lima beans, are included in the Starch/Bread List in amounts supplying approximately 15 g carbohydrate. Similarly, in the Fruit Exchange List the serving size of different fruits is varied, so that one exchange provides 15 g carbohydrate.

The relative proportions of sugars and starches in fruits and vegetables is determined by their degree of ripeness. Green bananas are high in starch and low in sugar, whereas ripe bananas have little starch and consist primarily of sugars. On the other hand, freshly picked and immature vegetables, for example, sweet corn, tender peas, and young carrots, contain more sugar and less starch than is found in mature vegetables.

Milk is the only animal food that contributes to the daily carbohydrate intake. Freshly opened oysters and scallops contain some glycogen, but the amount is of no practical significance. The glycogen in liver is rapidly converted to lactic and pyruvic acids when the animal is slaughtered.

Carbohydrates in the U.S. Diet In 1982 the national available food supply furnished about 390 g carbohydrate per day.[4] Of this total, simple carbohydrates furnished approximately 51 percent and starches 49 percent. This represents a significant shift in the consumption as compared with that early in this century when simple carbohydrate accounted for less than one third of the total carbohydrate. (See Figure 6-6.) This shift has occurred with an increase in the consumption of sugar and other sweeteners concomitant with a steady decline in the consumption of carbohydrate supplied by cereal grains and potatoes.

The total simple carbohydrates in the diet in 1982

Table 6-1. **Carbohydrate Content of Some Typical Foods**

Food	Per 100 g of Food (g)	Per Serving Portion		
		Measure	Weight (g)	Carbohydrate (g)
Complex Carbohydrates*				
Bread, all kinds	50–56	1 slice	25	13
Cereals, breakfast, dry	68–84	1 cup wheat flakes	30	24
Crackers, all kinds	67–73	4 saltines	11	8
Flour, all kinds	71–80	2 tablespoons	14	11
Legumes, dry	60–63	½ cup navy beans, cooked	95	20
Macaroni, spaghetti, dry	75	½ cup cooked	70	16
Nuts	15–20	¼ cup peanuts	36	7
Pie crust, baked	44	⅙ shell	30	13
Potatoes, white, raw	17	1 boiled	135	20
Rice, dry	80	½ cup cooked	105	25
Complex and Simple Carbohydrates (½ and ½)				
Cake, plain and iced	52–68	1 piece layer, iced	71	45
Cookies	51–80	1 chocolate chip	10	6
Simple Carbohydrates				
Beverages, carbonated	8–12	8 ounces cola	246	24
Candy (without nuts)	75–95	1 ounce milk chocolate	28	16
Fruit, dried	59–69	4 prunes	32	18
Fruit, fresh	6–22	1 apple	138	20
		1 orange	180	16
Fruit, sweetened, canned or frozen	16–28	½ cup peaches	128	26
		3 ounces frozen strawberries	85	24
Ice cream	18–21	½ cup	67	16
Milk	5	1 cup	244	12
Pudding	16–26	½ cup vanilla	128	21
Sugar, all kinds	96–100	1 tablespoon white	12	12
Syrups, molasses, honey	65–82	1 tablespoon molasses	20	13
Vegetables	4–18	½ cup green beans	63	4
		½ cup peas	80	10

* Foods are grouped according to the predominating type of carbohydrate present.

was 197 g, which accounted for approximately 23 percent of the available calories. The caloric contribution from each category was as follows:[4]

	Percent
Dairy products	2.6
Fruits	3.2
Sugars and other sweeteners	17.5
	23.3

The amount of sucrose in the food supply has fluctuated considerably. After reaching a peak in 1972, the amount of sucrose has decreased and in 1980 was 102 g per capita per day, 10 g more than at the beginning of the century.[5] By contrast, a marked increase has occurred in the use of corn syrup and high fructose corn syrups resulting in an overall increase in the use of sweeteners.

Today's consumer has less control of the use of sugar in foods. Before World War II most baking, canning, pickling, and jelly-making took place in the home and accounted for about two thirds of the refined sugar used. For the past 40 years most sugar is used by the food industry: baked foods and mixes, sugar-coated cereals, candy, fruits canned in syrups, sweetened juices and fruit drinks, sweetened beverage mixes, jellies, jams, pickles, ice cream, and soft drinks. The consumer is less aware of the sugar included in numerous products such as nondairy creamers, catsup, breading mixtures for meats, peanut butter, and others. By reading labels the consumer soon becomes aware of the uses of refined sugars and other caloric sweeteners. Thus, a single label might indicate the presence of not only cane sugar but also corn syrup and honey.

Soft drink consumption has more than doubled since 1960 and was equivalent to 400 12-ounce cans

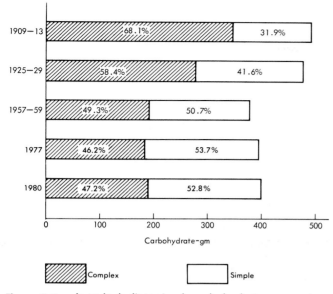

Complex ▨ Simple ▢

Figure 6-6. In today's diets simple carbohydrates account for over half of the carbohydrate and about 23 percent of the calories (see page 74). Early in the century complex carbohydrates (starchy foods) accounted for about two thirds of the carbohydrate intake. (Courtesy, Woteki, C. E., et al.: "Recent Trends and Levels of Dietary Sugars and Other Caloric Sweeteners," in Reiser, S., ed.: *Metabolic Effects of Utilizable Dietary Carbohydrates*, Marcel Dekker, New York, 1982.

Table 6-2. Carbohydrate Adjustment of the Basic Diet

	Carbohydrate (g)	Energy (kcal)
Basic Diet (page 38)	144	1,106
Potato, 1	20	90
Bread, 6 slices	76	380
	240	1,576
Fat, 9 teaspoons		300
Sugar, 1 ounce	30	120
	270	1,996
Complex carbohydrate, percentage of calories		48
Refined sugar, percentage of calories		6

per capita per year by 1979.[5] Soft drinks account for about 25 pounds of sweetener per capita annually and supply an estimated 4 percent of the calories in the food supply.

Adjustments to Conform to the Dietary Goals In view of the high proportion of sugars and also of fats in typical American diets, the following substantial modifications would be required if the Dietary Goals were applied:

Substantially increase the proportion of calories provided by breads, cereals, pastas, rice, and so on.
Increase the amounts of potatoes, legumes, fruits, and vegetables.
Decrease the consumption of sugar, sugar-containing beverages, cakes, cookies, candy, sugared cereals, and so on.

One way to adjust the Basic diet (page 38) for the woman who requires 2,000 kcal so that it furnishes 48 percent of the calories from complex carbohydrates and naturally occurring sugars, as recommended in the Goals, as shown in Table 6-2. This plan suggests the addition of 9 teaspoons of fat as an accompaniment for the bread equivalents and 1 ounce sugar that

could be consumed as such or in some sugar-containing food. As you can see, the total of nine slices of bread or its equivalent as rice, pastas, or other sources, in addition to the two potatoes and one serving of cereal are more than most women are accustomed to eating.

Artificial Sweeteners Saccharin and aspartame are the only noncaloric sweeteners currently approved for use. Saccharin is 350 times as sweet as sugar and has been extensively used during this century in foods for special dietary use and more recently in sugar-free soft drinks. Persons with diabetes mellitus, those who are trying to correct obesity, and others who are carbohydrate sensitive have long used saccharin as substitute sweeteners. Whether its use promotes dietary adherence is not certain.

In 1977 a Canadian study was reported that showed the occurrence of bladder cancer in male rats that had been fed a diet containing 5 percent saccharin over a 2-year period. Based on the requirement of the 1958 Delaney Amendment (see page 257) that the use of a substance must be prohibited if it is carcinogenic in any degree, the Food and Drug Administration moved to ban the use of saccharin. But there was great consumer resistance to this ban. It was argued that, based on body size, the dosages used to produce the cancers in the rats far exceeded the amounts that humans could ingest day by day over a lifetime. Also, many maintained that substituting sugar for saccharin could be a greater risk to health. In November 1977 Congress passed a law that placed a moratorium on the ban for 18 months; this moratorium has been extended several times.

Aspartame (e.g., Nutrasweet) is a dipeptide of phenylalanine and aspartic acid and thus can be metabolized by the body to provide energy. However, because it is 200 times as sweet as table sugar, the amount used is so small its caloric contribution is negligible. Although questions have been raised concerning the safety of aspartame, particularly if consumed in large amounts by children or pregnant women, insufficient evidence has been produced to convince the Food and Drug Administration to ban or restrict the use of aspartame.

An additional nonnutritive sweetener, cyclamate, was widely used for a number of years until Canadian studies in rats in the 1960s showed it to be slightly carcinogenic. Cyclamate was banned in 1970, and repeated efforts to have it reapproved have proved unsuccessful.

Dietary Fibers

"Roughage," "bulk," "residue," and "fiber" are imprecise terms that have long been applied to the indigestible substances of plant foods. The value of fiber in maintaining normal elimination of feces has been recognized for centuries.

Since the early 1970s there has been renewed interest in the role of fiber in the diet. This has come about because of the reports by some British clinicians that showed a correlation between fiber intake and the incidence of disease. Their epidemiologic studies showed that rural Africans who had a high-fiber intake had a low incidence of diverticulitis, irritable colon, hiatus hernia, hemorrhoids, cancer of the colon, coronary heart disease, obesity, diabetes, dental caries, and gallstones.[6,7] People in the Western world whose diets are low in fiber have a high incidence of these diseases. But it is important to keep in mind that fiber is only one of the many environmental factors that differ in the two groups, such as climate, pollutants, physical activity, fat and cholesterol intake, sugar intake, quality and amount of protein intake, and so on. Nonetheless, the British investigations have provided attractive hypotheses that require further testing. Although hundreds of reports have been published within the past decade, the results are often contradictory and confusing.

What Is Dietary Fiber DIETARY FIBERS include a number of polysaccharides and lignin that are not digested by the enzymes of the human gastrointestinal tract. These substances have specific chemical structures with varying physical and chemical properties. Their quantitative determination in foods is difficult, and the isolation of their effects on gastrointestinal function presents even greater problems to the investigator.

Cellulose is the most abundant molecule in nature and is the principal structure of cell walls. It is insoluble in water and is found abundantly in the bran of cereal grains.

Lignin, although classified with dietary fibers, is not a polysaccharide, since it contains no sugar units. This water-insoluble component makes up the woody part of plants. Legumes and fruits with seeds and the lignified cells of pears are important sources. Whole grain cereals are moderate in lignin content, whereas most vegetables are low.

Hemicelluloses are found in the cell walls of many plants. Some investigators include pectins, gums, and mucilages under this heading. The hemicelluloses are soluble in hot water and occur in a variety of plant foods: carrots, cabbage, celery, leafy vegetables, apples, melons, peaches, pears, and whole-grain cereals.

Pectin, unlike cellulose and lignin, does not have true fiber or threadlike characteristics. Nonetheless, it is an important structural material found in cell walls and functions as an intercellular cement. It is soluble in hot water and has the capacity to hold water and to form gels. Apples and citrus fruits are important sources, while cereals contain very little.

Mucilages and gums are nonstructural components of plant cells that are soluble in hot water.

Several indigestible polysaccharides are used in the food industry. Pectins are used in making fruit jellies. *Agar* obtained from seaweed is also useful for its gelling properties. *Carrageen* (Irish moss) and *alginates* from seaweed are often used to enhance the smoothness of foods such as ice cream and evaporated milk.

Effect of Fiber on Intestinal Physiology The effect of fiber on the gastrointestinal tract is influenced by the characteristics of the fiber itself, the particle size of the ingested fibers, the interaction between fibers, other dietary components, and bacterial flora. The following effects have been postulated. Some are well recognized while others remain speculative.[8,9]

1. Dietary fiber holds water so that stools are soft, bulky, and readily eliminated. Coarse bran is effective but fine bran often has little effect. It is generally agreed that a high-fiber intake prevents or relieves constipation although the amount of fiber required for this effect varies considerably among individuals. The large, bulky stool also represents a dilution of colon contents. Thus, any potential toxic substances such as carcinogens that might be present would become diluted and be less harmful.

2. Fiber generally increases motility of the small intestine and colon and decreases transit time. This could result from the stimulation of the mucosa by mechanical effect or perhaps by the by-products of bacterial fermentation. If transit time is shortened, then there could be less time for exposure of the mucosa to harmful toxicants. Also, there could be less time for bacteria to produce harmful substances. Transit time, however, is individually variable and unpredictable.

3. Pectins, mucilages, and gums retard gastric emptying. This can have two benefits: increased satiety so that less food is eaten, thus helping to keep energy intake within the requirement; and a smoother response by the blood circulation to absorbed glucose and hence decreased insulin secretion. This effect is one explanation for the lower insulin requirement observed in diabetic patients who consume a high-carbohydrate high-fiber diet.

4. High-fiber diets have been found to reduce intraluminal pressure in the colon of some persons who have diverticular disease or irritable colon. Yet, there is no evidence that low-fiber diets cause diverticulosis.

5. High-fiber diets, such as vegetarian diets, have somewhat lower coefficients of digestibility. Thus, the net energy realized to the body is a little less than that from diets containing high proportions of animal foods. Some forms of dietary fiber have the capacity to bind minerals such as calcium, magnesium, phosphorus, zinc, and others. This poses a possibility of nutritional deficiency, especially when diets contain marginal levels of mineral elements. For example, growth failure was observed in Iranian boys who consumed diets very high in fiber but low in zinc.[10] However, these diets also had a high content of phytic acid, which also binds minerals. The role of fiber in reducing mineral bioavailability remains controversial.

6. Pectins, mucilages, and gums chelate with bile acids and steroid materials. The chelating effect helps explain the reduction in blood cholesterol levels. But it must also be recognized that the lipid-lowering effect could be associated with the reduced level of fats that is characteristic of many high-fiber diets. Rolled oats and some legumes have been found effective in bringing about modest lowering of the blood cholesterol but the bran of wheat has not had such an effect.[11-13]

7. Pectins, hemicelluloses, gums, and mucilages are partially fermented by intestinal bacteria to volatile fatty acids, carbon dioxide, and methane. The caloric yield to the body by this fermentation is negligible and usually is of little practical significance. The extent to which the type or level of fiber intake can alter bacterial metabolism is not clear. Thus, it remains speculative as to whether fiber can modify intestinal flora so that harmful substances are detoxified or not produced.

8. Recent evidence suggests that vegetarians and other persons with high fiber intakes have blood pressures lower than those of persons with low fiber intakes. Possible mechanisms contributing to this effect have been postulated to include alterations in nutrient absorption, gastrointestinal function, and secretion of gastrointestinal and pancreatic hormones.[14]

Fiber Content of the Diet Many tables of food composition give data on "crude fiber" content of foods. By definition, CRUDE FIBER is the residue that remains after a food sample has been subjected to treatment by acid and then by alkali under standard conditions. The method excludes about 80 percent of the hemicelluloses, 50 to 90 percent of the lignin, and even up to 50 percent of the cellulose.[8] Because the proportions of fiber components vary from one food source to another, there is not practical way to convert crude fiber values to meaningful values of dietary fiber. In recent years more precise methods have been developed for identifying the various dietary fibers. Table A-3 gives values for fiber contents of foods.

The amount of fiber that should be present in the diet is not known. Most American diets could be improved by (1) substituting whole-grain for refined breads and cereals and (2) increasing the intake of fruits, vegetables, nuts, and legumes. Raw vegetables and fruits, including skins and seeds, are especially high in fiber.

An increase in the fiber intake should be accomplished gradually. This is especially important for those persons who choose to use bran daily for its extra fiber content (1 to 2 tablespoons is usually sufficient, starting with teaspoonful amounts). Initially many persons experience distention, cramping, and even diarrhea when the fiber intake is increased rapidly.

Excessive fiber intake should be avoided, not only because of the interference with absorption of mineral elements but also because it occasionally leads to intestinal obstruction.

Issues Related to Carbohydrate Intake

Low-Carbohydrate Reduction Diets From time to time claims are made for the effectiveness of low- or carbohydrate-free, high-protein, high-fat diets in bringing about weight loss. Such diets can be dangerous since they lead to ketosis with the associated clinical findings of excessive fatigue, dehydration, water loss, and electrolyte deficits. In susceptible individuals retention of uric acid sometimes leads to symptoms of gout. The increased supply of fat, especially saturated fat, may result in elevated blood lipids and increased risk of coronary heart disease. Low-carbohydrate diets are also low in fiber content. (See page 76.)

Hypoglycemia   Contrary to popular opinion, nonfasting reactive hypoglycemia is not common. The symptoms of hypoglycemia are hunger, weakness, trembling, sweating, headache, and, if severe, coma. People sometimes make a self-diagnosis based on what they have read or heard from a pseudo-scientist and attempt to treat themselves with a low-carbohydrate diet. The diagnosis, however, can be made only by a physician who relies not only on the presenting symptoms but also on the glucose tolerance test with multiple blood samples taken over a period of several hours.[15]

Nutritional Quality of High-Carbohydrate Diets   A high proportion of calories from carbohydrate is generally desirable provided that most of the carbohydrate is furnished by complex carbohydrates. Such diets furnish liberal intakes of minerals, vitamins, and fiber. By virtue of their lower fat content the risk of coronary heart disease is also reduced.

Sugar is useful as a concentrated source of energy and is valuable for contributing to diet palatability. However, excessive intake of sugars, candies, cakes, cookies, pastries, and sugar-containing soft drinks is likely to crowd out essential foods, thereby contributing to nutrient deficiencies as well as to problems of overweight. For example, the increasing use of soft drinks tends to reduce the intake of milk. The establishment early in life of habits of judicious consumption of sweets can scarcely be overemphasized.

Some people regard all refined sugar as harmful while regarding other forms of sugar—honey, raw sugar, molasses, maple syrup—as satisfactory substitutes. Although the substituted sweeteners may furnish some mineral elements, the amounts are too small to be of significance in the diet.

Dental Caries   The causes of tooth decay are many and complex. Yet, dentists agree that sugar is one of the important etiologic agents. Sugars provide the energy for bacterial growth, which leads to gradual buildup of plaque, a sticky carbohydrate–bacterial matrix that adheres firmly to the teeth. The acids formed by the bacteria from the sugar substrate gradually erode the tooth enamel and bring about decay. Two conditions accelerate the process: sticky carbohydrates that adhere to tooth surfaces for a long time; and frequent exposure of tooth surfaces to sugar. For example, sticky caramels are likely to be more harmful than a soft drink providing the same amount of sugar, since the latter is less likely to adhere to the tooth for a long period of time. But also, eating five caramels at five intervals during the day results in five exposures, while eating the five caramels at one time would reduce the total time of exposure.

Implication of Sugar in Other Problems   High-carbohydrate diets, per se, do not cause diabetes, nor is there convincing evidence that sugar will cause it.[16] But there is a high association between obesity and maturity-onset **diabetes** mellitus. Thus, caloric control rather than limitation of carbohydrate alone is the most important factor in delaying onset in susceptible individuals.

The contribution of high-carbohydrate intakes to elevation of blood triglycerides is controversial.[16,17] Again, persons who are obese are more likely to have elevated blood triglycerides. Some persons are genetically predisposed to hypertriglyceridemia and may be "carbohydrate sensitive." These individuals are usually advised to restrict their intake of sugar and of alcohol. (See Chapter 38.)

High intakes of sugar have been claimed to cause a variety of behavioral problems, particularly hyperactivity in children. The claims are based largely on anecdotal observations. The few controlled studies which have been conducted to evaluate the effects of sugar on hyperactivity produced conflicting results. Until additional scientific data are available, it is not possible to draw any conclusions about a relationship between sugar intake and adverse behavioral reactions.[18] (See page 315.)

Lactose Intolerance   Many adults other than those of northern European ancestry may be unable to tolerate milk because they have low levels of intestinal lactase activity causing malabsorption of lactose. As the unabsorbed lactose accumulates in the intestinal tract fermentation produces distention, cramping, and diarrhea. Although adults may be unable to drink milk, infants are usually lactose tolerant and will thrive on milk formulas. Children and teenagers can drink sufficient milk to meet their calcium requirements if the intake is well spaced throughout the day. To eliminate milk from the diet of all children belonging to ethnic groups having a high incidence of lactose intolerance is a nutritional disservice. When there is indication of some intolerance in children, a determination should be made of what levels of milk can be tolerated.[19] (See Chapter 31.)

Alcohol

Alcoholic beverages have been used throughout history. In the United States the consumption continues to increase, with wine especially gaining tremendously in popularity. On one hand is the social enjoyment and relief from tension that some people experience by consuming a cocktail, tankard of beer, or a glass of wine. At the other extreme is the problem of the alcoholic and the consequences of malnutrition and illness. Parents and educators are especially concerned about the increasing use of alcohol by teenagers.

Metabolism   Alcohol is rapidly absorbed from the stomach and small intestine and is promptly dispersed throughout the body fluids. There is no upper limit of absorption, but the rate of absorption is reduced when foods, especially those containing fat, are taken with the beverage.

Alcohol is oxidized almost exclusively by the liver to acetaldehyde, then to acetic acid. Because the muscles do not contain the enzymes necessary for the conversion to acetaldehyde, exercise is of no value in hastening the return to sobriety. The acetic acid formed is condensed with coenzyme A, and through the TCA cycle yields energy to the peripheral tissues as well as the liver.

Two pathways of the oxidation of alcohol to acetaldehyde by the liver have been described.[20] The first of these is the conversion to acetaldehyde in the presence of alcohol dehydrogenase and NAD$^+$:

$$CH_3CH_2OH + NAD^+ \xrightarrow{\text{alcohol dehydrogenase}}$$
ethanol
$$CH_3CHO + NADH + H^+$$
acetaldehyde

This is the primary pathway when the concentration of alcohol in the circulation is low. The availability of NAD$^+$ is the rate-limiting factor. About 0.1 g alcohol is metabolized per kilogram body weight per hour. Thus, it would require about 5 hours for a 70-kg man to completely metabolize the alcohol from 100 ml 86 proof (43 percent alcohol) whiskey.

The second pathway is accomplished by *mixed-function oxidase*, a system that requires two cytochrome enzymes:

$$CH_3CH_2OH + NADPH + H^+ \xrightarrow{\substack{\text{mixed-}\\\text{function}\\\text{oxidase}}}$$
$$CH_3CHO + NADP^+ + 2\ H_2O$$

This pathway is active when the ethanol concentration in the circulation is high. With chronic exposure to alcohol the amount and catalytic activity of this pathway increases, which helps explain the tolerance shown by alcoholics.

This pathway is called the mixed-function oxidase system because it also is responsible for the detoxification of a variety of substances including barbiturates. But the presence and interaction with one substance also reduces the activity toward the other. Obviously, barbiturates and alcohol become a dangerous mix!

Alcohol and Nutrition   Beer, wine, and distilled liquors contribute calories and these must be accounted for in maintaining caloric equilibrium. Each gram of alcohol yields 7.1 kcal (5.6 kcal per ml). Thus, 100 ml 86 proof whiskey would yield 241 kcal (43 ml alcohol × 5.6). Calories in excess of needs, regardless of source, will contribute to weight gain. Beer and wine contain minimal amounts of nutrients, and distilled liquors contain none.

Alcoholic beverages consumed in moderate amounts need not adversely affect nutritional status provided that foods are selected in recommended amounts from the essential food groups. In chronic alcoholism, however, alcohol often replaces essential foods in the diet because of reduced appetite or because the person does not have enough money to purchase both food and alcohol. With the reduced intake of nutrients, the stage is set for nutritional deficiency. Moreover, the metabolism of alcohol requires thiamin, niacin, and pantothenic acid, and the lack of these nutrients for other metabolic pathways may help explain the neuropathy that is sometimes present in alcoholism. In addition, alcohol impairs intestinal absorption and increases urinary losses of a number of vitamins and minerals. Other physiologic effects of alcohol consumption and diet counseling for alcoholics are discussed in Chapter 27.

SOME POINTS FOR EMPHASIS IN NUTRITION EDUCATION

1. Carbohydrates include sugars, starches, and fiber from plant foods. Milk, which contains lactose, is the only important source of carbohydrate from animal foods.
2. The principal function of carbohydrate is to furnish energy to the body. In the United States most diets furnish less than half the energy value of the diet from carbohydrate.
3. Only a small amount of carbohydrate is stored in the body in the form of glycogen. If there is an excess of carbohydrate beyond the body's immediate need, it is stored as fat.
4. The nutritive value of typical diets in the United States would be improved by including more complex carbohydrates and by reducing the intake of sugars.
5. Weight for weight, fresh fruits and vegetables contain much less carbohydrate than do breads and cereals. But breads and cereals furnish energy at low cost, and if selections are made from whole-grain or enriched products they contribute significant amounts of B-complex vitamins and iron to the diet.
6. Raw fruit and vegetables, legumes, nuts, and whole-grain breads and cereals should be emphasized for their fiber content.
7. Sugars and sweets should be used with discretion lest they replace essential foods in the diet. The trace amounts of nutrients other than sugar found in honey, brown sugar, raw sugar, and maple syrup are of little significance.
8. Palatable diets are possible when refined and processed sugars are restricted to less than 10 percent of the caloric intake.

Problems and Review

1. *Key terms*: adenosine triphosphate (ATP); aerobic metabolism; anaerobic metabolism; cellulose; citric acid cycle; coenzyme A; cytochrome; dietary fiber; disaccharide; electron transport; gluconeogenesis; glycogenesis; glycolysis; hemicellulose; lignin; lipogenesis; monosaccharide; oxidative phosphorylation; pectin; pentose shunt; polysaccharide.
2. Describe what happens during digestion to the carbohydrate in a breakfast consisting of orange juice, cereal sweetened with sugar and milk.
3. What advantages might be realized by increasing the intake of complex carbohydrates?
4. Drinking a glass of fruit juice removes feelings of hunger quickly but for a relatively short period of time. Explain this on the basis of physiologic and biochemical reactions that take place.
5. Even though you eat a diet that is high in carbohydrate the blood glucose will usually not reach the renal threshold. Explain the mechanisms whereby the blood sugar is maintained within such narrow limits.
6. If an individual is not eating, what mechanisms provide for the maintenance of a supply of glucose to the tissues?
7. If carbohydrate is eaten in excess of the energy requirement, what happens to it?
8. If a client's diet record revealed a high intake of sugar, what would be your reasons for recommending a reduced consumption of sugar?
9. What are some effects on gastrointestinal physiology of a high-fiber intake?
10. *Problem*. Calculate the carbohydrate and caloric content of your diet for one day. What percentage of calories are furnished by complex carbohydrates? By sugars? What steps could you take to increase the proportion of complex carbohydrate? The amount of fiber?
11. When counseling a client about his or her diet, why is it useful to know about the individual's consumption of alcohol?

References

1. Gray, G. M.: "Carbohydrate Absorption and Malabsorption," in Johnson, L. R., et al., eds.: *Physiology of the Gastrointestinal Tract*. Raven Press, New York, 1981, pp. 1063–72.
2. Food and Nutrition Board: *Recommended Dietary Allowances*, 10th ed. National Research Council–National Academy of Sciences, Washington, D.C., 1989.
3. U.S. Senate Select Committee on Nutrition and Human Needs: *Dietary Goals for the United States*, rev. ed. Government Printing Office, Washington, D.C., December 1977.
4. Marston, R. M., and Welsh, S. O.: "Nutrient Content of the U.S. Food Supply, 1982," *Natl. Food Review* (USDA), 7–13, Winter 1984.
5. Woteki, C. E., et al.: "Recent Trends and Levels of Dietary Sugars and Other Caloric Sweeteners," in Reiser, S., ed.: *Metabolic Effects of Utilizable Dietary Carbohydrates*. M. Dekker, New York, 1982, pp. 1–27.
6. Burkitt, D. P., et al.: "Dietary Fiber and Disease," *JAMA*, 229:1068–74, 1974.
7. Trowell, H.: "Ischemic Heart Disease and Dietary Fiber," *Am. J. Clin Nutr.*, 25:926–32, 1972.
8. Kelsay, J. L.: "A Review of Research on Effects of Fiber Intake on Man," *Am. J.Clin. Nutr.*, 31:142–59, 1978.
9. Eastwood, M. A., and Passmore, R.: "Dietary Fibre," *Lancet*, 2:202–6, 1983.
10. Prasad, A. S.: "Clinical, Biochemical and Nutritional Spectrum of Zinc Deficiency in Human Subjects: An Update," *Nutr. Rev.*, 41:197–208, 1983.
11. Kirby, R. M., et al.: "Oat-bran Intake Selectively Lowers Serum Low Density Lipoprotein Cholesterol Concentrations of Hypercholesterolemic Men," *Am. J. Clin. Nutr.*, 34:824–29, 1982.
12. Ullrich, I. H., and Albrink, N. J.: "Lack of Effect of Dietary Fiber on Serum Lipids, Glucose, and Insulin

in Healthy Young Men Fed High Starch Diets," *Am. J. Clin. Nutr.*, **36:**1–9, 1982.

13. Slavin, J. L.: "Dietary Fiber," *Diet. Currents* [Ross Laboratories], **10:**27–32, 1983.

14. Anderson, J. W.: "Plant Fiber and Blood Pressure," *Ann. Intern. Med.*, **98:**842–46, 1983.

15. American Diabetic Association: "Statement on Hypoglycemia," *Diabetes Care*, **5:**72–73, 1982.

16. Nuttall, F. Q., and Gannon, M. C.: "Sucrose and Disease," *Diabetes Care*, **4:**305–10, 1981.

17. Review: "Nutrition Update: Sugar," *Dairy Council Digest*, **55:**22–26, 1984.

18. Rapoport, J. L, and Kruesi, M. J. P.: "Behavior and Nutrition: A Mini Review," *Cont. Nutr.*, [General Mills], **8(10):**1982.

19. Lebenthal, E., and Rossi, T. M.: "Lactose Malabsorption and Intolerance," in Lebenthal, E., ed.: *Textbook of Gastroenterology and Nutrition in Infancy*. Raven Press, New York, 1981, pp. 673–88.

20. Lieber, C. S.: "Metabolism and Metabolic Effects of Alcohol," *Med. Clin. North Am.*, **68:**3–31, 1984.

7

Lipids

Fats are the most concentrated source of energy in foods and often supply two fifths or more of the total energy intake in typical American diets. They constitute the body's chief reserve of energy and are essential for diverse functions such as insulation and padding, integrity of cell membranes, synthesis of some hormones, and carriers of fat-soluble vitamins. Fats are valued for enhancement of food palatability.

Composition, Classification, and Characteristics

Composition   Lipids are a heterogeneous group of substances that includes fats, oils, and fatlike substances that share the characteristic of being soluble in certain organic solvents such as ether, alcohol, and benzene. Like carbohydrates, fats are organic compounds made up of carbon, hydrogen, and oxygen, but the resemblance ends there. Fats have a much smaller proportion of oxygen than do carbohydrates and differ in important ways in their structure and properties. Some lipids also contain carbohydrates, phosphates, or nitrogenous components.

Fatty Acids   The major constituent of many lipids is fatty acids. These compounds consist of chains of carbon atoms with a methyl (CH_3) group at one end and a carboxyl (COOH) group at the other end.

Most fatty acids in foods and in the body are straight even-numbered carbon chains. Fatty acids classified as short-chain contain 4 and 6 carbon atoms; medium-chain fatty acids contain 8 to 12; and long-chain contain more than 12. Most fatty acids found in animal tissues contain 16 to 26 carbon atoms.

Fatty acids are "saturated" or "unsaturated." A fatty acid in which each of the carbon atoms in the chain has two hydrogen atoms attached to it is saturated:

$$-\overset{\displaystyle H}{\underset{\displaystyle H}{C}}-\overset{\displaystyle H}{\underset{\displaystyle H}{C}}-$$

An unsaturated fatty acid is one in which a hydrogen atom is missing from each of two adjoining carbon atoms thus necessitating a double bond between the two carbon atoms:

CONTROVERSIAL ISSUES

Few issues in nutrition have created as much controversy as the fat content of the diet. Nutrition scientists, physicians, nutritionists, public health workers, politicians, and consumers have taken sides. Some segments of the food industry are aligned on one side and some on the other. Many years, perhaps decades, may be needed to fully resolve the controversy. Meantime Americans continue to ask:

Should we reduce our fat intake? Should we omit whole milk and eggs because they are high in saturated fats and cholesterol? What changes should we make in our consumption of meat?

What are the possible benefits of substituting special margarines and cooking oils for regular margarine, butter, and solid fats? Are there any adverse effects on nutritional status and health by such dietary adjustments?

Although final answers to these questions obviously cannot be provided, the reader of this chapter should be able to achieve an overall perspective and to provide responsible guidance to the public.

CH (CH)$_{16}$COOH Stearic acid (saturated) 18:0

CH$_3$(CH$_2$)$_7$ CH=CH (CH$_2$)$_7$COOH Oleic acid (monounsaturated) 18:1

CH$_3$(CH$_2$)$_4$ CH=CH CH$_2$ CH=CH (CH$_2$)$_7$COOH Linoleic acid (2 double bonds; polyunsaturated) 18:2

CH$_3$CH$_2$ CH=CH CH$_2$ CH=CH CH$_2$ CH=CH (CH$_2$)$_7$COOH Linolenic acid (3 double bonds; polyunsaturated) 18:3

Figure 7-1. These fatty acids contain 18 carbon atoms but differ in the level of saturation, having one, two, and three double bonds.

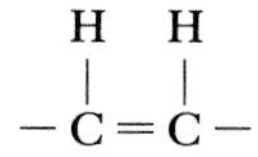

A MONOUNSATURATED FATTY ACID has one double bond. Oleic acid, the most important example, is widely distributed in food and body fats. A POLYUNSATURATED FATTY ACID (PUFA) contains two or more double bonds; linoleic, linolenic, and arachidonic acids are nutritionally important examples of this group. The formulas for these four fatty acids, which contain 18 carbon atoms but which differ in their saturation, are shown in Figure 7-1.

Unsaturated fatty acids can exist as geometric isomers. In the *cis* form the molecule folds back upon itself at each double bond. In the *trans* form the molecule extends to its maximum length.

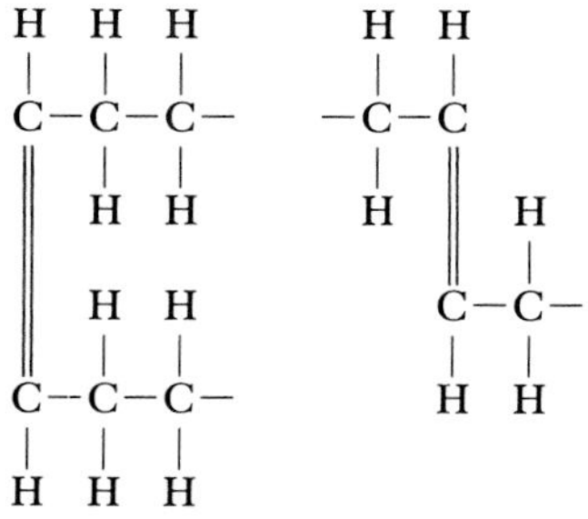

cis form   *trans* form

The form in which a fatty acid occurs can markedly influence its properties. Food and body fats exist principally in the *cis* form, although it has been estimated that the average consumption of *trans* fatty acids in the United States is about 8 percent of the fat. The primary sources of *trans* acids are margarines and shortenings made from partially hydrogenated vegetable oils.[1]

Classification Lipids are often classified in three groups:

1. *Simple lipids.* These are generally esters of fatty acids and alcohols, although free fatty acids some-

times also are included in this group. The most common esters are combinations of fatty acids with GLYCEROL, a 3-carbon alcohol with three hydroxyl groups. These compounds, also referred to as *neutral fats*, may contain one fatty acid (MONOGLYCERIDE or monoacylglycerol), two fatty acids (DIGLYCERIDES) or three fatty acids (TRIGLYCERIDES) combined with glycerol. A *simple triglyceride* is one in which the three fatty acids are the same. A *mixed triglyceride* is one in which at least two fatty acids are different. Mixed triglycerides account for 98 percent of fats in foods and over 90 percent of fat in the body. (See Figure 7-2.)

Figure 7-2. Formation of a triglyceride by condensation of three fatty acids and glycerol. Simple and mixed triglyceride.

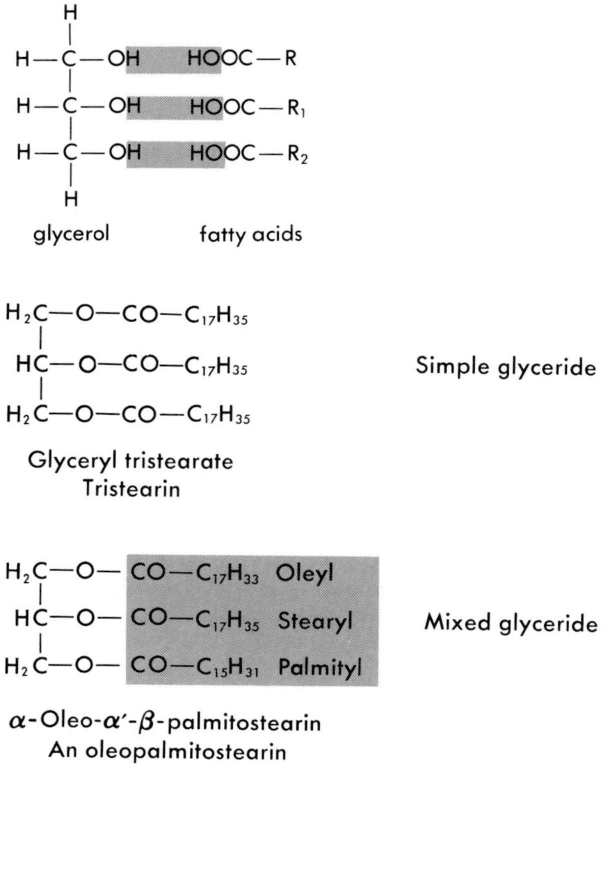

glycerol   fatty acids

H$_2$C—O—CO—C$_{17}$H$_{35}$
HC—O—CO—C$_{17}$H$_{35}$ Simple glyceride
H$_2$C—O—CO—C$_{17}$H$_{35}$

Glyceryl tristearate
Tristearin

H$_2$C—O— CO—C$_{17}$H$_{33}$ Oleyl
HC—O— CO—C$_{17}$H$_{35}$ Stearyl   Mixed glyceride
H$_2$C—O— CO—C$_{15}$H$_{31}$ Palmityl

α-Oleo-α'-β-palmitostearin
An oleopalmitostearin

Waxes are esters of fatty acids and long-chain or cyclic alcohols. This group includes the esters of cholesterol, vitamin A, and vitamin D.

2. *Compound lipids.* These are esters of glycerol and fatty acids, with substitution of other components such as carbohydrate, phosphate, and/or nitrogenous groupings. PHOSPHOLIPIDS such as lecithin and cephalin contain a phosphate and nitrogen grouping replacing one of the fatty acids in the molecule. (See Figure 7-3.) GLYCOLIPIDS such as the cerebrosides contain a molecule of glucose or galactose. LIPOPROTEINS include a variety of lipid molecules bound to protein molecules in order to facilitate transport in the aqueous medium of the blood.

3. *Derived lipids.* These include alcohols (glycerol and sterols such as cholesterol); carotenoids; and the fat-soluble vitamins, A, D, E, and K.

Characteristics of Fats The nature of fats—their hardness, melting point, and flavor—is determined by the length of the carbon chain and the level of saturation of the fatty acids as well as the order in which the fatty acids are attached to the glycerol molecule.

Although pure triglycerides are practically tasteless, they have the ability to hold flavors and aromas. A tremendous number of fats exist in nature. Each food fat—beef, lamb, chicken, olive oil, for example—has its distinctive flavor and hardness.

Hardness. The hardness of a fat is determined by its fatty acid composition. In turn, the fatty acid composition of body fat, and hence its hardness, can be modified by the diet. Fatty acids containing 12 carbon atoms or fewer and unsaturated fatty acids are liquid at room temperature. Saturated fatty acids containing 14 carbon atoms or more are solid at room temperature. Food and body fats contain mixtures of short- and long-chain fatty acids and of saturated and unsaturated fatty acids. No natural fat is made up completely of either saturated or unsaturated fatty acids.

The distribution of fatty acids in a number of fats is shown in Table 7-1. Only about 5 percent of fatty acids in food and body fats contain fewer than 14 carbon atoms, coconut oil being an exception.

Animal fats, often classified as "saturated" contain 30 to 60 percent saturated fatty acids, of which

Figure 7-3. In lecithin a phosphate group and choline replace one of the fatty acids of the glyceride. The composite benzene ring structure of cholesterol is typical of the structure of many steroids.

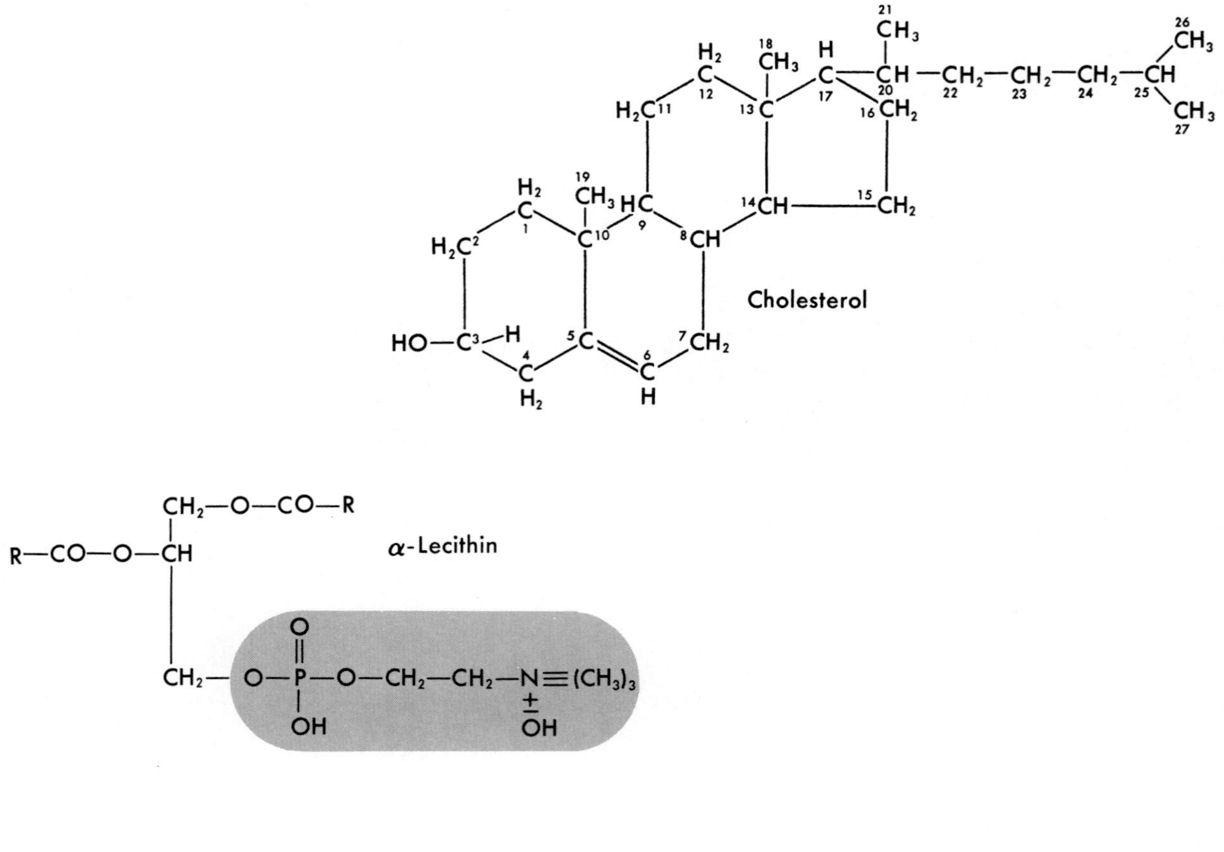

Table 7-1. Typical Major Fatty Acid Analyses of Some Fats of Animal and Plant Origin*†

	Saturated						Unsaturated				
	4–8	Capric 10.0	Lauric 12.0	Myristic 14.0	Palmitic 16.0	Stearic 18.0	Palmitoleic 16.1	Oleic 18.1	Linoleic 18.2	Linolenic 18.3	Arachidonic 20.4
Animal											
Lard		0.1	0.2	1.3	23.8	13.5	2.7	41.2	10.2	1.0	
Chicken			0.1	0.9	21.6	6.0	5.7	37.4	19.5	1.0	0.1
Egg				2.7	22.1	7.7	3.3	36.6	11.1	0.3	0.9
Beef		0.9	0.9	3.7	24.9	18.9	4.2	36.0	3.0	0.6	
Butter	6.3	2.5	2.8	10.1	26.3	12.1	2.2	25.2	2.2	1.5	
Human milk	0.1	1.1	4.1	5.6	22.4	9.2	3.8	35.0	10.8	0.4	0.4
Human adipose			0.7	3.5	20.0	3.4	10.7	53.0	7.1		
Vegetable											
Corn					10.9	1.8		24.2	58.0	0.7	
Peanut			0.1		9.5	2.2	0.1	44.8	32.0		
Cottonseed			0.8		22.7	2.3	0.8	17.0	51.5	0.2	0.1
Soybean			0.1		10.3	3.8	0.2	22.8	51.0	6.8	
Olive					11.0	2.2	0.8	72.5	7.9	0.6	
Coconut	8.1	6.0	44.6	16.8	8.2	2.8		5.8	1.8		

* Composition is given in weight percentages of the component fatty acids. The number of carbon atoms and the number of double bonds are indicated under the common name of the fatty acid.

† Sources of data:
  Human milk: Gibson, R. A., et al.: "Fatty Acid Composition of Human Colostrum and Mature Breast Milk," *Am. J. Clin. Nutr.*, **34**:252–57, 1981.
  Human adipose: Bray, G. A.: *The Obese Patient.* W. B. Saunders Co., Philadelphia, 1976, p. 97.
  Food: *Composition of Foods*, Agriculture Handbooks No. 8-1 (1976) and No. 8-4 (1979). U.S. Department of Agriculture, Washington, D. C.

palmitic and stearic acids predominate. Also, they contain about 25 to 50 percent oleic acid and small amounts of polyunsaturated fatty acids. In general, herbivora have harder fats than are found in carnivora, and land animals have harder fats than do aquatic animals. Lamb and beef fat, with their high content of palmitic and stearic acids, are much harder than pork and chicken fat, which contain somewhat more of the unsaturated fatty acids. Fats from fish have a high proportion of polyunsaturated fatty acids containing 20 to 24 carbon atoms. The proportion of saturated fatty acids is high in milk fat, but this fat is soft because of the presence of many short-chain fatty acids.

Oleic and linoleic acids predominate in vegetable fats, except for coconut oil. Safflower, corn, cottonseed, and soybean oils are very rich in linoleic acid, whereas peanut and olive oils are rich in oleic acid and correspondingly lower in linoleic acid. Of the vegetable fats, coconut oil is unique in that it is composed largely of the 12-carbon lauric acid, which is liquid at room temperature. Coconut oil is classified as a "saturated" fat and other vegetable fats as "unsaturated." Those fats that have a high proportion of fatty acids with two or more double bonds are referred to as "polyunsaturated."

Hydrogenation. In the presence of a catalyst such as nickel, liquid fats can be changed to solid fats by HYDROGENATION; this process consists of the addition of hydrogen at the double bonds of the carbon chain. In the manufacture of vegetable shortenings and margarines, some, but not all, of the double bonds in the oils are hydrogenated, thereby forming fats that are somewhat soft and plastic. During hydrogenation some of the fatty acids are changed from the *cis* to the *trans* form, but both forms are utilized by the body. Hydrogenation reduces the linoleic acid content of the fat.

Emulsification. Fats are capable of forming emulsions with liquids; that is, the fats can be dispersed into minute globules, thereby increasing the surface area and reducing the surface tension so that there is less tendency for the globules to coalesce. Bile salts and lecithin are essential biochemical emulsifiers in digestion and absorption. The property of emulsification is also utilized in the homogenization of milk and in the preparation of mayonnaise. Lecithin and other emulsifiers are widely used by the food industry.

Saponification. The combination of a fatty acid with a cation to form a soap is known as SAPONIFICA-

TION. In the alkaline medium of the intestine, for example, free fatty acid may combine with calcium to form an insoluble compound excreted in the feces. In certain diseases characterized by poor fat absorption—sprue, for example—the loss of calcium in this manner could be significant.

Rancidity. Air at room temperature can induce oxidation of fats, resulting in the changes in odor and flavor commonly known as rancidity. These changes are accelerated upon exposure to light and in the presence of traces of certain minerals. The oxygen attacks the double bonds of fatty acids to form *peroxides.* Thus, peroxidation occurs more readily in fats that have a high proportion of unsaturated fatty acids. Some fats are naturally protected by the presence of antioxidants, one of which is vitamin E. But in the process of preventing oxidation, the activity of vitamin E is lost. Commercially processed fats and oils are usually protected by the addition of small amounts of antioxidants.

Effect of Heat. Excessive heating of fats leads to the breakdown of glycerol, producing a pungent compound (acrolein) that is especially irritating to the gastrointestinal mucosa. Fatty acids are also oxidized by prolonged heating at high temperatures. Under ordinary conditions of home or commercial frying, few adverse effects on nutritional properties have been found.

Functions

Body Composition All body cells contain some fat. In healthy nonobese women fat makes up about 18 to 25 percent of body weight, and in healthy nonobese men about 15 to 20 percent of body weight. With aging the proportion of fat in the body generally increases as that of protoplasmic tissue decreases.

Adipose tissue, which consists principally of triglycerides, is stored in the subcutaneous tissues and in the abdominal cavity. It also surrounds the organs and is laced throughout muscle tissue. The predominant form of adipose tissue is white. Brown adipose tissue occurs in small amounts in the interscapular and axillary regions and at the nape of the neck. It is relatively more abundant in the newborn.

Cell membranes contain lipids that facilitate the transfer of nutrients. Cerebrosides, galactose-containing lipids, are components of the myelin sheath of nerves and the white matter of the brain. Gangliosides, glucose- and galactose-containing lipids, are constituents of brain tissue and of the synaptic membranes.

Insulation and Padding The subcutaneous layer of fat is an effective insulator that reduces losses of body heat in cold weather. Excessive layers of subcutaneous fat, as in obesity, interfere with heat loss during warm weather, thereby increasing discomfort. Vital organs such as the kidney are protected against physical injury by a padding of fat.

Energy The primary function of fat is to supply energy. Each gram of fat when oxidized yields approximately 9 kcal, or more than twice as much energy as a gram of carbohydrate or protein. The high density and low solubility of fats make them an ideal form in which to store energy. In fact, not only are fats as such stored in adipose tissue but any glucose and amino acids not promptly utilized are also synthesized into fats and stored.

A woman who weighs 55 kg, of which 20 percent is fat, has a store of about 85,000 kcal (7,700 kcal per kg of fat). Many examples could be cited of individuals who have survived starvation for 30 or 40 days or partial starvation for much longer periods of time. Their survival was possible only because of the energy available from the adipose tissue.

The small amount of brown adipose tissue is important in the production of body heat, perhaps including that which occurs after digestion of food. Abnormalities in brown adipose tissue have been shown to contribute to obesity in certain animal models, but their significance in human obesity is not known.[2]

Satiety Closely related to the provision of energy is the satiety value of fats. Because fats reduce gastric motility and remain in the stomach longer, the onset of hunger sensations is delayed. Diets that contain generous amounts of fat are sometimes described as "sticking to the ribs," "rich," or "satisfying"; that is, they have high satiety value.

Palatability How much food we eat as well as the kind of food we eat depend in part on our enjoyment of it. Fats lend palatability to the diet, whether it be as butter or margarine on bread, seasoning for vegetables, dressings on salads, or an ingredient of cakes, cookies, pastries, and other desserts. The fats in meats, poultry, and fish and the oils in fruits lend the characteristic flavors that we enjoy. If most fat is eliminated from the diet, as is necessary for some patients with disturbances of fat metabolism, the diet becomes very bulky; it is often difficult for these patients to ingest sufficient food to meet energy requirements.

Carriers of Fat-Soluble Vitamins Dietary fat is a carrier of the fat-soluble vitamins A, D, E, and K.

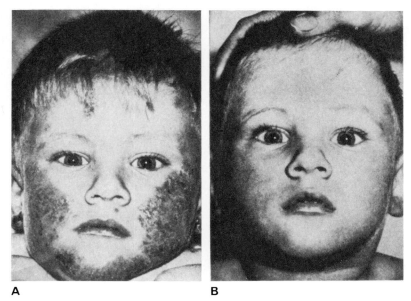

Figure 7-4. Child 2 ½ years old showing *(A)* eczema present since 2 months of age; *(B)* 1 month after adding a source of linoleic acid to the diet. (Courtesy, Dr. A.E. Hansen, Galveston, Texas.)

Some fat is also necessary for the absorption of vitamin A and its precursor, carotene.

Essential Fatty Acids LINOLEIC ACID, the 18-carbon acid with two double bonds, is an essential fatty acid; that is, it cannot be synthesized in the body and must be present in the diet. In the body linoleic acid is rapidly converted to ARACHIDONIC ACID, the physiologically functioning polyunsaturated fatty acid. In the absence of linoleic acid in the diet of animals growth retardation, skin lesions, and liver degeneration occur. Dryness and scaling of the skin have been observed in infants who received formulas lacking linoleic acid.[3] The eczemalike symptoms disappeared when a source of linoleic acid was provided. (See Figure 7-4.) Similar symptoms have been observed in patients maintained for long periods of time on intravenous feedings not containing fat.[4]

LINOLENIC ACID, another of the polyunsaturated fatty acids, has essential fatty acid properties in animals, although it does not cure the dermatitis that occurs in fatty acid deficiency. Its importance in human nutrition is not clear, but it generally is not considered essential. Linolenic acid is not a substitute for linoleic acid and cannot serve as a precursor for arachidonic acid.

The polyunsaturated fatty acids are constituents of phospholipids and thus have a role in regulating cell permeability. Others, particularly arachidonic acid, are precursurs of PROSTAGLANDINS, an important group of hormonelike compounds. Although the physiologic effects of the various prostaglandins differ, they include regulation of blood pressure, stimulation of smooth muscle contraction, stimulation of inflammation, modulation of the action of hormones, transmission of nerve impulses, and inhibition of gastric secretion and lipolysis. Some appear to enhance aggregation of blood platelets, while others inhibit aggregation. The effect of aspirin as an antiinflammatory drug probably relates to its inhibition of the biosynthesis of prostaglandins.

Phospholipids All cells contain phospholipids, but brain, nervous tissue, and liver are especially rich in these substances. The phospholipid level in the body is not reduced even in starvation, which suggests the vital role that they must play in metabolism. Phospholipids are powerful emulsifying agents and have an affinity for water. Hence, they are essential to the digestion and absorption of fats and they facilitate the uptake of fatty acids by the cells.

Phospholipids comprise a significant proportion of the blood lipoproteins, but their function in lipid transport is not clearly understood. They are manufactured and removed by the liver and apparently do not enter the tissue cells, which readily synthesize their own supply of phospholipid. Because of the ease with which the body synthesizes phospholipids there is no need for them in the diet.

Cholesterol The concentration of cholesterol is high in the liver, the adrenal, the white and gray matter of the brain, and the peripheral nerves. It is present in small amounts in almost all body tissues and constitutes an important fraction of the blood lipoproteins. It is synthesized by the liver to meet body needs regardless of dietary intake.

Cholesterol is a component of cell membranes and furnishes the nucleus for the synthesis of provitamin D, adrenocortical hormones, steroid sex hormones, and bile salts.

Digestion and Absorption

Digestion   Almost all the fats presented to the digestive tract for hydrolysis are triglycerides. Only a small fraction of dietary fat consists of cholesterol esters and phospholipids. Although fats are hydrolyzed primarily in the upper small intestine by the action of pancreatic lipase, some digestion of triglycerides may take place in the stomach. Much of the lipolytic activity of gastric contents is due to lipase secreted by the lingual serous glands located in the back of the tongue. This lingual lipase is most active on medium- and short-chain triglycerides. It also appears to prepare dietary fat for more efficient digestion in the small intestine.[5] Lingual lipase is believed to be particularly important in the digestion of fat in the newborn. Human breast milk also contains a lipase that contributes to fat digestion in the young infant. An additional lipase may be secreted by the stomach but appears to be insignificant in fat digestion.

As the chyme enters the duodenum, the presence of fat stimulates the release of the hormone *enterogastrone*. This hormone reduces motility and regulates the flow of chyme to correspond to the availability of the pancreatic secretions. The presence of fat in the duodenum also stimulates the intestinal wall to secrete CHOLECYSTOKININ, a hormone that is carried to the gallbladder by the bloodstream. Cholecystokinin stimulates the contraction of the gallbladder, thereby forcing bile into the common duct and thence into the small intestine.

Bile has several important functions in fat digestion and absorption: (1) it stimulates peristalsis; (2) it neutralizes the acid chyme so as to provide the optimum hydrogen ion concentration for enzyme activity; (3) it emulsifies fats, thereby increasing the surface area exposed to enzyme action; and (4) it lowers the surface tension so that intimate contact between the fat droplets and the enzymes is possible.

Hydrolysis of triglycerides by pancreatic lipase requires the presence of a protein factor called COLIPASE, also present in the pancreatic secretions. Colipase appears to bind to triglycerides in the presence of bile

acids and in some way facilitates interaction of lipase with its triglyceride substrate. The triglycerides are hydrolyzed stepwise by lipase; that is, one of the end fatty acids is removed at the time, yielding in turn a diglyceride and then a monoglyceride, with the fatty acid attached in the middle or number 2 position. Only about one fourth to one half of the triglycerides are completely hydrolyzed to glycerol and fatty acids. Some of the phospholipids are hydrolyzed by phospholipases that can attack several linkages of the molecule. Cholesterol esters are hydrolyzed by a *cholesterol esterase* present in the pancreatic secretions to form cholesterol and fatty acids. The end products of lipid hydrolysis that are presented for absorption include fatty acids, glycerol, monoglycerides, some di- and tri-glycerides, cholesterol, and phospholipids. (See Figure 7-5.)

Speed of Digestion   Fats reduce the motility of the gastrointestinal tract; consequently, any diet containing fat causes the food to remain in the stomach longer than does a diet low in fat. Fats that are liquid at body temperature are hydrolyzed more rapidly than are those that are solid at body temperature. Typical mixed diets contain complex mixtures of fats including short- and long-chain as well as saturated and unsaturated fatty acids. Adults normally experience no difficulty in digesting fats from any source. Infants and young children, as well as some elderly persons, seem to have somewhat better tolerance for the softer, more highly emulsified fats such as those in dairy products. They also may experience some discomfort after consuming meals high in fat.

Fried foods are digested somewhat more slowly than foods prepared by other methods of cookery because the food particles coated with fat must be broken up before they can be acted upon by enzymes. Properly fried foods do not normally cause digestive difficulties, even for persons who require therapeutic diets. When the frying temperature is too low, foods absorb excessive amounts of fat, lengthening the time required for their digestion. On the other hand, if foods are fried at too high a temperature the resulting decomposition products may be irritating to the intestinal mucosa.

Absorption   In the lumen of the small intestine the free fatty acids, monoglycerides, some diglycerides and triglycerides, and cholesterol are complexed with bile salts to form MICELLES; these water-soluble microscopic particles can penetrate the mucosal membrane. At the point of contact of the micelle with the brush border of the epithelial cell, the lipids are ap-

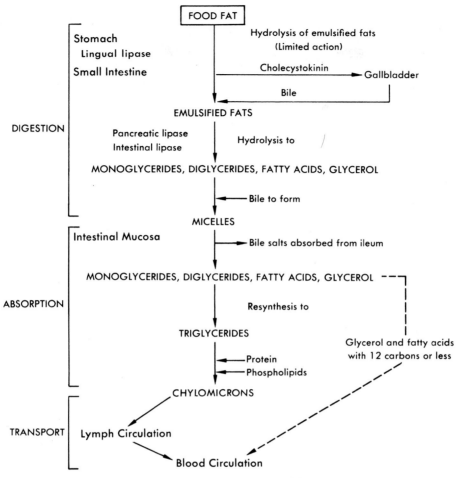

Figure 7-5. The digestion, absorption, and transport of fat.

parently released from the complex and enter the cell by mechanisms not fully understood. Most of the absorption of fats occurs from the jejunum.

Fatty acids that contain 12 carbon atoms or fewer are absorbed into the portal circulation without reesterification in the mucosal cell. They are attached to albumin for their transportation, and they may be used within the liver or released to other tissues in the body. The glycerol resulting from fat hydrolysis is also carried by the portal circulation.

Fatty acids that contain 14 carbon atoms or more are resynthesized to new triglycerides within the epithelial cell of the mucosa before they are extruded into the lymph circulation. The new fats are formed by the addition of two fatty acids to a monoglyceride molecule or by esterification of glycerol with three fatty acids. This is an energy-requiring process. Cholesterol is also reesterified within the epithelial cell. See page 92 for a further discussion of fat synthesis.

Chylomicrons. In order to penetrate the lipoprotein membrane of the epithelial cell for entrance to the lymph circulation, the newly formed fats are made soluble by surrounding them with a lipoprotein envelope consisting chiefly of phospholipids and a very small amount of protein. These particles are known as CHYLOMICRONS, having first been identified in chyle (lymph). They are of very low density and give the lymph a milky appearance. The chylomicrons enter the lymph circulation, which empties into the thoracic duct.

Enterohepatic Circulation. Bile salts are utilized over and over again through the cycle known as the *enterohepatic circulation.* This cycle consists of (1) the secretion of bile into the duodenum, (2) the complexing of bile with fat particles to form micelles, (3) the release of bile salts from the micelles at the brush border, (4) the reabsorption of bile salts by active transport from the ileum, (5) the entrance of the salts into the hepatic circulation, and (6) the secretion of bile once again into the duodenum. The total body pool of bile salts is estimated to be about 3 g, but this pool can be recirculated as much as 10 times in a day. This results in the effectiveness of 30 g bile salts per day. The liver normally synthesizes approximately 0.5 g bile salts per day, an amount that just about covers the excretion in the feces.

Completeness of Digestion and Absorption Normally about 95 percent of dietary fats and 10 to 50 percent of dietary cholesterol are absorbed.

A number of factors reduce the amount of fat that is digested and absorbed. Among these factors are (1) increased motility, so that food is moved along the tract too rapidly for complete enzyme action; (2) disease of the biliary tract so that the secretion of bile is deficient or does not reach the small intestine; (3) disease of the pancreas so that lipase is not secreted; and (4) reduction in the absorbing surfaces as in celiac disease or following surgery on the small intestine. When fat absorption is decreased, large amounts of fat are excreted in the feces (steatorrhea) with a consequent serious loss of calories, as well as impaired absorption of other fat-soluble substances. (See Chapter 31.)

Metabolism

The blood is the means of transportation of lipids from one site to another, and the liver and adipose tissues are the specialized organs that control lipid metabolism. The synthesis of new lipids (LIPOGENESIS) and the catabolism of lipids (LIPOLYSIS) are taking place continuously. These reactions are catalyzed by specific enzymes under the control of nervous and hormonal mechanisms. (See Figure 7-6.)

Blood Lipids The levels of cholesterol and of triglycerides in blood serum are frequently determined in the clinical laboratory and provide clues to the presence or absence of hyperlipidemia. In normal adults the serum cholesterol concentration ranges from 150 to 250 mg per dl. Many clinicians believe that a level below 225 mg and preferably at about 200 mg per dl reduces the risk of coronary disease.

The normal triglyceride level after a 12- to 14-hour fast is 140 mg per dl or less. Triglyceride levels vary widely during the day. They are increased when chylomicrons and very-low-density lipoproteins are being transported following a meal. The levels increase with lipolysis by adipose tissue as during weight loss. They decrease when fat is being synthesized by the adipose tissue or liver. The triglyceride levels increase gradually with age, but such an increase is not necessarily desirable.

Cholesterol and triglycerides do not exist in the free state in the circulation. Since fats are insoluble in water, proteins provide the mechanism for their transport in the aqueous medium of the blood. These protein–lipid complexes are known as lipoproteins. (See Table 7-2.) The chylomicrons are large particles consisting primarily of triglycerides. They are synthesized in the intestine and are the mechanism for transporting dietary lipids to adipose tissue and the liver. (See page 89.) Chylomicrons give a milky appearance to blood plasma shortly after a meal rich in fat. However, they are rapidly hydrolyzed by lipoprotein lipase, and the released triglycerides are taken up by the tissues. The blood plasma thus is "cleared."

Low-density or Beta-lipoproteins. Included in this group are the VERY-LOW-DENSITY LIPOPROTEINS (VLDL), a transient INTERMEDIATE-DENSITY LIPOPROTEIN (IDL), and LOW-DENSITY LIPOPROTEINS (LDL).

Figure 7-6. The liver and adipose tissue tissue are the principal organs of fat metabolism.

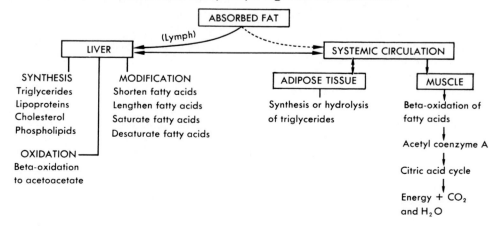

Table 7-2. Approximate Composition of Lipoproteins*

| | Protein (percent) | Lipids | | | |
		Triglycerides (percent)	Cholesterol (percent)	Phospholipids (percent)	Total (percent)
Chylomicrons	0.5–1.0	>85	2–5	3–6	99
Very-low-density lipoproteins (VLDL)	5–15	50–70	10–20	10–20	95
Low-density lipoproteins (LDL)	25	5–10	40–45	20–25	75
High-density lipoproteins (HDL)	45–55	2	18	30	50

* Adapted from Herera, G., and Nicolosi, R. J.: "A Clinician's Guide to Lipid Metabolism," in *Athero-sclerosis*, MEDCOM, Inc., New York, 1974, p. 27.

The bulk of VLDL is synthesized in the liver, although some synthesis occurs in the small intestine as well. VLDL are composed primarily of triglyceride, mostly of endogenous origin, which is transported to other tissues. Elevated VLDL are associated with carbohydrate-induced hyperlipidemia. (See Chapter 38.)

After removal of triglyceride from VLDL, the residues left are IDL; these lipoproteins are transported to the liver, where they are converted to LDL, the chief carriers of cholesterol in the blood. The concentration of LDL may be increased in persons consuming diets rich in saturated fatty acids, and to a lesser extent with diets containing substantial amounts of cholesterol. Elevated levels of LDL are considered a significant risk factor for cardiovascular disease.

High-density or Alpha-lipoproteins. Until recently little was known about the HIGH-DENSITY LIPOPROTEINS (HDL), except that they consist of about 50 percent protein and 20 percent cholesterol. This group has been found to have a protective effect; that is, increased HDL reduces the risk of coronary heart disease.

An important function of HDL is to transport cholesterol from peripheral tissues to the liver for excretion from the body. The effect of diet on HDL has not been clearly defined. Moderate alcohol consumption and moderate to strenuous exercise are associated with increased concentrations of HDL-cholesterol. Persons who are obese or sedentary, or who smoke cigarettes tend to have low plasma HDL.

Free Fatty Acids. The free fatty acids (FFA), also designated nonesterified fatty acids (NEFA), are the principal source of fatty acids made available to the cells for energy. They enter the circulation as the result of the hydrolysis of triglycerides, chiefly by adipose tissue. The fatty acids are attached rather tightly to plasma albumin and do not circulate in their free state. At the cell surfaces the fatty acid is released with ease from its carrier. The concentration of FFA in the blood at any given time is quite low, but the rate of turnover is so rapid that several thousand calories are transported daily in the circulation in this way. The concentration of free fatty acids is somewhat higher in the circulation during fasting, indicating more rapid release from adipose tissue. It is somewhat lower when carbohydrate is being absorbed, which indicates that carbohydrate is being used for energy as well as being synthesized to fat.

Adipose Tissue and Fat Metabolism The adipose cell is a specialized cell that provides for the synthesis, storage, and release of fats. It contains less water than is found in protoplasmic cells; as the cell size increases with the storage of fat the water content decreases. It is endowed with enzymes that bring about lipogenesis and lipolysis. Fat synthesis and breakdown take place continuously, but they are in equilibrium when the energy needs of the body are exactly met.

Several studies have shown that the number of adipose cells increases rapidly during infancy and childhood. The number usually remains constant during adult life, regardless of weight status, although some investigators have observed further hyperplasia. If the energy supplied to the body exceeds the body's needs, lipogenesis takes place and the cells enlarge (weight is gained) regardless of whether the calories were derived from fats, carbohydrates, or proteins. For the synthesis of fat, insulin is required.

When a calorie deficit exists, the adipose tissue will be catabolized more rapidly than it is being synthesized (weight is lost). The release of fatty acids from adipose tissue is accelerated by the same hormones that increase glucose breakdown: epinephrine, norepinephrine, glucagon, growth hormone, adrenocorticotropic hormone (ACTH), and thyrotropic hormone.

The Liver and Fat Metabolism   The liver is the key organ in the regulation of fat metabolism. It is able to accomplish the shortening or lengthening of the carbon chain of the fatty acids and to introduce double bonds into fatty acids. For example, a double bond can be introduced into stearic acid to yield oleic acid. On the other hand, a second double bond cannot be introduced into oleic acid to yield linoleic acid. With a dietary supply of linoleic acid, this essential fatty acid can be converted to arachidonic acid by adding a 2-carbon unit and by introducing two additional double bonds.

The liver hydrolyzes the triglycerides brought to it, re-forms new triglycerides, and again releases them to the circulation. It also synthesizes triglycerides from free fatty acids, glucose, or the carbon skeletons of amino acids. Phospholipids and lipoproteins are synthesized and released to the circulation or are removed from the circulation, thereby maintaining control over blood levels.

The liver is probably the chief regulator of the total body content of cholesterol and of the circulating blood cholesterol. It governs the endogenous synthesis of cholesterol, the removal of cholesterol from the circulation, the conversion of cholesterol to bile acids, and the excretion of cholesterol and bile acids by way of the bile into the intestine.

Certain LIPOTROPIC SUBSTANCES must be present to prevent the accumulation of fat in the liver. These substances include choline, vitamin B-12, betaine, and possibly inositol. Methionine, one of the essential amino acids, donates methyl groups for the synthesis of choline and is therefore a lipotropic substance.

Synthesis of Fats   Triglycerides are synthesized by the epithelial cells of the intestinal mucosa, by the adipose tissue, and by the liver. In order to synthesize triglycerides, a source of alpha-glycerophosphate is essential. This is furnished by the normal oxidation of glucose that occurs in each of these tissues through the glycolytic pathway (see page 71). A second source of alpha-glycerophosphate is available from the glycerol released from fat hydrolysis in the intestinal mucosa and in the liver. The glycerol so released combines with ATP in the presence of glycerokinase to form alpha-glycerophosphate. Adipose tissue does not contain glycerokinase and cannot convert glycerol to the active form.

The fatty acids for the triglyceride molecule are available from the hydrolysis of fats and also through synthesis from acetyl CoA derived through the oxidation of fats, glucose, and some amino acids.

The synthesis of fats from acetyl CoA is accomplished essentially by building up the carbon chain by successive additions of 2-carbon fragments. NADPH, a niacin-containing coenzyme, is required for this synthesis. It is made available through the pentose shunt of the glycolytic pathway. (See page 72.) The synthesis of fatty acids from acetyl CoA is thus seen to be dependent on normal carbohydrate metabolism and requires insulin. FFAs are not esterified directly with glycerophosphate but must first be converted to fatty acyl CoA. They are then attached in stepwise fashion to glycerophosphate to form the triglyceride.

Oxidation of Fatty Acids   All cells of the body except those of the central nervous system and red blood cells can oxidize fatty acids to yield energy. Although glucose is normally the only source of energy for the central nervous system, the brain cells after a period of total starvation can adapt to the utilization of ketone bodies derived from fat and amino acids.

The oxidation of fatty acids takes place in the cell mitochondria. BETA-OXIDATION is the major pathway for oxidation. By this process, oxidation occurs at the carbon that is beta from the carboxyl group. To prime the reaction, ATP is required. The oxidation is accomplished in five steps, the end result of which is a fatty acid that is two carbons shorter and also a molecule of acetyl CoA. Thus, the complete breakdown of an 18-carbon fatty acid requires 45 reactions.

$$CH_3(CH_2)_{16}COOH + CoA \longrightarrow$$
Stearic acid

$$CH_3(CH_2)_{14}COOCoA + CH_3COOCoA$$
Palmityl CoA   Acetyl CoA

Each molecule of acetyl CoA can (1) enter the TCA cycle for oxidation to energy, carbon dioxide, and water, or (2) be used for the synthesis of new fatty acids, cholesterol, and other compounds. (See Figure 6-4.)

The glycerol made available from the hydrolysis of fatty acids enters the glycolytic pathway by combining with ATP to form glycerophosphate. Thus, it is a potential source of glucose, glycogen, and energy or it may be the backbone for the new glyceride molecule.

Ketogenesis   Within the liver two molecules of acetyl CoA can condense to form acetoacetyl CoA, which in turn yields acetoacetic acid, beta-hydroxybutyric acid, and acetone. These compounds are known as KETONE BODIES and the process as KETOGENESIS. The ketone bodies are normally produced in small amounts by the liver. Although the liver cells do not possess the enzymes necessary for their further oxidation, muscle and other cells can utilize them to yield energy.

During rapid weight reduction using a starvation regimen or a low-calorie diet consisting of protein and fat but little or no carbohydrate, ketones are produced more rapidly than the tissues can use them. Carbohydrate metabolism is greatly reduced, while the production of acetyl CoA is sharply increased. The reduction in carbohydrate metabolism means that the amount of oxaloacetate available to combine with acetyl CoA in the TCA cycle is also reduced. The liver synthesizes vastly increased amounts of the ketones—far beyond the ability of the tissues to oxidize them. The principal effect of this increased production is a disturbance of the acid-base balance. Acetoacetic acid and beta-hydroxybutyric acid are fairly strong acids and combine with the available base. Their excretion in the urine (KETONURIA) is accompanied by loss of fluid and electrolytes. Acetone, being volatile, is excreted by the lungs. In normal persons small intakes of carbohydrate (approximately 50 g) are sufficient to reverse the ketosis.

In uncontrolled diabetes mellitus, ketosis occurs because of lack of insulin for the metabolism of carbohydrate. Ketosis is a serious complication that can lead to coma and even death; prompt measures are required to correct the acidosis and to restore normal carbohydrate metabolism.

Cholesterol Metabolism   The liver and intestine are the chief sites of cholesterol synthesis, but all cells are able to produce some cholesterol. The endogenous production of cholesterol has been variously estimated at 800 to 1,500 mg per day and is apparently independent of the dietary supply. Acetyl CoA is the direct precursor of cholesterol, and thus any donor of acetyl CoA—fatty acids, glucose, and some amino acids—is a potential source of cholesterol.

Cholesterol is transported in the blood in the various classes of lipoproteins. (See Table 7-2.) The body is unable to break down the cholesterol nucleus, but the liver converts it by enzyme action to bile acids. This is apparently rate limited[6] and therefore any excess supply poses problems of disposal. Cholesterol as such and bile acids are constituents of bile, and excretion occurs from the intestine.

Fat in the Diet

Dietary Allowance   People of the Orient consume diets that provide around 10 percent or less of the calories from fat, whereas Americans derive almost 40 percent of their calories from fat. These extremes of intake cannot be described categorically as being damaging to health or as affording promise of good health.

The Committee on Diet and Health of the Food and Nutrition Board has recommended that the total fat intake should not exceed 30 percent of the caloric intake. In addition less than 10 percent of the calories should be furnished by saturated fats.[10] By reducing the fat intake it becomes obvious that the carbohydrate intake would be increased to maintain caloric equilibrium.

The Dietary Goals for the United States[7] include the following recommendations:

Reduce overall fat consumption from approximately 40 percent to about 30 percent of energy intake.
Reduce saturated fat consumption to account for about 10 percent of total energy intake; and balance that with polyunsaturated and monounsaturated fats, which should account for about 10 percent of energy intake each.
Reduce cholesterol consumption to about 300 mg per day.

The Interim Dietary Guidelines to Prevent Cancer similarly recommend a reduction in fat intake to 30 percent of total calories.[8] The recommendation presented in the Dietary Guidelines is less specific: "Avoid too much fat, saturated fat, and cholesterol."[9]

Essential Fatty Acid Requirement.   Each diet must provide some linoleic acid. The signs of deficiency are prevented when 1 to 2 percent of dietary calories are provided by linoleic acid. For infants, a formula that supplies 3 percent of calories as linoleic acid is recommended. This level of linoleic acid is also satisfactory for persons who have a relatively low fat intake (less than 25 percent of calories). Most people in the United States consume diets in which the fat intake is 35 to 40 percent of calories and may benefit by a higher intake of linoleic acid.[10] Some persons at high risk for coronary disease often require a fat-controlled diet with fat restricted to 30 percent of calories or less. Of this fat intake, one fourth to one third, or 8 to 10 percent of total calories, should be supplied by polyunsaturated (essential) fatty acids.

Food Sources   In the United States the fat available for consumption in 1982 was 162 g.[11] The percentages contributed by each food group were as follows: fats and oils, including butter, 44.7; meat, poultry, and fish, 34.0; dairy products including butter, 11.7; legumes and nuts, 3.7; eggs, 2.6; flour and cereals, 1.3; fruits and vegetables, 0.8; and miscellaneous, 1.2.

The so-called "visible" fats include oils, lard, hydrogenated shortening, butter, margarine, fat back of pork, bacon, and salad dressings. A small amount of these concentrated sources of fat contributes importantly to the caloric level of the diet.

"Invisibile" fats include meat, poultry, fish, eggs, whole milk, cream, cheese, and baked products. Meats, poultry, and fish vary widely in fat content. The amount of fat ingested from meat will depend on the cut that was used, whether fat was carefully trimmed, whether fat drippings were used, and what the method of preparation was. Lean cuts of beef, pork, lamb, and veal differ little in their fat content. Fish is somewhat lower in fat than is meat. Fish that have a colored flesh are somewhat higher in fat than those with white flesh.

All the fat in the egg is in the yolk, about one third of this being in the form of phospholipid. Whole milk, cream, ice cream, and whole-milk cheeses furnish appreciable amounts of fat. Fruits, vegetables, legumes, cereals, and flours are low in fat. On the other hand, nuts contain an appreciable amount of fat.

Linoleic Acid.   Corn, cottonseed, safflower, and soy oils are good sources of linoleic acid. Some special margarines now available in food markets are processed by adding hydrogenated fat to oils, thereby retaining a greater proportion of linoleic acid. These margarines are much softer than regular margarines. In the labeling of such margarines the words *liquid oil* appear first, followed by a listing of hydrogenated oil as well as other ingredients. Fish and poultry furnish small amounts of linoleic acid.

Cholesterol.   Only animal foods furnish cholesterol. Liver, egg yolk, kidney, brains, sweetbreads, and fish roe are rich sources. Much smaller concentrations are found in whole milk, cream, butter, cheese, and meat. (See Table A-5.)

An individual who eats no eggs or organ meats probably ingests not more than 200 mg cholesterol daily; if, in addition, skim milk is used and vegetable margarine is substituted for butter, the intake will be further reduced to 100 to 150 mg per day. Each egg yolk adds about 250 mg cholesterol.

Fat Content of the Basic Diet   The contributions of the food groups to the fat content of the basic diet pattern are shown in Table 7-3. Note that the basic diet supplies approximately equal amounts of saturated and oleic acids, a proportion that is quite characteristic of American diets. The choice of additional foods to supply the needed energy requirements affords a wide range of possibilities for modifying the kind as

well as the amount of fat that is included. The two examples give important differences in the amounts of linoleic acid provided.

Dietary Fat and Health Issues

Fat in the U.S. Diet   Any consideration of the relationship of fat intake to health must begin with a review of the changing pattern of fat intake in the United States. The total fat content of the available food supply in the United States has increased from 125 g in 1909–13 to 163 g in 1982. (See Table 7-4.) During 1909–13 fat accounted for 32 percent of the total calories. The cholesterol content of the U.S. diet has varied only slightly since 1909–13 and in 1982 was 479 mg.[11]

The increase in total fat can be attributed to an increase in the amount of fat from vegetable sources, although animal sources still contribute the largest proportion. Greater use of salad and cooking oils in the home, by food processors, and by fast-food outlets has resulted in a rise in the linoleic acid content of the diet from 2 percent in 1909–13 to 7 percent of total calories in 1982.

It must be emphasized that data pertaining to available food supplies describe trends in consumption but do not indicate the actual amounts consumed. According to preliminary data from the 1977 Household Food Consumption Survey, the average fat intake for all age groups had declined since 1965—by as much as 20 percent for half the age–sex groups.[12] Even so, fat continued to account for two fifths or more of the total energy intake.

Fat and Nutritive Quality of the Diet   Although meat, poultry, fish, eggs, and dairy products furnish significant amounts of fat to the diet, these foods also supply many nutrients. On the other hand, visible fats and oils that contribute about 18 percent of the total available calories in the American food supply are of rather limited nutritive value. Butter and margarine provide about 9 percent of the vitamin A value of the food supply. Vegetable oils supply most of the linoleic acid and substantial amounts of vitamin E. The other nutrient contributions made by fats and oils are negligible. It was noted in Chapter 6 that sweets and sugars also make low nutrient contributions. Consequently, as the intake of fats and oils and sugars and sweets increases, the likelihood of meeting recommended allowances for nutrients decreases if the caloric intake is in balance with requirements.

Table 7-3. Fat Content of the Basic Diet*

| | | Total Fat (g) | Fatty Acids | | | Cholesterol (mg) |
			Saturated (g)	Oleic (g)	Linoleic (g)	
Basic Diet						
Vegetable–fruit group	4 servings	trace	trace	trace	trace	0
Bread–cereal group	4 servings	4	0.5	1.3	1.0	0
Milk, 2 percent	2 cups	10	5.8	2.4	0.2	44
Meat group	5 ounces	18	5.2	6.6	2.5	292
Total		32	11.5	10.3	3.7	336
Typical additions of fat to Basic Diet						
Margarine, soft	1 tablespoon	12	2.0	4.5	4.1	0
French dressing	1 tablespoon	6	1.1	1.3	3.2	0
Chocolate pudding	½ cup	6	3.8	1.7	0.2	30
Corn oil in cooked foods	1 tablespoon	14	1.7	3.3	7.8	0
Total additions		38	8.6	10.8	15.3	30
Totals (Basic Diet and additions)		70	20.1	21.1	19.0	366
Alternative additions of fat to Basic Diet						
Butter for table and cooking	2 tablespoons	24	14.4	5.8	0.6	70
Mayonnaise	1 tablespoon	11	2.0	2.4	5.6	10
Ice cream	½ cup	7	4.5	1.8	0.2	27
Total alternative additions		42	20.9	10.0	6.4	107
Totals (Basic Diet and alternative additions)		74	32.4	20.3	10.1	443

* See Table 4–1 for details of calculations.

Obesity This widely prevalent form of malnutrition results from a calorie intake that exceeds requirements, regardless of the source of the calories. Because fat contains more than twice as many calories per gram as carbohydrate and protein, it is easy to exceed one's caloric intake by consuming foods rich in fat. Moreover, many of the fats that add so much to palatability come in concentrated forms, so that their addition does not appreciably affect dietary bulk. A few examples of day-to-day uses of fat illustrate how easy it is to increase caloric intake.

	kcal
Baked potato, medium	145
Butter, 1 tablespoon	100
Lettuce and tomato salad	25
Mayonnaise, 2 teaspoons	65
Fresh peach, medium	40
Ice cream, ½ cup	135
Bread, whole wheat, 1 slice	65
Margarine, 2 teaspoons	65
Milk, skim, 1 cup	85
Milk, 2 percent, 1 cup	120
Milk, whole, 1 cup	150
Half milk, half cream, 1 cup	315

The Diet-Heart Disease Controversy Because cardiovascular diseases account for more than half of the deaths in the United States and also affect millions of others, it is not surprising that any factor that appears to reduce the risks will be widely acclaimed by the public.

Since 1960 the age-adjusted mortality rate from heart disease has declined about 20 percent.[13] How can this decline be explained: better medical supervision? more control of hypertension? reduced intake of saturated fat? increased intake of polyunsaturated fat? reduced intake of cholesterol? less cigarette smoking? weight reduction? more exercise? less stressful lifestyle? The answers are not known, but it is likely that a number of these factors rather than a single factor may have contributed.[14,15]

The diet–heart disease controversy has existed for about a quarter of a century and is destined to continue for many more years. Prominent nutrition scientists and clinicians have examined the evidence for and against the diet–heart disease hypothesis.[16-19]

Atherosclerosis is a disease process that begins early in life with the formation of cholesterol-containing plaques on the inner walls of the arteries. Smooth muscle fibers and connective tissue infiltrate these plaques. Gradually the lumen through which the

Table 7-4.   Fat in the U.S. Diet from Animal and Vegetable Sources (per-capita daily)*

Period	Meat Poultry, Fish (g)	Eggs (g)	Dairy Products Excluding Butter (g)	Butter Lard, Edible Beef Fat (g)	Total (g)	Other Fats and Oils (g)	Other Plant Foods (g)	Total (g)	All Fats (g)
	Animal Sources					**Plant Sources**			
1909–13	46.4	4.8	18.6	33.8	103.6	12.3	9.0	21.3	125
1947–49	46.8	6.0	24.5	27.4	104.7	25.1	10.6	35.7	140
1967–69	58.6	5.0	19.3	19.2	102.1	43.8	11.2	55.0	157
1981	58.4	4.2	18.6	13.3	94.5	57.1	11.4	68.5	163

* Adapted from Marston, R., and Page, L.: "Nutrient Content of the National Food Supply," *National Food Review*, U.S. Department of Agriculture, December 1978, p. 30, and Marston, R. M., and Welsh, S. O.: "Nutrient Content of the National Food Supply, 1981," *National Food Review*, U.S. Department of Agriculture, Winter 1983, p. 17.

blood flows is narrowed, and the heart must work harder to pump the blood through the arteries. When the condition is severe, the lumen may close, depriving a given tissue of its blood supply (ischemia). If the heart vessels are affected, the individual has a heart attack (myocardial infarction); if any of the vessels of the brain are affected, the person has a stroke or cerebrovascular accident.

All children and young adults have fatty streaks in the walls of the aorta. Under some circumstances not yet fully understood, these fatty streaks progress to form the disease lesions. Many studies have shown that persons with a serum cholesterol level above 225 mg per dl are at increased risk for coronary heart disease. As the hypercholesterolemia increases, so does the probability of a coronary event. Therefore, it is hypothesized that measures to reduce the serum cholesterol levels will also reduce risk. A number of measures will bring about lowering of the serum cholesterol: loss of weight by the obese, increased activity, reduced intake of total fat and of saturated fat, and increased intake of polyunsaturated fat. Dietary cholesterol, in the usual range of intake, appears to have a minimal effect on serum cholesterol levels.[20]

Dietary factors may be important in atherosclerotic cardiovascular disease because of effects other than alteration of blood cholesterol levels. Diets containing large amounts of marine oils decrease clotting and platelet aggregation and may explain the low prevalence of coronary heart disease in Greenland Eskimos. The major factor in the oil contributing to these effects is believed to be eicosapentaenoic acid, a 20-carbon fatty acid having five double bonds, with the first double bond at the third carbon.[21,22]

Dietary modification has been widely used for patients who have been identified as being at high risk or who have had a heart attack. The results have not always been as successful as anticipated. But one may argue that dietary adjustments, if they are to be effective, must begin early in life—not after pathologic changes have occurred.

The Diet-Cancer Hypothesis   The role of fat in the incidence of cancer is even less understood than its role in heart disease. Epidemiologic studies in different countries have demonstrated a strong association between the incidence of colon cancer and the per-capita consumption of total fat, saturated fat, and cholesterol. In animals dietary fat increases the incidence of chemically induced colon cancer. Several mechanisms have been proposed to explain this effect, including increased bile acid excretion and alterations in intestinal bacteria. Some evidence suggests that increased bile acids act to promote rather than initiate tumor formation. It has also been proposed that intestinal bacteria may convert bile acids to potential carcinogens.[23] No proof has been found to support or dispute the role of dietary fat in colon cancer.

A high incidence of breast and uterine cancer has also been associated with a high-fat diet and with obesity. Various mechanisms have been proposed, including changes in estrogen and prolactin synthesis or bacteria-induced changes in reabsorption and metabolism of estrogens in the gut. Although the hypothesis that dietary fat may influence breast cancer is reasonable, again there is no proof that it plays a major role in the etiology of cancer in humans.[24]

Toward Moderation in Diet Although it is important to avoid making exaggerated claims about the preventive aspects of diet, there is sufficient evidence to justify modifying the diet to provide not more than 35 percent of calories from fat. Such an adjustment can reduce the likelihood of excessive caloric ingestion, may improve the nutritional quality of the diet, and may be helpful as a preventive measure. There is no evidence that such a reduction in fat intake is harmful. The diet is palatable, affordable, and available from the American food supply. The following changes in food selection are designed to keep fat intake within 35 percent of calories and to reduce intake of saturated fat:

1. Select lean cuts of meat. Use poultry and fish more often instead of meat. Limit intake to 5 ounces per day. Trim off visible fat. Cook by broiling, roasting, or stewing rather than frying. Do not use fat drippings.
2. Use low-fat milk (2 percent, 1 percent, or skim) instead of whole milk. Use less cream, sour cream, ice cream and full-fat cheese.
3. Reduce the intake of visible fats. Substitute soft margarines for regular margarines and butter. Use oils for cooking instead of lard or solid shortenings.

SOME POINTS FOR EMPHASIS IN NUTRITION EDUCATION

1. Fats are essential constituents of all body cells and the principal source of energy stores within the body.
2. Fats are the most concentrated source of energy in the diet and furnish more than twice as many calories, gram for gram, as do carbohydrates and proteins. Consequently, a small volume of fatty food will increase the calorie intake considerably, and excessive intakes of fats and oils can rapidly contribute to obesity.
3. Linoleic acid is an essential fatty acid abundantly supplied by corn, cottonseed, soy, and safflower oils.
4. Lecithin and other phospholipids are essential constituents of nervous tissue and important for the transport of fats. The liver readily synthesizes the phospholipids so that their presence in the diet is not essential. An additional intake of lecithin does not convey unique benefits to health and is not necessary.
5. Cholesterol is an essential constituent of body tissues and is required for the regulation of important body functions. The liver synthesizes cholesterol so that body needs are not dependent on the dietary cholesterol. Daily intakes of 300 to 500 mg cholesterol do not appear to affect serum cholesterol levels adversely.
6. A diet that furnishes 30 to 35 percent of the calories as fat, and that is also designed to maintain normal weight contributes to maintaining a serum cholesterol level within desirable limits.

Problems and Review

1. *Key terms:* arachidonic acid; beta-oxidation; cholesterol; chylomicrons; enterohepatic circulation; high-density lipoprotein; ketones; ketogenesis; lecithin; linoleic acid; lipogenesis; lipolysis; low-density lipoproteins; micelles; peroxidation; phospholipid; polyunsaturated fatty acids; prostaglandins; triglyceride.
2. Prepare an outline showing the digestion, absorption, and metabolic fate of triglycerides supplied by the diet.
3. Give several reasons why fat is a useful constituent of the diet.
4. What is a hydrogenated fat? Give several examples. How does it compare in nutritional value with the fat from which it was made?
5. What effect will the inclusion of fatty foods such as fried potatoes and pork chops have on the digestion of the meal as a whole?
6. *Problem.* Compare the fat and calorie values of ½ cup ice cream; 1 tablespoon mayonnaise; 1 ounce cream cheese; 2 teaspoons butter; 1 cup milk.
7. *Problem.* Calculate your own fat intake for 1 day. Which of the foods you ate are good sources of linoleic acid? What percentage of the total calories in your diet was derived from fat?
8. A margarine may be manufactured from 100 percent vegetable oil but may still be a poor source of linoleic acid. Explain why this might be true.
9. *Problem.* Examine the labels of three or four brands of special types of margarine. What information do they give you about their value as sources of linoleic acid? How do these margarines compare with regular margarines in cost?
10. A patient tells you that he has not been eating butter, eggs, or whole milk because he read in a magazine that cholesterol causes heart disease. How would you respond to this?

References

1. Emken, E. A.: "Nutrition and Biochemistry of Trans and Positional Fatty Acid Isomers in Hydrogenated Oils," *Annu. Rev. Nutr.*, 4:339–76, 1984.
2. Himms-Hagen, J.: "Brown Adipose Tissue Thermogenesis in Obese Animals," *Nutr. Rev.*, 41:261–67, 1983.

3. Hansen, A. F.: "Essential Fatty Acids in Infant Feeding," *J. Am. Diet. Assoc.*, **34**:239–41, 1958.
4. Fleming, C. R., et al.: "Essential Fatty Acid Deficiency in Adults Receiving Total Parenteral Nutrition," *Am. J. Clin. Nutr.*, **29**:976–83, 1976.
5. Hamosh, M.: "A Review. Fat Digestion in the Newborn: Role of Lingual Lipase and Preduodenal Digestion," *Pediatr. Res.*, **13**:615–22, 1979.
6. Grundy, S. M.: "Absorption and Metabolism of Dietary Cholesterol," *Annu. Rev. Nutr.*, **3**:71–96, 1983.
7. U.S. Senate Select Committee on Nutrition and Human Needs: *Dietary Goals for the United States*, rev. ed. Government Printing Office, Washington, D.C., 1977.
8. Committee on Diet, Nutrition and Cancer: *Diet, Nutrition and Cancer*. National Research Council–National Academy of Sciences, Washington, D.C., 1982.
9. *Nutrition and Your Health: Dietary Guidelines for Americans*. U.S. Department of Agriculture and U.S. Department of Health, Education and Welfare, Washington, D.C., 1985.
10. Food and Nutrition Board: *Recommended Dietary Allowances*, 10th ed. National Research Council–National Academy of Sciences, Washington, D.C., 1989.
11. Marston, R. M., and Welsh, S. O.: "Nutrient Content of the U.S. Food Supply, 1982," *National Food Review*, U.S. Department of Agriculture, Winter 1984, pp. 7–13.
12. Pao, E. M.: "Nutrient Consumption Patterns of Individuals, 1977 and 1964," *Family Economics Review*. U.S. Department of Agriculture, Spring 1980, pp. 16–20.
13. Feinleib, M.: "The Magnitude and Nature of the Decreases in Coronary Heart Disease Mortality Rate," *Am. J. Cardiol.*, **54**:2C–6C, 1984.

14. Levy, R. I.: "Causes of the Decrease in Cardiovascular Mortality," *Am. J. Cardiol.*, **54**:7C–13C, 1984.
15. Brown, W. V., et al.: "Diet and the Decrease of Coronary Heart Disease," *Am. J. Cardiol.*, **54**:27C–29C, 1984.
16. Harper, A. E.: "Coronary Heart Disease—An Epidemic Related to Diet?," *Am. J. Clin. Nutr.*, **37**:669–81, 1983.
17. Reiser, R.: "A Commentary on the Rationale of the Diet–Heart Statement of the American Heart Association," *Am. J. Clin. Nutr.*, **40**:654–58, 1984.
18. Grundy, S. M., et al.: "Rationale of the Diet Heart Statement of the American Heart Association," *Circulation*, **65**:839A–54A, 1982. (See also *Nutr. Today*, **17**(5):16–20, **17**(6):15–19, 1982.)
19. Levy, R. I., et al.: "The Influences of Changes in Lipid Values Induced by Cholestyramine and Diet on Progression of Coronary Artery Disease: Results of NHLBI Type II Coronary Intervention Study," *Circulation*, **69**:325–37, 1984.
20. Keys, A.: "Serum Cholesterol Response to Dietary Cholesterol," *Am. J. Clin. Nutr.*, **40**:351–59, 1984.
21. Harris, W. S., et al.: "Dietary Fish Oils, Plasma Lipids and Platelets in Man," *Prog. Lipid Res.*, **20**:75–79, 1981.
22. Willis, A. L.: "Nutritional and Pharmacological Factors in Eicosanoid Biology," *Nutr. Rev.*, **39**:289–301, 1981.
23. Willett, W. C., and MacMahon, B.: "Diet and Cancer—An Overview," *N. Engl. J. Med.*, **310**:697–701, 1984.
24. Pariza, M. W.: "A Perspective on Diet, Nutrition, and Cancer," *JAMA*, **251**:1455–58, 1984.

8
Energy Metabolism

Conservation of energy resources and development of new sources of energy has become a crucial issue in our times. Although the primary focus of concern has been on the availability of resources such as oil, gas, coal, and electrical and atomic power, availability of sufficient food to meet the energy needs of the world's growing population is an equally critical issue. On a worldwide basis, the major nutritional deficiency is not a lack of any specific nutrient—it is a lack of sufficient food. When a reduction in available food leads to a moderate deficiency in energy intake, the capacity to work is reduced, and in children growth is retarded and ceases. As the energy available to the body continues to decrease, the body's own substance will be utilized until eventually no more of the body mass can be sacrificed. In marked contrast to the undernutrition in many parts of the world, the major nutritional problem in the United States is obesity arising as the consequence of excess energy intake in relationship to energy expenditure.

Energy Transformation

Energy is the capacity to do work. The sun is the original source of all energy, arising from nuclear reactions. Through the action of chlorophyll with sunlight, by the process known as photosynthesis, plants synthesize carbohydrates from carbon dioxide and water. The carbohydrates stored by the plants are then available as energy to animals and to humans. All of an individual's energy is derived from the plant and animal food she or he eats. Carbohydrates, fats, and proteins are the energy-yielding substances. In a typical American diet carbohydrate furnishes 45 to 55 percent of the calories, fats, 35 to 45 percent, and proteins about 15 percent.

Forms of Energy Potential (storage) energy is continuously available in the body from the small amounts of glycogen in muscle and liver, the sizable fat depots, and the cellular mass itself. This potential energy is transformed to other forms to accomplish the work of the body: for example, *mechanical* energy for muscle contraction; *osmotic* energy to maintain the transport of fluids and nutrients; *electrical* energy for the transmission of nerve impulses; *chemical* energy as in the synthesis of new compounds; and *thermal* energy for heat regulation.

Whenever one form of energy is produced, another form is reduced by exactly the same amount. This is known as the law of CONSERVATION OF ENERGY, which states that energy can be neither created nor destroyed. When foods supply more energy than is needed for the work of the body, the excess is stored as fat; the result is weight gain. This store of energy is available at such a time as the food supply might furnish too few calories for the body's activities.

ATP, the Currency for Energy ATP is used for all the work of the body: the synthesis of all cellular materials, the secretion of hormones and enzymes, the transport of nutrients and wastes in the circulation and across cell membranes, the contraction of muscles, and so on.

The formation of ATP occurs in the metabolic pathways described in the preceding chapters on carbohydrates, fats, and proteins. Initially these nutrients are oxidized independently to the "common denominators," namely, pyruvic acid, acetyl coenzyme A (CoA), and alpha-ketoglutaric acid. In this first phase some of the reactions require ATP for their initiation; other reactions release small amounts of energy so that ATP is regenerated from ADP, but the net yield is not great.

The common denominators enter the tricarboxylic acid (TCA) cycle, which is the common pathway for the oxidation of glucose, fatty acids, and amino acids. About 90 percent of the energy liberated from food occurs by this pathway. (See page 70 and Figure 6-4.) Oxidative phosphorylation is the mechanism whereby the hydrogens yielded by the TCA cycle are passed along the respiratory chain and energy is trapped as ATP. (See page 72 and Figure 6-5.)

Measurement: Units, Calorimetry, and Fuel Factors

Kilocalories The potential energy value of foods and the energy exchange of the body are expressed in terms of the calorie, which is a heat unit. By definition, a KILOCALORIE (kcal) is the amount of heat required to raise the temperature of 1 kg water 1°C (from 15 to 16°C). In the nutrition literature the kilocalorie is intended whether it is expressed as calorie, Calorie, or kilocalorie. The unit is 1,000 times as large as the small calorie used in the sciences of chemistry and physics.

Joules The joule (J) is the unit of energy used in the metric system. By definition, 1 J is the amount of energy expended when 1 kg is moved a distance of 1 m by a force of 1 newton; it is equal to 10^7 ergs. It is energy expressed in mechanical equivalents, not heat equivalents.

The eighth International Congress of Nutrition in Prague in 1969 and the Committee on Nomenclature of the American Institute of Nutrition in 1970 recommended the adoption of the joule in place of the calorie as the unit of energy. The conversion of energy values in food composition tables to joules will require some time. Students and practitioners in nutrition, however, must begin to think in terms of joules. To facilitate this, the joule equivalents in this chapter have been placed in parentheses whenever caloric values are given.

The following factors apply for the interconversion of calories and joules:

1 calorie (the unit used in physics) = 4.184 J
1 kcal = 4.184 kilojoules (kJ)
1,000 kcal = 4.184 megajoules (MJ)
1 kJ = 0.240 kcal
1 MJ = 240 kcal

Thus, a dietary allowance of 2,000 kcal is 8368 kJ, or 8.368 MJ. For approximate calculations the factor 4.2 may be used instead of 4.184.

Bomb Calorimeter The fuel values of foods are readily determined by means of an instrument known as a BOMB CALORIMETER. (See Figure 8-1.) A weighed sample of dried food is placed in a heavy steel container called a "bomb." The bomb is held in place in a well-insulated vessel and is surrounded by a known volume of water. After the bomb is filled with oxygen, the sample is ignited and the heat is dissipated into the water. By noting the change in the temperature of the water, one can calculate the energy value of the food

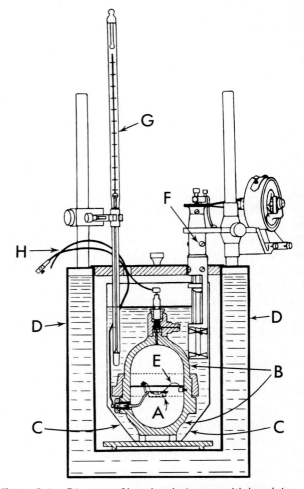

Figure 8-1. Diagram of bomb calorimeter with bomb in position. (Courtesy, the Emerson Apparatus Company.) *(A)* Platinum dish holding weighed food sample. *(B)* Bomb filled with pure oxygen enclosing food sample. *(C)* Can holding water of known weight in which the bomb is submerged. *(D)* Outer double-walled insulating jacket. *(E)* Fuse, which is ignited by an electric current. *(F)* Motor-driven water stirrer. *(G)* Thermometer calibrated to 1/1000°C. *(H)* Electric wires to send current through fuse.

by applying the definition for a calorie. The HEAT OF COMBUSTION for the energy-yielding nutrients is shown in the first column of Table 8-1.

Physiologic Fuel Factors Certain small losses occur in digestion so that it is necessary to reduce the values obtained in the bomb calorimeter to those that are physiologically available. For the typical American diet the coefficient of digestibility is 98 percent for carbohydrate, 95 percent for fat, and 92 percent for protein. In addition, the end products of protein metabolism such as urea and other nitrogenous prod-

Table 8-1. **Conversion of Bomb Calorimeter Values to Physiologic Values**

	Heat of Combustion (kcal)	Digestibility (percent)	Absorbed Energy Value (kcal/g)	Urinary Loss (kcal/g)	Physiologic Fuel Value (kcal)	Physiologic Fuel Value (kJ)
Carbohydrate	4.1	98	4.02		4.0	17
Fat	9.45	95	8.98		9.0	38
Protein	5.65	92	5.20	1.25	4.0	17
Alcohol	7.1	100	7.1 (5.6/ml)	0.1 (lungs)	7.0	29

ucts are combustible; their loss in the urine is equivalent to about 1.25 kcal per g protein. By applying these corrections, as shown in Table 8-1, the PHYSIOLOGIC FUEL FACTORS, first derived by Atwater are carbohydrate and protein, per gram, 4 kcal (17 kJ); fat, per gram, 9 kcal (38kJ); and alcohol, per gram, 7 kcal (29 kJ).

Specific Fuel Factors Each food has a specific coefficient of digestibility, and thus the fuel value likewise would be specific for each given food. For example, the coefficient of digestibility for the protein in milk, eggs, and meat is 97 percent, but for the protein of whole ground cornmeal it is only 60 percent; the coefficient of digestibility for the carbohydrate of wheat is 98 percent when white flour (70 to 74 percent extraction) is used, but is 90 percent when whole-wheat flour (97 to 100 percent extraction) is used. Specific fuel factors, rather than the average fuel factors, have been used for the caloric values stated in tables of food composition. Thus, students may find that their calculations using the physiologic fuel factors do not always agree exactly with caloric values given in the food tables. The error introduced by using the average values is small for typical mixed diets used in the United States.

Measurement of Energy Exchange of the Body

Direct and Indirect Calorimetry DIRECT CALORIMETRY is the measurement of the amount of heat produced by the body. By this method the individual is placed in a specially constructed chamber called a respiration calorimeter. The chamber is so well insulated that no heat can enter into or escape through the walls. The heat given off by the individual is picked up by water flowing through coils in the chamber. Measurements are made of the temperature of the water at the beginning of the study, at intervals, and at

the termination of the study. The volume of water flowing through the coils is also measured, and the calories expended can be calculated from these data. These calorimeters are very expensive to construct and require careful attention to many details of measurement. They are used only at a few research centers.[1]

The respiration calorimeter is so designed that the oxygen consumption and the carbon dioxide excretion can be measured at the same time as the heat production. The volume of oxygen consumed and the carbon dioxide expelled permit the calculation of the RESPIRATORY QUOTIENT (RQ) as follows:

$$RQ = \frac{CO_2}{O_2}$$

The RQ varies with the type of food being oxidized. For example, for pure glucose

$$C_6H_{12}O_6 + 6\,O_2 = 6\,CO_2 + 6\,H_2O$$
$$RQ = \frac{6\,CO_2}{6\,O_2} = 1.0$$

For a fatty acid such as palmitic acid

$$CH_3(CH_2)_{14}COOH + 23\,O_2 = 16\,CO_2 + 16\,H_2O$$
$$RQ = \frac{16\,CO_2}{23\,O_2} = 0.7$$

Proteins give an average RQ of 0.8. For an ordinary diet composed of mixed foodstuffs the RQ is approximately 0.85.

Numerous studies using the respiration calorimeter have established that each RQ has a caloric equivalent that can be used to determine the energy expenditure under given conditions. Thus, it becomes possible to determine the level of energy metabolism by the less time-consuming and far less costly procedures of indirect calorimetery.

INDIRECT CALORIMETRY measures the amount of oxygen consumed in a given time period and, in other than basal conditions, the amount of carbon dioxide excreted. Numerous experiments on people of all ages have shown that 1 liter of oxygen is equal to 4.825 kcal when the conditions for a basal metabolism test, described later, are met.

The energy expenditure at varying levels of activity can be measured by a respirometer under controlled conditions when the subject walks on a treadmill or rides on a stationary bicycle. (See Figure 8-2.) In other situations such as mountain climbing, or typing, or ironing, a portable apparatus is used. This light-weight piece of equipment consists of a meter for measuring the volume of expired air and a bag for collecting the sample of expired air. The air samples are analyzed for their amounts of oxygen and carbon dioxide, and from the data it is possible to determine caloric equivalents.

Basal Metabolism Test   The amount of energy required to carry on the involuntary work of the body is known as the *basal metabolic rate*. It includes the functional activities of the various organs such as the brain, heart, liver, kidneys, and lungs, the secretory activities of the glands, the peristaltic movements of the gastrointestinal tract, the oxidations occurring in resting tissues, and the maintenance of muscle tone and body temperature. The brain and nervous tissue account for about one fifth of the energy utilized in the basal state, and the liver, kidneys, lungs, and heart for an additional three fifths.

The basal metabolic rate is measured by indirect calorimetry under the following specific conditions.

1. Postabsorptive state: 12 to 16 hours after the last meal; usually performed in the morning.
2. Reclining, but awake: ½ to 1 hour of rest before the test is necessary if there has been any activity in the morning.
3. Relaxed and free from emotional upsets or fear of the test itself.
4. Normal body temperature.
5. Comfortable room temperature and humidity: about 21° to 24°C.

Under these conditions, normal individuals fall within ± 15 percent of standards established for their body size, sex, and age. Suppose a young woman consumes 1,200 ml oxygen in a 6-minute test period; in a 24-hour period her basal heat expenditure is calculated as follows:

$$\frac{10 \times 1,200 \times 24}{1,000} = \frac{288 \text{ liters oxygen}}{\text{in 24 hours}}$$

$$288 \times 4.825 \text{ kcal} = 1,390 \text{ kcal}$$

Factors Influencing the Basal Metabolic Rate   The adult basal metabolic rate is approximately 1 kcal (4.2 kJ) per kg per hour for men and about 0.9 kcal (3.8 kJ) per kg per hour for women. Thus, the range of basal metabolism for normal adults is about 1,300 to 1,700 kcal (5,439 to 7,113 kJ). This accounts for the largest proportion of the total energy requirement for most people. The rate of basal metabolism is influenced by size, shape, and weight of the individual, sex, age, rate of growth, the activity of the endocrine glands, sleep, body temperaure, and state of nutrition.

Surface Area.   About 80 percent of the energy from glucose and fat is lost as heat, all but 15 percent of heat loss being from the skin. The remaining heat loss occurs from the lungs and through the excreta. Since the heat loss is proportional to the skin surface, the basal heat production is directly proportional to the surface area. A tall, thin person has a greater surface area than an individual of the same weight who is short and fat, and the former therefore will have a higher basal metabolism.

In clinical practice the energy expenditure is expressed as kilocalories per square meter of body surface per hour. For convenience, charts have been developed by which surface area can be determined for any given height and weight.

The metabolic rate also has a linear relationship to metabolic body size, which is expressed as body weight to the three fourths power ($W^{0.75}$). For research purposes this is the preferred relationship. For practical purposes the calculations using surface area and those using metabolic size are comparable.

Sex.   Women have a metabolic rate about 6 to 10 percent lower than that of men. Formerly this was attributed to the fact that women have relatively higher proportions of adipose tissue, believed to be metabolically inert. However, this explanation is not fully satisfactory inasmuch as adipose tissue is now known to be metabolically active. The influence of the sex hormones may account for some of the difference.

Age.   Per unit of surface area the basal metabolic rate is at its highest during the first 2 years of life. It declines gradually throughout childhood and accelerates slightly in adolescence. Thereafter the decline continues throughout life and averages about 2 percent per decade after age 21. The rapid growth rate explains the high metabolic rate in early childhood. In the later years the lessened muscle tone and the reduction in muscle mass account for the lower rate.

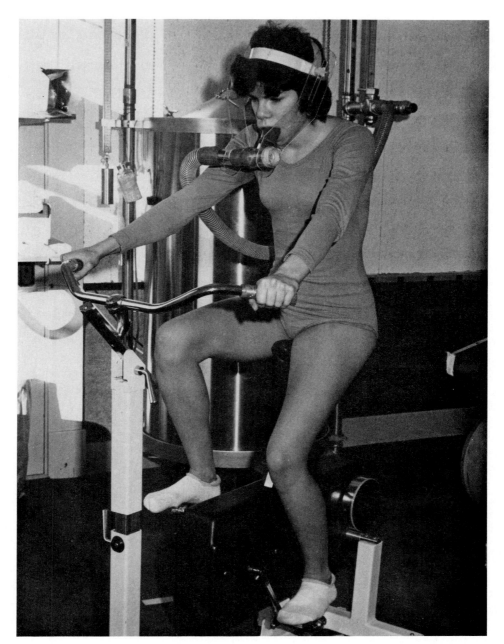

Figure 8-2. This student's energy expenditure while bicycling is being measured by using a respirometer under controlled conditions. (Courtesy, Department of Nutrition and Food Sciences, Texas Woman's University, Denton.)

Sleep. During the sleeping hours the basal metabolism is about 10 percent lower than in the waking state. However, this is quite variable depending on the amount of motion of the individual while asleep.

Body Temperature. An elevation of the body temperature above 37°C (98.6°F) increases the basal metabolism by 13 percent for each degree Celsius (7 percent for each degree Fahrenheit).

Endocrine Glands. The thyroid gland regulates the rate of energy metabolism, and any change in thyroid activity is reflected in the metabolic rate. If the thyroid is overactive (HYPERTHYROIDISM), the metabolism may be speeded up as much as 75 to 100 percent; if the activity of the gland is decreased (HYPOTHYROIDISM), the metabolism may be reduced by 30 to 40 percent.

Determination of the plasma concentration of thyroid hormones has now largely replaced the basal metabolism test as a measure of thyroid activity. (See page 128.) However, the basal metabolism test still may be used in research to evaluate energy expenditure in specific conditions, such as pregnancy or various disease states.

The growth hormones that stimulate new tissue formation are responsible in part for the higher metabolism that is observed in infants, children, and teenagers. Other endocrine secretions have a more transitory effect on the basal metabolism. An increased excretion of epinephrine during excitement or fear temporarily raises the metabolic rate. Disturbances of the pituitary gland may also modify the metabolic rate. At menstruation the basal metabolic rate decreases and falls to its lowest point approximately 1 week before ovulation, subsequently rising until the beginning of the next menstrual period.[2] These slight changes are of no overall significance in determining the energy requirement.

Pregnancy. During the last trimester of pregnancy the basal metabolism increases from 15 to 25 percent. This increase can be accounted for almost entirely by the increase in weight of the woman and the high rate of metabolism of the fetus.

State of Nutrition. Prolonged fasting or chronic undernutrition leads to a reduction in the basal metabolic rate. In some cases the decrease is proportional to the decrease in body weight, but in others the reduction is greater than can be explained on the basis of the loss of lean body mass. Although the mechanisms involved are not understood, the change is important in adaptation because it decreases the amount of nutrient stores that must be catabolized each day.

Physical Activity. During the night following a day of strenuous muscular work, the metabolic rate may be higher than after an inactive day. Although the trained athlete may have a slightly higher basal metabolic rate than that of a nonathlete, the difference is negligible and appears to be related to increased lean body mass.

Resting Metabolism The term RESTING METABOLISM should be differentiated from basal metabolism. It applies to energy expenditure under normal life conditions while at rest. In addition to the energy expenditure that occurs during a day in which there is no exercise and no exposure to cold, resting metabolism includes the calorigenic effect of foods (see page 105) and takes into account the decrease in metabolism that occurs during sleep.

Factors Influencing the Total Energy Requirement

Superimposed upon the energy expenditure for maintaining the involuntary activities of the body are such factors as voluntary muscular activity, the effect of food, and the maintenance of the body temperature.

Muscular Activity Next to the basal energy requirement, physical activity accounts for the largest energy expenditure; in fact, for some persons who are vigorously active, the energy needs for activity may exceed those for the basal metabolism. Sedentary work, which includes office work, bookkeeping, typing, teaching, and so forth, calls for less energy than more active and strenuous occupations such as nursing, homemaking, or gardening. A still greater amount of energy is required by those individuals who do hard manual labor such as ditch digging, shifting freight, and lumbering.

The energy expenditure for many activities has been measured in adults and children,[3] and the data serve as a guide in setting standards for various groups of people. A wide range of activities has been classified in five groups in Table 8-2. The calorie expenditures listed for each category include the basal metabolism and are representative for adults of average body size. The lower figure for each category would apply to women, and the higher figure to men. It must be realized that these vary from one individual to another not only on the basis of body size but especially because of variations of intensity of effort expended.

The figures in Table 8-2 illustrate the value of exercise in weight control, for it is quite evident that the student who sits quietly watching television, for example, is expending only half as many calories as one who is walking leisurely, and only one fourth as many calories as one who swims for an hour.

Not infrequently the question is raised as to the reason for the differing caloric needs of two people of the same build and body weight who are doing the same kind of work. The energy needs will be greater for the person who wastes many motions in the performance of a piece of work, who works under greater muscle tension, or who finds it difficult to relax completely even when at rest.

Mental Effort The nervous system is continuously active, and its energy requirement is about 20 percent of the basal rate. However, the energy expenditure beyond the basal rate for intense mental effort as in problem solving or writing examinations does not add appreciably to the caloric requirement. Some stu-

Table 8-2.   Calorie Expenditure for Various Kinds of Activity*

Type of Activity	Kilocalories per hour†
Sedentary	80–100
Reading; writing; eating; watching television or movies; listening to the radio; sewing; playing cards; typing; and miscellaneous office work and other acitvities done while sitting that require little or no arm movement	
Light	110–160
Preparing and cooking food; doing dishes; dusting; hand washing small articles of clothing; ironing; walking slowly; personal care; miscellaneous office work and other activities done while standing that require some arm movement; and rapid typing and other activities done while sitting that are more strenuous	
Moderate	170–240
Making beds; mopping and scrubbing; sweeping; light polishing and waxing; laundering by machine; light gardening and carpentry work; walking moderately fast; other activities done while standing that require moderate arm movement; and activities done while sitting that require more vigorous arm movement	
Vigorous	250–350
Heavy scrubbing and waxing; hand washing large articles of clothing; hanging out clothes; stripping beds; other heavy work; walking fast; bowling; golfing; and gardening	
Strenuous	350 or more
Swimming; playing tennis; running; bicycling; dancing; skiing; and playing football	

* Adapted from Page, L., and Raper, N.: *Food and Your Weight.* Home and Garden Bulletin No. 74, U.S. Department of Agriculture, 1977, p. 4.

† Lower figures apply to women, higher figures to men. The figures include the metabolism at rest as well as for the acitivity.

dents become tense and restless while solving problems, but the increased expenditure of energy in such a situation is not primarily that of mental work.

Calorigenic Effect of Food   The ingestion of food results in an increase in heat production known as the CALORIGENIC EFFECT OF FOOD or DIETARY-INDUCED THERMOGENESIS. Traditionally it has been referred to as the SPECIFIC DYNAMIC ACTION OF FOOD (SDA) or SPECIFIC DYNAMIC EFFECT. Although it may be related in part to the digestion and absorption of food, increased heat production also occurs when nutrients are given intravenously thus suggesting that stimulation of cellular metabolism may be of prime importance. Protein when eaten alone has been shown to increase the metabolic rate by 30 percent, whereas carbohydrates and fats produce much smaller increases. On the basis of mixed diets usually eaten, the calorigenic effect of food is approximately 10 percent of the total energy requirement.[4]

Maintenance of Body Temperature   Under normal conditions the temperature of the body is controlled by the amount of blood brought to the skin. Vasodilation of the blood vessels occurs when the environmental temperature is high and vasoconstriction occurs when the temperature is low. When the surrounding temperature is low, most of the heat is lost by radiation and convection, but when the environmental temperature is high, the body heat is lost chiefly through evaporation. It is a well known fact that more heat is lost by evaporation when the air is dry than when it is humid.

During cold weather, excessive heat losses from the body are avoided by the use of suitable clothing and the heating of the home or place of work. Moreover, body heat is conserved if there is a layer of adipose tissue under the skin. The subcutaneous fat serves to keep heat in the body rather than allowing it to be dissipated through the skin—an advantage in cold weather, but a disadvantage in warm weather. Infants and young children have a relatively large surface area and lose much heat from the body when they are exposed.

When the body is subjected to extreme cold, the body temperature is maintained by an increase in involuntary and often voluntary activity. The blood vessels constrict so that there is less blood reaching the skin surface, the muscles become tense, and shivering follows. These involuntary activities result in a considerable increase in the metabolic rate. As anyone knows who has been exposed to a cold winter day, one is not likely to stand still. In addition, then, to the increased energy expenditure occasioned by the involuntary activities, the individual increases voluntary activity.

Growth   The building of new tissue represents a storage of energy in one form or another; for example, every gram of protein in body tissue represents about

4 kcal. When growth is rapid, as during the first year of life, the energy allowance must be high. In fact, the energy need is greater per unit of body weight than at any other time of life. In pregnancy, likewise, the energy needs are increased to cover the building of new tissues. These needs are discussed in more detail in Chapters 19, 20 and 21.

Energy Allowances

Estimating Energy Requirements   One method for estimating the energy requirement of an individual is to keep a record of the amount of time spent for each activity during the day and calculate the energy equivalent. The calculation can be made by using the data from Table 8-2 or by referring to more precise tables of energy expenditure for given activities per kilogram of body weight.[3] An example of a woman's daily activities grouped according to the categories in Table 8-2 follows:

	Hours	kcal/Hour	Total kcal
Sleep	8	50	400
Sedentary	10	80	800
Light	3	110	330
Moderate	2	170	340
Vigorous	1	250	250
	24		2,120

Keeping a detailed record of activities is tedious and at best becomes only an approximation of actual caloric requirement inasmuch as wide variations occur from one individual to another within each category.

Another method widely used in clinical practice is to estimate an individual's activity to be sedentary, moderately active, or active. The approximate energy expenditure per kilogram of body weight is as follows:

Sedentary	30–35 kcal (126–147 kJ)
Moderately active	35–40 kcal (147–168 kJ)
Active	40–45 kcal (168–189 kJ)

Using these factors, a moderately active woman weighing 55 kg would require 1,925 to 2,200 kcal (8.1 to 9.2 MJ). Although these are only approximations, they provide a starting point for planning diets.

Recommended Allowances   The energy intake recommended by the Food and Nutrition Board,[5] for males and females of all ages is shown in Table 8-3. The bases for these allowances are described in the footnotes of the table.

Several adjustments may be required to take into account factors that increase or decrease an individual's energy requirement. The range of ± 20 percent for adults indicates customary variation in activity. For children, this range is greater. The declining requirements for adults over 50 years of age, takes into account the reduction in basal metabolism and also in activity.

Body Sizes.   People who are active and who are larger than the weight stated in the table will require more calories; those who are smaller will require less. Any activity that requires movement of the whole body, such as walking, entails more energy expenditure by an 80-kg (176 lb) person than by a 60-kg (132 lb) person. The differences are small with activities that involve only parts of the body—such as reading, typing, and so on.

Activity.   This is the greatest variable in the energy requirement. Today the average work week is 35 to 40 hours; sleep accounts for 50 to 60 hours; eating and travel to and from work consumes 20 hours, more or less; and leisure time amounts to 50 or 60 hours in a given week. The leisure activities may range from reading, watching television or movies, or stamp collecting, on the one hand, to such vigorous activities as tennis, gardening, golf, and swimming, on the other hand. Obviously, to set up an energy allowance in terms of one's activity at work alone is to ignore a large part of one's day.

For persons who are moderately active the allowances should be increased by about 300 kcal (1.26 MJ). Very active individuals such as athletes, military recruits, and construction workers may require 600 to 900 kcal (2.52 to 3.78 MJ) above the recommended allowances.

Adjustment for Climate.   In summer and winter most Americans live in an environmental temperature of 20° to 25°C (68°–77°F). In winter they wear warm clothing, live and work in well-heated buildings, and travel by heated means of transportation. Likewise, in summer many of them live and work in air-conditioned buildings. Therefore, adjustments for temperature are not usually necessary.

Table 8-3. Median Heights and Weights and Recommended Energy Intake*

Category	Age (years) or Condition	Weight[†] (kg)	Weight[†] (lb)	Height[†] (cm)	Height[†] (in)	REE[‡] (kcal/day)	Average Energy Allowance (kcal)[‡] Multiples of REE	Per kg	Per day[§]
Infants	0.0–0.5	6	13	60	24	320		108	650
	0.5–1.0	9	20	71	28	500		98	850
Children	1–3	13	29	90	35	740		102	1,300
	4–6	20	44	112	44	950		90	1,800
	7–10	28	62	132	52	1,130		70	2,000
Males	11–14	45	99	157	62	1,440	1.70	55	2,500
	15–18	66	145	176	69	1,760	1.67	45	3,000
	19–24	72	160	177	70	1,780	1.67	40	2,900
	25–50	79	174	176	70	1,800	1.60	37	2,900
	51+	77	170	173	68	1,530	1.50	30	2,300
Females	11–14	46	101	157	62	1,310	1.67	47	2,200
	15–18	55	120	163	64	1,370	1.60	40	2,200
	19–24	58	128	164	65	1,350	1.60	38	2,200
	25–50	63	138	163	64	1,380	1.55	36	2,200
	51+	65	143	160	63	1,280	1.50	30	1,900
Pregnant	1st trimester								+0
	2nd trimester								+300
	3rd trimester								+300
Lactating	1st 6 months								+500
	2nd 6 months								+500

*Food and Nutrition Board: *Recommended Dietary Allowances,* 10th ed. National Academy of Sciences—National Research Council, Washington, D.C., 1989.

[†]The heights and weights of adults represent the median heights and weights obtained from NHANES II (1976–1980) data.

[‡]REE = Resting Energy Expenditure

[§]The figures have been rounded. The actual energy output may vary by ±20 percent of the stated values.

During work at temperatures below 14°C (57°F) the energy expenditure is about 5 percent greater than in a warm environment. A small increase in calories (2 to 5 percent) may be necessary in winter for the person carrying a weight of heavy clothing. When a person is inadequately clothed, the energy expenditure increases considerably.

When people are physically active at high environmental temperatures, an increase in the calorie allowance of 0.5 percent for each degree above 30°C (86°F) is indicated. This increase is necessary to cover the slight increase that occurs in the metabolic rate and in the extra energy expenditure to maintain normal body temperature. In warm climates, most people tend to reduce their activity and thus their caloric needs.

Body Weight and Energy Requirement The energy intake by a given individual is that which is consistent with good health. This implies that desirable weight is maintained and that the individual experiences a sense of wellbeing. The caloric intake allows for growth during infancy, childhood, and adolescence, and provides for the additional needs during pregnancy and lactation.

Individuals can monitor their energy balance by weekly weighing on their home scales. Sudden changes in weight are usually explained by temporary changes in water balance rather than gains or losses of body tissue.

If the weight remains constant over a period of time, the caloric intake is appropriate for that individual. Weight loss signifies a negative caloric balance that might be prudently brought to the attention of a physician. Weight gain is, by far, the plight of many Americans in a society with labor-saving devices and sedentary leisure activities. The correction of such weight gain is a combination of reduced caloric intake and increased physical activity.

Foods for Energy The caloric value of the Basic Diet is shown in Table 8–4. This includes the recommended number of servings from the four essential food groups of the Daily Food Guide. The plan is suitable for a low-calorie diet for those who are overweight.

Typical additions for women and men of normal weight and whose energy requirement is 2,200 and 2,900 kcal, respectively, are also shown in Table 8-4. It should be especially noted that some of the typical additions are not high in nutrient density. To improve the nutrient density, additional servings of vegetables and fruits, breads and cereals, and lowfat milk would be preferable.

Foods that are high in fat, sugar, or starch content but low in water are concentrated sources of calories. By contrast, foods high in water content are low in calories. For example, a teaspoon of margarine contains 35 kcal, a tablespoon of sugar 45 kcal, and ½ cup tomatoes 25 kcal. Thus, the addition of small amounts of concentrated foods to the diet increases the calorie intake rapidly, and vegetables and fruits can be eaten in appreciable amounts without great increases in caloric intake.

Persons who use alcoholic beverages daily may derive 5 to 20 percent of their energy intake from this source.[5] It has been reported that some individuals consume up to 1,800 kcal from this source on a daily basis. Such consumption has an adverse effect on the nutritive adequacy of the diet since alcohol provides negligible amounts of other nutrients.

Problems Related to Energy Intake

Nutritive Quality of the Diet It has been emphasized in preceding chapters that sugars and sweets, fats and oils, and alcohol contribute substantial energy value to the diet but have limited if any nutrient

Table 8-4. Energy Values of the Basic Diet with Typical Additions*

Food Groups	Servings	Energy (kcal)
Basic Diet		
Vegetable–fruit	4	240
Bread-cereal	4	290
Milk, 2 percent	2 cups	240
Meat, lean	5 ounces	335
Total, Basic Diet		1,105
Typical additions by a woman		
Cream of mushroom soup	1 cup	135
Saltines	4	50
Margarine or butter	1 tablespoon	100
French dressing	2 tablespoons	130
Sugar, jam, jelly	1 tablespoon	45
Peanut butter	1 tablespoon	95
Blueberry pie	1 piece	325
Total additions		880
Total for the day (Basic + typical additions)		1,985
Further additions by a man		
Bread	2 slices	145
Margarine or butter	1 tablespoon	100
Meat group	2 ounces	135
French fried potatoes	10 strips	135
Whisky, 86 proof	2 jiggers	210
Total further additions		725
Total for the day (Basic + typical + further additions)		2,710

* See Table 4–1 for complete calculations of the Basic Diet. Refer to Table A-1 for caloric values of specific foods.

content. Numerous attractive snack foods that are high in calories but of low nutrient density are available in today's market. At the same time consumer concern about weight control has led to an increased selection of processed foods with lower calorie content. By reading labels on nutritional information, the consumer can learn to make wiser choices.

Healthy people can use foods of low nutrient density in moderation, and indeed some of these foods enhance diet palatability. However, when they are eaten in excessive amounts the result may be (1) an energy intake greater than energy output, which results in obesity, or (2) a reduced intake of essential nutrient-rich foods, which impairs nutritional status, or (3) both.

Weight Control The primary problem of malnutrition in the United States is obesity. Its prevention requires balance of energy intake and energy output. Such prevention must begin early in life when good food habits are being formed.

When the energy intake is less than 1,800 to 2,000 kcal, it is difficult to include all nutrients at recommended levels—especially for some of the trace elements. Thus, it is more appropriate to increase exercise than it is to decrease energy intake below 2,000 kcal if the goal is weight maintenance. For those who are obese, low-calorie diets ranging from 1,000 to 1,800 kcal are used, depending on individual needs. (See Chapter 25 for full discussion of obesity.)

SOME POINTS FOR EMPHASIS IN NUTRITION EDUCATION

1. Energy values in nutrition are expressed as kilocalories or kilojoules. The kilocalorie (1,000 times the small calorie) expresses energy in heat units. The kilojoule expresses energy in mechanical units. One kilocalorie equals 4.184 kilojoules.
2. A calorie is the same whether it comes from carbohydrates, fats, or proteins. Carbohydrates and proteins furnish 4 kcal (17 kJ) per gram and fats 9 kcal (38 kJ) per gram.
3. Weight for weight, foods that are dry or greasy are relatively high in calories: for example, cereals, cookies, cakes, pastries, sweets, butter, fatty meats. Foods that have a high concentration of water are much lower in calories: for example, fruits and vegetables.
4. The basal metabolism is the amount of energy the body uses at rest. It ranges from about 1,300 to 1,700 kcal (5.4 to 7.1 MJ) for adults and accounts for about half or more of the total calories needed by the average American.
5. The amount of physical activity is the important factor determining the number of calories needed above the basal metabolism. For the average young woman in America about 2,000 kcal (8.4 MJ) is needed daily; the average young man needs about 2,700 kcal (11.3 MJ). Sedentary young adults require less than this, and older persons require considerably fewer calories.
6. In addition to furnishing most of the needed amounts of protein, minerals, and vitamins, the Daily Food Guide in the recommended amounts provides 1,100 to 1,300 kcal. Thus, a young woman can use a reasonable amount of desserts, fats, and sugars without exceeding her energy requirement, but the older woman has very little leeway in using these foods if she is also going to meet her nutritional requirements.
7. The body is in energy balance when the calories supplied by food are equal to the energy needed for all the involuntary and voluntary activities of the body.
8. If the energy intake is greater than the body needs, weight is gained, and if the energy intake is less than the body needs, weight is lost.

Problems and Review

1. Define or explain what is meant by calorie; joule; calorimetry; bomb calorimeter; respiration calorimeter; indirect calorimetry; heat of combustion; physiologic fuel factor; basal metabolism; resting metabolism.
2. *Problem.* Using data from Table A-1, calculate the number of grams of each of the following foods to furnish 100 kcal: butter, whole milk, cheese, egg, potato, apple, banana, orange, sugar, bread, pork chop, cooked rice, chocolate cake.
3. What are the standard conditions for performing a basal metabolism test? What factors might make the basal metabolism of two adult individuals of the same age vary? How does age itself affect the basal metabolism?
4. Explain how the following factors affect the total energy requirement: muscular activity; food; climate; clothing; growth; muscle tension; endocrine secretions. Which of these has the greatest effect?
5. *Problem.* Calculate your own calorie intake for one day. What percentage of your calories was derived from each of the four food groups? What percentage from sweets, fats, desserts, and snack foods?
6. What is the best indication of adequate caloric intake?

7. In contrast to the recommended allowances for other nutrients designed to meet the needs of *most* healthy persons, why do the recommendations for energy represent the *average* needs of individuals in each age–sex category?

References

1. Jequier, E., and Schutz, Y.: "Long-term Measurements of Energy Expenditure in Humans Using a Respiration Chamber," *Am. J. Clin. Nutr.*, 38:989–98, 1983.

2. Solomon, S. J., et al.: "Menstrual Cycle and Basal Metabolic Rate in Women," *Am. J. Clin. Nutr.*, 36:611–16, 1982.

3. Durnin, J. V. G. A., and Passmore, R.: *Energy, Work and Leisure*. Heinemann Educational Books, London, 1967.

4. Horton, E. S.: "Introduction: An Overview of the Assessment and Regulation of Energy Balance in Humans," *Am. J. Clin. Nutr.*, 38:972–77, 1983.

5. Food and Nutrition Board: *Recommended Dietary Allowances*, 10th ed. National Research Council–National Academy of Sciences, Washington, D.C., 1989.

9

Mineral Elements

The function and requirements of trace minerals represents one of the most exciting and dominant topics of current nutrition research. Minerals once considered contaminants in foods are now known to be essential. Furthermore, the number of such minerals is expected to increase. Research related to minerals has been facilitated by the development of new analytical instruments and techniques that make it possible to detect trace concentrations or, as with the use of stable isotopes, to follow more precisely the utilization of the mineral in the human body. The findings of such research have emphasized the importance of the interrelationships in function that exist among all minerals as well as with other nutrients.

The major focus of this chapter is on calcium, phosphorus, sulfur, magnesium, iron, iodine, and zinc. A brief discussion is presented of several trace minerals for which specific recommended dietary allowances have not been set. Of these copper, manganese, fluorine, chromium, selenium, and molybdenum have had an "estimated safe and adequate daily dietary intake" suggested.[1] Sodium, potassium, and chlorine together with water balance and acid–base balance are discussed in Chapter 10.

Basic Concepts

Mineral Composition of the Body MINERALS are those elements that remain largely as ash when plant or animal tissues are burned. About 4 percent of the body weight consists of mineral matter. Seven MACRONUTRIENTS—that is, those occurring in appreciable amounts—account for most of the body content of minerals. Calcium and phosphorus account for three fourths of all mineral matter.

Some fifteen to twenty elements are present in such minute amounts that they are generally referred to as TRACE ELEMENTS or MICRONUTRIENTS. Many of these are known to be essential for humans, whereas the essentiality of others has been demonstrated only in animals. Several are considered only to be contaminants. Table 9-1 summarizes the mineral composition of the body, including approximate concentration of some minerals.

General Functions Mineral elements are present in organic compounds such as phosphoproteins, phospholipids, hemoglobin, and thyroxine; as inorganic compounds such as sodium chloride and calcium

Table 9-1. Mineral Composition of the Body

	Approximate Amount in Adult Body	
	percent	per 70 kg
Minerals for which an RDA has been set		
Calcium	1.75	1,200 g
Phosphorus	1.10	750 g
Magnesium	0.04	24 g
Iron	0.006	4 g
Zinc	0.002	1.7 g
Iodine	0.00004	28 mg
Minerals for which an Estimated Safe and Adequate Intake has been set		
Potassium	0.35	245 g
Sodium	0.15	105 g
Chlorine	0.15	105 g
Molybdenum	0.004	2.5 g
Selenium	0.003	1.8 g
Fluorine	0.001	1 g
Manganese	0.0002	150 mg
Copper	0.0002	150 mg
Chromium	trace	5 mg
Required minerals as constituents of other nutrients		
Sulfur	0.25	175 mg
Cobalt	trace	5 mg
Possibly essential (needed by some animals)		
Arsenic		
Cadmium		
Nickel		
Silicon		
Tin		
Vanadium		
No known function		
Aluminum		
Barium		
Boron		
Bromine		
Gold		
Lead		
Mercury		
Strontium		

phosphate; and as free ions. They enter into the structure of every cell of the body. Hard skeletal structures contain the greater proportions of some elements such as calcium, phosphorus, and magnesium, and soft tissues contain relatively higher proportions of potassium.

Mineral elements are constituents of enzymes such as iron in the catalases and cytochromes; of hormones such as iodine in thyroxine; and of vitamins such as cobalt in vitamin B-12 and sulfur in thiamin. Their presence in body fluids regulates the permeability of cell membranes; the osmotic pressure and water balance between intracellular and extracellular compartments; the response of nerves to stimuli; the contraction of muscles; and the maintenance of acid-base equilibrium.

The amount of an element present gives no clue to its importance in body functions. For example, the few milligrams of iodine in the body is just as critical to health as the approximate 1,200 g of calcium that is present.

Dynamic Equilibrium For the normal adult, a balance usually exists between the intake of an element and its excretion. Absorption and excretion are constantly adjusted to guard against an overload that might produce toxic effects. At the same time, however, precise mechanisms carefully conserve the amounts of minerals that are needed.

Homeostasis is maintained in spite of the fact that a continuous flow of nutrients into the cell and away from the cell is taking place. For example, bone, often thought of as being inert, is an exceedingly active tissue in its constant uptake and release of mineral constituents. Nevertheless, a state of balance or dynamic equilibrium is maintained provided that the supply of nutrients is adequate.

Foods as Sources of Mineral Elements When selecting foods for their mineral content, several factors must be considered: (1) the concentration of the mineral in the food; (2) how much of a given food is ordinarily consumed; (3) whether the food has lost some of its minerals through refinement or in cooking processes; and (4) whether the food contains the mineral in available form.

The best assurance that the diet will supply sufficient amounts of the essential mineral elements is to select a wide variety of foods, using the Basic Diet pattern (Table 4-1) as the basis. Fats and sugars are practically devoid of mineral elements, and highly refined cereals and flours are poor sources of most of them. Fabricated foods may lack important trace minerals for which no recommended allowances have been set. Many adolescent girls and women are unable to obtain sufficient iron even from a good diet and still keep within their caloric requirement.

Recommended Intakes Recommended daily allowances have been established only for calcium, phosphorus, magnesium, iron, iodine, and zinc. An "estimated safe and adequate daily dietary intake" has been set for several additional minerals; expression of recommended intake in this way emphasizes that these minerals are required but that sufficient data are not available to establish traditional recommended allowances.[1] Thus the safe and adequate intakes are more tentative and suggested ranges of intakes for maintaining health. The upper limit set on these ranges emphasizes the risk of possible toxicity for these nutrients. For many minerals the range between what is necessary and what becomes toxic is quite narrow. Although this danger is not widespread, it can become very real through the use of highly fortified products and supplements.

Evaluation of Mineral Nutriture   Methods to evaluate the adequacy of mineral intake are limited. Often blood levels of the mineral are maintained by homeostatic mechanisms that mobilize body stores of the mineral if intake is low. Because of such stores, a long time generally is required for clinical signs of deficiency to develop. For certain minerals the activity of enzymes containing the mineral can be measured in red blood cells or leukocytes and may provide a fairly reliable index of the adequacy of the mineral in body cells. Measurement of the concentrations of minerals in hair has attracted considerable attention, partly because of the noninvasive nature of this method of analysis. Results are influenced by many factors, including distance from the scalp that the hair sample is taken, color of hair, and products used on hair such as shampoos, sprays, and conditioners. Although measurement of hair concentrations of minerals such as zinc have provided useful information in some experimental studies, accepted standards of normal values have not been established for routine clinical use of hair analysis in nutritional assessment. Hair analyses, however, have proved useful in the detection of excessive exposure to toxic minerals such as arsenic, mercury, and lead.[2]

Calcium

Distribution and Functions   Of the approximately 1,200 g of calcium in the adult body, 99 percent is combined as the salts that give hardness to the bones and teeth. The bones not only provide the rigid framework for the body, but they also furnish the reserves of calcium to the circulation so that the concentration in the plasma can be kept constant at all times.

The remaining 1 percent of the calcium in the adult—about 10 to 12 g—is distributed throughout the extracellular and intracellular fluids of the body. It fulfills several important functions:

1. Activates a number of enzymes including pancreatic lipase, adenosine triphosphatase, and some proteolytic enzymes
2. Is required for the synthesis of ACETYLCHOLINE, a substance necessary for transmission of nerve impulses
3. Increases the permeability of cell membranes, thereby aiding in the absorptive processes
4. Aids in the absorption of vitamin B-12 from the ileum
5. Regulates the contraction and relaxation of muscles, including the heartbeat
6. Catalyzes several steps in the clotting of blood. The process of catalysis involves a cascade system in which a blood coagulation protein is converted from an inactive to an active form which then catalyzes the conversion of the next coagulation protein in the sequence. Final steps in the process involve

$$\text{Prothrombin} \xrightarrow{\text{Ca}^{2+}} \text{thrombin}$$
$$\downarrow$$
$$\text{fibrinogen} \longrightarrow \text{fibrin (the clot)}$$

Absorption   Calcium is absorbed by active transport, an energy-requiring process, chiefly from the duodenum. Passive diffusion of calcium across the intestinal mucosa also occurs from the jejunum and ileum. (See Figure 9-1.)

Factors Favoring Absorption.   Body need is the major factor governing the amount of calcium that is absorbed. Healthy adults receiving a diet that meets their requirements absorb approximately 30 to 40 percent of their dietary calcium. At higher levels of intake the proportion that is absorbed is lower, but the absolute amount that crosses the intestinal membranes depends on need. In many areas of the world, the diet supplies low amounts of calcium. People in these areas have adapted to these low levels and absorb a high proportion of the intake. During growth the absorption is increased to take care of increase in size and hardness of the skeleton. Thus children absorb proportionally more calcium than adults. Pregnancy and lactation are also two physiological states which trigger an increased absorption. Men generally absorb calcium more efficiently than do nonpregnant women. Elderly persons, especially women, absorb calcium less well than do younger individuals.

Several mechanisms control the amount of calcium that is absorbed. The two most important of these involve vitamin D and the parathyroid hormone (PARATHORMONE, or PTH). PTH is secreted when the

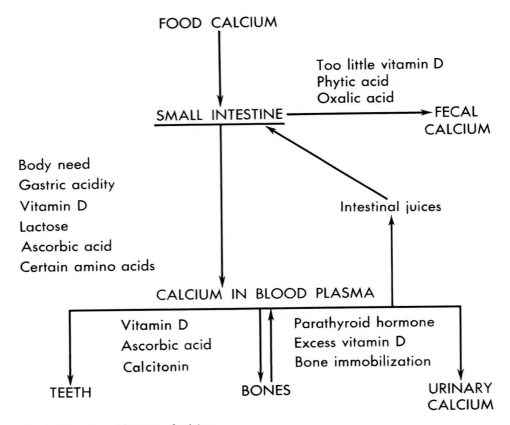

Figure 9-1. The utilization of calcium.

blood calcium concentration decreases. One of its functions is to stimulate the kidney to synthesize CALCITRIOL, the active form of vitamin D. This metabolite stimulates increased absorption from the intestine and, together with PTH, enhances mobilization of bone stores of calcium. (See the discussion of vitamin D, in Chapter 11.)

An acid milieu aids in the absorption of calcium because calcium salts are then more soluble. After bile and pancreatic juices have mixed with the chyme, it becomes strongly alkaline and the solubility of the calcium salts is reduced. The presence of ascorbic acid and certain amino acids may facilitate calcium absorption by increasing the solubility of calcium salts. Lactose is known to enhance calcium absorption, but the mechanism(s) involved are poorly understood.

Factors Interfering with Absorption. The lack of vitamin D seriously impairs the absorption of calcium. Such lack may arise from inadequate exposure to sunlight or failure to ingest vitamin D in some form. A reduction in the amount of acid, sometimes found in el-

derly persons, reduces the solubility of the calcium salts. A marked increase in gastrointestinal motility reduces the length of time that calcium remains in contact with the intestinal mucosa. Emotional stress also reduces the utilization of calcium.

The presence of oxalic acid or phytic acid in foods and an abnormal calcium-to-phosphorus ratio are known to result in the formation of insoluble calcium complexes and thus interfere with calcium absorption. These effects can be clearly demonstrated in experimental animals when a decidedly abnormal diet is fed. These factors are unlikely to be of sufficient magnitude to alter utilization of calcium significantly in typical American diets.

Oxalic acid is found in rhubarb, cocoa, and green leafy vegetables such as spinach, Swiss chard, and beet greens. Spinach, and probably other greens, contains sufficient calcium to bind its content of oxalic acid. Thus, the absorption of calcium in other foods eaten at the same time is not likely to be impaired.[3] The amount of cocoa that is ingested at one time is too small to reduce the absorption of calcium significantly. Consequently, one would expect chocolate-flavored milk to supply about the same amount of calcium as plain milk.

PHYTIC ACID is an organic phosphorous compound found in legumes and in the outer layers of cereal grains. Its effect in binding calcium into insoluble complexes would be important only when phytate-containing foods make up a major part of the diet and when calcium intake is low as well. These conditions may exist in some vegetarian diets in which unleavened bread, whole-grain cereals, or legumes provide most of the energy intake. The yeast fermentation that takes place during the preparation of leavened breads destroys much of the phytate present in whole-meal flour.[4]

High intakes of dietary fiber have been suspected of reducing calcium absorption, but experimental results have been conflicting.[3,5] Because many high-fiber foods also contain phytic acid or oxalic acid, often it is difficult to identify the effect that can be attributed specifically to fiber. Uronic acids present in certain types of fiber are thought to bind calcium and impair its absorption. However, most of the dietary uronic acids are fermented in the colon, so that conceivably the calcium would be released and become available for absorption.[3]

Excess phosphorus has been shown to impair calcium absorption in animals. In human diets a calcium-to-phosphorus ratio of 1:1 has been used in establishing recommended intakes, although it is recognized that a much wider range in ratios is tolerated.[1] Recent trends in food consumption involving decreased consumption of dairy products and increased consumption of meat and of processed foods with phosphate additives have resulted in decreased calcium intake relative to phosphorus. More research is needed to clarify the consequences of these changes.

Metabolism The concentration of calcium in the plasma is kept within the narrow range of 9 to 11 mg per dl (4.5 to 5.5 mEq per liter). About 40 percent of the calcium is bound to plasma protein and 60 percent is diffusible. The plasma level is regulated by (1) the active form of vitamin D synthesized by the kidney, (2) parathyroid hormone, and (3) CALCITONIN, a hormone secreted by the thyroid gland.

When the plasma concentration of calcium is lowered, increased secretion of parathyroid hormone occurs. This hormone then stimulates conversion of vitamin D to its active form in the kidney. The calcium level of the blood is increased by three actions: (1) increased absorption from the intestinal tract; (2) re-

lease of calcium from the bone (RESORPTION); and (3) increased reabsorption of calcium by the renal tubules. The excretion of phosphate in the urine is also increased, thereby maintaining a normal calcium-to-phosphorus ratio in the blood.

Calcitonin is antagonistic to parathyroid hormone and lowers the blood calcium when it becomes abnormally high. It does this by inhibiting bone resorption.

Bone. Bone consists of organic and inorganic substances. The principal organic substance is the protein COLLAGEN, and the ground substance consists of small amounts of mucoproteins and mucopolysaccharides, especially chondroitin sulfate. The formation of bone is initiated early in fetal life with the development of the cartilagenous matrix. During the latter part of pregnancy some mineralization of the fetal skeleton takes place so that the infant at birth has a body calcium content of about 28 g.

During growth the addition of mineral to bone exceeds the amounts that are removed. The bone hardness consists of a gradual addition of minerals by the process referred to as MINERALIZATION or OSSIFICATION. During fetal development and the first few months after birth the bones achieve sufficient mineralization so that the skeleton can support the weight of the baby when he or she walks. Throughout childhood and adolescence the bones increase in length and diameter. This increase in size is dependent upon adequate protein as well as mineral elements. The hardness of bones increases throughout the first 20 years—sometimes longer. About 165 mg calcium is added to the skeleton daily during the early growing years. At adolescence the retention is as high as 300 mg per day, with a yearly increase as high as 90 g.

The complex mineral substance in bone consists of an amorphous phase and a crystalline phase that is similar to HYDROXYAPATITE—$Ca_{10}(PO_4)_6(OH)_2$. Small amounts of calcium can be replaced by magnesium, sodium, potassium, lead, or strontium. Likewise, the anions sulfate, fluoride, citrate, carbonate, and chloride can enter the structure.

Bone is the principal reserve of calcium and phosphorus in the body. Contrary to popular belief, bones are continuously remodeled and reshaped by OSTEOBLASTS (bone-forming cells) and OSTEOCLASTS (bone-destroying cells). About 250 to 1,000 mg calcium enter and leave the bone each day in the adult.[6] Because of the turnover of calcium within the bone, widely varying intakes of calcium have no direct effect on the blood calcium.

In the well-nourished individual the readily available stores of calcium are in the ends of the long bones, and are known as TRABECULAE. In the absence of trabeculae calcium is withdrawn from the shaft of the long bone.

Teeth. Like bones, teeth are complex structures consisting of a protein matrix (keratin in the enamel, and collagen in the dentin) and mineral salts, principally calcium and phosphorus as hydroxyapatite. In the fetus the development of teeth begins by the fourth month and calcification proceeds during the growth of the fetus. Prenatally and during infancy and childhood tooth development requires adequate supplies of many diet factors including not only calcium and phosphorus, but also vitamins A and D, as well as protein. The deciduous teeth of the infant are fully mineralized by the end of the first year of life, but the calcification of permanent teeth is completed at various times during childhood and adolescence; for some teeth the mineralization is not completed until early adult years.

The turnover of calcium in teeth is very slow, but, unlike calcium in bone, once the calcium in teeth is lost it cannot be replaced. Thus, any factor that increases the solubility of mineral salts at the tooth surfaces will lead to decay: for example, the acids produced by microbial activity when sugars stick to the teeth. On the other hand, the presence of fluoride in the salts of tooth enamel increases the hardness, thereby reducing their decay. (See page 131.) Because of the slow rate of turnover of calcium in teeth, the fetus does not take much calcium from the mother's teeth, and the popular notion of the loss of "a tooth for every child" is false. (See Chapter 19.)

Excretion The urinary excretion for a given individual remains relatively constant regardless of calcium intake, but varies widely from one individual to another. The effect of dietary protein on urinary calcium excretion is greater than that of dietary calcium. Urinary calcium losses are increased as the protein intake is increased.[7-9] In one study adults were fed a diet containing 800 mg calcium and 47, 95, and 142 g protein.[7] The urinary calcium excretion on the three levels of protein intake was 217, 303, and 426 mg, respectively. The calcium balances were + 12, + 1 and − 85 mg, respectively. By contrast, little effect on calcium excretion was found in another study, in which meat was the primary source of the high-protein intake.[10] The high phosphorus content of the meat appears to be responsible for the differences in results.[11]

Fecal calcium includes endogenous calcium that is not reabsorbed from the digestive juices and dietary calcium. The fecal calcium varies directly with the dietary calcium. Under normal conditions the skin losses are small. When people work strenuously at very high temperatures and perspire profusely, the calcium losses could be considerable.

Daily Allowances The recommended allowance for calcium is 800 mg for adults and children aged 1 to 10 years; 1,200 mg for males and females aged 11 to 24 years and for pregnant and lactating women; and 400 to 600 mg during the first year of life.[1] The allowance for adults is based on obligatory losses in the urine, endogenous loss from digestive juices in the feces, and from the skin. These losses are estimated at 200 to 250 mg daily. Assuming absorption to be 35 to 40 per cent, this daily loss would necessitate an allowance of 800 mg.

A great deal of controversy exists concerning the requirement for calcium. The calcium balance technique for determining the calcium requirement has been criticized by many. People who ingest high levels of calcium are in negative balance if they suddenly shift to a lower intake, but in time most of them adjust to the lower level of intake. Adults throughout the world consume diets that often provide 400 mg or less of calcium, yet they do not show any adverse effects.

The FAO/WHO committee has recommended 400 to 500 mg calcium as a "practical allowance" for adults.[12] Such levels can be realized in most countries for the entire population, whereas higher levels would be impractical in terms of available food supplies. The Canadian allowance is 800 mg for men and 700 mg for women, with an additional 500 mg allowance for pregnancy and lactation.

Although the utilization of calcium may be altered by factors such as high intakes of protein, dietary fiber, or phytate, the range of intake of these dietary components by people in the United States usually is such that the RDA can still be used as a guide for nutritional adequacy. These factors pose a problem primarily when calcium intake is marginal or low.

Food Sources of Calcium The calcium content of some typical foods is shown in Table 9-2, and the calcium contribution of the basic diet pattern is charted in Figure 9-2. Milk is the outstanding source of calcium in the diet; without it, a satisfactory intake of calcium is extremely difficult. Whole or skimmed, homogenized or non-homogenized, plain or chocolate-flavored, sweet or sour milks are equally good. For the adult 2 to 3 cups milk daily and for the child 3

Table 9-2. Calcium Content of Some Typical Foods

	Household Measure	Calcium (mg)	Percentage of Adult Daily Allowance*
Yogurt, plain, low fat, added milk solids	1 cup	415	52
Milk, fresh, whole	1 cup	291	36
Milk, nonfat dry	⅓ cup	279	35
Yogurt, plain, whole milk	1 cup	274	34
Cheese, American processed	1 ounce	174	22
Salmon, pink, canned	3 ounces	167†	21
Collards, cooked from frozen	½ cup	150	18
Tofu	4 ounces	145	18
Turnip greens, cooked	½ cup	126	16
Clams or oysters	½ cup	113	14
Mustard greens, cooked	½ cup	97	12
Shrimp	3 ounces	98	12
Ice cream	⅛ quart	87	11
Kale, cooked	½ cup	78	10
Soybeans, mature, cooked	½ cup	73	9
Cottage cheese, creamed	½ cup	68	9
Broccoli, cooked	½ cup	68	9
Orange, whole	1 medium	54	7
Sweet potato, boiled	1 medium	48	6
Molasses, light	1 tablespoon	33	4
Egg, whole	1 medium	28	3
Cabbage, raw, shredded	½ cup	22	3
Carrots, cooked	½ cup	26	3
Bread, soft crumb type	1 slice	13	2

* Recommended Dietary Allowance of calcium for the adult is 800 mg.
† Includes bones packed with salmon.

to 4 cups daily will ensure adequate calcium intake. Cheddar cheese is an excellent source of calcium. Cottage cheese and ice cream are good sources but will not adequately substitute for milk. The dairy products, excluding butter, account for three fourths of the calcium in the American diet.

A diet excluding dairy products provides approximately 150 to 200 mg calcium per 1,000 kcal. Certain green leafy vegetables such as mustard greens, turnip greens, kale, and collards are important sources of calcium when they are eaten frequently. Canned salmon with the bones, as well as clams, oysters, and shrimp likewise are good sources, but they are not eaten with frequency. Meats and cereal grains are poor sources. The use of nonfat dry milk, dough conditioners, and mold inhibitors in bread enhances the calcium value of the diet. Calcium is also an optional enrichment ingredient in flours and breads.

Calcium Deficiency The evidence regarding the effect of a low intake of calcium on deficiency symptoms is contradictory. If a low calcium intake alone could cause deficiency, one would expect to see much more deficiency throughout the world than actually exists. There are, however, a number of disturbances of calcium metabolism that have serious consequences.

Bone resorption is increased during immobilization from illness or injury. The loss of calcium from bone occurs almost immediately, as demonstrated in the early space flights by the astronauts.[13] The release of calcium from the bones of those who are bedfast for long periods of time sometimes leads to calcium deposits in soft tissues and the formation of renal calculi.

Failure to provide vitamin D by exposure to sunshine or in the diet reduces the absorption and utilization of calcium. Eventually this leads to rickets in the young or osteomalacia in adults. (See also Chapter 11.) OSTEOMALACIA involves a reduction in the mineral content of the bone without reduction in bone size.

OSTEOPOROSIS is a reduction in the total bone mass. It occurs in millions of American women after age 50 and to a somewhat lesser extent in men. The role of dietary calcium in the etiology of osteoporosis is controversial. Whereas in the past diet was considered of little importance, recent evidence suggests that long-term low intakes of calcium may be a major risk factor. The efficiency of calcium absorption appears to decrease with age, and higher intakes are needed to achieve calcium equilibrium.[14] Generous intakes of calcium earlier in life may help prevent osteoporosis by promoting development of bones that are more resistant to the losses that accompany aging. In addition to dietary calcium, several other factors influence the development of osteoporosis: alterations in hormones, particularly estrogen; heredity; race; smoking; and level of physical activity. (See Chapter 22.)

Epidemiologic studies have shown that low dietary intakes of calcium also may be associated with high blood pressure or hypertension.[15] Healthy young adults given supplements of 1,000 mg calcium per day for 22 weeks showed a significant decrease in diastolic blood pressure.[16] Further research is needed to con-

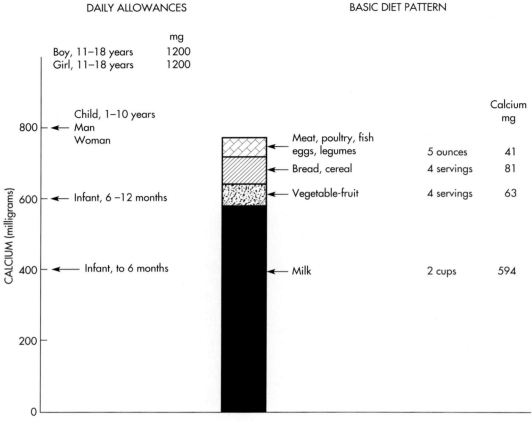

DAILY ALLOWANCES   BASIC DIET PATTERN

Figure 9-2. The milk group furnishes almost three fourths of the calcium allowance of the adult. The addition of 1 to 2 cups milk ensures sufficient calcium during periods of growth, in pregnancy, and in lactation. See Table 4-1 for complete calculation.

firm these results and elucidate the mechanism(s) involved.

In malabsorption disorders such as celiac disease large amounts of fat are excreted. The unabsorbed fat combines with calcium in the intestinal lumen to form insoluble soaps and the absorption of calcium as well as fat-soluble vitamins is greatly decreased. Hypocalcemia, tetany, and osteoporosis are frequently seen in these cases.

Chronic renal disease has long been recognized as contributing to hypocalcemia, osteitis, and osteomalacia. The cause of the metabolic disorder is the failure of the malfunctioning kidney to synthesize the metabolically active vitamin D_3. When calcitriol is given, the calcium absorption and utilization are improved.

TETANY is a condition characterized by a low blood calcium, increased excitability of the nerves, and uncontrolled contractions of the muscles. It is not caused by a dietary lack of calcium alone, although low intakes in combination with impaired absorption may lead to its occurrence. Tetany often is the consequence of lowered parathyroid function. Administration of parathyroid hormones brings the blood calcium level back to normal.

Hypercalcemia A number of conditions can cause HYPERCALCEMIA or increase in the blood calcium. It is accompanied by increased deposition of calcium in the soft tissues and increased calcium excretion in the urine. A high intake of calcium is not, in itself, a causative factor.

One of the situations in which hypercalcemia occasionally occurs is the milk-alkali syndrome in which patients with peptic ulcer have used excessive amounts of readily absorbed alkalies together with large amounts of milk over a period of years. The hypercalcemia in these patients was accompanied by vomiting, gastrointestinal bleeding, and increase in blood pressure.

Hypercalcemia occurs in persons who ingest an excess of vitamin D. Gastrointestinal upsets are noted and in infants the rate of growth becomes retarded. The condition is corrected by the removal of the excess vitamin from the diet. Hypercalcemia also has been reported in some cases of vitamin A toxicity.

Phosphorus

Distribution   Phosphorus accounts for about 1 percent of body weight or one fourth of the total mineral matter in the body. About 85 percent of the phosphorus is in inorganic combination with calcium as the insoluble apatite of bones and teeth. In bones the proportion of calcium to phosphorus is about 2 to 1. Soft tissues contain much higher amounts of phosphorus than of calcium. Most of this phosphorus is in organic combinations.

Functions   Perhaps no mineral element has as many widely differing functions as does phosphorus. In fact, reference has been made to phosphorus compounds at many points in preceding chapters of the text, and some of the many roles are listed here for review purposes.

1. Phosphorus is a constituent of the sugar–phosphate linkage in the structures of DNA and RNA, the substances that control heredity (see page 52).
2. Phospholipids are constituents of cell membranes, thus regulating the transport of solutes into and out of the cell. The phosphorus-containing lipoproteins facilitate the transport of fats in the circulation.
3. Phosphorylation is a key reaction in many metabolic processes: for example, the phosphorylation of glucose for absorption from the intestine, the uptake of glucose by the cell, and the reabsorption of glucose by the renal tubules. Likewise, monosaccharides are phosphorylated in the initial stages of metabolism to yield energy (see page 72).
4. Phosphorus compounds are essential for the storage and controlled release of energy—the ADP–ATP system (see page 99); in the niacin-containing coenzymes required for oxidation–reduction reactions—NADP—NADPH (see page 71); and for the active form of thiamin for decarboxylation reactions—TPP (see page 72).
5. Inorganic phosphates in the body fluids constitute an important buffer system in the regulation of body neutrality (see page 151).

Metabolism   Much of the phosphorus in foods is in organic combinations that are split by intestinal phosphatases to free the phosphate. The phosphorus is ab-

sorbed as inorganic salts. About 70 percent of dietary phosphorus is normally absorbed.

The inorganic phosphorus content of blood serum ranges from 2.5 to 4.5 mg. per dl and is slightly higher in children. The level is kept constant through regulation by the kidney. All of the plasma inorganic phosphate is filtered through the renal glomeruli but most of it is reabsorbed. Vitamin D increases the rate of reabsorption by the tubules, and parathyroid hormone decreases the reabsorption.

Daily Allowances   The phosphorus allowances recommended by the Food and Nutrition Board[1] are the same as those for calcium, except for infants. With ordinary diets, the phosphorus intake exceeds the calcium intake, but within a relatively wide range of calcium-to-phosphorus ratios there are no adverse effects in children or adults.

During the first 6 months of life the phosphorus allowance is 300 mg, and during the remainder of the first year the allowance is 500 mg. By keeping the phosphorous allowance below that of calcium during the first weeks of life, hypocalcemic tetany may be avoided.

Food Sources   Phosphorus is widely distributed in foods, the milk and meat groups being important contributors. Thus, a diet that furnishes enough protein and calcium will normally provide sufficient phosphorus. Whole-grain cereals and flours contain much more phosphorus than refined cereals and flours; however, much of this occurs as phytic acid, which combines with calcium to form an insoluble salt that is not absorbed. Vegetables and fruits contain only small amounts of phosphorus. Consumption of excessive amounts of phosphorus can change the Ca : P ratio and may decrease calcium availability. Large amounts of phosphorus without a balanced consumption of calcium can be obtained by consuming diets containing excessive amounts of meat and foods containing phosphorus additives. (See Table A-1.)

Magnesium

Distribution   The amount of magnesium in the body is much smaller than that of calcium and phosphorus. Of the 20 to 35 g in the adult body, about 60 percent is present as phosphates and carbonates chiefly at the surfaces of the bones. Most of the remaining magnesium is within the cells, where it ranks next to potassium in magnitude.

Extracellular fluids account for about 2 percent of the body's magnesium. The normal concentration of magnesium in blood serum is 2 to 3 mg per dl, about 80 percent of this being ionized; the remainder is bound to protein.

Functions Magnesium is essential for all living cells. In plants magnesium is present in chlorophyll in a chemical structure similar to the iron in hemoglobin. In addition to its function in the skeletal structures, magnesium is a catalyst in numerous metabolic reactions. It is involved in protein synthesis through its action on the aggregation of ribosomes. It is an activator for the enzymes involved in the oxidative phosphorylation of ADP to ATP (see page 70), and also for all enzymes that bring about the conversion of ATP to cyclic AMP, which in turn regulates parathyroid hormone secretion. These reactions are essential whenever energy is expended, as in active transport across cell membranes, and the accomplishment of physical work.

Magnesium, together with calcium, sodium, and potassium, must be in balance in the extracellular fluids so that transmission of nerve impulses and the consequent muscle contraction can be regulated. Magnesium is involved in muscle relaxation and thus has a function opposite that of calcium.

Metabolism Magnesium is absorbed by active transport and competes with calcium for carrier sites. Thus, a high intake of either element interferes with absorption of the other. Many of the factors that enhance calcium absorption such as acidity, or that interfere with calcium absorption such as oxalic and phytic acids, also affect the absorption of magnesium. Neither vitamin D nor parathyroid hormone is believed to influence magnesium absorption. The absorption of magnesium varies inversely with the intake; at low levels of intake it is as high as 75 percent, and at high levels of intake it may be as low as 25 percent. The absorption on typical intakes in America is about 45 percent.[17]

In magnesium deficiency the kidneys and the intestinal mucosa have a marked ability to retain magnesium. Thus, homeostasis can be maintained over a wide range of intake. The urinary excretion of magnesium in adults normally ranges between 100 and 200 mg. Almost all the magnesium in the feces represents unabsorbed dietary magnesium.

Daily Allowances The Food and Nutrition Board has recommended a daily allowance of magnesium for men at 350 mg and for women at 280 mg.[1] During pregnancy and lactation a daily allowance of 320 to 350 mg is recommended. The allowances range from 40 to 60 mg during the first year of life and thereafter gradually increase from 80 mg for the toddler to 270 mg for the child of 7 to 10 years.

Food Sources The food supply available for consumption in the United States supplies approximately 340 mg magnesium daily per capita. The percentage of this magnesium supplied by each food group is as follows: dairy products excluding butter, 20; vegetables, 20; grain products, 19; meat, poultry, fish and eggs, 15; dry beans, peas, soybeans, and nuts, 11; fruits, 7; and miscellaneous foods, 8.[18] (See Table 4-1 for calculations of the basic diet.) Green leafy vegetables are especially good sources as are also dry beans and peas, soybeans, nuts, and whole grains. High losses of magnesium occur in the refinement of foods, and some losses are sustained when cooking waters are discarded. (See Table A-2 for magnesium content of foods.)

The average mixed American diet supplies about 120 mg magnesium per 1,000 kcal.[1] Thus, if girls and women stay within their caloric requirements it would appear that they could not easily meet the recommended allowances. Indeed, the 1977–78 USDA Food Consumption Survey showed that 48 to 62 percent of females between the ages of 15 to 50 years consumed less than 70 percent of the RDA. The results in males of comparable ages were somewhat lower, 30 to 44 percent.[19] In spite of these reported low intakes there is little evidence of magnesium deficiency except in conditions such as those described below. Several factors undoubtedly contribute to this discrepancy between recommended intake and incidence of deficiency, including incomplete and possibly inaccurate data on food composition, lack of methods to detect a subclinical or marginal deficiency state, and limitation of methods used to quantify requirements.

Effects of Imbalance Under normal conditions of health and food intake, magnesium deficiency is not likely to occur. Unlike calcium, magnesium is only slowly mobilized from bone. Therefore, a generally poor intake of magnesium, if it is also accompanied by increased excretion, leads to rapid lowering of the plasma magnesium. The ionic imbalance thus produced in the extracellular fluid upsets the regulation of nervous irritability and muscle contraction. Characteristic symptoms of magnesium deficiency include muscle tremor, paresthesias, and sometimes convulsive seizures and delirium. These symptoms are characteristic of hypocalcemic tetany and may be the consequence of the hypocalcemia that also frequently accompanies magnesium deficiency. Administration of calcium without magnesium, however, will not correct the condition.

Among the circumstances under which magnesium deficiency is encountered are these: chronic alcoholism, cirrhosis of the liver, malabsorption syndromes such as sprue, kwashiorkor, severe vomiting, prolonged use of magnesium-free parenteral fluids, diabetic acidosis, and diuretic therapy. In most of these instances the deficiency has occurred because of curtailment of food intake or lowered absorption or both. The loss of magnesium from the body is increased during diuretic therapy, and also in diabetic acidosis.

High intakes of certain magnesium salts have a laxative effect but generally are not toxic unless kidney function is impaired. Symptoms of high blood concentrations of magnesium include extreme thirst, a feeling of excessive warmth, marked drowsiness, a decrease in muscle and nerve irritability, and atrial fibrillation. The early stages of hypermagnesemia are readily corrected by the administration of calcium gluconate.

Sulfur

Distribution   Sulfur accounts for about 0.25 percent of body weight, or 175 mg in the adult male. It is present in all body cells, chiefly as the sulfur-containing amino acids methionine, cystine, and cysteine. Sulfur is a constituent of thiamin and biotin, two vitamins that must be present in the diet. Connective tissue, skin, nails, and hair are especially rich in sulfur.

Functions and Metabolism   Sulfur is an essential element for all animal species inasmuch as they all require the sulfur-containing amino acid methionine. Almost all of the sulfur absorbed from the intestinal tract is in organic form, principally as the sulfur amino acids. Inorganic sulfates, present in only small amounts in foods, are poorly absorbed.

Sulfur is a structurally important constituent of mucopolysaccharides such as chondroitin sulfate found in cartilage, tendons, bones, skin, and the heart valves. Sulfolipids are abundant in such tissues as liver, kidney, the salivary glands, and the white matter of the brain. Other important sulfur-containing compounds are insulin (see page 70) and heparin, an anticoagulant.

Sulfur compounds are essential in many biochemical reactions. Included among these compounds are a number of coenzymes discussed elsewhere in this text: thiamin (see page 179); biotin (see page 191); coenzyme A (see page 72); and lipoic acid (see page 196). Glutathione, an important compound in oxidation-reduction reactions, is a tripeptide of glutamic acid, cysteine, and glycine. The concentration of glutathione is especially high in the red blood cells.

The metabolism of the sulfur amino acids within the cells yields sulfuric acid, which is immediately neutralized and excreted as the inorganic salts. One of the important reactions of sulfuric acid is the conjugation with phenols, cresols, and the steroid sex hormones, which thereby detoxifies compounds that would otherwise be harmful.

Excretion   About 85 to 90 percent of the sulfur excreted in the urine is in the inorganic form, being derived almost entirely from the metabolism of the sulfur amino acids.

The remaining sulfur is in the form of organic esters produced in the detoxification reactions. The fecal excretion of sulfur is about equal to the inorganic sulfur content of the diet.

Cystinuria is a relatively rare hereditary defect in which large amounts of cystine as well as lysine, arginine, and ornithine are excreted because of a failure of renal reabsorption. Being somewhat insoluble, the cystine forms renal calculi.

Requirements and Sources   The daily requirement for sulfur has not been determined. A diet that is adequate in methionine and cystine is considered to meet the body's sulfur needs.

The sulfur content of foods depends upon the concentration of methionine and cystine. Thus, meat, poultry, milk, and eggs may be considered to be important sources.

Trace Elements or Micronutrients

Iron

Distribution   The amount of iron in the body of the adult male is about 50 mg per kg, or a total of 3.5 g; in the woman it is about 35 mg per kg, or a total of 2.3 g. All body cells contain some iron. Approximately 70 percent of the iron is in the hemoglobin, 5 percent is held as myoglobin, 5 percent is present in cellular constituents including the iron-containing enzymes, and 20 percent is stored as FERRITIN or HEMOSIDERIN by the liver, spleen, and bone marrow. In healthy men the iron reserve is about 1,000 mg, but in menstruating women it is not more than 200 to 400 mg.

Iron circulates in the plasma bound to a betaglobulin, TRANSFERRIN. The concentration of iron in the serum for men ranges from 80 to 165 μg per dl, and for women from 65 to 130 μg per dl. Normally, the saturation of transferrin with iron ranges from 20 to 40 percent.

Functions   Hemoglobin is the principal component of the red blood cells and accounts for most of the iron in the body. It acts as a carrier of oxygen from the lungs to the tissues and indirectly aids in the return of carbon dioxide to the lungs.

MYOGLOBIN is an iron—protein complex in the muscle which stores some oxygen for immediate use by the cell. Enzymes such as the catalases, the cytochromes in hydrogen ion transport (see page 72), and xanthine oxidase contain iron as an integral part of the molecule. Iron is required as a cofactor for other enzymes.

Metabolism   The amount of iron that will be absorbed from the intestinal tract is governed by (1) the body's need for iron, (2) the conditions existing in the intestinal lumen, and (3) the food mixture that is fed. (See Figure 9-3.) Iron is absorbed into the mucosal cells as (1) nonheme iron from inorganic salts in foods, and (2) as heme iron. In the latter the porphyrin ring is split open in the cell and the iron is released into the blood circulation.

The absorption of iron is meticulously regulated by the intestinal mucosa according to body need. An increase in ERYTHROPOIESIS, the formation of red blood cells, leads to withdrawal of iron from the iron–transferrin complex in the circulation, and the lowering of transferrin saturation in turn brings about an increase in the amount of iron that is absorbed. Thus, growing children, pregnant women, and anemic individuals will have a higher rate of absorption than healthy males. The absorptive mechanism in normal individuals is also highly effective in preventing an overload of iron entering the body and causing toxic reactions. Although excess iron can be absorbed, extremely large intakes would be necessary for a long period of time before toxic reactions would result.

In the acid medium of the stomach and upper duodenum ferric iron is reduced to ferrous iron, a more soluble form that is readily absorbed. Achlorhydria, observed in many elderly persons and present in pernicious anemia, reduces the absorption of iron. Likewise, the surgical removal of the portion of the stomach that produces acid will result in lower absorption of iron. The alkaline reaction of pancreatic juice reduces the solubility of iron so that little absorption takes place from the jejunum and ileum. Absorption of iron is also hindered in malabsorption syndromes, and in the presence of excess phytates.

The absorption of iron from foods varies depending on whether HEME or NONHEME IRON is consumed.[20] The composition of the rest of the meal and the status of the individual's iron stores are also major influences on iron absorption. (See Table 9-3.) An individual with moderate iron stores would be expected to absorb about 23 percent of the heme iron consumed in a meal. Non-heme iron absorption can vary from 3 percent to 8 percent in the individual with moderate iron stores depending on the presence of absorption enhancing factors.

In addition to the increase in absorption that occurs when body iron stores are depleted, the most important factors enhancing iron absorption are the amounts of ascorbic acid and meat, fish, or poultry consumed with the meal. Inhibitory factors present with the meal such as tannins from tea, phytates from cereals, and antacids are recognized, but inadequate data are available to include these factors in absorption calculations.

Transport and Utilization.   Iron in the plasma is made available from three sources: (1) absorption from the intestinal tract, (2) release from body reserves, and (3) release from the breakdown of hemoglobin that takes place constantly. Within a 24-hour period the turnover of iron is about 35 to 40 mg.[21] Only 1 to 1.5 mg of this has been available from absorption.

Iron is withdrawn from the plasma into the bone marrow for the synthesis of HEMOGLOBIN, which is a complex substance composed of a basic protein, GLOBIN, linked to a prosthetic group, HEME. The heme molecule consists of protoporphyrin with reduced iron at its center; four heme molecules together with globin make up the hemoglobin. Copper and vitamin B-6 play a catalytic role in the incorporation of iron into the protoporphyrin molecule.

The body exercises amazing economy in the use of iron. When the red blood cell has fulfilled its life cycle of about 120 days, the cell is destroyed within the spleen, liver, and other reticuloendothelial tissues. The amino acids of the globin and cell structure, and the lipids are utilized again. Heme is disintegrated to release iron once again to the circulation, and the bile pigments are synthesized from the remainder of the molecule.

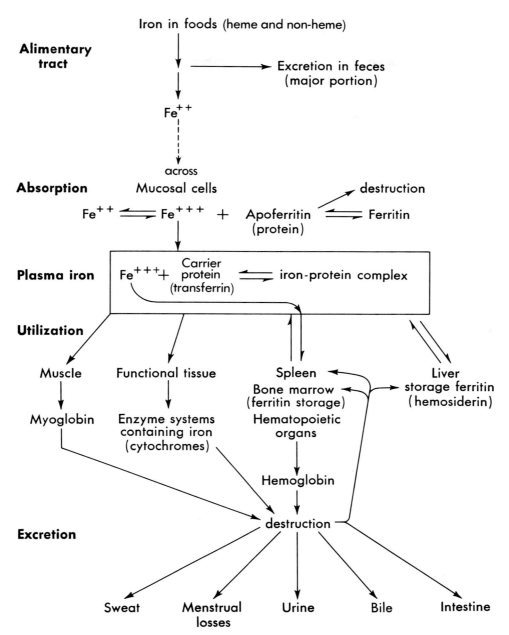

Figure 9-3. The utilization of iron.

Excretion. The daily excretion of body iron by adults is about 0.1 mg from the urine and 0.3 to 0.5 mg into the intestinal lumen. Small amounts of iron are also lost in the perspiration and by exfoliation of the skin. The iron losses through menstruation range from 0.3 to 1.0 mg on a daily basis, but about 5 percent of women have losses in excess of 1.4 mg per day.[1] Thus, the total iron losses by women are 1 to 2 mg per day.

Most of the iron in the feces represents the unabsorbed iron from the diet. A small amount of fecal iron is of endogenous origin, namely, that derived from the sloughing off of mucosal cells, bile pigments, and other digestive juices.

Daily Allowances Dietary iron is required for (1) replacement of the daily losses of all individuals; (2) an expanding blood volume and increasing amounts

Table 9-3.   Available Nonheme and Heme Iron in Different Meals*

Meal Description	Percentage of Iron Available for Absorption at Each Meal†	
	Nonheme Iron	Heme Iron

Low availability of nonheme iron
  a. <30 g (1 oz) lean, raw weight, of meat, poultry, or fish
    OR
  b. <25 mg ascorbic acid
	3	23

Medium availability of nonheme iron
  a. 30–90 g (1–3 oz) lean, raw weight, of meat, poultry, or fish
    OR
  b. 25–75 mg ascorbic acid
	5	23

High availability of nonheme iron
  a. >90 g (3 oz) lean, raw weight, of meat, poultry, or fish
    OR
  b. >75 mg ascorbic acid
    OR
  c. 30–90 g lean meat, poultry, or fish *plus* 25–75 mg ascorbic acid
	8	23

* Adapted from Monsen, E. R., et al.: "Estimation of Available Dietary Iron," *Am. J. Clin. Nutr.*, **31**:134–41, 1978.

† The factors cited here assume that a woman has a 500-mg store of iron. It is recommended that these factors be used for dietary calculations. For men with larger iron stores, the percentage of iron absorbed is lower; for women with iron stores below 500 mg the percentage of iron absorbed is higher. For appropriate factors when iron stores are known, see cited publication.

of hemoglobin in growing children; (3) replacement of the varying losses through menstruation; (4) development of the fetus and to avoid anemia in pregnant and lactating women; and (5) a reserve of iron that is available when blood loss occurs from any cause whatsoever.

The amount of iron needed by various age groups for replacement of losses and synthesis of essential iron compounds is listed in Table 9-4. Also shown are the recommended allowances of the Food and Nutrition Board. For women during pregnancy it is assumed that the diet should be supplemented with iron. Likewise, some menstruating women need supplements if they achieve their recommended intake of 15 mg. The iron content of typical diets adequate in other respects is estimated to be 6 mg per 1,000 kcal.[1] Thus, in order to get 15 mg iron, a woman would need to consume 2,500 kcal, which obviously is in excess of the energy needs of most women. One objective for setting the allowance at this level is to try to achieve iron stores in women similar to those in men.

The issue of whether or not iron intakes of less than 18 mg, which may be sufficient to maintain normal hemoglobin status but not iron stores, are detrimental is the basis for the controversy that has long been associated with the allowance for women. Whereas some authorities believe the allowance is unrealistic, others strongly support an allowance of 18 mg as a desirable nutritional goal in spite of the difficulty in achieving the allowance by diet.

Food Sources   Meat, fish, and poultry are good sources of iron and contribute approximately 30 percent of the iron available for consumption in the United States.[18] Liver is a particularly rich source of iron. Other foods having a relatively high iron content include whole grain and enriched cereals, legumes, green leafy vegetables, eggs, and dried fruit. Cereal and grain products contribute about 32 percent of the iron available for consumption. Part of this iron is added as enrichment and fortification. (See page 262.) Depending on the type of cereal product, the form of iron added is usually metallic iron or ferrous sulfate. The bioavailability of both forms is considered acceptable. An attempt several years ago to require an increase in the amount of iron used in enrichment was defeated partly because of lack of evidence that such a measure would substantially improve the intake of those at risk of deficiency. There also was concern that some persons in the population might become at risk of excess intake.[22]

Much more research is required to determine the

Table 9-4.   Daily Iron Requirements*

	Absorbed Iron Requirement (mg/day)	Recommended Dietary Allowance† (mg/day)
Men and nonmenstruating women	0.5–1	10
Menstruating women	0.7–2	15
Pregnant women	2.0–4.8	15+‡
Adolescents	1.0–2	12–15
Children	0.4–1	10
Infants	0.5–1.5	6–10

*Adapted from Committee on Iron Deficiency, Council on Foods and Nutrition: "Iron Deficiency in the United States," *JAMA*, **203**:407–14, February 5, 1968; and Food and Nutrition Board: *Recommended Dietary Allowances*, 10th ed. National Academy of Sciences—National Research Council, Washington D.C., 1989.

†Assuming an absorption of 10 percent.

‡This amount of iron cannot be derived from diet and should be met by iron supplementation during pregnancy.

availability of iron in foods, especially those of plant origin, as well as the conditions that enhance or detract from that availability. The iron contained in lean meats, poultry, and fish is present as about 40 percent heme iron, which is absorbed intact. The remaining 60 percent of iron in animal tissues and the iron in plant foods is nonheme iron. Even though absorption of nonheme iron is lower than that of heme iron, the amount of nonheme iron consumed is much greater. Thus, nonheme iron usually makes the larger contribution to available iron in the average diet.

Cooking procedures may also influence the amount of iron that is actually ingested. Some mineral salts are leached out when large amounts of water are used and subsequently discarded. Cooking foods, particularly those with a high acid content, in iron pots or skillets increases their iron content.[23]

Calculation of Available Dietary Iron Absorption availability of iron can be estimated by the computation of five variables for *each meal*.[24]

1. Total iron consumed from each food item in the meal (from food composition table),
2. Estimating heme iron (40 percent of total iron in animal tissues, that is, meat, poultry, and fish),
3. Estimating nonheme iron (variable 1 minus variable 2),
4. Estimating total amount of vitamin C in the meal as consumed (estimated from food composition table),
5. Estimating total amount of meat, poultry, and fish consumed. Each meal can then be determined to have high, medium, or low nonheme iron avail-

ability and the total iron for the meal can be calculated. (See Tables 9-3 and 9-5.) For these estimation purposes, moderate iron stores are assumed. At these storage levels it is assumed that 23 percent of the heme iron is absorbed. The heme iron absorption does not vary, as it is not influenced by the composition of the meal.

Effects of Imbalance If dietary intakes of iron are low in relationship to need, depletion of iron stores will occur followed by a decrease in serum iron and transferrin saturation. Clinical symptoms may not be present in the early stages of iron deficiency or may be nonspecific such as weakness and easy fatigue. Severe iron deficiency leads to anemia and various clinical manifestations. Because iron deficiency is the most common cause of nutritional anemia, it will be described in greater detail in the separate section on anemias that follows.

Iron imbalance involving excess rather than deficient iron occurs in HEMOSIDEROSIS and HEMOCHROMATOSIS, two disorders of iron metabolism in which there are large deposits of iron in the liver, pancreas, and other organs that store iron. The term hemosiderosis generally is reserved for excess iron stores without tissue damage. In hemochromatosis the excess iron produces complications such as cirrhosis of the liver or diabetes. One form of hemochromatosis appears to be a congenital disorder in which iron is absorbed much more efficiently than normal.

Iron overload has been shown to affect a high proportion of the adult Bantu population in South Africa and is believed to be caused by an overload of die-

Table 9-5.   Sample Calculation of Iron Availability from a Meal

Food	Weight (g)	Ascorbic Acid (mg)	Total Iron (mg)	Heme Factor	Heme Iron (mg)	Nonheme Iron (mg)
Roast pork, 2 ounces*	56	0	2.2	0.4	0.9	1.3
Mashed potato, ½ cup	105	10.5	0.4			0.4
Buttered carrots, ½ cup	78	4.5	0.45			0.45
Dinner roll, 1	26		0.5			0.5
Milk, 2 percent, 1 cup	244	2	0.1			0.1
Cantaloupe, ⅓ 5-in. melon*	180	60	0.7			0.7
		77	4.35		0.9	3.45
High availability of iron*						
Percentage of iron absorbed					23	8
Amount of iron absorbed					0.21	0.28
Total available for absorption (0.21 + 0.28)						0.49

* If a fruit low in ascorbic acid were substituted for the cantaloupe in this example, the rating would be medium availability.

tary iron.[25] Bantu men commonly ingest 30 mg iron daily and frequently as much as 100 mg per day. The beer that they drink is fermented in iron pots, and likewise the acid-fermented cereal foods and sour porridge are cooked in these pots. The resulting foods have a high iron content.

Hemosiderosis also occurs when there is abnormal destruction of the red blood cells as in hemolytic anemia. It may also occur following prolonged iron therapy when it is not needed.

Anemias and Iron Deficiency

General Characteristics of Anemias ANEMIA is a condition in which there is a reduction in the total circulating hemoglobin. Anemias may be described biochemically in terms of lowered hemoglobin, hematocrit (packed red cell volume), and number of red blood cells. Normal values for these blood indices are listed in Table 9-6. Additional useful information can be obtained by expressing these indices in relationship to each other. Thus, the average volume or size of red blood cells is indicated by the mean corpuscular volume (MCV) calculated as follows:

$$MCV = \frac{\text{packed red cell volume } (\%) \times 10}{\text{red cell count } (\times 10^{12}/\text{liter})}$$

The mean corpuscular hemoglobin (MCH) describes the amount of hemoglobin contained in the cells, and the mean corpuscular hemoglobin concentration (MCHC) the hemoglobin concentration in the "average" red cell.

Anemias are also differentiated on the basis of the size and appearance of the red blood cells: normo-cytic, macrocytic or microcytic; nucleated or nonnucleated; normochromic, hyperchromic, or hypochromic. Other laboratory tests may be used to aid in the identification of the cause(s) of the anemia.

Etiology. Anemias may be caused by several factors including a blood loss, bone marrow failure, increased destruction of red blood cells and deficiencies of nutrients that play a critical role in hemoglobin and red cell synthesis. Vitamin B-12 and folacin are required for the synthesis of DNA, which is essential for the growth and normal division of cells. When either or both of these vitamins are deficient, fewer red blood cells can be produced, and they are released into the circulation as large, nucleated cells called megaloblasts. (See also Chapter 13, pages 193 and 195.) Hemoglobin synthesis requires a constant source of iron for the formation of heme and of protein for the formation of globin. The rate of synthesis can be no more rapid than the supply of iron. Anemias seen in severe deficiencies of other nutrients such as copper and ascorbic acid may be related to their role in the body's utilization of iron.

Symptoms. Mild anemias diagnosed by laboratory studies are not closely associated with clinical symptoms. When anemias become more severe, however, the symptoms are more consistent and include skin pallor, weakness, easy fatigability, headaches, dizziness, sensitivity to cold, paresthesia, and reduced physical work capacity as determined by treadmill testing. Cheilosis, glossitis, loss of appetite, and loss of gastrointestinal tone with accompanying symptoms of distress are seen in severe anemias. Concave "spoon"

Table 9-6. **Red Cell Values in Normal Adults***

	Male	Female
Red blood cell count, × 10¹²/liter	4.5–6.3	4.2–5.5
Hemoglobin, g/dl	14.0–18.0	12.0–16.0
Volume of packed red cells (VPRC) or hematocrit (Hct), percent	40–54	37–47
Reticulocytes, percent	0.8–2.5	0.8–4.1
Mean corpuscular volume (MCV), femtoliters (f1 = 10⁻¹⁵ liters)†	80–94	
Mean corpuscular hemoglobin (MCH), pg/cell†	26–32	
Mean corpuscular hemoglobin concentration (MCHC), g/dl RBCs†	32–36	

* Adapted from Wintrobe, M. M., et al.: *Clinical Hematology*, 8th ed. Lea & Febiger, Philadelphia, 1981.

† $MCV = \dfrac{\text{hematocrit (percent)} \times 10}{\text{red cell count } (\times 10^{12}/\text{liter})}$ $MCHC = \dfrac{\text{hemoglobin (g/dl)} \times 100}{\text{hematocrit (percent)}}$

$MCH = \dfrac{\text{hemoglobin (g/dl)}}{\text{red cell count } (\times 10^{12}/\text{liter})}$

fingernails (koilonychia) with longitudinal ridging of the nails is sometimes present. With increasing severity of anemia, the oxygenation of tissues is reduced—hence the feeling of fatigue. The heart rate increases, palpitation occurs, and there is shortness of breath.

Iron-Deficiency Anemia Iron-deficiency anemia is widely prevalent throughout the world. Generally the incidence is high in preschool children, adolescents, and women in the child-bearing years. It also occurs more frequently among persons of low economic status. In some developing countries iron deficiency has been reported in 50 percent of adult menstruating women, more than half of whom have detectable anemia.[26] By contrast, the prevalence of iron deficiency in women in developed countries is 10 percent. The Second National Health and Nutrition Examination Survey (1976–1980) found that approximately 6 percent of infants, teenage girls, and young women had hemoglobin values below the 95 percent reference range. Iron deficiency appeared to be the major cause of the low hemoglobin.[27]

Diagnosis. Iron deficiency generally follows a sequence that makes certain tests useful in its diagnosis. First, the iron stores become depleted accompanied by a drop in serum ferritin concentrations. As the iron reserves are used up, the serum transferrin level increases, followed by a decrease in serum iron. These changes result in a decrease in transferrin saturation and indicate that inadequate iron is being supplied to tissues. The increase in red cell free protoporphyrin that also occurs likewise indicates a deficient iron supply to the developing red cell. Finally, the hematocrit and hemoglobin concentration fall and the red cells are pale and reduced in size. Thus, the designation for the anemia is microcytic, hypochromic.

Laboratory values associated with severe iron-deficiency anemia are as follows:[28]

serum iron, less than 50 μg per dl
iron-binding capacity, more than 400 mg per dl
transferrin saturation, less than 15 percent
serum ferritin, less than 10 μg per dl.

In mild iron-deficiency anemia serum ferritin is usually diminished but changes in the other constituents are not necessarily seen. In this stage, microcytic, hypochromic cells are not characteristic.

Etiology. Among the factors to be considered as initiating iron-deficiency anemia are these:

1. Blood loss (most common cause in adults)
   a. Accidental hemorrhage
   b. Chronic diseases, such as tuberculosis, ulcers or intestinal disorder, when accompanied by hemorrhage
   c. Excessive menstrual losses
   d. Excessive blood donation
   e. Parasites such as hookworm
   f. In infants, introduction of whole milk before about 6 months
2. Deficiency of iron in the diet during period of accelerated demand
   a. Infancy—rapidly expanding blood volume
   b. Adolescence—rapid growth, and onset of menses in girls
   c. Pregnancy and lactation
3. Inadequate absorption of iron
   a. Diarrhea, as in sprue, pellagra
   b. Lack of acid secretion by the stomach
   c. Antacid therapy in chronic renal disease
4. Nutrition deficiencies such as severe protein depletion
   a. Protein-calorie malnutrition

Treatment. For iron-deficiency anemia the primary emphasis in treatment is a supplement of iron salts such as ferrous sulfate, gluconate, or fumarate. Oral therapy is as effective as parenteral therapy except where there is severe interference with absorption as in ulcerative colitis or regional enteritis. Some individuals have an initial intolerance to iron salts but usually become adjusted to the medication. It is helpful to take the salts after meals.

Iodine

Distribution and Function About one third of the iodine in the adult body, variously estimated from 25 to 50 mg, is found in the thyroid gland, where it is stored in the form of THYROGLOBULIN. The concentration of iodine in the thyroid gland is about 2,500 times as great as that in any other tissues.

The only known function of iodine is as a constituent of the thyroid hormones, THYROXINE (T_4) and TRIIODOTHYRONINE (T_3). These hormones are composed of two molecules of tyrosine combined with three or four atoms of iodine. The thyroid hormones regulate the rate of oxidation within the cells and in so doing influence physical and mental growth, the functioning of the nervous and muscle tissues, circulatory activity, and the metabolism of all nutrients.

Metabolism Iodine is ingested in foods as inorganic iodides and as organic compounds. In the digestive tract iodine is split from organic compounds and is rapidly absorbed as inorganic iodide. The degree of absorption is dependent upon the level of circulating thyroid hormone.

Iodine is transported by the circulation as free iodide and as PROTEIN-BOUND IODINE. The protein-bound fraction (PBI) is sensitive to changes in the level of thyroid activity; it rises during pregnancy and with hypertrophy of the gland and falls with hypofunction of the gland. Another measure of thyroid activity is the uptake of radioactive iodine 24 hours after a measured dose of ^{131}I has been given. Tests using PBI and ^{131}I uptake to evaluate thyroid function have been replaced almost entirely by newer assays that determine blood T_3 and T_4 concentrations directly.

Thyroid activity is controlled by the thyroid-stimulating hormone (TSH) secreted by the anterior lobe of the pituitary. TSH synthesis and release in turn are stimulated by thyroid-releasing hormone (TRH), which is synthesized in the hypothalamus and secreted into the pituitary. When the blood concentration of thyroid hormones is low, TSH and presumably TRH secretion are stimulated, leading to increased activity of the thyroid gland. By this action the thyroid gland removes iodide from the circulation, concentrates it and eventually uses it to synthesize T_3 and T_4.

After thyroid hormones are used in the body tissues for cellular oxidation, iodine is released into the circulation. About one third of the released iodine is again incorporated into thyroid hormones, and the remainder is excreted in the urine.

Daily Allowances The recommended allowance for men and women over the age of 11 is 150 μg. Infants should receive 40 to 50 μg during the first year, and children up to 10 years, 70 to 120 μg. The allowances in pregnancy and lactation are 175 and 200 μg, respectively.[1]

Sources The most important dietary source of iodine is iodized salt. The concentration of iodine used in salt is 1 part sodium or potassium iodide per 10,000 parts of salt. One-fourth teaspoon of salt (1.25 g) would furnish about 95 μg iodine. About one half the table salt sold in the United States is iodized. Salt used in the processing of food and bulk salt for institutional use are not likely to be iodized.[1]

Seaweed, saltwater fish, and shellfish contain important amounts of iodine for people who consume these foods on a regular basis. The iodine content of eggs, dairy products, and meats depends upon the io-

dine content of the animal's diet. Some milk may have an especially high content, partly because of the use of iodine supplements for cattle. Vegetables grown on iodine-rich soils near the seacoast are good sources of iodine; those grown on iodine-poor soils, generally inland, contain little iodine. Because of widespread food distribution, the iodine content of foods purchased in stores is variable and unpredictable. Although a recent analysis of the iodine content of representative diets in the United States showed the average intake to exceed recommended allowances, authorities generally agree that the use of iodized salt should continue to be recommended.

Effects of Deficiency ENDEMIC GOITER, the iodine-deficiency disease, occurs in those areas in which the iodine content of the soil is so low that insufficient iodine is obtained through food and water, and when no provision is made for supplying iodized salt. Among the areas of iodine-poor soils are the Great Lakes region, the Pacific Northwest, Switzerland, Central American countries, mountainous areas of South America, New Zealand, and the Himalayas. The World Health Organization has estimated that up to 200 million people throughout the world may be affected. The iodine intake in the United States is generally adequate, and deficiency is no longer considered to be a problem.[29]

Lack of iodine leads to an increase in the size and number of epithelial cells in the thyroid gland and thus an enlargement of the gland. This condition known as simple or endemic goiter, presents no other abnormal physical findings. The basal metabolism remains normal. The deficiency is more prevalent in females than males and is more frequent during adolescence and pregnancy.

The most urgent reason for stressing iodine as a preventive measure is not the goiter itself but the cretinism which is its ultimate sequel in areas severely deficient in iodine. Cretinism occurs in the infant when the pregnant woman is so severely depleted that she cannot supply iodine for the development of the fetus. CRETINISM is characterized by a low basal metabolism, muscular flabbiness and weakness, dry skin, enlarged tongue, thick lips, arrest of skeletal development, and severe mental retardation. Thyroid hormone given early enough to the infant results in marked improvement of physical development; mental retardation may be less severe, but any damage that has occurred to the central nervous system cannot be reversed. Endemic cretinism is rare or nonexistent in the United States today.

Goitrogens Certain substances called GOITROGENS are known to interfere with the use of thyroxine and will produce goiters, at least in experimental animals, even though the iodine intake would normally be adequate. Goitrogens are present in the *Brassica* family, which includes a number of widely used vegetables—cabbage, turnips, rutabagas, radishes, cauliflower, and Brussels sprouts. Goitrogens are also present in peanuts and oilseeds, such as rape seed. Oilseed proteins may become more important in our food supply as these products are developed as alternative protein sources. The substances are inactivated by cooking, and there is currently no evidence that goiters in endemic regions are caused by them.

Zinc

Distribution in the Body About 2 to 3 g zinc is present in the adult body. It is distributed widely in all tissues but not evenly. High concentrations are found in the eye, especially the iris and retina, in the liver, bone, prostate and prostatic secretions, and in the hair. In the blood about 85 percent of the zinc is in the red blood cells; however, each leukocyte contains about 25 times as much zinc as each red blood cell.

Functions Zinc is essential for all living organisms. Its numerous functions include the following:

1. Integral part of at least 70 enzymes that belong to a large group known as metalloenzymes, which include the following:

   CARBONIC ANHYDRASE, which is as essential to the transport of carbon dioxide to the lungs as hemoglobin is to the transport of oxygen

   LACTIC DEHYDROGENASE involved in the interconversion of pyruvic and lactic acid in the glycolytic pathway

   ALKALINE PHOSPHATASE required in bone metabolism; concentration especially high in white blood cells

   CARBOXYPEPTIDASE and AMINOPEPTIDASE, which bring about removal of the terminal carboxyl and amino groups in the digestion of proteins

   ALCOHOL DEHYDROGENASE in the liver, which oxidizes not only ethanol but other primary and secondary alcohols as well, including methanol and ethylene glycol, thus serving as a major detoxifying mechanism

2. Cofactor in the synthesis of DNA and RNA, and thus of proteins. In this role it is especially important in cellular systems that undergo rapid turnover, as in the gastrointestinal tract including the taste buds. Thus, zinc plays a role in the sensory systems that control food intake.

3. Mobilization of vitamin A from the liver to maintain normal concentrations in the blood circulation

4. Enhancement of the action of follicle-stimulating hormone and luteinizing hormone

5. Essential for normal cellular immune functions

6. Necessary for spermatogenesis and normal testicular function

7. Contributing factor in the stabilization of membrane structure

Metabolism Absorption of zinc takes place primarily from the duodenum and jejunum. The presence of a zinc-binding compound found in pancreatic secretions and human breast milk facilitates absorption.[30] Absorbed zinc can be transported through the intestinal cell into the portal bloodstream, it can enter into cell functions, or it can combine with a sulfur-rich protein called *thionein* to form *metallothionein*. This protein appears to have an important role in the homeostatic regulation of zinc absorption. Zinc absorption is impaired by high intakes of calcium, vitamin D, phytate, and possibly dietary fiber.

Zinc is transported in the plasma, mostly bound to albumin. The normal serum concentration is about 80 to 140 μg per dl. The rate of turnover in the liver, pancreas, kidney, and pituitary is rapid. Zinc is excreted primarily in pancreatic and intestinal juices. The normal urinary loss is about 500 μg per day.

Recommended Allowances As the importance of zinc in human nutrition has become better understood, increasing numbers of studies are being conducted to determine zinc requirement. The present recommended allowance is 15 mg for males, 12 mg for females, 5 mg for infants, 10 mg for children, 15 mg during pregnancy, and 19 mg for the lactating woman.[1]

Food Sources Data on food composition are sparse, and there is little information on the variability from sample to sample. Rich sources include oyster, liver, high-protein foods, and whole-grain cereals. Beef, lamb, and pork contain three to four times as much as fish; and dark meat of chicken furnishes about three times as much as light meat. Legumes, peanuts, and peanut butter are good sources, but fruits and most vegetables are poor sources. The zinc in plant proteins is less available than that in animal proteins.[30] Vegetarian diets and low-protein diets are likely to be low in zinc. (See Table A-2).

Deficiency The first description of human deficiency of zinc was reported from Iran and Egypt.[31] Dwarfed adolescent boys in those countries were observed to consume a diet in which more than half of the calories were furnished by unleavened whole-grain bread. Although the whole-grain cereals are good sources of zinc, practically all of the mineral is tied up by the high concentration of phytate in the unleavened bread. In addition to growth failure, other abnormalities were hypogonadism, enlarged liver, and severe anemia. Serum zinc levels were about 50 μg per dl. With the addition of zinc to the diet there was considerable improvement in growth and development of the sexual organs.

As research on zinc status has accumulated, the list of clinical manifestations associated with zinc deficiency has become long and varied: growth retardation, hypogonadism in males, poor appetite, mental lethargy, delayed wound healing, increased susceptibility to infections, abnormal dark adaptation, skin lesions, loss of hair, and disturbances in taste and smell acuity. HYPOGEUSIA is a decrease in taste acuity; DYSGEUSIA is an unpleasant or perverted taste. Reports of marginal zinc status in the United States are becoming more frequent. Several studies have found low plasma and hair concentrations of zinc in children of short stature, poor nutritional status and with hypogeusia.[32,33] Zinc supplementation was accompanied by an increase in the linear growth velocity of children with evidence of mild zinc deficiency.[34] Problems in zinc nutriture have been identified in patients with malabsorption, kidney disease, pancreatic insufficiency, sickle cell anemia, and inflammatory bowel disease.[31,35-38] Acrodermatitis enteropathica is a rare genetic disorder occurring in infants characterized by severe dermatitis, chronic diarrhea, emotional disturbances and growth retardation. The condition appears to be due to a defect in zinc absorption.

The identification of zinc deficiency is hindered by lack of satisfactory methods to evaluate zinc nutriture. Plasma zinc levels may reflect dietary intake but do not necessarily reflect tissue concentrations of zinc. Measurement of hair concentrations of zinc frequently are made, but a number of variables may influence the results, so that hair zinc alone is not considered an acceptable basis for evaluating zinc status. Future tests may include leukocyte zinc concentrations, salivary zinc, or measurement of activity of zinc-containing enzymes.

Toxicity In spite of no evidence to support the value of increased zinc intake in persons with adequate zinc nutriture, zinc supplements have become popular for a variety of purposes, including the treatment of acne and improvement of sexual function. Fortunately zinc is one of the least toxic of the trace elements. Zinc salts in very large amounts, 60 to 120 times the recommended allowances, will induce vomiting, cramps, and diarrhea within 3 to 12 hours, but the symptoms subside shortly. High intakes of zinc interfere with the utilization of copper and have been shown to have a deleterious effect on copper nutriture.[39]

Copper

Distribution The presence of copper in blood was first recognized in 1875, but the nutritional significance was not established until Hart and Elvehjem at the University of Wisconsin found that traces of copper were essential for the formation of hemoglobin. The body of the human adult contains about 100 to 150 mg copper. Traces of copper are found in all tissues, but by far the highest concentrations are found in the liver, brain, heart, and kidney. In the fetus and at birth the levels in these organs are several times higher, and they decrease during the first year.

Metabolism Copper is absorbed from the stomach and from the upper gastrointestinal tract.

Absorbed copper is readily taken up by the liver and other tissues. Copper in the liver is then incorporated into CERULOPLASMIN and released into the plasma and bile or stored temporarily in the liver. About 95 percent of the copper in blood plasma is firmly bound in ceruloplasmin, and 5 percent is loosely bound to albumin and amino acids. Copper in red blood cells is mostly in the form of superoxide dismutase, a copper-containing enzyme. Almost all of the excretion of copper is in the feces, chiefly through the excretion of bile. Molybdenum, zinc, and cadmium are antagonistic to copper; thus, an increased intake of these elements increases the requirement for copper. Large amounts of ascorbic acid impair copper absorption and have been shown to decrease plasma ceruloplasmin levels.

Functions Copper is the essential element of several enzymes involved in oxidative reactions:

1. Ceruloplasmin is necessary for the oxidation of iron in the plasma for binding to transferrin and thus plays a role in transport of iron to sites where

hemoglobin synthesis can occur. It may also be involved in mobilization of iron from storage sites in the liver.

2. Cytochrome c oxidase, another copper-containing protein, is one of the enzymes involved in the electron transport system and thus is essential for energy production. (See page 72.)

3. Superoxide dismutase contains two copper and two zinc atoms per molecule. This enzyme has an important role in protecting the cell against oxidative damage.

4. Lysyloxidase is involved in the synthesis of elastin and collagen. Consequently connective tissues, including those in bones and blood vessels, may be defective in the presence of copper deficiency.

5. Tyrosinase participates in the conversion of tyrosine to melanin, which is essential to the pigmentation process. Other amine oxidases involved in the metabolism of norepinephrine and serotonin may be copper dependent.

Estimated Safe and Adequate Intake   The intake of copper considered adequate and safe for adults is 1.5 to 3 mg per day. For infants an intake of 0.4 to 1 mg is considered satisfactory. One to 2.5 mg per day is the suggested intake for children, increasing with age.[1]

Food Sources   Typical diets furnish from less than 1 to 5 mg copper. The copper content of foods is somewhat dependent on the copper content of soil. Among rich sources are organ meats, shellfish, chocolate, whole-grain cereals, legumes, and nuts. Milk is a poor source. (See Table A-2.)

Effects of Imbalance   Dietary deficiency of copper is not common in humans, although recent surveys have shown that many persons appear to have intakes below the recommended levels. Low blood levels of copper have been observed in kwashiorkor, the nephrotic syndrome, and sprue, and occasionally in patients with iron-deficiency anemia or treated with total parenteral nutrition. Severe copper deficiency is characterized by an anemia similar to that seen in iron deficiency. Neutropenia (decreased neutrophils in the blood), leukopenia, neurologic abnormalities, decreased skin pigmentation, and demineralization of bones may also be present. Copper deficiency in some animals produces hypercholesterolemia and damage to blood vessels. It has been proposed that low copper intake in humans may contribute to the development of atherosclerosis.[40] Menke's disease, or *kinky hair* syndrome, is a rare congenital disorder in copper me-

tabolism occurring in male infants. Symptoms include failure to thrive, mental retardation, sparse "steely" hair, and changes in elastic fibers in blood vessels. Whereas some symptoms resemble those of copper deficiency, anemia and neutropenia usually are not present.

In excessive amounts copper is toxic. A rare hereditary disorder known as Wilson's disease is characterized by a marked reduction of blood ceruloplasmin and greatly increased deposits of copper in the liver, brain, and other organs. The excess copper in these tissues leads to hepatitis, lenticular degeneration, renal malfunction, and neurologic disorders.

Fluorine

Distribution and Function   Fluoride occurs normally in the body primarily as a calcium salt in the bones and teeth. Small amounts of fluoride bring about striking reductions in tooth decay, probably because the tooth enamel is made more resistant to the action of acids produced in the mouth by bacteria.

Carefully controlled studies in a number of cities for more than 10 years have established that fluoridation of the water supplies at a level of 1 part fluoride per million (1 ppm or 1 mg/liter) may be expected to reduce the incidence of dental caries in children by approximately 50 to 60 percent. Several thousand communities in the United States have now initiated water fluoridation as an effective public health measure. Children who have been drinking fluoridated water since infancy show the greatest benefits; those who begin the ingestion of fluoridated water in later school years are helped to a lesser extent.

Fluorides may be involved in some way in the maintenance of bone structure. Some studies have shown that osteoporosis occurs less frequently in elderly persons who live in areas supplied with fluoridated water.[41] The fluoride salts of calcium are less readily lost from bone during immobilization or following the menopause.

Metabolism   Fluorides are absorbed readily from the gastrointestinal tract. They replace the hydroxyl groups in the calcium phosporus salts of bones and teeth to form fluoroapatite. The fluoride crystals are less readily resorbed than are crystals of hydroxyapatite. Most of the fluoride ingested is excreted in the urine. An average daily excretion is about 3 mg.

Estimated Safe and Adequate Intake   The intake of fluorine considered adequate and safe for adults is

1.5 to 4.0 mg per day. For children and adolescents a range of 0.5 to 2.5 mg per day is recommended, depending on age. Infants should have a daily intake of 0.1 to 1.0 mg.[1] For breast-fed infants, supplementation may be considered.

Food Sources Fluoride occurs in all soils, water supplies, plants, and animals, and is a normal constituent of the diet. The amounts present are in direct correlation with the fluoride concentration of water and soils. In low-fluoride areas the daily diet furnishes only 0.3 mg; in high-fluoride areas the daily intake from food is about 3.1 mg.[1] Six glasses of water containing 1 ppm will provide an additional 1.2 mg.

Effects of Excess Chronic dental FLUOROSIS results when the concentration of fluoride in drinking water is in excess of 2.5 ppm. The teeth become MOTTLED; that is, the tooth enamel becomes dull and unglazed with some pitting. At higher concentrations of fluoride some dark-brown stains appear. Although esthetically undesirable, such teeth are surprisingly free of dental caries.

Large excesses of fluorine—20 to 80 mg daily for several years—lead to skeletal fluorosis, which is characterized by chalky, brittle bones that fracture easily.

Other Trace Elements

Manganese, molybdenum, selenium, chromium, and cobalt are essential trace elements. Their principal functions are as integral constituents of enzymes or as activators of enzymes.

For these minerals, estimated safe and adequate daily intake ranges have been recommended because of sparse experimental data on the human requirements. Data on the distribution and the availability of these elements in foods are also sparse. A diet that is adequate in other nutrients, and that does not contain a high proportion of refined foods, is considered to satisfy the needs for these trace elements. Dietary deficiency is not likely in human beings.

Experimental studies on animals have shown that the mineral elements are closely interrelated. Thus, an excess of one element may increase the need for another. Excessive amounts of trace elements produce symptoms of toxicity in animals.

Manganese About 2.5 to 7 mg manganese is supplied in the daily diet of the adult.[1] Seeds of plants— nuts, legumes, and whole-grain cereals—are good

sources, but animal foods are much lower in their content.

The intake of manganese considered adequate and safe for people over 11 years is 2.5 to 5.0 mg per day. Recommendations range from 0.5 to 3.0 mg per day for infants and younger children.[1]

Manganese is rather poorly absorbed from the small intestine by a mechanism similar to that for the absorption of iron. It is loosely bound to a protein and transported as TRANSMANGANIN. Tissues that are rich in mitochondria take up manganese readily from the blood. A dynamic equilibrium exists between the intracellular and extracellular manganese. Most of the metabolic manganese is excreted into the intestine as a constituent of bile, but much of this is again reabsorbed, indicating an effective body conservation. Very little manganese is excreted in the urine.

Studies on experimental animals have shown that manganese is required for normal bone growth and development, normal lipid metabolism, reproduction, and regulation of nervous irritability. Manganese is an activator for a number of enzymes, including arginase, which is required for the formation of urea; a number of peptidases that bring about hydrolysis of proteins in the intestine; enzymes involved in the synthesis of mucopolysaccharides, which are important for bone development; and an enzyme that regulates utilization of pyruvate. Manganese can substitute for magnesium in a number of enzymes required for oxidative phosphorylation.

Molybdenum A precise balance of molybdenum is essential for plant and animal life. Nitrogen-fixing bacteria require this metal for their growth, and thus the synthesis of proteins and ultimately of animal life are affected. A deficiency of molybdenum will adversely affect the growth of legumes. Also, in molybdenum deficiency the growth of certain fungi that produce mycotoxins is favored. These mycotoxins have been shown to be carcinogenic in animals. (See also Chapter 17.)

The concentration of molybdenum in food is highly variable. Intake has been estimated at between 0.1 and 0.46 mg.[1] Molybdenum is found especially in legumes, whole-grain cereals, and organ meats. It is absorbed as molybdate and is concentrated especially in the liver, adrenal, and kidney. It is a cofactor for a number of flavoprotein enzymes and is found in XANTHINE OXIDASE, an enzyme that brings about the oxidation of xanthine to uric acid. High molybdenum intakes have been linked to goutlike symptoms in a human population.[1] The estimated safe and adequate intake for people over 7 years is 50 to 150 μg with

15 to 150 μg suggested for infants and younger children.[1] Most diets of mixed foods should supply adequate amounts of molybdenum. One case of deficiency was reported in a patient during prolonged intravenous feeding.[42]

Molybdenum competes with copper for the same metabolic sites, and an excess of molybdenum will result in symptoms of copper deficiency. Cattle grazing on lands that have a high molybdenum content develop a condition known as *teart*, characterized by diarrhea, brittle bones, loss of pigmentation, and weight loss. When the sulfate content of the diet is increased, the symptoms of toxicity are avoided inasmuch as the excretion of molybdenum is increased. This affords an interesting example of the interrelationship of sulfur, copper and molybdenum.

Selenium Some selenium is present in all tissues, with the highest concentrations in kidney, liver, spleen, pancreas, and testes. In whole blood the average concentration of selenium is about 25 μg per dl.

For many years it has been known that selenium and vitamin E could spare each other. Both nutrients can behave as antioxidants and have a role in preventing cellular damage by lipid peroxidases. Lipid peroxides are strong oxidizing agents that can injure cell membranes. Selenium is an integral component of the enzyme GLUTATHIONE PEROXIDASE, which is believed to deactivate lipid peroxides. It is hypothesized that vitamin E functions to prevent the formation of these peroxides. Selenium also functions in the oxidative phosphorylation of energy compounds.

Selenium occurs in food mostly as organic compounds in which it is combined with sulfur-containing amino acids, methionine or cysteine. Meat and seafoods are rich sources of selenium. The selenium content of plant foods varies considerably depending on the soil concentration. Regions with low selenium are in the northeastern, Pacific northwest, and extreme southeastern United States, eastern Finland, parts of New Zealand and much of the People's Republic of China.[43] Cereals generally are a good source of selenium, and unlike some elements there is relatively little loss in the milling of grains. Vegetables and fruits are poor sources. The concentration of selenium in foods correlates closely with the protein content.

The recommended dietary allowance ranges from 30 to 70 μg for people over the age of 7 years. For infants and younger children, an intake of 10 to 20 μg is suggested. Diets in the United States provide a range of 85 to 129 μg per day without difficulty.[1]

It has been known for many years that some people have very low intakes of selenium, but a deficiency of selenium in humans has been documented only recently. Keshan disease, a condition characterized by abnormalities in the heart muscle, claimed the lives of thousands of children in China each year until it was discovered that selenium supplements are extremely effective in reducing its prevalence. Although a second factor may be involved, this conquest of Keshan disease is considered one of the most significant public health achievements of this century.[44] Selenium deficiency also has been identified in patients fed intravenously for long periods of time.[45]

Excess selenium is toxic. Many cattle grazing in areas in which the soil has a high selenium content suffer from "alkali disease" characterized by stiffness, blindness, deformity of the hooves, loss of hair and sometimes death. The amount of selenium needed to cause toxicity in humans is not known, but habitual intakes greater than 0.2 mg per day are not recommended.[1]

Selenium has been of particular interest in relationship to cancer. Limited epidemiologic evidence suggests that the risk of certain types of cancer is inversely related to selenium intake. A growing body of experimental data indicate that pharmacologic amounts of selenium can inhibit carcinogenesis in some animal models. Much more research is needed, however, to establish the value of selenium, particularly amounts exceeding usual dietary intake, in preventing cancer. Because of the potential for toxicity, indiscriminate, unsupervised use of selenium supplements for cancer prevention is strongly advised against.

Chromium The adult body contains about 5 mg chromium. There are high concentrations in the hair, spleen, kidney, and testes, and lower concentrations in the heart, pancreas, lungs, and brain. The plasma chromium is about 3 parts per billion. With age there is a decline in body chromium, possibly caused by an accumulated dietary deficit. Chromium functions in the body primarily in the form of the GLUCOSE TOLERANCE FACTOR (GTF), an organic compound containing glycine, glutamic acid, cysteine, and niacin. The absorption of the trivalent chromium in GTF is about 10 to 25 percent; only 1 percent of inorganic chromium is absorbed.

Glucose tolerance factor is essential for the efficient use of insulin. It appears to facilitate the attachment of insulin to cell membranes, ultimately enhancing the uptake of glucose by the cells[46]. It also stimulates fatty acid and cholesterol synthesis. It has been found to be associated with RNA and may have a role in protein synthesis. Chromium is also an activator of several enzymes.

The estimated safe and adequate intake ranges from 50 to 200 μg chromium per day for people over the age of 7 years. For infants and younger children, an intake of 10 to 120 μg is suggested.[1]

Diets in the United States furnish about 50 to 100 μg chromium,[1] a level that is lower than in Italy, Egypt, South Africa, and India. Yeast, beer, liver, whole-grain cereals and breads, meat, and cheese are good sources. The milling of grains removes up to 83 percent of chromium. Milk, white flour and bread, chicken breast, fish and vegetables are low in chromium. Even diets that are considered to be adequate in other respects may be marginal in chromium. One of the problems that arises in assessing chromium intake is the lack of knowledge about the different forms of chromium in foods and their utilization relative to the GTF.

Chromium deficiency is believed to occur in the United States and may be manifested by impaired glucose tolerance. It is seen especially in older persons, in maturity-onset diabetes, and in infants with protein-calorie malnutrition. Supplements of chromium have been found to improve glucose tolerance in some, but not all, patients with diabetes. Chromium obviously can not replace insulin therapy in insulin-dependent diabetics[46].

Cobalt   This element is an essential constituent of vitamin B-12 and must be ingested in the form of the vitamin molecule inasmuch as humans cannot synthesize the vitamin. No other function of cobalt has been established.

CASE STUDY 1

Young Boy with Iron-Deficiency Anemia

Juan, age 5, awoke in the middle of the night crying because of an earache and fever. The next day, his mother took him to the Migrant Health Care Clinic. In addition to otitis media, iron-deficiency anemia was diagnosed. Juan's hemoglobin was 9.5 g per dl (normal range, 10.5 to 14.0 g/dl); mean corpuscular volume (MCV), 70 fl. Mrs. X mentioned that Juan had less energy than usual this summer. Juan was placed on antibiotics and ferrous sulfate. The nurse practitioner also conducted a diet history and discussed the need for iron-rich foods in Juan's diet.

Juan is the youngest of four children. The X family's home base is in Texas, but they move through the Central States during the summer doing seasonal farm work. Significant factors that influence the X family's food habits include their Mexican–American cultural background, poverty-level income, and lack of adequate food storage and preparation facilities. Tortillas, pinto beans, lentils, and rice are staples in their diet. Mrs. X prepares her own masa from corn. Chilies, both hot and sweet, onions, garlic, and tomatoes are used in food preparation whenever they are available. The X family eats meat infrequently, rarely drinks milk, and has fresh fruits and vegetables only when they are in season. Juan usually drinks sweetened fruit-flavored beverages instead of milk.

Questions:
1. What findings in Juan's history contributed to the development of iron-deficiency anemia?
2. What role did symptoms play in the identification of the anemia?
3. What changes in red blood cells are characteristic of iron deficiency? What laboratory finding was consistent with such changes?
4. What other laboratory tests could have been used to document that the anemia was caused by lack of iron?
5. What is the recommended intake of iron for a child Juan's age?
6. Which foods appeared to supply most of the iron in the family's diet?
7. What is the iron content of an average serving of pinto beans and lentils? What factors affect the bioavailability of that iron?
8. Develop a list of diet recommendations to increase Juan's iron intake that takes into consideration his family's economic status, lifestyle, and traditional food habits.
9. What dietary factors enhance the availability of iron in plant foods? What practical recommendations could be included in your list that would take advantage of the effects of these factors?

Other Minerals Deficiencies of nickel, vanadium, and silicon have been produced in experimental animals. This suggests that they are essential for some animals but to date, this cannot be established for humans. Experimental data on the need for tin, arsenic, and cadmium is even more sparse. Further research is necessary before it can be determined if they are needed by humans.

A summary of mineral elements and review questions appear at the end of Chapter 10.

References for the Case Study

DALLMAN, P. R., et al.: "Iron Deficiency in Infancy and Childhood," *Am. J. Clin. Nutr.*, 33:86–118, 1980.

KENNEDY-CALDWELL, C.: "Metabolism of Vitamins and Trace Minerals," *Nurs. Clin. North Am.*, 18:29–45, 1983.

MANDELBAUM, J. K.: "The Food Square: Helping People of Different Cultures Understand Balanced Diets," *Pediatr. Nurs.*, 9 (Jan/Feb): 20–21, 1983.

O'BRIEN, M. E.,: "Reaching the Migrant Worker," *Am. J. Nurs.*, 83:895–97, 1983.

References

1. Food and Nutrition Board: *Recommended Dietary Allowances*, 10th ed. National Research Council–National Academy of Sciences, Washington, D.C., 1989.
2. Hambidge, K. M.: "Hair Analysis: Worthless for Vitamins, Limited for Minerals," *Am. J. Clin. Nutr.*, 36:943–49, 1982
3. Allen, L. H.: "Calcium Bioavailability and Absorption: A Review," *Am. J. Clin. Nutr.*, 35:783–808, 1982.
4. Harland, B. F., and Harland, J.: "Fermentative Reduction of Phytate in Rye, White, and Whole Wheat Breads," *Cereal Chem.*, 57:226–29, 1980.
5. Kelsay, J. L., and Prather, E. S.: "Mineral Balances of Human Subjects Consuming Spinach in a Low-Fiber Diet and in a Diet Containing Fruit and Vegetables," *Am. J. Clin. Nutr.*, 38:12–19, 1983.
6. Avioli, L. V.: "Calcium and Phosphorus," in Goodhart, R. S., and Shils, M. E., eds.: *Modern Nutrition in Health and Disease*, 6th ed. Lea & Febiger, Philadelphia, 1980, pp. 294–309.
7. Walker, R. M., and Linkswiler, H. M.: "Calcium Retention in the Adult Human Male as Affected by Protein Intake," *J. Nutr.*, 102:1297–1302, 1972.
8. Allen, L. H., et al.: "Protein-induced Hypercalcemia: A Longer Term Study," *Am. J. Clin. Nutr.*, 32:741–49, 1979.
9. Allen, L. H., et al.: "Reduction of Renal Calcium Reabsorption in Man by Consumption of Dietary Protein," *J. Nutr.*, 109:1345–50, 1979.
10. Spencer, H., et al.: "Further Studies of the Effect of a High Protein Diet as Meat on Calcium Metabolism," *Am. J. Clin. Nutr.*, 37:924–29, 1983.
11. Zemmel, M. B., and Linskwiler, H. M.: "Calcium Metabolism in the Young Adult Male as Affected by Level and Form of Phosphorus Intake and Level of Calcium Intake," *J. Nutr.*, 111:315–24, 1981.
12. FAO: *Handbook on Human Nutritional Requirements.* FAO Nutritional Studies Report No. 28, FAO, Rome, 1974.
13. Mack, P. B., and LaChance, P. A.: "Effects of Recumbency and Space Flight on Bone Density," *Am. J. Clin. Nutr.*, 20:1194–1205, 1967.
14. Heaney, R. P., et al.: "Calcium Nutrition and Bone Health in the Elderly," *Am. J. Clin. Nutr.*, 36:986–1013, 1982.
15. Parrott-Garcia, M., and McCarron, D. A.: "Calcium and Hypertension," *Nutr. Rev.*, 42: 205–13, 1984.
16. Belizian, J. M., et al.: "Reduction of Blood Pressure with Calcium Supplementation in Young Adults," *JAMA*, 249:1161–65, 1983.
17. Schwartz, R., et al.: "Measurement of Magnesium Absorption in Man Using Stable ^{26}Mg as a Tracer," *Clin. Chim. Acta*, 87:265–73, 1978.
18. Marston, R. M., and Welsh, S. O.: "Nutrient Content of the U.S. Food Supply, 1982," *National Food Review.* U.S. Department of Agriculture, Winter 1984, pp. 7–13.
19. Pao, E. M., and Mickle, S. J.: "Problem Nutrients in the United States," *Food Technol.*, 35:58–69, 1981.
20. Bjorn-Rasmussen, E.: "Iron Absorption: Present Knowledge and Controversies," *Lancet*, 1:914–16, 1983.
21. Beutler, E.: "Iron," in Goodhart, R. S., and Shils, M. E., eds.: *Modern Nutrition in Health and Disease*, 6th ed. Lea & Febiger, Philadelphia, 1980, pp. 324–54.
22. "Anatomy of a Decision," *Nutr. Today*, 13(1):6–10, 28–29, 1978.
23. Sharon, G. S.: "Of (Iron) Pots and Pans," *Nutr. Today*, 7(2):34–35, 1972.
24. Monson, E. R., et al.: "Estimation of Available Dietary Iron," *Am. J. Clin. Nutr.*, 31:134–41, 1978.
25. deBruin, E. J. P., et al.: "Iron Absorption in the Bantu," *J. Am. Diet. Assoc.*, 57:129–31, 1970.
26. Finch, C. A., and Cook, J. D.: "Iron Deficiency," *Am. J. Clin. Nutr.*, 39:471–77, 1984.
27. Dallman, P. R., et al.: "Prevalence and Causes of Anemia in the United States, 1976 to 1980," *Am. J. Clin. Nutr.*, 39:437–45, 1984.
28. Pisciotta, A. V.: "The Anemic Patient," *Am. Fam. Physician*, 18:144–52, November 1978.
29. Allegrini, M., et al.: "Total Diet Study: Determination of Iodine Intake by Neutron Activation Analysis," *J. Am. Diet. Assoc.*, 83:18–24, 1983.
30. Solomons, N. W.: "Biological Availability of Zinc in Humans," *J. Am. Clin. Nutr.*, 35:1048–75, 1982.
31. Prasad, A. S.: "Clinical, Biochemical and Nutritional Spectrum of Zinc Deficiency in Human Subjects: An Update," *Nutr. Rev.*, 41:197–208, 1983.
32. Buzina, R., et al.: "Zinc Nutrition and Taste Acuity in Schoolchildren with Impaired Growth," *Am. J. Clin. Nutr.*, 33:2262–67, 1980.
33. Hambidge, K. M., et al.: "Low Levels of Zinc in Hair, Anorexia, Poor Growth and Hypogeusia in Children," *Pediatr. Res.*, 6:868–74, 1972.
34. Walravens, P. A., et al.: "Linear Growth of Low Income School Children Receiving a Zinc Supplement," *Am. J. Clin. Nutr.*, 38:195–201, 1983.

35. Crofton, R. W., et al.: "Zinc Absorption in Celiac Disease and Dermatitis Herpetiformis: A Test of Small Intestinal Function" *Am. J. Clin. Nutr.*, **38**:706–12, 1983.

36. Tsukamoto, Y., et al.: "Disturbances of Trace Element Concentrations in Plasma of Patients with Chronic Renal Failure," *Nephron*, **26**:174–79, 1980.

37. Boosalis, M. G., et al.: "Impaired Handling of Orally Administered Zinc in Pancreatic Insufficiency," *Am. J. Clin. Nutr.*, **37**:268–71, 1983.

38. Fleming, C. R., et al.: "Zinc Nutrition in Crohn's Disease," *Dig. Dis. Sci.*, **26**:865–70, 1981.

39. Fischer, P. W. F., et al.: "Effect of Zinc Supplementation on Copper Status in Adult Man," *Am. J. Clin. Nutr.*, **40**:743–46, 1984.

40. Klevay, L. M., and Forbush, J.: "Copper Metabolism and the Epidemiology of Coronary Heart Disease," *Nutr. Rept. Int.*, **14**:221–25, 1976.

41. Schamschula, R. G.: "Fluoride and Health: Dental Caries, Osteoporosis, and Cardiovascular Disease," *Annu. Rev. Nutr.*, **1**:427–35, 1981.

42. Abumrad, N. N., et al.: "Amino Acid Intolerance During Prolonged Total Parenteral Nutrition Reversed by Molybdate Therapy," *Am. J. Clin. Nutr.*, **34**:2551–59, 1981.

43. Combs, G. F., and Combs, S. B.: "The Nutritional Biochemistry of Selenium," *Annu. Rev. Nutr.*, **4**:257–80, 1984.

44. Mertz, W.: "The Significance of Trace Elements for Health," *Nutr. Today*, **18**(5):26–31, 1983.

45. Fleming, C. R., et al.: "Selenium Deficiency and Fatal Cardiomyopathy in a Patient on Home Parenteral Nutrition," *Gastroenterology*, **83**:689–93, 1982.

46. Uusitupa, M. I. J., et al.: "Effect of Inorganic Chromium Supplementation on Glucose Tolerance, Insulin Response, and Serum Lipids in Noninsulin-dependent Diabetes," *Am. J. Clin. Nutr.*, **38**:404–10, 1983.

10

Fluid and Electrolyte Balance

Precise regulation of the volume and composition of body fluids is essential for maintenance of the interchange that constantly takes place between the body and its external environment as well as among cells, tissues, and organs within the body. The electrolytes and nonelectrolytes held in solution in the aqueous media of the body maintain normal osmotic pressure relationships, control nervous irritability and muscle contraction, regulate acid–base balance, and facilitate movement of nutrients into cells and removal of wastes from cells.

Water is the main solvent of the body. Often its role as an essential nutrient is overlooked until it becomes a problem such as during scarcity. With increased participation in exercise programs to improve physical fitness, many persons are becoming more conscious of fluid and electrolyte requirements. To understand the body's need for water, one must understand the important interrelationships that exist among water balance, the metabolism of sodium, potassium, and chloride; the role of the kidney; and the maintenance of acid–base balance in the body.

Water

The body's need for water is second only to that for oxygen. One can live for weeks without food, but death is likely to follow a deprivation of water for more than a few days. A 10 percent loss of body water is a serious hazard, and death usually follows a 20 percent loss.

Distribution Water makes up 50 to 65 percent of the weight of the adult human body. Lean individuals have a higher percentage of body water than do obese individuals. Men have a higher proportion of body water than women inasmuch as even women of normal weight have more adipose tissue. In infants water makes up 70 to 75 percent of the body weight, thus making adequate fluid intake even more critical than in adults.

All body tissues contain water, but the variations in tissue contents are wide. For example, the approximate percentage of water in teeth is 5; fat and bone, 25; and striated muscle, 80.

Fluid Compartments. Body fluids exist in two so-called compartments that are disseminated throughout the entire body. The INTRACELLULAR FLUID is that which exists within the cells. It accounts for about 45 percent of body weight. The EXTRACELLULAR FLUID is subdivided as follows: (1) the plasma fluid, accounting for 5 percent of body weight, which contains protein as well as numerous substances that easily penetrate the capillary membrane; and (2) the interstitial fluid, representing about 15 percent of body weight,

IMPORTANT ISSUES

Most current guidelines for good nutrition recommend a reduction in sodium chloride intake as a measure to prevent high blood pressure. (See Chapter 3.) For many Americans such a reduction represents a significant change in eating habits and food choices. On what types of evidence is such a recommendation based? Are some people more likely than others to benefit from reduced salt intake? What are the food sources of sodium and what changes in food selection and preparation are necessary to achieve recommended intakes? These questions will be addressed briefly in this chapter with further discussion and details of sodium-restricted diets given in Chapter 39.

which is similar to plasma fluid except in its much lower concentration of protein. Also included in the extracellular fluids are the lymph circulation and secretions such as those of the lacrimal glands, pancreas, liver and gastrointestinal mucosa. (See Figure 10-1.)

Functions   Most of the many functions of water are self-evident. Water is a structural component and a cushion of all cells. Each gram of protein holds about 4 g water, and each gram of fat is associated with about 0.2 g water. In some instances, as in bone, water is tightly bound, but in most tissues a constant interchange takes place between intracellular and extracellular fluid in order to maintain osmotic pressure relationships.

Water is the medium of all body fluids, including digestive juices, lymph, blood, urine, and perspiration. All the physiochemical changes that occur in the cells of the body take place in the precisely regulated environment of the body fluids. Water enters into many essential reactions, such as hydrolysis that occurs in digestion. In oxidation–reduction reactions water is often the end product as in the oxidation of glucose.

Water is a solvent for the products of digestion, holding them in solution and permitting them to pass through the absorbing walls of the intestinal tract into the bloodstream. Because nutrients and cellular wastes are soluble in water, it is the means whereby nutrients are carried to the cells and wastes are removed to the lungs, kidney, gut, and skin. The metabolic wastes are diluted by water, thereby preventing cellular injury.

Water is essential as a body lubricant: the saliva that makes possible the swallowing of food; the mucous secretions of the gastrointestinal, respiratory, and genitourinary tracts; the fluids that bathe the joints; and so on.

Water regulates body temperature by taking up the heat produced in cellular reactions and distributing it throughout the body. About 25 percent of the heat lost from the body occurs by evaporation from the lungs and skin. Each liter of water lost in perspiration represents a heat loss of about 600 kcal. When there is an increase in body temperature, centers in the hypothalamus stimulate increased sweating and hence greater evaporation and loss of body heat.

Sources of Water to the Body   Water to meet the body's needs is supplied by (1) the ingestion of water and beverages, (2) the preformed water in foods, and (3) the water resulting from the oxidation of foodstuffs.

As may be seen in the following list, water is the principal constituent by weight of almost all foods, pure sugars and fats being the important exceptions.

	Water (percent)
Milk	87
Eggs	74
Cooked meat, poultry, fish	
Well done	40–50
Medium to rare	50–70
Cheese, hard	35–40
Fruits and vegetables	70–95
Bread	35
Dry cereals, crackers	3–7
Cooked cereals	60–85
Nuts, fats, sweets	0–10

The oxidation of glucose, fatty acids, and amino acids yields water; for example

$$C_6H_{12}O_6 + 6\,O_2 \rightarrow 6\,H_2O + 6\,CO_2$$

The following amounts of water are produced in the oxidation of foodstuffs:

	Water (ml)
100 g fat	107
100 g carbohydrate	56
100 g protein	41

Using these equivalents, the water of oxidation for a 2,000-kcal diet consisting of 80 g protein, 80 g fat, and 240 g carbohydrate is approximately 253 ml.

Daily Losses of Water   The daily losses of water include

	(ml)
Feces	100–200
Urine	1,000–1,500
Lungs	250–400
Insensible perspiration	400–600
Visible perspiration	None to 10,000

Some losses of water are OBLIGATORY, that is, they are essential for the maintenance of physicochemical equilibrium. The losses in the feces, through the lungs, and in insensible perspiration occur regardless of intake.

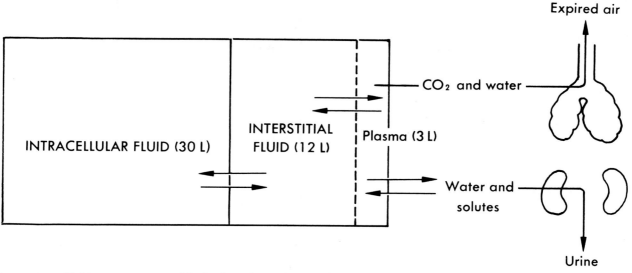

Figure 10-1. Fluid compartments of the body and interchanges from one compartment to another.

Renal Losses. The amount of water loss from the kidney that is obligatory depends upon the amount of wastes that must be dissolved. Under normal circumstances it is about 600 ml. Urea and sodium chloride are the principal solids that are excreted, and thus any reduction in their production will correspondingly reduce the obligatory loss of water in the urine. A diet that is high in carbohydrate to minimize tissue catabolism and low in protein is one that reduces the formation of urea and thus will spare body water. Facultative water excretion by the kidney is in addition to the obligatory losses, and varies according to body needs and water intake.

Skin. Insensible perspiration accounts for a relatively constant amount of water loss that is proportional to the surface area of the body. It is so called because the evaporation takes place from the skin immediately and the water loss is not noticeable. This evaporation is an important means by which body temperature is maintained. Infants have a much greater surface area relative to body weight than do adults; consequently they are much more vulnerable to water losses from the skin and rapid changes in body temperature.

The water losses by visible perspiration are highly variable, ranging from zero in cool weather to several liters during very warm weather under conditions of strenuous activity. Whenever a great deal of water is lost by perspiration, body water is conserved by the elimination of a much more concentrated urine.

Lungs. Air expired from the lungs also contains water. Any condition that would increase the rate of respiration—for example, fever—likewise increases the water loss by this route. The individual engaged in vigorous activity will lose more water by this route than the one who is sedentary.

Requirement The 24-hour water requirement is that amount that replaces the losses by the kidneys, lungs, skin, and bowel. Ordinarily, thirst is an accurate guide to supplying the necessary amounts of water. Under ideal conditions including a low-solute diet, a minimum of physical activity, and the absence of sweating, the water need for the adult is about 1.5 liters from beverages, food, and water of oxidation. Although conditions are variable, the daily requirement is about 1 ml per kcal for adults and 1.5 ml per kcal for infants.[1]

Table 10-1 illustrates a typical balance between water intake and water losses from the body. The mecha-

Table 10-1.   Normal Water Balance for an Adult*

Available Water	g	Excreted Water	g
Water, coffee, tea, etc.	1,200	In urine	1,350
Water in foods, including milk	900	In stool	200
		In vapor from lungs	400
Water of oxidation	250	From skin	400
Total	2,350	Total	2,350

* Assumes light activity and no visible sweating.

nisms for the regulation of fluid balance and some of the problems of imbalance are discussed on pages 146 through 149.

Electrolytes

Definitions and Measurement   An ION is an atom or group of atoms that carries an electrical charge. CATIONS (Na^+, K^+, Ca^{2+}, Mg^{2+}) carry positive electrical charges; they are electron donors. ANIONS (Cl^-, HCO_3^-, HPO_4^{2-}, SO_4^{2-}) carry negative electrical charges; they are electron acceptors. Because proteins in body fluids have a net negative charge, they also act as anions. In any solution the total cations are exactly equal to the total anions.

An ELECTROLYTE is any substance that dissociates into its component ions when dissolved in water. It is so named because an electrical current can be transmitted by a solution containing any one of these substances. The dissociation for a given substance is constant, but the degree of dissociation varies widely from one substance to another. Strong electrolytes are those substances such as inorganic acids or bases that dissociate almost completely.

The concentrations of physiologic solutions are expressed, and most easily compared, in milliequivalents (mEq) rather than in weights per dl or per liter. A MILLIEQUIVALENT is the weight in milligrams of an element that combines with or replaces 1 mg of hydrogen. Harry Statland[2] used a dance analogy to describe this concept. For a dance one would invite equal numbers of boys and girls—not 1,400 pounds of boys and 1,400 pounds of girls. It is the number of boys to pair off with girls that is important, not their weight. With an equal number of boys and girls, any boy could dance with any girl.

Likewise, with cations and anions; any cation can pair off with any anion. For example, 1 mEq of sodium combines with 1 mEq of chloride. Expressed in weight, 23 mg sodium have combined with 35 mg chloride. But 1 mEq of potassium can also combine with 1 mEq of chloride; in this instance, 39 mg potassium have combined with 35 mg chloride. Another example: calcium, with two positive charges, can pair off with two chloride ions; it can, instead, pair off with one phosphate ion, since phosphate carries two negative charges. Thus, it is the *chemical combining power* rather than the weights of the substances that is most convenient in measuring electrolyte concentrations. The calculation of milliequivalents of an electrolyte, when the concentration in milligrams is known, may be expressed as follows:

$$mEq/liter = \frac{mg \text{ per liter}}{Equivalent \text{ weight}}$$

$$Equivalent \text{ weight} = \frac{atomic \text{ weight}}{valence \text{ of the element}}$$

Suppose the concentration of calcium in blood serum is 9.5 mg per dl (100 ml). Since the atomic weight of calcium is 40 and the valence is 2, the equivalent weight is $40 \div 2 = 20$.

$$mEq/liter = \frac{9.5 \times 10}{20} = 4.75$$

Electrolyte Composition of Body Fluids   The electrolyte balance of the body is studied principally by determining the electrolyte concentrations in blood plasma. The electrolyte compositions of plasma and of cellular fluid are compared in Table 10-2. The electrolyte patterns for plasma and interstitial fluid are almost identical except for the much greater concentration of protein in the plasma. Note that within each fluid compartment the total milliequivalents of cations exactly balance the total milliequivalents of anions. There are marked differences in the electrolyte composition of plasma and intracellular fluid, yet the concentrations are such that osmotic balance is maintained. Because of the higher protein within the cell, the total of all electrolytes is higher than that in extra-

Table 10-2.   Electrolyte Composition of Body Fluids*

	Blood Plasma		Intracellular Fluid
	mg/dl	mEq/liter	mEq/liter
Cations			
Sodium (Na^+)	327	142	10
Potassium (K^+)	20	5	150
Calcium (Ca^{2+})	10	5	
Magnesium (Mg^{2+})	3.6	3	40
Total cations		155	200
Anions			
Chloride (Cl^-)	366	103	
Bicarbonate (HCO_3^-)	165	27	10
Phosphate (HPO_4^{2-})	10.6	2	150
Sulfate (SO_4^{2-})	1.6	1	
Organic acids⁻	17.5	6	
Proteinate⁻		16	40
Total anions		155	200

* Adapted from Table 35-1 in Frisell, W. R.: *Human Biochemistry.* Macmillan Publishing Co., Inc., New York, 1982, p. 552.

cellular fluid. Each protein molecule carries eight negative charges, thus combining with eight potassium ions; the protein molecule and the eight potassium ions would thus yield only nine osmotically active particles.

Extracellular Fluid. Sodium accounts for over 90 percent of the cations in plasma and interstitial fluid; potassium, magnesium, and calcium are found in very small, though physiologically important, concentrations. The principal anion of plasma is chloride; there are smaller concentrations of bicarbonate and proteinate and very small amounts of phosphate, sulfate, and organic acids.

Wide variations in electrolyte concentrations are found in the digestive juices. For example, in the acid gastric juice, the concentration of sodium is low, and that of chloride is high and is balanced by hydrogen ions. Intestinal juice and bile compare with plasma in their principal electrolytes.

Intracellular Fluid. Potassium is the principal cation in intracellular fluid, with magnesium, sodium, and calcium accounting for the remainder. Phosphate as the organic phosphate in adenosine triphosphate, creatine phosphate, and sugar phosphate as well as inorganic phosphate is the principal balancing anion. Proteinate accounts for about one fourth of the anions in intracellular fluid, and the amounts of bicarbonate, chloride, and sulfate are small.

Sodium

Throughout human history salt has occupied a unique position. Moasic law prescribed the use of salt with offerings made to Jehovah, and there are frequent biblical references to the purifying and flavoring effects of salt. Greek slaves were bought and sold with salt, and a good slave was said to be "worth his weight in salt." Because salt was scarce and greatly prized, the Via Salaria of Rome was a carefully guarded artery for the transport of salt. Salt served as a medium of exchange; thus the word *salary* from the Latin *salaria*. To own salt was a privilege, and royal banquet halls had imposing salt cellars. Important persons were invited to "sit above the salt" and those of lesser importance were seated "below the salt." Today salt is so commonplace that only those who are denied its free use give more than casual thought to it.

Distribution About 50 percent of the body's sodium is present in the extracellular fluid, 40 percent in bone, and 10 percent or less in intracellular fluid.

Much of the sodium in bone is readily interchangeable with extracellular fluid, but some of it is located deeply in dense long bones. In terms of concentration, the sodium content of blood plasma is about 14 times that of intracellular fluid. (See Table 10-2.)

Functions Sodium is the principal electrolyte in extracellular fluid for the maintenance of normal osmotic pressure and water balance. It functions mutually with some and antagonistically with other ions in maintaining the normal irritability of nerve cells and the contraction of muscles, and in regulating the permeability of the cell membrane. The sodium "pump" maintains electrolyte differences between intracellular and extracellular fluid compartments. (See page 148.)

Metabolism Most of the sodium in the diet is in the form of inorganic salts, principally sodium chloride. The absorption of sodium from the gastrointestinal tract is rapid and practically complete, there being only small amounts of sodium in the feces. The kidneys regulate the sodium level in the body. When the intake of sodium is high, the excretion is likewise high. But if the intake of sodium is low, the excretion of sodium is likewise decreased. An analysis of a 24-hour collection of urine is a good measure of the level of intake in the normal individual. When sodium is drastically restricted in the diet, the excretion of sodium by the normal kidney practically reaches the vanishing point, and sodium is almost completely conserved. (The mechanisms for these controls will be discussed further on page 148.)

The losses of sodium in perspiration depend on the concentration and the total volume of sweat. In very warm weather the initial losses may be so high that the sodium depletion syndrome occurs unless compensation is made by increasing salt and fluid intake. With acclimatization there is a gradual reduction in the concentration of sodium in perspiration, and consequently less sodium will be lost through the skin. Concentrations of sodium in sweat ranging from 12 to 104 mEq per liter have been reported.[3]

Requirements In the absence of visible perspiration the need for sodium is very low. Healthy adults living in a temperate climate and without visible sweating can maintain sodium balance with an intake of as little as 115 mg. To allow for variations in activity and climate, a minimum intake of 500 mg is safe. No known advantage pertains to higher intakes.

The minimum daily requirement for sodium is 120 to 200 mg per day (23 mg per kg) for infants, and

225-400 mg for children. Pregnant and lactating women require additional sodium, the needs of which are easily met by the usual diet.

Average Sodium Intakes. From 6 to 15 g salt is consumed daily by Americans. This is equivalent to 2,500 to 6,000 mg sodium (108 to 260 mEq). Such intakes are more than twice the estimated safe and adequate intake and are far in excess of physiologic requirements. They reflect an acquired taste for salt. Some people desire so much salt that they add salt to food without tasting it, whereas others prefer only a light salting of food.

Guidelines for the Public. In view of the high sodium intake by many Americans and its possible role in the development of hypertension (see below), recent dietary guidelines make the following recommendations:

Senate Select Committee on Nutrition and Human Needs: "Limit the intake of sodium by reducing the intake of salt to about 5 g a day."[4] A subsequent clarification of this goal stated that the limit of 5 mg sodium chloride referred to the salt added to raw foods, whether in commercial processing, home preparation, or at the table. This is in addition to the sodium occurring naturally in foods equivalent to about 3 g sodium chloride.[5]
U.S. Department of Agriculture: "Avoid too much sodium."[6]
Food and Nutrition Board: "Use salt in moderation; adequate but safe intakes are considered to range between 3 to 8 g of sodium chloride daily."[7]

Food Sources The principal source of sodium in the diet is sodium chloride by virtue of its universal use in food preservation, in cookery, and at the table. One teaspoon of salt contains almost 2,000 mg sodium. The basic diet pattern (Table 4-2) furnishes about 500 mg sodium if all foods are processed, prepared and cooked without the addition of salt or other sodium-containing compounds. Some foods have a natural high sodium content: milk, egg white, meat, poultry, fish and certain vegetables such as spinach, beets, celery and chard. Most vegetables, fruits, cereals, and legumes are naturally low in sodium. Most drinking waters contain less than 20 mg sodium per liter, but in some areas the sodium content is considerably higher, particularly if home-softened water is used. (See also Table A-2.)

Many sodium-containing compounds are used in processed foods. These may be ingredients or additives. The sodium content of processed foods is frequently listed on the label. In the absence of this labeling information, the user should look for the word "sodium" in the ingredient listing. Commonly used sodium compounds in prepared foods are baking soda, baking powder, monosodium glutamate, sodium citrate, and sodium propionate. An increasing number of processed foods with reduced salt content are becoming available. (See also Chapter 39.)

Reducing Sodium Intake To keep sodium intakes within the recommended safe and adequate range, the following changes are compatible with a palatable diet:

1. Use no salt at the table.
2. Reduce the amount of salt used in food preparation. Try ½ to ¾ teaspoon when a recipe specifies 1 teaspoon. Many cookies, cakes and desserts can be prepared without adding salt.
3. Substitute herbs and spices for salt in flavoring meats and vegetables.
4. Use salty foods sparingly, such as salted meats and fish, pickles, soy sauce, salted nuts, potato chips, and many other snack foods.
5. Read label for information on sodium and salt content.

Sodium Depletion, Retention, and Hypertension An imbalance in sodium intake or retention in the body may result in a number of changes affecting fluid balance, blood pressure, membrane permeability, and neuromuscular function.

Sodium Depletion. Athletes and persons at heavy labor lose significant amounts of sodium in sweat, and these sodium and fluid losses must be replaced. Salt tablets are not recommended. The individual who experiences these losses should be advised to increase salt intake at meals by using salt at the table and by eating more salty foods. The amount of body weight lost during an athletic event can be used as guide to the amount of fluid that should be replaced.[8]

A deficiency of adrenocorticotropic hormone that is characteristic of Addison's disease leads to such large losses of sodium that the patient hungers for salt. With persistent vomiting and diarrhea, sodium is drawn into the gastrointestinal tract, and ultimately the extracellular fluid is depleted of its normal sodium content.

The symptoms of sodium depletion include weakness, mental confusion, nausea, lethargy, muscle cramps, and, in severe depletion, circulatory failure.

Sodium Retention. When sodium excretion is reduced, water accumulates as excess extracellular fluid, a condition known as *edema*. The acid-base balance is also disrupted. Excessive sodium or fluid intake is not the primary cause, and restricting either the water or sodium intake will not solve the underlying problem. Cardiac and renal failure are among the principal causes of reduced sodium excretion. An excessive secretion of cortical hormones, as by adrenal tumors, leads to increased retention of sodium. Likewise, adrenocorticotropic hormone used therapeutically in a variety of conditions also increases the retention of sodium.

Hypertension. Development of hypertension (high blood pressure) may involve a variety of factors, including genetic predisposition, obesity, smoking, stress, cardiovascular and renal pathology and a lifetime history of high sodium intake. Data from various epidemiologic studies have shown that among populations there is a direct correlation between the incidence of hypertension and the average daily salt intake.[9,10] Although a cause-and-effect relationship cannot be demonstrated, these results suggest that sodium intake may be an environmental factor influencing development of hypertension.

It is strongly suggested that the risk of high sodium intakes is genetically determined. If animal models hold true for humans, the consumption of high sodium levels from infancy in genetically susceptible individuals can increase the risk of hypertension. An imbalance of the sodium-to-potassium ratio can also affect blood pressure, and increased intake of potassium may partially offset the effect of high sodium intakes.[11,12] Some evidence suggests chloride also may be involved.[13]

Lower intakes of salt over a lifetime may benefit about 20 percent of the population believed to be genetically predisposed. Unfortunately, it is not yet practical to identify early in life those 40 million or so persons who are so predisposed. Although moderation of salt intake by the rest of the population may not be of value, there is no known harm resulting from reduced intakes, nor is there any known benefit of excessive intakes.

Potassium

Distribution The total potassium content of the adult body is about 250 g. Of this, about 97 percent is within the tissue cells with the remainder being distributed in the extracellular fluid compartment.

From Table 10-2 it may be seen that the concentration of potassium in cellular fluid is about thirty times that in the plasma.

Functions Potassium is an obligatory component of all cells and increases in proportion to the increase in the body's cell mass. Because a fixed proportion of potassium is bound to protein, the measurement of body potassium is often used to determine the total lean body mass.

Within the cell potassium is the principal cation for the maintenance of osmotic pressure and fluid balance, just as sodium is the principal cation in extracellular fluid.

Potassium is required for enzymatic reactions taking place within the cell. Some potassium is bound to phosphate and is required for the conversion of glucose to glycogen; this potassium is released during glycogenolysis.

The small concentration of potassium in extracellular fluid is essential, together with other ions, for the transmission of the nerve impulse and for contraction of muscle fibers. Maintenance of normal potassium concentration in the body fluid is especially important for normal functioning of the myocardium.

Metabolism Potassium is readily absorbed from the gastrointestinal tract. Although the digestive juices contain relatively large amounts of potassium, most of this is reabsorbed and the losses in the feces are small.

Under conditions of protein synthesis, glycogen formation, and cellular hydration, potassium is rapidly removed from the circulation. With the removal of sodium from the cell to the extracellular fluid by the sodium pump, potassium ions move in, thus balancing the cations between the fluid compartments. Potassium leaves the cell during protein catabolism, dehydration, or glycogenolysis.

Excess potassium is excreted by the kidney. Aldosterone secretion increases potassium excretion. Although the normal kidney readily excretes excess potassium, the ability to conserve potassium in the face of a deficit is much less rigid than that for sodium. Even in the absence of any potassium intake and with low tissue levels, the urinary losses may be 15 to 30 mEq per day.[14]

Requirements For the adult the minimum need for potassium is 2,000 mg. For infants less than 1 year 500 to 700 mg is recommended. Children 1 year to adulthood should consume between 1,000 and 2,000 mg depending on their age.[1]

Food Sources Because potassium is widely distributed in foods, the daily intake increases as the caloric intake increases. Typical diets furnish 50 to 150 mEq (2 to 6 g) daily.[1] Meats, poultry, and fish are good sources. Fruits, vegetables, and whole-grain cereals are especially high in potassium. Bananas, potatoes, tomatoes, carrots, celery, oranges, and grapefruit are rich sources. (See Table A-1 for potassium values in foods.)

Potassium Deficiency Potassium deficiency is not primarily of dietary origin, but there are numerous circumstances under which it can occur. One of these is defective food intake such as that in severe malnutrition, chronic alcoholism, anorexia nervosa, low carbohydrate diets for weight reduction, or some illness that seriously interferes with the appetite. Any condition that reduces the availability of nutrients for absorption can lead to potassium depletion: for example, prolonged vomiting, gastric drainage, and diarrhea. Adrenal tumors that increase aldosterone secretion lead to potassium loss. Losses may exceed replacement in severe tissue injury, following surgery, in burns, and during prolonged fevers. Some therapeutic measures may also initiate potassium deficiency: for example, prolonged parenteral feeding without potassium in the parenteral fluids; excessive adrenocortical steroid therapy; or some diuretics used in the treatment of hypertension and edema. Rapid infusions of glucose and insulin in diabetic acidosis bring about such rapid shifts of potassium into the cell that the plasma potassium levels may be reduced to levels that could bring about cardiac failure.

Potassium deficiency is characterized by low plasma levels of potassium (hypokalemia). The symptoms of deficiency include nausea, vomiting, listlessness, apprehension, muscle weakness, paralytic ileus, hypotension, tachycardia, arrhythmia, and an altered electrocardiogram. The heart may stop in diastole.

Potassium Excess Hyperkalemia is a frequent complication in renal failure, in severe dehydration, following too rapid parenteral administration of potassium, and in adrenal insufficiency. Hyperkalemia is characterized by paresthesias of the scalp, face, tongue, and extremities; muscle weakness; poor respiration; cardiac arrhythmia; and changes in the electrocardiogram. Cardiac failure may follow, with the heart stopping in systole. Hyperkalemia is corrected by using a low-potassium, low-protein, liberal-carbohydrate diet. Carbohydrate intake results in the formation of glycogen and the movement of potassium into the cells.

Chloride

Distribution Chlorine exists in the body almost entirely as the chloride ion. Most of the 100 g or so of chloride in the body is present in the extracellular fluid but it also occurs to some extent in the red blood cells and to a lesser degree in other cells.

Functions Chloride accounts for two thirds of the total anions of extracellular fluid. It is important in the regulation of osmotic pressure, water balance, and acid–base balance. It is the chief anion of gastric juice and is accompanied by the hydrogen ion rather than the sodium ion, thereby providing the acid medium for the activation of the gastric enzymes and the digestion in the stomach. Chloride is one of several activators of amylases.

Metabolism For the secretion of gastric juice chloride is withdrawn from the blood circulation, and changes in dietary intake do not modify its production. The gastric juice mixes with foods and moves along the intestinal tract. The chloride from foods and that from the gastric juice is readily absorbed into the circulation.

The CHLORIDE SHIFT between the red blood cells and the plasma is a mechanism whereby changes in pH are minimized. When the blood reaches the lungs, the blood CO_2 tension is decreased, the bicarbonate ions in the red blood cells decrease, bicarbonate ions move from the plasma into the cells, and chloride and OH ions move from the cells into the plasma. When the blood returns to the tissues, the partial pressure of CO_2 increases and these ionic shifts are reversed.

Chloride, like other ions, is filtered by the glomerulus and selectively reabsorbed from the renal tubules. Excess chloride is readily excreted. The chloride excretion usually parallels the excreton of sodium, but when it is essential to conserve sodium the kidney will substitute the ammonium ion. Sweat and feces contain variable amounts of chloride accompanied by sodium or potassium.

Dietary Intake Most of the chloride intake is from table salt. The amount consumed usually parallels sodium intake and is not deficient under normal circumstances. The estimated minimum requirement for adults has been set at 750 mg per day.

Chloride Imbalance Severe vomiting, drainage, or diarrhea will lead to large losses of chloride, and alkalosis develops because of the replacement of chloride with bicarbonate.

Role of the Kidney

Structural Unit The NEPHRON, of which there are approximately 1 million in each kidney, is the functioning unit of the kidney. (See Figure 10-2.) Each nephron consists of the GLOMERULUS, which is a tuft of capillaries surrounded by a capsule (Bowman's capsule), and a TUBULE, including (1) the proximal convoluted tubule, (2) the loop of Henle, and (3) the distal convoluted tubule. The nephrons finally empty into collecting tubules.

Blood flows into the glomerulus through an *afferent arteriole* and leaves through an *efferent arteriole* and then flows through a system of *peritubular capillaries* that surround the tubules.

Functions of the Kidney Every meal we eat would seriously upset metabolic balances were it not for the function of the kidneys. The primary function of the kidneys is to maintain the constant composition and volume of the blood. This includes the regulation of (1) the osmotic pressure, (2) the electrolyte and water balance, and (3) the acid–base balance. By regulation of the composition of the blood, homeostasis in the interstitial and intracellular fluid compartments of the body is achieved.

The production of urine permits the elimination of excess water and solutes such as sodium, chloride, and others, the byproducts of metabolism such as urea, and ingested substances that may be toxic.

Glomerular Filtration About 1,200 ml of blood flow through the kidneys each minute, this being about one fourth of the total cardiac output. The total amount of glomerular filtrate produced is about 125 ml per minute for a 24-hour total of 180 liters. The glomerular filtrate has essentially the same composition as the blood plasma except that it contains no protein or other large colloidal particles.

The many branching capillaries in the glomerulus

Figure 10-2. *(A)* The cut section of the kidney shows its parts. *(B)* The nephron is the functioning unit of the kidney. (Courtesy, Pansky, B.: *Dynamic Anatomy and Physiology*, Macmillan Publishing Co., Inc., New York, 1975, page 479.)

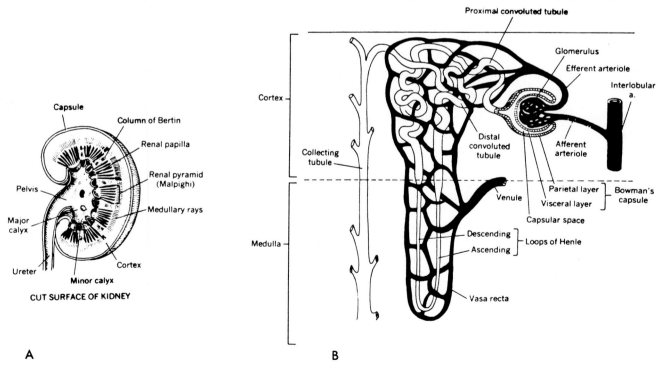

reduce the rate of renal flow, thus promoting filtration. These capillary branches unite to form the efferent arteriole, which has a much smaller diameter. This further resists flow and increases filtration.

Functions of the Tubules There are two broad functions of the tubules: (1) selective reabsorption, and (2) secretion. If it were not for reabsorption from the tubules, the body would lose all of its water, sodium, bicarbonate, glucose, and other filtered substances within half an hour and death would ensue.

As the glomerular filtrate moves through the proximal convoluted tubules, all of the glucose, amino acids, acetoacetic acid, and a number of other substances are reabsorbed if blood levels are within normal limits. For example, when glucose loads in the blood are within normal limits, all the glucose will be reabsorbed. Only when glucose levels in the blood exceed normal limits—as in diabetes mellitus—is some glucose not reabsorbed.

About 80 percent of the water and electrolytes are reabsorbed from the proximal tubule. Since the tubular epithelium is almost impermeable to waste products such as urea, these substances continue to pass along the tubule.

By the time the filtrate has reached Henle's loop, marked changes in composition have occurred. Most of the remaining sodium and some of the remaining water are reabsorbed into the circulation from Henle's loop.

About 3 percent of the electrolytes and 13 percent of the water still remain in the filtrate that reaches the distal convoluted tublule. At this point the final adjustments in the concentration of water and solutes are made by mechanisms described in more detail following. (See Figure 10-3.)

Energy Requirements. Only the liver exceeds the kidney in its metabolic activities. Water and urea move across the membranes by passive diffusion, which does not require energy. However, most substances are reabsorbed by active transport, thus entailing considerable energy expenditure. Fatty acids are the principal source of energy in the aerobic oxidations occurring in the cortex, but glucose, fructose, and other substrates can also be oxidized. In the renal medulla oxidation is principally by anaerobic glycolytic pathway, glucose being the chief substrate. (See page 71.)

Secretory Activities. The final control of acid–base balance is brought about by the distal portion of the tubule. Hydrogen ions are continually released from

carbonic acid by the action of carbonic anhydrase into the tubules. The tubules synthesize ammonia (NH_3), which then combines with the hydrogen ions to form the ammonium (NH_4^+) ion, thus releasing bicarbonate ions to the blood, thereby replacing the alkaline reserve.

Formation of 1,25-dihydroxy vitamin D_3 takes place in the kidney. This form of the vitamin enhances intestinal absorption of calcium and mobilization of calcium from bone. (See page 164.)

Composition of Urine As the glomerular filtrate passes through the tubules, the metabolic wastes—unlike water and electrolytes—are poorly reabsorbed. Their concentration therefore increases as the filtrate moves along the tubules with the resultant formation of urine. Urine consists of about 95 percent water and 5 percent solids. The kidney can produce a urine varying in specific gravity from about 1.008 to 1.035 depending on the proportions of water and solids to be excreted. The average daily excretion of solids is about 50 to 70 g, with three fifths of this being nitrogenous and two fifths inorganic salts. Urea is the predominating nitrogenous substance in the urine, along with much smaller amounts of uric acid, ammonia, and creatinine. (See Table A-28.)

Inorganic ions in the urine include Na^+, K^+, Ca^{2+}, Mg^{2+}, Cl^-, SO_4^{2-}, and PO_4^{2-}. These are not true wastes inasmuch as they are essential to cellular function. They are excreted only when they are in excess of body needs, and the quantity excreted depends upon dietary intake.

With an increase in solid wastes, the fluid required for their excretion would also be increased. Among the situations in which increased solid wastes are produced are the following: (1) protein intake in excess of tissue needs so that large amountsof amino acids are deaminized and the urea production is increased; (2) increased tissue catabolism following any stress such as surgery, injury, burns, or fever; and (3) increased intake of salt. Whenever the kidney is unable to concentrate urine, the fluid requirement for excretion of wastes is greatly increased.

Regulation of Fluid and Electrolyte Balance

Fluid Exchange Although the sources of water to the body and the losses from the body are in balance, the fluid exchanges that take place in a 24-hour period are of tremendous magnitude and impressive in the precision of their regulation. For the digestive pro-

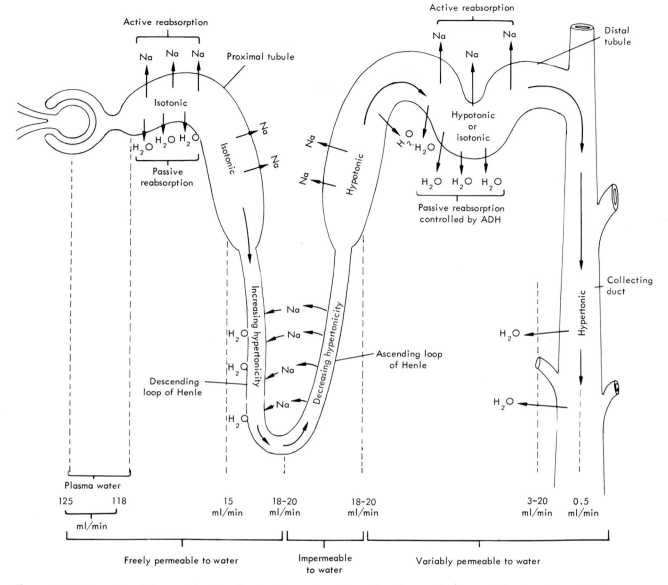

Figure 10-3. Function of the nephron in adjusting the reabsorption of sodium and water, and the formation of urine. (Courtesy, Pansky, B.: *Dynamic Anatomy and Physiology,* Macmillan Publishing Co., Inc., New York, 1975, page 488.)

cess alone the estimated daily volume of fluid that enters and leaves the gastrointestinal tract is estimated to be about 9 liters and is made up of the following[15]:

	(ml)
Water intake as beverage and in food	2,000
Saliva	1,500
Gastric juice	2,000
Bile	500
Pancreatic juice	1,500
Intestinal juice	1,500

The fluid exchanges between the gastrointestinal tract and the blood circulation are variable from hour to hour; yet they are so balanced that normally the volume of the blood and the fluids within the tract are in equilibrium. Inasmuch as the daily losses from the bowel are no more than 100 to 200 ml, it is evident that the outpouring of digestive juices into the intestinal tract is continuously balanced by the reabsorption of water from the gut. That the kidneys are highly efficient conservators of body water has been pointed out earlier. (See page 146.) The magnitude of water exchange that occurs between the blood circulation, the interstitial fluid, the lymph vessels, and the cells is no doubt very great.

Factors Influencing Fluid and Electrolyte Balance

The movements of water and solutes from one compartment to another are influenced by many factors: (1) the permeability of membranes to water and other substances; (2) the hydrostatic pressure within the capillaries; (3) the colloid osmotic pressure exerted by large molecules such as proteins; (4) the osmotic effect of electrolytes in the fluids of extracellular and intracellular fluids; (5) the lymph flow; (6) the mechanisms for active transport; (7) the competition of substances for carriers to transport materials across cell membranes; and (8) the hormonal and nervous controls influencing each of these factors.

The transport of most solutes across cell membranes has been described earlier. (See page 24.) Water can move in and out of cells by OSMOSIS, which is the passage of fluid from the less concentrated to the more concentrated side of the membrane. Osmotic pressure is the difference in the force exerted on each side of the membrane. Thus, the solution that is more concentrated exerts a pull on the water in the more dilute solution.

Sodium has little effect on the osmotic pressure between the capillaries and the interstitial fluid because its concentration in the two fluids is about equal. However, sodium is the principal cation in intercellular fluid and potassium in intracellular fluid so that these electrolytes effect important osmotic controls between these fluid compartments. A reduction of extracellular sodium, for example, results in the entrance of fluid into the cell, whereas an increase in extracellular sodium results in the withdrawal of fluid from the cell.

Proteins are large molecules that form colloidal (gluelike) solutions. They cannot pass through membranes and exert COLLOIDAL OSMOTIC PRESSURE within the blood vessels. Plasma albumin is the principal force that maintains fluid equilibrium between the interstitial fluid and the plasma. The plasma albumin exerts a constant pull of fluid from the interstitial fluid to the plasma. Thus, the colloid osmotic pressure opposes and balances the flow of materials out of the capillaries that is exerted by filtration pressure. When the concentration of plasma albumin is reduced, the osmotic pressure is reduced and the fluid remains in the tissue spaces.

Mechanisms to Regulate Water Balance

The sensation of thirst is one means whereby the body meets its water need. When the ionic concentration of the extracellular fluid is increased, the cells in the *thirst center* of the hypothalamus become dehydrated and the desire to drink water is initiated.

Water reabsorption from the renal tubule is modified according to the extracellular fluid concentration. This depends upon the *osmoreceptor system*, which is effective in two ways. One of these is the change in osmotic pressure that occurs in the interstitial fluid of the renal medulla. The loops of Henle of the renal tubules extend into the medulla. Because rapid, active absorption of sodium and chloride occurs, the interstitial fluid of the medulla has a high concentration of sodium and chloride and hence exerts increased osmotic pressure. As the tubular fluid passes into the collecting ducts located in the medulla, water is rapidly absorbed from the ducts.

Water reabsorption by the tubules is also controlled by the secretion of antidiuretic hormone by the posterior pituitary gland. Osmoreceptors especially in the supraoptic nuclei of the hypothalamus are sensitive to increases in the osmolarity of the extracellular fluid. Under conditions of increased concentration, impulses are initiated that stimulate production of ADH. The hormone enters the circulation and passes to the kidney where it increases the permeability of the distal and collecting tubules so that the amount of water that is reabsorbed is greatly increased. If the concentration of electrolytes is low, no stimulation of the osmoreceptors occurs and hence the hormone is not produced. The cell permeability is then decreased so that more water will be excreted, thereby restoring normal electrolyte concentration. (See Figure 10-4.)

Regulation of Ionic Balance

The regulation of sodium concentration in the extracellular fluid is better understood than that of other ions, but it is believed that the mechanisms that control the concentrations of other electrolytes are similar. These mechanisms are under nervous and hormonal control.

A low concentration of sodium in the extracellular fluid stimulates the secretion of aldosterone and, to a lesser extent, other mineralocorticoids by the adrenal cortex. The sequence for the stimulation of the adrenal is believed to be as follows: with a drop in blood pressure of the juxtaglomerular cells, the kidney is stimulated to produce RENIN, an enzyme, which in turn acts on a globulin substance in blood, ANGIOTENSINOGEN, to convert it to ANGIOTENSIN I, an inactive substance. An enzyme in the plasma converts angiotensin I to angiotensin II; the latter substance in the blood circulation stimulates the production of aldosterone by the adrenal cortex. Upon reaching the renal circulation, aldosterone increases the permea-

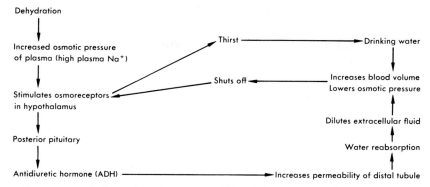

Figure 10-4. The regulation of water balance by thirst and antidiuretic hormone mechanisms.

bility of the distal and collecting tubules so that more sodium is reabsorbed into the peritubular capillaries. When the extracellular sodium concentration is high, the adrenal cortex stops secreting aldosterone, and thus greater amounts of sodium will be excreted. When sodium is reabsorbed it carries positive electrical charges which draw negative ions, principally chloride, through the tubular membrane. Thus, the reabsorption of chloride closely parallels that of sodium. (See Figure 10-5.)

Potassium ions are passively secreted into the distal and collecting tubules. This secretion is greater when the potassium content of the extracellular fluid is high. The retention of sodium under the influence of aldosterone is accompanied by an increased loss of potassium.

Fluid Imbalance A deficiency of fluid, dehydration, may occur because of inadequate intake, or abnormal loss, or a combination of the two. Abnormal loss of water occurs from prolonged vomiting, hemorrhage, diarrhea, protracted fevers, burns, excessive perspiration, drainage from wounds, and so on. It leads to decrease in peristaltic action, reduced blood volume, poor absorption of nutrients, impairment of renal function, and circulatory failure. Loss of fluid is accompanied by electrolyte losses as well. Thus, the adjustment of fluid balance requires also the consideration of electrolyte concentration.

In some pathologic conditions the body is in *positive* water balance; that is, the intake of fluids is greater than the excretion, and the patient is said to have an edema. The effect of the lowered plasma al-

Figure 10-5. The regulation of sodium concentration in extracellular fluid.

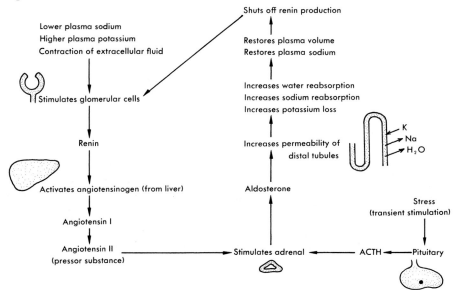

bumin has been mentioned. (See page 61.) Congestive heart failure, cirrhosis of the liver, nephritis, and nephrosis are examples of cardiovascular and renal disturbances in which sodium excretion is reduced, thereby contributing to the retention of water.

Acid-Base Balance

Acid–base balance refers to the regulation of the hydrogen ion concentration of body fluids. Normal metabolic processes result in the continuous production of acids that must be eliminated. The mechanisms for maintaining body neutrality are so efficient that the healthy individual does not need to give any thought whatsoever to the nature of his or her diet insofar as acid-producing or alkali-producing elements are concerned.

Many pathologic conditions, however, are characterized by serious disturbances in acid–base balance: for example, acidosis in uncontrolled diabetes mellitus, or fasting for weight reduction, following severe dehydration, and in renal failure. Through the study of physiology and biochemistry the student has gained an understanding of electrolyte and fluid balance, the chemistry of respiration, and the regulation of acid-base balance. Several references at the end of the chapter may be consulted by the student who desires a review or more extensive study than is provided in the following brief summary.

Definitions and Measurements   An ACID is a substance that gives off or donates protons (H$^+$ ions); a BASE is a substance that combines with or accepts protons. The acidity of a fluid is measured by its concentration of hydrogen ions; the greater the concentration of hydrogen ions, the greater the acidity. The pH designation is used to describe the acidity or alkalinity of solutions. The pH is a logarithmic function of the actual hydrogen ion concentration, and a pH difference of one unit represents a tenfold difference in the actual hydrogen ion concentrations. Thus a pH of 4 represents ten times as many hydrogen ions as a pH of 5. Neutrality is an equal concentration of hydrogen and hydroxyl ions and is designated pH 7. Alkaline solutions have pHs between 7 and 14 while acid solutions are designated with pHs below 7. The further the pH is from 7, the more acid or alkaline the solution.

The pH of blood plasma is maintained within very narrow limits of 7.35 to 7.45—a slightly alkaline reaction. The extremes of pH compatible with life are 6.8 and 7.8; obviously, at these extremes individuals are very ill and prompt therapeutic measures must be instituted if the person is to survive.

Acids Formed in Metabolism   The principal end products of metabolic activities are acid, chiefly carbonic acid. The oxidation of carbohydrates, fatty acids, and amino acids in the tricarboxylic acid cycle (see page 72) yields carbon dioxide and water; carbonic acid is the hydrated form of carbon dioxide. Intermediate products in metabolism are also acid, such as lactic and pyruvic acid formed in carbohydrate metabolism, keto acids formed in fatty acid oxidation, and amino acids resulting from the hydrolysis of proteins. Urea synthesis is an acid-producing process, and nucleoproteins give rise to uric acid. Sulfuric acid is formed in the body from the sulfur-containing amino acids and phosphoric acid from the phospholipids and phosphoproteins.

Acid and Alkaline Ash Foods   If the cations (Na$^+$, K$^+$, Mg^{2+}, and Ca^{2+}) remaining in the body on the metabolism of a food exceed the anions (PO$_4^{2-}$, and Cl$^-$), the food is said to produce an ALKALINE ASH and the excess cations will allow the body to retain more bicarbonate ions, thus producing an alkaline reaction. Vegetables, fruits, milk, and some nuts yield excess cations.

Meat, fish, poultry, eggs, cheese, cereals, and some nuts when metabolized yield an excess of anions that are not removed from the body immediately. These foods are said to produce an ACID ASH. The excess anions carrying a negative charge must be balanced approximately with some cations. This yields an acid reaction because less bicarbonate, which also carries a negative charge, can exist in the body. The excess bicarbonate ions form carbonic acid, increasing the acidity.

Fats, sugar, and starches contain no mineral elements and are metabolized quickly to carbon dioxide and water which are rapidly removed from the body. These foods, therefore, do not form excess cations or anions which would disturb the neutrality regulation.

Although lemons, oranges, and certain other fruits contain some free organic acids that give them a taste of acid (sour), they yield an alkaline ash because the body quickly oxidizes the anions of the acid to carbon dioxide and water and leave excess cations that are removed more slowly from the body. Plums, cranberries, and prunes contain aromatic organic acids that are not metabolized in the body, and therefore they increase the acidity of the body fluids.

The Regulation of Body Neutrality   The reaction of the body fluids is kept within a narrow range by the following mechanisms:

1. Dilution is an important defense against the effects of the metabolic acids. The total volume of body

fluid, representing about two thirds of body weight, is so great that the considerable amounts of carbon dioxide produced result in only a slight increase in the bicarbonate concentration because of the distribution throughout the fluid system.

2. Acid–base buffer systems are an important mechanism for the regulation of acid–base balance. A BUFFER is a substance that will react chemically with either acids or alkalies so that there is not a marked change in the pH of the solution. The bicarbonate-carbonic acid (HCO_3^-/H_2CO_3) system is one important buffer of the blood in maintaining neutrality. The ease and speed with which the body can get rid of carbon dioxide obtained from this buffer mixture constitute one of the first lines of defense. The plasma bicarbonate is an indicator of the alkaline reserve of the body. Serious disturbances may occur if the alkaline reserve is depleted to a low level. Other buffer systems include the following:

$$\frac{\text{Protein}}{\text{H}\cdot\text{protein}} \quad \frac{HPO_4^{2-}}{H_2PO_4^-} \quad \frac{Hb-}{HHb} \quad \frac{HbO_2^-}{HHbO_2}$$

3. In addition to its buffer action, hemoglobin aids in the transport of carbon dioxide from the cells to the lungs, where it can be excreted from the body in the expired air. This loss represents part of the functioning of the bicarbonate–carbonic acid buffer system.

4. The respiratory rate regulates the losses of carbon dioxide and the intake of oxygen. If the hydrogen ion concentration is increased, the respiratory center in the brain causes an increase in the rate of pulmonary ventilation. The increased respiratory rate increases the loss of carbon dioxide, and the hydrogen ion concentration of the body fluids returns to normal. If the hydrogen ion concentration is lowered, the respiratory center is inhibited and the rate of ventilation is reduced; thus, the carbonic acid concentration of the body fluids rises.

5. The kidney makes the final adjustment that keeps the body pH within normal limits. The glomerular filtrate has a pH of 7.4, but the kidney can excrete a urine that is as acid as pH 4.5 or as alkaline as pH 8; normally, the average urine pH is 6.0. Bicarbonate ions are filtered into the tubular fluid and their loss from plasma represents loss of alkali. Hydrogen ions are secreted into the tubules, and their loss from plasma represents a loss of acid. When the hydrogen ions of the plasma are increased, the secretion of the hydrogen ions into the tubular fluid also increases and exceeds the loss of bicarbonate, thus permitting the return of plasma to its normal pH. The urine excreted is then more acid.

Conversely, in alkalosis the hydrogen ion secretion into the tubules is decreased, thus allowing greater loss of bicarbonate. The urine then becomes more alkaline.

The kidney cannot excrete strong acids such as HCl and H_2SO_4. The hydrogen ions secreted into the lumen of the tubule are excreted by combining with disodium phosphate to form monosodium acid phosphate. By excreting practically all of the phosphate as acid phosphate ($H_2PO_4^-$, instead of HPO_4^{2-}) only one phosphate is lost instead of two, thus reducing by half the number of milliequivalents of fixed anions that are excreted; this permits the return of more fixed anions to the circulation.

The kidney is also able to synthesize ammonia from glutamine and other amino acids. The ammonia combines with hydrogen ions to form the ammonium ion (NH_4^+), which can then replace cations such as sodium or potassium.

Acidosis and Alkalosis The acid-base balance of the body can be upset by an increase in hydrogen ions, a loss of hydrogen ions, an increase in base, or a loss of base. In each instance the treatment can be instituted only after evaluation of symptoms that are present, the determination of the pH and the carbon dioxide content of the blood plasma, and the cause of the imbalance. (See Figure 10-6.)

ACIDOSIS is a condition in which the hydrogen ion concentration is increased or there is an excessive loss of base (mineral cations); the ratio of bicarbonate to carbonic acid is less than 20:1, and the pH is below 7.35. ALKALOSIS is a condition in which the hydrogen ion concentration is decreased or the base is increased; the ratio of bicarbonate to carbonic acid is greater than 20:1, and the pH is above 7.45.

With changes in concentrations of hydrogen ions and base, the lungs and kidneys attempt to compensate. Ventilation by the lungs is increased when there is an increase in hydrogen ions, and the kidney attempts to adjust by excreting a more acid urine and conserving base with the synthesis of more ammonia. When there is an increase in base, the respiration is depressed, and the hydrogen ions are retained and more base is excreted by the kidneys. If these adjustments succeed in keeping the bicarbonate–carbonic acid ratio at 20:1, the pH remains at 7.35 to 7.45; the acidosis or alkalosis is said to be "compensated." When the pH is outside these limits, the acidosis or alkalosis is "uncompensated."

Respiratory acidosis or alkalosis results from an abnormality of the control of the normal CO_2 tension. Hypoventilation such as that seen in pneumonia, pulmonary edema, suppression of breathing as with mor-

Table 10-3. Summary of the Minerals

Minerals	Functions in the Body	Metabolism	Food Sources	Daily Allowances
Calcium	Hardness of bones, teeth Transmission of nerve impulse Muscle contraction Normal heart rhythm Activate enzymes Increase cell permeability Catalyze thrombin formation	*Absorption:* about 15 to 40 percent, according to body need; aided by gastric acidity, vitamin D, lactose; excess phosphate, fat, phytate, oxalic acid interfere *Storage:* trabeculae of bones; easily mobilized *Utilization:* needs parathyroid hormone, vitamin D *Excretion:* 60 to 85 percent of diet intake in feces; small urinary excretion; high protein intake increases urinary excretion *Deficiency:* retarded bone mineralization; fragile bones; stunted growth; osteoporosis.	Milk, hard cheese Ice cream, cottage cheese Greens: turnip, collards, kale, mustard, broccoli Oysters, shrimp, salmon, clams	Infants: 400–600 mg Children: 800 mg Teenagers: 1,200 mg Adults: 800 mg Pregnancy: 1,200 mg Lactation: 1,200 mg
Chlorine	Chief anion of extracellular fluid Constituent of gastric juice Acid–base balance; chloride–bicarbonate shift in red cells	*Absorption:* rapid, almost complete *Excretion:* chiefly in urine; parallels intake *Deficiency:* with prolonged vomiting, drainage from fistula, diarrhea	Table salt	Estimated minimum requirement Infants: 180–200 mg Children: 350–600 mg Teenagers: 750 mg Adults: 750 mg Daily diet contains in excess of need
Chromium	Efficient use of insulin in glucose uptake; glucose oxidation, protein synthesis, stimulation of fat, and cholesterol synthesis Activation of enzymes	Usable form in organic compound: glucose tolerance factor	Liver, meat Cheese Whole-grain cereals	Estimated safe and adequate intake: Infants: 0.01–0.06 mg Children: 0.02–0.20 mg Teenagers: 0.05–0.20 mg Adults: 0.05–0.20 mg
Copper	Aids absorption and use of iron in synthesis of hemoglobin Electron transport Melanin formation Myelin sheath of nerves Purine metabolism	*Transport:* chiefly as protein, ceruloplasmin *Storage:* liver, central nervous system *Excretion:* bile into intestine *Deficiency:* rare; occurs in severe malnutrition Abnormal storage in Wilson's disease	Liver, shellfish Meats Nuts, legumes Whole-grain cereals Typical diet provides 1 to 5 mg	Estimated safe and adequate intake: Infants: 0.4–0.7 mg Children: 0.7–2.0 mg Teenagers: 1.5–2.5 mg Adults: 1.5–3.0 mg
Fluorine	Increases resistance of teeth to decay; most effective in young children Moderate levels in bone may reduce osteoporosis	*Storage:* bones and teeth *Excretion:* urine Excess leads to mottling of teeth and skeletal fluorosis	Fluoridated water: 1 ppm	Estimated safe and adequate intake: Infants: 0.1–1.0 mg Children: 0.5–2.5 mg Teenagers: 1.5–2.5 mg Adults: 1.5–4.0 mg
Iodine	Constituent of triiodothyronine, thyroxine; regulate rate of energy metabolism	*Absorption:* controlled by blood level of protein-bound iodine *Storage:* thyroid gland; activity regulated by thyroid-stimulating hormone *Excretion:* in urine *Deficiency:* simple goiter; if severe, cretinism—rarely seen in United States	Iodized salt is most reliable source Seafood Foods grown in nongoitrous coastal areas	Infants: 40–50 μg Children: 70–120 μg Teenagers: 150 μg Adults: 150 μg Pregnancy: 175 μg Lactation: 200 μg
Iron	Constituent of hemoglobin, myoglobin, and oxidative enzymes: catalase, cytochrome, xanthine oxidase	*Absorption:* about 3 to 23 percent, depending on food source and body need; aided by gastric acidity, ascorbic acid *Transport:* bound to protein, transferrin *Storage:* as ferritin in liver, bone marrow, spleen *Utilization:* chiefly in hemoglobin; daily turnover about 27 to 28 mg; iron used over and over again *Excretion:* men, about 1 mg; women, 1 to 2 mg; in urine, perspiration, menstrual flow; fecal excretion is from unabsorbed dietary iron *Deficiency:* anemia; frequent in infants, preschool children, teenage girls, pregnant women	Liver, organ meats Meat, poultry Egg yolk Enriched and whole-grain breads, cereals Dark-green vegetables Legumes Molasses, dark Peaches, apricots, prunes, raisins Diets supply about 6 mg per 1,000 kcal	Infants: 6–10 mg Children: 10 mg Teenagers: 12–15 mg Men: 10 mg Women: 15 mg Pregnancy: 15+ mg Lactation: 15 mg

Mineral	Functions	Absorption, Utilization, Excretion, Deficiency	Food Sources	Requirements
Magnesium	Constituents of bones, teeth; Activates enzymes in carbohydrate metabolism; Muscle and nerve irritability	*Absorption:* parallels that of calcium; competes with calcium for carriers; *Utilization:* slowly mobilized from bone; *Excretion:* chiefly by kidney; *Deficiency:* seen in alcoholism, severe renal disease; hypomagnesemia, tremor	Whole-grain cereals; Nuts; legumes; Meat; Milk; Green leafy vegetables	Infants: 40–60 mg; Children: 80–170 mg; Women: 280 mg; Men: 350 mg; Pregnancy and lactation: 320–355
Manganese	Activation of many enzymes; oxidation of carbohydrates, urea formation, protein hydrolysis	*Absorption:* limited; *Excretion:* chiefly in feces; *Deficiency:* not known	Legumes, nuts; Whole-grain cereals	Estimated minimum requirement; Infants: 0.3–1.0 mg; Children: 1.0–3.0 mg; Teenagers: 2.0–5.0 mg; Adults: 2.0–5.0 mg
Molybdenum	Cofactor for flavoprotein enzymes; present in xanthine oxidase	Absorbed as molybdate; Stored in liver, adrenal, kidney; Related to metabolism of copper and sulfur	Organ meats; Legumes; Whole-grain cereals	Estimated minimum requirement; Infants: 15–40 μg; Children: 25–150 μg; Teenagers: 75–250 μg; Adults: 75–250 μg
Phosphorus	Structure of bones, teeth; Cell permeability; Metabolism of fats and carbohydrates: storage and release of ATP; Sugar–phosphate linkage in DNA and RNA; Phospholipids in transport of fats; Buffer salts in acid–base balance	*Absorption:* about 70 percent; aided by vitamin D; *Utilization:* about 85 percent in bones; controlled by vitamin D, parathyroid hormone; *Excretion:* about one third of diet in feces; metabolic products chiefly in urine; *Deficiency:* poor bone mineralization; poor growth; rickets	Milk, cheese; Eggs, meat, fish, poultry; Legumes, nuts; Whole-grain cereals	Infants: 300–500 mg; Children: 800 mg; Adults: 800 mg; Pregnancy: 1,200 mg; Lactation: 1,200 mg
Potassium	Principal cation of intracellular fluid; Osmotic pressure; water balance; acid–base balance; Nerve irritability and muscle contraction, regular heart rhythm; Synthesis or protein	*Absorption:* readily absorbed; *Excretion:* chiefly in urine; increased with aldosterone secretion; *Deficiency:* following starvation, correction of diabetic acidosis, adrenal tumors; some diuretics; muscle weakness, nausea, tachycardia, glycogen depletion, heart failure	Widely distributed in foods; Meat, fish, fowl; Cereals; Fruits, vegetables	Estimated minimum requirement; Infants: 500–700 mg; Children: 1,000–1,600 mg; Teenagers: 2,000 mg; Adults: 2,000 mg; Diet adequate in calories supplies ample amounts
Selenium	Antioxidant; Constituent of glutathione peroxidase	Stored especially in liver, kidney; Spares vitamin E	Meat and seafoods; Cereal foods	Recommended allowance: Infants: 10–15 μg; Children: 20–30 μg; Teenagers: 40–70 μg; Adults: 55–70 μg
Sodium	Principal cation of extracellular fluid; Osmotic pressure; water balance; Acid–base balance; Regulate nerve irritability and muscle contraction; "Pump" for active transport such as for glucose	*Absorption:* rapid and almost complete; *Excretion:* chiefly in urine; some by skin and in feces; parallels intake; controlled by aldosterone; *Deficiency:* rare; occurs with excessive perspiration and poor diet intake: nausea, diarrhea, abdominal cramps, muscle cramps	Table salt; Processed foods; Milk; Meat, fish, poultry	Estimated minimum requirement: Infants: 120–200 mg; Children: 225–400 mg; Teenagers: 500 mg; Adults: 500 mg; Diets supply substantial excess
Sulfur	Constituent of proteins, especially cartilage, hair, nails; Constituent of melanin, glutathione, thiamin, biotin, coenzyme A, insulin; High-energy sulfur bonds; Detoxification reactions	Absorbed chiefly as sulfur-containing amino acids; Excreted as inorganic sulfate in urine in proportion to nitrogen loss	Protein foods rich in sulfur-amino acids; Eggs; Meat, fish, poultry; Milk, cheese; Nuts	Not established; Diet adequate in protein meets need
Zinc	Constituent of enzymes: carbonic anhydrase, carboxypeptidase, lactic dehydrogenase; DNA synthesis; immune system function	*Absorption:* limited; competes with calcium for absorption sites; *Storage:* liver, muscles, bones, organs; *Excretion:* chiefly by intestine; *Deficiency:* marginal occurs in United States; skin lesions, growth retardation; hypogeusia, hypogonadism	Seafoods; Liver and other organ meats; Meats, fish; Wheat germ; Yeast; Plant foods are generally low; Usual diet supplies 10 to 15 mg	Infants: 5 mg; Children: 10 mg; Teenagers: 15 mg; Adults: 12–15 mg; Pregnancy: 15 mg; Lactation: 16–19 mg

153

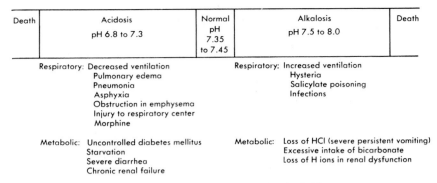

Death	Acidosis pH 6.8 to 7.3	Normal pH 7.35 to 7.45	Alkalosis pH 7.5 to 8.0	Death

Respiratory: Decreased ventilation
      Pulmonary edema
      Pneumonia
      Asphyxia
      Obstruction in emphysema
      Injury to respiratory center
      Morphine

Respiratory: Increased ventilation
      Hysteria
      Salicylate poisoning
      Infections

Metabolic: Uncontrolled diabetes mellitus
      Starvation
      Severe diarrhea
      Chronic renal failure

Metabolic: Loss of HCl (severe persistent vomiting)
      Excessive intake of bicarbonate
      Loss of H ions in renal dysfunction

Figure 10-6. Normal and abnormal pH ranges in body fluids.

phine, and asphyxia lead to acidosis. The kidneys partially compensate by increasing the excretion of hydrogen ions and the synthesis of ammonia, thereby increasing the return of bicarbonate to the blood.

Respiratory alkalosis occurs when there is overventilation of the lungs so that excessive amounts of carbonic acid are lost. This may result from hysteria, from salicylate poisoning, in fevers and infections, and at high altitudes. By reducing the excretion of hydrogen ions and the synthesis of ammonia and by increasing the excretion of sodium, the kidneys compensate in part.

Metabolic acidosis or alkalosis refers to changes resulting from faulty intake or output of acids or bases other than carbonic acid. Metabolic acidosis occurs in a variety of circumstances: the rapid production of ketones in uncontrolled diabetes mellitus; the inability of the kidney to excrete acid phosphates in chronic renal failure; the ketosis of starvation; or the loss of bicarbonate and sodium with severe diarrhea. Ventilation of the lungs is greatly increased. The synthesis of ammonia by the kidney may increase tenfold in an effort to conserve base.

Metabolic alkalosis occurs when there is a severe loss of hydrochloric acid as a result of vomiting, or by the ingestion of soluble alkalinizing salts such as sodium bicarbonate.

SOME POINTS FOR EMPHASIS IN NUTRITION EDUCATION

1. Mineral elements perform varied and interrelated functions in the body. Among these functions are the following:
   a. Provide structure and hardness for bones and teeth: calcium and phosphorus
   b. Associate with proteins in numerous ways; for example, potassium with cellular proteins, iron with hemoglobin, many minerals with enzymes
   c. Regulate transmission of the nerve impulses and the contraction of muscles
   d. Maintain a proper environment around and within all cells and tissues of the body; maintain acid-base balance
2. Mineral elements do not yield energy, as do carbohydrates, fats, and proteins; yet they are essential in the processes whereby the body derives its energy from foods.
3. Only calcium and iron require particular attention in the planning of diets for normal individuals. Diets that are adequate in protein, calories, and these minerals and that include a variety of foods, can be expected to supply the other mineral elements in satisfactory amounts.
4. For most persons the calcium allowance can be met only when the diet includes 2 to 4 cups of milk, depending upon age. Cheese or yogurt may be substituted for part of the milk allowance.
5. A deficiency of calcium may not become apparent for a long time because the bones supply the blood with its needs. Eventually, sufficient calcium is withdrawn from bones so that they may become brittle and break easily, and osteoporosis may occur later in life.
6. Iron deficiency is widely prevalent, especially in infants, preschool children, teenage girls and pregnant women. The only practical way by which these groups can obtain their iron needs is through the use of foods highly fortified with iron or by oral supplements of iron.
7. Iodine deficiency leads to endemic goiter. It can be prevented by the use of iodized salt.
8. Water is the body's universal solvent and must be supplied in adequate amounts.

9. Variations in the intake of acid-producing or alkali-producing foods do not result in acidosis or alkalosis in healthy individuals.

Problems and Review

1. Give several examples of the ways in which minerals function together in the body structure; in regulatory activities.
2. List four functions of calcium; of phosphorus.
3. What substances may combine with calcium in the intestinal tract and thus interfere with absorption? In which foods do these predominate? Of what practical significance is this in American diets?
4. Many adults believe that their needs for calcium are low because their bones are fully developed. Explain why this reasoning is wrong.
5. *Problem*. Calculate your daily intake of calcium, iron and zinc for two days. Compare your intake with the recommended allowances. What were the important sources of calcium in your diet? of iron? of zinc? What percentage of your total intake of these minerals came from animal foods?
6. *Problem*. Using the basic diet calculation on page 38, calculate the amount of iron available for absorption.
7. What dietary factors impair the absorption of iron? of zinc?
8. What is the principal function of iodine? What happens if the intake is inadequate?
9. What is the significance of fluorine in nutrition? What levels of fluorine are recommended in drinking water?
10. What is meant by dental fluorosis? At what levels of intake does it occur?
11. What problems are associated with an inadequate intake of zinc?
12. What is the principal function of selenium? Why might there be concern about indiscriminate use of selenium supplements?
13. Why has there been interest in chromium in relationship to diabetes?
14. *Problem*. Go to a grocery or drug store and examine labels on various supplements. What minerals are included in a typical multivitamin–mineral product? How do the amounts contained in each tablet or capsule compare with the recommended allowances for those minerals?
15. Name the principal mineral elements that contribute to an alkaline ash. Which foods are classified as alkali producing?
16. Name the principal mineral elements that contribute to an acid ash. Which foods are classified as acid producing?
17. What is the metabolic effect of an excess of acid-producing or of alkali-producing foods?
18. Describe the water compartments of the body in terms of (a) relative size; (b) electrolyte composition.
19. What are the daily sources of water to the body? What are the routes of excretion by the healthy individual?
20. What hormones control the excretion of water? Of sodium and potassium?
21. What is meant by obligatory water loss? If you found yourself in a situation where drinking water was extremely limited in supply, how could you reduce the loss of water from your body?

References

1. Food and Nutrition Board: *Recommended Dietary Allowances*, 10th ed. National Research Council–National Academy of Sciences, Washington, D.C., 1989.
2. Statland, H., cited by Snively, W. D., Jr., and Brown, B. J.: "In the Balance," *Am. J. Nurs.*, 58:55–57, 1958.
3. Consolazio, C. F.: "Nutrition and Performance. Sweat Losses," *Prog. Food Nutr. Sci.*, 7(1/2):113–128, 1983.
4. U.S. Senate Select Committee on Nutrition and Human Needs: *Dietary Goals for the United States*, rev. ed. Government Printing Office, Washington, D.C., December 1977.
5. "Addendum to Commentary: Dietary Goals for the United States, Second Edition," *J. Am. Diet. Assoc.*, 74:533, 1979.
6. *Nutrition and Your Health: Dietary Guidelines for Americans*. U.S. Department of Agriculture and U.S. Department of Health, and Human Resources, Washington, D.C. 1985.
7. Food and Nutrition: *Toward Healthful Diets*. National Research Council–National Academy of Sciences, Washington, D.C., 1980.
8. American Dietetic Association: "A Statement. Nutrition and Physical Fitness," *J. Am. Diet. Assoc.*, 76:437-43, 1980.
9. Altschul, A. M., and Grommet, J. K.: "Sodium Intake and Sodium Sensitivity," *Nutr. Rev.* 38:393–402, 1980.
10. Tobian, L.: "The Relationship of Salt to Hypertension," *Am. J. Clin. Nutr.*, 32:2739–48, 1979.
11. Bulpitt, C.: "Is There a New Member in the High Blood Pressure Mafia?," *Nutr. Today*, 17:6–11, 1982.
12. MacGregor, G. A.: "Sodium and Potassium Intake and Blood Pressure," *Hypertension*, (Suppl. III) 5:79–84, 1983.
13. Whitescarver, S. A., et al.: "Salt-Sensitive Hypertension: Contribution of Chloride," *Science*, 223:1430–32, 1984.
14. Krehl, W. A.: "The Potassium Depletion Syndrome," *Nutr. Today*, 1:20, 1966.
15. Luciano, D. S., et al.: *Human Anatomy and Physiology*, 2nd ed. McGraw-Hill Book Company, New York, 1983.

11

The Fat-Soluble Vitamins

Introduction to the Study of the Vitamins

The story of the vitamins—their discovery, their functions in maintaining health, and their usefulness in healing deficiency diseases—is fascinating and deserving of considerable study. Popular interest was early aroused by the discovery of the role of vitamins in preventing such severe deficiency diseases as scurvy, pellagra, and beriberi. It is now known that most of the water-soluble vitamins function primarily in enzyme systems which facilitate the metabolism of amino acids, fats, and carbohydrates. Those who understand the functions of vitamins do not minimize their importance in relationship to the utilization of food. However, it is important that no one be misled into believing that vitamins are "cure-alls" for disease. The properties of vitamins, their functions in metabolism, their distribution in foods, and the effects of deficiency will be discussed in the following sections.

Definition and Nomenclature The term *vitamins* was first coined in 1912 by Funk, a Polish chemist, who believed that the water-soluble antiberiberi substance he was describing was a "vital amine"; that is, an amine with life-giving properties. The final "e" was soon dropped because the substance was found, in reality, to be a group of essential compounds not all of which were amines. VITAMINS is the name given to a group of potent organic compounds other than protein, carbohydrate, and fat that are essential in minute quantities for specific body functions of growth, maintenance, and reproduction. With the exception of vitamin D, vitamins cannot be synthesized by the body and must be supplied by food.

Early classifications listed two groups of vitamins: fat soluble and water soluble. This classification is still used although within each of the classes the vitamins differ widely in their properties, functions, and distribution. Vitamins were first named for their cu-

rative properties and were given a convenient letter name according to the order of their discovery; for example, antiscorbutic vitamin or vitamin C. The nomenclature used today includes chemically descriptive terms, but letter designations are also used.

Measurement Before the chemical nature of vitamins was discovered, their potency could be measured only by their ability to promote growth or to cure a deficiency when test doses were fed to experimental animals such as rats, guinea pigs, pigeons and chicks. Such measurement is known as *bioassay* and has been expressed in units. Vitamins A, D, and E still may be expressed in international units (IU). Other vitamins are measured by their ability to promote the growth of microorganisms; this is known as *microbiologic assay*. Many vitamins formerly measured by bioassay are now measured by *chemical assay* in units of weight. Some vitamins are measured in milligram (mg) amounts; for example, the adult allowance for vitamin C is 60 mg. Other vitamins are measured in microgram (μg) amounts; the adult allowance for vitamin B-12 is 3 μg. Thus, the weight of ascorbic acid needed is 20,000 times that for vitamin B-12.

Selection of Foods for Vitamin Contents

In selecting the foods to furnish vitamins in the diet it is well to keep in mind the following points: (1) under normal circumstances it is better to use common food sources than concentrates, because foods furnish other essential factors as well; (2) it is important to consider the amount of a food that is ordinarily consumed and the frequency of its use in the diet; (3) the effects of processing and preparation of foods on the vitamin retention must be clearly understood; and (4) economic factors such as availability and cost must be considered. For example, 100 g of parsley furnish about 7,500 IU of vitamin A, whereas 100 g of milk supply only 130 IU of vitamin A. The small amount of parsley used occasionally as a garnish, however, will provide an insignificant amount of vitamin A compared with the 2 cups of milk a day, essential in an adequate diet, which furnish about 620 IU or 12 percent of the day's allowance for adults.

Vitamin Supplementation of the Diet Diets that are selected on the basis of the Daily Food Guide and that include a variety of foods usually provide the recommended amounts of vitamins. Although intakes of a few vitamins may not consistently reach the recommended level, the lack of evidence of overt or subclinical deficiency may indicate that the allowances are unrealistically high. Claims for the need and value of vitamin supplements are often exaggerated, and the popularity of megadose supplements is worrisome. Enthusiasm for vitamin pills frequently is based on the erroneous ideas that foods in the United States are depleted of vitamins or that excessive intakes will produce "super" health. In addition to concern about the unnecessary expense associated with purchase of the vitamins, often by those least able to afford them, the possibility of toxicity must be considered. Excessive intakes of vitamins A and D are known to have adverse effects. Traditionally water-soluble vitamins have been assumed to be nontoxic because the excess vitamin is excreted in the urine. This assumption, however, may not be appropriate in view of the number of undesirable side effects of ascorbic acid that have been reported since megadose consumption has become common. Self-medication with vitamins also creates the possibility of delay of proper medical care until a disease state is difficult or impossible to treat.

The value of appropriate use of vitamin supplementation cannot be disputed. Vitamin D supplementation for infants, growing children, and pregnant or lactating women is needed if fortified milk is not available or if exposure to sunlight is inadequate. With diets providing less than 1,400 kcal, it is difficult to select foods that provide the recommended intakes of all vitamins. Thus, vitamin supplements usually are desirable for persons consuming low calorie diets to lose weight or for elderly persons with reduced energy needs.

Vitamin supplements are also needed in some clinical situations, for example, illness characterized by inability to consume a normal diet, following surgery or severe injury, such as burns, in diseases of malabsorption, and so on. Sometimes supplements are needed to restore reserves when the diet has been inadequate because of ignorance, poor eating habits, or inability to obtain the necessary foods.

Vitamin A

Discovery In 1913 McCollum and Davis of the University of Wisconsin[1] and Osborne and Mendel of Yale University[2] independently discovered that rats consuming purified diets with lard as the only source of fat failed to grow and developed soreness of the eyes. When butterfat or ether extract of egg yolk was added to the diet, growth resumed and the eye condition was corrected. The term *fat-soluble A* was applied by McCollum to the organic complex present in the ether extract that was necessary for normal growth.

A few years later Steenbock at the University of Wisconsin[3] demonstrated that the yellow pigments in plants, the carotenes, had vitamin A activity. Because these carotenes and certain other carotenoid compounds can be converted to vitamin A in the body, they are now often referred to as PRECURSORS of vitamin A or as PROVITAMIN A.

Chemistry and Characteristics Vitamin A is active in many forms, the nomenclature being as follows[4]:

RETINOL—vitamin A, vitamin A alcohol (See Figure 11-1.)
RETINYL ESTERS—vitamin A esters
RETINALDEHYDE—vitamin A aldehyde, retinene, retinal
RETINOIC ACID—vitamin A acid

Collectively, these forms may be referred to as vitamin A.

In its pure form vitamin A is a pale-yellow crystalline compound. It occurs naturally in the animal kingdom and has been synthesized so that it is available commercially. It is soluble in fat and fat solvents. It is insoluble in water, but water-miscible forms are available for use in pharmaceutical products and food fortification. Vitamin A is relatively stable to heat and alkali. It is unstable to light and acid and is easily oxidized. Rapid destruction occurs with exposure at high temperatures in the presence of air, with ultraviolet irradiation, or in rancid fats.

The ultimate source of all vitamin A is the carotenoids which are synthesized by plants. Animals, in turn, and humans as well, convert a considerable proportion of the carotenoids in the foods they eat into vitamin A. The carotenoids are dark red crystalline compounds that give a deep yellow coloration to plants such as carrots and sweet potatoes. In deep green plants, also rich in carotenoids, the color is masked by chlorophyll. The carotenoids having vita-

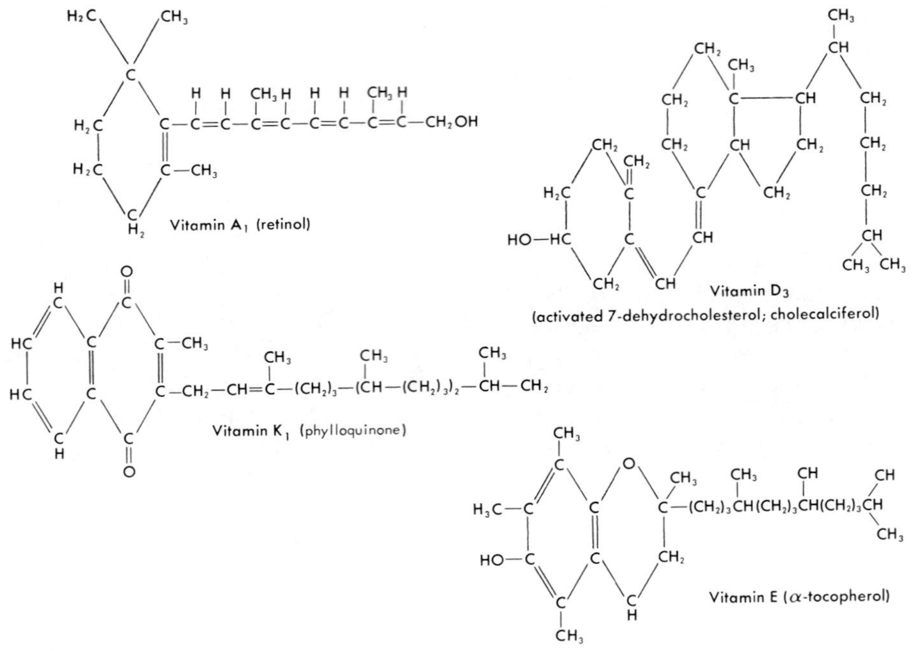

Figure 11-1. Each of the fat-soluble vitamins exists in several forms, only one of which is shown here. Note the similarity of structure of vitamin D to that of cholesterol.

min A activity include alpha-, beta-, and gamma-carotene and cryptoxanthin. Of these precursors, beta-carotene is the most plentiful in human foods and has the highest biologic activity. Upon hydrolysis each molecule of beta-carotene theoretically yields two molecules of vitamin A. Because of physiologic inefficiency in this conversion, however, the biologic activity of beta-carotene on a weight basis is only half that of vitamin A. The other carotenoid precursors are about half as active as beta-carotene.

Measurement   Vitamin A is measured in international units. The equivalents are

1 IU = 0.3 μg retinol
1 IU = 0.6 μg beta-carotene
1 IU = 1.2 μg other carotenoids

The Food and Nutrition Board had recommended that RETINOL EQUIVALENTS (RE) replace the international unit.[5] This system of measurement takes into account the amount of absorption of the carotenes as well as the degree of conversion to vitamin A, and thus is a more precise system of measures. The equivalents are

1 RE = 1 μg retinol (3.33 IU)
1 RE = 6 μg beta-carotene (10 IU)
1 RE = 12 μg other carotenoids (10 IU)

Values for vitamin A in this chapter will be expressed in RE with the corresponding values in IU placed in parentheses. Tables of food values at present express the values for vitamin A in international units.

Absorption, Storage, and Transport   Preformed vitamin A present in food as retinyl esters is hydrolyzed by pancreatic and intestinal enzymes to form free retinol. After absorption into the mucosal cell, retinol is reesterified to retinyl esters and incorporated into the chylomicrons for transport through the lymphatic system by way of the thoracic duct to the blood stream. Carotenes are split in the intestinal mucosa to form retinaldehyde which is then reduced to retinol. Although the principal conversion of carotenes to vitamin A takes place in the intestine, some carotenes are absorbed intact and converted in other tissues such as liver or kidney. The small amount of retinoic acid that may be present in the intestine is transported directly into the general circulation through the portal vein.

The absorption of vitamin A and the carotenes, like that of fat, is facilitated by bile. When a diet is very low in fat, or when there is an obstruction of the bile duct, the absorption of vitamin A and the carotenes is seriously impaired.

The simultaneous presence of vitamin E in the intestinal tract prevents the excessive oxidation of vitamin A that would otherwise occur. On the other hand, the presence of mineral oil reduces the absorption. Since mineral oil itself is not absorbed, it carries with it vitamin A and other fat-soluble vitamins. If used as a laxative, mineral oil should not be taken at or near mealtime.

Retinol is assumed to be completely absorbed from the gastrointestinal tract but the absorption of carotenes is about one third. Since about half of the absorbed beta-carotene is converted to retinol, only one sixth of the intake in food is actually utilized. For other carotenoids only one fourth is converted to retinol; thus, only one twelfth of the intake in foods is available. (See retinol equivalents, page 158.)

Vitamin A transported to the liver by the chylomicrons is removed for storage. About 90 percent of body stores of vitamin A are found in the liver, with the remainder being present in the kidney, lungs, adrenal glands, and adipose tissue. The healthy adult has reserves that are adequate for several months to a year. Infants and young children have not built up such reserves and therefore are much more susceptible to the effects of deficiency.

When vitamin A is released from the liver stores for use by other tissues, it is transported in the circulation as part of a complex with a specific transport protein called retinol-binding protein (RBP) and prealbumin. Normal concentrations of vitamin A in blood serum range form 20 to 80 μg per dl. The liver maintains the level in the blood as long as there is an adequate reserve. Only when the liver reserves are depleted will the blood concentration be lowered.

Vitamin A and products formed from its breakdown are excreted primarily in the bile. Some reabsorption occurs but most of the vitamin is lost in the feces. Some breakdown products may be excreted in the urine.

Functions   Although the existence of vitamin A has been known for over 60 years, its functions have not been fully explained. Retinyl esters, retinol, and retinaldehyde are readily converted from one form to the other, but retinoic acid cannot be converted to other forms. Retinoic acid appears to be the active form of the vitamin in some tissues but it cannot function in the visual cycle or support reproduction in most species. Retinoic acid also cannot be stored in the body.

Vision.   The best understood function of vitamin A is related to the maintenance of normal vision in dim light. The retina of the eye contains two kinds of light receptors: the rods for vision in dim light and the cones for vision in bright light and color vision. The rods produce a photosensitive pigment, RHODOPSIN or VISUAL PURPLE, and the cones produce IODOPSIN or VISUAL VIOLET.

In both these pigments vitamin A in the form of retinaldehyde is the prosthetic group, but the proteins to which the aldehyde is attached are different. When light strikes rhodopsin, changes occur in the chemical configuration of retinaldehyde and the pigment splits into its component parts, retinaldehyde and protein. These changes initiate a nerve impulse that is then transmitted to the brain by way of the optic nerve. Regeneration of rhodopsin occurs in the dark, but some retinaldehyde is lost in each cycle so that a constant supply from the blood must be present. A simplified diagram of the visual cycle is shown in Figure 11-2.

Other Functions.   Retinol and retinoic acid have a marked effect on the differentiation and proliferation of cells. Data from many studies suggest that vitamin A influences the expression of genes or gene products involved in these processes.[6]

Figure 11-2.   Metabolism of vitamin A for vision in dim light.

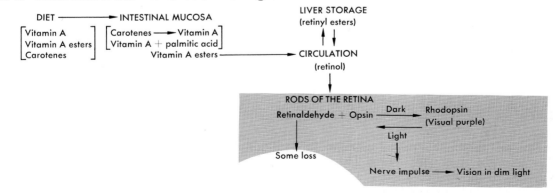

Vitamin A is required for healthy epithelium, whether covering the body externally or lining the mucous membranes. Because of the rapid turnover of epithelial cells, the need for vitamin A may relate to its role in cell differentiation and proliferation. Another way in which vitamin A influences epithelial tissues is through its role in the synthesis of constituents of mucus, such as the mucoproteins. The mucus secretions maintain the integrity of the epithelium, especially the membranes lining the eyes, the mouth, and the gastrointestinal, respiratory, and genitourinary tracts. These membranes provide resistance to bacterial invasion, and tissues weakened by a lack of vitamin A are more susceptible to infection. Large intakes of vitamin A exceeding amounts needed for normal functions, however, will not confer additional protective benefits against infection.

Vitamin A is essential for normal skeletal and tooth development. With a deficiency of vitamin A bones do not grow in length and the normal remodeling process does not take place. The precise function of vitamin A in these processes is not known but may relate to its role in the synthesis of glycoproteins, in cellular differentiation and proliferation, and in maintenance of the stability of cellular membranes. Studies in experimental animals have shown that vitamin A is essential for spermatogenesis in the male and normal estrous cycle in the female. If vitamin A is not available to the animal during fetal development, many malformations result.

Daily Allowances The recommended allowances for vitamin A are stated in retinol equivalents and international units.[5] When international units are calculated to retinol equivalents (see page 158), it is assumed that one half of the vitamin A is retinol and one half is beta-carotene. Thus, in the sample calculation 5,000 IU = 1,000 RE:

$$
\begin{array}{rl}
2,500 \text{ IU} \div 3.33 = & 750 \text{ RE} \\
2,500 \text{ IU} \div 10 \ = & \underline{250 \text{ RE}} \\
& 1,000 \text{ RE}
\end{array}
$$

The vitamin A allowance for males over 10 years is 1,000 RE or 5,000 IU and for females over 10 years it is 800 RE or 4,000 IU. The allowances for infants over 6 months and children up to 10 years are 375 to 700 RE, for pregnancy 800 RE, and for the first 6 months of lactation 1,300 RE.

Food Sources Only animal foods contain vitamin A as such, fish-liver oils being outstanding. These oils are generally not classified with common foods, but milk, butter, fortified margarines, whole-milk cheese, liver, and egg yolk contain vitamin A.

The principal source of vitamin A in the diet is likely to be from the carotenes, which are widespread in those plant foods that have high green or yellow colorings. There is a direct correlation between the greenness of a leaf and its carotene content. Dark-green leaves are rich in carotene, but the pale leaves, in lettuce and cabbage for example, are insignificant sources. Abundant sources of carotene are found in foods such as

Green leafy vegetables—spinach, turnip tops, chard, beet greens
Green stem vegetables—asparagus, broccoli
Yellow vegetables—carrots, sweet potatoes, winter squash, pumpkin
Yellow fruits—apricots, peaches, cantaloupe

The vitamin A contribution of the Daily Food Guide is indicated in Figure 11-3. The meat group contributes only when liver or an organ meat is served once every week to 10 days. One egg provides about one tenth of the daily allowance.

Retention of Food Values Since vitamin A is stable to the usual cooking temperatures, only slight losses are likely to occur in food preparation. The wilting of vegetables or dehydration of foods results in considerable losses. Canned and frozen foods retain maximal values for 9 months or longer. Vitamin A activity is rapidly lost in rancid fats.

Effects of Vitamin A Deficiency In the United States vitamin A deficiency should be practically nonexistent inasmuch as there are abundant dietary sources of vitamin A available. Results of the Nationwide Food Consumption Survey of 1977–78 showed that the average intake of vitamin A met or nearly met the recommended allowance for all sex–age groups.[7] However, 31 percent of individuals had intakes less than 70 percent of the recommended allowances, with the greatest numbers of low intakes occurring in persons 19 to 22 years of age. Evaluated on a nutrient-density basis, vitamin A intakes per 1,000 kcal for white and black individuals averaged 46 to 88 percent higher than that for individuals of Hispanic origin.[8] Average intakes of vitamin A in the 1976–80 Health and Nutrition Examination Survey essentially met the recommended allowances except in females 15 to 17 years of age with average intake of low income females being only about 66 percent of the recommended allowance.[9] Because the 1971–1974 HANES survey had shown little evidence of problems in vitamin A nutriture in older individuals, determinations of serum vitamin A in 1976 were made only in children aged 3 to 11 years. Serum vitamin A values

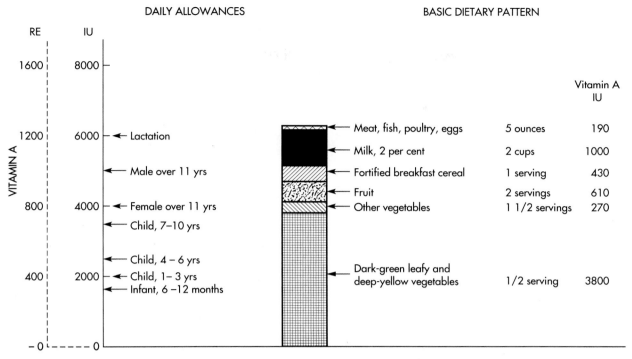

DAILY ALLOWANCES   BASIC DIETARY PATTERN

Vitamin A
IU

			Vitamin A IU
Meat, fish, poultry, eggs	5 ounces		190
Milk, 2 per cent	2 cups		1000
Fortified breakfast cereal	1 serving		430
Fruit	2 servings		610
Other vegetables	1 1/2 servings		270
Dark-green leafy and deep-yellow vegetables	1/2 serving		3800

RE / IU scale labels: Lactation (6000 IU), Male over 11 yrs, Female over 11 yrs (4000 IU), Child, 7–10 yrs, Child, 4–6 yrs, Child, 1–3 yrs (2000 IU), Infant, 6–12 months

Figure 11-3   The four food groups of the Basic Diet provide a liberal allowance of vitamin A for all age categories. Note the contributions made by dark green leafy and deep yellow vegetables. Some cereals are fortified with vitamin A but the bread-cereal group is not an important source. See Table 4-1 for complete calculations.

less than 20 μg per dl were found in about 2.5 percent of the boys and 3.2 percent of the girls.[10] The greatest number of low values occurred in black boys and white girls aged 3 to 5 years.

In other parts of the world vitamin A deficiency is the most prevalent vitamin deficiency and ranks second only to protein-energy malnutrition in its incidence. When the two conditions are present in the same child, the prognosis is very poor. Severe forms of vitamin A deficiency are practically nonexistent in the United States, but throughout the world up to 100,000 persons, chiefly children, become blind each year because of xerophthalmia caused by a lack of vitamin A.[11] The predominant regions of severe deficiency are the Middle East, India, Malaysia, Latin America, and South America.

It is ironic that the most severe forms of vitamin A deficiency occur in areas where there is an abundance of green plant foods. Through ignorance the young child is not given these foods. Vitamin A deficiency has been a major problem in areas in which famine has occurred such as Bangladesh and Africa. Vitamin A deficiency also results from faulty absorption in such diseases as sprue, celiac disease, and other malabsorptive disorders.

Night Blindness.   One of the earliest signs of vitamin A deficiency is night blindness, or NYCTALOPIA. This is a condition in which the individual is unable to see well in dim light, especially on coming into darkness from a bright light as in entering a darkened theater. Drivers who are easily blinded (glare blindness) by the headlights of other automobiles and who consequently see road markers, pedestrians, and so on, with difficulty constitute a special traffic hazard.

Night blindness occurs when there is insufficient vitamin A to bring about prompt and complete regeneration of visual purple. Blood carotene and vitamin A levels and a substantiating dietary history are useful in establishing a diagnosis of vitamin A deficiency. Other causes of night blindness must be ruled out. If a therapeutic dose of vitamin A does not bring about relief of night blindness after a few weeks' trial, it may be assumed that the condition is not a vitamin A deficiency.

Epithelial Changes.   An inadequate supply of vitamin A may lead to definite changes in the epithelial tissues throughout the body: KERATINIZATION, or a noticeable shrinking, hardening, and progressive degeneration of the cells, occurs, which increases the susceptibility to severe infections of the eye, the nasal passages, the sinus, middle ear, lungs, and genitourinary tract.

Skin changes in severe vitamin A deficiency known as FOLLICULAR HYPERKERATOSIS have been described. The skin becomes rough, dry, and scaly. The keratinized epithelium plugs the sebaceous glands so that goose-pimple-like follicles appear first along the upper forearms and thighs, and then spread along the shoulders, back, abdomen, and buttocks.

Xerophthalmia The term XEROPHTHALMIA means dryness of the eye. Development of the condition passes through various stages that may ultimately lead to irreparable damage.[12] The first mild symptoms of epithelial changes in the eye are suggested by night blindness. The young child, most likely to be affected, is unable to describe this condition, but the mother, upon questioning, may be aware that the child does not see well at dusk. Then XEROSIS of the conjunctiva occurs, characterized by dryness and dullness. BITOT'S SPOTS, which are grayish plaques appearing on the conjunctiva, may or may not be seen. This is followed by xerosis of the cornea, which becomes dry and opaque. At this stage the condition is reversible if properly treated. The corneal xerosis rapidly progresses to involvement of the deeper layers of the cornea, perforation, keratomalacia, scarring, and loss of sight. (See Figure 11-4.)

Prevention and Treatment Much vitamin A deficiency could be prevented if carotene-rich foods were included in the diet. A very low fat intake, common in many dietaries, reduces the efficiency of absorption. When skim milk is used for the correction of protein-calorie malnutrition, it is essential that it be fortified with vitamin A; such fortification is now prevalent.

When deficiency occurs, treatment is rapidly effective with large doses of vitamin A provided that the eye conditions have not become irreversible. In parts of the world with a high incidence of blindness, strategies to prevent deficiency include intermittent administration of massive oral doses of vitamin A (100,000 to 300,000 IU), fortification of one or more foods that are widely consumed, increased production of vitamin-A-rich foods as well as nutrition education.

Hypervitaminosis A Excessive intakes of vitamin A are toxic to both children and adults and should be avoided. Toxicity in adults is seen with intakes more than 50,000 IU for months or years.[13] In young children administration of doses of 20,000 to 60,000 IU per day for periods of 1 to 3 months has produced vitamin A intoxication.[14] The common symptoms of toxicity are anorexia, hyperirritability, drying and desquamation of the skin. Loss of hair, bone and joint pain, bone fragility, headaches, hypercalcemia, and

Figure 11-4.   Indonesian girl, 2 years of age, with xerophthalmia. There is extensive xerosis and wrinkling of the conjunctiva. The cornea is dry, dull and opaque. From: Oomen, H. A. P. C.: "Vitamin A Deficiency, Xerophthalmia and Blindness," *Nutr. Rev.*, **32:**161, 1974. (Courtesy, The Nutrition Foundation, Inc.)

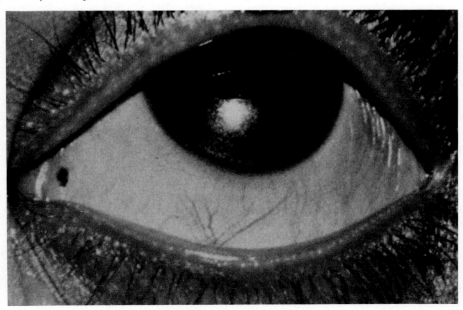

enlargement of the liver and spleen are other manifestations of toxicity. When vitamin A is discontinued, recovery takes place. Excessive intake of carotenes does not produce toxicity but may produce a yellow discoloration of the skin that disappears when the intake is reduced.

Vitamin A and Cancer The possibility of an important relationship between vitamin A and cancer is supported by experimental and epidemiologic data. Many years ago it was observed that a deficiency of vitamin A leads to cellular changes similar to those that occur when a normal cell is transformed to a precancerous cell.[15] In animals vitamin A also has been shown to have a preventive effect on the appearance of certain types of tumors induced by chemical carcinogens. Because cancer is basically a disorder of cell differentiation, it is easy to postulate that the vitamin A status of a cell may influence its potential for cancer development.[6] Several epidemiologic studies have shown an inverse correlation between plasma retinol levels and cancer risk, although findings in a recent study failed to support such a relationship.[16] Other epidemiologic studies have shown that high intakes of foods rich in retinol and beta-carotene are associated with decreased cancer risk. The protective effect of beta-carotene may be independent of its ability to be converted to retinol.[17] Because of the toxicity of retinol, research efforts have focused on development of synthetic retinoids that will have similar anticancer properties without the undesirable side effects. Clinical studies have been initiated to evaluate some of these products and also beta-carotene in protecting against cancer. The Interim Dietary Guidelines to Prevent Cancer emphasize the consumption of carotene-rich vegetables. (See Table 3-4.)

Vitamin D

Cod liver oil has been recommended as a remedy for rickets ever since the Middle Ages but does not appear to have been used with any consistency until the present century. During World War I, Hess and Unger noted the effect of cod liver oil in protecting black children in New York City against rickets. Then in 1919 Mellanby found that the skeletal structure of puppies was influenced by some fat-soluble substance in food. McCollum, Steenbock, and Drummond simultaneously reported that cod liver oil in which vitamin A had been destroyed still retained its antirachitic properties, and hence it was shown that vitamin A was not the antirachitic factor. Steenbock and Hess in 1924 independently found that foods that had

been exposed to ultraviolet rays possessed antirachitic properties. Pure vitamin D was isolated in crystalline form in 1930 and was called calciferol.

Chemistry and Characteristics Vitamin D is a group of chemically distinct sterol compounds possessing antirachitic properties. The two forms of the vitamin which are of significance nutritionally are vitamin D_2 (ERGOCALCIFEROL, CALCIFEROL, or VIOSTEROL) and vitamin D_3 (CHOLECALCIFEROL). Vitamin D_2 is formed when ergosterol found in plants is exposed to ultraviolet light. Vitamin D_3 is the chief form occurring in animal cells and develops in the skin on exposure of 7-DEHYDROCHOLESTEROL to ultraviolet light from sunshine. (See Figure 11-1.) Pure D vitamins are white, odorless crystals that are stable to heat, alkalies, and oxidation. They are insoluble in water but soluble in fat and fat solvents.

Measurement Traditionally vitamin D has been measured in international units (1 IU = 0.025 μg pure crystalline vitamin D). Based on the recommendations of an international expert committee, the Food and Nutrition Board has decided to express intakes of vitamin D as micrograms of cholecalciferol.[5]

For many years, the LINE TEST was used to measure the potency of vitamin D in materials. The test was based on changes in the line of calcification in the ends of the long bones of young vitamin D-deficient rats after administration of the test material for 7 to 10 days. Standard cod liver oil was fed to a similar group of animals and was used as the basis for comparison. For most purposes the line test has been replaced by newer methods that determine the concentration of the vitamin itself as well as its metabolites. However, these methods may not be practical for routine clinical use.

Absorption and Excretion Dietary vitamin D is absorbed along with food fats from the jejunum and ileum and is transported in the chylomicrons through the lymph circulation. Bile is essential for effective absorption, and anything that interferes with fat absorption, such as pancreatitis, sprue, and malabsorption disorders, also affects the completeness of vitamin D absorption. Vitamin D made in the skin enters the blood, where it circulates attached to a specific protein that also transports metabolites of the vitamin formed in other tissues. The major pathway for excretion of vitamin D appears to be through the bile.

Functions Although the importance of vitamin D in calcium and phosphorus metabolism has been recognized for many decades, the mechanisms involved in its actions were poorly understood. Exciting research in the past 15 years by DeLuca and co-workers at the University of Wisconsin[18] and others[19-21] has contributed significantly not only in elucidating the functions of vitamin D but also in making available new forms of the vitamin which have had important applications in the treatment of serious bone diseases.

Vitamin D itself is an inactive, storage form of the vitamin that is concentrated in the liver and to a lesser extent in the skin, spleen, lungs, brain, and kidney. In the liver vitamin D is rapidly hydroxylated to 25-HYDROXYVITAMIN D_3 (25-OH-D_3), also known as 25-HYDROXYCHOLECALCIFEROL or CALCIDIOL. The 25-OH-D_3 released from the liver is the principal form of vitamin D circulating in the blood, but at physiological concentrations it does not appear to act directly on any target tissue. In the kidney 25-OH-D_3 is further hydroxylated to form a number of metabolites, the most important being 1,25-DIHYDROXYCHOLECALCIFEROL [1,25(OH)$_2D_3$] or CALCITRIOL. This compound, considered the active form of vitamin D, circulates to the intestine where it stimulates synthesis of proteins necessary for the transport of calcium across the intestinal mucosa. It also promotes absorption of phosphorus. Formation of 1,25(OH)$_2D_3$ in the kidney occurs in response to the increase in the blood level of parathyroid hormone that is initiated whenever there is a fall in serum calcium. Low serum phosphorus also enhances 1,25(OH)$_2D_3$ formation. In addition to affecting intestinal absorption, 1,25(OH)$_2D_3$ stimulates mobilization of calcium, and consequently phosphorus, from bone and may improve renal reabsorption of calcium. These actions increase the calcium and phosphorus levels of the blood, thereby permitting normal mineralization of the bone matrix and cartilage as well as maintaining the correct concentration of calcium in extracellular fluids for muscle contraction and nerve irritability.

Because of its effect on distinct target tissues and the feedback control on its formation mediated by changes in serum calcium and phosphorus, 1,25(OH)$_2D_3$ may be considered a hormone and vitamin D a prohormone. (See Figure 11-5.) Nevertheless, vitamin D still can be considered a vitamin, because many individuals would be unable to meet their requirement for this essential substance if it were not supplied at least in part by the diet.

Daily Allowances   As little as 2.5 μg (100 IU) will promote bone development and prevent rickets. The recommended allowance of 10 μg (400 IU) is well documented for full-term and premature infants. Vita-

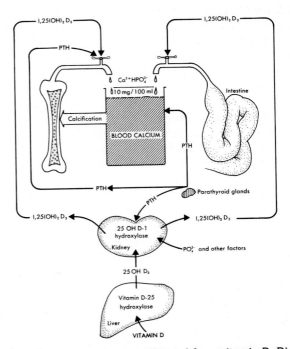

Figure 11-5.   Hormonal loop derived from vitamin D. Diagram shows calcium homeostatic system. In the intestine 1.25(OH)$_2D_3$ functions without the presence of parathyroid hormone: in bone the presence of parathyroid hormone is essential. (Reprinted from *Federation Proceedings* **33:**2215. 1974. Courtesy, Dr. H. F. DeLuca and *Federaton Proceedings*.)

min D should be supplied to bottle-fed infants either in fortified milk or in supplements. Supplements of vitamin D also are frequently recommended for breast-fed infants.[22]

The allowances for persons of other ages are difficult to establish because of exposure to sunlight, but 10 μg (400 IU) is recommended daily for children and young adults through 24 years of age. The allowance is reduced to 5 μg (200 IU) for men and women. To meet the increased needs occurring in pregnancy and lactation, an intake of 10 μg (400 IU) is recommended.

Sources   Exposure to sunlight, fortified foods, fish-liver oils, and commercial vitamin D preparations are the sources of vitamin D. Natural foods are poor sources of vitamin D, although small amounts are present in egg yolk, liver, and fish such as herring, sardines, tuna, and salmon.

About 85 percent of fresh milk and almost all evaporated milk are fortified with 10 μg (400 IU) vitamin D per quart. Milk is especially suitable for fortification since it contains the calcium and phosphorus whose absorption it facilitates and because it is an important food consumed by children. The fortification of foods other than milk is of dubious value, since the ingestion of several foods so treated could lead to excessive intake.

Exposure of the skin to sunlight brings about the synthesis of vitamin D from the precursor 7-dehydrocholesterol. Sunlight cannot always be depended upon to supply the body with adequate ultraviolet rays to manufacture vitamin D, because these rays are so easily strained out by dust, smoke, fog, clothing, and ordinary window glass—all of which act as barriers to prevent the rays from reaching the skin.

The tolerance for vitamin D varies widely. As little as 45 μg (1,800 IU) over a long period of time may be mildly toxic to children, whereas massive doses of 2500 μg (100,000 IU) are tolerated and may be required by those rare individuals who have vitamin D-resistant rickets. The symptoms of toxicity include nausea, vomiting, diarrhea, excessive thirst, weight loss, polyuria, and nocturia. As the toxicity becomes more severe, renal damage and calcification of the soft tissues such as the heart, blood vessels, bronchi, stomach, and tubules of the kidney occur. Diagnosis is based on history of excess intake and laboratory tests showing hypercalcemia.

A deficiency of vitamin D leads to inadequate absorption of calcium and phosphorus from the intestinal tract and to faulty mineralization of bone and tooth structures. The inability of the soft bones to withstand the stress of weight results in skeletal malformations.

Rickets.   Infantile rickets is rarely seen in the United States because of the widespread use of fortified milk or of vitamin D preparations in prophylaxis. When such preventive measures are not taken, rickets is more prevalent in northern regions than in warm, sunny climates. It is more likely to develop in dark, overcrowded sections of large cities where the ultraviolet rays of sunshine, especially in the winter months, cannot penetrate through the fog, smoke, and soot. Poverty and ignorance may account for failure to obtain enough vitamin D from concentrates, fortified milk, or skin exposure. Dark-skinned children are more susceptible to rickets than those of the white race. Premature infants are more susceptible to rickets than full-term infants since the growth rate and the calcification of the skeleton impose additional demands for vitamin D.

Fully developed cases of rickets present the following characteristics (see Figure 11-6):

1. Delayed closure of the fontanelles, softening of the skull (craniotabes), and bulging or bossing of the forehead, giving the head a boxlike appearance
2. Soft, fragile bones leading to widening of the ends of the long bones; bowing of the legs; enlargement of the costochondral junction with rows of knobs or beads forming the RACHITIC ROSARY; projection of the sternum as in "pigeon breast"; narrowing of the pelvis; spinal curvature
3. Enlargement of wrist, knee (knock-knees), and ankle joints
4. Poorly developed muscles; lack of muscle tone—pot belly—being the result of weakness of abdominal muscles; weakness, with delayed walking
5. Restlessness and nervous irritability
6. High serum alkaline phosphatase; low inorganic blood phosphorus; normal or low serum calcium

Early skeletal deformities of rickets often persist throughout life. Bowlegs that curve laterally, as shown here, indicate that the weakened bones have bent after the second year, as a result of standing. (Courtesy, Dr. Rosa Lee Nemir, Professor of Pediatrics, New York University—Bellevue Medical Center, and the Upjohn Company, *The Vitamin Manual* published by The Upjohn Company.)

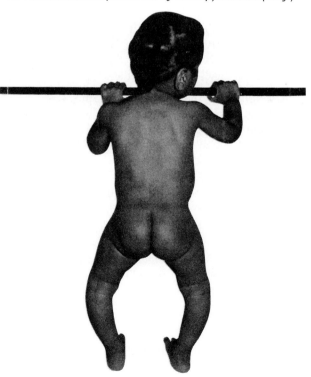

Rickets is treated by giving relatively large amounts of vitamin D concentrates, the dosage being prescribed by the physician.

Tetany. Tetany is characterized by a low serum calcium (7.5 mg per dl or less), muscle twitchings, cramps, and convulsions. It results from insufficient absorption of calcium or vitamin D, or from a disturbance of the parathyroid gland. The physician prescribes calcium salts to control the acute spasms, a diet liberal in calcium, and vitamin D.

Dental Health. In rachitic infants and children there may be delayed dentition and malformation of the teeth. Permanent teeth forming in the jaw are more subject to decay.

Osteomalacia. Frequently referred to as "adult rickets," OSTEOMALACIA literally means bone softening. It occurs when there is lack of vitamin D and calcium. In the Orient it is seen in women who have had many pregnancies, who subsist on a meager cereal diet, and who have little exposure to sunshine.

Osteomalacia may occur when there is interference with fat absorption, and hence also vitamin D absorption. The steatorrhea also reduces the absorption of calcium. In chronic renal disease patients often complain of bone pain, and osteodystrophy may be severe. There is little absorption of calcium apparently because the kidney is unable to produce $1,25(OH)_2D_3$. Bone abnormalities also are associated with some diseases of the liver because of impaired formation of $25\text{-}(OH)\text{-}D_3$.

The following changes take place in osteomalacia:

1. A softening of the bones, which may be so severe that the bones of the legs, spine, thorax, and pelvis bend into deformities.
2. Pain of the rheumatic type in bones of the legs and lower part of the back.
3. General weakness with difficulty in walking, and especially difficulty in climbing stairs.
4. Spontaneous multiple fractures.

Availability of $25\text{-}(OH)\text{-}D_3$ and $1,25(OH)_2D_3$ has led to significant advances in the treatment of these bone disorders. The effective dosages are much smaller than those of vitamin D_3.

Vitamin E

Discovery Evans and Bishop established the fact that a fat-soluble factor was necessary for reproduction in rats. They showed that absence of vitamin E, or the antisterility factor, as it was designated, led to irreparable damage of the germinal epithelium in male rats, and female rats which had diets deficient in vitamin E were unable to carry their young to term. In severe deficiency the fetus dies and is reabsorbed completely. In the female the damage is not permanent; that is, normal reproduction could again take place if the diet were once more adequate in this factor. The name TOCOPHEROL was suggested for this factor based on the Greek words *tokos* meaning "birth" and *phero* "to carry." The ending *-ol* indicates that the substance is an alcohol.

Chemistry and Characteristics Vitamin E is a generic term for a group of lipid-soluble compounds, the tocopherols and tocotrienols, that possess varying degrees of vitamin activity. Alpha-tocopherol is the most active of these compounds. (See Figure 11-1.) The tocopherols and tocotrienols differ in the chemical structure of their side chains.

High temperatures and acids do not affect the stability of vitamin E, but oxidation takes place readily in the presence of rancid fats or lead and iron salts. Decomposition occurs in ultraviolet light. Vitamin E itself acts as an antioxidant.

Measurement Vitamin E is expressed in international units or in milligrans of alpha-tocopherol. One international unit of vitamin E is equal to 1 mg synthetic *dl*-alpha-tocopherol acetate. The activity of the natural form, *d*-alpha-tocopherol acetate, is 1.36 IU per mg; and that of the free alcohol, *d*-alpha-tocopherol, is 1.49 IU per mg.[5] Dietary evaluations are concerned primarily with alpha-tocopherol. The other tocopherols and tocotrienols in foods contribute vitamin E activity equal to about 20 percent of the alpha-tocopherol content of the diet.

Physiology Vitamin E requires the presence of fat and of bile salts for absorption into the intestinal wall. The vitamin is taken up from the intestine into lymph and transported to the circulation in chylomicrons. In the blood vitamin E in chylomicrons equilibrates with other plasma lipoproteins. Thus there is no specific transport protein for vitamin E in plasma. Small amounts of vitamin E are present in all body tissues, with the bulk of the body stores of vitamin E in the muscle, liver, and adipose tissue. There is little transfer of vitamin E across the placenta to the fetus. Hence, newborn infants have low tissue stores.

The total plasma tocopherol ranges from 0.5 to 1.2 mg per dl. A level below 0.5 is undesirable. In normal individuals there is a high correlation between plasma total lipids and plasma tocopherol concentration. Thus, conditions that alter blood lipids may lead to changes in plasma tocopherol that may not necessarily reflect changes in tissue concentrations of the vitamin.[23]

Functions The metabolic roles of vitamin E are poorly understood. The principal role appears to be as an antioxidant. By accepting oxygen, vitamin E helps to prevent the oxidation of polyunsaturated fatty acids and phospholipids thereby helping to maintain the integrity of cellular membranes. As a constituent of the enzyme glutathione peroxidase, selenium shares a role with vitamin E in preventing destruction of lipids by oxidation. In animal experiments selenium has been shown to prevent some of the symptoms associated with vitamin E deficiency. Vitamin E has a sparing effect on vitamin A by protecting it against oxidation. Many other functions have been proposed for vitamin E as well but have not received wide acceptance.

Daily Allowances Intakes of vitamin E recommended by the Food and Nutrition Board are expressed as alpha-tocopherol equivalents in which 1 mg d-alpha-tocopherol = 1α-TE.[5] Total vitamin E activity (mg α-TE) in a mixed diet is calculated as follows:

$$\begin{array}{ll} \text{mg alpha-tocopherol} & \\ + \text{ mg beta-tocopherol} & \times 0.5 \\ + \text{ mg gamma-tocopherol} & \times 0.1 \\ + \text{ mg alpha-tocotrienol} & \times 0.3 \end{array}$$

These are the only vitamers present in the United States diet that have significant vitamin activity. If only the alpha-tocopherol content of a mixed diet is known, the value in milligrams should be multiplied by 1.2 to account for the other tocopherols that are present.

Recommended intakes are 3 to 4 mg α-TE during the first year of life, 8 mg α-TE for women and 10 mg α-TE for men. An additional 2 and 4 mg α-TE are recommended for women during pregnancy and lactation, respectively.

The need for vitamin E is higher when the intake of polyunsaturated fatty acids is increased. Since the principal source of vitamin E is from vegetable oils and margarines, the increased intake of linoleic acid from these fats is accompanied by the satisfactory intake of vitamin E. At the present time there is no fixed ratio of vitamin E to polyunsaturated fatty acids that can be recommended.[24]

Sources The principal sources of vitamin E in the diet are vegetable oils (corn, soy, cottonseed, safflower), hydrogenated fats from these oils, whole grains, and dark green leafy vegetables, nuts, and legumes. Foods of animal origin are low in vitamin E. Human milk provides adequate vitamin E for the infant, but cow's milk is low. See Table A-2 for alpha-tocopherol content of foods.

The content of tocopherols in foods varies widely. In general, the tocopherol level in oils increases as the linoleic acid content increases. There is considerable loss in fried foods that are frozen and also in the heating of oils. The milling of grains removes about 80 percent of the vitamin E. Destruction of the remaining vitamin occurs if chlorine dioxide is used in the bleaching process. Typical diets in the United States provide 7 to 9 mg alpha-tocopherol or a total vitamin E activity of 8 to 11 mg α-TE.[25] In view of the absence of signs of dietary deficiency of vitamin E, the diets in the United States are presumed to meet body needs.

Effects of Deficiency Vitamin E deficiency is extremely rare. In the United States deficiency in adults has been observed only in individuals with chronic fat malabsorption. Changes occurring in severe deficiency include increased hemolysis of red blood cells, creatinuria, and deposition of brownish ceroid pigment in smooth muscle. Recent evidence has established that vitamin E deficiency is a cause of the impaired neuromuscular function sometimes seen in patients with disorders that interfere with absorption or transport of the vitamin.[23,26] Symptoms include poor reflexes, impaired locomotion, decreased sensation in the hands and feet, and changes in the retina. This evidence indicates that vitamin E has an important role in the maintenance of normal neurologic structure and function.

Normal men fed experimental diets extremely low in vitamin E over a period of several years showed an increased hemolysis of red blood cells but no clinical symptoms. The length of time to bring about the onset of hemolysis was shortened when the intake of polyunsaturated fats was increased.[27]

Premature and low-birth-weight infants show an extremely low level of tocopherol in the serum and increased hemolysis of red blood cells. When such infants were fed a diet high in polyunsaturated fat and low in vitamin E, they developed a syndrome characterized by edema, skin lesions, and hemolytic anemia. These abnormalities disappeared when vitamin E supplements were given.[28] Evidence of vitamin E deficiency also has been observed in children with cystic fibrosis.

Other Claims for Vitamin E. When animals are placed on diets devoid of vitamin E a wide range of symptoms is observed, with considerable variation from one species to another. Among the changes observed have been reproductive failure, macrocytic anemia, shorter life span of the red cells, creatinuria, liver necrosis, encephalomalacia, and muscular dystrophy. The results of these studies have been widely misinterpreted and applied to human nutrition. The fact that human diets generally provide ample amounts of vitamin E is ignored.

Vitamin E has been recommended for such widely varying conditions as heart disease, muscular dystrophy, acne, ulcers, habitual abortion, disorders of the menopause, and sexual impotence. Objective studies, however, have failed to support most of these exaggerated claims. Vitamin E treatment may lead to improvement in some patients with intermittent claudication, a condition that causes pain in the calves of the legs while walking. Administration of vitamin E also appears to be beneficial in preventing retinal damage in premature infants receiving oxygen therapy. However, further research is needed to evaluate these and other therapeutic uses which have been proposed for vitamin E.[23]

Toxicity In view of the widespread popularity of megadose supplementation with vitamin E, it is fortunate that the vitamin appears to be relatively nontoxic. Most adults appear to be able to tolerate doses as high as 100 to 1,000 IU per day. However, several reports of adverse effects such as elevation of serum lipids, impaired blood coagulation, and reduction of serum thyroid hormones would suggest that indiscriminate ingestion of excessive amounts of the vitamin over long periods of time should be discouraged.[13,23]

Vitamin K

The existence of vitamin K was first suggested by Dr. Dam of Copenhagen, who in 1935 found that a "Koagulations Vitamin" was necessary to prevent fatal hemorrhages in chicks by promoting normal blood clotting.

Chemistry and Characteristics Vitamin K consists of a number of related compounds known as *quinones*; vitamin K_1, also known as *phylloquinone*, was first isolated from alfalfa, and vitamin K_2 also termed *menaquinone*, was produced from putrefied fishmeal and is also the form synthesized by intestinal bacteria. (See Figure 11-1.)

Menadione is a synthetic compound that is two to three times as potent as the natural vitamin. Vitamin K is fat soluble, resistant to heat, but easily destroyed by acids, alkalies, light, and oxidizing agents.

Measurement The activity of test materials has traditionally been measured by their ability to prevent hemorrhage in young chicks. New methods are available which measure the amount of the different vitamin K compounds directly.

Physiology Being fat soluble, dietary vitamin K requires the presence of bile for its absorption, most of which occurs in the upper part of the small intestine. Vitamin K also can be synthesized by bacteria in the lower intestinal tract. It is estimated that approximately 50 percent of the daily requirement is derived from plant sources and the rest from bacterial synthesis.[29] Limited stores of vitamin K are maintained but the concentration is not as high in any tissues.

The newborn infant has a very limited supply of vitamin K, and synthesis by the relatively sterile intestinal tract does not take place for several days. Human milk supplies about one fourth as much vitamin K as does cow's milk. Thus, the first few days may be critical for the infant.

Function Vitamin K is essential for the formation of PROTHROMBIN and other clotting proteins by the liver. (See page 113.) It acts as a cofactor for an enzyme in the liver which converts glutamic acid residues in a precursor protein to gamma-carboxyglutamic acid, this reaction being necessary before prothrombin can function in blood coagulation. A high prothrombin level indicates good ability to coagulate blood, whereas low blood levels of prothrombin are associated with a slow rate of clotting. Vitamin K also is assumed to be required for the synthesis of other proteins containing gamma-carboxyglutamic acid which have been identified in bone and kidney. More research is needed to clarify the functions of these proteins.[30]

Daily Allowances For the first time vitamin K allowances have been listed in the table of allowances. The maintenance of a normal plasma prothrombin concentration of 80 to 120 μg per ml is the primary basis for setting an allowance. Human milk is low in vitamin K and will supply about one fifth the daily infant's allowance of 5 μg. The recommended allowance for children ranges from 15 to 30 μg, for teenagers and young adults from 45 to 70 μg. The recommended intake for adults, 65 to 80

Table 11-1. Summary of the Fat-Soluble Vitamins

Nomenclature	Important Sources	Physiology and Functions	Effect of Deficiency	Daily Allowances*

Vitamin A
Retinol
Retinal
Retinyl ester
Retinoic acid
Provitamin A
Alpha-, beta-,
gamma-carotene,
cryptoxanthin
	Animal
	Fish-liver oils
	Liver
	Butter, cream
	Whole milk
	Whole-milk cheeses
	Egg yolk
	Plant
	Dark-green leafy vegetables
	Yellow vegetables
	Yellow fruits
	Fortified margarines
		Bile necessary for absorption
		Stored in liver
		Maintains integrity of mucosal
		  epithelium, maintains visual
		  acuity in dim light
		Large amounts are toxic
			Faulty bone and tooth development
			Night blindness
			Keratinization of epithelium—
			  mucous membranes and skin
			Xerophthalmia
				Children: 400–700 RE
				  (2,000–3,300 IU)
				Men: 1,000 RE (5,000 IU)
				Women: 800 RE (4,000 IU)
				Pregnancy: 800 RE (4,000 IU)
				Lactation: 1,200 RE (6,000 IU)

Vitamin D
Vitamin D_2
Ergocalciferol
Vitamin D_3
Cholecalciferol
Antirachitic factor
	Fish-liver oils
	Fortified milk
	Activated sterols
	Exposure to sunlight
	Very small amounts in butter, liver,
	  egg yolk, salmon, sardines
		Synthesized in skin by activity of
		  ultraviolet light
		Liver synthesizes $25(OH)D_3$
		Kidney synthesizes $1,25(OH)_2 D_3$
		Functions as steroid hormone to
		  regulate calcium and phosphorus
		  absorption, mobilization, and
		  mineralization of bone
		Large amounts are toxic
			Rickets in children
			Soft, fragile bones
			Enlarged joints
			Bowed legs
			Chest, spinal, pelvic, bone
			  deformities
			Delayed dentition
			Tetanic convulsions in infants
			Osteomalacia in adults
				Infants, 6 months: 7.5 μg
				Children 1–18 years: 10 μg
				Adults 19–24 years: 10 μg
				Adults: 5 μg
				Pregnant or lactating
				  women: 10 μg

Vitamin E
Alpha-, beta-, gamma-tocopherol
Antisterility vitamin
	Plant tissue—vegetable oils; wheat
	  germ, rice germ; green leafy
	  vegetables; nuts; legumes
	Animal foods are poor sources
		Not stored in body to any extent
		Related to action of selenium
		Humans: reduces oxidation of
		  vitamin A, carotenes,
		  polyunsaturated fatty acids, and
		  phospholipids
		Animals: normal reproduction;
		  utilization of sex hormones,
		  cholesterol
			Humans: hemolysis of red blood
			  cells; mild anemia; impaired
			  neuromuscular function;
			  deficiency is not likely
			Animals: sterility in male rats;
			  resorption of fetus in female rats;
			  muscular dystrophy; creatinuria;
			  macrocytic anemia
				Infants: 3–4 mg α-TE
				Men: 10 mg α-TE
				Women: 8 mg α-TE
				Pregnancy: 10 mg α-TE
				Lactation: 11 mg α-TE

Vitamin K
Phylloquinone
  (K_1)
Menaquinone
Menadione
	Green leaves such as alfalfa,
	  spinach, cabbage
	Liver
	Synthesis in intestine
		Bile necessary for absorption
		Formation of prothrombin and other
		  clotting proteins
		Sulfa drugs, large amounts of
		  vitamins A and E, and antibiotics
		  interfere with absorption
		Large amounts are toxic
			Prolonged clotting time
			Hemorrhagic disease in new born
			  infants
				Infants: 5–10 μg
				Children: 15–30 μg
				Teenagers: 45–65 μg
				Adults: 65–80 μg

* See Recommended Dietary Allowances (inside front cover) for complete listing.

μg per day, is easily supplied by diet in the United States, and dietary deficiency is not believed to be a problem.

Sources Green leaves of plants such as spinach and kale are excellent sources of vitamin K as are also cabbage, cauliflower, and pork liver. Cereals, fruits, and other vegetables are poor sources.

Effects of Deficiency A low blood level of prothrombin and other clotting factors leads to increased tendency to hemorrhage. Premature infants, anoxic infants, and those whose mothers have been taking anticoagulants are most susceptible to deficiency. The hemorrhagic disease of the newborn can be prevented by a single dose of vitamin K_1 administered to the infant immediately after birth. The practice of giving vitamin K to the mother before delivery has been questioned since too much may lead to hemolytic anemia in the infant.

Dietary deficiency of vitamin K is not likely. Deficiency may occur in adults because of a failure in absorption, or interference with the synthesis in the intestine, or inability to form prothrombin by the liver. Oral therapy with sulfa drugs and antibiotics interferes with the synthesis of the vitamin in the intestine. Obstruction of the biliary tract and severe diarrhea as in sprue, celiac disease, and colitis may seriously interfere with absorption. Large amounts of vitamins A and E may interfere with the absorption or metabolism of vitamin K. In severe disease of the liver, the synthesis of the clotting factors is impaired even though the source of vitamin K is adequate.

If absorption is inadequate, vitamin K may be prescribed orally together with bile salts. Parenteral administration may be required when there is severe intestinal disease.

Dicumarol is an anticoagulant often used to treat coronary thrombosis. It is antagonistic to the action of vitamin K and prevents the formation of prothrombin. Anticoagulant therapy carries the risk of hemorrhage. When an excessive amount of anticoagulant is given, vitamin K may be administered to counteract it.

Problems and Review

1. What is the relationship of carotene to vitamin A? What are the important sources of carotene?
2. Why are young children more susceptible than adults to deficiency of vitamin A or D? Describe the signs of deficiency that may be seen in children.
3. *Problem.* Calculate the vitamin A content of your own diet for two days. What percentage of your daily allowance is provided by sources rich in vitamin A? By sources rich in the provitamin?
4. A diet supplies 2,000 IU retinol and 3,000 IU beta-carotene. To how many RE are these equivalent? Does the diet meet the need of the pregnant woman?.
5. Why is the fortification of milk with vitamin D generally recommended? Why is the fortification of other foods not desirable?
6. What interrelationship exists between these factors: vitamin A and E; vitamin D and phosphorus; vitamin D and calcium; vitamin E and selenium; vitamin E and polyunsaturated fatty acids; vitamin E and vitamin K?
7. What is the relationship of vitamin K to blood clotting? Under what circumstances is a deficiency of vitamin K likely to occur?
8. What is the principal function of vitamin E? What conditions are necessary to produce a deficiency of vitamin E? What abnormalities are associated with vitamin E deficiency in humans?
9. Which of the fat-soluble vitamins functions as a hormone? How is the hormone formed? What is the role of the parathyroid hormone?
10. Describe the mechanism by which retinaldehyde participates in night vision.
11. What problems are associated with excess intakes of the fat-soluble vitamins? What levels of intake are likely to lead to toxicity?
12. What functions of vitamin A make it especially important in relationship to cancer?

References

1. McCollum, E. V., and Davis, M.: "The Necessity of Certain Lipids in the Diet During Growth." *J. Biol. Chem.*, 15:167–76, 1913. See " Nutrition Classic," *Nutr. Rev.*, 31:280–81, 1973.
2. Osborne, T. B., and Mendel, L. B.: "The Relation of Growth to the Chemical Constituents of the Diet," *J. Biol. Chem.*, 15:311-26, 1913.
3. Steenbock, H.: "White Corn Versus Yellow Corn and a Probable Relation Between the Fat Soluble Vitamin and Yellow Plant Pigments," *Science*, 50:352–53, 1919.
4. "Nomenclature Policy: Generic Descriptions and Trivial Names for Vitamins and Related Compounds." *J. Nutr.*, 110:8–15, 1980.
5. Food and Nutrition Board: *Recommended Dietary Allowances*, 10th ed. National Research Council–National Academy of Sciences, Washington, D.C., 1989.
6. Goodman, D. S.: "Vitamin A and Retinoids in Health and Disease," *N. Engl. J. Med.*, 310:1023–31, 1984.
7. Pao, E. M., and Mickle, S. J.: "Problem Nutrients in the United States," *Food Technol.*, 35:58–69, 1981.
8. Windham, C. T., et al.: "Nutrient Density of Diets in the USDA Nationwide Food Consumption Survey, 1977–1978: 11. Adequacy of Nutrient Density Consumption Practices," *J. Am. Diet. Assoc.*, 83:34–43, 1983.
9. Carrol, M. D., et al. (National Center for Health Statistics): *Dietary Intake Source Data: United States, 1976–80.* Vital and Health Statistics, Series 11, No. 231. DHHS Pub. No. (PHS) 83–1681, 1983.
10. Fulwood, R., et al. (National Center for Health Statis-

tics): *Hematological and Nutritional Biochemistry Reference Data for Persons 6 Months—74 Years of Age: United States, 1976–80.* Vital and Health Statistics, Series 11, No. 232. DHHS Pub. No. (PHS) 83-1682, 1981.

11. Bauernfeind, J. S.: *The Safe Use of Vitamin A.* The Nutrition Foundation, Inc., New York, 1980.

12. Tielsch, J. M., and Sommer, A.: "The Epidemiology of Vitamin A Deficiency and Xerophthalmia," *Annu. Rev. Nutr.*, 4:183–205, 1984.

13. Committee on Safety, Toxicity, and Misuse of Vitamins and Trace Minerals, National Nutrition Consortium, Inc.: *Vitamin–Mineral Safety, Toxicity and Misuse.* American Dietetic Association, Chicago, 1978.

14. Committee on Drugs and on Nutrition, American Academy of Pediatrics: "The Use and Abuse of Vitamin A," *Nutr. Rev.*, (Suppl. 1) 32:41–43, 1974.

15. Bollag, W.: "Vitamin A and Retinoids: From Nutrition to Pharmacotherapy in Dermatology and Oncology," *Lancet*, 1:860–64, 1983.

16. Willett, W. C., et al.: "Relation of Serum Vitamins A and E and Carotenoids to the Risk of Cancer," *N. Engl. J. Med.*, 310:430–34, 1984.

17. Wolf, G.: "Is Dietary β-Carotene an Anti-Cancer Agent?," *Nutr. Rev.*, 40:257–61, 1982.

18. DeLuca, H. F.: "The Vitamin D System in the Regulation of Calcium and Phosphorus Metabolism," *Nutr. Rev.*, 37:161–93, 1979.

19. Fraser, D. R., and Kodicek, E.: "Unique Biosynthesis by Kidney of a Biochemically Active D Metabolite," *Nature (Lond.)*, 228:764–66, 1970.

20. Haussler, M. R., and McCain, T. A.: "Basic and Clinical Concepts Related to Vitamin D Metabolism and Action," *N. Engl. J. Med.*, 297:974–83, 1041–50, 1977.

21. Henry, H. L., and Norman, A. W.: "Vitamin D: Metabolism and Biological Actions," *Annu. Rev. Nutr.*, 4:493–520, 1984.

22. Fomon, S. J., et al. "Recommendations for Feeding Normal Infants," *Pediatrics*, 63:52–59, 1979.

23. Bieri, J. G.: "Medical Uses of Vitamin E," *N. Eng. J. Med.*, 308:1063–71, 1983.

24. Scott, M. L.: "Vitamin E," in DeLuca, H. F., ed.: *The Fat-Soluble Vitamins.* Plenum Press, New York, 1978, pp. 133–210.

25. Bauernfeind, J. C.: "The Tocopherol Content of Food and Influencing Factors," *Crit. Rev. Food. Sci. Nutr.*, 8:337–82, 1977.

26. Muller, D. P. R., et al.: "Vitamin E and Neurological Function," *Lancet*, 1:225-28, 1983.

27. Horwitt, M. K.: "Vitamin E and Lipid Metabolism in Man," *Am. J. Clin. Nutr.*, 8:451–61, 1960.

28. Ehrenkranz, R. A.: "Vitamin E and the Neonate," *Am. J. Dis. Child.*, 134:1157–66, 1980.

29. Olson, R. E.: "The Function and Metabolism of Vitamin K," *Annu. Rev. Nutr.*, 4:281–337, 1984.

30. Suttie, J. W.: "Vitamin K," in DeLuca, H. F., ed.: *The Fat-Soluble Vitamins.* Plenum Press, New York, 1978, pp. 211–77.

12

The Water-Soluble Vitamins:

Ascorbic Acid

Ascorbic acid (vitamin C) was identified more than 50 years ago as the component in foods that cured scurvy, but much remains to be learned about the extent and manner of its involvement in chemical reactions taking place in the body. Controversial claims about the importance of ascorbic acid in preventing or treating the common cold and cancer have led to new questions regarding desirable dietary intakes of the vitamin as well as the value and safety of supplements.

Discovery   Scurvy has been known as a dread disease since ancient times. It was described as early as 1500 B.C. by the Egyptians in the Papyrus Ebers, a treatise on medicine. It particularly plagued the seagoing adventurers of the sixteenth and seventeenth centuries, who lost thousands of men to scurvy. Jacques Cartier in his explorations in Canada was slightly more fortunate, for the Indians showed him how a brew of pine needles and bark could cure scurvy, and many men were thus saved.

In 1747, Dr. James Lind, a British physician, tested six remedies on 12 sailors who had scurvy. He found that oranges and lemons were curative. But it took another 50 years before the British navy required rations of lemons or limes on the sailing vessels. From that day to the present the British sailor has been known as a "limey." During this same period Captain Cook was able to reduce the incidence of scurvy on his seagoing voyages by stocking up on fresh fruits and vegetables whenever he was in port and also by including sauerkraut as part of the rations. The sauerkraut kept well and was a good preventive of scurvy.

The scientific era of vitamin C began in 1907 when two Norwegian scientists, Holst and Frölich, produced scurvy in guinea pigs. The isolation and chemical nature of vitamin C, or ascorbic acid, was accomplished by Dr. Charles G. King and his co-workers at the University of Pittsburgh and by Dr. Szent-Györgyi of Hungary in the early 1930s.

Chemistry and Characteristics   ASCORBIC ACID is a white crystalline compound of relatively simple structure, and closely related to the monosaccharide sugars. It is synthesized from glucose and other simple sugars by plants and by most animal species. It can be prepared synthetically at low cost from glucose. Vitamin C activity is possessed by two forms: L-ascorbic acid (the reduced form) and L-dehydroascorbic acid (the oxidized form). (See Figure 12-1.) The latter is oxidized further with complete loss of activity. Isoascorbic acid, a compound often used as a preservative in foods, appears to have little or no biologic value in humans.

Of all vitamins, ascorbic acid is the most easily destroyed. It is highly soluble in water. The oxidation of ascorbic acid is accelerated by heat, light, alkalies, oxidative enzymes, and traces of copper and iron. Oxidation is inhibited to a marked degree in an acid reaction, and when the temperature is reduced.

Figure 12-1.   Ascorbic acid and dehydroascorbic acid are biologically active. These forms are easily converted to diketogulonic acid which is inactive. Note the similarity of the structure of ascorbic acid to that of glucose.

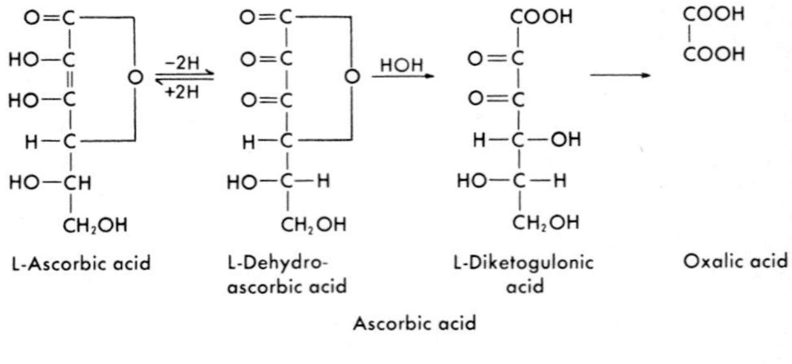

Measurement Ascorbic acid is determined by chemical assay, and the concentration in tissues and foods is expressed in milligrams.

Metabolism Only a few species are known to require a dietary source of ascorbic acid: humans, monkeys, guinea pigs, Indian fruit bats, the red-vented bulbul bird, and certain fish such as trout and carp. Ascorbic acid is rapidly absorbed from the gastrointestinal tract and distributed to the various tissues of the body. The adrenal gland and the retina contain an especially high concentration of vitamin C, but other tissues such as the spleen, intestine, bone marrow, pancreas, thymus, liver, pituitary, and kidney also contain appreciable amounts.

A plasma concentration of greater than 0.6 mg ascorbic acid per dl indicates tissue saturation and a body pool equivalent to 1,500 mg in the adult. Plasma concentrations in the range of 0.1 to 0.39 mg per dl are considered low, and values of less than 0.1 mg per dl suggest deficiency.[1] Plasma concentrations of ascorbic acid tend to be lower in cigarette smokers and women using oral contraceptive agents.[2,3]

The kidney exercises some control over the excretion of ascorbic acid. If tissues are saturated, most of a large dose of vitamin C will be excreted. If tissues are depleted, only a small amount of vitamin C will be excreted. Ascorbic acid is excreted as such, or as metabolites including oxalic acid and ascorbic acid sulfate.

The body efficiently utilizes either synthetic L-ascorbic acid or the vitamin in its natural form as in orange juice.[4]

Functions One of the principal functions of ascorbic acid is the formation of collagen, an abundant protein that forms the intercellular substance in cartilage, bone matrices, dentin, and the vascular epithelium. In the synthesis of collagen, ascorbic acid is necessary for the HYDROXYLATION (introduction of —OH groups) of proline and lysine to hydroxyproline and hydroxylysine. These hydroxyamino acids are important constituents of collagen. This function helps explain the importance of vitamin C in wound healing and the ability to withstand the stress of injury and infection.

Ascorbic acid also may play an important role in other hydroxylation reactions. Conversion of tryptophan to serotonin, an important neurotransmitter and vasoconstrictor, and formation of norepinephrine from tyrosine involve hydroxylation reactions that may utilize ascorbic acid. These reactions may explain some of the abnormalities in vascular and neu-

rologic activity that are observed in persons deficient in the vitamin. Conversion of cholesterol to bile acids is another hydroxylation reaction that may require vitamin C.

Ascorbic acid is an important antioxidant and thus has a role in the protection of vitamins A and E and the polyunsaturated fatty acids from excessive oxidation. Ascorbic acid enhances iron absorption by reducing ferric iron to ferrous iron, the form which is absorbed most efficiently. It may also bind with iron to form a complex that facilitates transfer of iron across the intestinal mucosa. In the circulation, ascorbic acid aids in the release of iron from transferrin so that it can be incorporated into tissue ferritin. Evidence also exists to support a role of vitamin C in biosynthesis of mucopolysaccharides, microsomal drug metabolism, leukocyte function and synthesis of anti-inflammatory steroids by the adrenal glands.[5] It does not appear that vitamin C functions as a coenzyme in these reactions or the hydroxylation reactions described above.

Recommended Allowances As little as 10 mg ascorbic acid will prevent scurvy. This level may be regarded as a minimum requirement, but it does not ensure fully satisfactory tissue levels. Each day the adult male removes about 30 mg ascorbic acid from body stores. The recommended allowance has been set at 60 mg for males and females over 14 years, 30 to 35 mg for infants, 40 to 45 mg for children, 70 mg for pregnancy and 95 mg for lactation.[5] During infections such as tuberculosis, rheumatic fever, and pneumonia and severe stress such as burn injuries the ascorbic acid requirement is increased.

Food Sources Almost all the daily intake of ascorbic acid is obtained from the vegetable-fruit group. (See Figure 12-2.) In the American diet the vitamin C in the available food supply is furnished from food groups in these percentages: citrus fruits, 27; other fruits, 13; potatoes and sweet potatoes, 14; dark green and deep yellow vegetables, 11; other vegetables including tomatoes, 27; all other foods, 8.

Vitamin C has been called the "fresh-food vitamin," since it is found in highest concentrations just as the food is fresh from the plant. In general, the active parts of the plant contain appreciable amounts, and mature or resting seeds are devoid of the vitamin.

Raw, frozen, or canned citrus fruits such as oranges, grapefruit, and lemons are excellent sources of the vitamin. Orange sections including the thin white peel contain more vitamin C than an equal weight of strained juice.

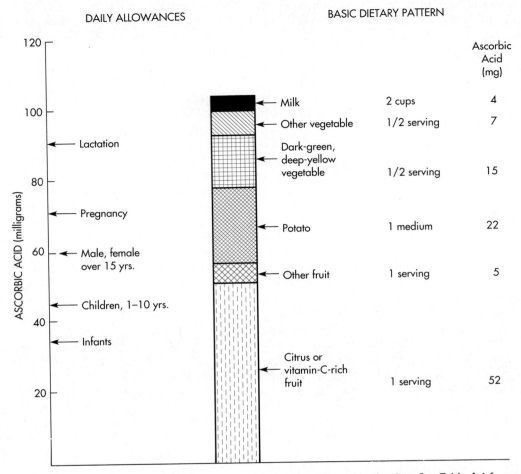

Figure 12-2. The vegetable-fruit group accounts for almost all the ascorbic acid in the diet. See Table 4-1 for complete calculation of the Basic Diet.

Fresh strawberries, cantaloupe, pineapple, and guavas are also excellent sources. Other nonacid fresh fruits such as peaches, pears, apples, bananas, and blueberries contribute small amounts of the vitamin; when eaten in large amounts these fruits may be an important dietary source. The concentration of ascorbic acid in the nonacid canned fruits is considerably reduced.

Broccoli, brussels sprouts, spinach, kale, green peppers, cabbage, and turnips are excellent-to-good sources even when cooked. The use of potatoes and sweet potatoes as staple food items enhances the vitamin C intake considerably, provided that appropriate methods of preparation are used to avoid destruction of the vitamin.

Milk, eggs, meat, fish, and poultry are practically devoid of vitamin C as they are consumed. If the mother's diet has been adequate, human milk contains four to six times as much ascorbic acid as cow's milk and is able to protect the infant from scurvy. Liver contains a small amount of vitamin C, but most of this is lost during cooking.

Retention of Food Values Heat, exposure to air, solubility in water, alkali, and dehydration are detrimental to the retention of ascorbic acid in foods. The cutting of vegetables releases oxidative enzymes and increases the surfaces exposed to leaching by water. Since the vitamin is so soluble, losses are considerable when large amounts of water are used. Vegetables should be added to a small quantity of boiling water, covered tightly, and cooked until just tender for high retention of ascorbic acid. Retention is also good when a pressure cooker is used, provided that the cooking time is carefully controlled. The practice of adding baking soda to retain green color of vegetables not only reduces the vitamin C level but may also modify the flavor and texture of the vegetable. Leftover vegetables lose a large proportion of the ascorbic acid, although losses are reduced somewhat when the container is tightly covered in the refrigerator. Retention of the vitamin is good in properly refrigerated citrus juices and tomatoes.

Effects of Deficiency Results of the Nationwide Food Consumption Survey showed that average intakes of ascorbic acid in 1977 were considerably higher than intakes in 1965 and met or exceeded recommended intakes for all sex–age groups. This increased intake was attributed to fortification of beverages and other foods with vitamin C and increased consumption of citrus fruit and juice.[7]

In spite of high average intakes, substantial percentages of persons in a few sex–age categories had intakes of ascorbic acid that might be considered low. Intakes were poorest in women aged 19 to 22 years, with 43 percent of the group consuming less than 70 percent of the recommended allowance for vitamin C.[8] Results of the first Health and Nutrition Survey (1971–72) likewise showed that the average intake of persons aged 1 to 74 years exceeded the standard. In that survey the highest prevalence of low intake was found in low-income white men aged 45 to 54 years.[9] Without biochemical or clinical data, however, conclusions cannot be made with respect to the prevalence of problems in vitamin C nutriture.

A deficiency of ascorbic acid results in the defective formation of the intercellular cement substance. Fleeting joint pains, irritability, retardation of growth in the infant or child, anemia, shortness of breath, poor wound healing, and increased susceptibility to infection are among the signs of deficiency, but none of these can establish a diagnosis. A dietary history, the concentration of ascorbic acid in the blood plasma and in the white blood cells, and a measure of the excretion of a test dose in the urine help establish the diagnosis.

Scurvy. The classic picture of scurvy is rarely seen in adults in the United States. The incidence is also uncommon in infants, but a gross deficiency of ascorbic acid results in scurvy during the second 6 months of life. Infections, fevers, and hyperthyroidism may precipitate the symptoms when the intake has been inadequate. The symptoms are related to the weakening of the collagenous material.

Pain, tenderness, and swelling of the thighs and legs are frequent symptoms of severe infantile scurvy. The baby shows a disinclination to move and assumes a position with legs flexed. He is pale and irritable and cries when handled. Loss of weight, fever, diarrhea,

and vomiting are frequently present. If the teeth have erupted, the gums are likely to be swollen, tender, and hemorrhagic. Bone calcification is faulty because of degeneration or lack of proper development of the bone matrix. The cartilage supporting the bones is weak, and bone displacement results. The ends of the long bones and of the ribs are enlarged somewhat as in rickets, but tenderness is a distinguishing characteristic in scurvy.

Scurvy in adults results after several months of a diet devoid of ascorbic acid. The symptoms include petechiae or hemorrhagic spots on the skin; swelling, infection, and bleeding of the gums; tenderness of the legs; and anemia. (See Figure 12-3.) The teeth may become loose and eventually may be lost. As the disease progresses the slightest injury produces excessive bleeding, and large hemorrhages may be seen beneath the skin. There may be general degeneration of the muscle structure and of the cartilage.

Acute scurvy responds within a few days to the administration of 100 to 200 mg ascorbic acid given in synthetic form or as orange juice. Chronic changes that have occurred, such as bone deformities and anemia, require much longer periods for their correction.

Use of Supplements After the publication of Dr. Linus Pauling's book in 1970,[10] thousands of people began taking large doses of ascorbic acid to prevent or treat colds, or both. Although use of the vitamin for this purpose is less popular now, some individuals continue to claim benefits. The dosages used to prevent or treat colds often are 20 to 100 times the recommended allowances and should be regarded as pharmaceutic agents. Although the results of some controlled studies have suggested that supplements of vitamin C have an effect in reducing the incidence and severity of cold symptoms, other studies have shown little or no effect.[11,12] In a study of Navajo children in a boarding school in Arizona, administration of 1,000 mg vitamin C resulted in 26 percent fewer symptomatic days in the younger children receiving the vitamin than in placebo recipients. In older girls receiving 2,000 mg of vitamin C per day a 33 percent reduction in symptomatic days was observed. Repetition of the study the next year using supplements of 1,000 mg, however, showed only 9 percent fewer symptomatic days overall in children receiving the vitamin. Average duration of a cold was slightly less in vitamin C recipients in the first study, but was about the same in the two groups in the second study.[13]

Claims have also been made for the value of megadose supplements of ascorbic acid in treating cancer patients. In one study, administration of ascorbic acid

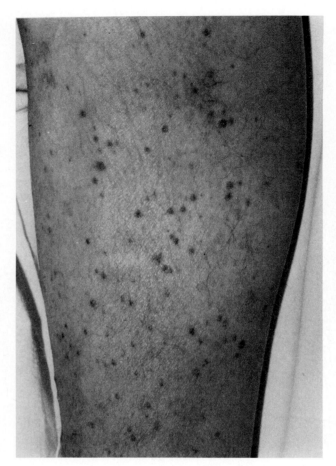 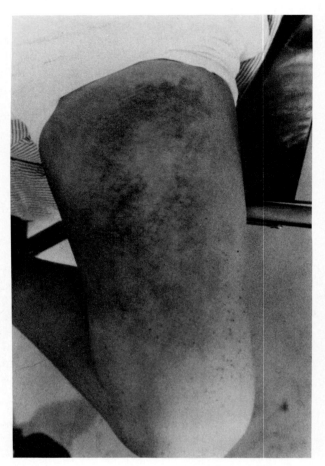

Figure 12-3. *(A)* Tiny petechial hemorrhages around hair follicles are early signs of ascorbic acid deficiency. *(B)* Large areas of hemorrhages are also characteristic of ascorbic acid deficiency. (Courtesy, Dr. A. J. Bollet, Clinical Professor of Medicine, Yale University Danbury Hospital, and *Medical Times,* **109:**67-79, 1981.)

was reported to prolong survival time in patients with terminal cancer.[14] However, other investigators were unable to confirm these results in a controlled study using similar doses of the vitamin.[15]

The value of ascorbic acid in prevention of cancer is based on limited epidemiologic data. The data also are indirect because they are based on the consumption of foods, such as fruits and vegetables that are assumed to have a high concentration of vitamin C, rather than on actual measurements of vitamin intake. Consumption of vitamin C-rich foods has been shown to be associated with a lower risk of certain cancers such as gastric and esophageal cancer.[16] Because of such evidence, the Interim Dietary Guidelines to Prevent Cancer include the recommendation to emphasize consumption of citrus fruits. (See Chapter 3.) Promotion of large supplements of vitamin C to prevent cancer, however, can not be justified based on available evidence.

Supplements of ascorbic acid also have been advocated to treat hypercholesterolemia because of results in deficient guinea pigs showing an increase in blood cholesterol concentrations. However, human subjects fed diets deficient in vitamin C for 34 to 96 days showed no change for plasma total cholesterol, triglycerides, or distribution of cholesterol in various lipoprotein fractions.[17]

Effects of Excess Intakes. In view of the widespread use of large amounts of vitamin C, often without medical supervision, the possibility of adverse effects of excessive intakes needs to be considered. Although in the past large doses were generally assumed to be nontoxic, a growing list of complications is now being identified. Formation of kidney stones may be enhanced in certain individuals because of an increase in urine acidity or because of increased oxalate excretion arising from breakdown of the vitamin.

An abrupt decrease in intake may precipitate symptoms of scurvy, and the possibility of conditioned deficiency occurring in infants of mothers ingesting large amounts of the vitamin is of special concern. Other problems associated with megadoses of vitamin C include gastrointestinal disturbances, interference with anticoagulants, destruction of red blood cells, excessive absorption of iron, and impaired utilization of copper.[18-20] Since many of the claims for megadose use of ascorbic acid have not been documented, and since excessive intakes may have adverse effects, routine use of large supplements of vitamin C does not appear to be advisable.

A summary of ascorbic acid appears at the end of Chapter 13.

Problems and Review

1. In what way is ascorbic acid related to the functioning of each of these substances: iron, collagen, folacin, cholesterol, vitamin A, tryptophan?
2. What are the clinical manifestations of a deficiency of ascorbic acid?
3. What is the effect of an intake of ascorbic acid in excess of the body's needs?
4. List the instructions you would give for the preparation and service of these foods in order that the maximum ascorbic acid would be retained: tossed green salad, cooked cabbage?
5. *Problem.* Calculate the ascorbic acid content of your own diet for two days. Compare your intake with the recommended allowances.
6. *Problem.* Calculate the amounts of each of the following foods necessary to furnish 25 mg of ascorbic acid: orange juice, tomato juice, sweet potato, cabbage, grapefruit, endive, strawberries, cantaloupe, apple, lettuce.
7. Mashed potatoes served in a restaurant probably should not be relied upon as a source of ascorbic acid. Give several reasons why this is true.
8. *Problem.* Check the label on vitamin supplements advertised for "stress" or as having "mega" dosages. How does the amount of ascorbic acid in these products compare with the recommended allowance?
9. Why is vitamin C added to commercial infant formula or recommended as a supplement for infants given evaporated milk formula? Are such supplements necessary for the breast-fed infant?

References

1. Hodges, R. E.: "Ascorbic Acid," in Goodhart, R. S., and Shils, M. E., ed.: *Modern Nutrition in Health and Disease*, 6th ed. Lea & Febiger, Philadelphia, 1980, pp. 259–73.
2. Kallner, A. B., et al.: "On the Requirements of Ascorbic Acid in Man: Steady-State Turnover and Body Pool in Smokers," *Am. J. Clin. Nutr.*, **34**:1347–55, 1981.
3. Rivers, J. M.: "Oral Contraceptives and Ascorbic Acid," *Am. J. Clin. Nutr.*, **28**:550–54, 1975.
4. Pelletier, O., and Keith, M. O.: "Bioavailability of Synthetic and Natural Ascorbic Acid." *J. Am. Diet Assoc.*, **64**:271–75, 1974.
5. Food and Nutrition Board: *Recommended Dietary Allowances*, 10th ed. National Research Council–National Academy of Sciences, Washington, D.C., 1989.
6. Marston, R. M., and Welsh, S. O.: "Nutrient Content of the U.S. Food Supply, 1982," *National Food Review*, U.S. Department of Agriculture, Washington, D.C., Winter 1984, pp. 7–13.
7. Pao, E. M.: "Nutrient Consumption Patterns of Individuals, 1977 and 1965," *Family Econ. Rev.*, Spring 1980, pp. 16–20.
8. Pao, E. M., and Mickle, S. J.: "Problem Nutrients in the United States," *Food Technol.*, **35**:58–69, 1981.
9. *Caloric and Selected Nutrient Values for Persons 1–74 Years of Age: First Health and Nutrition Examination Survey, U.S., 1971–1974.* U.S. Dept. of Health, Education and Welfare, DHEW Publ. No. (PHS) 79–1657, 1979.
10. Pauling, L.: *Vitamin C and the Common Cold.* W. H. Freeman and Company, San Francisco, 1970.
11. Anderson, T. W.: "Large-scale Trials of Vitamin C," *Ann. N.Y. Acad. Sci.*,**258**:498–504, 1975.
12. Chalmers, T. C.: "Effects of Ascorbic Acid on the Common Cold: An Evaluation of the Evidence," *Am. J. Med.*, **58**:532–36, 1975.
13. Coulehan, J. L.: "Ascorbic Acid and the Common Cold: Reviewing the Evidence," *Postgrad. Med.*, **66** (September):153–60, 1979.
14. Cameron, E., and Pauling, L.: "Supplemental Ascorbate in the Supportive Treatment of Cancer: Prolongation of Survival Times in Terminal Human Cancer," *Proc. Natl. Acad. Sci. U.S.A.*, **73**:3685–89, 1976.
15. Creagan, E. T., et al.: "Failure of High-Dose Vitamin C (Ascorbic Acid) Therapy to Benefit Patients with Advanced Cancer," *N. Engl. J. Med.*, **301**:687–90, 1979.
16. Committee on Diet, Nutrition, and Cancer: "Diet, Nutrition, and Cancer: Interim Dietary Guidelines," *J. Natl. Cancer Inst.*, **70**:1153–70, 1983.
17. Duane, W. C., and Hutton, S. W.: "Lack of Effect of Experimental Ascorbic Acid Deficiency on Bile Acid Metabolism, Sterol Balance, and Biliary Lipid Composition in Man," *J. Lipid Res.*, **24**:1186–95, 1983.
18. Committee on Safety, Toxicity, and Misuse of Vitamins and Trace Minerals, National Nutrition Consortium, Inc.: *Vitamin–Mineral Safety, Toxicity and Misuse.* American Dietetic Association, Chicago, 1978.
19. Alhadeff, L., et al.: "Toxic Effects of Water Soluble Vitamins," *Nutr. Rev.*, **42**:33–40, 1984.
20. Finley, E. B., and Cerklewski, F. L.: "Influence of Ascorbic Acid Supplementation on Copper Status in Young Adult Men," *Am. J. Clin. Nutr.*, **37**:353–56, 1983.

13

The Water-Soluble Vitamins:

The Vitamin B Complex

In areas of the world where polished rice is a staple food, beriberi, a serious disease affecting the nerves, has been known for generations. Takaki, a Japanese medical officer, studied the high incidence of the disease among men of the Japanese navy during the years 1878–83. Among 276 men serving on one sailing vessel he found 169 cases of beriberi, including 25 deaths at the end of 9 months, but only 14 cases with no deaths occurred among a similar number of men on a second vessel who had received more meat, milk, and vegetables in their diet. Takaki believed this difference was related to the protein content of the diet.

About 15 years later (1897), Eijkman, a Dutch physician in the East Indies, noted that illness in fowls that ate scraps of hospital food consisting chiefly of polished rice was similar to beriberi seen in humans. He subsequently showed that the addition of rice polishings to the diet would cure the disease. He theorized that the starch of the polished rice was toxic to the nerves, but that the outer layers of the rice kernel were protective. Another Dutch physician, Grijns, interpreted the findings as a deficiency of an essential substance in the diet.

A number of chemists demonstrated the effects of extracts from rice. Funk in 1912 coined the term *vitamine* for the substance which he found to be effective in preventing beriberi. McCollum and Davis applied the term *water-soluble B* to the concentrates that cured beriberi.

The water-soluble vitamin B described by Funk and others was soon discovered to be not a single substance, but a group of compounds that we now designate as the vitamin B complex. Most of these have been synthesized, and their chemical and physical properties are fairly well understood. Principally these vitamins combine with specific proteins to function as parts of the various enzyme systems which are concerned with the breakdown of carbohydrate, protein, and fat in the body. Thus, they are interrelated and are intimately involved in the mechanisms that release energy, carbon dioxide, and water as the end products of metabolism.

Thiamin

Discovery Crystalline thiamin (vitamin B-1) was isolated from rice bran in 1926. Identification of the structure and synthesis of the vitamin were accomplished in 1936 by Dr. R. R. Williams, who had worked for a quarter of a century on studies of beriberi and on the factor in rice polishings, which brought about cure of the disease. Because of the presence of sulfur in the molecule, the vitamin was named THIAMIN.

Chemistry and Characteristics Thiamin is available commercially as thiamin hydrochloride in a crystalline white powder. (See Figure 13-1.) It has a faint yeastlike odor and a salty nutlike taste and is readily soluble in water. The vitamin is stable in its dry form, and heating in solutions at 120°C in an acid medium (pH 5.0 or less) has little destructive effect. Cooking foods in neutral or alkaline reaction, however, is very destructive. Thiamin is now measured in milligrams or micrograms. It is determined by chemical or microbiologic methods.

Physiology The thiamin ingested in food is available in the free form or bound as thiamin pyrophosphate or in a protein–phosphate complex. The bound forms are split in the digestive tract, after which absorption takes place principally from the first part of the duodenum. The amount of thiamin present in the body is not great—probably about 50 mg in all. The liver, kidney, heart, brain, and muscles have somewhat higher concentrations than the blood.

178

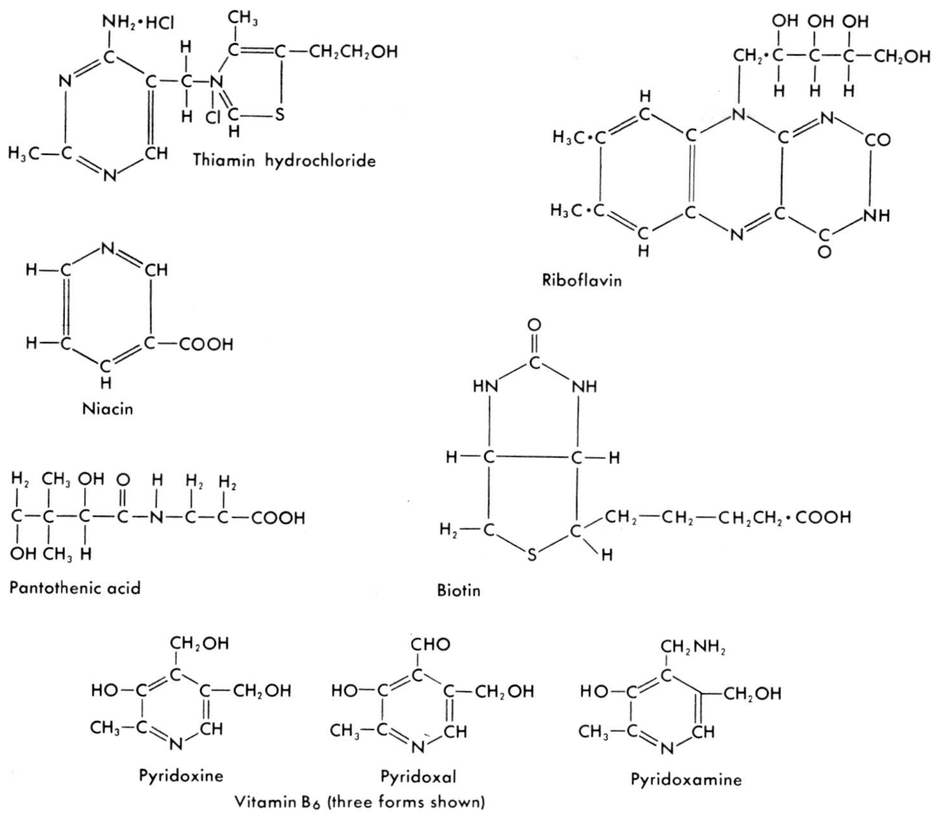

Figure 13-1. These B-complex vitamins are converted to essential coenzymes in metabolic reactions involving carbohydrates, fats and proteins. Note the wide variations in structure.

The principal functioning form of thiamin is THIAMIN PYROPHOSPHATE (TPP), also formerly known as cocarboxylase. Conversion of thiamin to this active form requires ATP. Thiamin pyrophosphate acts as a coenzyme for a number of important enzyme systems.

If thiamin is ingested in excess of tissue needs, it is excreted in the urine. With a low dietary intake, the urinary excretion promptly falls.

Functions   One of the critical points at which TPP functions in carbohydrate metabolism is in the oxidative decarboxylation of pyruvic acid and the subsequent formation of acetyl CoA, which in turn enters the TCA cycle. (See Figure 6-4.) This is one of the most complex reactions in carbohydrate metabolism and, in addition to TPP, also requires these cofactors: coenzyme A, which contains pantothenic acid (see page 190); nicotinamide adenine dinucleotide (NAD), which contains niacin (see page 185); magnesium ions; and lipoic acid (see page 196).

Another point in carbohydrate metabolism that involves oxidative decarboxylation is in the TCA cycle

in the conversion of alpha-ketoglutaric acid to succinic acid. Because breakdown products of fats and proteins as well as carbohydrate can contribute to alpha-ketoglutaric acid, thiamin, and the other factors listed here are involved in the metabolism of the three energy-producing nutrients.

Thiamin pyrophosphate is also a cofactor for TRANSKETOLASE, an enzyme required to produce active glyceraldehyde through the pentose shunt. (See Figure 6-4.) In addition to its coenzyme function, thiamin may be involved in some aspect of the function of nerve cell membranes or in some way influence the action of neurotransmitters such as acetylcholine or serotonin.[1]

Daily Allowances   The thiamin requirement is proportional to the calorie requirement. The minimum requirement is about 0.33 to 0.35 mg of thiamin per 1,000 kcal, and the recommended allowance has been set at 0.5 mg per 1,000 kcal.[2] This provides a margin of safety for individual variation and affords some protection during periods of stress.

The daily allowance for men aged 25 to 50 years is 1.5 mg, and for women of the same age it is 1.1 mg. Elderly persons utilize thiamin somewhat less efficiently, and therefore an allowance of at least 1.0 mg. is recommended, even though the calorie requirement may be below 2,000. The allowance for pregnant and lactating women is increased by 0.4 and 0.5 mg, respectively. Infants should receive 0.3 to 0.4 mg per day, and children up to 10 years are allowed 0.7 to 1.0 mg per day.

Sources Thiamin is widely distributed in many foods, but most foods do not furnish especially high concentrations. Although brewers' yeast and wheat germ are rich sources, they do not form an important part of most diets. The American food supply provides 2.07 mg per capita.[3] Of this, about 43 percent is furnished by whole-grain or enriched cereals, flours, and breads.

The meat group supplies approximately one fourth of the daily intake of thiamin. Lean pork—fresh and cured—is especially high in its thiamin concentration; its frequent inclusion in the diet thus makes it a highly significant source. Liver, dry beans and peas, soybeans, and peanuts are also excellent sources. The thiamin in egg, a fair source, is concentrated in the yolk.

Although the concentration of thiamin in vegetables and fruits is low, the quantities of these foods eaten may be such that important contributions are made to the daily total. Milk is likewise a fair source because of the amounts taken in the daily diet and because milk is not subjected to treatment other than pasteurization, which does not materially reduce the thiamin level. The thiamin contribution of the basic diet pattern is shown in Figure 13-2.

Uncooked clams, some fishes, and shrimp contain THIAMINASE, an enzyme that splits the thiamin molecule, thereby inactivating it. In most situations this presents no problem, since cooking inactivates thiaminase. Tea and a few other foods contain compounds that act as thiamin antagonists. Persons on marginal diets consuming large amounts of tea may have an increased risk of developing deficiency.

Retention of Food Values Little loss of thiamin occurs in the preparation of cooked breakfast cereals inasmuch as the water used in preparation is consumed. Losses are considerable when rice is washed before cooking and when it is cooked in a large volume of water that is later drained off. Losses are minimized if rice is cooked in just enough water so that all of it is absorbed by the grains. "Converted" rice retains more

of the thiamin than does regular rice because in its processing the water-soluble nutrients are distributed throughout the grain. In the baking of bread about 15 to 20 percent of the thiamin content is lost.

Thiamin losses are 25 percent or less when meats are broiled or roasted. When meats are cooked in liquid, the losses approach 50 percent if the liquid is discarded. If the liquid in which meat is cooked is consumed, the loss is about 25 percent.

Thiamin losses in vegetable cookery are minimal if vegetables are cooked in a small amount of water for a short time without the addition of baking soda. In general, when the principles for retention of ascorbic acid are observed in food preparation, the maximum thiamin content will also be preserved.

Effects of Deficiency Severe thiamin deficiency is rare in the United States. The incidence of mild deficiency is not known. Deficiency may arise following gastrointestinal disturbances accompanied by persistent vomiting or diarrhea or subsequent to febrile diseases or surgery when the dietary intake is poor. One group that is especially susceptible is the alcoholic population. The neurologic disorder, Wernicke-Korsakoff syndrome, which is seen most often in alcoholics, is due primarily to a deficiency in thiamin.

Beriberi still occurs in the Orient where high-carbohydrate diets are common and where enrichment of rice and wheat is not practiced.

Diagnosis. The symptoms of mild deficiency are so vague that a diagnosis of thiamin deficiency is difficult. The activity of an enzyme, erythrocyte transketolase, which is found in the red blood cells, correlates closely with thiamin nutrition,[4] and is believed to be useful in detecting marginal deficiency before clinical symptoms have become apparent. An elevated level of pyruvic and lactic acids in the blood, especially after exercise and the administration of a standard amount of glucose, together with a low concentration of thiamin in the urine is suggestive of deficiency. If such tests are further substantiated with a dietary history of thiamin lack plus the appearance of peripheral neuritis and disorders of the cardiovascular system, thiamin deficiency is apparent.

Symptoms. The individual who daily receives less than the minimum amount of thiamin builds up an increasing deficiency that affects the gastrointestinal, cardiovascular, and peripheral nervous systems. The early symptoms are nonspecific for thiamin lack and include fatigue, lack of interest in ones's affairs, emotional instability, irritability, depression, anger and

DAILY ALLOWANCES   BASIC DIETARY PATTERN

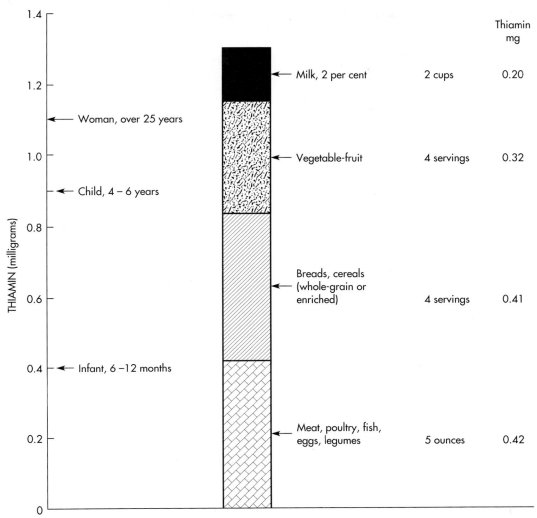

Figure 13-2. Recommended amounts from each of the food groups will provide the thiamin allowances for women and children. The slightly increased allowances for teenagers and men are easily met by increased amounts from one or more of these food groups. See Table 4-1 for complete calculation of the basic dietary pattern.

fear, and loss of appetite, weight, and strength. As the deficiency becomes more marked, the patient may complain of indigestion, constipation, headaches, insomnia, and tachycardia after moderate exercise. There appears a feeling of heaviness and weakness of the legs, which may be followed by cramping of the calf muscles and burning and numbness of the feet—an indication of the development of peripheral neuritis.

The neuritic effects are first noted in the foot, then the muscles of the calf, and then the thigh. The muscle degeneration may be so pronounced that coor-

dination is impossible and a characteristic high-stepping gait results. This form of the disease characterized primarily by emaciation and multiple neuritic symptoms often is referred to as "dry" beriberi.

Thiamin deficiency also leads to enlargement of the heart, tachycardia, dyspnea, and palpitations on exertion. In the acute type of beriberi, acute cardiac failure may be fatal before the seriousness of the disease has been fully appreciated. This state of the disease is known as "wet" beriberi because the chief manifestation is a severe edema that masks the emaciation that is also present.

Infantile Beriberi. In the Far East infants are especially susceptible to beriberi because the mother has had a deficient intake of thiamin and the milk she supplies to the infant consequently contains a very low level of thiamin. The onset is often sudden and is characterized by pallor, facial edema, irritability, vomiting, abdominal pain, loss of voice, and convulsion. The infant may die within a few hours. With thiamin therapy, recovery is dramatic.

Treatment. Because beriberi is a complex vitamin deficiency disease, patients make the greatest improvement when B-complex vitamins, rather than thiamin alone, are prescribed. In addition to the B-complex concentrates, it is customary to prescribe a diet that is high in protein and calories.

Riboflavin

Discovery As early as 1879 a pigment that possessed a yellow-green fluorescence had been discovered in milk. Other workers later obtained it from such widely varying sources as liver, yeast, heart, and egg white. The pigments that possess these fluorescent properties were designated "flavins."

During the early 1920s the substance in yeast which prevented polyneuritis was shown to be more than one vitamin. The antineuritic fraction which was destroyed by heat was called vitamin B-1. Another fraction not destroyed by heat did not prevent or cure polyneuritis but it was needed for growth. It was designated as vitamin B-2 or vitamin G; it is now known as RIBOFLAVIN.

In 1932 a yellow enzyme necessary for cell respiration was isolated from yeast by Warburg and Christian, who also discovered that a protein and the pigment component were two factors in the enzyme. It then remained for Kuhn and his co-workers in 1935 to report on the synthesis of riboflavin and to note the relation of its activity to the green fluorescence, thereby establishing that lactoflavin and the vitamin are one and the same thing. This was the first example of a vitamin functioning as a coenzyme.

Chemistry and Characteristics Riboflavin was so named because of the similarity of part of its structure to that of the sugar ribose and because of its relation to the general group of flavins. (See Figure 13-1.) In its pure state, this vitamin is a bitter-tasting, orange-yellow, odorless compound in which the crystals are needle shaped. It dissolves sparingly in water to give a characteristic greenish-yellow fluorescence. In solu-

tion it is quickly decomposed by ultraviolet rays and visible light and is sensitive to strongly alkaline solutions. This vitamin is stable to heat, to oxidizing agents, and to acids. Riboflavin is measured in terms of milligrams or micrograms by chemical and microbiologic methods.

Physiology Riboflavin is present in the free state in foods, or in combination with phosphate, or with protein and phosphate. During digestion these combinations are broken down and the free riboflavin that is released is absorbed in the upper part of the small intestine. Rephosphorylation occurs in the intestinal cell before transport into the portal circulation. Riboflavin is present in body tissues as the coenzyme or as flavoproteins.

The body guards carefully its stores of riboflavin so that even in severe deficiency as much as one third of the normal amount has been found to be present in the liver, kidney, and heart of experimental animals. Apparently the flavin content of the body tissues cannot be increased beyond a certain point since the urinary excretion increases markedly if intake exceeds 0.75 mg per 1,000 kcal.[5] A decided reduction in the intake leads to restriction or even curtailment of the urinary excretion.

Functions Riboflavin is a constituent of two coenzymes: riboflavin monophosphate or FLAVIN MONONUCLEOTIDE (FMN) and FLAVIN ADENINE DINUCLEOTIDE (FAD). Both these coenzymes are prosthetic groups for aerobic dehydrogenases that act as hydrogen acceptors. The enzymes are required for the completion of several reactions in the energy cycle by which ATP is generated and in which hydrogen is transferred from one compound to another until eventually it reaches oxygen and forms water. Functionally, these enzymes are closely associated with the niacin-containing enzymes.

Riboflavin is also a component of L- and D-amino acid oxidases that oxidize amino acids and hydroxy acids to alpha-keto acids, and of xanthine oxidase, an enzyme that catalyzes the oxidation of a number of purines.

Daily Allowances At various times the allowances for riboflavin have been based on the calorie intake, the protein allowance, and the metabolic size. Regardless of the base used, the calculated allowance is about the same. The present recommendation of the Food and Nutrition Board is 0.6 mg per 1,000 kcal for persons of all ages.[2]

The recommended allowance for males 25 to 50

years is 1.6 mg and for females 1.2 mg. For pregnancy and lactation, the allowances are increased by 0.3 and 0.5 mg, respectively. The infant's allowance is 0.4 to 0.6 mg, and for children to 10 years 0.8 to 1.4 mg are recommended.

Hyperthyroidism, fevers, the stress of injury or surgery, malabsorption, and increased physical activity are among the factors that increase the requirement. Achlorhydria may precipitate deficiency because the vitamin is so quickly destroyed in an alkaline medium.

Food Sources On a per-capita basis the American food supply furnishes 2.28 mg riboflavin daily; 37 percent of this is supplied by dairy products, 27 percent by meat, fish, poultry, and eggs; and 24 percent by cereal and flour products.[3] A diet that supplies 2 cups milk and a serving of meat daily is not likely to be deficient in riboflavin.

Liver, kidney, and heart contain considerable quantities of riboflavin, and other meats, eggs, and green leafy vegetables supply smaller, but nevertheless im-

portant, amounts. Cereals and flours are ordinarily low in riboflavin; their enrichment adds significantly to the riboflavin content of the diet.

Fruits, roots, and tubers are poor sources of riboflavin, and fats and oils are practically devoid of the vitamin. The contribution of the basic diet is shown in Figure 13-3.

Retention of Food Values Pasteurization, irradiation for vitamin D, evaporation, or drying of milk accounts for loss of not more than 10 to 20 percent of the initial riboflavin content of milk. On the other hand, milk that is bottled in clear glass loses up to 75 percent with 3½ hours exposure in direct sunlight. The distribution of milk in opaque containers prevents this loss.

Meats that have been stewed, roasted, or braised retain more than three fourths of the riboflavin; most of the remainder can be accounted for in the drippings. Because riboflavin is sparingly soluble, the usual cooking procedures for vegetables do not contribute to much loss, but the addition of sodium bicarbonate to preserve green color is destructive.

Figure 13-3. Note the important contribution of milk to the total riboflavin content of the diet. See Table 4-1 for complete calculations of the basic dietary pattern.

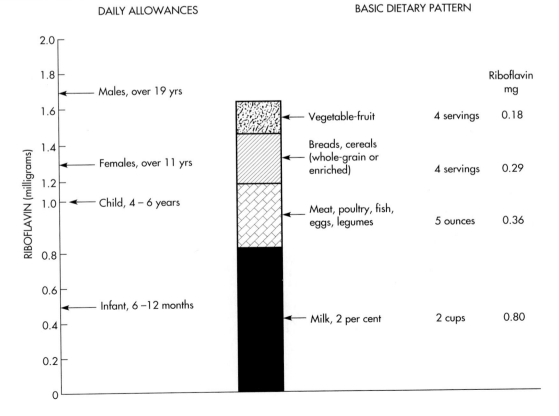

DAILY ALLOWANCES

BASIC DIETARY PATTERN

	Riboflavin mg
Vegetable-fruit 4 servings	0.18
Breads, cereals (whole-grain or enriched) 4 servings	0.29
Meat, poultry, fish, eggs, legumes 5 ounces	0.36
Milk, 2 per cent 2 cups	0.80

Males, over 19 yrs
Females, over 11 yrs
Child, 4 – 6 years
Infant, 6 –12 months

RIBOFLAVIN (milligrams)

Effect of Deficiency   Riboflavin nutriture is evaluated by determining the activity of the riboflavin-dependent enzyme, glutathione reductase, in red cells. Enzyme activity is measured in vitro both in the absence and in the presence of added FAD. Erythrocytes from persons depleted in riboflavin show a marked stimulation in glutathione reductase activity in response to added FAD. Urinary excretion of riboflavin also has been used to evaluate riboflavin nutriture but is not considered a good test because it reflects primarily recent dietary intake rather than tissue levels of the vitamin.

Little is known about the prevalence of ariboflavinosis. An individual rarely seeks medical advice for this condition alone, but it may accompany other deficiencies especially of the B-complex vitamins. Based on determination of erythrocyte glutathione reductase activity, a deficiency of riboflavin was found in 26 percent of of an adolescent population of low socioeconomic status in New York City. Prevalence of deficiency was highest among those consuming less than 1 cup of milk per week.[6] Depletion of tissue riboflavin may be produced temporarily in babies receiving phototherapy as treatment of hyperbilirubinemia, but no long-term effects are believed to occur.

Symptoms.   When a group of women were fed a diet extremely low in riboflavin they developed over the course of 94 to 130 days such symptoms as greasy dermatitis around the folds of the nose, a cracking of the lips at the corners (CHEILOSIS), glossitis, and increased vascularization of the cornea.[7] The lips and tongue assumed a purplish red and shiny appearance in contrast to the scarlet color seen in niacin deficiency. (See Figure 13-4.)

Ocular manifestations may be among the earliest signs of riboflavin deficiency. The eyes become sensitive to light and easily fatigued. Blurring of the vision, itching, watering, and soreness of the eyes occur as well. An increased number of capillaries may develop in the cornea, and the eye becomes bloodshot in appearance. Some of these changes in the eye and appearance of the tongue have not been observed in other controlled studies.[8]

Growth failure is characteristic in young animals, and would also apply if children fail to receive minimum requirements for riboflavin. The appetite, attitude, and activity are not adversely affected with riboflavin lack as they are thiamin deficiency. No human deaths have been reported because of riboflavin deficiency.

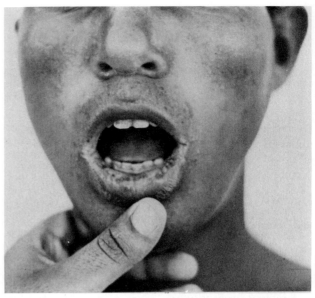

Figure 13-4.   Cheilosis—lesions of the lips and fissures at the angles of the mouth. (Courtesy, Nutrition Section, National Institutes of Health.)

Niacin (Nicotinic Acid and Nicotinamide)

Early Studies   In 1735 a Spanish physician, Casals, described a disease, *mal de la rosa* which came to be known as PELLAGRA, a term of Italian origin meaning "rough skin." In the early part of this century it was one of the leading causes of mental illness and of death in this country. Its causes had been variously ascribed to toxic substances present in corn, infections from microorganisms, of toxicity produced by exposure to the sun, lack of tryptophan in the diet, and amino acid imbalance.

Goldberger, a physician in the U.S. Public Health Service, who was assigned to study the problem of pellagra in the South, early noted that the disease was almost always associated with poverty and ignorance and that hospital attendants who worked with the patients never contracted the disease. In 1915 he performed a classic experiment on 12 prisoners, who were promised release in return for their cooperation in eating a diet representative of the poorer classes in the southern states.[9] The diet consisted of sweet potatoes, corn bread, cabbage, rice, collards, fried mush, brown gravy, corn grits, syrup, sugar biscuits, and black coffee. After a few weeks the prisoners developed headache, abdominal pain, and general weakness, and in about 5 months the typical dermatitis of pellagra appeared. Goldberger then suggested the existence of a pellagra-preventing ((P-P) factor and related it to the B vitamins.

Identification of the Vitamin   Goldberger in 1922 concluded that blacktongue in dogs was similar to pellagra in humans. Nicotinic acid had been know as a chemical substance since 1867, but it remained for Elvehjem and his co-workers in 1937 to discover its effectiveness as a curative agent for blacktongue in dogs.[10] After this discovery, Smith, Spies, and others were soon making reports of dramatic clinical improvement in pellagrous patients who had been given nicotinic acid. The term *niacin* was suggested by Cowgill to avoid association with the nicotine of tobacco.

Chemistry and Characteristics   Nicotinic acid and niacinamide (see Figure 13-1) are organic compounds of relatively simple structure with equal biologic activity. Niacin is the generic term that includes both forms. The two forms are white, bitter-tasting compounds, moderately soluble in hot water but only slightly soluble in cold water. Niacin is very stable to alkali, acid, heat, light, and oxidation; even boiling and autoclaving do not decrease its potency. Niacin is measured in milligrams by using chemical methods or microbiologic assay.

Physiology   Niacin is readily absorbed from the small intestine. Some reserves are found in the body, but, as with other B-complex vitamins, the amount appears to be limited so that a day-to-day supply is desirable. Any excess of niacin is excreted in the urine as N-methylnicotinamide and N-methyl pyridone. In a deficiency such as pellagra the metabolites in the urine diminish markedly or are absent.

Tryptophan, one of the essential amino acids, is a precursor of niacin so that a diet that contains a liberal amount of tryptophan will likely provide enough niacin, even though the diet is low in preformed niacin. Milk and eggs are excellent sources of tryptophan but poor sources of preformed niacin; their pellagra-preventive characteristics have long been known.

Niacin is not toxic in amounts that considerably exceed recommended allowances. In pharmacologic doses, nicotinic acid, but not nicotinamide, brings about some vasodilation and consequent flushing of the skin and tingling sensations. Other adverse effects of long-term use that may occur are elevation of serum uric acid, impairment of glucose tolerance, and liver damage. From 3 to 6 g of nicotinic acid have

been prescribed to reduce the blood levels of cholesterol, beta-lipoproteins, and triglycerides.[11] Although use of nicotinamide would be preferable because of its lack of toxicity, it unfortunately is ineffective in lowering blood lipids.

Functions   Like other B-complex vitamins, niacin is a constituent of coenzymes involved in glycolysis, tissue respiration, and fat synthesis. Nicotinamide adenine dinucleotide (NAD) contains nicotinamide, ribose, two phosphate groups, and adenine; it is also referred to in the literature as diphosphopyridine nucleotide (DPN) or coenzyme I. Nicotinamide adenine dinucleotide phosphate (NADP) is similar to NAD except that it contains three phosphate groupings; it was formerly known as triphosphopyridine nucleotide (TPN) or coenzyme II.

NAD and NADP are hydrogen acceptors involved in many reactions. For example, the complex reaction required for the decarboxylation of pyruvic acid and the formation of acetyl coenzyme A requires dehydrogenation by NAD (see also page 71); NAD and NADP are involved in dehydrogenation reactions in the TCA cycle; hydrogen is transferred from NAD to FAD to cytochrome c in the respiratory chain in which ATP is liberated. (See page 72.)

In the pentose shunt (see page 72), NADP is the hydrogen acceptor for two reactions, thereby forming NADPH. The latter is required for the synthesis of fatty acids and cholesterol, and for the conversion of phenylalanine to tyrosine.

Daily Allowances   Recommended intakes of niacin are expressed as niacin equivalents (NE) in which 1 NE is equal to 1 mg niacin or 60 mg of dietary tryptophan. Symptoms of pellagra can be prevented by a daily intake of 4.4 mg niacin per 1,000 kcal. The recommended allowances provide about 50 percent margin of safety and are based on 6.6 mg NE per 1,000 kcal.[2]

For the reference man, 25 to 50 years, the allowance is 19 mg NE and for the reference woman it is 15 mg NE. Additions of 2 and 5 mg NE are recommended during pregnancy and lactation, respectively. From 5 to 6 mg NE are recommended during the first year, and 9 to 13 mg NE for children up to 10 years. For boys and girls 11 to 14 years, allowances are 17 and 15 mg respectively.

As with the other B-complex vitamins, the niacin requirements are increased whenever metabolism is accelerated as by fever and the stress of injury or surgery.

Sources A diet that furnishes the recommended allowances for protein also provides enough niacin inasmuch as protein will supply tryptophan for conversion to niacin, and the protein-rich foods are generally, except for milk, rich sources of preformed niacin. Animal proteins contain about 1.4 percent tryptophan, and plant proteins about 1 percent tryptophan.[2] If one assumes that a mixed diet provides 1 percent of the protein as tryptophan, then an intake of 65 g protein is equivalent to 650 mg tryptophan, or 10.8 mg niacin.

Poultry, meats, and fish constitute the most important single food group insofar as preformed niacin is concerned. (See Figure 13-5.) Organ meats, peanuts, peanut butter and brewers' yeast are rich sources, but are not ordinarily consumed in sufficient amounts to greatly affect the dietary level.

Whole grains are fair sources of niacin, but most of this is in a bound form that appears to be mostly unavailable.[12] Treatment of cereals with alkali, which some population groups have traditionally done in making corn tortillas, releases much of the bound niacin. Cooking does not appear to increase availability.[12]

Potatoes, legumes, and some green leafy vegetables contain fair amounts of preformed niacin, but most fruits and vegetables are poor sources—as are also milk and cheese.

Retention of Food Values The cookery of foods does not result in serious losses of niacin, except insofar as part of the soluble vitamin may be discarded in cooking waters which are not used. The application of principles for the retention of ascorbic acid and thiamin, which have been discussed earlier, will result in maximum retention of niacin as well.

Effect of Deficiency Pellagra appears after months of dietary deprivation. The phenomenal decrease in the incidence of pellagra in the United States may be attributed to several factors, including the enrichment program, which is mandatory in some states; the concerted efforts in nutrition education; and the

Figure 13-5. Preformed niacin and the niacin equivalents from protein provide the recommended allowances for niacin for all age-sex categories when recommended amounts of foods in the basic dietary pattern are consumed. Note the important contribution made by the meat group. Note also that milk contributes little preformed niacin but, through its tryptophan content, makes a substantial contribution. See Table 4-1 for calculation of the basic dietary pattern. (Calculations based on tryptophan as 1 percent protein. See Table 4-1.)

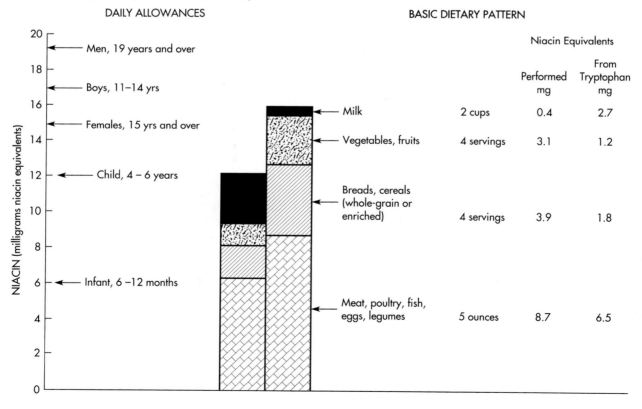

improvement in income. Pellagra is still a public health problem in some countries such as Spain, Yugoslavia, and certain areas of Africa. It tends to occur most often in areas where corn is the major source of protein and calories in the diet.

Symptoms and Clinical Findings. Pellagra involves the gastrointestinal tract, the skin and the nervous system. Although no two cases of pellagra are exactly alike, the following symptoms are characteristic:

1. Early signs include fatigue, listlessness, headache, backache, loss of weight, loss of appetite, and general poor health.
2. Sore tongue, mouth, and throat, with glossitis extending throughout the gastrointestinal tract, are present. The tongue and lips become abnormally red in color. The mouth becomes so sore that it is difficult to eat and swallow.
3. A deficiency of hydrochloric acid with a resultant anemia similar to pernicious anemia may be found.
4. Nausea and vomiting are followed by severe diarrhea.

5. A characteristic symmetric dermatitis especially on the exposed surfaces of the body—hands, forearms, elbows, feet, legs, knees, and neck—appears. (See Figure 13-6.) The dermatitis is sharply separated from the surrounding normal skin. At first, the skin becomes red, somewhat swollen, and tender, resembling a mild sunburn; if the condition is untreated, the skin becomes rough, cracked, and scaly and may become ulcerated. Sunshine and exposure to heat aggravate the dermatitis.
6. Neurologic symptoms, which include confusion, dizziness, poor memory, and irritability, and leading to hallucinations, delusions of persecution, and dementia, are noted as increases in severity.

The classic "Ds" are the final stages of the disease—dermatitis, diarrhea, dementia, and death.

Treatment and Prophylaxis. Treatment includes 300 to 500 mg nicotinamide daily in divided doses as well as supplements of other nutrients, which frequently are deficient.[13] Initially the diet should be soft so that it can be easily eaten while the person is acutely ill.

Figure 13-6. Dermatitis of pellagra.

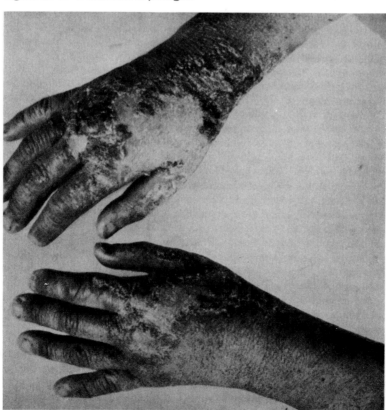

Obviously, prophylaxis must include careful and persistent education in dietary improvement, emphasis upon enrichment programs, and efforts to improve the economic status of affected populations.

Vitamin B-6

Discovery Goldberger and Lillie in 1926 provided a description of dermatitis in rats that was recognized several years later to be characteristic of vitamin B-6 deficiency. In 1934 György reported that vitamin B-2 consists of two factors—riboflavin, and another factor that he named vitamin B-6 that prevented skin lesions (acrodynia) in rats. In 1938 the isolation of a crystalline compound with vitamin B-6 activity was reported by several laboratories, followed by identification of the chemical structure and its synthesis in 1939.

Chemistry and Characteristics Vitamin B-6 consists of a group of related pyridines: PYRIDOXINE, PYRIDOXAL, and PYRIDOXAMINE. (See Figure 13-1.) These may appear in tissues and foodstuffs in the free form, or combined with phosphate, or with phosphate and protein. The preferred terminology is vitamin B-6; pyridoxine, being only one of the three active forms, is not entirely synonymous.

Vitamin B-6 is soluble in water and relatively stable to heat and to acids. It is destroyed in alkaline solutions and is also sensitive to light. Of the three forms, pyridoxine is more resistant to food processing and storage conditions and probably represents the principal form in food products. Vitamin B-6 concentrations are expressed in milligrams or micrograms. The vitamin is determined in tissues and foods by chemical or fluorometric procedures. Because the vitamin occurs in various bound forms, some difficulties have been experienced in providing acceptable tabulations for food values.

Physiology The active form of vitamin B-6 is the coenzyme pyridoxal phosphate, which can be formed from any of the three compounds. Since vitamin B-6 is water soluble, the body stores are small; about half of it is present as part of the structure of the enzyme glycogen phosphorylase. All forms of the vitamin may be excreted in the urine, but the principal metabolite is pyridoxic acid.

Functions Pyridoxal phosphate is the coenzyme for a large number of enzyme systems, most of which are involved in amino acid metabolism. Following are a few examples:

Decarboxylation. The removal of the carboxyl group from amino acids requires enzymes that contain pyridoxal phosphate. Each of the amino acids is decarboxylated by a specific enzyme. For example, the decarboxylation of tryptophan produces tryptamine and carbon dioxide. Serotonin is also produced by decarboxylation of tryptophan and is a potent vasoconstrictor as well as an agent in the regulation of brain and other tissues.

Transamination. Each of the many transaminases involves a distinct protein for which pyridoxal phosphate is the coenzyme. An example of transamination is shown on page 53. In the reaction, the amino group is removed from an amino acid and transferred to a ketoacid, thus forming a new amino acid. This reaction is important in the formation of the nonessential amino acids.

Transulfuration. This involves the removal and transfer of sulfur groups from the sulfur-containing amino acids such as cysteine by transulfurases.

Tryptophan Conversion to Niacin. The importance of tryptophan as a source of niacin has been described on page 185. Several steps are required in this conversion, one of which is catalyzed by vitamin B-6.

Pyridoxal phosphate is also required for glycogen phosphorylase, an enzyme by which glycogen is broken down to glucose; for the formation of antibodies; for the synthesis of a precursor of the porphyrin ring, which is part of the hemoglobin molecule; and possibly for the conversion of linoleic acid to arachidonic acid.

Daily Allowances The need for vitamin B-6 is proportional to the amount of protein metabolized. A vitamin B-6 level of 0.016 mg per gram of protein intake is satisfactory. The recommended allowances are 2.0 mg per day for adult men and 1.6 mg for women.[2] These amounts provide a reasonable margin of safety and permit a protein intake of 100 g or more.

The allowance for infants is 0.3 to 0.6 mg; for children 1 to 10 years, it increases gradually from 1.0 to 1.4 mg; and for adolescents, recommended intakes are 1.4 to 2.0 mg. During pregnancy an additional 0.6 mg is recommended, which is decreased to 0.5 mg during lactation.

Food Sources The vitamin B-6 available in the American food supply per capita is 1.97 mg. The principal source is meat, poultry, and fish, with this group accounting for 40 percent of the total amount available. Potatoes, sweet potatoes, and vegetables account for about 23 percent of the total supply; dairy products, 11 percent; and flour and cereals, 11 percent.[3] Whole grains are good sources of pyridoxine, but most of this is lost in the milling of the grains. In addition, availability of the vitamin in cereals and legumes may be limited because of binding to other components such as plant fiber.[14]

Effects of Deficiency Results of the Nationwide Food Consumption Survey of 1977–78 showed that 51 percent of individuals had intakes of vitamin B-6 less than 70 percent of their recommended intake.[15] The average intake of females over 15 years of age ranged between 58 to 63 percent of their 1980 RDA for the vitamin. In spite of these low intakes, there is little clinical or biochemical evidence suggesting problems in vitamin B-6 nutriture. However, satisfactory methods for assessing the vitamin B-6 status of large population groups are not available.

Traditionally the TRYPTOPHAN LOAD TEST has been used to measure vitamin B-6 adequacy. In this test a measured dose of tryptophan is given, after which the 24-hour urinary excretion of xanthurenic acid is measure. XANTHURENIC ACID is an intermediary metabolite of tryptophan metabolism that is excreted when there is insufficient vitamin B-6 to catalyze the reactions throughout the normal pathway. Reduced levels of serum and red blood cell transaminases and lowered excretion of pyridoxic acid are also found in vitamin B-6 deficiency. With the availability of improved methods of analyses, a reduction in plasma and erythrocyte concentrations of pyridoxal phosphate likewise has been demonstrated.

Deficiency in Infants. During the 1950s vitamin B-6 deficiency was reported in infants who had received a commercial formula in which the pyridoxine had been inadvertently destroyed in the processing of the milk. The infants showed nervous irritability and convulsive seizures. Other related symptoms included anemia, vomiting, weakness, ataxia, and abdominal pain. The convulsive seizures responded dramatically to the administration of pyridoxine.[16,17]

Deficiency in Adults. A number of studies in college students fed vitamin B-6 deficient diets have shown a rapid fall in urinary excretion of vitamin B-6 and pyridoxic acid as well as decreased blood concentrations of pyridoxal phosphate. Soon after these changes appeared, increased excretion of xanthurenic acid was found with the tryptophan load test.[18] Despite this biochemical evidence of deficiency, no clearcut symptoms have been observed in adults. However, when an antagonist such as deoxypyridoxine is fed together with a diet deficient in vitamin B-6, seborrheic dermatitis around the eyes, eyebrows, and angles of the mouth has been described.[19] Large doses of vitamin B-6 will counteract the effect of the antagonist.

Isonicotinic acid hydrazide (INH) is widely used in the treatment of tuberculosis. It is chemically related to pyridoxine and acts as an antagonist to vitamin B-6 activity. Patients who have been treated with this drug have experienced neuritic symptoms believed to be caused by the imposed vitamin B-6 deficiency; the condition was corrected when additional vitamin supplements were prescribed. Penicillamine, a drug used in the treatment of Wilson's disease and cystinuria, is also an antagonist of vitamin B-6. Vitamin B-6 supplements are usually prescribed for patients receiving this drug.

Pregnant women and those who are using the steroid contraceptive pill are found to have increased excretion of xanthurenic acid as measured by the tryptophan load test, as well as lower blood transaminase activity. The biochemical changes are readily corrected by increasing the intake of vitamin B-6, but there is little indication of physiologic advantage.[2]

Vitamin B-6 Dependency. An inborn error of metabolism has been described in which convulsive seizures are controlled by up to 200 to 600 mg pyridoxine hydrochloride per day.[20]

Adverse Effects The effect of megadoses of pyridoxine was tested on normal individuals by giving 200 mg pyridoxine daily for 33 days. When these large doses were withdrawn, the individuals required greater-than-normal intakes of vitamin B-6 to maintain normal biochemical levels.[2] Because of the possibility of inducing vitamin B-6 dependency, use of such megadoses is contraindicated as a routine measure. A report of sensory-nervous system dysfunction in women taking 2 to 6 g of vitamin B-6 per day, in most cases as a self-imposed supplement, further emphasizes the potential adverse effects of excess intakes of the vitamin.[21]

Pantothenic Acid

Discovery Pantothenic acid was isolated in 1938 by Dr. R. J. Williams and synthesized by other investigators in 1940. Although its vitamin nature was demonstrated by its ability to prevent certain deficiencies in animals, little interest was shown in this vitamin until about a decade later. In 1946 Lipmann and his associates showed that coenzyme A was essential for acetylation reactions in the body, and in 1950 reports from this same laboratory showed pantothenic acid to be a constituent of coenzyme A. The name for this vitamin is derived from the Greek worked *pan-thos*, meaning "everywhere." The universal distribution of this vitamin in biologic materials suggests the key role that it plays in metabolism.

Characteristics PANTOTHENIC ACID, as the free acid, is an unstable, viscous yellow oil, soluble in water. (See Figure 13-1.) Commercially, it is available as the sodium or calcium salt, which is slightly sweet, water soluble, and quite stable. There is little loss of the vitamin with ordinary cooking procedures, except in acid and alkaline solutions.

The pantothenic acid content of tissues and foods is determined by microbiologic, chemical, or radio-immunoassay methods; values are expressed in milligrams or micrograms.

Functions Pantothenic acid functions in the body as a component of COENZYME A (CoA) and as a prosthetic group on the acyl carrier protein. CoA is a complex molecule consisting of a sulfur-containing compound, adenine, ribose, phosphoric acid, and pantothenic acid. The sulfur linkage is highly reactive. The part of the acyl carrier protein containing pantothenic acid has a structure similar to part of CoA.

CoA functions in reactions that accept or remove the acetyl group ($-CH_3CO$). One of these reactions is the formation of acetylcholine, a substance of importance in the transmission of the nerve impulse. CoA participates in the oxidation of pyruvate, α-ketoglutarate, and fatty acids. (See Figure 6-4 and page 72.) CoA reacts with pyruvic acid to form acetyl CoA, which, in turn, combines with oxaloacetate to form citrate, thus initiating the TCA cycle for the release of energy. CoA is also involved in the synthesis of cholesterol and other sterols, and porphyrin in the hemoglobin molecule. The acyl carrier protein has an essential role in fatty acid synthesis.

CoA is synthesized in all cells and apparently does not cross cell membranes. Liver, kidney, brain, adrenal, and heart tissues, being metabolically active, contain high concentrations.

Requirement The daily requirement is not known, but the Food and Nutrition Board has estimated the safe and adequate daily intake to be 4 to 7 mg for adults. The customary intake of pantothenic acid from ordinary foods in the United States is approximately 5 to 10 mg per day.[3] Intakes of 2 to 3 mg for infants and 3 to 5 mg for children are believed to be satisfactory.

Food Sources Most of the pantothenic acid in animal tissues is in the form of coenzyme A. As its name indicates, pantothenic acid is widely distributed in animal foods and in whole grains and legumes. Liver, yeast, egg yolk, and meat are particularly good sources. Fruits, vegetables, and milk contain smaller amounts. About 50 percent of the pantothenic acid of grains is lost in their milling, and dry processing of foods also leads to significant losses.

Effects of Deficiency No clear-cut demonstration of pantothenic acid deficiency has been afforded by experimental diets low in pantothenic acid. When an antagonist, omega methyl pantothenic acid, was fed with deficient diets, the following symptoms were observed: loss of appetite, indigestion, abdominal pain; sullenness, mental depression; peripheral neuritis with cramping pains in the arms and legs; burning sensations in the feet; insomnia; and respiratory infections. In these subjects there was an increased sensitivity to insulin, and increased sedimentation rate for erythrocytes, and marked decrease in antibody formation.[22,23]

The neuropathy observed in alcoholics is possibly related to pantothenic acid deficiency. However, when diets are deficient in pantothenic acid, they are also deficient in many other factors, and therefore the separation of symptoms attributable to the lack of various nutrients becomes exceedingly difficult.

Biotin

Discovery During the 1920s a factor essential for the growth of yeast was described and named *bios*. A decade later, Dr. Helen Parsons and her co-workers and others reported on the symptoms observed in rats that were fed a diet including raw egg white. The animals lost their fur, particularly around the eyes, giving a spectacle-like appearance; there was rapid loss of weight, paralysis of the hind legs, and eventual cyanosis and death. The symptoms did not occur when cooked egg white was used.[24]

Small quantities of the active factor were isolated from egg yolk in 1936 and were later established as being identical with the yeast growth factor and the anti-egg-white injury factor.

The substance in raw egg white has been found to be a glycoprotein that binds biotin and thereby prevents its absorption from the intestinal tract. It is called AVIDIN, which means "hungry albumin." Heating of egg white inactivates the binding capacity of avidin.

Characteristics   BIOTIN is a relatively simple compound, a cyclic urea derivative, which contains a sulfur grouping. (See Figure 13-1.) In its free form it is a crystalline substance, very stable to heat, light, and acids. It is somewhat labile to alkaline solutions and to oxidizing agents. In tissues and in foods it is usually combined with protein.

Functions and Metabolism   Biotin is a coenzyme of a number of enzymes that participate in carboxylation, decarboxylation, and deamination reactions. For example, it is required in the synthesis of fatty acids. Another reaction catalyzed by biotin-containing enzymes is the fixation of CO_2 in the conversion of pyruvate to oxaloacetate, an important reaction that generates the TCA cycle. (See Figure 6-4.) Within the TCA cycle, biotin is also required for the conversion of succinate to fumarate and oxalosuccinate to ketoglutarate.

Biotin is essential for the introduction of CO_2 in the formation of purines, these compounds being essential constituents of DNA and RNA. The deaminases for threonine, serine, and aspartic acid also require biotin as a coenzyme.

Biotin is stored in minute amounts principally in the metabolically active tissues such as the kidney, liver, brain, and adrenal. The biotin content of the feces and likewise of the urinary excretion is considerably greater than the dietary intake. This indicates the intestinal synthesis of biotin and the absorption of the vitamin from this source.

Dietary Needs   A recommended dietary allowance for biotin has not been established. The estimated safe and adequate daily intake of 30 to 200 μg recommended by the Food and Nutrition Board for adults is based on reports indicating that diets supplying 28 to 42 μg did not lead to deficiency. Similar estimates are 10 to 15 μg for infants and 20 to 30 μg for children.

Good dietary sources of biotin include organ meats, egg yolk, legumes, and nuts. Cereal grains, muscle meats, and milk contain only small amounts.

Effects of Deficiency   Biotin deficiency has been described in humans when large amounts of raw egg whites were fed. Four volunteer subjects were fed an experimental diet containing approximately 3,000 kcal, low in biotin, and including 928 of the total calories from egg white (equivalent to about 60 egg whites!) for a period of 10 weeks. Beginning with the third to fourth weeks symptoms appeared approximately in this order: scaly desquamation, lassitude, muscle pains, hyperesthesia, pallor of skin and mucous membranes, anorexia, and nausea. The hemoglobin levels were lowered, the blood cholesterol levels were increased, and the urinary excretion of biotin dropped to about one tenth of the normal levels. All these abnormalities were cured within 5 days when 150 μg biotin was given daily.[25]

Biotin deficiency has been reported in patients maintained for long periods of time on intravenous feeding. Characteristic symptoms were loss of hair (alopecia) and dermatosis.[26,27] Considerable evidence exists indicating that a type of seborrheic dermatitis in young infants is due to biotin deficiency. Blood levels and urinary excretion of the vitamin are depressed. Prompt improvement is achieved by administration of 5 mg biotin daily for 10 days either intravenously or intramuscularly.[28]

Vitamin B-12

Discovery   Until the 1920s pernicious anemia was an invariably fatal disease. Then came the dramatic announcement by Minot and Murphy[29] that large amounts of liver—about a pound a day—could control the anemia and prevent the neurologic changes.

Castle set forth the hypothesis that liver contains a substance that he termed the EXTRINSIC FACTOR (now known to be vitamin B-12) and that its absorption requires another principle in normal gastric secretion that he called the INTRINSIC FACTOR. Patients with pernicious anemia were lacking the intrinsic factor. Nevertheless, when very large amounts of liver were consumed, some absorption of the extrinsic factor took place by simple diffusion.

The active principle in liver was extracted during the 1930s and provided the basis for the treatment of patients by injection. Then in 1948 came the announcement of the isolation of a few micrograms of a red crystalline substance that was shown to be dramatically effective in the remission of pernicious anemia. The structure of this complex molecule was elucidated in 1955, but synthesis of the vitamin by Woodward and others was not accomplished until 1973—25 years after its isolation.[30]

Characteristics   Vitamin B-12 is the most complex of all vitamin molecules; it contains a single atom of

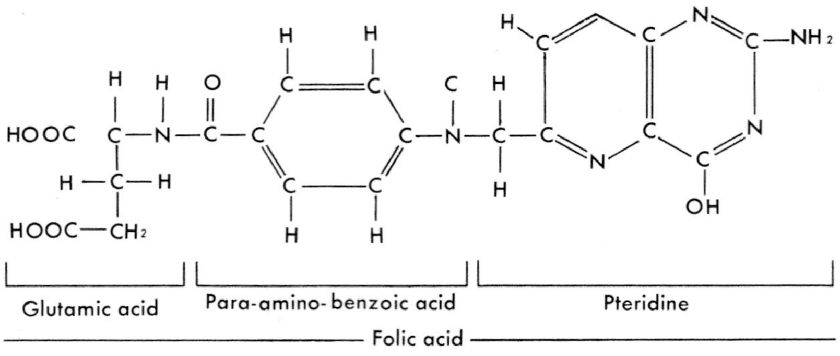

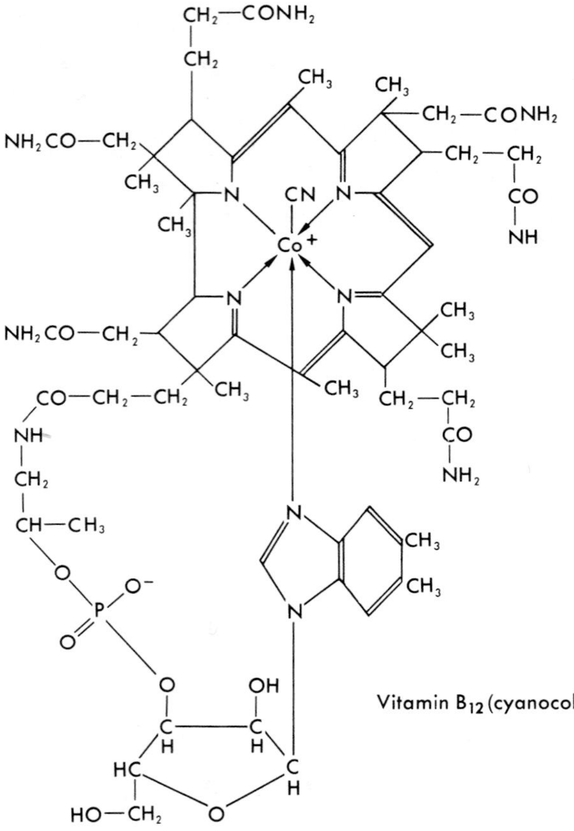

Vitamin B_{12} (cyanocobalamin shown)

Figure 13-7. Folic acid and vitamin B-12 are essential for the regeneration of red blood cells. Vitamin B-12 has the most complex structure of any of the vitamins. Note the similarity of the position of cobalt in the structure to the position of iron in hemoglobin and of magnesium in chlorophyll.

cobalt held in a structure similar to that which holds iron in hemoglobin and magnesium in chlorophyll. (See Figure 13-7.) It occurs in several forms designated as COBALAMINS. Cyanocobalamin, the form available commercially, is the most stable form but is present in the body only in small amounts. Forms found in plasma and tissues include methylcobalamin, hydroxycobalamin, and adenosylcobalamin.

Cyanocobalamin forms deep red needle-like crystals that are slightly soluble in water, stable to heat, but inactivated by light and by strong acid or alkaline solutions. Large amounts of ascorbic acid present in a meal or added to serum samples may lead to destruction of vitamin B-12. There is little loss of vitamin B-12 in food by ordinary cooking procedures.

Vitamin B-12 is assayed microbiologically or by radioassay, and is measured in micrograms or picograms, (pg, $\mu\mu$g, micromicrograms).

Metabolism   Vitamin B-12, being a very large molecule, requires a special, rather complex mechanism for absorption: (1) vitamin B-12 is separated from its polypeptide linkages in food by the gastric acid and enzymes; (2) in the stomach vitamin B-12 binds with proteins called *R proteins* present in salivary and gastric secretions; (3) the vitamin B-12–R protein complex is cleaved in the duodenum by pancreatic proteolytic enzymes; (4) vitamin B-12 then binds to the intrinsic factor, which is secreted by the parietal cells of the stomach; (5) the vitamin B-12–intrinsic factor complex, which is resistant to digestive enzymes, passes to the ileum and in the presence of calcium binds to receptor sites on the mucosal cells; (6) the vitamin is released from the complex and transferred across the mucosal epithelium; (7) vitamin B-12 enters the portal blood circulation and is transported bound to a protein TRANSCOBALAMIN II.[31]

Intrinsic factor regulates the amount of absorption to about 2.5 to 3 μg daily.[32] When the dietary intake is only 1 to 2 μg daily, 60 to 80 percent is absorbed. With good diets young men averaged 10 percent absorption and elderly men about 5 percent. Absorption is greater if the vitamin is present in three meals than if it is all provided in a single meal.

The liver is the principal site of storage for vitamin B-12. Storage in the bone marrow is limited, and amounts to only 1 to 2 percent of that in the liver. The enterohepatic circulation varies from 0.6 to 6 μg per day vitamin B-12 with practically complete reabsorption taking place. Thus, the normal liver store of 2,000 to 5,000 μg is sufficient to take care of body needs for 3 to 5 years.

The serum concentration of vitamin B-12 is 200 to 900 pg per ml. A level of 80 pg per ml represents unequivocal deficiency.

Functions   Vitamin B-12 functions in all cells, but especially those of the gastrointestinal tract, the nervous system, and the bone marrow. Within the bone marrow a vitamin B-12 coenzyme participates in the synthesis of DNA. When DNA is not being synthesized, the erythroblasts do not divide but increase in size, becoming megaloblasts which are released into the circulation. Whether the influence of vitamin B-12 is a direct action or a facilitation of the use of folic acid is not well understood.

Vitamin B-12 is required for enzymes that accomplish the synthesis and transfer of single-carbon units such as the methyl group, for example, the synthesis of methionine and choline. Conversion of methylmalonate, which is formed during degradation of certain amino acids and odd-chain fatty acids, to succinate also requires vitamin B-12 coenzymes. An increase in urinary excretion of methylmalonate occurs in vitamin B-12 deficiency and may be useful in diagnosis.

Dietary Needs   A daily intake of 2.0 μg of vitamin B-12 per day is sufficient for normal hematopoiesis and good health and will replenish liver stores. The recommended allowance for children ranges from 0.7 to 1.4 μg per day, and 2.2 μg for pregnancy and lactation.[2] For infants from birth to 6 months 0.3 μg is recommended daily. The allowance is 0.6 μg for older infants, 0.7 μg for children 1 to 3 years, and 1.0 μg for those 4 to 6 years.

The vitamin B-12 available per capita in the American food supply is 8.7 μg, of which 70 percent is supplied by meats, poultry, and fish, 20 percent by dairy foods excluding butter, and 9 percent by eggs.[3] Plant foods do not supply vitamin B-12.

Effect of Deficiency   Vitamin B-12 deficiency usually occurs because of a defect in absorption rather than due to inadequate dietary intake. Pernicious anemia is a disease, probably of genetic origin, in which intrinsic factor is not produced, and consequently, vitamin B-12 is not absorbed. The bone marrow is unable to produce mature red blood cells, but releases fewer large cells (macrocytes) into the circulation. Thus, the capacity to carry hemoglobin is reduced. The characteristic symptoms include pallor, anorexia, dyspnea, prolonged bleeding time, abdominal discomfort, loss of weight, glossitis, neurologic disturbances including unsteady gait, and mental depression. Patients respond to as little as 1 μg given parenterally; usually, initial therapy provides 50 to 100 μg until the anemia is corrected, after which maintenance therapy usually consists of monthly injections of approximately 100 μg.[33]

Megaloblastic anemia from vitamin B-12 deficiency also occurs following surgical removal of the part of the stomach that produces intrinsic factor, or the part of the ileum where the absorption sites are located. Such deficiency occurs 3 to 5 years following the surgery and can be prevented by injections of vitamin B-12 at periodic intervals. Malabsorption syndromes such as sprue may also be characterized by megaloblastic anemias resulting from deficient absorption of vitamin B-12 as well as folic acid.

Dietary deficiency of vitamin B-12 has been described in vegetarians who consumed no animal foods whatsoever.[34] They showed low serum levels of vitamin B-12, glossitis, paresthesias, and some changes in the spinal cord but did not have the characteristic anemia. Vitamin B-12 deficiency also has been reported in a breast-fed infant whose mother was a strict vegetarian.[35]

Diagnosis of vitamin B-12 deficiency is usually based on low serum concentrations of the vitamin. The size and appearance of the red blood cells can be used initially to differentiate the anemia from that caused by a lack of iron. Increased urinary excretion of methylmalonate also supports a diagnosis of vitamin B-12 deficiency. Deficiency due to lack of intrinsic factor and impaired absorption can be identified by the Schilling test. In this test radioactive vitamin B-12 is given orally and is followed by a parenteral injection of the nonradioactive vitamin. Excretion of the radioactive vitamin in a 24-hour urine sample is monitored; low excretion implies vitamin B-12 deficiency. The test is then repeated with an oral dose of intrinsic factor in addition to the vitamin B-12. Improved absorption when intrinsic factor is added indicates pernicious anemia. If improvement does not occur, other factors are responsible for the impaired absorption.

Folacin (Folic Acid)

Discovery During the 1930s and 1940s many investigators had described water-soluble factors required by various animal species and microorganisms and given them names such as factor U (unknown factor required for chick growth); vitamin B_c (antianemia factor for chicks); Wills factor for treatment of tropical macrocytic anemia of pregnancy described by Dr. Lucy Wills; vitamin M, essential for monkeys; L-casei factor, citrovorum factor, and SLR factor for growth of various microorganisms. Folic acid was named in 1941 by Mitchell and his associates. The name was chosen because of the factor's prevalence in green leaves: *folium* is the Latin word for leaf. In 1945 the identification of the structure and the synthesis of folic acid by Angier and his co-workers established that these variously named factors were one and the same substance. That same year Dr. Tom Spies showed that folic acid was effective in the treatment of megaloblastic anemia of pregnancy and of tropical sprue.

Characteristics FOLACIN is the generic term for folic acid, pteroylglutamic acid, and other compounds having the activity of folic acid. It consists of three linked components: a pteridine grouping, para-aminobenzoic acid, and glutamic acid, an amino acid. (See Figure 13-7.)

Polyglutamate forms of folacin having from two to eight glutamic acid groups are common in foods and body tissues.[36] The major form in cabbage, for example, has seven groups and is known as heptapteroylglutamic acid.

Pure folic acid occurs as a bright yellow crystalline compound, only slightly soluble in water and quite stable at pH 5 and above even with heating at 100°C. It is easily oxidized in an acid medium and is sensitive to light.

Folic acid is measured in micrograms or nanograms (ng, millimicrograms) and is assayed microbiologically or by colorimetric or fluorometric methods.

Metabolism About 25 percent of folacin in foods is in free form and is readily absorbed. Before the polyglutamate forms can be absorbed, the extra glutamate groups must be removed by conjugase, an enzyme present in the mucosal cells of the proximal intestine. Efficiency of absorption of dietary folacin varies considerably depending on the presence of conjugase inhibitors or other unidentified interfering factors in foods.

Folacin is stored principally in the liver. The active form is TETRAHYDROFOLIC ACID. Ascorbic acid prevents the oxidation of this active form and thus maintains an adequate level of the folate for metabolic needs.[37]

Functions After absorption folacin undergoes a series of reactions to form coenzymes known as tetrahydrofolates. These are linked to single carbon groupings: methyl ($-CH_3$); hydroxymethyl ($-CH_2OH$); formyl ($-OCH$); and formimino ($-CH=NH$). The ability to link up with and to donate these single carbon units forms the basis for the biochemical functions of folacin. Tetrahydrofolates, together with vitamin B-12, are essential for DNA snythesis and thus are necessary for the synthesis and maturation of red blood cells in the bone marrow. The interrelationship of these two vitamins in DNA synthesis is shown in Figure 13-8. Folacin also is necessary for the synthesis of serine, a 3-carbon amino acid, from glycine, a 2-carbon amino acid; the formation of choline; and conversion of homocysteine to methionine.

Because of the importance of folacin in protein synthesis, folacin inhibitors such as methotrexate have been used successfully in the chemotherapy of various types of cancer to inhibit tumor growth and cell proliferation.

Recommended Allowances 200 μg is recommended for men, and 180 μg for women. For pregnancy the allowance is 400 μg and for lactation it is 280 μg; during

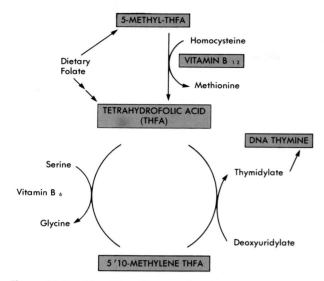

Figure 13-8. Simplified diagram showing interrelationship of folic acid and vitamin B-12 in DNA synthesis. Continuous regeneration of tetrahydrofolic (THFA) acid requires vitamin B-12. The vitamin acts as a coenzyme by taking a methyl group from 5 methyl THFA and donating it to homocysteine to form methionine. The THFA that remains is converted to 5, 10-methylene THFA, which is needed for thymine formation. Deficiency of either vitamin B-12 or folic acid interferes with the cycle.

the first year of life the needs are met with 30 to 45 μg per day.

Food Sources Folic acid is widely distributed in foods in both free and conjugate forms. The availability of the latter to meet body needs is not known. Liver, kidney, yeast, and deep green leafy vegetables are excellent sources; lean beef, veal, eggs, and whole-grain cereals are good sources; and root vegetables, dairy foods, pork, and light green vegetables are relatively low in the vitamin. As much as 50 to 95 percent of the folacin content of food may be destroyed by extended cooking or other processing.[33]

Effects of Deficiency Folic acid deficiency results from inadequate dietary intake or is secondary to disease. In many instances dietary surveys have shown the intake to be considerably below the recommended allowances, but without accompanying biochemical or subjective signs of deficiency. This suggests that utilization of conjugated forms may be higher than anticipated in setting up the recommended intakes or that the margin of safety is high.

With a deficiency the serum folate level is reduced and changes take place in the production of red blood cells in the bone marrow. The anemia that results from folic acid deficiency is characterized by a reduction in the number of red blood cells, the release into the blood circulation of large nucleated cells (hence the designation macrocytic, or megaloblastic, anemia), low hemoglobin levels, but a high color content of each cell, and lowered leukocyte and platelet levels. Diagnosis of folacin deficiency usually is based on serum and/or red cell concentrations of the vitamin. Values for serum folacin equal to or greater than 6.0 nanograms (ng) per ml generally are considered acceptable; normal values for red cell folacin are 160 to 650 ng per ml.

Anemia due to lack of folacin has been observed in elderly patients who have had poor diets and who have various organic diseases, in pregnant women, in some women using contraceptive pills, and in infants whose formulas may be inadequate in folic acid or ascorbic acid. Because of the prevalence of low serum folacin and megaloblastic anemia during pregnancy, supplements frequently are recommended. Folic acid deficiency frequently accompanies disease conditions in which the requirement for the vitamin is greatly increased, as in Hodgkin's disease and leukemia. Malabsorption syndromes, notably tropical sprue, are characterized by the presence of megaloblastic anemias.

The administration of folic acid to patients with megaloblastic anemia brings about dramatic reversal of the changes in the bone marrow. The red blood cells become normal in size, their number increases, the total hemoglobin increases, and the leukocyte levels return to normal. Many of the patients have a glossitis and diarrhea especially associated with malabsorption; these too are improved.

Folacin will bring about remission of the anemia in vitamin B-12 deficiency. However, it is not effective in preventing or correcting the neurologic disturbances. Therefore, folacin is not administered to a person with megaloblastic anemia until tests, such as determinations of serum concentrations of the vitamins, are done to document that the condition is due to folacin deficiency rather than to vitamin B-12 deficiency. Similarly, the amount of folacin in vitamin supplements is regulated to avoid masking the existence of vitamin B-12 deficiency and delaying its diagnosis by curing the anemia.

Toxicity High intakes of folic acid have been reported to interfere with various anticonvulsant drugs and produce increased seizures in patients receiving these drugs. Very high serum concentrations of folic acid in animals following intravenous administration of the vitamin have been shown to have a convulsive effect, but the levels were higher than those that would likely occur in humans following oral ingestion of the vitamin.[33]

Other Factors

Choline All living cells contain CHOLINE, principally in phospholipids such as phosphotidylcholine (lecithin), which is essential for the structure and function of cell membranes and serum lipoproteins. Another choline-containing phospholipid, sphingomyelin, is found in high concentrations in nervous tissues. As a component of acetylcholine, choline is essential in the transmission of nerve impulses. One of the important functions of choline is the donation of methyl groups that can be utilized in numerous reactions.

Choline has been shown to be essential for various animal species, but the need for it by humans has not been clearly established. Probably synthesis of choline within the body is sufficient. Large doses of choline have been tried in a number of disorders including fatty liver and cirrhosis and, more recently, memory deficits in the elderly and tardive dyskinesia, a condition characterized by involuntary muscular twitching. Results of such use have been equivocal and any effects probably should be regarded as pharmacologic rather than physiologic.

Egg yolk is especially rich in choline, but legumes, organ meats, milk, muscle meats, and whole-grain cereals are also good sources. A typical diet furnishes from 200 to 600 mg per day. These relatively large amounts indicate that choline is probably not a true vitamin.

Myo-inositol MYO-INOSITOL, also known as inositol or mesoinositol, is a water-soluble, sweet-tasting substance distributed in fruits, vegetables, whole grains, meats, and milk. It possesses lipotropic activity, but its significance in human nutrition has not been established.

Lipoic Acid LIPOIC ACID is a sulfur-containing, fat-soluble substance also known as *thioctic acid* and *protogen*. Strictly speaking, it is not a vitamin because it is not necessary in the diet of animals. It functions, however, in the same manner as many of the B-complex vitamins. It is a component of the complexes involved in the decarboxylation of ketoacids such as pyruvic acid and alpha-ketoglutaric acid. (See page 71.)

Carnitine Because carnitine can be synthesized in human liver and kidney it is not considered a vitamin, although growing evidence suggests that dietary sources may be important in certain situations. Carnitine has an essential role in the transport of long-chain fatty acids from the cytosol of the cell to the mitochondria, where the enzymes necessary for oxidation are located. Abnormalities seen in patients with genetic disturbances in carnitine metabolism include muscle weakness, lipid accumulation between muscle fibers, and hypoglycemia. Evidence of carnitine deficiency has been reported in premature infants maintained on intravenous feeding, and low serum carnitine levels have been found in infants fed soy formula.[38-40]

Bioflavinoids The BIOFLAVINOIDS are a group of chemical substances comprised primarily of flavine and flavinoid compounds found in citrus fruits as well as other fruits and vegetables. In 1936 it was reported that bioflavinoids exerted a synergistic effect on vitamin C in curing scurvy. Because of their effect on capillary permeability they became known as vitamin P. Despite a tremendous amount of work done with these compounds there is no evidence that they are essential for humans or animals and deficiency states have never been produced.

Para-Aminobenzoic Acid PARA-AMINOBENZOIC ACID (PABA) is an integral part of the structure of folic acid. Although some microorganisms may be able to utilize PABA to synthesize folacin, a role for PABA in human nutrition has not been documented in spite of frequent claims for its value.

Nonnutrients LAETRILE and AMYGDALIN, sometimes referred to as vitamin B-17, are part of a group of cyanide-containing glycoside compounds found in the pits of apricots, peaches, bitter almonds, and apple seeds. Laetrile has been widely promoted for the prevention and cure of cancer but scientific evidence does not exist to support either its effectiveness or lack of adverse effects. Similarly, there is no evidence that physiologic or biochemical abnormalities develop when these substances are not included in the diet. Thus, the use of the term "vitamin" is erroneous and misleading.

Another substance erroneously promoted as a vitamin is PANGAMIC ACID or vitamin B-15. Products called vitamin B-15 vary considerably in chemical composition, and the Food and Drug Administration considers pangamic acid an unidentifiable substance. None of the many claims for its value in treating such diverse conditions as allergies, schizophrenia, hepatitis, or autism in children has been documented in controlled studies.

SOME POINTS FOR EMPHASIS IN NUTRITION EDUCATION (A GENERAL SUMMARY)

1. Vitamins are compounds of known chemical nature occurring in minute amounts in foods. They have precise functions in the body for the use of carbohydrates, fats, and proteins for energy and for the synthesis of tissues, enzymes, and other body regulators. Thus, vitamins help to maintain healthy tissues and normal functions of all organs.
2. Each vitamin has specific functions and cannot substitute for another. Many reactions in the body require several vitamins; a lack of any one can interfere with the function of another.
3. Synthetic vitamins and the vitamins occurring naturally in foods have the same chemical formulas and, weight for weight, are of equal use in the body.
4. A diet that includes recommended amounts of the Daily Food Guide selected from a variety of foods generally will furnish sufficient amounts of the vitamins to meet the needs of nearly all healthy persons without the use of supplements.
5. Each food group makes a special vitamin contribution to the diet. All the vitamin needs are not easily met if one or more of these food groups are omitted. For example, fruits and vegetables are the principal sources of ascorbic acid; dark green leafy vegetables and deep yellow vegetables and fruits are a major source of carotene; milk is a principal source of riboflavin; meats, poultry, and fish are outstanding for niacin, vitamin B-6, vitamin B-12, and thiamin; and whole-grain and enriched breads and cereals are especially important for thiamin and niacin.
6. Vitamin D is present in natural foodstuffs in only small amounts. Infants, children, pregnant and lactating women, and people who have little exposure to sunlight should use vitamin D milk or a supplement.
7. All vitamins are susceptible to destruction under certain conditions. However, for practical purposes, if the homemaker observes rules for the preservation of ascorbic acid, thiamin and riboflavin, all other vitamins are likely to be satisfactorily retained. For riboflavin, the principal destruction comes about when milk in clear containers is allowed to stand in direct sunlight. The retention of ascorbic acid, thiamin, and other vitamins is assured if (1) some raw foods such as salads are freshly prepared and used daily, (2) cutting and exposure of surfaces are reduced to the shortest possible period of time, (3) cookery takes place in a small volume of liquid, (4) the use of alkali to retain green color is avoided, (5) foods are cooked only to the point of tenderness, and (6) foods are served promptly after preparation.
8. Vitamins A and D are toxic, and high-potency supplements should be used only when prescribed by a physician for specific deficiencies.
9. If taken in greater amounts than the body needs, the water-soluble vitamins are excreted in the urine; hence, supplements in addition to a good diet are probably an economic waste. Long-term intake of excess amounts of certain water-soluble vitamins also may have adverse effects and megadose usage is not advisable without medical supervision.
10. Vitamin deficiencies can be diagnosed only by means of accurate dietary and medical history, physical examination, and laboratory studies. Self-diagnosis and therapy are wasteful and can be dangerous.
11. Vitamin deficiency diseases can occur (1) if the dietary intake is generally poor, (2) if a food group is consistently omitted without making appropriate compensation for such omission, and (3) when there is too little money to buy an adequate diet.
12. A large proportion of vitamin deficiencies in the United States are secondary to disease, including anorexia and vomiting and failure to eat, malabsorption as in diarrhea, sprue, and other conditions, and increased metabolic requirements because of fever and other stress factors.
13. Specific vitamin deficiencies require therapy with the vitamins that are lacking. Usually, synthetic vitamins are used to correct the deficiency inasmuch as large dosages can bring about rapid improvement.

Problems and Review

1. Explain how the following nutrients are interrelated: riboflavin and niacin; vitamin B-6 and protein; cobalt and vitamin B-12; tryptophan and niacin; tryptophan and vitamin B-6; folic acid and ascorbic acid; glucose and thiamin.
2. What is the effect on carbohydrate metabolism of a deficiency of thiamin? What are clinical signs of such deficiency?
3. What is the role of niacin in metabolism? What clinical symptoms are observed in a niacin deficiency?
4. How can you explain the fact that milk is a pellagra-preventive food even though it contains very little niacin?

Table 13-1. Summary of Water-Soluble Vitamins
(see also Points for Emphasis, page 197)

Nomenclature	Important Sources	Physiology and Function	Effects of Deficiency	Daily Allowances*
Ascorbic acid Vitamin C	Citrus fruits; tomatoes; melons; cabbage, broccoli; strawberries; fresh potatoes; green leafy vegetables	Very little storage in body Formation of intercellular cement substance; synthesis of collagen Absorption and use of iron Prevents oxidation of folacin	Weakened cartilages and capillary walls Cutaneous hemorrhage; sore, bleeding gums, anemia Poor wound healing Poor bone and tooth development *Scurvy*	Men: 60 mg Women: 60 mg Pregnancy: 70 mg Lactation: 95 mg Infants: 35 mg Children under age 11: 45 mg Boys and girls: 50–60 mg
Thiamin Vitamin B-1	Whole-grain and enriched breads, cereals, flours; organ meats, pork; other meats, poultry, fish; legumes, nuts; milk; green vegetables	Limited body storage Thiamin pyrophosphate (TPP) is coenzyme for decarboxylation and transketolation; chiefly involved in carbohydrate metabolism	Poor appetite; atony of gastrointestinal tract, constipation Mental depression, apathy, polyneuritis Cachexia, edema Cardiac failure *Beriberi*	Men: 1.5 mg Women: 1.1 mg Pregnancy: +0.4 mg Lactation: +0.5 mg Infants: 0.3–0.4 mg Children under age 11: 0.7–1.0 mg Boys and girls: 1.1–1.5 mg
Riboflavin Vitamin B-2	Milk; organ meats; eggs; green leafy vegetables	Limited body stores, but reserves retained carefully Coenzymes for removal and transfer of hydrogen; flavin mononucleotide (FMN) and flavin adenine dinucleotide (FAD)	Cheilosis (cracks at corners of lips) Scaly desquamation around nose, ears, Sore tongue and mouth Burning and itching of eyes Photophobia	Men: 1.7 mg Women: 1.3 mg Pregnancy: +0.3 mg Lactation: +0.5 mg Infants: 0.4–0.5 mg Children under age 11: 0.8–1.2 mg Boys and girls: 1.3–1.8 mg
Niacin Nicotinic acid Nicotinamide	Meat, poultry, fish; wholegrain and enriched breads, flours, cereals; nuts; legumes Tryptophan as a precursor	Coenzyme for glycolysis, fat synthesis, tissue respiration. Coenzymes NAD and NADP accept hydrogen and transfer it	Anorexia, glossitis, diarrhea Dermatitis Neurologic degeneration *Pellagra*	Men: 19 mg NE Women: 15 mg NE Pregnancy: +2 mg NE Lactation: +5 mg NE Infants: 5–6 mg NE Children under age 11: 9–13 mg NE Boys and girls: 15–20 mg NE
Vitamin B-6 Three active forms: pyridoxine, pyridoxal, pyridoxamine	Meat, poultry, fish; potatoes, sweet potatoes, vegetables	Pyridoxal phosphate is coenzyme for transamination, decarboxylation, transulfuration of amino acids Conversion of tryptophan to niacin; conversion of glycogen to glucose Requirement related to protein intake	Nervous irritability, convulsions Weakness, ataxia, abdominal pain Dermatitis; anemia	Men: 2.0 mg Women: 1.6 mg Pregnancy: +0.6 mg Lactation: +0.5 mg Infants: 0.3–0.6 mg Children under age 11: 1.0–1.4 mg Boys and girls: 1.4–2.0 mg

Vitamin	Food Sources	Functions	Deficiency	Recommended Allowances
Pantothenic acid	Meat, poultry, fish; whole-grain cereals; legumes. Smaller amounts in fruits, vegetables, milk	Constituent of coenzyme A: oxidation of pyruvic acid, alpha-ketoglutarate, fatty acids; synthesis of fatty acids, sterols, and porphyrin	Deficiency seen only with severe multiple B-complex deficits; gastrointestinal disturbances, neuritis, burning sensations of feet	Adolescents and adults: 4–7 mg Infants: 2–3 mg Children: 3–4 mg
Biotin	Organ meats, egg yolk, nuts, legumes	Avidin, a protein in raw egg white, blocks absorption; large amounts of raw eggs must be eaten. Coenzyme for deamination, carboxylation, and decarboxylation	Deficiency only when many raw egg whites are consumed for long periods of time. Dermatitis, anorexia, hyperesthesia, anemia	Adolescents and adults: 30–100 μg Infants: 10–15 μg Children: 20–30 μg
Vitamin B-12 Cyanocobalamin Hydroxycobalamin	In animal foods only: organ meats, muscle meat, fish, poultry; eggs; milk	Requires intrinsic factor for absorption. Biosynthesis of methyl groups. Synthesis of DNA and RNA. Formation of mature red blood cells	Lack of intrinsic factor leads to deficiency: pernicious anemia, following gastrectomy. Macrocytic anemia. Neurologic degeneration	Adults: 2 μg Pregnancy: 2.2 μg Lactation: 2.6 μg Infants: 0.3–0.5 μg Children: 0.7–1.4 μg Boys and girls: 2 μg
Folacin Folic acid Pteroylglutamic acid	Organ meats, deep green leafy vegetables; muscle meats, poultry, fish, eggs; whole-grain cereals	Active form is tetrahydrofolic acid; requires ascorbic acid for conversion. Coenzyme for transmethylation; synthesis of nucleoproteins; maturation of red blood cells. Interrelated with vitamin B-12	Megaloblastic anemia of infancy, pregnancy, tropical sprue	Adults: 180–200 μg Pregnancy: 400 μg Lactation: 280 μg Infants: 25–35 μg Children under age 11: 50–150 μg Boys and girls: 180–200 μg
Choline	Egg yolk, meat, poultry, fish, milk, whole grains	Probably not a true vitamin. Donor of methyl groups: lipotropic action. Component of acetylcholine, lecithin, sphingomyelin	Has not been observed in humans	Not known; typical diet supplies 200–600 mg
Lipoic acid Thioctic acid Protogen		Probably not a true vitamin. Coenzyme for decarboxylation of ketoacids	Not known	Not known
Inositol	Widely distributed in all foods	Lipotropic agent. Vitamin nature not established	Has not been observed in humans	Not known

* See also Table inside front cover for a complete listing of allowances.

5. The dietary intake of vitamins may appear to be satisfactory when compared with recommended allowances, but a physician may prescribe a vitamin supplement. Under what circumstances would you expect such a supplement to be necessary?

6. What is the possible significance of each of the following in human nutrition: folacin; choline; biotin; pantothenic acid; vitamin B-6; inositol; vitamin B-12?

7. *Problem.* Compare the label information on three packages of dry cereal, including whole grain, enriched or restored, and fortified. Which of these would give the highest nutritional value for an expenditure of 10 cents? Show your calculations.

8. *Problem.* Mrs. Smith has asked for your guidance in the selection, storage, and preparation of food so that maximum nutritive value will be retained. On the basis of your information concerning the stability of vitamins, indicate briefly a set of instructions for guiding Mrs. Smith. Show how these rules apply to the preparation of a meal that includes roast beef, potatoes, green beans, cole slaw, milk, and fruit cup. Which vitamin or vitamins are especially concerned in each rule you have laid down?

9. *Problem.* Calculate the thiamin, riboflavin, and niacin content of your own diet for 2 days. Compare your intake with the recommended allowances. If there are any deficits, show how you could correct them.

10. *Problem.* A dietary calculation showed an intake of 80 g protein and 12 mg niacin. Calculate the total niacin equivalent of this diet.

11. *Problem.* Calculate the percentage of your own daily requirement for thiamin and riboflavin that 2 cups milk would supply. For each of these nutrients list two foods that would serve as effective supplements to the milk in supplying your daily needs.

12. Compare the label information and price on different vitamin supplement products. Are the amounts of vitamins in multivitamin products different in store brands than in name-brand products? How does the amount of vitamin in single-vitamin products compare with that in mulitvitamin products? Give an example of an ingredient included in some products that has not been established as an essential vitamin for humans.

References

1. Dreyfus, P. M.: "Thiamin and the Nervous System: An Overview," *J. Nutr. Sci. Vitaminol, (Suppl.)*, **22**:13–16, 1976.

2. Food and Nutrition Board: *Recommended Dietary Allowances*, 10th ed. National Research Council–National Academy of Sciences, Washington, D.C., 1989.

3. Marston, R. M., and Welsh, S. O.: "Nutrient Content of the U.S. Food Supply, 1982," *National Food Review*, U.S. Department of Agriculture, Winter 1984, pp. 7–13.

4. Wood, B., et al.: "A Study of Partial Thiamin Restriction in Human Volunteers," *Am. J. Clin. Nutr.*, **33**:848–61, 1980.

5. Horwitt, M. K., et al.: "Correlation of Urinary Excretion of Riboflavin with Dietary Intake and Symptoms of Ariboflavinosis," *J. Nutr.*, **41**:247–64, 1950.

6. Lopez, R., et al.: "Riboflavin Deficiency in an Adolescent Population in New York City," *Am. J. Clin. Nutr.*, **33**:1283–86, 1980.

7. Sebrell, W. H., and Butler, R. E.: "Riboflavin Deficiency in Man," *Publ. Health Rep.*, **54**:2121–31, 1939.

8. Horwitt, M. K., et al.: "Effects of Dietary Depletion of Riboflavin," *J. Nutr.*, **39**:357–73, 1949.

9. Goldberger, J.: "The Prevention of Pellagra: A Test Diet Among Institutional Inmates," *Publ. Health Rep.*, **30**:3117–31, 1915; nutrition classic reproduced in part in *Nutr. Rev.*, **31**:152–53, 1973.

10. Elvehjem, C. A., et al.: "The Isolation and Identification of the Anti-Black Tongue Factor," *J. Biol. Chem.*, **123**:137–49, 1938; nutrition classic reproduced in part in *Nutr. Rev.*, **32**:48–50, 1974.

11. Kudchodkar, B. J., et al.: "Mechanisms of Hypolipidemic Action of Nicotinic Acid," *Clin. Pharmacol. Ther.*, **24**:354–73, 1978.

12. Carter, E. G. A., and Carpenter, K. J.: "The Bioavailability for Humans of Bound Niacin from Wheat Brans," *Am. J. Clin. Nutr.*, **36**:855–61, 1982.

13. Sandstead, H. H.: "Clinical Manifestations of Certain Classical Deficiency Diseases," in Goodhart, R. S., and Shils, M. E., eds.: *Modern Nutrition in Health and Disease*, 6th ed., Lea & Febiger, Philadelphia, 1980, pp. 685–96.

14. Gregory, J. F., and Kirk, J. R.: "The Bioavailability of Vitamin B$_6$ in Foods," *Nutr. Rev.*, **39**:1–6, 1981.

15. Pao, E. M., and Mickle, S. J.: "Problem Nutrients in the United States," *Food Technol.*, **35**:58–69, 1981.

16. Snyderman, S. E., et al.: "Pyridoxine Deficiency in the Human Infant," *Am. J. Clin. Nutr.*, **1**:200–207, 1953.

17. Coursin, D. B.: "Convulsive Seizures in Infants with Pyridoxine-Deficient Diet," *JAMA*, **154**:406–408, 1954.

18. Linkswiler, H. M.: "Vitamin B$_6$ Requirements of Men," in Food and Nutrition Board: *Human Vitamin B$_6$ Requirements*, National Academy of Science–National Research Council, Washington, D.C., 1978, pp. 279–90.

19. Mueller, J. R., and Vilter, R. W.: "Pyridoxine Deficiency in Human Beings Induced with Desoxypyridoxine," *J. Clin. Invest.*, **29**:193–201, 1950.

20. Frimpter, G. W., et al.: "Vitamin B$_6$-Dependency Syndromes: New Horizons in Nutrition," *Am. J. Clin. Nutr.*, **22**:794–805, 1969.

21. Schaumburg, H., et al.: "Sensory Neuropathy from Pyridoxine Abuse," *N. Engl. J. Med.*, **309**:445–48, 1983.

22. Glusman, N.: "The Syndrome of 'Burning Feet' (Nutritional Melalgia) as a Manifestation of Nutritional Deficiency," *Am. J. Med.*, **3**:211–23, 1947.

23. Hodges, R. E., et al.: "Human Pantothenic Acid Deficiency Produced by Omega-Methyl Pantothenic Acid," *J. Clin. Invest.*, **38**:1421–25, 1959.

24. Parson, H. T., et al.: "Interrelationship Between Dietary Egg White and Requirements for Protective Factor in Cure of Nutritional Disorder Due to Egg White," *Biochem. J.*, **31**:424–32, 1937.

25. Sydenstricker, V. P., et al.: "Preliminary Observation in 'Egg White Injury' in Man and Its Cure with a Biotin Concentration," *Science*, **95**:176–77, 1942.

26. McClain, C. J., et al.: "Biotin Deficiency in an Adult During Home Parenteral Nutrition," *JAMA*, **247**:3116–20, 1982.

27. Innis, S. M., and Allardyce, D. B.: "Possible Biotin Deficiency in Adults Receiving Long-term Total Parenteral Nutrition," *Am. J. Clin. Nutr.*, 37:185–87, 1983.

28. Bonjour, J. P.: "Biotin in Man's Nutrition and Therapy—A Review," *Int. J. Vit. Nutr. Res*, 47:107–18, 1977.

29. Minot, G. R., and Murphy, W. P.: "Treatment of Pernicious Anemia by a Special Diet," *JAMA*, 84:470–76, 1926; nutrition classic reproduced in part in *Nutr. Rev.*, 36:50–52, 1978.

30. Staff report: "Discovery and Synthesis of Vitamin B_{12} Celebrated," *Nutr. Today*, 8:24–27, January–February, 1973.

31. Lau, K. S.: "Cobalamins in Man," *Pathology*, 13:189–95, 1981.

32. Heyssel, R. M., et al.: "Vitamin B_{12} Turnover in Man," *Am. J. Clin. Nutr.*, 18:176–84, 1966.

33. Herbert, V., et al.: "Folic Acid and Vitamin B_{12}," in Goodhart, R. S., and Shils, M. E., eds. *Modern Nutrition in Health and Disease*, 6th ed. Lea & Febiger, Philadelphia, 1980, pp. 229–59.

34. Smith, A. D. M.: "Veganism: A Clinical Survey with Observations on Vitamin B_{12} Metabolism," *Br. Med. J.*, 1:1655–58, 1962.

35. Clinical Nutrition Cases: "Vitamin B_{12} Deficiency in the Breast-fed Infant of a Strict Vegetarian," *Nutr. Rev.*, 37:142–44, 1979.

36. Stokstad, E. L. R., et al.: "Distribution of Folate Forms in Food and Folate Availability," in Food and Nutrition Board: *Folic Acid*, National Academy of Science–National Research Council, Washington, D.C., 1977, pp. 56–68.

37. Stokes, P. L., et al.: "Folate Metabolism in Scurvy," *Am. J. Clin. Nutr.*, 28:126–29, 1975.

38. Borum, P.: "Possible Carnitine Requirement of the Newborn and the Effect of Genetic Disease on the Carnitine Requirement," *Nutr. Rev.*, 39:385–90, 1981.

39. Schmidt-Sommerfeld, E., et al.: "Carnitine Deficiency in Premature Infants Receiving Total Parenteral Nutrition: Effect of L-Carnitine Supplementation," *J. Pediatr.*, 102:931–35, 1983.

40. Slonim, A. E., et al.: "Dietary-Dependent Carnitine Deficiency as a Cause of Nonketotic Hypoglycemia in an Infant," *J. Pediatr.*, 99:551–56, 1981.

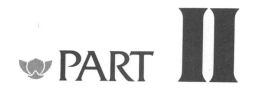

PART II

Practical Applications
of the Principles
for Normal Nutrition

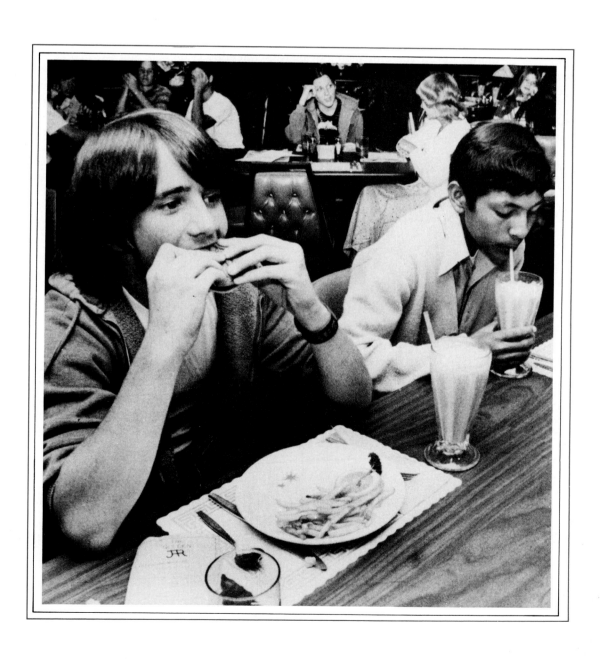

Applying nutrition science to the needs of individuals will be one of your future challenges. Part II provides guidelines for using what is currently known about normal nutrition to help individuals meet optimal nutritional goals.

People eat because they are hungry, they enjoy good food, they find food to be an important part of social interaction, they feel better if they eat when they are under some stress at work or in their personal lives, and so on. People eat those foods that will satisfy their emotional, psychologic, social, and cultural patterns within the constraints of the environment in which they live. People eat, too, to keep healthy and to lead productive, vigorous, and happy lives.

Nowhere in the world can one find such a diversity of cultural food patterns nor so varied a supply of food as in North America. The abundance of foods, the high nutritive values of most foods, and the wholesomeness and safety of the food supply are accomplishments of agriculture, food science, and food technology that comsumers far too often take for granted. Laws that pertain to the quality of the food supply are enforced through federal, state, and local governmental agencies.

The maintenance of good nutrition is a lifelong goal that includes a successful outcome of pregnancy, desirable levels of growth and development for infant, child, and teenager, and physical fitness for the adult years into the later years of life. In recent years many people have improved their physical fitness through exercise that promotes cardiovascular health and through dietary balance that controls weight, provides essential amounts of nutrients, and avoids the exesses of fats, sugars, salt, alcohol, and highly refined foods.

The tragic consequences of a limited food supply, poverty, and ignorance in many of the developing countries of the world are all too common. Children and the elderly in these countries are especially vulnerable to hunger, starvation, and finally death. Even in the affluent countries poverty and ignorance remain as obstacles to a healthy life for some people.

The nurse, dietitian, and other health professionals are able to help meet the nutritional needs of indivduals by making nutritional assessments and by developing plans for implementation that incorporate nutrition education and dietary counseling techniques. The health professional is, in fact, an important link between nutrition science and the practical applications that can promote health in individuals.

14

Food Selection and Meal Planning for Nutrition and Economy

Foods are complex substances that should be evaluated for the variety of nutritive contributions that they make to meeting nutritional needs. The Daily Food guide provides a practical basis for planning meals that are nutritionally balanced and appetizing. A recent survey by the Economics and Statistics Service of the U.S. Department of Agriculture showed that 64 per cent of the American households studied had made changes in their diets during the preceding three years for reasons of health and nutrition.[1] Most nutritionists agree that changes with respect to the levels of fat, cholesterol, sugar, and salt, as well as weight control are desirable. Such changes can be made within the framework of the Daily Food Guide.

Up to this point the reader has become familiar with the important sources for individual nutrients (Chapters 5–13). But meal planning requires consideration of the broad package of nutrients supplied by each food and food group. By referring to the calculation for the Basic Diet (Tables 4-1 and 4-2, page 38), the reader can see how each food group makes rather unique contributions to the whole. Another evaluation of the nutritive contribution made by major food groups is that provided annually by the U.S. Department of Agriculture. Based upon the food supply available in the United States, the percentage contribution made by each major food group to each nutrient can be calculated. (See Table 14-1.)

A major consideration in meal planning for most families is the cost of food and the amount of money that is available for food purchase. Food expenditures are controlled by the best available purchase information, by menu adjustments, by adequate storage facilities, by appropriate preparation techniques, and by control of waste from the point of purchase to the plate at the table.

Characteristics of Food Groups

Vegetable-Fruit Group

No group of foods lends greater variety to the diet in terms of color, flavor, and texture than the vegetable–fruit group. This group includes practically every part of the plant—leaves, stems, roots, tubers, bulbs, flowers, and seeds. Mature seeds of the grasses are included in the cereal group, and those of leguminous plants such as peas and beans are included in the meat group.

Daily Choices In order to ensure optimum vitamin and mineral contributions, the daily recommendation of four servings from the vegetable–fruit group should be governed as follows:

1 serving daily of a good source of vitamin C such as citrus fruits
1 serving frequently of dark green or deep yellow vegetables for vitamin A
1 serving frequently of unpeeled fruits and vegetables and those with edible seeds such as berries for fiber

A serving is equivalent to ½ cup cooked vegetable, salad, or a whole piece of vegetable or fruit such as a banana, an apple, or medium-sized potato. Teenagers should have larger servings of each, and young children may have smaller-size servings.

Nutritive Characteristics Based on the national food supply, fruits and vegetables are the only important source of ascorbic acid. (See Table 14-1.) They furnish about half of the vitamin A in the form of carotene. About one fifth of the dietary iron is supplied by this group, although the bioavailability of the iron

Table 14-1. Contribution of Major Food Groups to Nutrient Levels, 1982 (expressed as percentage)*

Food Group	Food Energy	Protein	Fat	Carbo-hydrate	Cal-cium	Phos-phorus	Iron	Magne-sium	Vitamin A Value	Thia-min	Ribo-flavin	Niacin	Vitamin B-6	Vitamin B-12	Ascorbic Acid
Meat, poultry, and fish	20.1	42.4	34.0	0.1	4.1	27.9	30.7	13.7	21.0	26.0	22.2	45.2	40.0	70.0	1.9
Eggs	1.8	4.8	2.6	0.1	2.3	5.1	5.1	1.2	5.6	1.9	4.9	0.1	2.0	8.5	0
Dairy products, excluding butter	10.2	21.3	11.7	5.7	72.4	33.7	2.6	20.2	13.2	7.4	37.3	1.3	10.8	19.7	3.3
Fats and oils, including butter	19.1	0.1	44.7	+	0.4	0.2	0	0.4	8.4	0	0	0	0.1	0	0
Citrus fruits	1.0	0.5	0.1	2.0	1.0	0.8	0.8	2.4	1.6	2.8	0.5	0.8	1.4	0	26.7
Noncitrus fruits	2.2	0.7	0.3	4.8	1.3	1.3	4.0	4.5	6.0	1.9	1.8	1.7	7.5	0	12.5
Potatoes and sweet potatoes	2.9	2.4	0.1	5.5	1.1	3.8	4.9	7.4	4.8	5.0	1.5	6.3	10.0	0	14.3
Dark-green, deep-yellow vegetables	0.2	0.5	+	0.5	1.4	0.7	1.5	2.1	22.9	0.8	1.1	0.6	2.3	0	10.7
Other vegetables including tomatoes	2.2	3.1	0.3	4.2	4.8	4.8	9.2	10.4	13.5	6.1	4.5	5.1	10.6	0	27.0
Dry beans and peas, nuts, soy products	2.8	5.0	3.7	1.7	2.7	5.7	5.9	11.2	+	4.6	1.8	6.5	4.3	0	+
Grain products	20.0	18.9	1.3	36.7	3.8	13.4	32.1	19.2	0.4	43.4	23.8	28.9	10.9	1.7	0
Sugar and other sweeteners	16.9	+	0	38.2	4.0	0.8	0.7	0.2	0	+	+	+	+	0	+
Miscellaneous‡	0.7	0.4	1.2	0.5	0.9	1.7	2.4	7.0	2.4	0.1	0.6	3.4	0.1	0	3.5

* Marston, R. M., and Welsh, S. O.: "Nutrient Content of the U.S. Food Supply, 1982," *Natl. Food. Rev.*, U.S. Department of Agriculture, Washington, D.C., Winter 1984, p. 8.

† Less than 0.05 percent.

‡ Includes coffee, chocolate liquor equivalent of cocoa beans, and fortification of products not assigned to a food group.

is low. The composition of vegetables and fruits covers a wide range depending upon the part of the plant represented. Moreover, the handling of the food from farm to table can be so variable that the amounts of vitamins and minerals retained may be high or low. The vitamin concentration is affected by the season, the degree of maturity, the temperature and length of storage, and the preparation techniques.

Water. As the chief constituent of fruits and vegetables, water constitutes 75 to 95 percent of the weight. Foods relatively high in carbohydrate, such as bananas and potatoes, are lower in water content than those that are low in carbohydrate such as tomatoes, lettuce, and melons.

Energy. As a group, these foods are not important contributors to the caloric value of the diet, although potatoes and sweet potatoes, when eaten in large quantities, make an appreciable contribution. Many vegetables, such as tomatoes, celery, asparagus, salad greens, and others, furnish no more than 25 kcal per serving. Potatoes, lima beans, fresh corn, and bananas, for example, are slightly below 100 kcal per serving unit. Other vegetables and fruits range from 40 to 80 kcal per average serving. The caloric value of this group is greatly increased by additions of sugar, butter, cream, and sauces.

Protein and Fat. The protein concentration of most fresh vegetables ranges from 1 to 2 percent and is even lower in fruits. Fresh peas and lima beans are slightly above these levels. All foods of this group are extremely low in fat with the exception of avocados and olives. Vegetables and fruits contain no cholesterol.

Carbohydrate. The carbohydrate composition of this group ranges widely, from as low as 3 to 5 percent for rhubarb, greens, summer squash, tomatoes, and others, to more than 30 percent for a few foods such as sweet potatoes. Dried fruits contain about 65 percent carbohydrate.

The carbohydrate in fruits and vegetables occurs as sugars—glucose, fructose, and sucrose, dextrins, starches, and dietary fiber. The starch in immature fruits such as bananas and pears is converted to sugars during ripening. By contrast, the sweetness of young peas and tender corn is lost as these vegetables become more mature.

The exchange lists (Table A-4) provide a convenient classification of fruits and vegetables according to carbohydrate content. Fruit exchanges (list 4) are stated in amounts required to furnish 15 g carbohydrate. Most vegetables (list 2) contain about 5 g carbohydrate per ½ cup serving. Some vegetables, such as chicory, Chinese cabbage, endive, escarole, lettuce, parsley, radishes, and watercress, do not contribute significant amounts of carbohydrate. The so-called starchy vegetables, including lima beans, corn, lentils, peas, potato, plantain, winter squash, and sweet potatoes, are comparable to a slice of bread in carbohydrate, protein, and energy value (list 1).

Minerals. Turnip greens, dandelion greens, mustard greens, collards, kale, and broccoli are excellent sources of calcium. The calcium of spinach, poke, dock, beet greens, chard, and lamb's quarters is not nutritionally available because the oxalic acid of those plants combines with calcium to form insoluble salts that are not absorbed. Some fruits contribute small amounts of calcium, but the daily contribution cannot be considered important.

The dark green leafy vegetables are fair-to-good sources of iron. Likewise, fresh and dried apricots, raisins, prunes, dates, figs, peaches, and berries are good sources of iron. The availability of the iron is enhanced in the presence of ascorbic acid or in a meal that includes meat.

Fruits and vegetables are rich sources of potassium, but the sodium content is negligible except for a few vegetables such as beets, carrots, spinach, celery, and chard.

Fruits and vegetables contribute to an alkaline ash. The acid or sour taste of some fruits, including citrus fruits, peaches, and others, is accounted for by several organic acids (citric, malic, tartaric) that are fully oxidized in the body. Because of the preponderance of cations in fruits, the net yield is an alkaline ash. Plums, prunes, rhubarb, and cranberries, on the other hand, contain benzoic acid, which cannot be metabolized in the body; hence they contribute to an acid reaction.

Vitamins. Among the best contributors to ascorbic acid are the citrus fruits, fresh strawberries, cantaloupe and honeydew melon, broccoli, kale, spinach, turnip greens, sweet green peppers, and cabbage. Potatoes and sweet potatoes contain lesser concentrations of this vitamin, but the amounts eaten daily by some people may appreciably add to the total intake. Dried fruits supply little vitamin C.

Dark-green leafy vegetables and deep yellow vegetables and fruits are outstanding for their carotene content. The concentration of the vitamin is directly proportional to the depth of the color. Lightly colored foods such as lettuce, cabbage, and white peaches are poor sources of the vitamin, although the outer green leaves of lettuce may contain 30 times as much vitamin A as the inner pale leaves.

Vegetables and fruits are fair sources of the B-complex vitamins, but do not contain vitamin B-12.

Selection and Care If purchased in season, green beans, broccoli, cabbage, salad greens, tomatoes, apples, citrus fruits, grapes, peaches, and pears are generally good buys in terms of nutritional values for money spent. Asparagus and most berries are examples of foods in this group that are likely to be expensive.

Crisp, ripe, but not overmature vegetables that are firm in texture and free from blemishes should be selected. As vegetables become too mature, the lignocellulose that is formed gives the characteristic stringy or woody texture which cannot be overcome with cookery. Wilted vegetables are lower in carotene and ascorbic acid content, and recrisping the vegetables will not restore these values.

Fruits improve in flavor and aroma with ripening. Some fruits such as peaches and pears bruise so easily that they are customarily picked before they are fully ripe. They should be allowed to ripen at room temperature before refrigeration.

Bananas are high in starch content when green. During ripening at room temperature, this starch is changed to more digestible sugars. Bananas have the best flavor when the skin shows speckles of brown.

Most fruits and vegetables should be stored in the hydrator of the refrigerator. Some root vegetables such as potatoes can be kept for a short time in a cool room. Berries, being highly perishable, should be kept under refrigeration and used within a day or two.

Frozen vegetables are likely to be less expensive than fresh vegetables out of season and compare favorably with fresh vegetables in nutritive values. Frozen citrus juices are more economical than the juices squeezed in the home from fresh oranges. Frozen foods should be kept in the freezer or freezer compartment of the refrigerator at $-18°C$ ($0°F$).

Canned fruits and vegetables are usually sold by grade. Grade A products are uniform in color and size of pieces, practically free of blemishes, and of the proper maturity. Grade B fruits and vegetables are less uniform in color and size of pieces, slightly less tender, and less free of defects. However, they are just as nutritious as grade A vegetables and fruits.

Commercially canned fruits and vegetables closely approximate cooked fresh products in their nutritive values since vacuum closure of the cans reduces the rate of oxidation. There is some unavoidable loss of as-corbic acid and thiamin. These losses are accelerated with storage at high temperatures for long periods of time.

The water-soluble nutrients distribute themselves in canned foods so that the concentration is about equal in the liquid and solid phases. Thus, if the contents are two-thirds solid and one-third liquid, two thirds of the vitamin C, for example, would be in the solids and one third in the liquid. Thus, the maximum nutritive value is obtained when liquid as well as solid is consumed.

Bread-Cereal Group

Importance in World Diets Today, in nearly every country of the world, some cereal grain is regarded as the "staff of life."

By reason of its availability, high yield per acre, low production cost, and excellent keeping qualities, grain is used more abundantly than any other food material. Rice is the chief dietary staple for half the world's population and constitutes as much as 80 percent of the calories for most of Asia's peoples. Wheat ranks second to rice in worldwide use but is the principal cereal grain used in the United States and in some European countries. Corn is widely used in Central and South America. Millet, sorghum, rye, and barley are important in some parts of the world.

Daily Choices The bread–cereal group includes all products made with whole-grain or enriched cereals, flours, and meals: bread, biscuits, muffins, pancakes, waffles; ready-to-eat or cooked breakfast cereals; rice; noodles, spaghetti, macaroni, and other pastas; grits; cornmeal, flours, barley, and bulgur.

Four servings are recommended each day. Additional servings are desirable to meet caloric requirements and to make adjustments for the Dietary Goals. One serving is one slice of bread, or ½ to ¾ cup cooked cereal, macaroni, rice, and so on, or 1 ounce of ready-to-eat cereal.

Nutritional Value of Cereal Foods In the national food supply (Table 14-1) the flour–cereal group takes first place as a source of thiamin and second place as a source of calories, iron, and niacin. This group becomes increasingly important for these nutrients as the income is lowered and the consumption of them is increased.

The seed or kernel of the cereal grain (see Figure 14-1) is divided into three parts, the bran, germ, and endosperm. The aleurone layer just below the bran

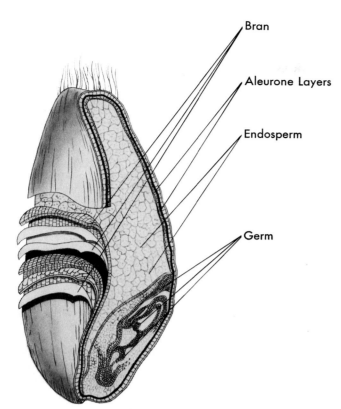

Bran

Aleurone Layers

Endosperm

Germ

Figure 14-1.   Whole wheat—cross section of grain. (Courtesy, the Ralston Purina Company.)

The Bran. The brown outer layers. This part contains:
1. Bulk-forming carbohydrates
2. B vitamins
3. Minerals, especially iron

The Aleurone Layers. The layers located right under the bran. They are rich in:
1. Proteins
2. Phosphorus, a mineral

The Endosperm. The white center. This consists mainly of:
1. Carbohydrates (starches and sugars)
2. Protein

This is the part used in highly refined white flours. Less refined flours and refined cereals are made from this part and varying amounts of the aleurone layer.

The Germ. The heart of wheat (embryo). It is this part that sprouts and makes a new plant when put into the ground. It contains:
1. Thiamin (vitamin B-1). Wheat germ is one of the best food sources of thiamin.
2. Protein. This protein is of value comparable to the proteins of meat, milk, and cheese.
3. Other B vitamins
4. Fat and the fat-soluble vitamin E
5. Minerals, especially iron
6. Carbohydrates

layer is sometimes identified as a fourth part. Although cereal grains vary somewhat in their composition, the average percentage composition of the whole grain is protein, 12; fat, 2; carbohydrate, 75; water, 10; minerals, especially phosphorus and iron, and the B-complex vitamins, especially thiamin, 1. Cereal grains contribute importantly to every nutrient need except calcium, ascorbic acid, vitamin A, vitamin B-12, and vitamin D.

In the exchange lists (Table A-4), one slice of bread or one serving cooked or ready-to-eat unsweetened cereal is one exchange, and provides 3 g protein and 15 g carbohydrate.

Energy.   Cereal foods, it is well known, are the primary source of energy for most of the world's people. Many people infer from this fact that cereals per se are fattening, and so they omit this group of foods from their diets. By such omission they lose the many nutrient benefits provided by whole-grain and enriched products. The average serving of a cereal food furnishes from 65 to 100 kcal. (See Figure 14-2.)

Protein.   Lysine is a limiting amino acid in wheat, rice, and corn, whereas tryptophan and threonine are limiting in corn and rice, respectively. Beans, peas, or soybeans served in the same meal with foods from the cereal group will supply the limiting amino acids. Thus, rice and kidney beans or brown bread and baked beans are effective combinations. The protein quality of whole grains is somewhat superior to that in refined grains, since the aleurone layer and the germ have a better assortment of amino acids.

Minerals and Vitamins.   The greater part of the minerals, iron and phosphorus, as well as the B-complex vitamins occurs in the bran and germ of the grain. Consequently, most of these nutrients are lost when cereals are highly milled. Enrichment replaces the thiamin, riboflavin, and niacin as well as iron, which are lost in refining. However, whole grains are superior in zinc, copper, vitamin B-6, pantothenic acid, biotin, folacin, and vitamin E.[1]

Selection   Label reading is important in the selection of foods from the bread-cereal group. The consumer should look for information on enrichment, nutrient fortification, and sugar content.

Bread.   About 85 percent of white bread and rolls sold to the American public are enriched. Thiamin, riboflavin, niacin, and iron are included at levels to equal whole wheat bread.

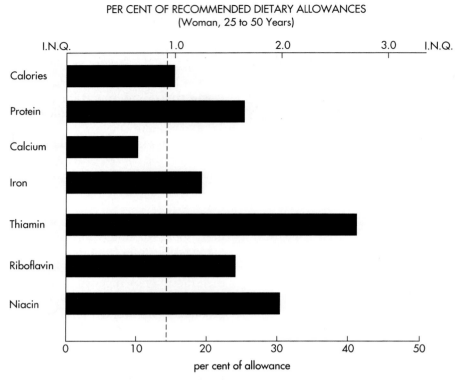

PER CENT OF RECOMMENDED DIETARY ALLOWANCES
(Woman, 25 to 50 Years)

Figure 14-2. Contribution of three slices white enriched or whole wheat bread plus one serving breakfast cereal to the day's allowance for a woman aged 25 to 50 years. Note the Index of Nutritional Quality (INQ) over 1.0 for protein, iron, thiamin, riboflavin, and niacin. See Table 4-1 for calculations.

Whole wheat flour is the only flour that may be used in bread labeled as "whole wheat," "graham," or "entire-wheat" bread. Breads labeled as "cracked wheat," "wheaten," "wheat," and "rye" are made with varying proportions of these flours and white flour.

Specialty breads are often advertised as possessing greater nutritional values. Soy flour, wheat germ, molasses, and nonfat milk increase the nutritive value in relation to the amounts used in the bread formula. The greater cost of some of these breads may not justify their selection if the increase in nutritive value is small.

Breakfast Cereals. Cereals vary widely in their protein, mineral, and vitamin content. Refined, unenriched cereals supply but a small percentage of the daily allowances for minerals and vitamins. Many breakfast cereals are fortified beyond the usual mineral–vitamin contents of the whole-grain cereal. Indeed, fortification often includes vitamins A, B-12, C, and D, none of which are constituents of the whole grain.

An increasing number of breakfast cereals are presweetened, presumably to appeal especially to children. In some products sugar accounts for as much as 50 percent of the total weight. It is preferable to select unsweetened cereals so that the amount of sugar added can be controlled.

Generally, cereals that require cooking are more economical than ready-to-eat cereals. Among the more costly breakfast cereals are those that are sugar coated, with raisins and/or nuts, "natural," and precooked instant cereals, as well as those packaged in individual portions.

Other Cereal Foods. Brown rice is the whole-grain rice with the hull and a little of the bran removed. White rice is milled to remove the hull, bran, and germ. Since white (polished) rice is a staple food for so many of the world's people, enrichment is of major importance. Rice should not be washed prior to cooking since the enrichment premix coats the surface of the grain. The amount of water used for cooking should be no more than can be absorbed by the rice kernels.

Parboiled rice is steamed by a special process so that the thiamin and other vitamins and minerals are distributed throughout the kernel with only a slight loss taking place in washing and cooking. *Converted rice* is parboiled by a patented process. *Precooked rice* requires the addition of hot water and a short period of standing before it is ready to be served; it is more costly than uncooked rice.

Bulgur is a wheat product of whole or cracked grains with a nutlike flavor and a slightly chewy texture. The wheat is parboiled and dried, and some of the bran is removed. Present methods of processing retain 75 percent or more of the minerals and vitamins in the wheat.

A special kind of hard wheat flour—durum—is used in the manufacture of some 150 different shapes of pastas, including macaroni, spaghetti, vermicelli, and noodles. The pastas are used in many side dishes for the main meal or as a main dish in combination with cheese, meat, fish, or poultry.

Milk Group

Milk serves as the sole food for the young during the most critical period of life for some 8,000 species. Cow's milk is by far the most commonly used in the United States.

Daily Choices The milk group includes all forms of milk: whole, 1 or 2 percent fat, nonfat, evaporated—whole or skim, buttermilk or other cultured milks, and chocolate milk. It also includes nonfat dry milk, yogurt, ice cream or ice milk, sour cream, cream, and half-and-half (half whole milk and half light cream), and some 400 varieties of cheese.

One serving of milk is an 8-ounce cup or its equivalent. (See Daily Food Guide, page 30, for equivalents.) The recommended servings of milk are

2 cups for adults
3 cups for school children and pregnant women
4 cups for teenagers and lactating women

To reduce the fat intake, the following adjustments can be made:

1. Substitute skim or 1 or 2 percent milk for whole milk to reduce the intake of saturated fat.
2. Use low-fat cheeses more frequently and whole-milk cheeses less often.
3. Omit cream and ice cream. Use milk in coffee, and ice milk for desserts. Dairy toppings for desserts are acceptable substitutes for whipped cream.

The per-capita consumption of milk and cheese has changed greatly during this century, as shown by the following data[2]:

	1909–13	1947–49	1980
Whole milk, lb	265	299	171
Low-fat milk, lb	61	36	106
Cheese, lb	5	10	22

These changes, at least in part, have resulted from the consumer's awareness of the advantage of reducing fat intake. Also, improvements in milk processing technology have produced more highly acceptable products.

Nutritive Characteristics In the national food supply (Table 14-1), milk and dairy products far exceed other food groups as a source of calcium and riboflavin. They are second only to the meat group for the protein contribution.

Milk is a complex substance in which more than 100 separate components have been identified. The exact composition of milk varies with the breed of cattle, the feed used, and the period of lactation. Pooled market milk, however, has a uniform composition that may vary slightly according to local or state regulations for butterfat and solids content.

One cup of skim milk is the basis for the milk exchanges (Table A-4), each exchange supplying 8 g protein and 12 g carbohydrate. Adjustments are made for low-fat and whole milk.

Energy. From Figure 14-3 it may be seen that milk has a high nutrient density. Two cups of 2 percent milk furnish about 12 percent of the calories for the woman, but the percentage of contribution for most nutrients is considerably greater. By adjusting the fat level of milk, caloric modifications can be made for low-calorie and high-calorie diets.

1 cup skim milk = 85 kcal
1 cup 2 percent milk = 120 kcal
1 cup whole milk = 150 kcal
1 cup half-and-half milk and cream = 315 kcal

Protein. One cup of whole, skim, or diluted evaporated milk contains 8 g protein. Thus, 2 cups daily furnish about one third of the adult protein allowance.

Casein accounts for four fifths of the protein in cow's milk, and various whey proteins, including lactalbumins and lactoglobulins, constitute the remain-

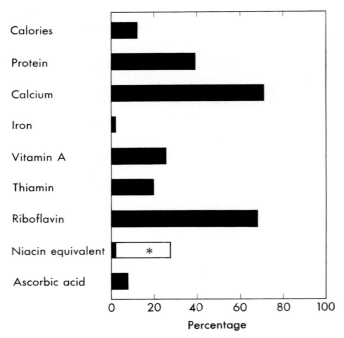

Figure 14-3. Percentage contribution of 2 cups of milk (2 percent fat) to the recommended dietary allowances for the woman of 25 to 50 years. *Unshaded area represents niacin equivalent from tryptophan.

ing protein fractions. The essential amino acids present in milk proteins are supplied in almost ideal proportions for maximum tissue synthesis.

Fat. The fat of milk is highly emulsified and is easily digested. About 60 to 75 percent of the fatty acids in milk are saturated, 24 to 40 percent are monounsaturated, and 2 to 10 percent are polyunsaturated.

Carbohydrate. Lactose is a carbohydrate occurring only in milk. This sugar is much less sweet, less soluble, and more stable than sucrose and other sugars. It gives to milk a bland flavor. Lactose favors the growth of lactic acid–producing bacteria which are believed to retard or prevent the growth of putrefying bacteria. Lactose probably favors the absorption of calcium and phosphorus and the synthesis of some B-complex vitamins in the small intestine. Some persons, especially adults, have a lactase deficiency and therefore a poor tolerance for milk. (See Chapter 31.)

Minerals and Vitamins. Only the milk group provides a practical basis for meeting the recommended allowance for calcium. Phosphorus occurs in correct proportions with calcium to support optimum skeletal growth. Milk contains appreciable amounts of sodium, potassium, and magnesium, but it furnishes

very little iron, so that the infant's diet must be supplemented at an early age to prevent anemia.

Milk is an outstanding dietary source of riboflavin, and also supplies fair amounts of vitamin A, thiamin, vitamin B-6, and vitamin B-12. It is low in niacin but is an excellent source of tryptophan, which functions as a precursor of niacin. Most market milk today is fortified with vitamin D to a level of 400 IU per quart. Vitamin A is usually added to liquid and dry nonfat milks. Processed cow's milk contains only traces of ascorbic acid.

Cheese The composition of cheese depends on the kind of milk used—whole or skim—and the amount of water present. A pound of hard cheese contains the casein and fat of 1 gallon of milk. Cheeses, except cream cheese, are excellent sources of protein. The proteins contain all the essential amino acids and are therefore of high biologic value. Only a trace of the lactose in milk remains in the cheese. Some of the water-soluble minerals and vitamins are removed in the whey. Hard cheeses are an important source of calcium, but soft cheeses, such as cottage cheese, supply much less. See equivalents for 1 cup of milk, page 30. Cheeses also furnish significant amounts of phosphorus, vitamin A (if made with whole milk,) riboflavin, and vitamins B-6 and B-12.

Process cheese is a blend of mild cheeses, followed by pasteurization. An emulsifying agent, such as disodium phosphate or sodium citrate, gives a smooth texture and keeps the fat from separating out.

Selection and Care Fresh milk is more economical when purchased in half-gallon or gallon containers at a food or dairy store. Nonfat dry milk costs one half to two thirds as much as fresh milk. When reconstituted it makes an acceptable beverage if well chilled. It may also be mixed with an equal part of whole milk to give a beverage containing about 2 percent fat. Evaporated milk is less expensive than fresh milk, does not require refrigeration until opened, and lends itself especially to the preparation of cooked dishes. Ultrasterilized milk can be kept at room temperature until the carton is opened, after which it requires refrigeration.

Cultured milks have a nutritive value equal to that of the milk from which they are made. The fermentation of the milk results in the splitting of some of the lactose to lactic acid and in some coagulation of casein. Yogurt is prepared from whole, skim, or partially skimmed milk and is fermented with a mixed culture of microorganisms.

Ice cream supplies the nutrients of cream, milk,

and any fruits, nuts, and sugar that are added. Most ice creams contain about 10 percent fat.

Imitation milk is a product resembling milk, but it contains no milk products such as skim milk or nonfat dry milk. Typical constituents of imitation milk are a protein source such as sodium caseinate or soy protein, corn syrup solids, sugar, and a vegetable fat (usually coconut oil). Additives for color, flavor, and stability are normally present. The nutritive values vary from brand to brand, but they are generally lower in protein, calcium, and vitamins than milk and are not a replacement for whole milk.

Coffee whiteners contain a protein source such as casein, vegetable fat (usually coconut oil), corn syrup solids, emulsifiers, stabilizers, and coloring. Although convenient for use in coffee, a coffee whitener should not be used as a substitute for milk, as on breakfast cereals, since the nutritive values are much lower than they are for milk.

For the best buys in cheese select domestic cheddar, Swiss, process, or cottage cheese, rather than imported cheese. Buy cheese in wedges or sticks, rather than in slices, chunks, or grated. Aged cheeses, imported cheeses, cream, and ice cream are the more expensive items in the milk group. Cheese should be kept refrigerated. When it is to be served as an accompaniment to fruit or crackers, cheese should be brought to room temperature for best flavor.

Meat Group

Daily Choices The meat group includes beef, veal, lamb, pork, poultry, fish, shellfish, dry beans or peas, soybeans, lentils, eggs, seeds, nuts, peanuts, and peanut butter. The daily recommendation from this group is two servings. One serving is 2 to 3 ounces of edible portion of lean cooked beef, veal, pork, lamb, poultry or fish. The equivalents for 1 ounce of meat are as follows:

1 egg
½ to ¾ cup cooked dry beans, dry peas, soybeans, or lentils
2 tablespoons peanut butter
¼ to ½ cup sesame or sunflower seeds, or nuts

Place of Meat in the Diet The often-heard comment "It doesn't seem like a meal without meat" attests to the popular and psychologic importance of meat. All over the world, as economic positions improve, people are increasing their consumption of meat. In fact, the consumption of meat within a country is probably an indicator of its economic position.

The aromas and flavors provided by meat extractives stimulate the appetite. The protein and fat content increase the satiety value of the meal.

The per capita consumption of foods from the meat group for three time intervals was as follows[2]:

	1909–13	1947–49	1980
Beef, lb	54	52	78
Pork, lb	62	64	69
Poultry, lb	18	22	62
Fish, lb	13	13	17
Eggs, lb	37	47	35
Dry beans, peas, nuts, soy products, lb	16	17	18

Pork and beef are the principal foods consumed in this group. Note especially that beef consumption, when compared with 1909–13, is about half again as high, while poultry consumption has more than tripled. Veal, lamb, and mutton account for less than 5 percent of the meat consumed. Egg consumption at the present time has declined from the 1947–49 period—perhaps as a result of the consumer's concern about the cholesterol content of the egg yolk. The consumption of legumes and nuts remains low and fairly stable.

Nutritive Characteristics In the national food supply (Table 14-1) the meat group, including eggs and dry beans, peas, and nuts as well as meat, poultry, and fish, ranks first as a source of protein, phosphorus, magnesium, iron, thiamin, niacin, vitamin B-6 and vitamin B-12. Because of the high level of consumption, this group ranks second for vitamin A and riboflavin. Variations in the composition of meat from one cut to another are due largely to the proportion of lean and fatty tissue. The nutritive value of meat as consumed depends on whether (1) fat was trimmed off before cooking, (2) fat in drippings was used, and (3) surrounding fat on meat was eaten.

Protein. On a cooked basis, 30 g (1 oz) lean meat, one egg, ½ cup cooked dried beans or peas, and 2 tablespoons peanut butter furnish about 7 g protein.

Regardless of the species, the amino acid composition of the proteins of flesh foods is relatively constant and of such balance and quality that meats, fish, and poultry rank only slightly below eggs and milk in their ability to effect tissue synthesis. The protein differences between so-called red and white meats are insignificant.

The proteins in beans and nuts are somewhat lower

in quality because the amounts of methionine and cystine are below optimum levels. However, when eaten in combination with cereal grains, or with small amounts of milk, eggs, or meat, these deficiencies are corrected.

Fat. In the Exchange Lists (Table A-4, list 5) meat cuts or their equivalents are grouped according to fat content:

1 ounce low-fat meat: 3 g fat
1 ounce medium-fat meat: 5 g fat
1 ounce high-fat meat: 8 g fat

The fatty acids in meat are more saturated than those in poultry and fish. Peas, beans, and lentils are very low in fat. Seeds, nuts, and soybeans contain significant amounts of fat, with high proportions of polyunsaturated fatty acids.

Only animal foods contain cholesterol. Egg yolk, liver, and brains are high in cholesterol content. The lean and fat portions of muscle meats contain approximately equal concentrations of cholesterol. Fish and shellfish (except shrimp) are relatively low in cholesterol. (See Table A-5.)

The following adjustments can be made in fat content of the meat group to comply with dietary guidelines:

1. Restrict the total meat intake to 4 to 5 ounces cooked edible portion each day.
2. Select only lean cuts of meat and trim off visible fat.
3. Discard drippings from roasts or broiled meats.
4. Use poultry, fish, and legumes frequently in place of meat.
5. Use eggs 3 to 4 times a week if cholesterol is restricted.

Minerals. The meat group is valuable for its biologically available iron. The inclusion of meat in a meal also enhances the availability of iron from the vegetable–fruit and bread–cereal groups. Red meats and oysters are especially valuable for their zinc content, and dry beans, peas, soybeans and nuts for magnesium. Meats are also rich in phosphorus, sulfur, and potassium and are moderately high in sodium, but they are poor in calcium content. Some shellfish and canned salmon with the bones contain appreciable amounts of calcium. Saltwater fish is a good source of iodine.

Vitamins. All foods of the meat group are good sources of the B-complex vitamins. Pork, liver, and other organ meats and legumes are excellent for their thiamin content; poultry, dry peas, and peanuts are rich in niacin. Vitamin B-12 is supplied by organ meats, muscle meats, poultry, and eggs, but it is not found in the plant foods of this group.

Extractives and purines. Various non-protein nitrogenous substances give meat its characteristic flavor. They are readily extracted from meat with water, as in the preparation of broth. They have very little nutritive value.

Selection The meat group accounts for a significant part of the food budget. In many families the expenditure for this group is too great, thereby reducing the amount of money that can be spent for the other groups.

The standards for various grades of beef, veal, and lamb established by the U. S. Department of Agriculture are based on the amount of surface fat and marbling (fat interspersed among the muscle fibers), color, firmness of flesh, texture, and maturity.

Prime beef, which is very tender and has a considerable amount of surface fat and generous marbling, is sold in some meat specialty markets and to restaurants and hotels. Most of the meat sold in retail markets is graded *choice* or *good*. These grades are less generously marbled, but they are juicy and flavorful. *Standard*-grade beef has very little fat, is less tender and juicy, but quite rich in flavor.

For many years Americans preferred meats that were generously marbled. To bring about marbling, animals must be fed grains for a period of time before marketing. Some concerned people consider this an extravagant use of grain in a world where severe shortages of food exist for some people. More recently the American public has been demanding leaner meat because of their concern about the fat and cholesterol levels, and the meat industry has responded to this demand.

The costs of protein vary widely according to the following factors:

1. *Market supply.* In recent years veal and lamb, which account for only a small part of the total meat consumed in the United States, have been far more costly than beef and pork. In general, poultry has been less expensive than beef or pork. Fresh fish is no longer among the low-cost sources of protein.
2. *Cuts of meat and quality.* For example, compare frozen beef liver and fresh calf's liver; ground beef and rib roast or steak; pink or red salmon.
3. *Amount of processing before sale.* Note, for example, the differences between dry and canned

beans; whole chicken or chicken breasts; kinds of cheese; pizza.

4. *Amount of food needed to provide a given quantity of protein.* Note that just over half a pound of bacon or of cream cheese would need to be consumed to supply 20 g protein—not a likely amount to be consumed at one time.

Brown or white eggs are equal in nutritive value, and there is no merit in paying additional amounts for one color or the other. Grade A eggs are best for table use, while grade B eggs can be used for cooking and for some table purposes. Small eggs are often a better buy in the fall, whereas large eggs may cost only a few cents more during winter and spring months.

Dried beans and peas, lentils, cowpeas, chickpeas, and peanuts or peanut butter are inexpensive alternatives for meat. Dry beans and peas require a long time for cooking, but are lower in cost than the corresponding canned product.

Textured vegetable proteins are the basis for a number of meat analogs, especially useful for vegetarian diets. To produce textured vegetable protein, the protein is extracted from grains or legumes, soy protein being widely used. The protein is solubilized and forced through spinnerets to form fibers, which are then coagulated. The fibers are further processed to simulate beef, pork, ham, chicken, or fish by appropriate flavorings, coloring, and texture modification. Minerals and vitamins may be added to correspond to the composition of the product it replaces.

Fats, Sweets, and Alcohol Group

Choices This group includes butter, margarine, mayonnaise, salad dressings, vegetable oils, and solid shortenings; sugar, syrups, candy, jelly, jams, sweet toppings, honey; soft drinks; and beer, wine, and distilled liquors. It also includes bakery products made with refined, unenriched flours.

There are no recommendations for daily allowances. This group furnishes variety and interest to the meal; for example, dressing on a tossed salad, butter or margarine in a baked potato or on a piece of bread, jelly or preserves with a piece of meat or on a biscuit; or wine with dinner.

This is the group that must be especially restricted to avoid obesity, but it can be used in greater amounts by those who need to gain weight. Several dietary guidelines emphasize reduced intake of sugars, and replacement of saturated fats with those that are rich in polyunsaturated fatty acids.

Nutritive Characteristics In the national food supply (Table 14-1) sugars and sweets and fats and oils each contribute about one sixth of the energy value of the diet but do not add appreciably to the protein, mineral, or vitamin levels. This group is a concentrated source of calories: 4 kcal per g for sugar, 9 kcal per g for fat, and 7 kcal per g for alcohol.

Despite a slight decline in recent years in the amount of sucrose (cane and beet sugar) consumed, this has been more than compensated for by a great increase in the use of corn sugars, especially high-fructose corn syrup. The latter is used in soft drinks, canned foods, bakery products, and other processed foods. Soft drink consumption has more than tripled in the last quarter century.

Margarines are fortified with 15,000 IU vitamin A to correspond to the value in butter. Soft type margarines and vegetable oils are good sources of polyunsaturated fatty acids and vitamin E.

Meal Planning and Budgeting

Essentials of Meal Planning

The nutritive value of a basic diet for the adult using recommended amounts of food from the Daily Food guide is shown in Tables 4-1 and 4-2 (pages 38–39). The basic diet serves as a foundation upon which meals can be planned to meet a great variety of circumstances. In addition to meeting nutritive needs, successful meal planning depends on many factors that are summarized in Table 14-2.

Begin with a Good Breakfast A great number of adults and children eat an inadequate breakfast or skip it altogether. Studies conducted many years ago at the State University of Iowa[3] showed that (1) efficiency in physiologic performance as measured by bicycle ergometer, treadmill, and maximum grip strength, decreased in late morning hours when breakfast was omitted; (2) attitude toward schoolwork and scholastic achievement was poorer when breakfast was omitted; (3) the content of the breakfast did not determine its efficiency so long as it was nutritionally adequate; (4) a breakfast providing one fourth of the daily caloric and protein allowances was superior to smaller or larger breakfasts for maintaining efficiency in the late morning hours; (5) a protein intake of 20 to 25 g maintained the blood glucose level during the late morning hours; and (6) the omission of breakfast was of no value in weight reduction. In fact,

Table 14-2. Factors to Consider in Meal Planning

Essential Factors	Interpretation
Family composition	Adjust amounts for children, teenagers, pregnant and lactating women. For persons with low energy requirements (women and elderly persons) select foods high in nutritive value
Food habits	Consider psychologic and cultural meanings of food. See Chapters 15 and 16 for full discussion
Food costs	Budgeting and food selection for economy are discussed on page 217.
Time for food preparation	Budget time for best use, by planning menus for several days; shopping once a week, planning for leftovers; using some convenience foods if homemaker is also employed outside the home
Variety in meals	*Daily Food Guide:* establish menu pattern that includes recommended amounts of each group for each member of the family. Keep selection of sweets, fats, and alcohol to a minimum. *Variety of choice:* vary the choice of foods within each group from day to day; do not use the same meats, vegetables, fruits every day *Color:* be sensitive to color combinations. Avoid meals that are all white, or all one color tone. Use garnishes for a touch of color; for example, paprika, pepper rings, radishes, parsley *Texture:* include some crisp and chewy foods with soft foods *Flavor:* combine bland foods with those that are more strongly flavored; do not use all spicy or all bland foods at one meal *Preparation:* use a variety of preparation methods, for example, boiling, roasting, baking, frying; with or without sauces; various combinations of foods
Season	Hearty foods such as stews and soups are favored in cold weather; lighter foods in hot weather, but including the same nutrients
Satiety	Provide some protein and fat in each meal to allay sense of hunger
Meal spacing	Arrange meal times so that family can be together whenever possible. Plan snacks to include nutrients for the day. Be discriminate in use of high-carbohydrate, high-calorie foods for snacks

those who omit breakfast while on a weight reduction regimen experience greater hunger in addition to being physiologically inefficient.

A change to better breakfast habits means (1) planning simple, easy-to-prepare, but varied meals; (2) arising sufficiently early so that there is time for eating breakfast; (3) eating breakfast with the family group so that it, like other meals, has pleasant social associations.

Breakfast may include some protein food such as egg or milk, cereal or breadstuff, or both, and a beverage. Children and teenagers should include milk for breakfast. If citrus fruit or another good source of ascorbic acid is included at breakfast, the day's allowance is ensured. Cereal may be hot or cold; breads may vary from plain white enriched or whole grain to muffins, griddle cakes, waffles, or sweet rolls, as the occasion warrants. A breakfast may be light or heavy depending upon the individual's activity and preferences.

Lunch Is Often Neglected Thousands of workers eat lunches that are limited to the choices in a fast-food restaurant or to the sandwich carried from home. The hamburger on a bun, French fries, and a soft drink or coffee is a common pattern. This can be improved by including a salad and a glass of milk or by carrying a piece of fruit from home.

Through school food services lunches that supply about one third of the recommended allowances are available to children and teenagers in most of the nation's schools. Older Americans, too, in many cities and rural communities are able to receive a noon meal at centers for group feeding.

Often the lunch eaten by homemakers and preschool children consists of a day-to-day monotony of leftovers because the homemaker does not take time for adequate planning or preparation. Sometimes this leads to indiscriminate snacking throughout the day. The following are examples of luncheons in varying circumstances:

At Home with Preschool Children
Tomato soup
Chicken sandwich on whole wheat bread with chopped celery, lettuce, and mayonnaise
Fresh fruit cup
Peanut butter cookies
Milk

Fast-Food Restaurant
Hamburger on bun
Salad from salad bar
Milk shake

Brown Bag
Egg salad sandwich
Whole cherry tomatoes
Fresh fruit such as apple, orange
Beverage: milk, coffee, tea—brought in thermos or purchased at work

Dinner Patterns The evening meal is the only meal over which most homemakers have control. For many families it is the only time when all members are together. This meal must make up for any deficiencies that might have occurred earlier in the day.

Meat, fish, fowl, cheese, eggs, or legumes comprise the main dish at dinner. Potatoes or a starchy food and a green or yellow vegetable are generally included. If no salad has been provided in the luncheon, it should be served here. Dessert may consist of fruits, simple puddings, cake, or pastries. Milk should be given to children.

Snacks Most people consume snacks and beverages between meals and in the evening. When they are selected as part of the total food pattern for the day, and consist primarily of nutrient-rich foods, they can enhance the nutritive quality of the diet. Far too often, snacks consist of high-calorie foods that are low in nutritive value. This means that some people will exceed their caloric requirements and that others, especially children, may not consume sufficient amounts of essential nutrients.

Some good snack selections for children are listed on page 273.

Meal Patterns The Daily Food Guide together with adjustments for dietary guidelines provides the foundation for planning meals. In the following example, note how the items in the center column conform to the basic food groups, and how this pattern is adjusted to meet caloric requirements, to provide additional nutrients, and to increase menu appeal.

Planning the Food Budget

Factors to Consider in Budgeting Meal planning, food purchase, and meal preparation are common tasks that must be performed by each household. But the way in which they are accomplished is as variable as the persons involved. Among the factors to consider are these:

1. Number of family members, their age distribution, increased needs during pregnancy and lactation and adolescence, or special needs for modified diets.
2. Family income. On a national average about 16 percent of income is spent for food. But this average can give a false impression. When the income is low the proportion of money spent for food is likely to be 25, 30, or 40 percent or even more.
3. Where meals are eaten. Of expenditures for food in 1983 in the United States, 72 cents of every dollar was spent for food eaten at home, and 28 cents of each dollar was spent for food eaten in restaurants and away-from-home snacks.[4]
4. The availability of supplementary programs when income is limited. Food stamps, free or reduced-cost school lunches and breakfasts, the WIC program for women, infants, and children, and congregate meal programs for the elderly are important ways to increase the available food supply.
5. The location of markets. Although supermarkets generally provide food at less cost than small, neighborhood markets, transportation to these large markets is a problem for some people.
6. Alternative marketing choices. Some community groups have organized cooperatives; that is, they arrange to purchase food in wholesale lots and sell them at cost to the members of the group. Usually these cooperatives are restricted to certain foods; for example packaged goods or farm produce. Another alternative is the discount food store that eliminates the frills of merchandising.
7. The choice of foods within each major food group. The variations within the food groups have been discussed in the preceding pages. (See Figure 14-4.)

Ways to Effect Economy The following suggestions can result in appreciable savings for the food budget.

1. Eat meals at home or carry meals to work whenever practical. Meals purchased in restaurants cost several times as much as comparable meals prepared at home.

Food Groups	Sample Menu Using Food Groups	Completed Menu with Typical Additions
BREAKFAST		
Fruit, rich in viamin C	Orange juice	Orange juice
Cereal, whole-grain or enriched	Oatmeal	Oatmeal with milk and sugar
Bread, whole-grain or enriched	Muffin	Muffin with soft-type margarine
Milk	Milk—2 percent fat	Milk—2 percent fat
		Coffee or tea for adults; cream and sugar
LUNCHEON		
Meat—1 to 2 ounces	Sandwich:	Sandwich:
	Tuna fish—2 oz	Tuna fish—2 ounces
Bread—2 slices	Whole wheat bread—2 slices	Whole wheat bread—2 slices
		Chopped celery
Fat—2 teaspoons	Mayonnaise—2 teaspoons	Mayonnaise—2 teaspoons
Fruit—1 serving	Fresh plums	Fresh plums
		Spice cupcake
Milk—1 cup	Milk, 2 percent—1 cup	Milk, 2 percent—1 cup
DINNER		
Meat—3 to 4 ounces	Meat loaf	Meat loaf with gravy
Potato—1 medium	Mashed potatoes	Mashed potatoes
Leafy green or deep yellow vegetable	Carrots	Parsley carrots with margarine
Raw vegetable or fruit	Lettuce and tomato salad	Lettuce and tomato salad
Fat—3 teaspoons		Italian dressing
		Margarine on vegetables
		Fresh fruit cup
		Milk for children
		Coffee or tea for adults
		SNACK
		Apple slices with cheese

2. Read newspaper reports for foods in plentiful supply. Watch advertisements for items featured as specials for the week.

3. Plan meals several days in advance. To ensure good nutrition use the Daily Food Guide as a basis for planning.

4. Plan meals that the family will eat. Uneaten foods are no bargain, but the wise homemaker introduces new foods attractively prepared from time to time so that the family learns to enjoy a wide variety.

5. Use smaller portions of meat. Select less expensive cuts of meat. Learn to use meat in combination dishes. Use poultry, fish, peanut butter, and legumes in place of meat two or three times a week.

6. Determine when to make foods from scratch and when to use convenience foods. Some convenience foods compare favorably in cost with home-prepared products: canned soups, fruits, vegetables, and citrus juices; frozen citrus juices and vegetables; muffin, cake, and pudding mixes. Many convenience foods are appreciably more expensive than those prepared at home: ready-to-eat salads, packaged salad greens, many seasoned salad dressings; ready-to-bake rolls, pastries, frozen entrees, and frozen vegetables in sauces.

7. Restrict the amount of money spent for snack items and beverages. This category of foods can substantially increase the food expenditure without great returns in nutrition.

8. Use a market list. Be prepared to make substitutions when other foods of equal value are cheaper. Avoid buying foods on impulse.

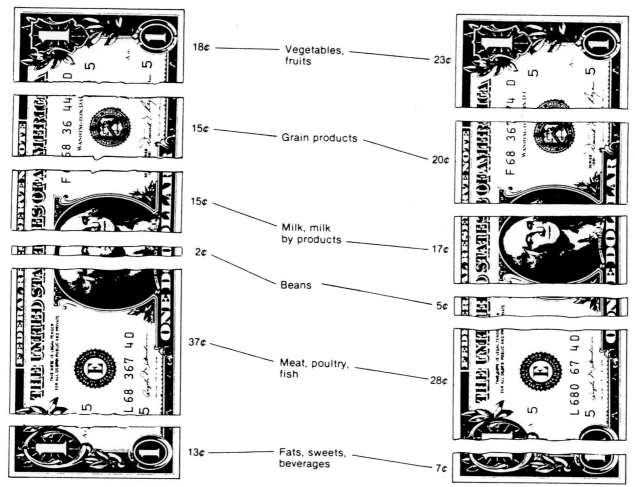

Figure 14-4. (Left) How the food dollar was spent by families in the 1977-78 National Food Consumption Survey. (Right) Better nutrition could be achieved by reducing the proportion of the food dollar spent for meat, poultry, fish, and fats, sweets, beverages and by increasing the proportion spent for the other food groups. (Courtesy, *Family Economics Review*, U.S. Department of Agriculture, 1983.)

9. Read labels. Look for information on dates and nutritive values. Purchase the grade appropriate for the intended use. Compare unit prices of various brands. (See page 260 for a discussion of labeling.)
10. Use discount coupons only if they represent saving for a product and brand that you would ordinarily use.
11. Buy large-size packages only if the price per unit is less, if there is space to store the food properly, and if the food can be used while it is still fresh.
12. Avoid home waste:
    a. Store foods to maintain their freshness and use at peak of quality.
    b. Avoid loss of nutrients from vegetables by excessive peeling.
    c. Cook vegetables in minimum quantities of water until just tender to preserve maximum nutritive value.
    d. Season foods and serve attractively so that they are well accepted and plate waste is kept to a minimum.
    e. Use leftovers within 24 horus.

Master Food Plans

Although the Daily Food Guide is a convenient tool for planning diets that will be nutritionally satisfactory, it does not provide the quantitative basis for estimating the full cost of a diet. Nutritionists, nurses, and other health workers must be able to help families

Table 14-3. Low-Cost Food Plan, 1983: Quantities of Food for a Week (expressed in pounds)[*][a][c]

	Child				Male				Female[b]		
Food Group	1–2 years	3–5 years	6–8 years	9–11 years	12–14 years	15–19 years	20–50 years	51 years or more	12–19 years	20–50 years	51 years or more
Vegetables											
Potatoes (fresh weight)	0.50	0.73	1.16	1.28	1.55	1.88	1.97	1.71	1.19	1.19	1.11
High-nutrient vegetables	.55	.50	.86	.98	1.30	1.34	1.91	2.00	1.19	1.86	2.17
Other vegetables	.82	.88	1.20	1.41	1.41	1.54	2.12	2.19	1.54	2.30	2.04
Mixtures, mostly vegetable; condiments	.06	.10	.14	.17	.18	.20	.29	.30	.15	.24	.15
Vitamin C-rich fruit[d]	1.51	1.43	1.79	1.94	2.03	2.16	1.62	1.75	1.76	1.79	1.91
Other fruit	1.97	1.58	2.30	2.44	2.07	1.45	1.98	2.21	1.81	1.53	2.19
Grain products											
Whole-grain/high-fiber breakfast cereals	.35[e]	.27	.31	.35	.36	.28	.14	.22	.33	.21	.31
Other breakfast cereals	.38[e]	.26	.33	.38	.39	.31	.16	.25	.36	.23	.22
Whole-grain/high fiber flour, meal, rice, pasta	.11	.07	.08	.09	.10	.10	.11	.10	.09	.09	.12
Other flour, meal, rice, pasta	.86	.83	1.04	1.17	1.32	1.34	1.40	1.34	.95	1.01	.83
Whole-grain/high-fiber bread	.12	.17	.22	.26	.31	.39	.42	.30	.28	.30	.25
Other bread	.41	.79	1.08	1.28	1.52	1.95	2.08	1.45	1.19	1.24	.84
Bakery products, not bread	.09	.36	.62	.75	.96	.85	.86	.71	.44	.46	.19
Grain mixtures	.15	.20	.18	.30	.33	.34	.29	.13	.23	.22	.14
Milk, cheese, cream[c]											
Milk, yogurt (quarts)[f]	3.41	3.23	4.26	4.69	5.02	4.86	2.49	2.07	4.64	1.85	2.16
Cheese	.17	.17	.20	.19	.22	.30	.36	.28	.34	.34	.35
Cream, mixtures mostly milk	.13	.44	.57	.69	.67	.75	.51	.50	.65	.34	.55
Meat and alternates											
Lower-cost red meats, variety meats	.71	.52	.60	.74	.99	1.23	1.65	1.23	1.13	1.57	1.67
Higher-cost red meats, variety meats	.37	.38	.47	.57	.79	.94	.86	1.04	.70	.95	1.21
Poultry	.42	.43	.63	.67	.85	.77	.94	.98	.83	.91	.95
Fish, shellfish	.09	.07	.14	.11	.16	.14	.25	.23	.17	.21	.19
Bacon, sausage, luncheon meats	.15	.39	.48	.51	.58	.57	.34	.58	.29	.41	.21
Eggs (number)	3.34	3.24	2.50	2.99	3.02	2.97	3.38	3.93	3.82	4.23	4.02
Dry beans, peas, lentils (dry weight)[g]	.22	.09	.12	.15	.20	.19	.27	.19	.24	.34	.14
Mixtures, mostly meat, poultry, fish, egg, legume	.08	.08	.11	.15	.19	.20	.22	.15	.16	.17	.16
Nuts (shelled weight), peanut butter	.09	.20	.20	.22	.20	.22	.14	.08	.11	.07	.04
Other foods[h]											
Fats, oils	0.9	.27	.43	.50	.55	.54	.68	.54	.25	.32	.26
Sugar, sweets	1.5	.46	.57	.62	.74	.77	.84	.83	.43	.35	.43
Soft drinks, punches, ades (single strength)	1.53	1.96	2.72	3.25	3.35	4.63	3.67	1.19	3.96	3.33	.96

[*] *USDA Family Food Plans, 1983: Low-Cost, Moderate-Cost, and Liberal,* Consumer Nutrition Division, Human Nutrition Information Service, U.S. Department of Agriculture, 1983.

[a] Quantities are for food as purchased or brought into the household from garden or farm. Food is for preparation of all meals and snacks for a week. About 10 percent of the edible parts of food above quantities needed to meet kcal needs is included to allow for food assumed to be discarded as plate waste, spoilage, etc.

[b] Pregnant and lactating females usually require added nutrients and should consult a doctor for recommendations about diet and supplements.

[c] Quantities in pounds except milk, which is in quarts and eggs, which are by number.

[d] Frozen concentrated juices are included as single-strength juice.

[e] Cereal fortified with iron is recommended.

[f] Quantities of dry and evaporated milk and yogurt included as their fluid whole milk equivalents in terms of calcium content.

[g] Count 1 pound of canned dry beans—such as pork and beans, kidney beans—as 0.33 pound.

[h] Small quantities of coffee, tea, and seasonings are not shown. Their cost is a part of the estimated cost for the food plan.

set up food plans that are nutritionally adequate within their incomes. The Consumer Nutrition Division of the U.S. Department of Agriculture has set up master food plans at four cost levels: thrifty; low cost; moderate cost; and liberal cost. Each of the plans was designed to furnish the recommended dietary allowances as foods are actually consumed. The plans include recommendations for men, women, and children of differing ages, and for pregnant and nursing women. See Table 14-3.

The 1983 food plans generally contain more grain products, legumes, fruits, and vegetables and less cheese, eggs, fats, oils, sugars, sweets, and soft drinks than the averages reported by the households in 1977. By these adjustments the food plans meet the dietary guidelines, providing

35 percent or less fat
350 mg cholesterol per day
12 percent of calories or less from caloric sweeteners
1,600 mg sodium per 1,000 kcal

The low-cost food plan includes more foods that are the most economical sources of nutrients. Also, in the low-cost plan it is expected that choices from each of the food groups will be made from lower cost foods within that group—for example, ground beef instead of steak. As the cost of the plan increases, the amounts of fruit, vegetables, meat, poultry, and fish generally increase and the quantities of grain products, legumes, and eggs generally decrease. Within moderate- and liberal-cost food plans the users are also able to select from a wider variety of foods as well as some more expensive foods within each food group.

The Consumer Nutrition Division estimates food costs for each plan monthly and releases this information through the USDA's news service. The costs are also released periodically in *Family Economics Review*.

Problems and Review

1. *Problem.* Calculate the nutritive values for three foods that you eat regularly. Which of these provides the greatest nutritive value per 100 kcal?
2. *Problem.* Select a series of menus from a popular magazine. Check the menus against the Daily Food Guide for dietary adequacy. Point out examples of good menu planning. What adjustments in these menus would be necessary to reduce fat and sugar levels?
3. *Problem.* Plan a breakfast for a teenager who does not like cereal. Include some food from each of the groups of the Daily Food Guide.
4. Why are each of the following poor examples of menu planning? How could you improve each combination?

   a. Meat loaf, mashed potatoes, mashed winter squash, baked custard
   b. Macaroni and cheese, roast pork, buttered spinach, cheese cake
   c. Broiled flounder, creamed onions, spicy cole slaw, pickles
5. Compare the nutritive values of these snacks: 1 small bag (20 g) potato chips; one apple; 1 ounce salted peanuts; 4 chocolate chip cookies; 10 thin pretzel twists. How would you rate these for snacks for yourself?
6. *Problem.* Calculate the cost of 25 mg ascorbic acid from each of five fresh fruits available in the market.
7. *Problem.* Compare the unit prices for various size packages of the following cereals: puffed wheat; cornflakes; two brands of sugar-coated cereals; two brands of cereals that are fortified with minerals and vitamins. Tabulate the nutritive value for 1 ounce of each of the cereals, according to information on the label. List the cereals in order of best buys, nutritive values being considered.

References

1. Putnam, J. J., and Weimer, J.: "Nutrition Information—Consumer's Views," *Natl. Food Rev.*, 14:18–20, Spring 1981.
2. Welsh, S. O., and Marston, R. M.: "Review of Trends in Food Use in the United States, 1909 to 1980," *J. Am. Diet. Assoc.*, 81:120–25, 1982.
3. *Breakfast Source Book*, Cereal Institute, Chicago.
4. Gallo, A. E.: "Food Spending and Income," *Natl. Food Rev.*, 24:27, 1983.

Publications for the Consumer

PUBLICATIONS BY THE UNITED STATES DEPARTMENT OF AGRICULTURE:

BEEF AND VEAL IN FAMILY MEALS, G 118.
BREADS, CAKES, AND PIES IN FAMILY MEALS, G 186.
CEREALS AND PASTAS IN FAMILY MEALS, G 150.
CHEESE IN FAMILY MEALS, G 112.
EAT A GOOD BREAKFAST, Leaflet 268.
EGGS IN FAMILY MEALS, G 103.
FAMILY FARE: A GUIDE TO GOOD NUTRITION, G 1.
FAMILY FOOD BUDGETING FOR GOOD MEALS AND NUTRITION, HG 94.
FOOD, HG 228.
FOOD GUIDE FOR OLDER FOLKS, G 17.
FOOD FOR FAMILIES WITH SCHOOL CHILDREN, G 13.
FOOD FOR FAMILIES WITH YOUNG CHILDREN, G 5.
FOOD FOR THE YOUNG COUPLE, G 85.
FRUITS IN FAMILY MEALS, G 125.
LAMB IN FAMILY MEALS, G 124.
MILK IN FAMILY MEALS, G 127.
MONEY SAVING MAIN DISHES, G 43.
NUTRITION: FOOD AT WORK FOR YOU, GS-1.
NUTS IN FAMILY MEALS, G 176.
PORK IN FAMILY MEALS, G 160.
POULTRY IN FAMILY MEALS, G 110.
VEGETABLES IN FAMILY MEALS, G 105.
YOUR MONEY'S WORTH IN FOODS, HG 183.

15

Factors Influencing Food Intake and Food Habits

Food has nutritional and nonnutritional values. The intake of food depends on complex interrelated body signals, environmental factors, and behavioral influences. Food habits are derived from the earliest experiences in life and are influenced by sensory, esthetic, economic, geographic, social, and cultural factors. The term "habit" suggests a static condition, but habits can change according to the need to adapt to a new environment, to new attitudes, and to new values. Health professionals need to be aware of the many meanings of food so that they can adjust their counseling to the clients individual values and behavior.

Physiologic Factors That Determine Food Intake

Hunger The word "hunger" carries painful visions of the need for food—for example, the hungry children in a poverty-stricken countryside. HUNGER in a physiologic sense has been defined as "that set of internal signals that stimulate the acquisition and consumption of food."* SATIETY is the reciprocal of hunger. Most of the research on the internal factors involved in hunger and appetite have been conducted on animals. For humans, hunger and appetite are far more complex. (See Figure 15-1.) Within the past two decades studies have shown that circulating nutrients, monoamines, and neurotransmitters are interrelated in producing the hunger or satiety signals.[1,2]

Early in this century two famous physiologists, Walter B. Cannon and Anton Carlson, observed that hunger increases the contractions of the stomach while satiety occurs when the stomach was filled. A link between the stomach and the brain was postulated. Later observations showed that persons who had suffered surgical removal of the stomach continued to express sensations of hunger; therefore the stomach could no longer be considered as having the leading role in initiating the hunger sensation.

Later studies established the important role of the hypothalamus in hunger. The destruction of the ventromedial center of the hypothalamus in experimental animals led to overeating. On the other hand, if the lateral nucleus of the hypothalamus was destroyed, the animals stopped eating and starved to death. Thus, the ventromedial center became known as the satiety center and the lateral nucleus as the feeding center. Together, these centers were referred to as the "appestat" in popular literature.

The hypothalamus is only one of several centers in the brain associated with hunger and satiety. It has been likened to a computer that receives messages from the periphery and integrates them to send out a signal of what to do.[2] Several theories have been proposed concerning the role of nutrients in hunger and satiety.

Glucostatic Theory. Mayer[3] observed in experimental animals that chemoreceptors in the ventromedial center of the hypothalamus have an affinity for glucose and are activated by it. When glucose utilization is high, these receptors act as a brake on the lateral nucleus so that feeding ceases. When glucose utilization is low, there is no stimulation of the receptor in the ventromedial center and the subsequent sensation of hunger causes the animal to eat.

Lipostatic Theory. According to this theory, a metabolite, such as the enzyme *lipoprotein lipase* circulating in the blood, is linked with the hypothalamus to establish a set point that determines caloric intake. This set point can be readjusted from time to time to new levels of adipose tissue.[1]

---

* Castonguay, T.W., et al: "Hunger and Appetite: Old Concepts/New Distinctions," *Nutr. Rev.*, 41:101, 1983.

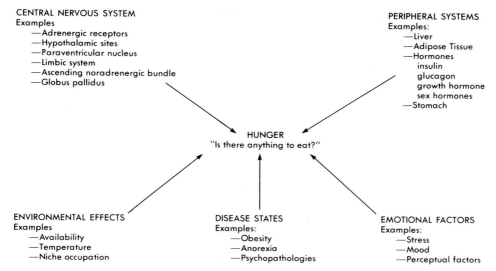

Figure 15-1. A partial listing of the ever-growing number of factors that are known to influence the onset of hunger. (Courtesy, Dr. T. W. Castonguay and *Nutrition Reviews*, **41:**102, 1983.)

Aminostatic Theory. The level of amino acids in the circulation can determine the initiation or cessation of hunger. Animals will eat more of a diet that is low in protein and show a preference for a diet that is balanced in its amino acid composition.[1]

Thermostatic Theory. According to Brobeck,[4] animals that are exposed to cold increase their intake of food, while animals in a warm environment decrease their intake.

In addition to these factors regulating hunger are many monoamines and neurotransmitters. From 20 to 30 gastrointestinal peptides have been found to behave as hormones and neurotransmitters.[2] These internal signals are now known to be bewildering in their complexity and interrelatedness. Only a few examples are listed below. Among the internal signals are the following:

Gastrin increases stomach contractions, while cholecystokinin decreases contractions and reduces food intake.
A low liver glycogen content can lead to hunger sensations.
Insulin lowers blood sugar and increases food intake.
Glucagon raises the peripheral blood sugar and increases food intake.
Dopamine, a monoamine, enhances feeding, while serotonin, another monoamine, inhibits feeding.

Temperature is an environmental factor that influences feeding. With cold temperatures food intake increases, and with hot temperatures the intake decreases. Perhaps this helps explain why patients with a high fever do not feel like eating.

Exercise has a variable influence on food intake. Immediately after acute exercise the food intake is decreased, but moderately active humans engaging in chronic exercise increase their food intake.[1] Thus, laborers who exert much physical activity eat more to satisfy their energy needs than do sedentary workers who are not so stimulated.

Appetite Appetite commonly refers to the pleasurable sensations provided by food and to the choices made for specific food items. The term is also used "to refer to that set of signals that guide selection and consumption of specific foods and nutrients."* It is influenced not only by metabolic factors but also by hedonic factors, environmental and social influences, cultural factors, and learned preferences. Drugs used in various therapies may have an influence on inhibiting or enhancing appetite. (See Figure 15-2.)

Early in this century Osborne and Mendel showed laboratory rats to prefer a diet providing sufficient nutrients to a diet similar in all respects except for a low protein content. Other studies have shown rats to have a specific sensitivity to salt. If deprived of salt rats show a preference to a salt solution over one that contains no salt. Patients with Addison's disease, a condition characterized by adrenal insufficiency, have a hunger for salt. (See page 142.)

* Castonguay, T.W., et al: "Hunger and Appetite: Old Concepts/New Distinctions," *Nutr. Rev.*, **41:**101, 1983.

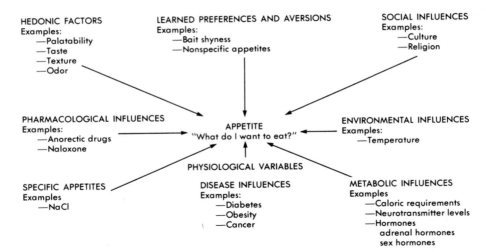

Figure 15-2. Some of the factors that determine appetite. (Courtesy, Dr. T. W. Castonguay and *Nutrition Reviews*, **41**:106, 1983.)

Appetite sometimes refers to the craving for certain foods. For example, some pregnant women say they have a craving for a food such as pickles or ice cream. Such cravings are poorly understood. Also, some pregnant women crave and eat nonfood items such as clay or laundry starch—a condition known as PICA. Some investigators believe that these cravings could indicate a mineral deficiency.

BAIT SHYNESS is an aversion to food that results from some unpleasant circumstance. An animal that is made sick by a nausea-producing drug while sampling a particular food will later refuse to eat that food item. Perhaps some teenager's aversion to certain drinks may be explained by the unpleasant tasting medicine taken with that drink in earlier years.

Hedonic Factors in Food Choice. The palatability of food is a composite of taste, smell, texture, and temperature. It is further conditioned by the surroundings in which food is consumed.

Sweet, sour, salty, and bitter are terms used to describe the sensations that result when foods placed in the mouth produce specific stimuli to the taste buds on the tongue. (See Figure 15-3.) The sense of taste is more highly developed in some individuals than in others; foods may be too salty for one person's taste and just right for another. Some persons can detect slight differences in taste, others cannot. The number of taste buds varies not only from individual to individual, but also from age to age. Preschool children who had low taste sensitivities were found to accept a greater variety of foods than did those with high taste sensitivities.[5] As the taste buds diminish in number

later in life, foods that are more highly flavored tend to be preferred, whereas children voluntarily select bland or sweet foods. Taste sensitivity is decreased in those who smoke.

Figure 15-3. The upper surface of the tongue, showing kind of papillae and areas of taste. (Courtesy, Miller, M.A., and Leavell, L.C.: *Kimber-Gray-Stackpole's Anatomy and Physiology*, 16th ed. Macmillan Publishing Co., Inc. New York, 1972.)

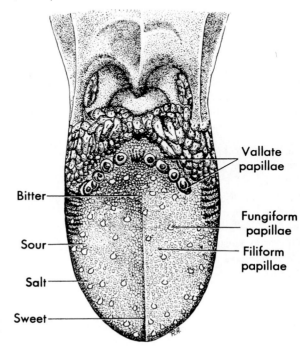

The taste and smell of foods are directly linked. If one were to hold the nose while eating a piece of fruit, much of the enjoyment would be lost. As a matter of fact, smell is the most important component of flavor, and an individual would derive limited pleasure from food if the tongue were the sole source of the sensations. The stimulation of the olfactory organs is brought about by certain volatile oils. Foods may be accepted because of their aromas, or they may be rejected because of their repulsive odors. No doubt, the odors of certain cheeses, for example, are the determinants in their acceptance by some and their rejection by others.

The sense of touch is highly developed in the tongue. Temperature, pain, and variations in texture or "feel" are experienced. Steaming hot foods are necessary to enjoyment by some, but children usually prefer foods that are lukewarm. A choice of ice cream may be influenced as much by its texture—smooth, creamy, and velvety, or crystalline and grainy—as by its other flavor qualities. Children may reject foods that are slippery such as baked custard or a gelatin dessert only later to learn to enjoy this texture sensation. The stringiness of certain vegetables, the stickiness of some mashed potatoes, the greasiness of fried foods may be important factors in rejection.

Environmental and Behavioral Factors Influencing Food Acceptance

Animals stop eating when satiated, but humans often continue to eat because they derive pleasure from food. Social pressures, habits, prejudices, and the communications media are among the many factors that can obscure the internal signals of hunger and satiety. But in unpleasant situations humans may cease eating even though they are not satiated.

Role of Culture Humans do not chose by instinct that which is best for them. In different environments humans eat what is available and sometimes learn by experience that some foods are better for them than others. The circumstances under which one eats are largely determined by one's culture. Used in this sense, CULTURE is "the sum total of ways of living built up by a group of human beings and transmitted from one generation to another."*

The food culture or foodways may have existed among a given ethnic group for centuries, and such a heritage accounts for great conservatism in accepting

* *Random House Dictionary.*

change. These patterns reflect the social organization of the people, including their economy, religion, beliefs about the health properties of food, and attitudes toward the various members of the family. The emotional reactions to the consumption of certain foods may be so deeply rooted that effecting acceptance of them is almost impossible.

Food Taboos and Folklore. In every group of people customs have arisen concerning foods that should and should not be eaten. Although there is little or no scientific basis for these taboos, they are rigidly held so that change is likely to be resisted. Among people in the developing nations these taboos often accentuate malnutrition. For example, in one ethnic group in Nigeria children are rarely given meat or eggs. These are expensive foods, and it is thought that giving them to children will encourage them to steal. Coconut milk is taboo for children since it is believed to make them unintelligent. Similar taboos prevail for the pregnant woman. She should not eat snails so that her baby will not salivate too much. She should not eat pounded yams because the pounding is likely to have an effect on the child's brain. On the other hand, the pregnant woman is encouraged to eat food left by rats, since this will help ensure an easy delivery such as rats are supposed to have.[6]

An example of folklore is the belief system held by many Chinese, especially those who are older.[7] These beliefs have their origin in Eastern philosophy, which holds that the universe is regulated by two opposing components, *yin* and *yang.* To maintain health these forces must be in balance. When illness is caused by an excess of yang, "cold" or yin foods should be used, and vice versa. Among the yin or "cold" foods are winter melon, white turnips, and bean sprouts; yang or "hot" foods include scrambled eggs and ginger root.

The Family. The mother has often been referred to as the "gatekeeper" or the one who controls the food that reaches the table. In many families this role is diminishing. Food selection and meal preparation are often shared by parents and older children, and each of these influence the food that is presented to the family. Also, many meals, especially noon meals, are eaten away from home.

Within the home the food choices may reflect the environment in which the parents grew up, including the geographic region from which they came, their level of education, income, and beliefs about food. An atmosphere of security and contentment reinforces the positive values of food. On the other hand, in an environment of hostility, anger, and tension unpleasant images are created for food, often leading to their rejection. In this atmosphere, also, there may be excessive concern about "pure" foods, "pure" morals, and so on.[8]

Meal Patterns. Nutritional planning is usually based on a three-meal pattern. Although many people in the United States eat three meals a day, others eat only two, and still others four or five. The coffee break is prevalent in business and industry, and is, for many, a replacement of breakfast. Midafternoon and evening snacks are commonplace.

Breakfasts tend to be light and informal. Family members often eat this meal at different times depending upon the time they must leave for work or school. Such a casual arrangement does not always provide the share of essential nutrients, nor is there the enjoyment that should be experienced at mealtime. In rural areas breakfast is still a substantial meal. Elderly people often enjoy breakfast more than other meals.

A good deal of ritual is part of the mealtime in some homes. Bread becomes the "staff of life" to some people; rice is the basic food for others, and corn to still others. The meal would not be complete if these foods were not included. The art of food preparation is exercised, and food is highly valued for its many properties. Meals are to be enjoyed and relaxation is encouraged. A siesta following meals is customary in some countries. In other homes, mealtime is hurried. It may become the time when members of the family air their problems and when tensions are created.

Communications. The influence of the mass media on food habits can scarcely be overestimated. Those who enjoy an abundant variety of food can no longer be ignorant of the malnutrition and hunger that exist even in the United States as well as in the underdeveloped nations of the world. By these media the poor are also exposed to food products which they are unable to purchase. The affluent and the poor alike know that the distribution of food is decidedly uneven and that the capability exists to feed all people better.

Manufacturers usually create desires for their products by appealing to the emotions. Foods are pictured in forms highly appealing to the eye and in situations that suggest fun, social status, and group acceptance. Foods will consequently be purchased to fulfill these emotional needs rather than for their nutritional content.

Political Significance. Many food programs exist in the United States and throughout the world to help the poor meet their nutritional needs. Such programs are important in determining agricultural policies and food prices, on the one hand, and impose regulations for participation by the poor, on the other hand.

During a war food supplies may be rationed and people are forced to substitute one food for another. The scarcity of a given food sometimes creates a tremendous pressure to possess that food. The collapse of a government may indeed be brought about by its failure to provide food for its people.

Throughout history people have gone on "hunger strikes" to achieve some political goal. Gandhi, the great Indian leader, comes to mind for his many fasts. Not many years ago, some people who protested the involvement of the United States in the Vietnam war fasted for brief or long periods of time.

Food Movements. Millions of Americans today have adopted eating patterns that differ widely from those of their childhood and that are at variance with so-called typical American diets. Among these groups are (1) those who are vegetarians for ecologic, philosophic, or religious reasons (see also pages 230–33); (2) those who oppose the use of any additives in foods or the use of chemical fertilizers, and who consume only "natural" or "organic" foods (see also page 239); and (3) those who subscribe to the healthful properties of some foods and who proscribe other foods. It is not always possible or even necessary to change these beliefs, but the counselor for nutrition should recognize what is good in the individual's diet and should attempt to improve the diet within the framework of the beliefs.

Economic Influences on Food Intake A major change in the United States in recent years has been the increasing number of women in the labor force. About 60 percent of all women who are heads of families are working. A significant number of these women have children under school age as well as those who are attending school. Generally, the income of these women is about half of that for family units that include a father. These women are restricted not only in the amount of money that they can spend for food, but also in the amount of time they have to shop and prepare food.

Income influences the variety of foods from which people can choose, and also the amount of food that may be purchased from each of the food groups. Generally, people with limited incomes depend on lower cost foods from the bread-cereal group to supply much of the caloric and nutrient needs. They use smaller amounts of the meat and milk groups. Also, the selection from the meat group is restricted to less expensive cuts. From the fruit–vegetable group the selection must be made from a more limited variety of lower cost items.

The meat group, to many people, is essential to meal satisfaction, and the ability to buy it also has a connotation of status. Thus, when the income of poor people improves, the amount of meat purchased is usually increased. Not infrequently, a disproportionate part of the food dollar is spent for meat, leaving too little money for milk and vegetables and fruits.

When the income is liberal, people have the freedom to choose from an almost unlimited variety of foods—in or out of season, locally produced or from some distant state or country, fresh or processed. The cost of food is often equated with status. Lobster, prime ribs of beef, fresh asparagus, and champagne are examples of items that one might choose in an expensive restaurant. But beef stew instead of steak, cabbage instead of asparagus, and applesauce instead of fresh strawberries might be more typical choices by people with limited income. Thus, in the hierarchy of food status, these choices may be considered less desirable even though nutritive values might be equal.

People eat more frequently in restaurants. Those who are affluent choose expensive restaurants for the creative menus that sometimes emphasize ethnic gourmet foods, for the excellence of food preparation, for the ambience of the dining room and even for the association with other persons of affluence. By contrast, persons with low income can afford to eat in restaurants only infrequently or not at all. For them the fast-food restaurant is often the only affordable choice. (See page 239.)

Social Values of Food "To break bread" together has been from time immemorial an act of friendship. One provides food for friends during a visit in the home; one likewise extends friendship to the stranger by inviting him to share food. The food served to guests is the best that one can afford and the table appointments are as beautiful as one can make them. Important family events are joyously celebrated with meals: the wedding breakfast or reception; birthday parties; Christmas dinner; a Fourth of July picnic. To eat together, whatever the occasion, is to provide friendly relaxation and conversation. The loneliness of eating by oneself, day after day, is not appreciated by those who have never tried it.

Eating together also has connotations of status. Throughout history one's place at the table has been governed by his or her social standing. To be placed "above the salt" at a medieval banquet, to sit at the "head" table at a banquet today, and to be invited to eat at the captain's table while on board ship are marks of social distinction. In some societies women are considered to be inferior to men and must wait to eat until the men and boys have finished the meal. In other authoritarian situations, children may not be permitted to eat until the father has had his meal; in such a society, the father is always served the choicest foods. Many bonds of business or of politics are cemented at businessmen's luncheons or political dinners.

Children too are highly influenced by the foods that are popular with their peer groups. Sometimes they come to scorn certain foods that they have liked because they are different from the prevailing pattern of other children. On the other hand, they are also susceptible to the suggestions of their teachers and classmates and learn to like foods with which they have not been familiar in their homes.

Some people delight in being epicures or gourmets. They derive a certain satisfaction from adventurous eating of food which is unusual to most people—rattlesnake meat, for example. Or they serve food that is difficult to obtain, distinctive in flavor, or exacting and time consuming in preparation.

Religious and Moral Values Attributed to Foods Almost all religions place some regulations on the use of foods. The association of a food with religion gives some clue to its importance in daily living. In the Middle East, bread becomes a symbol in the religious ceremonies of the people; to the Indians of Mexico, corn, the staple food, is invested with religious significance. Christians use bread and wine as symbols of Christ's body and blood in the Eucharist (Lord's Supper or Holy Communion). Religious significance is attached to a number of foods by the Jewish people. (See page 233.)

Certain foods are forbidden by religious regulation. Pork is forbidden to the Orthodox Jews and to the Muslims. Strict Hindus and Buddhists are vegetarians; they will eat no flesh of any animal, and many of them also abstain from eggs, and milk. Seventh Day Adventists are lactovegetarians; that is, they will eat milk, cheese, eggs, nuts, and legumes but they eat no flesh foods. (See also Chapter 16.)

Fasting is common to most, if not all, religions. On fast days one food may be substituted for another or foods may be abstained from altogether. A substitute food, such as fish for meat, is likely to be associated with denying oneself, and so when one wishes enjoyment, one doesn't choose to eat fish!

Moral attributes—"good" and "bad"—are often ascribed to foods. A child may be told to eat liver even if she does not like it because it is "good" for her; she may also be told not to eat candy, which she does like, because it is "bad" for her. Or she might be told that she may have candy if she eats some liver!

Food is often used as a reward, punishment, or means of bribery. Thus, a child who has behaved well is rewarded with a prized food—candy, ice cream, cake; but one who has behaved badly may be punished by being deprived of a food such as dessert. Adults, too, may reward themselves after a strenuous day or a trying experience by eating a special food or an expensive meal, saying as they do so, "I certainly earned this today!" The family may feel a sense of reward, as well as the expression of a mother's love, when they sit down to a meal of their favorite foods; they may feel punished and unloved when the meal includes foods they dislike.

Age and Sex Influence Food Choices Some foods are categorized as being suitable for a given age group, or as more suitable for one sex than the other. Peanut butter, jelly, and milk are looked upon as foods for children, but olives and coffee are appropriate for adults! Teenagers adopt current fashions in foods— hot dogs, hamburger, pizza, ice cream with many sauces and toppings. Women are said to prefer light foods such as soufflés, salads, fruits, and vegetables, whereas filling meals such as meat, potatoes, and pie represent the more usual choice of men.

Emotional Outlets Provided by Food Eating provides gratification for life stresses—the difficult examination in school; the homely adolescent who has no date to take her to the movies; the quarrel with a friend; the frustration and loneliness of having no friends; the profound grief at the death of a dear one; and countless others.

Food is a symbol of security to many. Milk, the first food of the infant, is associated with the security of the infant held lovingly in his mother's arms. A person away from home, or ill, looks upon milk as expressing the comfort and security of the home; or, milk might be refused because the individual drinking it experiences a feeling of dependence which he does not want to admit, and so he says he does not "want to be treated like a baby."

Food may be used as a weapon. An insecure child refuses to eat food so that his mother will be concerned about him. The ill and the lonely impose dietary demands upon those caring for them in an effort to gain as much attention as possible.

Illness Modifies Food Acceptance Disease processes and drug therapy often modify the appetite. The anxiety of illness, the loneliness experienced if one eats from a tray alone, the lack of activity, and perhaps a modified diet are likely to interfere with food intake. (See also Chapter 26.)

Problems and Review

1. *Key terms*: appetite; food culture; food folklore; food taboos; food habits; glucostatic theory; hot-cold theory; hunger; satiety; thermostatic control.
2. How do you feel about food? List insofar as you are able the meanings you clearly associate with foods. List the foods you especially like; those you especially dislike. Can you give any specific reason for placing the food in one category or another?
3. Note for one day the comments made by people around you about food. Do any of these fall within the physiologic or psychologic categories discussed in this chapter?
4. Suppose you were trying to introduce nonfat dry milk to a group of people who were entirely unfamiliar with it. How would you go about gaining their acceptance?
5. Describe the physical factors in food acceptance.

References

1. Castonguay, T. W., et al.: "Hunger and Appetite: Old Concepts/New Distinctions," *Nutr. Rev.*, 41:101–110, 1983.
2. Levine, A. S., and Morley, J. E.: "The Shortening Pathways to Appetite Control," *Nutr. Today*, 18:6–14, January 1983.
3. Mayer, J.: "Why People Get Hungry," *Nutr. Today*, 1:2–8, June 1966.
4. Brobeck, J. R.: "Food Intake as a Mechanism of Temperature Regulation," *Yale J. Biol. Med.*, 20:545–52, 1948.
5. Korslund, M., and Eppright, E. S.: "Taste Sensitivity and Eating Behavior of Preschool Children," *J. Home Econ.*, 59:168–70, 1967.
6. Ogbeide, O.: "Nutritional Hazards of Food Taboos and Preferences in Mid-west Nigeria," *Am. J. Clin. Nutr.*, 27:213–16, 1974.
7. Chang, B.: "Some Dietary Beliefs in Chinese Folk Culture," *J. Am. Diet. Assoc.*, 65: 436–38, 1974.
8. Bruch, H.: "The Allure of Food Cults and Nutritional Quackery," *J. Am. Diet. Assoc.*, 57:316–20, 1970.

16

Cultural Food Patterns in the United States

The food patterns for a given group of people have their origin in the variety and availability of foods in the country in which they live. With individual mobility, rapid communication with all parts of the world, extensive advertising of food through the national media, changes in agricultural and food technology, advances in education, and adoption of new life-styles, it is not surprising that food habits also change.

Dietary counselors need to recognize that even within a cultural group the individual food habits often vary considerably from group patterns. Moreover, counselors must avoid being judgmental of patterns that differ widely from their own. They must understand the many concerns that people have about diets and nutritive values and be able to give reliable answers to questions that are asked.

Regional Food Patterns in the United States

There is no typical American diet. Perhaps nowhere in the world can one find so great a variety of foods and methods of preparation as in the United States. The dietary patterns are an amalgamation of the foods native to the region and of the habits and customs handed down generation by generation. With each influx of people from other parts of the world new dishes are introduced. The foods vary from the wheat of the North Central plains to the rice of Louisiana, the potatoes of Maine and Idaho to the citrus fruits of Florida, the dairy products of Minnesota and Wisconsin to the beef of the western ranges, the fish of the seacoast to the fruits of the Far West. One might associate baked beans with New England, chile con carne with the Southwest, and fried chicken with the South, but today these dishes are served everywhere in the United States.

New England. In addition to the baked beans and brown bread on a Saturday night, in New England one is likely to encounter such favorite dishes as codfish cakes, lobster, clam chowder, and other seafood specialties. Pumpkin pie, squash, Indian pudding, and turkey originated with the Pilgrim fathers, who made adaptations of foods used by the American Indian.

Pennsylvania Dutch. The Pennsylvania Dutch are known for many rich foods including potato pancakes, many kinds of sausage, Philadelphia scrapple, sticky cinnamon buns, pickles and relishes ("seven sweets and seven sours"), and shoofly pie.

The South. Fried chicken, country ham, and hot biscuits are specialties of the South. Green vegetables such as turnip tops, collards, kale, and mustard greens are well liked; they are likely to be cooked for a relatively long time with fat pork as a flavoring agent. Sweet potatoes are preferred to white potatoes, and corn is the cereal of choice, although rice and wheat are also widely used. Corn appears in such forms as corn pone, corn bread, hominy grits, spoon bread and hush puppies—especially in South Atlantic states and Florida.

New Orleans is noted for its fine restaurants, which show the influence of French and Creole cookery. Soups and fish dishes are often highly seasoned, and sauces are used for many meats and vegetables.

Middle West. Dairy products, meat, and eggs abound in the Middle West. Here one finds dietary patterns similar to those of Scandinavia, Germany, Poland, England, and other northern European countries.

South West. The Mexican and Spanish influences are felt in the Southwest where pinto beans, tortillas

229

made from flour or lime-treated corn, and chili, a hot pepper, are important constituents of the diet. Usually these staple food items are served with highly seasoned sauces.

Far West.   The abundance of luscious fruits and vegetables in the Far West leads to a much greater consumption of salads as main dishes as well as accompaniments of the meal. The Oriental influence is especially noted in the delicious vegetables of Japanese and Chinese cookery. Seafoods abound in great variety on the West Coast, as in the East, but the salmon of the Pacific Northwest is especially prized.

Vegetarian Diets

What Is Vegetarianism?   A vegetarian is a person who uses a diet that includes plant foods but eliminates one or more of these groups of foods: meat; poultry; fish; milk; eggs.

Lactovegetarians include plant foods and milk and other dairy products in their diet. They do not use meat, poultry, fish or eggs.

Lacto-ovo-vegetarians include plant foods, milk, and eggs, but do not use meat, fish, or poultry.

Pure vegetarians (vegans) include only plant foods in their diets. Some use all plant foods, whereas others avoid one or more food groups such as processed foods, cooked foods, legumes, cereals, grains, or fruits. Fruitarians limit their food intake to raw and dried fruits, nuts, honey, and oil.

Reasons for Vegetarianism   Probably fewer than 1 percent of Americans adhere to a vegetarian diet of one kind or another.[1] Vegetarians, like omnivores, have widely varying beliefs and educational, economic, and cultural backgrounds. Their reasons for adopting a vegetarian diet include health, religious beliefs, land and water resources, humanitarian concerns, and economics. Many vegetarians give more than one reason for adherence to vegetarian diets.

The Seventh Day Adventists and the Trappist monks are lacto-ovo-vegetarians. They also abstain from alcohol, tobacco, and caffeine-containing beverages. Their diet is one of self-discipline but also one that improves health. Studies on males who are Seventh Day Adventists have shown that serum cholesterol levels were lower and that the first heart attack occurred at least a decade later than average. The incidence of heart disease was 60 percent as high as that of a control group in California. The difference was attributed to the low intake of cholesterol and satu-

rated fat and the higher intake of fiber.[2] Abstinence from tobacco and alcohol might also have contributed to this difference.

People of all ages adopt vegetarian diets, but they are more widely used by young people. They are often well educated and self-reliant. They often say that they feel better and are "less groggy" when they abstain from animal foods. Those who cite health as a reason for vegetarianism avoid foods that contain additives or hormones or that have been grown on chemically fertilized soils. They also are concerned that animal foods contain toxins, too much uric acid, or are infected with *Salmonella*.[3]

Ecologic reasons are cited by some. In a world where population threatens to exceed the ability to provide food, the rationale is that consuming foods directly is a more efficient use of land resources than feeding plant foods to animals that are subsequently consumed by humans.

Economic reasons are given by some, since vegetarian diets can be less expensive than permitting animal foods. Still others object to the large agri-business in the United States and choose not to buy their foods from markets that are controlled by giant corporations.

Nutritional Characteristics   Nutritional adequacy is not a problem for lacto- and lacto-ovo-vegetarians. Because meat, poultry, and fish are not used, the diet includes greater amounts of legumes, nuts, seeds, grains, meat analogs, and milk, or milk and eggs. (See Table 16-1.)

Pure vegetarian diets can also be made adequate by using a wide variety of foods from each plant food group and by adding appropriate mineral and vitamin supplements. Risk of nutritional inadequacy is greatly increased when the individual imposes limitations on the kinds of plant foods that he will accept.

Vegetarian diets are more bulky than those that contain animal foods. They are relatively high in carbohydrate and dietary fiber. The bulkiness of the diet helps prevent overeating and obesity as well as constipation. Most of the fat is contributed by vegetable oils and margarines which are higher than animal fats in polyunsaturated fatty acids. Milk and cheese, if they are used, are the only sources of cholesterol. These changes in the types and amounts of fat are considered by many to aid in reducing the risks of cardiovascular diseases and cancer.

Energy.   The caloric requirement must be met in order to ensure efficient use of protein. Only minimal amounts of fats and sweets can be consumed if all nu-

Table 16-1. Nutritive Values for a Lacto-ovo-vegetarian Diet for the Adult

Food	Measure	Weight (g)	Energy (kcal)	Protein (g)	Fat Total (g)	Fat Saturated (g)	Fat Linoleic (g)	Carbohydrate (g)	Minerals Ca (mg)	Minerals P (mg)	Minerals Fe (mg)	Vitamins A IU	Vitamins Thiamin (mg)	Vitamins Riboflavin (mg)	Vitamins Niacin (mg)	Vitamins Ascorbic Acid (mg)
Vegetables																
Dark leafy green or deep yellow*	½–⅔ cup	100	30	2	trace			6	28	32	0.8	7,620	0.06	0.08	0.6	30
Potato	1 medium	135	90	3	trace			20	8	57	0.7	trace	0.12	0.05	1.6	22
Other vegetable†	½–⅔ cup	100	40	4	trace			8	22	36	0.8	540	0.06	0.06	0.8	14
Fruits																
Vitamin-C-rich	1 cup	250	110	1	trace			28	44	44	0.8	532	0.22	0.06	0.8	104
Other‡	1 serving	100	60	trace	trace			15	8	15	0.4	340	0.03	0.03	0.4	5
Bread–cereal group																
Cereal grains§	2 servings	210 (cooked)	182	5	1	0.1	0.2	37	18	124	1.5	trace	0.17	0.07	1.9	0
Bread, whole-wheat	4 slices	112	260	12	4	0.4	0.8	56	96	284	3.2	trace	0.36	0.12	3.2	0
Milk Group																
Milk (2 percent fat)	2 cups	488	240	16	10	5.8	0.2	24	594	464	0.2	1,000	0.20	0.80	0.4	4
Protein group																
Legumes#	¼ cup dry	50	180	13	3			29	62	198	3.6	trace	0.34	0.12	1.0	0
Nuts, seeds‖	1 ounce	30	207	7	16	2.4	6.5	5	32	195	1.7	trace	0.19	0.08	2.0	0
Egg	4 per week	30	46	3	3	1.0	0.2	1	16	52	0.6	149	0.02	0.09	trace	0
Fats																
Margarine	1 tablespoon	14	100	trace	12	2.0	4.1	0	3	3		470	0	0	0	0
Oil (corn)	1 tablespoon	14	120	0	14	1.7	7.8	0	0	0		0	0	0	0	0
Totals			1,665	66	63	13.4	19.8	229	931	1,504	14.3	10,651	1.77	1.56	12.7	179
Recommended Daily Allowances																
Women (25–50 years)			2,200	50					800	800	15.0	4,000	1.1	1.3	15	60
Men (25–50)			2,900	63					800	800	10.0	5,000	1.5	1.7	19	60

* Includes broccoli, carrots, escarole, kale, green peppers, pumpkin, spinach.
† Includes snap beans, lima beans, cabbage, cauliflower, celery, corn, cucumbers, lettuce, onions, peas, tomatoes.
‡ Includes fresh, canned, and frozen fruits: apples, apricots, bananas, cherries, grapes, peaches, pears, pineapple, plums.
§ Includes oatmeal, grits, rolled wheat, pastas, rice, bulgur.
" Includes chick peas, navy beans, lentils, soybeans, split peas.
‖ Includes almonds, peanuts, English walnuts, pumpkin seeds, sunflower seeds.

trient requirements are to be met. Children are sometimes unable to consume sufficient amounts of bulky foods to meet their energy needs.

Protein. All plant foods lack sufficient amounts of one or more essential amino acids. But if a food low in a given amino acid is combined with another food that is a good source of that amino acid, the combination is satisfactory. (See Figure 16-1.) Such foods are complementary only if both of them are eaten in the same meal. To illustrate:

	Low in	High in
Grains	Lysine	Methionine
+		
Legumes	Methionine	Lysine

Other good plant food combinations are the following:

Grains + milk, cheese
Seeds + legumes

Each group provides many choices:

Legumes—dry beans: black, broad, kidney, lima, navy, pea, soy; dry peas: blackeye, chick, split

Lentils
Grains—barley, corn, oat, millet, rye, wheat—whole grains better than refined
Seeds—sesame, sunflower, squash, pumpkin
Nuts—black walnut, Brazil, cashew, peanut, peanut butter, pistachio; pecans, English walnuts, and coconut lower in protein content

Fortified soy milk should be used for infants and children who are fed a pure vegetarian diet. The fortification should include calcium, riboflavin, thiamin, vitamin B-12, and vitamin D.

Minerals. Calcium is furnished by liberal intakes of dark green leafy vegetables that do not contain oxalate (see page 114), broccoli, okra, rutabaga, peanuts, almonds, sesame seeds, and fortified soy milk.

Although the amount of iron ingested from a varied vegetarian diet may be equal to that consumed by people who eat meat, the availability of that iron is lower. The availability is improved with the simultaneous ingestion of ascorbic acid-rich foods.

The bioavailability of zinc from plant foods is also low. Whole grains, legumes, peanuts, and peanut butter are good sources of zinc but fruits and vegetables are poor sources.

The high phytate content of whole grains also inter-

Figure 16-1. High school students study the food combinations that will provide the essential amino acids in a lactovegetarian diet. (Courtesy, Harry Broder and Marple Newtown School District, Newtown Square, Pennsylvania.)

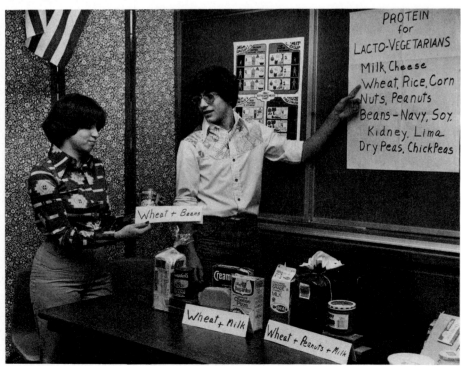

feres with the absorption of iron and zinc, but this effect is greatly reduced in yeast-leavened breads. Iodized salt should be used in food preparation.

Vitamins. Vitamin B-12 deficiency is characteristic of all pure vegetarian diets since vitamin B-12 is found only in animal foods. The signs of deficiency are not likely to show up until after several years use of the diet and then correction may be too late. In infants and young children the lack of vitamin B-12 may lead to growth failure. A vitamin B-12 supplement or fortified cereal or soy milk is indicated for pure vegetarian diets.

Except for vitamin B-12 the requirements for B-complex vitamins are met by a diversified selection of whole grains, legumes, nuts, seeds, and vegetables and fruits. Deep yellow and dark green vegetables ensure an ample supply of carotene. Vitamin D should be furnished as a supplement unless there is ample exposure to sunshine.

Orthodox Jewish Food Patterns

Outstanding Characteristics Orthodox Jews observe dietary laws based on biblical and rabbinical regulations (the rules of Kashruth). These laws pertain to the selection, preparation, and service of food. Many Conservative Jews are as observant of dietary laws as are Orthodox Jews. But some conservative Jews nominally observe the laws but make distinctions within and without the home, while Reform Jews minimize the significance of dietary laws. Food habits of the Jewish people are also influenced by the country of origin—for example, Russia, Poland, or Germany.

Religious festivals include certain food restrictions. No food is cooked or heated on the Sabbath. Yom Kippur (Day of Atonement) is a 24-hour period of fasting from food and drink. The Passover, sometimes also referred to as "The Feast of Unleavened Bread," lasts for eight days and commemorates the release of the Israelites from the slavery of Egypt. Only utensils and dishes that have made no contact with leavened foods are used during this time. Thus, the Orthodox Jewish home would have four sets of dishes: one for meat and one for dairy meals during the Passover, and one for meat and one for dairy meals during the rest of the year when leavened breads and cakes may be used.

TYPICAL FOODS AND THEIR USES

Milk Group Milk, cottage and cream cheese, sour cream used abundantly. Milk and its products may not be used at same meal as meat (Exod. 23:19; 34:26; Deut. 14:21). Milk may not be taken until 6 hours after eating meat. Separate dishes and utensils must be used for milk and meat dishes.

Meat Group *(Allowed Foods).* All quadruped animals that chew the cud and divide the hoof (Lev. 11:1-3; Deut. 14:3-8); cattle, deer, goats, sheep. Organs of these animals may be used.

Animals must be killed in prescribed manner for minimum pain to animal and for maximum blood drainage. Blood is associated with life and may not be eaten (Gen. 9:4; Lev. 3:17; 17:10-14; Deut. 12:23-27). Meat is made *kosher* (clean) by soaking it in cold water, thoroughly salting it, allowing it to drain for an hour, and then washing it in three waters.

Hindquarters of meat may be used only if the part of the thigh with the sinew of Jacob is removed (Gen. 32:33).

Poultry: chicken, duck, goose, pheasant, turkey. Chicken is common for Sabbath eve meal.

Fish with fins and scales (Lev. 11-9; Deut. 14:9-10): Cod, haddock, halibut, salmon, trout, tuna, whitefish, and so on.

Eggs: Fish and eggs may be eaten at both meat and milk meals.

Dried beans, peas, lentils, in many soups.

Corned beef, smoked meats, herring, lox (smoked, salted salmon) are well liked.

Cholent: casserole of beef, potatoes, and dried beans. Served on the Sabbath.

Gefilte fish: chopped, highly seasoned fish; a first course for the Sabbath meal.

Kishke: beef casings stuffed with rich filling and roasted.

Knishes: pastry filled with ground meat or potatoes.

Kreplach: noodle dough filled with ground meat or cheese filling.

(Prohibited Foods): Animals that do not chew the cud or divide the hoof (Lev. 11:4-8): pork.

Diseased animals or animals dying a natural death (Deut. 14:21).

Birds of prey (Lev. 11:13-19; Deut. 14:11-18).

Fish without fins or scales (Lev. 11:10-12): eels, shellfish such as oysters, crab, lobster.

Egg with blood spot.

Vegetable-Fruit Group All kinds used without restriction.

Cucumber, lettuce, tomato very frequently used.

Cabbage, potatoes, and root vegetables are often cooked with the meat.

Borscht: soup with meat stock and egg, or without meat stock and with sour cream; includes beets, spinach, cabbage.

Dried fruits are used in many pastries.

Bread-Cereals Group All kinds used without restriction.

Rye bread (pumpernickel), white seed rolls; noodles and other egg and flour mixtures.

Bagel: doughnut-shaped hard yeast roll.

Blintzes: thin rolled pancakes filled with cottage cheese, ground beef, or fruit mixture; served with sour cream.

Bulke: light yeast roll.

Challah: braided loaf or light white bread.

Farfel: noodle dough grated for soup.

Kasha: buckwheat groats served as cooked cereal or as potato substitute.

Kloese: dumplings, usually in chicken soup.

Latkes: pancakes.

Matzoh: flat, unleavened bread.

Other Foods

Unsalted butter preferred.

Chicken fat or vegetable oils for cooking.

Rich pastries are common.

Cheese cake.

Kuchen: coffee cake of many varieties.

Leckach: honey cake for Rosh Hashana (New Year).

Strudel: thin pastry with fruit, nut filling.

Teiglach: small pieces of dough cooked in honey, with nuts.

Sponge cake and macaroons at Passover.

Many preserves, pickled cucumber, pickled green tomatoes, relishes.

Many foods are highly salted.

Food Patterns of Native Americans

Native Americans include diverse ethnic groups such as American Indians who are integrated into the general population, Indians who are relatively isolated on vast reservations, and Eskimos in Alaska. The American Indians live in areas that are vastly different from one another—from Maine to Florida, from Wisconsin to Washington and Oregon and to Arizona, New Mexico, and other states. The Eskimos live on islands, in coastal villages, in mountainous areas, and the Arctic tundra of Alaska and Canada.

American Indians Many foods used throughout the world were probably first used by the Indians of North, Central, and South America. These foods include beans, corn, cranberries, peanuts, peppers, potatoes, pumpkin, wild rice, squash, and tomatoes. Because of the diversity of regions in which Indians live there is no single typical diet.

Today traditional dishes are prepared infrequently except for ceremonial occasions. Among such dishes still used are *wasna* (a combination of dried berries, powdered dried meat, fat, and sugar), *wojapi* (a fruit pudding), and *fry bread* (biscuit dough fried in deep fat). Even the Arizona Hopi who still live in old villages that their ancestors inhabited use their native dishes infrequently.[4]

Dietary changes have occurred partly because of the relocation of the tribes on reservations where the food resources are different. Unemployment and poverty have contributed to a decline in the quality of the diet. Knowledge is often lacking of the foods that will meet nutritional needs at low cost. Excessive use of soft drinks, sweets, potato chips, and other snack foods contribute to the low nutrient density of the diet. Folklore pertaining to the use of foods for health still abounds. The nutrients most likely to be deficient in the American Indian diet are calcium, iron, ascorbic acid, and vitamin A.

In many Indian diets corn is the staple food. It is eaten fresh roasted or broiled, as hominy, or as cornmeal in a variety of dishes. Meat is eaten when it can be obtained by hunting or fishing, but because of its cost it is used sparingly if it must be purchased in the market. Milk is little used. Lactose intolerance occurs commonly among adult Indians, but children can usually consume enough milk to meet their needs. Berries, wild plants, and roots are used when available, but the intake of fruits and vegetables requires more emphasis. White flour is gradually replacing cornmeal. When corn is soaked in lime and ground it is a good source of calcium. However, the lime treatment is less frequently used, thus bringing about another decline in diet quality.

Eskimos The traditional diet of nomadic Eskimos consisted almost entirely of frozen, dried, or fresh game and fish.[5] Inland Eskimos hunted for caribou while coastal Eskimos caught sea mammals and fish. Fowl, polar bear, musk ox, rabbits, and foxes were eaten depending on local supply. Berries, leafy greens, roots, and seaweed were seasonally available.

For one meal a day meat might be cooked as soup over a seal-oil lamp, using seawater and seaweed for seasoning. During the remainder of the day the family would nibble on raw *muktuk* (whale skin), caribou, or char (fish). The protein intake was extremely high (average over 300 g daily) and the carbohydrate intake was insignificant. The meat and fish supplied the minerals and vitamins, including vitamin C from raw liver.

With the transition from a nomadic life to the recent settlements of the white man, the Eskimos were suddenly thrown into a new civilization for which they had no preparation. In the villages the Eskimos still hunt some game and fish. Most of them are unemployed or employed only part time. Profound changes in the composition of the diet have occurred. Store-bought foods were found to be appealing to the taste and also conveyed status.

Sugar, candy, soft drinks, and processed foods are consumed throughout the day and thus contribute to a high intake of simple, rapidly absorbed carbohydrate. The protein intake remains liberal (about 100 g daily). The adoption of the least desirable aspects of the white culture's diet has led to health problems that did not exist in earlier times. Eskimos had perfect teeth, but dental decay is now rampant. Obesity, gallbladder disease, and acne—hitherto unknown—are now prevalent. Diabetes mellitus occurs more often and there is a diabetic-type response to the glucose tolerance test. Blood lipid and cholesterol levels are elevated, which suggests that change in physical activity rather than diet may be responsible. Infections and allergic reactions are seen in infants who are bottle fed.[5]

Black American Food Patterns

Outstanding Characteristics   There is no typical food pattern for all black Americans. The foods eaten by black and white people of a given geographic area tend to be similar. As black Americans have migrated from the South to northern cities they have gradually adopted the foods typical of the areas in which they live. Some favorite dishes, often termed "soul foods," are retained; these foods signfiy well-being and the caring of the provider. Many of them originated in pre-Civil War days.

When income permits, black Americans spend increasing amounts of money for meat. Too little money is spent for vegetables, fruits, and milk. Although lactose tolerance is poor in many adults, most children can drink sufficient milk to meet their calcium needs without untoward symptoms. Meat, poultry, fish, and sweet potatoes are often fried. Greens are usually cooked for a long time and seasoned with salt pork, bacon, or bits of meat. Generally the diet is high in fat and in sweets.

Obesity, hypertension, and anemia are frequent nutritional problems seen in black Americans. Dietary counseling should include emphasis on ways to increase the iron content of the diet and to reduce the salt intake.

TYPICAL FOODS AND THEIR USES

Milk Group   Little milk is consumed. Most children can tolerate milk well and should be given moderate amounts spaced throughout the meals for the day.

Meat Group
Fried chicken and fish are well liked; also catfish stew.
Meat from every part of the pig: bacon, ham hocks, pork chops, salt pork, spareribs (often barbecued); chitterlings (lining of pig stomach boiled and then fried); and pig's feet, tail, and ears.
Wild game when available: beaver, coon, possum, rabbit, squirrel.
Blackeyed peas with molasses and bacon or salt pork: kidney beans; marrow fat beans.

Vegetable-Fruit Group
Greens: collards, dandelion, kale, mustard, turnip—boiled in salt water with bacon or ham hocks or bits of salt pork; "pot likker" is consumed as well as the greens.
Stewed corn, okra, tomatoes, sweet potatoes.
Fruit sometimes used as snack; needs more emphasis.

Bread-Cereals Group
Baking powder biscuits, served hot.
Corn bread in many ways: crackling bread, hoecakes, hush puppies, spoon bread.
Hominy grits, rice.

Puerto Rican Food Patterns

Outstanding Characteristics   Rice, legumes, and viandas (starchy vegetables) are basic to all diets. Rice and beans offer a combination of high nutritive quality at low cost and their use should be encouraged. When served at the same meal, the rice and beans are complementary in supplying the essential amino acids. The combination also is an important source of calories and B-complex vitamins. Neither milk nor fruits and vegetables are eaten as much as they should be.

Some Puerto Ricans subscribe to the *hot-cold* theory of foods. This refers to inherent properties of heating or cooling that given foods are supposed to possess and is not related to the spiciness or temperature at which food is served. It is believed that some disease conditions are benefited by "hot" foods and others by "cold" foods. Since the foods placed in each category are likely to vary from person to person, the dietary counselor must determine the client's beliefs about specific foods.

TYPICAL FOODS AND THEIR USES

Milk Group

Milk is well liked, but very little is used. Children especially should be encouraged to drink more milk.

Most of the milk is used in strong coffee (*café con leche*): 2-5 ounces milk per cup. Many drink this beverage several times a day.

Cocoa and chocolate used widely.

Meat Group

Chicken, pork especially well liked.

Chicken often cooked with rice (*arroz con pollo*).

Codfish used frequently; served with viandas.

Legumes (*granos*): chick peas, kidney beans, navy beans, dried peas, pigeon peas, and other varieties. Stewed and dressed with sauce (*sofrito*). About 3-4 ounces legumes eaten daily.

Vegetable-Fruit Group

Viandas (starchy vegetables): sweet potatoes (*batata amarillo*) and white potatoes should be emphasized.

Other viandas used on the island may be imported: plantain, white *name*; white *tanier*; *panapen* (breadfruit); yautia; *yuca* (cassava). Viandas are boiled and served hot with oil, vinegar, and some codfish—often as a one-dish meal.

Beets and eggplant most commonly used vegetables. Some spinach and chard, but insufficient succulent vegetables. Small amounts of carrots, green beans, okra, and tomatoes. Yellow squash (*calabaza*) used in soups or fritters.

Fruits are eaten irregularly, and usually between meals. Preference often shown for canned peaches, pears, apples, and fruit cocktail. Citrus fruits should be emphasized.

Bread-Cereals Group

Rice (*arroz*) used once or twice daily by all (about 7 ounces per capita). May be boiled and dressed with lard, or combined with legumes, chopped pork sausages, dry codfish, or chicken.

Cornmeal mush made with water or milk is popular.

Oatmeal may be cooked in thin gruel for breakfast.

Cornmeal may substitute for rice and may be eaten with beans and codfish.

Whole-grain or enriched breads should be encouraged.

Other Foods and Seasonings

Sofrito: sauce made of tomatoes, onion, garlic, thyme, and other herbs, salt pork, green pepper and fat. This is basis for much of cooking.

Annato: yellow coloring used with rice.

Lard, oil, salt pork, or ham butts used in cooking. Butter and margarine are not used.

Sugar in large amounts in coffee, cocoa, chocolate; molasses.

Coffee (Mocha, never a blend) is very strong; usually served with hot milk. Carbonated beverages are used more frequently.

Pastries and other desserts not widely used.

Mexican-American Food Patterns

Outstanding Characteristics Most Mexican Americans live in the southwestern states—Texas, New Mexico, Arizona, and California. They have introduced many dishes that have become popular throughout the United States, such as tacos, enchiladas, and chili con carne.

The chief foods of the Mexican-American diet are dried beans, chili peppers, corn, and tomatoes. Many families eat one good meal daily such as lentil-noodle vegetable soup. Breakfast and supper are often light. If the income is low, very little meat is used—usually in combination with beans, soups, or vegetable stews.

The National Nutrition Survey in the Southwest showed low blood levels of vitamin A, riboflavin, and hemoglobin to be prevalent among Mexican-Americans. When meat intake is low, it is especially important to emphasize vitamin C-rich foods at each meal, in order to improve the utilization of iron from vegetables and legumes. For children there needs to be increased emphasis on milk in the diet.

Mexican Americans often cite causes for illness as being of a magical nature, of emotional origin, or of an imbalance between "hot" and "cold" foods. An example of food classification according to the hot-cold theory is as follows:

"*Hot*" *foods*: chili pepper, green and red pepper, garlic, onion, potatoes, sweet potatoes; goat milk; fish, turkey, capon; white beans, chick peas, rice, wheat bread, sweet roll, wheat tortillas, honey, sugar, and salt.

"*Cold*" *foods*: green beans, beets, cabbage, carrots, cauliflower, cucumber, coriander, parsley, peas, pumpkin, radish, spinach, squash, tomato, turnip; cow's milk, donkey milk, human milk; beef, hen, lamb, mutton, rabbit, red beans, lentils; oatmeal, corn tortillas, vermicelli.[6]

TYPICAL FOODS AND THEIR USES

Milk Group

Very little milk is used. Milk for children needs emphasis. Milk intolerance is fairly prevalent in adults, but usually tolerated well by children.

Meat Group

Beef and chicken well liked; meat used only two to three times weekly.

Eggs: two or three times a week.

Fish: infrequently.

Pinto or calico beans: refried (*frijoles refritos*); used daily by some; two or three times weekly by others.

Chile con carne: beef with garlic seasoning, beans, chili peppers.

Enchiladas: tortilla filled with cheese, onion, shredded lettuce, and rolled.

Taco: tortilla filled with seasoned ground meat, lettuce, and served with chili sauce.

Tamales: seasoned ground meat placed on masa, wrapped in corn husks, steamed, and served with chili sauce.

Topopo: corn tortilla filled with refried beans, shredded lettuce, green or ripe olives.

Vegetable - Fruit Group

Corn: fresh or canned; *chicos*; corn steamed while green and dried on the cob; *posole*, similar to hominy.

Chili peppers: fresh, canned, or frozen are good source of ascorbic acid.

Beets, cabbage, many tropical greens, peas, potatoes, pumpkin, squash, string beans, sweet potatoes, turnips.

Bananas used frequently. *Chayotes* (cactuslike fruit), oranges.

Nopalitos; leaf or stem of prickly pear cactus; diced as vegetable.

Bread-Cereals Group

Corn is staple cereal, with wheat gradually replacing it. Rice, macaroni, spaghetti. Some yeast bread; sweet rolls very popular. Increasing use of ready-to-eat cereals.

Atole: cornmeal gruel.

Masa: dried corn that has been heated and soaked in lime water, washed, and ground while wet into puttylike dough; contains appreciable amounts of calcium.

Sopaipillas: puffs of deep-fried dough. Used as bread or dessert, usually with honey.

Tortilla: thin, unleavened cakes baked on hot griddle, using masa; wheat now replacing lime-treated corn.

Other Foods and Seasoning

Ground red chili powder is essential to most dishes; garlic and onion very common; salt in abundance.

Cinnamon, coriander, lemon juice, mint, nutmeg, oregano, parsley, saffron.

Butter rarely used.

Coffee with much sugar used in large amounts.

Sugar and sweets in large amounts.

Food Patterns of the Vietnamese

Adjustments to Living in the United States   Of the tens of thousands of Vietnamese who have resettled in the United States, the largest number are living in California. There are also many Vietnamese living in midwestern, southern, and eastern cities. They find themselves cut off from their own cultural roots. They have had to face problems of finding employment, learning English, managing their money, and becoming accustomed to new life styles.

Characteristics of Diet   Kaufman has described the dietary characteristics of the Vietnamese and the adjustments that are possible for a nutritious diet.[7] In Vietnam three meals a day are preferred, with breakfast being the least important meal. Soup (*pho*) made with rice noodles, thin slices of beef or chicken, and greens or bean sprouts is a popular breakfast dish. Another breakfast pattern includes fried eggs, French bread, and café-au-lait.

Rice with mixtures of vegetables and meat or seafood is used for other meals. The universally used fermented fish sauce (*nuoc mam*) is high in sodium and iodine and also contributes some protein. Poultry, pork, and fish are well liked and used when income permits. Soybeans and peanuts are also important sources of protein. Cabbage, corn, spinach, squash, sweet potato, and watercress are widely used. Bananas, grapefruit, pineapple, mango, lichee, and jackfruit are used for dessert. Tea is drunk daily, but soft drinks and beer are also popular. Lactose intolerance occurs frequently in adults, and milk is little used. Children can usually tolerate milk if the amounts given are spaced throughout the day.

The Vietnamese are not familiar with American markets. Although they can purchase the fish sauce, herbs, tea, and rice noodles to which they are accustomed in Oriental food stores in major cities, these imported items are expensive. The Vietnamese are accustomed to buying foods daily, since in Vietnam they did not have refrigeration. Steaming, braising, stir-frying, deep-fat frying, and grilling are used. In Vietnam ovens were rare, so baked goods were purchased.

Dietary Patterns of the Middle East— Armenia, Greece, Syria, Turkey

TYPICAL FOODS AND THEIR USES

Milk Group
Cow's, goat's, or sheep's milk; fermented preferred to sweet (yogurt); little used by adults. Often served hot and sweetened to children.
Soft and hard cheeses.

Meat Group
Lamb is preferred; also pork, poultry, mutton, goat, beef.
Fish: fresh, salted, or smoked; octopus, squid, shellfish, roe.
Eggs often used as main dish but not at breakfast.
Beans, peas, and lentils.
Nuts may be used with wheat and rice in place of meat; pignolias, pistachios.
Ground or cut meat often cooked with wheat or rice, or in stews with cereal grains and vegetables. For example:
Breast of lamb stuffed with rice, currants.
Squash stuffed with chopped meat, onions, rice, parsley.
Cabbage rolls with ground meat, rice, and baked in meat stock; served with lemon juice.
Barbequed meats on special occasions: skewered meats are broiled.
Shashlik: mutton or lamb marinated in garlic, oil, vinegar; roasted on skewers with tomato and onion slices.

Vegetable - Fruit Group
Eggplant, greens, onions, peppers, tomatoes; also cabbage, cauliflower, cucumbers, okra, potatoes, zucchini.
Vegetables cooked with olive oil and served hot or cold; cooked in meat or fish stews; stuffed with wheat, meat, nuts, beans; salads with olive oil, vinegar.
Grapes, lemons, oranges; also apricots, cherries, dates, figs, melons, peaches, pears, plums, quinces, raisins. Fresh fruits widely used in season; fruit compotes.

Bread - Cereals Group
Bread is staff of life; used at every meal. Baked on griddles in round, flat loaves
Cracked whole wheat (*bourglour*) and rice used as starchy food, or with vegetables, or with meat (*pilavi*).
Corn in *polenta*.

Other Foods and Seasonings
Olive oil and seed oils used in cooking. Butter is not much used.
Nuts (hazel, pignolia, pistachio) used for snacks, in desserts, pastries.
Baklava: pastry with nuts and honey.
Black olives.
Herbs, honey, sugar, lemon juice, seeds of caraway, pumpkin, and sesame.
Apricot candy, Turkish paste.
Wine, coffee.

Dietary Patterns of the Chinese

Characteristics Adaptations of the Chinese cuisine have become very popular in the United States. Depending on the geographic region in China, there are variations in the availability of foods, the methods of preparation, and the seasoning of foods.

Northern characteristic of Beijing, includes sweet and sour dishes; duck; noodles; and steamed breads.

Coastal as in Shanghai includes greater amounts of seafoods.

Inland (Szechuan) includes greater use of spicy, hot seasonings.

Southern (Cantonese) includes pork, chicken, dumplings. Many Chinese restaurants in the United States serve Cantonese foods.

Rice is a staple food throughout China, but more so in the southern parts of the country where it is widely grown. Wheat is also an important staple cereal grain and is grown in the northern regions of China. Only small amounts of meat, poultry, and fish are served. Usually meat—preferably pork—is cut in small pieces and combined with vegetables.

TYPICAL FOODS AND THEIR USES

Milk Group
Milk and cheese are well liked but need to be emphasized. When soybean milk is substituted for infants and children, it should be fortified.

Meat Group
Pork, lamb, goat, chicken, duck, fish, and shellfish, eggs, and soybeans. Organ meats including brain and spinal cord, blood, and bone are used.
Egg rolls: shrimp or meat and vegetable filling rolled in thin dough, and fried in deep fat.
Egg foo young: combination of eggs, chopped chicken, mushrooms, scallions, celery, bean sprouts cooked similar to an omelet.
Sweet and pungent pork: pork cubes coated with batter and fried in oil; then simmered in a sauce

of green pepper, cubed pineapple, molasses, brown sugar, vinegar, and seasonings.

Stir-fried fish with vegetables: diced white meat fish fillets are coated with egg white and fried quickly in deep fat; drained. Sauce of chicken stock, soy sauce, rice wine or sake combined with peas. Scallion, and garlic stir-fried in small amount oil. Bamboo shoots, sauce, and fish added and blended thoroughly. Often served on bed of stir-fried spinach.

Tofu: soybean curd; used in many dishes. An excellent source of protein, iron, and calcium if made with calcium salts.

Vegetable - Fruit Groups

Bok choy (Chinese cabbage), broccoli, cabbage, carrots, onions, peas, cucumbers, many greens, mushrooms, bamboo shoots, soybean sprouts, sweet potatoes.

Stir-fried vegetables are thinly sliced or chopped; cooked in a little oil for a short time before water is added to seal in flavor, preserve crispness, and fresh green color. Any juice remaining is served with vegetable.

Apples, dates, lichee, oranges, peaches, plums, and pineappple are used.

Bread-Cereals Group

Rice is staple food served with every meal.
Wheat and millet are widely used; noodles.

Other Foods and Seasonings

Lard, soy, sesame, and peanut oils used in cooking.

Soy sauce present in almost every meal contributes to high salt intake.

Almonds, ginger, sesame seeds, garlic, fresh herbs, for flavoring.

Tea is beverage of choice.

NUTRITIONAL CONCERNS ABOUT SOME AMERICAN FOOD PATTERNS

"Junk Food"   The term "junk food" has been applied indiscriminately to hamburgers, pizzas, hot dogs, and other foods from a fast-food restaurant, numerous snack-type crackers, pretzels, chips, cakes, cookies, pies, sweets, and soft drinks. Such a designation ignores the wide variation that exists among these foods insofar as nutrient content is concerned. The nutrient density of some of these foods is good while that of others is low. But even foods such as sweets and fats as well as some snack items that supply few nutrients are sources of energy and can be used in moderation in an otherwise well-balanced and varied diet. Foods of low nutrient density are harmful only when they replace foods that supply the needed nutrients and when they are superimposed on an adequate diet so that the caloric intake exceeds the caloric requirement. No food should be labeled "junk food" but perhaps the individual who uses a given food to the exclusion of others is making a "junk" use of that food!

Fast Foods   The phenomenal growth of the fast-food industry continues not only in the United Sates but in other countries as well. Fast-food restaurants appeal to persons of all ages, but especially to the young. Rapid service, convenience, moderate cost, taste, and a place to be with one's peers are some reasons given for their popularity. Lack of variety, high caloric content in relationship to nutrient contribution, high sugar content, high salt content, and lack of fiber are frequent criticisms of fast foods. (See Figure 16-2.)

What is the impact of fast foods on nutrition? For those who eat a meal or a snack in a fast-food restaurant once a week or so, the effect on dietary adequacy is not great. But for workers and teenagers who might eat a meal every day at these places the nutritive contribution must be carefully considered.

A typical meal in a fast-food restaurant (hamburger, french fries, milk shake) furnishes about half the caloric requirement for a teenage boy, 40 percent or more of his protein allowance, and up to one third of his thiamin, riboflavin, and niacin allowances. The meal also provides significant amounts of calcium and iron. Buf if coffee or a soft drink is substituted for the milkshake, the calcium content of the meal is very low.

Many fast-food restaurants are responding to their customer's tastes and health concerns by introducing breakfast items, juices, frozen yogurt, ice cream, and salad bars. There are choices of beef, pork, seafood, and poultry, and an increasing range of beverages and desserts. (See Table A-6 for the nutritive values of some fast foods.)

"Organic," "Natural," and "Health" Foods   These terms are used loosely and often interchangeably. Many people use foods so described believing them to be more healthful. "Organically grown" foods are those grown on soils enriched with compost and manure and in the absence of chemical fertilizers and pesticides. The term "organic foods" is a poor choice for two reasons: (1) manures and composts used to enrich the soil must be degraded by bacteria to inorganic phosphates and nitrates, since the plant utilizes only the inorganic substances just as it would from the commercial fertilizer, and (2) all foods consist of the organic compounds protein, fat, and carbohydrate, so that all foods, regardless of the soil on which they were grown, are actually "organic." The nutritive values of food grown on so-called organically enriched soils and those grown on chemically

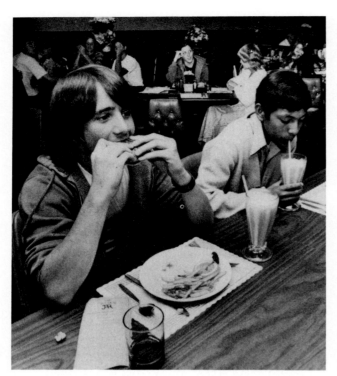

Figure 16-2. Hamburger on bun, French fries, and a milk shake are popular foods for teenagers. They provide substantial amounts of energy and many nutrients. A salad such as coleslaw or a piece of fruit would furnish missing nutrients such as ascorbic acid. (Courtesy, U.S. Department of Agriculture.)

fertilized soils are of equal value. The foods are equally safe and wholesome. Efficient agricultural practices fully utilize the humus resulting from manures and composts together with chemical fertilizers.

"Natural foods" are those that are used in the form in which they are produced and with a minimum of processing. They contain no additives and usually are "organically grown." Raw sugar, raw milk, stone ground meals, and raw vegetables are examples. Those who subscribe to the use of natural foods believe that processed foods have lost much of their nutritive value and that additives are harmful. (See page 253 for discussion of the uses of additives.) Food technologists have developed processing techniques that retain most of the nutrients present in the freshly harvested food. In fact, a food that is canned or frozen immediately after harvesting may retain a higher nutrient level than a raw product in the market that has remained on unrefrigerated shelves too long. (See page 208.)

"Health foods" are those to which special virtues are assigned for the prevention or cure of disease. Blackstrap molasses, honey and vinegar, seaweed, fertilized eggs, and various soy products

are often cited for their special virtues. Also, dietary supplements such as garlic, parsley, brewer's yeast, sea salt, and herbal teas are included in this category. All foods are healthful insofar as they contribute to the body's energy and nutrient needs. It is dangerous to rely on a particular food or food combination for the treatment of disease because the individual may fail to seek needed medical advice for the condition.

Macrobiotic Diets This system of diet derived from Zen Buddhism was introduced into the United States some years ago by George Ohsawa. Adherents to this regimen believe that it promotes physical, emotional, and spiritual well-being. They also believe that illness can be prevented or cured by the use of this diet.

The diet maintains a balance between yin and yang. (See page 225.) It consists of 10 stages that progress from one that can be planned to be nutritionally adequate to one that is grossly inadequate in many nutrients. The first stage, Diet − 3, consists of these percentages from the food groups: cereal, 10; vegetables, 30; soup, 10; animal foods, 30; salads and fruits, 15; and desserts, 5. With each progression the amount of cereal is increased by 10 percent with corresponding decreases in the percentage of other groups. Diet 7 consists of 100 percent cereal foods. All levels of diet pose a restriction of fluids.

Fluid restriction poses the risk of dehydration. Most people who subscribe to a macrobiotic diet do not follow through to the final stages. If they adhere to lower stages that include a variety of foods from all groups, good nutrition is possible. Usually, the foods used in this diet are "organic" or "natural."

References for the Case Study

AMERICAN DIETETIC ASSOCIATION: "Position Paper on the Vegetarian Approach to Eating," *J. Am. Diet. Assoc.*, 77:61–69, 1980.

BURR, M. L., AND SWEETMAN, P. M.: "Vegetarianism, Dietary Fiber, and Mortality," *Am. J. Clin. Nutr.*, 36:873–77, 1982.

NARINS, D. M., AND BELKENGREN, R. P.: "Nutrition and the Growing Athlete," *Pediatr. Nurs.*, 9:163–68, May/June 1983.

References

1. Dwyer, J.: "Vegetarianism," *Contemp. Nutr.*, 4 (6): June 1979.
2. Register, U. D., and Sonnenberg, L. M.: "The Vegetarian Diet," *J. Am. Diet. Assoc.*, 62:253–61, 1973.

CASE STUDY 2

High School Student on a Vegetarian Diet

Phil, age 15, the eldest of three boys, lives with his family in a middle-income area of Chicago. His father is a fireman and his mother works part time in a bakery.

Phil is a good student who excels in the sciences and mathematics. As a result of his studies about ecology and limited natural resources, Phil strongly believes that the people of the United States consume too much meat and are wasting their natural resources. He and several of his friends have decided to become vegetarians.

Phil is in good health and is physically fit. He weighs 52.3 kg (115 lb) and is 162 cm (64 in) tall. A skillful athlete, he particularly enjoys soccer and tennis. In the last three soccer games Phil has not scored as well as usual. He has not lasted the game and the coach has had to send in replacements. The coach thinks that Phil's fad diet is ruining his health and his game and has told him to see the school nurse.

Phil refuses to eat meat, poultry, fish, and eggs but will drink milk and eat other dairy foods. Since the school lunch menus usually include animal protein, Mrs. S. prepares bag lunches for Phil. She includes two cheese sandwiches, an apple or orange, and graham crackers. Phil buys milk at school.

At first Phil's mother was openly critical about his insistence on following a vegetarian diet and there were many arguments at home. Since none of the other family members is interested in following such a diet, preparing another menu for Phil places an extra burden upon Mrs. S. She is upset that Phil will not eat many of the foods she prepares and thinks that his refusal to eat meat will stunt his growth.

After Phil consistently avoided animal protein foods (except milk) for over two months, Mrs. S. decided to talk with a friend of hers who is a dietitian. Phil has lost 2.3 kg (5 lb) since he started this new diet. Mrs. S. has many questions about food preparation and meal patterns that will be tasty, varied, and provide adequate nutrients, especially protein. Mrs. S.'s friend offered several tips on meal planning and loaned her a cookbook on vegetarian diets.

Physiologic Correlations

1. In what ways might a carefully selected vegetarian diet be beneficial to health?

2. List some adverse effects of vegetarian diets if not carefully planned.
3. What is the likelihood that Phil's recent performance in soccer games is due to his diet?

Nutritional Assessment

4. What is meant by each of the following: vegans; lacto-vegetarian; lacto-ovo-vegetarian?
5. Which nutrients are likely to be in short supply in a strict vegetarian diet? In Phil's lacto-vegetarian diet?
6. Suggest some practical ways of including the missing nutrients in the strict vegetarian diet.
7. For a project in biology, Phil studied protein quality of plant foods by feeding four groups of weanling rats. All rats received the same quantity of protein and their diets were adequate in all other respects. What results would you expect on growth for these diets:
   a. Navy beans
   b. Rice
   c. Beans plus rice
   d. Milk (control group)
8. Which essential amino acids are provided in limited supply in wheat; rice; beans; chickpeas; corn?

Planning the Diet

9. Using the food groups in Table 16-1, plan a day's menu for Phil.
10. Why is the inclusion of foods supplying at least 25 mg ascorbic acid at each meal desirable?
11. Phil and his friends have suggested to the school lunch committee that occasional lacto-vegetarian lunches be served as examples of the studies they have made in their biology class. List five main dishes that the dietitian might include.

Dietary Counseling

12. Suggest some nutritious snacks that Phil's mother might keep on hand to boost his caloric intake.
13. Mrs. S. is concerned that vegetable proteins are not as good as animal proteins. What would you tell her?
14. Mrs. S. believes Phil should take vitamin B-12 injections, but Phil says he does not need them. Who is right? Explain.
15. Phil has read about the macrobiotic diet but has decided that it was not the best diet for him. What are the characteristics of the macrobiotic diet? What nutrients are lacking in the final stages of this diet? Why is this diet dangerous?

3. Dwyer, J. T., et al.: "The New Vegetarians: The Natural High?," *J. Am. Diet. Assoc.*, **65**:529–36, 1974.
4. Kuhnlein, H. V., et al.: "Composition of Traditional Hopi Foods," *J. Am. Diet. Assoc.*, **75**:37–41, 1979.
5. Schaefer, O.: "When the Eskimo Comes to Town," *Nutr. Today*, **6**:8–16, 1979.
6. Smith, L. K.: "Mexican-American Views of Anglo Medical and Dietetic Practices," *J. Am. Diet. Assoc.*, **74**:463–64, 1979.
7. Kaufman, M.: "Vietnam, 1978: Crisis in Food, Nutrition, and Health," *J. Am. Diet. Assoc.*, **74**:310–16, 1979.

17

Safeguarding the Food Supply

Illness Caused by Food

Foodborne Diseases as a Public Health Problem
The number of cases of food-related illness is not known, since only a small proportion is ever reported to the Centers for Disease Control in Atlanta, Georgia. Of these, *Salmonella*, *Clostridium perfringens*, and *Staphylococci*, often referred to as the "big three," are responsible for up to two thirds of all instances of food-related illness. Estimates indicate that millions of persons are afflicted each year by foodborne infections.

For most people in good health, the illness is of short duration, leading to discomfort and absence from work or school for a day or two. But for the very young, the elderly, and those debilitated from other illness, these seemingly mild infections can lead to serious fluid and electrolyte imbalances and other complications that are sometimes fatal. The outbreak of an infection in a child-care institution or in a nursing home is especially life threatening.

Other diseases transmitted by foods are typhoid fever, bacillary dysentery, tuberculosis, scarlet fever, streptococcic sore throat, botulism, undulant fever, amebic dysentery, trichinosis, infectious hepatitis, and cholera.

Some illnesses are enteric in that the symptoms are confined to the gastrointestinal tract with mild to severe nausea, vomiting, abdominal pain, and diarrhea. Other foodborne diseases are systemic; that is, the organisms invade the circulation and produce symptoms in organs and tissues.

Foodborne diseases result from eating food (1) from an animal or plant that has been infected, (2) that has been contaminated by organisms transmitted by insects, flies, roaches, or rodents, (3) that has had contact with sewage-polluted water (shellfish, for example), or (4) that has been contaminated by a food handler who has not observed good personal hygiene or acceptable food-handling practices. A single egg that is infected can contaminate a whole batch of eggs being frozen or dried. A butcher block or kitchen counter with which infected meat has been in contact is a source of contamination for any food placed upon it.

Bacterial Food Infections A bacterial *infection* results from the ingestion of food that has been contaminated with large numbers of bacteria. The bacteria continue to grow in the favorable intestinal environment and produce irritation of the mucosa with symptoms occurring in 12 to 36 hours after ingestion of the food.

Salmonellosis. About 1,300 serotypes of the *Salmonella* genus have been identified, each of which is capable of causing infections in humans. The organisms are easily killed by boiling for 5 minutes, but survive in foods that are inadequately heated. Paratyphoid fever (enteric fever) occurs frequently. The symptoms usually last for 2 to 3 days, but the organisms may be present in body wastes for 2 or 3 weeks thereby providing a continuing source of contamination for others.

Typhoid fever, fortunately rare in the United States, is the most serious of the *Salmonella* infections. The symptoms of the gastrointestinal tract may be severe with ulcerations of the mucosa occurring. Unlike most infections by *Salmonella*, typhoid fever is systemic. The organisms particularly affect the liver and gallbladder, but they may also localize in the bone marrow, kidney, spleen, and the lungs, where bronchitis and pneumonia may result.

Meat, poultry, fish, eggs, and dairy products that are eaten raw or that have been inadequately heated are most frequently implicated in salmonellosis. Contaminated cake mixes, bakery foods, coloring agents, powdered yeast, and chocolate candy have also caused outbreaks of the infection.

Shigellosis (Bacillary Dysentery). The *Shigella* genus includes pathogenic organisms widely distributed and

243

FOOD SAFETY—A CONSUMER CONCERN

Many people today are uncertain about the safety of the U.S. food supply. Some question the objectivity of the food industry in giving assurances that foods are indeed safe. Others wonder whether governmental regulators are doing all that they can or should be doing to ensure food safety. News media often give dramatic emphasis to current problems, sometimes creating exaggerated fears and misplaced direction. Discussions of food safety are often highly emotional rather than being related to findings from research. People wonder:

How safe is the American food supply?
What are the chief causes of illness from foods?
Why are additives needed in our foods?
Are most vitamins destroyed when foods are processed?
Nitrosamines, EDB, PCBs, and many other chemical compounds—aren't all of these carcinogenic?
Wouldn't the population be better off if all pesticides were banned for use on crops?
What precautions should be observed by food preparers in the home or in institutions to ensure food safety?

A Perspective on Food Safety Health professionals must be able to provide answers to the questions listed above and to many others, and must be able to assist consumers to place food safety into the perspective of benefits and risks. Let us consider several commonly used terms.

SAFETY is freedom from the occurrence or risk of injury, danger or loss.
BENEFIT is anything that is advantageous to the good of a person or thing.
RISK is the exposure to the chance of injury or loss.

In any of life's endeavors there is no absolute safety. Riding in an automobile carries some risk of accident, but you choose to do it because the benefit outweighs the risk. Surgery carries some risk, but usually its benefit of prolonging life leads people to accept the risk. Eating food carries some risk, whether it be the excess leading to obesity or the imbalance leading to malnutrition or the ingestion of some substance that causes illness. Some risks are acceptable, but we must be certain that the ratio of benefit to risk is substantial.

TOXICITY is the capacity of a substance, when tested by itself, to harm the living organism.
HAZARD is the capacity of a substance to produce injury under conditions of use.

For example, vitamin A is potentially toxic, but it is a hazard only when ingested in amounts that are 10 to 20 times the recommended allowances. Salt is potentially toxic; it is a hazard when ingested in three to five times normal amounts. For hypertensive patients salt may be hazardous at much lower levels.

To consider food safety in perspective, one might begin by examining a list of priorities set up by the Food and Drug Administration.[1]

1. Food-borne infections. These are, by far, the most important problems related to food safety.
2. Nutrition. With new products replacing other foods in the diet, are the essential nutrients being provided for dietary adequacy?
3. Environmental contamination. What are the problems of water and soil pollution relating to the food supply? How can they be detected? How can they be corrected?
4. Natural toxicants in food. Which foods contain them? What are the tolerance levels?
5. Pesticides.
6. Intentional additives.

Note that the pesticides and additives that so often create headlines rank low on the totem pole of priorities. Because of regulations concerning their use, they are not important causes of human illness.

People often forget that they are a fantastically complex organization of chemical substances—the organic compounds such as amino acids, lipids, carbohydrates, and vitamins; the inorganic mineral salts; and that marvelous chemical combination of hydrogen and oxygen—water. People forget, too, that their entire living environment—the food they eat, the air they breathe, the clothes they wear, the houses in which they live, the earth on which they walk—all are chemical in nature. Life itself requires a chemical environment. The science of chemistry and the applications by nutrition scientists and food technologists have vastly improved our food supply and extended the quality of our lives. But for all good things there must be limits and safeguards to avoid abuse. See Chapter 18 for further details.

capable of producing severe illness. Bacillary dysentery is characterized by fever, abdominal pain, vomiting, and diarrhea. The intestinal mucosa may become ulcerated, and stools often contain blood and mucus. Fatalities from the infections are ordinarily low, but in tropical countries where sanitation is poor and malnutrition is prevalent the disease is fatal to as many as 20 percent of persons affected.

Infected human feces are the source of the infection, which is transmitted by the direct fecal-oral route or through contamination of food or water.

Clostridium Perfringens. This gas gangrene organism appears normally in the soil, in the intestinal tract of humans and animals, and in sewage. The usual numbers in the gastrointestinal tract do not produce illness. However, when a food is consumed that has been contaminated with large numbers of bacteria, nausea, vomiting, and diarrhea for 24 hours can occur. The bacteria are destroyed by heat, but the spores they produce will survive boiling for as long as 5 hours. If foods are allowed to remain at temperatures between 10 and 60°C (50 and 140°F) for several hours, the spores germinate and prodigious numbers of bacteria are then present in the food. Food should be refrigerated immediately after heating to prevent rapid germination of spores. Shallow containers are preferred since a large food mass in a deep container cools so slowly that considerable bacterial growth occurs.

Bacterial Food Intoxications Food poisoning frequently results from the ingestion of a food in which a bacterial toxin has been produced. The preformed toxin is responsible for the symptoms, which may be mild to severe. Usually the symptoms are apparent from 1 to 6 hours following a meal.

Staphyloccal Poisoning. Ingestion of food containing the *staphylococcal* enterotoxin causes gastrointestinal symptoms that are often severe but usually the illness lasts for only 1 to 3 days.

Staphylococci are found in the air and occur especially in infected cuts and abrasions of the skin, boils, and pimples. They may be present in the nose and throat of food handlers. Food becomes contaminated through failure to observe rules of hygiene. Rapid growth of the bacteria occurs in contaminated food if it is held at temperatures ranging between 10 and 60°C (50 and 140°F) for 3 to 4 hours. Semisolid foods such as custards, cream fillings in pastries, cream puffs, cream sauces, mayonnaise, chicken and turkey salads, croquettes, potato salad, ice cream, poultry dressing, ham, ground meat, stews, and fish provide the ideal culture media for bacterial growth.

Staphylococci are killed at high temperatures, but the toxin is not inactivated with temperatures ordinarily used in food preparation. The contaminated food usually does not smell, taste, or appear to be spoiled. The best safeguard against staphylococcal poisoning is prompt refrigeration of food so that bacterial growth is retarded and toxin formation does not take place.

Botulism. Each year there are ten to twenty outbreaks of botulism in the United States with two to five deaths. Most instances of botulism are traced to the ingestion of inadequately processed home-canned nonacid vegetables and meats. A few outbreaks in recent years have been reported from commercially processed tuna fish, whitefish, soup, and smoked fish.

The symptoms of botulism occur 8 to 72 hours after ingestion of the contaminated food and usually begin in the gastrointestinal tract. Headache, dizziness, double vision, difficulty in swallowing, speech difficulty, and paralysis occur. Death is usually the result of respiratory paralysis and cardiac failure. With early diagnosis and prompt treatment with antitoxin, the death rate is about 25 percent. Failure to initiate early treatment increases the death rate to about 65 percent.

Clostridium botulinum is present in soils all over the world and in the sediment at the bottom of rivers and lakes. Consequently, vegetables grown on these soils and fish become contaminated. The bacteria do not grow in the presence of oxygen; that is, they are anaerobic. They will grow within a few millimeters below the surface of the foods, however. The bacteria are sporeformers that are resistant to ordinary boiling temperature. As the spores germinate, the deadly neurotoxin is produced.

Canned foods that contain little or no acid (pH above 4.6) such as meat, beans, asparagus, corn, and peas are very good media for the growth of the bacillus botulinus, whereas acid-containing foods such as tomatoes and certain fruits are not favorable to growth. Some recently developed varieties of tomatoes, however, do not contain sufficient acid to prevent the growth of the bacteria. The use of sterilization with steam under pressure is absolutely necessary in the home for any nonacid food products, as well as for those processed commercially.

Botulinus-infected foods do not necessarily taste or smell spoiled, so home-canned vegetables should be brought to a vigorous boil and kept boiling for 10 minutes. Any toxin that may be present will thereby be inactivated. Any can of food that shows gas production, change in color or consistency, bulging ends, or leaks should be discarded without even tasting. "When in doubt, throw it out" is a good axiom. The foods must be disposed of so that animals do not have access to them since they too might be poisoned.

Parasitic Infestations of Foods Many protozoa and helminths (worms) gain admission to the body by means of food and parasitize the bowel, thereby causing injury to the intestinal lining. Some of them also invade other tissues of the body.

Among the parasitic protozoa are *Endamoeba histolytica*, which causes amebic dysentery. The source of infection is human feces, and infection is transmitted by a food handler who is a carrier or by contaminated water supplies. The symptoms may be acute, chronic, or intermittent. Erosion of the intestinal mucosa sometimes occurs with profuse bloody diarrhea. The individual with a chronic infection may experience only mild discomfort of diarrhea or constipation. The liver, lung, brain, and other tissues may be infected and abscesses may form. Preventive measures include maintenance of sanitary controls of the water supply and sewage disposal, as well as supervision of public eating places by health agencies.

The helminths that frequently invade the intestinal tract include *nematodes* (roundworms), *cestodes* (tapeworms), and *trematodes* (liver, intestinal, and lung flukes). Trichinosis, one of the more serious infestations, results from the ingestion of raw or partially cooked pork infected with *Trichinella spiralis*, a very minute roundworm barely visible to the naked eye. In the intestinal tract the larvae are set free from their cysts during digestion of the meat and develop into adults within a few days. The females deposit larvae in the mucosa and invade the lymph and blood circulation. The muscles of the diaphragm, the thorax, the abdominal wall, the biceps, and the tongue are frequently involved, there being muscular pain, chills, and weakness.

Trichinella is destroyed by cooking pork until no trace of pink remains. The recommended internal temperature for cooked pork is 77°C (170°F), which allows a margin of about 17°C (30°F) above the lethal point of the organisms. *Trichinella* is also destroyed by freezing at $-18°C$ (0°F) or below for at least 72 hours. The widely adopted regulation that all garbage fed to hogs be cooked has gone a long way toward reducing *Trichinella* infestation.

Hookworm infestation is a serious problem in children in tropical countries of the world, and in some parts of the United States. The larvae penetrate the exposed skin and reach the lymphatics and blood circulation. They are carried to the lungs and migrate into the alveoli, trachea, epiglottis, and pharynx and are swallowed. They may also be carried from soil to hands to mouth.

A single hookworm removes almost 1 ml blood per day as it carries on its blood-sucking activity in the intestine. The loss of blood produces an anemia with symptoms of weakness, fatigue, and growth retardation. Usually the infestation is present in children who also are malnourished. A good nutritious diet is always important for these children, but the eradication of hookworm infestation depends on sanitary measures for disposal of feces so that the cycle of parasite growth in the soil is broken.

Naturally Occurring Toxicants in Foods Foods are exceedingly complex mixtures of chemicals. The naturally occurring chemicals in the food supply probably number in the hundreds of thousands. For example, potatoes, often considered to be a simple food, contain at least 150 chemical substances including not only the nutritionally important protein, carbohydrate, minerals, and vitamins, but oxalic acid, tannins, solanine, arsenic, and nitrate as well.

Foods contain thousands of compounds that are potentially toxic. The hazards are minimal because of several factors: (1) the body has metabolic mechanisms for degrading, detoxifying, and eliminating some substances; (2) some toxic substances are modified by processing—for example, the heating of soybeans to destroy trypsin inhibitor; and (3) some toxic compounds are antagonistic to other toxic compounds, and the net effect is one of neutralization. Molybdenum, an essential nutrient, is toxic in excess; copper, another essential nutrient which is also toxic, is antagonistic to molybdenum. Thus, together they reduce the toxicity of the pair.

Poisoning from natural food toxicants often occurs in times of stress such as famine or war when abnormally large amounts of single foods containing toxic materials are ingested daily for prolonged periods of time.

Alkaloids. The alkaloids such as strychnine, atropine, scopalamine, solanine, and others have long been known as poisonous compounds. Varieties of hemlock have been mistaken for parsley, horseradish, or wild parsnip and eaten in salads and soup only to produce immediate, often fatal, illness. Monkshood, foxglove and deadly nightshade have from time to time been mistaken for edible plants and have caused violent illness.

The Food and Drug Administration has recently called attention to the possible hazard of consuming some herbal teas in excessive amounts.[2] Some herbs contain alkaloids (morphine, nicotine) and glycosides (digitalis) that dissolve readily in hot water. A case of excessive bleeding in a young woman who drank large quantities of a herbal tea containing coumarin has been described. Among the unsafe herbs listed were: absinthe, bloodroot, heliotrope, jimson weed, lily of the valley, mandrake, mistletoe, morning glory, and periwinkle.

SOLANINE, representing a series of glycosides, occurs in the stems and leaves of the potato plant and in the green part of sprouting potatoes. When potatoes are stored in bright light, significant amounts of solanine are produced in the skin, evidenced by greening. When ingested in sufficient amounts, solanine produces pain, vomiting, jaundice, diarrhea, and prostration. Ordinarily the green parts of the potato are removed with the peel.

Legumes and Seeds. Because legumes are important sources of protein and energy in some parts of the world, the presence of toxic factors in them is of nutritional and economic importance. Soybeans are a most valuable source of protein when they are heated. Raw soybeans contain a TRYPSIN INHIBITOR and probably some other factors that interfere with the metabolism and with growth in animals. In addition, the phytic acid content of soybeans binds zinc, so that animals fed a diet in which soybeans are the source of protein develop a severe zinc deficiency. This can be corrected by supplementing the diet with zinc. Soybeans also contain a goitrogen, but this is not believed to be a factor in endemic goiter.

Cassava and lima beans contain LINMARIN, a glycoside that can be split to hydrocyanic acid. People in West Africa, Jamaica, and Malaysia consume up to 750 g cassava daily. It is thought that the incidence of blindness and tropical ataxic neuropathy, a degenerative disease, may be caused by chronic cyanide poisoning from the cassava.

LATHYRISM has been known since the time of Hippocrates. It is observed in India and in Mediterranean countries following the ingestion for 6 months or more of large amounts of the seeds of *Lathyrus sativus*, a legume. These legumes grow under adverse conditions of drought and hence they may be ingested extensively during a famine. Lathyrism is a neurologic disease characterized by weakness of the leg muscles, dragging of the feet, loss of sensation of heat and pain, and spinal cord lesions.

FAVISM is an inherited sensitivity to fava or broad beans and is fairly common in the Mediterranean area, and in Asia and Formosa. Sensitive individuals have a deficiency of glucose 6-phosphate dehydrogenase and reduced glutathione content of the red blood cells. An unidentified substance in the fava beans leads to hemolysis of the red blood cells and thus hemolytic anemia in the sensitive individuals.

GOSSYPOL is a toxicant in cottonseed that must be removed before the meal can be used in protein mixtures. Some strains of cottonseed are now being developed that are free of this toxic substance.

Mushroom Poisoning. A few species of mushrooms are so toxic that eating them may be fatal, others are mildly toxic, and many species are harmless and greatly enjoyed. The *Amanita* is the most poisonous of the mushrooms and produces severe abdominal pain, prostration, jaundice, and death in more than half the people who ingest it. This source of poisoning can be eliminated if people use only the commercially grown mushrooms.

Mycotoxins. In medieval times a poisoning known as "St Anthony's Fire" was a terrible scourge.[3] It was caused by ergot, a toxic fungus, growing on cereal grains. Ergotism is almost unknown today. Deaths of thousands of people in Russia in times of war and famine have been attributed to the consumption of moldy millet.

Many molds growing on grains and nuts can produce illness in animals and probably in humans. AFLATOXINS produced by the mold *Aspergillus flavus* are a class of substances of extreme toxicity to swine, cattle, poultry, and laboratory animals. The aflatoxins are potent hepatocarcinogens. The only practical way to prevent the development of the mold is through prompt drying of grains and nuts to a moisture content not over 15 percent. Allowing crops to remain in fields over winter invites mold growth.

Paralytic Shellfish Poisoning. A toxin produced by oysters, clams, mussels, and scallops has caused many fatal illnesses. The shellfish ingest large quantities of "red tide," the plankton *Gonyaulaux catennela*. Saxitoxin, an extremely toxic metabolite, is produced from the plankton. The toxin resists ordinary cooking procedures.

Tyramine Toxicity. TYRAMINE is produced by the decarboxylation of tyrosine. It is a potent vasopressor substance that is normally metabolized in the body by the action of MONOAMINE OXIDASE.

Patients with depressive states are frequently

treated with monoamine oxidase inhibitor because of the ability of this agent to produce euphoria. Since the inhibitor interferes with the metabolism of tyramine, the ingestion of tyramine-containing foods leads to nausea, vomiting, headache, severe hypertension, and sometimes death. Aged cheeses, yeast extracts, bologna, pepperoni, salami, and Chianti wine are high in tyramine and should be avoided when the inhibitor is being used. A single glass of Chianti wine or as little as an ounce of aged cheese contains enough tyramine to produce toxic effects.

Interference with Nutritive Properties Some chemical substances interfere with the utilization of a nutrient, resulting in a nutritional deficiency. One of the best-known examples of this is OXALIC ACID found in certain green leafy vegetables such as spinach, beet tops, and chard. Oxalic acid interferes with the absorption of calcium. The occasional use of these vegetables with an adequate intake of calcium is of no concern whatsoever. However, if the calcium intake is low and the vegetables are eaten frequently, a problem of calcium deficiency could arise. Rhubarb leaves are so high in oxalic acid that their ingestion leads to gastrointestinal upsets, and in severe intoxications to hematemesis, hematuria, noncoagulability of the blood and convulsions.

PHYTATES interfere with the absorption of calcium, magnesium, iron, and zinc. They are present in whole grains. The effect is not important when (1) a varied diet contains recommended levels of these mineral elements, (2) moderate amounts of fiber are consumed, and (3) the phytates are present in yeast-leavened breads. A diet that consists primarily of whole grains in the form of unleavened breads is likely to result in deficiency.

Goiter is a major public health problem affecting 200 million people throughout the world. GOITROGENS, which are antithyroid compounds, are held responsible for about 4 percent of the goiter incidence, representing a total of 8 million persons. Goitrogens are found in broccoli, Brussels sprouts, cabbage, cauliflower, kale, kohlrabi, rutabagas, and turnips. There is no adverse effect when eating normal amounts of these vegetables, but when they become a major part of the diet for extended periods of time, the antithyroid effect becomes evident. Additional iodine does not counteract this effect.

THIAMINASE, an enzyme antagonistic to thiamin, is present in bracken fern, raw fish, and a variety of fruits and vegetables. In an ordinary mixed diet this is of no concern. The enzyme is destroyed by heat.

Influence of Excessive Nutrient Intakes The toxic effects of vitamins A and D are well known. The ingestion of seal or polar bear liver leads to symptoms of acute vitamin A toxicity, inasmuch as 1 pound of the liver contains about 10 million IU of vitamin A. On a practical basis in the United States the hazards of vitamin A toxicity relate to the indiscriminate use of vitamin supplements and not to excesses in the diet itself. If several foods that are fortified with vitamin D are consumed each day, the intake could be in excess of requirements, and hypercalcemia is a possible outcome. Excessive intake of iron can interfere with vitamin E activity, while excessive intake of vitamin E can inhibit the action of vitamin K.

Poisoning by Trace Mineral Elements A number of essential trace mineral elements are also potent toxicants. These include iodine, copper, fluorine, manganese, molybdenum, selenium, and zinc. Lead, mercury, and cadmium are serious environmental pollutants. These minerals modify metabolism in several ways: (1) by inactivating enzymes such as ribonuclease, alkaline phosphatase, catalase, and others; (2) by chelating with a nutrient so that the latter is unavailable; (3) by altering cell permeability; and (4) by replacing a structural element—for example, lithium in place of sodium.

Many nutrient–toxicant interactions exist. A few examples follow. Calcium, iron, and protein interact with lead to reduce absorption and thus to lessen the toxic effects. The presence of selenium protects against the toxicity of mercury and cadmium. When a copper deficiency exists, the susceptibility to toxic reactions from cadmium, mercury, and zinc is increased. A zinc deficiency increases the susceptibility to toxicity of cadmium, copper, and mercury.

Lead is a particularly serious contaminant since it accumulates in the body and results in chronic illness characterized by severe anemia, changes in the arteries and kidneys, and serious effects on the nervous system. A minute quantity of lead occurs naturally in food and is ingested daily, but when the daily intake is 1 mg or more, the eventual accumulations may become toxic. Toddlers who chew lead-based paint from woodwork may ingest as much as 3 mg per day. Deficiencies of calcium and iron increase the amount of lead that is absorbed.

Food becomes contaminated with lead when it is exposed to dust containing lead or when it is kept in containers in which solder, alloys, or enamel containing lead have been used.

Severe mercury poisoning leading to death occurred in Japan some years ago when fish from waters heavily polluted by industrial mercury wastes was eaten. Accidental poisonings also occur when chemicals have been mistaken for flour, powdered milk, or baking powder. In one such instance, 47 deaths resulted when roach powder containing sodium fluoride was mistakenly used as dry milk powder.[4] In another instance boric acid was mistaken for lactic acid for the preparation of infant formulas, again resulting in infant deaths. It goes without saying that insecticides, lye, mothballs, and numerous other poisons should be well labeled, kept away from foodstuffs, and out of the reach of small children.

The metals used in cooking utensils and in food containers have been a source of much controversy. Many studies have shown that glass, stainless steel, aluminum, agate, and tin are suitable containers for food, since these materials are practically insoluble or, when dissolved to a slight degree, are not harmful to health. Acid foods may dissolve some of the tin from cans so that a change of flavor results from the iron underneath the tin coating, but the ingestion of these foods is not harmful. It is recommended that acid foods be transferred from the can to a covered glass container if the food is to be refrigerated after opening.

Radioactive Fallout   People have always been exposed to the radiation of naturally occurring radioisotopes in the environment. Potassium-40 and ^{14}C are the major contaminants of food from natural sources. The danger from these is slight because ^{14}C is absorbed into the body in very small amounts and ^{40}K remains in the body for only short periods of time.

With the advent of the nuclear bomb and nuclear-powered generator plants the potential for harmful exposure has increased. Following a nuclear detonation the radionuclides are ingested by humans by eating contaminated plants or animal foods from animals that have eaten the contaminated plants. Strontium-90 is related to calcium and is deposited chiefly in the bones; ^{137}Ce, like potassium, is distributed throughout the body in the soft tissues; and within 48 hours of ingestion ^{131}I is accounted for in the thyroid gland and in the urine. Excessive deposits of radioactive elements carry the threat of cancer—of the thyroid with ^{131}I, and of the bone with ^{90}Sr.

Each radioisotope has a specific *physical half-life*. This is the amount of time that elapses before half of the element is decayed. The element thus emits radiations to the external environment with consequent exposure of humans, animals, and plants over this pe-

riod of time. Strontium-90 and ^{137}Ce have a physical half-life of 28 years.

The *biologic half-life* refers to the length of time before half of the element is excreted from the body. Some elements are excreted rapidly, thus causing little harm. Strontium-90 is of serious biologic consequence since its rate of turnover is slow in the body, whereas ^{137}Ce has a biologic half-life of 140 days.

The U.S. Public Health Service and the U.S. Department of Agriculture periodically analyze foods from all over the country to determine levels of radioactivity. About one third to one half of the dietary ^{90}Sr is present in milk; however, the high calcium intake helps ensure a preferential use of calcium rather than strontium by the body. The current levels in foods present no risks whatsoever.

Preservation of Foods

Factors Contributing to Food Deterioration and Spoilage   Foods are made unsafe to eat or become aesthetically undesirable or both by the actions of bacteria, yeasts, and molds; by enzymatic action; by chemical or physical changes; and by contact with insects and rodents. In food spoilage these factors often coexist. Unsafe foods do not necessarily show any changes in appearance and palatability, and hence the danger from them is great. Foods that are rancid, moldy, or rotting are less likely to be consumed and therefore may not be a direct threat to health, but the economic waste is considerable.

Temperature and Growth of Organisms.   Bacteria, yeasts, and molds grow rapidly at temperatures of 10° to 60°C (50° to 140°F); within this range the rate of growth increases tenfold for each 10°C (18°F) increase in temperature. Thus, the bacteria produced in a food left at room temperature for 3 or 4 hours can reach astronomical numbers.

Growth of microorganisms is retarded at refrigerator temperatures and is stopped at freezing temperatures. Many molds and some bacteria known as *psychrophils* grow even at refrigerator temperatures, leading to spoilage of food. Pathogenic bacteria do not grow at these temperatures. Many bacteria are not killed by freezing—an important fact to remember when frozen foods are thawed and allowed to stand at room temperatures. (See Figure 17-1.)

Some bacteria known as *thermophils* thrive at relatively high temperatures. They are responsible for the "flat sour" which occurs in some home-canned foods.

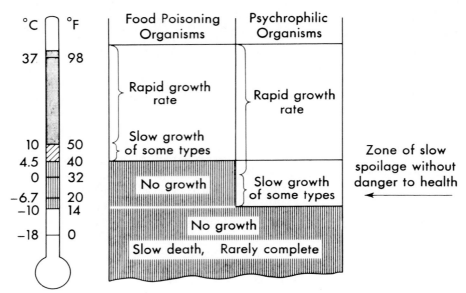

Figure 17-1. Low-temperature limits on growth of food poisoning and psychrophilic organisms. (Courtesy, Dr. Horace K. Burr and the *Journal of the American Medical Association*.)

Many bacteria produce spores that are very resistant to heat. In fact, several hours of boiling do not destroy them. Under favorable conditions such spores will germinate rapidly.

Physical and Chemical Changes. Appearance, texture, flavor, and the chemical constituents of foods are modified by the influence of air, heat, light, moisture, and time. These changes are accelerated by enzyme action and by the presence of minute traces of mineral catalysts such as copper and iron. All plant and animal tissues contain enzymes that are highly active at room temperatures and above.

The rate of chemical change doubles for each 10°C (18°F) rise in temperature. Rancidity of fats is one example of undesirable oxidation and contributes to the deterioration of flavor even in foods that contain only small amounts of fat. Oxidation also leads to loss of ascorbic acid.

Plant and animal tissue fibers are softened, and the surface of cut nonacid fruits is oxidized and becomes darkened as a result of enzyme action, thereby changing the texture, color and nutritive value. Some nutrients may be lost by discarding fluids in which they have been dissolved. The exposure of milk to sunlight leads to a tallowy flavor and loss of riboflavin and vitamin B-6. With storage, changes in texture also occur: sugar may crystallize out of jellies; ice cream becomes gummy and granular; and frozen meats and poultry become dry.

Food Preservation Methods The criteria for successful food preservation, whether it be for a day or two or for months, are these: (1) safety from contamination by pathogenic organisms or toxicity through chemicals; and (2) maintenance of optimum qualities of color, flavor, texture, and nutritive value.

Methods of food preservation that destroy bacteria are *bactericidal*; these include the application of heat by cooking, canning, preserving, and irradiation sterilization. Other methods such as dehydration, freezing, treatment with antibiotics, salting, and pickling retard the growth of bacteria, molds, and yeasts; they are *bacteriostatic*.

Food preservation is accomplished by one or more of these methods:[5]

1. Moisture removal—drying by sun, hot air, vacuum, spray drying, freeze drying: dried fruits, dry milk, instant coffee
2. Acidity control—fermentation, acid addition: yogurt, buttermilk, sauerkraut
3. Chemical processing—salt, sugar, nitrates, sodium benzoate, and other additives: salted fish and meat; jams, jellies, candied fruit; cured meat, fish, and poultry; dried fruits treated with sulfite to prevent discoloration
4. Heat treatment—pasteurization, cooking, blanching, sterilization, ultrahigh-temperature processing
5. Low temperature treatment—refrigeration, freezing, cool storage

6. Irradiation—exposing foods to gamma and x-rays that kill spoilage-causing microoganisms.

Food Preservation by Heat Bacterial destruction by heat depends upon the degree of heat and the length of time it is applied.

Pasteurization. Milk is pasteurized by (1) the *holding* process in which milk is heated to at least 62°C (143°F) and kept at that temperature for at least 30 minutes, or by (2) the *high-temperature short-time* method in which milk is heated to 71°C (160°F) and kept at that temperature for at least 15 seconds.

Pathogenic bacteria are destroyed by pasteurization, but nonpathogenic bacteria remain in the milk. These do not grow rapidly when milk is kept under refrigeration. Milk may be sterilized by boiling as in the preparation of infant formulas or by heat as in the processing of evaporated milk. Ultrasterilized milk that does not require refrigeration is now available in many markets. Once the container is opened the milk must be kept under refrigeration.

Cooking. Boiling of food (100°C) kills bacteria but will not destroy the spores of *Clostridium botulinum* or *perfringens*. Toxins formed by staphylococci are not inactivated even with prolonged boiling, but botulin is destroyed with boiling for 10 minutes. Cooking with a pressure cooker will kill bacteria and also destroy the spores of *Clostridium perfringens* and *botulinum*.

Low-heat cookery as for custards and sauces does not destroy *Salmonella* and other bacteria. Likewise the heat produced in the interior of casseroles and stuffed poultry is inadequate for the destruction of bacteria. Poultry should be stuffed just before it is placed in the oven for roasting. Any leftover stuffing should be removed from the poultry promptly, kept under refrigeration, and used within 24 hours.

Canning. Exact procedures for commercial canning have been developed for each food. Sterilization is brought about by steam under pressure for specified lengths of time.

Home Canning. When foods are canned at home, a pressure cooker should always be used for low-acid foods, including most vegetables, poultry, and meat, in order to destroy bacteria and their heat-resistant spores. Fruits and tomatoes, being acid foods, may be safely canned using the boiling-water bath method.

Nutritive Values of Canned Foods. Commercial processes for canning generally result in optimal nutrient retention. Small losses of the heat labile thiamin and ascorbic acid occur. The greater losses occur when canned foods are held for long periods of time at high temperatures. As much as 25 percent of ascorbic acid and thiamin may be lost from fruits and vegetables stored for a year at 27°C (80°F), but with storage at 18°C (65°F) these losses are reduced to 10 percent. Meats, likewise, lose 20 to 30 percent of their thiamin content after 6 months' storage at 21°C (70°F), but the riboflavin content is not adversely affected. Carotene losses in fruits and vegetables are small even after months of storage. Water-soluble nutrients distribute themselves evenly throughout the solids and liquids; thus, if the solids constitute two thirds of the total, one third of these watersoluble nutrients will be lost if the liquid is not used.

Food Preservation at Cold Temperatures Modern refrigeration has been largely responsible for the tremendous variety of foods available all over the country, in season and out. By means of refrigeration foods can be kept for long periods of time in commercial cold-storage rooms at the proper humidity or transported from coast-to-coast without danger of loss from spoilage or freezing, and they can be kept in the home refrigerator to reduce the number of trips the homemaker makes to the market.

Cool storage is being gradually extended to canned and dehydrated foods to retain optimum color, flavor, and nutritive values.

Freezing. In the quick freezing of foods, bacteria are unable to grow and enzymes are inactivated.

Care and Use of Frozen Foods. Because frozen foods contain bacteria and enzymes in a dormant state, it is essential that foods be maintained at −18°C (0°F), or lower, until they are to be used. Bacteria begin to multiply and enzymes begin to bring about oxidative changes as soon as foods begin to thaw. These changes can be rapid if foods are allowed to stand for some time at room temperature. Fully thawed foods should not be frozen again since further deterioration in quality will occur. Fruits retain their best color if they are thawed in the container in which they are packed. Most vegetables are cooked by dropping the frozen product directly into a small quantity of boiling water and rapidly bringing it to the boiling point. Meat and poultry should be thawed in the refrigerator, and not at room temperature. This requires transfer from the freezer to the refrigerator a day or two in advance of cookery.

Nutritive Values of Frozen Foods.   Before freezing, vegetables must be blanched to inactivate oxidative enzymes. The losses of water-soluble minerals and vitamins can be appreciable with hot-water blanching, but these losses are kept to a minimum with present-day commercial techniques. The nutritive values of frozen foods compare favorably with those of fresh foods. In fact, the vitamin content of food frozen at the peak of quality may be higher than that of fresh food that is overripe or that has remained for hours in a warm market.

Nonacid foods kept for a year at $-18°C$ may lose an appreciable amount of ascorbic acid and thiamin, but the losses are much less when freezer temperature is kept at $-23°$ to $-28°C$. Citrus fruits and juices kept in the freezer for a year lose not more than 6 percent of their ascorbic acid content.

Food Irradiation   The use of ionizing radiation to preserve foods has been studied especially by the U.S. Army for about 40 years. Ionizing radiation includes x-rays, gamma-rays, and beta-rays (high-velocity electrons). Low-dose irradiation can kill insects that infest grains, fruits, and vegetables; can inhibit the sprouting of potatoes and onions; and can retard mold growth as on strawberries. Foods subjected to low-dose irradiation are completely safe to eat and are not changed in appearance or flavor. Irradiation of grains has been suggested as a substitute for spraying grains with EDB. (See page 253.)

High-dose radiation can kill all microorganisms so that foods so treated can be kept in sealed containers for years at room temperature. Such sterilized foods have been used by American astronauts and by some patients such as recipients of organ transplants who are confined to a sterile environment. Meat, poultry, and fish have been successfully sterilized, but undesirable flavor changes occur in dairy products. With high-dose sterilization the vitamin losses are similar to those that occur in canning. Studies on animals have shown no health hazards using high-dose irradiation of feeds.

Each food must be individually tested to determine the appropriate dose of irradiation. The regulation of the use of food irradiation is a responsibility of the Food and Drug Administration under the 1958 Additives Amendment, although irradiation is a process, not an additive. The equipment required for irradiation requires a considerable outlay of capital and thus the use, at least initially as approval is given by FDA, is likely to be limited to large food processors.

Food Additives

An ADDITIVE, broadly defined, is any substance added directly or indirectly to any food product. Additives have been used throughout history, salt and spices being a primary reason for the travels of early explorers from the days of Marco Polo and thereafter. Today about 3,000 substances are classed as additives,[6] but they make up less than 1 percent of the weight of the food we eat. Sugar, corn syrup, and salt account for the largest amount of additives in our food supply by far. Leavening agents, spices, and herbs are used daily in our kitchens, though we may not think of these as additives.

Intentional Additives   An INTENTIONAL ADDITIVE is a substance of known composition that has been added to food to enhance the quality of the food; for example,

1. Improve the nutritional quality by the addition of minerals and/or vitamins
2. Maintain or improve the keeping quality of a product; for example, prevent molding, rancidity
3. Improve texture of the product; for example, use of yeast to give lightness to bread; an emulsifier to keep oil from separating out as in peanut butter or mayonnaise; a stabilizer to prevent crystal formation in ice cream.
4. Make food more appealing in appearance or taste; for example, a red or yellow coloring in a gelatin product; sugar added to sour fruit to improve its taste.

Some additives perform a single function and others perform several. For example, salt is both a preservative and flavoring agent. Ascorbic acid prevents the discoloration of cut fruit and also adds to the nutritive value. Table 17-1 lists some examples of additives and the functions that they perform.

The Nitrite Dilemma   Nitrates and nitrites have been used for centuries in the curing of bacon, frankfurters, sausages, ham, and smoked fish. These compounds impart color and flavor to the product. More important, they protect the product against botulism.

Under certain conditions nitrites can combine with amines that are also present in meat and in the stomach to form NITROSAMINES. Animal studies have shown that nitrosamines are potent carcinogens, although there is no existing evidence that nitrosamines have caused cancer in humans.[7] The formation of nitrosamines is inhibited if ascorbic acid is consumed at the same meal as the nitrite-containing food.

Nitrates occur naturally in water and in many foods: broccoli, beets, carrots, celery, collards, let-

Table 17-1. **Typical Uses of Some Intentional Additives**

Function	Chemical Compounds	Examples of Food
Acids, alkalies, buffers		
Enhance flavor	Acetic acid	Cheese, catsup, corn syrup
	Sodium hydroxide	Pretzel glaze
Leavening	Baking powder, baking soda	Cakes, cookies, quick breads, muffins
Antioxidants		
Prevent darkening	Ascorbic acid	Fruit to be frozen
	Sulfur dioxide	Apples, apricots, peaches to be dried
Prevent rancidity	Butylated hydroxyanisole (BHA); butylated hydroxytoluene (BHT)	Lard, potato chips, meat pies, cereals, crackers
	Lecithin	Margarine, candy
	Tocopherol	Candy, oils
Coloring	Annatto; carotene	Butter, margarine
	Certified food colors	Baked foods, soft drinks
Flavoring (over 300 compounds in use)	Aromatic chemicals, essential oils, spices	
Nutritional fortification	Mineral salts, vitamins	Iodized salt; enriched breads and cereals; fortified milk and margarine; see p. 000.
Preservatives	Sodium chloride	Brined pickles, salted meats
	Sodium benzoate	Dried codfish; maraschino cherries
Inhibit mold	Calcium propionate	Bread, rolls
	Sorbic acid	Cheese wrappers
Sweeteners, nonnutritive	Saccharin; aspartame	Dietetic foods and beverages
Texture	Alum	Firm pickles
Anticaking agents, retain moisture, emulsifiers, give body, jelling, thickening, binding	Disodium orthophosphate	Evaporated milk, cheese
	Mono- and diglycerides	Margarine, chocolate
	Sodium alginate	Cream cheese, ice cream
	Pectin	Jelly, French dressing
Whipping agents	Carbon dioxide	Whipped cream in pressurized can
Yeast foods and dough conditioners	Calcium phosphate; calcium lactate	Bread

tuce, radishes, and spinach. Moreover, saliva also contains nitrates. Whether the elimination of nitrates for the curing of meats is useful remains to be determined. The Food and Drug Administration and the Department of Agriculture continue to study this problem, and have lowered the levels of nitrates that may be used. Irradiation of foods may be an alternative to the use of nitrates. (See page 252.)

Incidental Additives Foods sometimes contain minute traces of a chemical as a result of contact with a substance used in its production, processing, or packaging. Since its presence serves no useful purpose in the final product, such a chemical is considered to be an INCIDENTAL ADDITIVE. For example, food may have picked up a substance from a wrapper or container, either through dissolving it out or by abrasion from the container into the food. Or food may contain a residue of detergents remaining on dishes, or a residue of pesticides used in crop control. Dirt, hairs, and insect fragments are also included in this group.

The farmer uses chemicals that destroy insects, control plant diseases, and kill weeds. Without the use of these pesticides it is doubtful that enough food could be produced to feed the population. Nevertheless, these chemicals, if improperly used, pose some hazards.

Ethylene Dibromide (EDB). A recent example of public concern about a pesticide, EDB has been widely used to spray citrus fruits and grains that are stored in order to reduce pest infestation. In 1984 residues of these sprays were detected in various mixes containing flour, and the products were removed from the market. About 90 percent of the EDB is destroyed in baking. The occasional ingestion of traces of EDB is probably not harmful, but whether there might be a long-term buildup of this pesticide in the tissues so as to produce cancer is not known. The Environmental Protection Agency has now banned the use of EDB on grains and citrus fruits.

Polychlorinated Biphenyls. A group of organic compounds known as polychlorinated biphenyls (PCBs) are widely used in paints, rubber, plastics, asphalt, adhesives, lubricants, and electric insulators. They enter the food chain through industrial accidents or improper disposal. A random sample of people in the United States showed that 30 percent had significant amounts (over 1 ppm) of PCBs in adipose tissue.[8] The cumulative effect is not known.

Monkeys fed diets containing 300 ppm PCBs for 3 months developed hyperplasia of the gastric mucosa together with skin and liver changes.[8] The dosage used was ten times the concentration reported by the Food and Drug Administration present in milk and fish. Environmental control of these compounds is essential, and much study is required to determine the possibility of hazard to humans.

Antibiotics.   Penicillin and tetracycline are widely used in animal foods. They reduce infections in animals and poultry and increase the rate of growth as well as the amount of weight gain per unit of feed consumed. There is a theoretical risk in the use of antibiotics: (1) some persons who consume foods that contain residues of these additives may be allergic to them, and (2) the ingestion of the antibiotic residues may result in bacterial resistance so that treatment of a human infection by such an antibiotic may be unsuccessful.

The American Council on Science and Health in a position statement indicates that "an immediate health hazard is lacking."[9] The Council believes that the restrictions on low-dose antibiotic use are presently not warranted, but there should be review from time to time of the low-dose use of antibiotics in animal feeds.

The pesticide residues remaining on foods should be at levels that do not constitute any danger to health of

---

CASE STUDY 3

Children's Picnic Ends with *Salmonella* Outbreak

For several days the children in the day-care center had been looking forward to the annual family picnic. Each child brought a note home to the parents explaining that hot dogs and beverages would be provided. Each family was asked to bring a favorite salad or dessert to share with the other families.

When the big day finally arrived, the excitement of the children was not dampened in the least by the oppressively hot and humid weather. All kinds of playground equipment awaited the children at the park where the families and staff met for the pot-luck picnic. The excitement was complemented by tasty salads that included spinach–mushroom, potato, and chicken–rice creations, in addition to fruited gelatins and a taco salad with sour cream topping. The youngsters were particularly delighted with all the desserts, which included watermelon, brownies, chocolate chip cookies, angel food cake, and a banana cream pie.

The next morning, however, several children and two staff members were absent from the day-care center. Parents and teachers were calling in with reports of flulike symptoms. The affected people were experiencing varying degrees of headache, nausea, abdominal cramps, and diarrhea.

The director of the center suspected food poisoning and contacted the local health officer. The resulting investigation confirmed the existence of food poisoning caused by *Salmonella*. In response to parent requests, the director of the center invited a dietitian to speak at the next parent group meeting on food safety.

Questions for Case Study
1. What organisms should be considered as possible causes of the illness?
2. On what basis did the health officer suspect that this was a bacterial infection?
3. What differentiates a bacterial infection from a bacterial intoxication?
4. Which of the foods listed in the study were most likely to be contaminated with *Salmonella*?
5. Explain your reasons for selecting these foods as possible causes of the illness.
6. What circumstances might have led to other foods becoming contaminated?
7. One of the parents who had eaten the spinach–mushroom salad wondered whether the mushrooms might have been responsible for the illness. What is the basis for such speculation?
8. What conditions probably contributed to the growth of the salmonella?
9. Why is illness from contaminated food particularly dangerous for young children?
10. List the principal points that you think the dietitian should emphasize when she talks with the parents.

the consumer either immediately or through gradual buildup in the body over a long period of time. It is equally important that there be no appreciable increase from year to year in the concentration of pesticides in the environment to endanger animal, fish, or bird life or to increase the levels in soils and water so that future food supplies contain levels that are toxic. Some pesticides meet these criteria but others do not. The kinds and amounts of pesticides that may be used and the residues that may remain in foods are established by regulations formulated by the Food and Drug Administration, the U.S. Department of Agriculture and the Environmental Protection Agency.

References for the Case Study

Lecos, C.: "Determining When a Food Poses a Hazard," *FDA Consumer*, June 1983, pp. 25–28.
Available from Food Safety and Inspection Service, U.S. Department of Agriculture:
Food-Borne Bacterial Poisoning
Food Safety for the Family
Holiday Food Safety
Safe Brown Bag Lunches
Summertime Food Safety

References

1. Schmidt, A. M.: "Food and Drug Law: A 200-year Perspective," *Nutr. Today*, 10(4):29–32, 1975.
2. Larkin, T.: "Herbs Are Often More Toxic than Magical," *FDA Consumer*, 17(8):15–17, October 1983.
3. Strong, F. M.: "Toxicants Occurring Naturally in Foods," *Nutr. Rev.*, 32:225–31, 1974.
4. Lidbeck, W. L., et al.: "Acute Sodium Fluoride Poisoning," *JAMA*, 121:826–27, 1943.
5. Roberts, T.: "Food Preservation and Nutrition," *Natl. Food Rev.* 20:2–6, February 1983.
6. Lehmann, P.: "More Than You Ever Thought You Would Know about Food Additives," *FDA Consumer*, April 1979.
7. IFT Expert Panel on Food Safety and Nutrition: "Nitrites, Nitrates, and Nitrosamines in Foods—A Dilemma," *J. Food Sci.*, 37: 989–92, 1972.
8. Allen, J. R., and Morback, D. H.: "Polychlorinated Biphenyl- and Triphenyl-induced Gastric Mucosal Hyperplasia in Primates," *Science*, 179:198–99, 1973.
9. *Antibiotics in Animal Feed: A Threat to Human Health?*. Report from American Council on Science and Health, New York, November 1983.

18

Controls for the Safety and Nutritive Value of the Food Supply

You shall not eat anything that dies of itself.

DEUT. 14:21

You shall not have in your bag two kinds of weights, a large and a small. You shall not have in your house two kinds of measures, a large and a small. A full and just weight you shall have, a full and just measure you shall have.

DEUT. 24:13–15

These biblical quotations are but two of the many laws concerning the use of food set down by Moses and others. Throughout history laws have been enacted to protect consumers against fraud and to enhance the safety of the food supply. The most notable advances have occurred in the present century through the passage of food laws by the U.S. Congress and the enforcement of these laws by federal agencies.

The Need for Food Laws

The Changing Food Environment The twentieth-century developments in microbiology have provided the rationale for good practices in handling food and

PUBLIC CONCERNS ABOUT FOOD

Education by various media, advertising, and concern about the environment in which we live have sensitized the public to issues of food and nutrition as never before. People are requesting an accounting from the food industry and from regulatory agencies. The major issue pertains to the right to know what is in the food that is eaten. They want to know what ingredients are present in foods and also the amounts of principal ingredients. They wonder whether enriched, fortified, and fabricated foods are safe and of high nutritional quality. They also are concerned about the amounts and types of fat, cholesterol, sugar, salt and additives that are present in foods. Many seek information on the nutritive values of the product. But they are often confused by the information that appears on labels and don't know how to interpret it. Those who require modified diets are frequently unable to decide whether a given food product is appropriate for their needs.

The consumer has a role to play in legislation and in the regulations that result from the laws pertaining to the food supply. First, there is a need to be informed: to know what is required for an adequate diet; what is essential for a safe food supply; and how to read and interpret the information on labels. Second, the consumer should be alert to new legislation and/or regulations that are proposed, and should make his position known by testimony to the appropriate legislators or agencies. Third, the consumer in his self interest will include a wide variety of foods in his diet, thereby ensuring the intake of the widest assortment and quantity of needed nutrients, as well as minimizing the influence of any potential hazard in a given food.

The sections that follow in this chapter will include discussion of important laws that pertain to food safety and quality, to regulations that apply to the enforcement of these laws, and to the interpretation of the label.

have served as the basis for setting up controls that might be exercised for a safe food supply. The chemist's laboratory has opened hitherto undreamed-of possibilities for variety in the food supply, preservation, and improvement of nutritional quality, but it has also created vast problems in controls from farm, to factory, to warehouse, and to market. Today's farmer fertilizes the soil with products purchased from a chemical plant; dusts and sprays crops; sometimes uses antibiotics and antibacterials to accelerate the growth of animals. The manufacturer chooses from hundreds of chemical products to improve the color, flavor, texture, nutritional quality, and keeping properties of the product. Chemicals of some sort enter into the numerous steps in food production—from the sanitation of the plant machinery to the package in which the food is sold. Without these aids from the chemical industry, this country could not produce its abundant supply of high-quality food.

There are systems developed for the quality grading of food as it is received, complex machinery for handling food from raw product to package, continuous emphasis upon sanitation, and attractiveness of the finished product. The laboratories in such a plant are at the very center of the successful operation. On the one hand, they are concerned with quality control; on the other, they are developing products for tomorrow's market basket.

Food Legislation One of the principal crusaders in the movement to secure legislation for a wholesome food supply was Dr. Harvey W. Wiley, who was a chief chemist in the U.S. Department of Agriculture. Through his writings and public appearances he sought the cooperation of women's groups and was instrumental in the enactment in 1906 of the first "pure food" law, the Food and Drug Act. The law, signed by President Theodore Roosevelt, has been represented by some as the most significant peacetime legislation in the history of the country.

Food, Drug, and Cosmetic Act. With rapid advances in food technology and industry, the manufacture and distribution of food grew increasingly complex and broader in scale so that the original law became inadequate. Many consumer pressures in the 1930s led to the enactment of the Food, Drug, and Cosmetic Act of 1938. The objectives of the law have been summarized as "safe, effective drugs, and cosmetics; pure, wholesome foods; honest labeling and packaging."*

* Larrick, G. P.: "The Role of the Food and Drug Administration in Nutrition," *Am. J. Clin. Nutr.*, 8:377–82, 1960.

Meat and Poultry Inspection Act. The "pure food" law of 1906 did not include meat and meat products. The Meat Inspection Act was passed in 1906, the Poultry Inspection Act in 1957, and the Egg Products Inspection Act in 1970. These laws provide for (1) the inspection of animals intended for slaughter; (2) the inspection of carcasses and all meat and poultry products; (3) enforcement of sanitary regulations; and (4) guarding against the use of harmful preservatives.

Additive Amendments. The Food, Drug, and Cosmetic Act has been amended a number of times to meet new problems of control as they have arisen. Although additives are essential for high-quality food in sufficient supply for a rapidly expanding population, the introduction of thousands of such products on the market necessitates legal controls for safety and usefulness. For such protection, these amendments to the 1938 laws have been enacted:

1954: Pesticides Amendment
1958: Food Additives Amendment, including intentional and incidental additives
1960: Color Additive Amendments

An important regulation in the additives amendment is the Delaney clause. This states that an additive is prohibited if at any level of feeding whatsoever it induces cancer in an experimental animal.

Fair Packaging and Labeling Act. In 1966 the Congress authorized the FDA to set up requirements for complete information in labeling and for packaging that is not deceptive in terms of the contents. This act supplements the 1938 law.

Law Enforcement and Specific Regulations

Responsibility The Food and Drug Administration (FDA) in the Department of Health and Human Services is responsible for the control of food products (except meat, poultry, and eggs) that move in interstate commerce and in import and export trade. The U.S. Department of Agriculture is responsible for enforcing laws pertaining to meat, poultry, and eggs. The Federal Trade Commission protects the consumer by preventing advertising that is false or deceptive or that is claimed to prevent or treat a disease. To avoid inconsistency in advertising and labeling, close cooperation between the several agencies is essential.

The newest of these regulatory agencies is the Environmental Protection Agency, founded in 1970. It develops and enforces standards for the quality of the air and water and for the levels of noise pollution and toxic substances and pesticides in the environment.

U.S. Public Health Service.   One of the concerns of the Public Health Service is the effect of diet on nutritional status and health, and it has sponsored research to make these determinations. The safety of the food supply is another concern that leads to the promulgation of sanitary codes and ordinances. During outbreaks of food poisoning, the Centers for Disease Control conduct tests to determine the source and nature of the poisoning.

The Public Health Service has defined standards for milk production and quality that provide the basis for the codes used in most states and communities. It also certifies interstate milk shippers.

Food Protection Committee.   To study the legitimate uses of chemical additives, the Food Protection Committee was established in 1950 as a permanent committee of the Food and Nutrition Board. The membership of the committee includes specialists who are qualified to establish criteria for the evaluation of additives on the basis of their chemical and physical properties, their toxicologic aspects when tested in several species, and their metabolic and nutritional aspects.

The Food Protection Committee acts as a clearing house for information on pesticides and intentional additives; it reviews the information and makes it available; it assists in the integration and promotion of research on foods; it aids regulatory agencies such as the Food and Drug Administration in the formulation of principles and standardized procedures; it aids in the dissemination of accurate information to the public.

State and Local Regulations.   Food that is produced and sold within state boundaries does not come under control of federal agencies. Therefore, states and communities must establish their own regulations for the safety and quality of foods. The identity of foods, the labeling, and the inspection of plants, markets, and public eating places are subject to controls set up by the state departments of agriculture and health. Some cities and states require periodic medical examination of food handlers. Most of the regulations are patterned after those of federal laws, but considerable variations exist, nevertheless, from state to state.

Functions   Among the many functions, especially of the USDA and FDA are these:

1. Development of regulations to implement the law.
2. Inspection of factories and warehouses to determine compliance with the law: the raw materials used; the manufacturing process; the packaging and storage practices; and plant sanitation.
3. The approval of products for use in manufacture, for example, new additives.
4. Research to determine the physical and chemical characteristics of products; development of methods to detect deviation from standards.
5. Educational programs for the industry and also for consumers.

Standards for Processed Foods   The Food and Drug Administration has published a guide *Good Manufacturing Practices* that describes regulations for sanitation, inspection of materials and finished products for specific food categories.

Adulteration of food has occurred if the food contains any substance injurious to health; it contains any filthy, putrid, or decomposed substance; it is prepared, handled, or stored under unsanitary conditions; diseased animals have been used in preparation; the container is made of a poisonous substance which will render the contents harmful; valuable constituents have been omitted; substitutes have been used to conceal inferiority; it contains colors other than those permitted by law; it contains pesticide residues or additives not recognized as safe.

A *standard of identity* establishes what a food product really is. A product that has been so defined must include specified ingredients, with amounts within designated minimum–maximum ranges. For example, the standard of identity for Cheddar cheese specifies a minimum of 50 percent milk fat (on a moisture-free basis) and not more than 25 percent moisture.

In addition to the required ingredients in a food standard, certain optional ingredients may be used. Any ingredient not mentioned either in the required or optional category is prohibited.

Among the products for which standards of identify have been established are: chocolate and cocoa products; cereal flours and related products; bakery products; milk and cream; cheese and cheese products; frozen desserts; dressings for foods—mayonnaise, French dressing, salad dressing; canned fruit and canned fruit juices; fruit butters—jellies, preserves; shellfish; canned tuna; eggs and egg products; oleomargarine—margarine; vegetables and vegetable products.

Standards of quality indicate the minimum quality below which foods must not fall. Foods that do not meet the quality specifications must be labeled "Below Standard in Quality" followed by a statement such as "Good Food—Not High Grade" or "Excessively Broken," and so on. Canned foods that do not meet standards of quality are seldom seen on the market.

Standards for fill aim to protect the customer against deception through the use of containers that appear to contain more food than they actually do. Specifications are set up for foods that tend to shake down in the package, or for number of pieces of food within a container.

Standards for Meat, Poultry, and Eggs. The Department of Agriculture has authority to seize meat and poultry products that are moved illegally or that are adulterated or misbranded after leaving official premises. An important aspect of the laws permits a cooperative arrangement between state and federal inspection programs, thus providing better protection for the consumer for meat products sold within the state.

Federal inspection stamps are placed on the surface of an animal carcass if the meat is wholesome, declaring "U.S. Inspected and Passed." The flesh of an animal that is diseased is stamped "Inspected and Condemned" and the carcass must be destroyed or may be used for nonfood purposes if warranted.

Additives The Additives Amendment defines what an additive is and authorizes the Food and Drug Administration to issue permission to the food manufacturer to use the additive under specified conditions.

The GRAS List. At the time the Food Additives Amendment was enacted, about 600 substances were excluded from testing since they had been used over long periods of time, and they were "generally recognized as safe" (GRAS). Among the items on the GRAS list are salt, baking powder, baking soda, spices, and minerals and vitamins for nutritional purposes as well as preservatives, flavorings, and so on.

Cyclamate, a widely used noncaloric sweetening agent in the 1960s, was included in the GRAS list. But a Canadian study had shown that rats developed bladder cancers when given huge doses of cyclamate. Based on the Delaney clause it was necessary to remove cyclamate from the GRAS list and to ban its use. Since that time the National Academy of Sciences has been conducting a thorough study of the items on the GRAS list.[1] They are retained or removed from the list according to the findings.

Animal studies showed saccharin to be weakly carcinogenic. To comply with the Delaney clause it was necessary for FDA to issue a ban on its use. But saccharin had been used for many decades and there was

a great public outcry against this ban. Therefore, Congress extended the time that it could be used. The label for any product containing saccharin must now include the following statement: "Use of this product may be hazardous to your health. This product contains saccharin, which has been determined to cause cancer in laboratory animals."

Another sweetener, *aspartame*, was approved by the Food and Drug Administration in 1981. It is about 180 times as sweet as sugar. In many products currently on the market aspartame is combined with small amounts of saccharin.

Antibiotics and Antibacterials. The FDA requires animal drug manufacturers to test the safety and efficacy of antibiotics and antibacterials that are used in animal feeds. (See the following.) The FDA establishes tolerance levels and conditions for use, and is responsible for ensuring that livestock and poultry producers and manufacturers of drugs and feeds comply with the law. An important function of the FDA is to develop educational programs for drug manufacturers, farmers that produce animals, and meat packing plants.

Introduction of a New Additive. Before an additive may be marketed approval must be secured from the Food and Drug Administration, which has spelled out in some detail the requirements that must be met. Essentially, the law places the burden of proof for usefulness and safety of a food additive upon the manufacturer, who is required to submit full data which includes name, chemical properties, methods for manufacture, quantities to be used, the conditions for use, the effect of additions on the food, methods for detecting residues in foods, safety, and recommended tolerances. Data pertaining to safety must include toxicity tests on two or more species of animals, usually for a 2-year period; estimates of the maximum amounts that might be consumed in a day; and the cumulative effects on the body.

The Food and Drug Administration may conduct further tests after examination of the manufacturer's data. Approval will include specific limits for amounts and conditions of use. The tolerance level for a proposed additive is set at "1/100 of the maximum amount demonstrated to be without harm to the experimental animals." If a request for use of an additive is denied, the manufacturer may appeal the decision, submit additional data, and request a hearing.

Pesticide Regulation Pesticide residues sometimes remain on foods at the time of purchase. What are the tolerable limits for such residues? Industrial pollutants may contaminate soil and water as demonstrated some years ago when some fish contained mercury in excess of tolerances.

The 1954 Miller Pesticide Amendment provided for the establishment of acceptable tolerances for residues on foods. The law provides that the manufacturer must establish to the U.S. Department of Agriculture the usefulness of the product and to the Food and Drug Administration the safety of the product. More than 2,000 tolerance levels for pesticides have been established by the FDA. The use of pesticides is of worldwide importance for crop yields can be greatly increased, so that populations everywhere can more nearly meet their nutritional requirements. Therefore, the World Health Organization (WHO) and the Food and Agriculture Organization (FAO) of the United Nations have also established criteria for the use of pesticides and acceptable daily intakes of residues.

The Food Label

Regulations Under the regulations applicable to the Fair Packaging and Labeling Act, the label most provide the following information:

1. The common name of the product such as *peaches* or *beets*; the form of packing such as "whole," "sliced," or "chopped."
2. The name and address of the manufacturer, packer, or distributor.
3. The net contents in terms of standard measures.
4. The size of serving portion if the number of servings is stated.
5. If ingredient listing is required, the ingredients shall be listed by common name in decreasing order of prominence.

Misbranding Foods are misbranded if the label is false or misleading; the food is sold under another name; imitations are not clearly indicated; the size of the container is misleading; statement of weight, measure, or count is not given or is wrong; manufacturer, packer, or distributor is not listed on the package forms; it is below standard without indication of substandard quality on the label; it fails to list nutrient information when nutrients have been added or when claims are made for nutritional properties; it fails to list artificial colorings, flavorings, and preservatives.

Open-Date Labeling There are no federal regulations that pertain to date labeling. The practices vary from state to state. Food processors are gradually replacing private codes with one of these methods of date labeling:

Date when product was packed—usually applied to foods that have a long shelf life
Last date at which a product should be sold—usually used for perishable foods such as cold cuts and milk
Last date at which quality of the product can be assured

Universal Product Code Labels on many packaged foods now include a symbol unique for each product that consists of a linear bar system and a 10-digit number. These codes are being used in some supermarkets at the checkout counter. The code is placed over a scanner that reads the line pattern and feeds it into a computer coupled with a cash register. As each food is checked out, the description of the item and the price is printed on the customer's receipt. The system also maintains a constant inventory for each product.

Food Fortification and Fabrication

The central reason for adding nutrients to foods is to enhance the nutritive value of a product so that the nutrient intake of the population will be at levels that promote better health.

Definitions and Purposes ENRICHMENT is a "quantitative increase in content of one or more important nutrients present in lower than desirable amounts."* Generally it has included the addition of thiamin, riboflavin, niacin, and iron to flour and grain products.

FORTIFICATION is the "addition to a food of significant quantities of a nutrient that was initially not present in the food."* Milk fortified with vitamin D, margarine fortified with vitamin A, and salt fortified with iodine are examples.

RESTORATION is the "addition of nutrients to conventional foods in order to restore the level of those nutrients that were present naturally but have been destroyed or lost in processing."*

General Policies The Food and Nutrition Board of the National Research Council and the Council on Foods and Nutrition of the American Medical Association adopted jointly a statement of general policy re-

* Darby, W. J., and Hambraeus, L.: "Proposed Nutritional Guidelines for Utilization of Industrially Produced Nutrients," *Nutr. Rev.*, 36:65–71, 1974.

garding addition of specific nutrients to foods. They endorse

> The enrichment of flour, bread, degerminated cornmeal, corn grits, whole-grain cornmeal, white rice, and certain other cereal grain products with thiamin, riboflavin, niacin, and iron; the addition of vitamin D to milk, fluid skim milk, and nonfat dry milk; the addition of vitamin A to margarine, fluid skim milk, and nonfat dry milk; and the addition of iodine to table salt. The protective action of fluoride against dental caries is recognized and the standardized addition of fluoride to water in areas in which the water supply has a low fluoride content is endorsed. *

The Food and Nutrition Board has developed these guidelines for the improvement of conventional foods by nutrient additions:

1. The potential intake of a nutrient considered for addition to food should be judged to be below a desirable quantity in the diets of a significant number of people.
2. The food that is to carry the nutrient should be consumed by the segment of the population in need, and the added nutrient should make an important contribution to the diet.
3. The addition of the nutrient should not create a dietary imbalance.
4. The nutrient added should be stable under customary conditions of storage and use.
5. The nutrient should be physiologically available from the food.
6. There should be reasonable assurance that an excessive intake to a level of toxicity will not occur.
7. The additional cost should be reasonable for the intended consumer. †

Food Fabrication Food technologists have developed many products that are substitutes for conventional foods such as nondairy creamer, margarine, instant breakfast drink, imitation milk, and soy protein products that resemble meat. Other products are formulations for special purposes such as infant formulas, tube feedings, and substitute or supplementary feedings for modified diets.

A food must be labeled *imitation* if it resembles another food but is inferior in nutritive value to the food that it replaces in the diet. Nutritional inferiority is defined as a reduction in the amount of an essential nutrient such as protein, minerals, or vitamins when compared with the food it replaces. Thus, analyses of imitation low-fat dry milk showed that the protein

content was only one third to one half as much as that in regular milk.[2] The imitation product also supplied less calcium, phosphorus, magnesium, zinc, thiamin, and niacin equivalents. Since milk is an important source of these nutrients, the substitution of imitation milk on a regular basis could compromise nutritional adequacy. Another example: an orange-flavored instant breakfast drink supplies the vitamin C and caloric levels of orange juice but is not necessarily fortified with potassium, vitamin A, thiamin, and folacin—all of which are supplied by orange juice.[2]

Nutritional quality guidelines have been developed for frozen TV dinners, breakfast cereals, main dishes such as macaroni and cheese, vitamin C-fortified fruit or vegetable juices, and meal replacements. For example, if a product such as a frozen dinner replaces a meal, it should furnish 25 to 50 percent of the daily nutrient needs. Fabricated foods that are analogs of conventional foods should supply the same variety and quantities of the essential nutrients that are present in the foods they replace.[3]

Nutrition Labeling

Purposes Served The principal reason for nutrition labeling is that the consumer has a right to know what is in the foods being purchased in order to be able to make better decisions for personal well-being and that of his or her children. A consumer can compare one product with another to determine which product offers the best nutritive values for the money. One important result of such comparisons is that the consumer gradually becomes aware of the good and poor sources of nutrients. Labeling also leads food processors to be constantly aware of the nutritive values of the foods that they produce. Nutrition labeling is a useful teaching tool in the classroom and in education of the public. Labeling will help persons who require modified diets to select those foods appropriate for their needs. One urgent reason for labeling is the identification of the nutritive values of the numerous fabricated foods that food technology has made possible. With such information the consumer can decide whether the fabricated food is an appropriate replacement for an ordinary food.

The Labeling Standard For labeling purposes the FDA has developed the U.S. Recommended Dietary Allowances (USRDA). (See Table 18-1.) There are four standards:

Adults and childen over 4 years; this standard will be used for most food labeling

---

* "General Policies in Regard to Improvement of Nutritive Quality of Foods," *Nutr. Rev.*, 31:324–26, 1973.
† "Proposed Nutritional Guidelines," p. 69.

Table 18-1.   United States Recommended Daily Allowances (USRDA) for Labeling Purposes

Nutrients	Adults and Children (4 years or older)	Pregnant or Lactating Women	Infants (to 12 months)	Children (under 4 years)
Mandatory				
Protein—quality equal to or greater than that of casein, g	45	45	18	20
Protein—quality less than that of casein, g	65	65	25	28
Vitamin A, IU	5,000	8,000	1,500	2,500
Vitamin C, mg	60	60	35	40
Thiamin, mg	1.5	1.7	0.5	0.7
Riboflavin, mg	1.7	2.0	0.6	0.8
Niacin, mg	20	20	8	9
Calcium, mg	1,000	1,300	600	800
Iron, mg	18	18	15	10
Optional				
Vitamin D, IU	400	400	400	400
Vitamin E, IU	30	30	5	10
Vitamin B-6, mg	2.0	2.5	0.4	0.7
Folacin, mg	0.4	0.8	0.1	0.2
Vitamin B-12, μg	6	8	2	3
Phosphorus, mg	1,000	1,300	500	800
Iodine, μg	150	150	45	70
Magnesium, mg	400	450	70	200
Zinc, mg	15	15	5	8
Copper, mg	2	2	0.6	1
Biotin, mg	0.3	0.3	0.05	0.15
Pantothenic acid, mg	10	10	3	5

Pregnant and lactating women, with reference especially to mineral and vitamin supplements that are recommended

Infants under 12 months

Children under 4 years with special reference to labeling for baby foods and mineral–vitamin supplements.

The USRDA are intended for labeling purposes only. They should not be confused with the RDA of the Food and Nutrition Board. For labeling purposes it was not practical to have separate standards for each of the 17 age–sex categories. Moreover, the RDA are revised at approximately 5-year intervals so that label changes based on such revisions would be confusing to the consumer and costly to manufacturers.

The USRDA for adults and children over 4 years of age is based on the highest level for a given nutrient (usually the adult male) in the 1968 RDAs. For example, the vitamin A level of 5,000 IU for the adult male was adopted; the iron level of 18 mg for the female was chosen.

Two standards are given for protein. When the quality of protein is equivalent to that found in ca-

sein, the standard has been set at 45 g; this would include milk, eggs, poultry, meat, and fish, and also combinations of vegetable protein that equal casein in value. Single-plant protein foods or combinations of plant foods that have a quality less than that of casein are evaluated at a higher standard—65 g.

For healthy adults the standards afford a margin of 30 to 50 percent to allow for individual variations. Many adults need only two thirds to three fourths of the USRDA and many children about half. The standards include some nutrients not listed in the 1968 recommended dietary allowances but for which requirements have been estimated. The nutrient information listed by the manufacturer on a label must be based upon laboratory analyses of the product; calculations of nutritive values are not adequate.

Mandatory and Optional Labeling   Labeling for nutrition information is mandatory for (1) any food to which a nutrient has been added—enrichment, fortification, or restoration, and (2) any food for which a claim is made for nutritional properties either on the label or in advertising. All foods for special dietary use require labeling.

Manufacturers may voluntarily provide nutrition labeling for products that are not enriched or for which no nutritional properties are claimed. By 1978 it was estimated that 44 percent of the dollar volume in retail stores for packaged processed foods carried nutrient labeling.[4] If nutrition labeling is used, it must follow a specified format (see Figure 18-1):

1. Serving size and number of servings in container
2. Calories in one serving
3. Protein, carbohydrate, and fat in grams per serving
4. Percentages of the USRDA provided by one serving for protein, vitamins A and C, thiamin, riboflavin, niacin, calcium, and iron

Optional vitamins and minerals may also be declared on the label. When they are declared they shall be stated in the percentages of the USRDA for these nutrients. Except where claims are made for specific nutritional properties, the declaration of cholesterol and fatty acids is optional. When the information is included, it shall list the following:

1. Percentage of calories from fat
2. Amounts of saturated and polyunsaturated fatty acids in grams per serving
3. Amount of cholesterol in milligrams per serving and per 100 g of food

Special Dietary Foods Full nutritional labeling is mandatory for any food that claims a use in modified diets; for example, fat controlled, diabetic, weight control, or sodium restricted.

A food may be called "low calorie" only if it provides 40 kcal or less per serving, and if it has a caloric density of no more than 0.4 kcal per g.

A food may be called "reduced calorie" only if the food is not nutritionally inferior to the compared food and the calories are at least one third lower than the food with which it is compared.

Any food that contains a nonnutritive sweetener must be labeled to indicate such use. If a food contains both a caloric and nonnutritive sweetener, both must be indicated.

A food represented for use in diabetic diets, in addition to nutritional labeling, must include the following statement: "Diabetics: This product may be useful in your diet on the advice of a physician. This food is not a reduced calorie food." The statement is not required on foods that are labeled for reduced calories.

Labeling for the sodium content of foods, effective after July 1985, must be stated in milligrams per serving of food for all products that carry a nutrition label as well as for products that do not carry a nutrition label but for which claims are made for sodium. The following are the standards required for various labeling claims:

"Sodium free"—less than 5 mg per serving
"Very low sodium"—35 mg or less per serving
"Low sodium"—140 mg or less per serving
"Reduced sodium"—processed to reduce the usual level of sodium by 75 percent

Figure 18-1. Regulations for nutrition labeling are established by the Food and Drug Administration. When nutrition labeling is used, it must provide information on the sodium content of the product but potassium labeling remains voluntary.

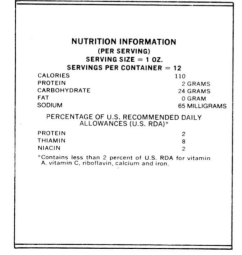

This is the minimum information that must appear on a nutrition label.

A label may include optional listings for cholesterol, fats, and potassium.

"Unsalted"—processed without salt when the food normally is processed with salt

Labeling regulations for special dietary foods include the following prohibitions[5,6]:

1. Any claim or promotional suggestion that products are sufficient in themselves to prevent, treat, or cure disease
2. Claims that a diet of ordinary foods cannot supply adequate nutrients
3. Claims that inadequate or insufficient diet is due to the soil in which it is grown
4. Claims that transportation, storage, or cooking of foods may result in inadequate or deficient diet
5. Nutritional claims for nonnutritive ingredients such as rutin, other bioflavinoids, para-amino-benzoic acid, inositol, and similar ingredients and prohibits their combination with essential nutrients

Problems and Review

1. *Key terms*: adulteration; enrichment; fabricated food; fortification; GRAS list; misbranding; restoration.
2. What is the aim of the Food, Drug, and Cosmetic Act? Under its provisions what is meant by misbranding? Adulteration?
3. What provisions are included in the Meat Inspection Act?
4. Where does the primary responsibility for proving the safety of an additive rest? What information is essential for establishing this safety?
5. What purposes are served by nutrition labeling?
6. Compare the nutritional labeling for three brands of ready-to-eat cereals. Which is the best buy? Why?
7. Compare two margarines that carry nutritional labeling for fat and cholesterol. Which supplies the greater amount of polyunsaturated fatty acids? On the basis of cost is such a difference justified?
8. *Problem*. Watch television advertising for three food products. Note especially the words used to describe products and the claims for the products. Look for labels on the packages of these products in a market. What conclusions can you make regarding this advertising?
9. Determine the governmental agency in your community that is responsible for controlling the sale of milk; the sale of meat within your state; the inspection of public eating places.
10. *Problem*. Prepare a short paper (about 300 words) that describes the activities of any one of the following organizations in promoting a safe food supply: Food Protection Committee; your state department of health; your state department of agriculture; the U.S. Public Health Service; the Federal Trade Commission; the Environmental Protection Agency.

References

1. Irving, G. W.: "Safety Evaluations of the Food Ingredients Called GRAS," *Nutr. Rev.*, **36**:351–56, 1978.
2. Kotula, K., and Briggs, G. M.: "The Nutritional Aspects of Imitation and Substitute Foods," *Nutr. News* (National Dairy Council), **46(1)**, February 1983.
3. Darby, W. J., and Hambraeus, L.: "Proposed Nutritional Guidelines for Utilization of Industrially Produced Nutrients," *Nutr. Rev.*, **36**:65–71, 1978.
4. Reidy, K.: "A New Nutrient Label?" *Natl. Food Rev.*, **22**, Spring 1983, pp. 14–19.
5. Food and Drug Administration: "The New Look in Food Labels," DHEW Pub. (FDA) **73**:2036, Washington, D.C., 1973.
6. Stephenson, M.: "Making Food Labels More Informative," *FDA Consumer*, **9(8)**:13–17, 1975.

Publications for the Consumer

DEUTSCH, R.: *Nutrition Labeling—How It Can Work for You*, The Nutrition Consortium, The American Dietetic Association, Chicago, 1976.

FOOD AND DRUG ADMINISTRATION, U.S. DEPARTMENT OF HEALTH, EDUCATION AND WELFARE:
Additives in Our Foods, Pub. 43.
Metric Measures in Nutrition Labels, Pub. 74-2022.
FDA—What It Is and Does, Pub. 1.
How Safe Is Our Food? Pub. 41.
Nutrition Labeling—Terms You Should Know, Pub. 74-2010.
Nutrition Labels and U.S. RDA, Pub. 73-2042.
We Want You to Know About the Laws Enforced by FDA, Pub. 73-1031.
We Want You to Know About Nutrition Labels on Food, Pub. 74-2039.

PETERKIN, B., et al.: *Nutrition Labeling—Tools for Its Use*, Information Bull. 382, U.S. Department of Agriculture, Washington, D.C., 1975.

19

Nutrition During Pregnancy and Lactation

The object of maternity care is to ensure that every expectant and nursing mother maintains good health, learns the art of child care, has a normal delivery, and bears healthy children. Maternity care in the narrower sense consists in the care of the pregnant woman, her safe delivery, her postnatal care and examination, the care of her newly born infant, and the maintenance of lactation. In the wider sense, it begins much earlier in measures aimed to promote the health and well-being of the young people who are potential parents and to help them to develop the right approach to family life and to the place of the family in the community. It should also include guidance in parentcraft and in problems associated with infertility and family planning.*

* World Health Organization: *The Organization and Administration of Maternal and Child Health Services.* Fifth Report of the World Health Organization Expert Committee on Maternal and Child Care, WHO Tech. Rep. Serv. NO. 428, Geneva, 1969.

IMPORTANT CONCERNS

The position of the World Health Organization just cited is a comprehensive statement of the objective of maternity care. According to the 1984 report by the United States Department of Health and Human Resources, the infant mortality for whites is 10.5 per 1,000 births and for blacks is 20.0 per 1,000 births. The national goal set by the U.S. Surgeon General is to bring the national rate of infant deaths down to 9 per 1000 by the year 1990. Despite steady progress in improving the outcome of pregnancy, several problems still exist.

About 1 million pregnancies (1 in 10 teenage girls) occur each year in adolescents; of these, 600,000 babies are born. A quarter of a million births are to girls 17 years and under; 13,000 are to girls under 15 years. The mortality rate is higher in pregnant adolescents; the younger the girl, the greater the risk.

For nonwhite women the mortality rate is higher and appears to be associated with low income. Nonwhite and white women of similar income show no such difference.

Of all births in the United States, 7.1 percent have a low birth weight (2500 g or less).[1] Low-birth-weight infants are 20 times as likely to die as are their normal-weight counterparts. Almost two thirds of infants who die in the first year are of low birth weight. Even when the low-birth-weight infant survives, there remains a long period of costly care and a continuing concern about establishing normal physical and mental growth.

About two thirds of infant deaths occur within the first month of life. Prematurity, congenital anomalies, anoxia and hypoxia, and difficult labor and delivery account for most of these. The mortality rate is higher in infants born to mothers of low income and to teenage mothers. The differences reflect the adverse effects of poverty, limited education, faulty nutrition, and other environmental factors.

Alcohol, cigarette smoking, and drug addiction increase the likelihood of low birth weight, problems of growth and development, congenital defects, and mental retardation.

Oral contraceptives are widely used. They bring about biochemical changes, but their effects on nutritional status are not yet fully understood.

Physiologic and Biochemical Changes in Pregnancy

Growth Processes   Growth of any organ or tissue involves HYPERPLASIA, an increase in cell number, HYPERTROPHY, an increase in cell size, and development of the INTERCELLULAR MATRIX, the material between the cells. Initially, a single cell divides to form two identical cells; these divide again and again, increasing geometrically in numbers. As hyperplasia continues, the cells gradually increase in size. Then there is rapid deceleration of the increase in cell numbers while the increase in cell size continues.

Each organ is governed by a CRITICAL TIME for its growth and development; that is, the full increase in cell numbers must take place within the given time frame. Any environmental factors that might interfere with such growth could lead to permanent deficiency in the given organ. For example, most of the brain development takes place during fetal life and in the first 5 to 6 months after birth. If there is a severe insult to the developing fetus—for example, severe malnutrition or chronic alcoholism, the optimal development of the brain might be compromised with little if any opportunity for later catchup.

Three Stages of Pregnancy   Pregnancy may be considered in three stages.

1. *The first 2 weeks following conception:* the fertilized ovum becomes implanted in the endometrium of the uterus and rapid cell proliferation occurs. Initially the uterine glands and the outer layers of the germ plasm nourish the embryo, and the placenta begins to develop.
2. *About 2 to 8 weeks:* all the major organs are formed during this period—heart, kidneys, lungs, liver, and skeleton. At the end of 8 weeks the embryo is about 2.5 cm long and weighs about 4 g. Studies on experimental animals have shown that congenital malformations occur during this stage when the pregnant animal has had a diet grossly deficient in vitamin A, riboflavin, vitamin B-6, vitamin B-12, or folacin. However, it is difficult to correlate these findings with malformations that are sometimes seen in human infants.
3. *Eighth week to term:* rapid growth of the fetus occurs. Most of the increase in length of the fetus takes place during the second trimester, while most of the increase in weight occurs in the third trimester. Also during this period the maternal reserves are established in preparation for labor, the puerperium, and the production of milk. During each

of these stages, both cell hyperplasia and hypertrophy are occurring, with the rate of each varying from organ to organ.

The Placenta   There is no direct connection between the mother's circulation and that of the fetus. The placenta is the organ to which the fetus is attached by means of the umbilical cord and by which the transfers between the two circulatory systems occur. The placenta achieves its maximum size early in gestation. Its large surface area is estimated to be between 10 and 13 m^2.

Some nutrients such as water, oxygen, and electrolytes diffuse through the placental membrane to the fetal circulation. Others such as glucose and amino acids require active transport from the maternal to the fetal circulation. Just as nutrients are transported to the fetus, so metabolic wastes from the fetus are returned to the maternal circulation.

The placenta also has synthetic functions and regulates selectively the transfer of nutrients and hormones according to the changing needs of the fetus. Many drugs such as tranquilizers, sedatives, and some antibiotics are not filtered out by the placenta and thus have access to the fetal circulation. The pregnant woman should consult her physician about the possible effects of any prescribed or proprietary drug that she might use.

Undernourishment leads to smaller placental size. Fewer cells are available for the transfer of nutrients and oxygen to the fetus, thus leading to lower birth weight. Also the placenta is less able to dispose of any toxic substances including catabolites, the effects of smoking, and so on.

Hormones   Progesterones, the estrogens, and the gonadotropins are the hormones primarily involved in reproduction. PROGESTERONE is secreted by the corpus luteum and brings about increased secretion by the endometrium, as well as developing glycogen and lipid stores. It also inhibits contraction of the uterine smooth muscle layers thereby preventing expulsion of the embryo. In these ways progesterone has prepared for the implantation of the fertilized ovum and its early growth. Between the second and third months of gestation the formation of progesterone is taken over by the placenta.

GONADOTROPINS are especially concerned with organ formation up to about the fourth month of pregnancy and with fetal growth. Chorionic gonadotropin is produced by the *trophoblastic cells* (outer layer of cells of the dividing ovum) and has the same effects on the corpus luteum as the luteinizing hormone and the luteotropic hormone from the pituitary gland. It keeps the corpus luteum from degenerating and keeps it secreting large quantities of estrogen and progesterone. The endometrium remains in the uterus and is gradually phagocytized by the growing fetal tissues, thereby furnishing a major portion of the nutrition to the fetus during the first weeks of pregnancy.

ESTROGEN production increases appreciably after about the one-hundredth day of gestation. Estrogen and progesterone stimulate the growth of the mammary glands and also inhibit the lactogenic function of the pituitary gland until birth of the infant.

Steroid hormones are produced in greater amounts with the result that water and sodium are more readily retained in the body. The thyroid gland is less active during the first four months of pregnancy, and thereafter is somewhat more active than normal.

Body Fluids During pregnancy a gradual increase in the volume of intracellular and extracellular fluids accounts for several pounds of the total increase in body weight. Late in pregnancy some fluid retention is fairly common.

The total blood volume is increased by as much as one third by the end of pregnancy. With the increase in blood volume, the concentration of serum albumin, hemoglobin, and other blood constituents is reduced. The average hemoglobin level of 13.7 g per 100 ml (range, 12.0 to 15.4 g) for healthy nonpregnant women drops to about 12.0 g per 100 ml despite the ingestion of supplemental iron.[2] Although the concentration of hemoglobin is lower, with the increase in blood volume the total circulating hemoglobin is much greater. A level of 11.0 g hemoglobin per 100 ml blood is considered the border below which true anemia exists.

Gastrointestinal Changes Pregnant women sometimes have cravings for some foods and aversions to others. Whether there is an alteration in taste sensitivity is not known. Especially during the first half of pregnancy some women experience distaste for meat, poultry, sauces flavored with oregano, coffee, soda, beer, wine, and alcoholic spirits.[3] Coffee provokes nausea in some, while the elimination of sodas and alcoholic beverages may be linked more closely with concern for the developing fetus. Women often express cravings for foods such as milk, ice cream, sweets, chocolate candy, and fruits.

Less acid and pepsin are produced by the stomach, and regurgitation of stomach contents into the esophagus (heartburn) sometimes occurs. This may become more pronounced with the increasing pressure of the growing fetus.

The motility of the intestinal tract is reduced, thus contributing to constipation. The absorption of important nutrients, however, is enhanced.

Cardiovascular and Renal Changes An accelerated heart rate and stroke volume lead to increased cardiac output. The flow of blood to the uterus, kidneys, and the skin is increased. The glomerular filtration rate increases to take care of the elimination of additional wastes. Occasionally because of this accelerated filtration rate there may be some glucosuria, which must be distinguished from that occurring in diabetes mellitus. Late in pregnancy with an increase in venous pressure there may be pooling of fluid in the legs. This fluid disappears when the woman is supine, and may account for nocturia. Urinary urgency sometimes occurs late in pregnancy because of the pressure of the fetus against the bladder.

Weight Gain The weight gain is accounted for by the weight of the full-term infant, the increase in size of the uterus, the placenta, amniotic fluid, breast tissue, expanding blood circulation, and the reserves of nitrogen and lipids that help to meet the needs during parturition and lactation. (See Table 19-1.)

The gain in weight for the healthy woman who enters pregnancy at a normal weight for her height and body frame should average 11 kg (24 pounds).[4] Gains in weight vary widely, being somewhat greater in young women than in those who are older, and greater in those who are having their first babies. According to a recent study by Naeye,[5] optimal weight

Table 19-1. **Average Components of Weight Gain in Pregnancy***

	Cumulative Gain (kg) at End of Each Trimester		
	First	Second	Third
Fetus	Negligible	1.0	3.4
Placenta	Negligible	0.3	0.6
Amniotic fluid	Negligible	0.4	1.0
(Fetal subtotal)		(1.7)	(5.0)
Increased uterine size	0.3	0.8	1.0
Increased breast size	0.1	0.3	0.5
Increased blood volume	0.3	1.3	1.5
Increased extracellular fluid	0	0	1.5
(Maternal subtotal)	(0.7)	(2.4)	(4.5)
Total gain accounted for	0.7	4.1	9.5

* Pitkin, R. M., et al.: "Maternal Nutrition. A Selective Review of Clinical Topics," *Obstet. Gynecol.,* **40**:777, 1972.

gain during pregnancy, that is, the weight resulting in the lowest perinatal mortality, was related to the woman's weight prior to pregnancy. These weight gains were 13.6 kg (30 pounds) for the underweight woman; 9.1 kg (20 pounds) for the woman of normal proportions; and 7.3 kg (16 pounds) for the overweight woman.

The pattern of weight gain is as important as the total weight gain. During the first trimester there is little or no increase in weight; from 0.7 to 1.4 kg (1.5 to 3.0 pounds) is appropriate. Thereafter, a steady gain of 0.35 to 0.40 kg (0.8 to 0.9 pounds) per week is desirable. In addition to the expected gains for pregnancy, the adolescent girl should also increase her weight by an amount appropriate for the nonpregnant girl of her age. (See Figure 19-1.)

Faulty patterns of weight gain cannot be fully corrected. For example, a woman who has gained 8 to 10 kg during the first trimester should not be held down to the recommended 11 kg. Such restriction could seriously interfere with the supply of nutrients to the fe-

Figure 19-1. Weight is checked at each clinic visit. After the first trimester the weekly gain should be about 0.8 pound. (Courtesy, School of Nursing, University of Pennsylvania, Philadelphia, and Gates Rhodes, photographer.)

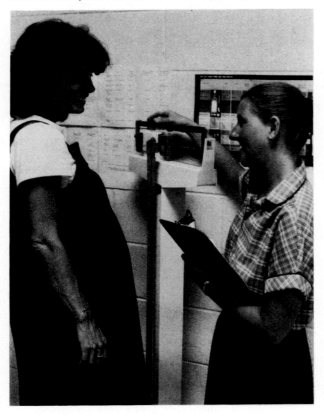

tus. On the other hand, a woman who has gained little during most of her pregnancy cannot expect to make up entirely for this deficiency by considerable increase in weight during the last trimester.

For obese women, restriction of caloric intake to maintain weight or even to lose weight is no longer advocated. Although obesity increases the risk of pregnancy, the correction of it during pregnancy imposes even greater risks on the fetus. If a woman is fasting or is restricting her caloric intake, her blood glucose will be lower, glycogenesis will be reduced, and ketosis will be increased. With a reduced supply of glucose, the fetus is unable to synthesize glycogen and fat. Ketosis may interfere with neurologic development.[6]

Assessment and Nutritional Status During Pregnancy

Factors Influencing the Outcome of Pregnancy On a probability basis, a mother who is well nourished before and during pregnancy is likely to have an uncomplicated pregnancy and to deliver a healthy infant. A poorly nourished woman is more likely to have complications during pregnancy and to bear a small infant in poor physical condition. There are, of course, exceptions. Some well-nourished mothers have problems during pregnancy and may not bear a healthy infant. Also, some poorly nourished mothers may have a successful pregnancy. Such exceptions are understandable when one considers the numerous factors influencing the outcome of pregnancy. (See Figure 19-2.)

Many nutritional and nonnutritional factors interact to determine the outcome of pregnancy. An assessment of the nutritional status of the pregnant woman must include an evaluation of the factors that increase the risk of complications during pregnancy and of a low-birth-weight infant with its attendant high rate of mortality. Among these are the following[2,7]:

Biologic immaturity (under 17 years of age)
High parity (3 or more pregnancies within 2 years)
History of unsuccessful pregnancy: spontaneous abortion, still birth, low-birth-weight infant, toxemia
Multiple births
Small stature
Low prepregnancy weight for height (85 percent or less of standard)
High prepregnancy weight (above 120 percent of standard)
Low weight gain or poor pattern of weight gain during pregnancy
Heavy use of alcohol, cigarettes, or tobacco

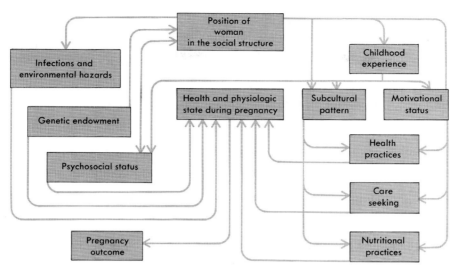

Figure 19-2. Factors influencing pregnancy outcome: a theoretic model. (Reprinted with permission of *Nutrition Today.* Copyright Summer 1970 by *Nutrition Today,* Inc; chart adapted by permission of the Food and Nutrition Board.)

Poor socioeconomic status (women who have income below the poverty level; women who are on local, state, or federal assistance programs)

Faddist: consuming bizarre, nutritionally inadequate diet

Has a chronic disease and requires a modified diet (diabetes mellitus, cardiovascular disease, phenylketonuria)

Low hemoglobin (below 11.0 g per dl) and low hematocrit (below 33 percent)

Premeternal Nutrition Fewer complications in pregnancy, fewer premature births, and healthier babies result when the mother is well nourished prior to pregnancy. The health professional who first sees the pregnant woman can do nothing about past weight status or past reproductive history. However, a recognition of the premeternal risks is useful in planning the strategy for prenatal care. It also brings to the fore the lesson that good nutrition in childhood and the later growing years can improve the prospects for success of the woman as she enters upon pregnancy.

The influence of the quality of premeternal nutrition was strikingly demonstrated in World War II.[8] In Holland pregnant women on reasonably good diets before conception but who were on diets that furnished 1,000 kcal or less during the pregnancy had babies that were shorter and of lower birth weight. However, there was no increase in the rate of still births, prematurity, and malformations. By contrast, in Leningrad women had severely deficient diets before conception as well as during the pregnancy. There was a marked increase in prematurity and still-births. The infants had low vitality, had poor resistance to infection, and did not suckle well. The better results in Holland were ascribed to the better diets the women had enjoyed before conception.

Another study at Vanderbilt University showed that women who weighed 85 percent or less of standard produced smaller babies and prematurity occurred more often. Women who weighed more than 120 percent of the standard had more stillborn infants and a threefold increase in preeclampsia.[9]

Difficult deliveries are more frequent in short than in tall women, according to a study reported from Scotland.[10] The more frequent occurrence of "flat pelvis" in short women was believed to be related to inadequate diet in childhood. Thus, a short stature may mean that a woman has not achieved the full genetic possibilities of body structure because of dietary inadequacy.

Prenatal Nutrition A classic study by Burke in Boston showed that infants born to women who had poor to very poor diets during pregnancy were more likely to be premature, have congenital defects, or be stillborn.[11] Almost invariably in this study women with good diets bore infants in good physical condition. Moreover, toxemia in varying degrees of severity occurred in women with poor diets but not in women with good diets. In the Vanderbilt study cited above, women who had diets that furnished less than 1,500 kcal and less than 50 g protein had greater frequency of complications during pregnancy and of the newborn.[9]

Food supplements provided to high-risk women who had low incomes resulted in increased weight gains and to higher birth weights of the infants.[12] Thus, such supplements are cost effective because they reduce the care required for the low-birth-weight infant in the hospital.

Some Habits that Inferfere with Successful Pregnancy During assessment the health professional should determine whether the client drinks alcoholic beverages, smokes, or eats some abnormal substances (pica).

Alcohol. Although the harmful effects of alcohol have been known for centuries, the description of FETAL ALCOHOL SYNDROME (FAS), first made in the early 1970s, has focused on the seriousness of the problem.[13,14] The syndrome, which is specific for alcohol abuse, is ranked as one of the greatest contributors to mental impairment in the western world. FAS is characterized by subnormal prenatal and postnatal growth, defective craniofacial development, and mental insufficiency. The infant has a small head circumference, small eyes close together, a flat nasal bridge, short nose, and a thin upper lip. There are vertical folds at the inner canthus of the eyes, similar to the folds seen in normal children of Mongolian origin. The grooves between the nose and upper lip are indistinct. None of the symptoms observed in the infant are corrected as the child grows.

Fetal alcohol syndrome occurs in 30 to 45 percent of infants born to chronic heavy users of alcohol. Heavy drinkers consume 3 or more ounces of absolute alcohol daily: 8 beers or 1 pint whisky or more than one bottle wine. They obtain as much as one half their calories from alcohol thereby displacing the protein, minerals, and vitamins they would obtain from food. The potential for an increase in FAS is just beginning to be realized, for of women of child-bearing age one in twenty is a confirmed alcoholic, seven of 10 drink regularly, and one in 10 drink occasionally.

Pregnant women may ask whether one or two cocktails a day, or an occasional alcoholic drink, or even a binge once in awhile is harmful to the fetus. Whether there is a minimum safe intake, or a particular time during pregnancy when there is a greater potential for harm is not known. Until these questions can be answered with authority, clearly the safe advice to the pregnant woman is to abstain from all alcohol.

Tobacco. In the United States and Canada it is estimated that 20 to 40 percent of low-birth-weight incidence is caused by maternal smoking. The greater the number of cigarettes smoked the lower is the infant's birth weight. Nicotine and carbon monoxide act together to produce chronic hypoxia (oxygen deficiency) in the fetus. Smoking is also associated with a greater risk of spontaneous abortion as well as neonatal death for the infant.[1,15]

Maternal complications such as vaginal bleeding are 25 percent more common in women who smoke less than a pack per day and 92 percent more common in women who smoke more than a pack per day. If a woman stops smoking during pregnancy, her chances of having a low-birth-weight baby are no greater than that of the nonsmoking woman.[15]

Caffeine. Coffee, tea, cocoa, chocolate, and cola beverages as well as many over-the-counter drugs contain caffeine, a methylxanthine. When ingested, caffeine readily crosses cell membranes including the placental membranes, is a central nervous system stimulant, and has various other pharmacologic effects. What is the influence of caffeine ingestion on the development of the fetus?

Studies on animals have shown that very high doses of caffeine can result in low birth weight and in some birth defects. When very high doses were given by stomach tube to experimental animals (equal to 56 and 87 cups of coffee by humans) some birth defects such as missing toes were observed.[16] No such defects were observed in the animals when they had intakes equal to 4, 8, and 28 cups of coffee.

Studies on more than 12,000 women failed to show any association between caffeine intake and malformations, gestation period, and low birth weight.[17] Although there is no conclusive evidence that caffeine consumption in moderate amounts has any adverse effects on the fetus, good advice to the pregnant woman should place emphasis on this moderation, especially during the third trimester when caffeine is more slowly metabolized.

Pica. When making a nutritional assessment, the health professional should ask women about any cravings that they have. Ice cream, pickles, milk, and other food cravings can be indulged when they contribute to the nutritional needs of the woman. However, abnormal cravings for substances that have little or no nutritional value, known as PICA, are harmful. Dirt and clay (geophagia), laundry starch (amylophagia), and ice are the most frequent. The amounts consumed vary from a handful of clay to as much as a quart, or a few pieces of laundry starch to a box or more daily.[18] Other substances less frequently ingested include wall plaster, toilet bowl air freshener, charcoal, coffee grounds, cigarette ashes, and baking soda.

The abnormal cravings occur most commonly but not exclusively in blacks of low income in the southern states. They have been variously explained as originating from psychologic, cultural, or physiologic needs, such as relief from nausea, although none of these explanations are fully satisfactory.

Eating these abnormal substances in sizeable amounts is likely to displace some of the foods that are needed. Each box of laundry starch supplies about 1,600 kcal and thus is likely to contribute to excessive weight gain. Among other adverse effects are interference with absorption of nutrients, intestinal blockage as by clay, and lead intoxication from wall plaster.

Pregnancy During Adolescence   Pregnant adolescents are "medically, nutritionally, and socially at risk."[19] The adolescent girl has not achieved her full growth, and superimposed upon her own needs are the considerable requirements for a successful pregnancy. Those who have become pregnant within 2 years of menarche, which normally occurs at about 12.5 years, are at far greater risk than are those who become pregnant at 17 to 19 years. If they have two or more babies during their teens the risk is extremely high. Among the frequent undesirable outcomes for the mother are anemia, preeclampsia and toxemia, premature labor, prolonged labor, and an increased rate of maternal deaths. For the infant the risks are greatly increased for premature birth, low birth weight, and neonatal death.

In addition to the physical risks, the pregnant adolescent often has serious psychologic, social, and economic problems. Some teenagers view the pregnancy favorably because it confers grown-up status and gives them something (the baby) of their very own. But others try to hide the pregnancy as long as they can, often by bizarre dieting and weight loss. When the girl encounters disapproval of her family and friends, she becomes isolated from the support she needs. She may be unable to continue her education and is in no economic position to support herself either during the pregnancy or later after the birth of the child. If she lives with a family that has a low income she may not be able to get the food that she needs for a successful pregnancy.

Most pregnant adolescents do not receive prenatal care until the second or even third trimester, yet are in desperate need of counseling for serious physical, psychologic, and social problems. Many teenagers have poor food habits and are poorly nourished. They often skip meals, eat snack foods of low nutrient density, and pursue unwise weight-reducing regimens. Their intake of calories, calcium, iron, and vitamin A, and sometimes even protein has frequently been inadequate to meet the growth needs of their own bodies. If the pregnant girl is under severe emotional stress, the nutrient balances such as calcium and nitrogen are often negative, even though an adequate diet may be consumed. Many teenagers smoke; of those who do, about two thirds continue to do so during pregnancy.

Nutritional Considerations

The recommended allowances for nutrients are listed in Table 19-2. The recommended intakes for protein, calcium, phosphorus, magnesium, folacin, and vitamin D are increased by 50 percent or more.

Energy   The total caloric cost of producing the fetus, the placenta, and other maternal tissues and of establishing reserves is about 80,000 kcal. For most women an extra allowance of 300 kcal per day during the second and third trimester will permit satisfactory weight gain. An allowance of at least 36 kcal per kg pregnant weight is needed for satisfactory utilization of protein, with 40 kcal per kg being an average intake.[4]

The caloric requirement may vary as much as 800 to 900 kcal, depending on the activity of the woman. Some adolescent pregnant girls are so sedentary that their caloric need is increased by only 150 kcal. But women who have several children and the associated household duties or women whose employment involves body movement require more than the 300 kcal per day increase. The adequacy of the caloric requirement can be evaluated by maintaining a desirable rate of weight gain.

Protein   About 925 g protein is deposited in the fetus and maternal tissues during pregnancy. The rate of deposit in these tissues averages 1.3, 6.1 and 10.7 g per day during the trimesters of pregnancy.[4] Protein may be stored in the body at a uniform rate during the entire pregnancy and is made available to the specialized tissues as needed.

The recommended allowance during pregnancy is increased by 10 g. Nonpregnant girls 15 to 18 years should have an intake of 0.8 protein per kg, and girls 11 to 14 years an intake of 0.9 g per kg. To this allowance, an additional 10 g protein per day should be included during pregnancy.

Minerals   The efficiency of absorption of minerals such as calcium and iron improves during pregnancy,

Table 19-2. Recommended Dietary Allowances Before and During Pregnancy and Lactation*

Nutrient	11–14 Years	15–18 Years	19–24 Years	25–50 Years	Pregnancy	Lactation
Energy, kcal	2,200	2,200	2,200	2,200	+300	+500
Protein, g	46	44	46	50	+10	+15
Vitamin A						
RE	800	800	800	800	+500	+400
IU	4,000	4,000	4,000	4,000	+2,500	+2,000
Vitamin D, μg	10	10	10	5	+5	+5
Vitamin E, mg α-TE	8	8	8	8	+2	+4
Ascorbic acid, mg	50	60	60	60	+10	+25
Thiamin, mg	1.1	1.1	1.1	1.1	+0.4	+0.5
Riboflavin, mg	1.3	1.3	1.3	1.3	+0.3	+0.5
Niacin, mg equiv.	15	15	15	15	+2	+5
Vitamin B-6, mg	1.4	1.5	1.6	1.6	+0.6	+0.5
Folacin, μg	150	180	180	180	+220	+100
Vitamin B-12, μg	2.0	2.0	2.0	2.0	+0.2	+0.6
Calcium, mg	1,200	1,200	1,200	800	+400	+400
Phosphorus, mg	1,200	1,200	1,200	800	+400	+400
Magnesium, mg	280	300	280	280	+40	+75
Iron, mg	15	15	15	15	†	†
Zinc, mg	12	12	12	12	+3	+7
Iodine, μg	150	150	150	150	+25	+50

*Recommended Dietary Allowances, 10th ed. Food and Nutrition Board, National Academy of Sciences—National Research Council, Washington, D.C., 1989.
†Supplemental iron, 30–60 mg per day, is recommended.

but the demands of the fetus and other developing tissues necessitate increases in the diet during the second and third trimester. The full-term fetus contains about 28 g calcium. Some calcium and phosphorus deposition takes place early in pregnancy, but most of the calcification of bones occurs during the last 2 months of pregnancy. The first set of teeth begins to form about the eighth week of prenatal life, and they are well formed by the end of the prenatal period. The 6-year molars, which are the first permanent teeth to erupt, begin to calcify just before birth.

If the mobile reserve of calcium is lacking in the mother, the demands of the fetus can be met, perhaps inadequately, only at severe expense to the mother. For many women it is advisable to increase the calcium intake early in pregnancy even though fetal calcification does not occur until later. The phosphorus allowance should be about equal to that for calcium and will be readily supplied through the calcium-rich and protein-rich foods.

Iron. The prematernal store of iron is about 300 mg or less. For women who have had several pregnancies in rather close succession, the stores are especially depleted. With the cessation of menstruation during pregnancy there is a saving of 120 to 240 mg iron.

Against this saving and the iron stores of the mother are needs for about 300 mg for the full-term fetus, about 500 mg in anticipation of the expanding blood volume and the losses at delivery, and about 300 mg through normal excretion from the skin, hair, urine, and stools. The net need throughout the pregnancy is thus about 1,000 to 1,200 mg, or a daily average absorption of 3.5 to 4 mg. Many factors determine the bioavailability of iron in the diet. (See Chapter 9.) But assuming a 10 to 15 percent rate of absorption, the diet would need to contain 20 to 40 mg per day. Since well-chosen diets furnish only about 6 mg per 1,000 kcal, it becomes evident that the iron needs could be met from diet only if the caloric intake were high. There is wide agreement that an iron supplement furnishing 30 to 60 mg per day be prescribed, especially for the second and third trimesters and during the first month after delivery.

Zinc. Intakes of zinc by pregnant women, whether of moderate or low income, are likely to be about half of the recommended allowance of 20 mg.[20,21] To achieve the recommended allowance the diet would need to be very high in both protein and calories. Zinc is known to be important for normal growth. However there is no firm evidence that the levels of zinc usually provided by well-chosen diets are inadequate to meet maternal and fetal needs, even though such diets do not furnish the recommended allowance. Whether a zinc supplement is indicated has not been established.

Iodine. The daily allowance of 175μg iodine is easily met by using iodized salt. If sodium restriction is required for any reason, the physician may prescribe a supplement.

Sodium. During pregnancy the sodium requirement increases to take care of fetal needs, the enlarging maternal tissues, and the expanding blood volume. The homeostatic mechanisms spare sodium loss that might otherwise occur because of the increased glomerular filtration rate. There is no convincing evidence that sodium restriction has any effect on the incidence of preeclampsia. The woman should be permitted to salt food to her taste.

Vitamins The thiamin, riboflavin, and niacin allowances are slightly increased to correspond to the increase in calories. There is also an increased allowance for vitamins A and D.

Folacin deficiency manifested as megaloblastic anemia occurs occasionally in women whose dietary intakes have been low. The recommended allowance is 400 μg, a level that can be easily achieved by food selection. An oral supplement is not needed with a well chosen diet.

Blood levels of vitamin B-6 are often low in pregnant women. Although supplementation with vitamin B-6 will restore blood levels to the normal range, there is no evidence that such supplementation confers any physiologic advantage.

DIETARY COUNSELING

Attitudes Toward Counseling Although most women believe strongly that diet is important for a successful outcome of pregnancy, many of them do not feel the need for dietary counseling.[22] Negative attitudes are expressed in this way: "it makes you feel bad"; "difficult to follow"; "like being sent to the principal"; "feel guilty." Women especially view the dietary advice given by physicians as being restrictive inasmuch as recommendations are still being made for caloric and sodium restriction. Women who have the least education and the least income often do not attend classes concerning prenatal care for a variety of reasons. Obviously, the dietary counselor must give advice that emphasizes the positive aspects of diet, real-

istic suggestions for food choices according to available income, and adaptations to individual needs.

Dietary counseling of the adolescent is especially important but not always well accepted. The counselor must be sensitive to the adolescent's needs and be supportive. With a nonjudgmental approach the counselor can show the teenager how to improve her diet for her own physical wellbeing and that of her baby. An interdisciplinary approach through an educational component within the school curriculum, together with prenatal care and counseling, delivery, family planning and child care can be effective.[19]

The Basic Diet The basic diet plan (Table 4-1) furnishes about half of the calories needed by the pregnant woman and provides ample amounts of protein, vitamin A, and ascorbic acid. The addition of 1 to 2 cups milk ensures satisfactory intakes of calcium, thiamin, and riboflavin as well as additional protein. (See Table 19-3 and Figure 19-3.)

Good sources of vitamin B-6, folacin, magnesium, iron, and zinc should be emphasized, since the diets of many pregnant women do not meet the recommended allowances.

The kinds of foods and meal patterns for some ethnic groups—for example, Asians, Hispanics, and blacks, often differ considerably from the typical middle class American diet. The counselor must determine what differences exist, and make recommendations that are compatible with the client's habits. Some of these women may be lactose intolerant, and should be advised about the use of milk treated with lactase and of other calcium-rich sources.

Lacto- and lacto-ovo-vegetarians can provide high-quality protein at each meal without difficulty. Strict vegetarians need to know the complementary value of plant foods and the need to supply these at each meal.

Supplements to Diet Many physicians routinely prescribe multivitamin-mineral supplements to pregnant women. For women who are well nourished, vitamin-mineral supplementation does not change the blood levels of various nutrients.[23] When the nutritional status is poor, the primary emphasis should be placed on dietary improvement. In addition, a supplement may be prescribed to hasten the improvement of nutritional status.

Iron supplementation—30 to 60 mg per day—is recommended, since even a carefully planned diet cannot meet both the maternal and fetal needs for iron. (See page 272.) Unfortunately, many women do not take the iron because of nausea, constipation, or, in some cases, diarrhea.[22] Thus, the die-

Table 19-3. **Food Allowances for Pregnancy and Lactation**

	Pregnant Woman	Pregnant Teenage Girl	Lactating Woman
Milk, whole or low-fat	3–4 cups	4–5 cups	4–5 cups
Meat, fish, poultry (liver once a week), cooked weight	4 ounces	4 ounces	4 ounces
Eggs	3 to 4 per week	3 to 4 per week	3 to 4 per week
Vegetables, including			
Dark green leafy or deep yellow	½ cup	½ cup	½ cup
Potato	1 medium	1 medium	1 medium
Other vegetables	½–1 cup	½–1 cup	½–1 cup
One vegetable to be raw each day			
Fruits, including			
Citrus	1 serving	1 serving	1 serving
Other fruit	1 serving	1 serving	1 serving
Cereal, whole grain or enriched	1 serving	1 serving	1 serving
Bread, whole grain or enriched	4 slices	4 slices	4 slices
Butter or fortified margarine	To meet caloric needs	To meet caloric needs	To meet caloric needs
Desserts, cooking fats, sugar, sweets			
An iron supplement is usually prescribed.			
Iodized salt			

Figure 19-3. The Basic Diet (page 38) furnishes sufficient protein, riboflavin, and ascorbic acid for the pregnant woman. It also provides ample amounts of vitamin A and niacin (not shown in the chart). The addition of 1 to 2 cups of milk supplies the needed calcium as well as additional protein and riboflavin. The iron intake can be increased by including liver weekly and by eating more meat, dark green leafy vegetables, and enriched bread. An iron supplement prescribed by the physician will be less costly and also helps the woman to keep her caloric intake at the desired level.

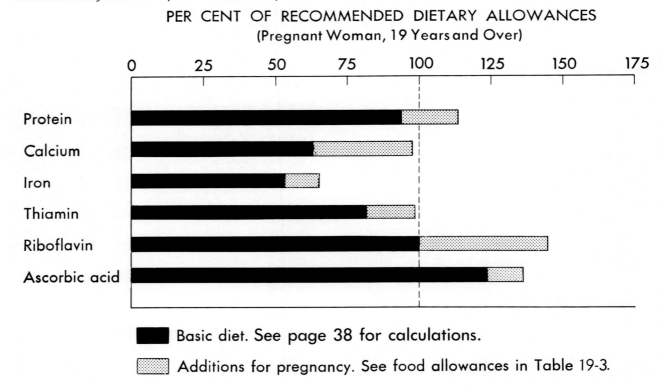

PER CENT OF RECOMMENDED DIETARY ALLOWANCES
(Pregnant Woman, 19 Years and Over)

■ Basic diet. See page 38 for calculations.

▨ Additions for pregnancy. See food allowances in Table 19-3.

tary counselor should monitor and promote compliance by explaining the need for iron and by suggesting the correction of constipation through fiber and fluid intake. (See the following.)

When there is biochemical and clinical evidence of deficiency, a supplement of folacin (200 to 400 μg) may be recommended. A calcium supplement is required only for those who have intolerance to milk or who are strict vegetarians. Vitamin B-12 supplementation is required for strict vegetarians.

Nutrition Programs The Supplementary Food Program for Women, Infants, and Children (WIC) administered by the Food and Nutrition Services of the U.S. Department of Agriculture and available in designated health centers and clinics throughout the country is intended for pregnant women who are at risk and who qualify on the basis of low income. Nutritional anemia, a history of miscarriage or premature births, underweight, obesity, or poor food habits place women in the at-risk category. The supplemental foods are available throughout pregnancy and for 6 months postpartum; for the lactating woman they are available for 1 year. The foods provided are milk and cheese, iron-fortified cereals, eggs, and vitamin C-rich fruit or vegetable juices.

The Maternal and Infant Care Projects (MIC) provide a comprehensive range of prenatal services, including screening for nutritional problems and dietary counseling. Eligible clients may be referred to the WIC program for supplemental foods or to the Food Stamp Program.

Complications of Pregnancy

Mild Nausea and Vomiting During the first trimester, the physiologic and biochemical balances are often disturbed, possibly because of excessive hormone production. Gastrointestinal upsets, including loss of appetite, nausea, and vomiting, are relatively frequent; loss of weight occasionally takes place because of an inability to eat sufficient food.

Mild early morning nausea may usually be overcome by the use of high-carbohydrate foods such as crackers, jelly, hard candies, and dry toast before arising. Frequent small meals rather than three large ones are preferable. Fluids should be taken between meals rather than at mealtime. Fatty, rich foods such as pastries, desserts, fried foods, excessive seasoning, coffee in large amounts, and strongly flavored vegetables may be restricted or eliminated if the nausea persists or if the patient complains of heartburn or gastric distress.

Constipation The occurrence of constipation especially during the latter half of pregnancy is common. The amount of pressure exerted by the developing fetus on the digestive tract, the limitation of exercise, and insufficient bulk may be contributing factors. The normal diet outlined in Table 19–3 provides a liberal allowance of whole-grain cereals, fruits, and vegetables, and consequently of fiber. It is also necessary to stress the importance of adequate fluid intake and of regular habits of exercise, elimination, sleep, and recreation.

Anemia About 15 to 20 percent of pregnant women have anemia. Women who have had repeated pregnancies and young girls who are still maturing are most likely to become anemic and to bear infants who have low iron reserves. Most anemia is the result of iron deficiency. The anemia should be differentiated from the lower hemoglobin and hematocrit levels that result from the increase in the blood volume—the so-called "physiologic anemia of pregnancy." Blood levels below 11 g hemoglobin per dl and 33 percent hematocrit should be corrected by iron salts such as ferrous sulfate. Dietary counseling is also essential so that these women will select foods that are rich in iron, ascorbic acid, and protein. Megaloblastic anemia caused by folacin deficiency is comparatively rare in the United States. It is corrected by prescribing a folacin supplement.

Hyperemesis Gravidarum About 2 percent of pregnant women experience severe nausea and vomiting during the first trimester. Hyperemesis gravidarum is characterized by dehydration, electrolyte imbalance, ketonuria, and weight loss. The condition is life threatening, and prompt hospitalization is essential.

Nutritional care involves the physician, nurse, dietitian, and psychiatrist.[24] The dietitian obtains a detailed diet history, with particular emphasis on any past food problems, allergies, and food likes and dislikes. Initially, electrolyte and fluid balances are corrected. Some nutritional needs are met by intravenous glucose, minerals, and vitamins. Thereafter small feedings of clear fluids are given for 24 hours. If tolerated small amounts (20 ml) of a blended formula* that provides the recommended allowances is given six to eight times a day.[24] It is recommended that the formula be placed on the tray with medications so

---

* Meritene (Doyle Pharmaceutical Co., Minneapolis), whole milk, Lipomul (Upjohn Company, Kalamazoo), ice cream, and flavoring.

that the patient regards it as medical therapy rather than as food. The patient must never be told: "You must eat." When the formula is well tolerated, three small meals of easily digested food are given. The patient is on the road to recovery when there is gain in weight, electrolyte and fluid balances have returned to normal, and ketonuria is no longer present.

Toxemia By toxemia is meant that combination of symptoms including hypertension, edema, and albuminuria. Preeclampsia is the appearance of hypertension, edema of the face and hands, and/or albuminuria about the twentieth week of pregnancy. It should be suspected when there is a sudden gain in weight, indicating fluid retention rather than tissue building. Eclampsia is the end result of preeclampsia; it includes the earlier symptoms but may culminate in convulsions.

The treatment of toxemias is highly controversial. In fact, toxemia has been called the "disease of theories."[2] Protein and calorie restriction are no longer recommended, and sodium restriction should be used with caution.

Chronic Conditions Preexisting conditions such as diabetes mellitus, heart disease, hypertension, inborn errors of metabolism, and others increase the risks of pregnancy just as pregnancy adds to the stress of these conditions. With good prenatal care and adjustment of the diet to meet the dual requirements of the pregnancy and the disease condition, a successful outcome is likely. See chapters pertaining to specific disease conditions in Part III.

Lactation

With a resurgence of interest in breast feeding, three of every four women in middle and upper socioeconomic groups breast feed their babies, at least for a short time. But in lower socioeconomic groups the rate of breast feeding is more nearly one of every four women. The advantages as well as disadvantages are discussed fully in Chapter 20.

Nutritive Requirements When one considers the nutritive value of human milk, and that the nursing mother will produce 20 to 30 ounces each day, it becomes apparent that the requirements for protein, minerals, vitamins, and energy are even greater than they were during pregnancy. See Tables 19-2 and 19-3 for recommended dietary allowances and suggested food intake.

Energy. Each 100 ml breast milk supplies 67 to 77 kcal. The conversion of food energy to milk energy is 80 to 90 percent efficient, thus necessitating 95 kcal to produce 100 ml milk. The average daily production of 750 ml milk, representing 525 kcal, necessitates an expenditure of 640 kcal.[4]

If weight gain followed recommended levels during pregnancy, the fat deposits will furnish 100 to 150 kcal for the first 100 days of lactation. Thus, an added allowance of 300 kcal to the diet is recommended.

Protein. Each 100 ml of human milk contains 1.2 g protein. Thus, 750 ml milk daily would yield 9 g protein. Since the efficiency of conversion of dietary protein to milk protein is about 70 percent, and individual variations also occur, the recommended allowance for lactation is an additional 15 g protein.[4]

The need for protein is greatest when lactation has reached its maximum, but it is a need that should be anticipated and planned for during pregnancy.

Minerals. Even liberal intakes of calcium may not be successful in completely counteracting a negative calcium balance. Consequently, a high level of calcium intake and the building of reserves during pregnancy cannot be overemphasized. Four to five cups of milk daily is recommended during lactation.

The infant is born with a relatively large reserve of iron, since milk is not a good source of iron. A good allowance of iron in the mother's diet during lactation does not convey additional iron to the infant. Nevertheless, iron-rich foods are essential for the mother's own health, and supplements are included early in the infant's diet.

Vitamins. The adequacy of the mother's intake of vitamins is reflected to some extent in the vitamin levels of the milk she produces. For example, low levels of intake of thiamin and vitamin B-6 have been shown to result in low levels of these vitamins in the milk. Ascorbic acid is transferred to the milk, and the needs of the infant are fully met if the mother's diet is adequate.

DIETARY COUNSELING

Successful lactation is dependent not only on an adequate diet but on a desire to nurse the baby, freedom from anxiety, and sufficient rest as well. The decision to nurse the baby should be made early in pregnancy, and the woman needs the support and counseling of her physician, nurses, nutritionists, and family.

The choice of foods during lactation should be wide. No specific foods need to be omitted unless there is evidence of distress caused by them. Occasionally strongly flavored vegetables or highly seasoned or spicy foods may be implicated.

Alcohol, tobacco, marijuana and other street drugs, and some proprietary and prescribed medications are transmitted to the milk and infants may be adversely affected. The lactating woman is well advised to omit these except on the specific recommendation of her physician.

Oral Contraceptives

With the widespread use of oral contraceptives there is much interest in the possible effects of these compounds on nutritional status. The preparations in common use contain varying proportions of estrogens and progestogens. In some respects the metabolic effects are similar to those observed in pregnancy.

Reports of numerous studies on the metabolic changes resulting from the use of oral contraceptives are often contradictory. Although biochemical changes occur, clinical manifestations of nutritional deficiency are rare. The significance of the observed biochemical changes is by no means clear.

The biochemical changes are more likely to be observed in women whose nutritional status is poor than in those who are well nourished. Among these changes are the following:[4,25-26]

Impaired glucose tolerance
Increased blood concentrations:
    Phospholipids, cholesterol, triglycerides
    Plasma vitamin A; plasma retinol-binding protein
    Plasma copper; plasma ceruloplasmin
    Serum iron; total iron-binding component
Decreased blood concentration:
    Ascorbic acid in leukocytes, platelets
    Riboflavin in red blood cells
    Serum folacin (megaloblastic anemia is rarely seen)
    Red blood cell folacin
    Serum vitamin B-12
    Plasma pyridoxal phosphate
    Plasma zinc
Changes in urinary excretion:
    Decrease in riboflavin
    Increase in xanthurenic acid and kynurenine

Particular emphasis has been placed on vitamin B-6 deficiency and its relationship to changes in tryptophan metabolism and also to the occasional incidence of mental depression. If the vitamin B-6 intake is deficient, the excretion of xanthurenic acid and kynurenine is increased, indicating interference with the normal pathways of tryptophan metabolism. For example, conversion of tryptophan to niacin does not occur.

The changes observed for vitamin B-6 and other nutrients can be reversed by improvement of the diet alone so that it meets the RDA. Routine supplements of vitamin B-6 and other nutrients are not justified.[4]

CASE STUDY 4

Pregnant Adolescent

Linda B., age 16, is an attractive, slender, and well-groomed girl. She is an above-average student in school where she is active in extracurricular affairs including band and gymnastics. She is the only child in her family. Her father is a banker and her mother is an interior decorator. Both of her parents are involved in their careers and enjoy their work. The B's live in a spacious home in the suburbs.

Linda is very weight conscious and has tried several fad diets to lose a few pounds. She is also a finicky eater. She does not drink milk and does not like many vegetables. She rarely eats breakfast; when she does, it consists of a glass of orange juice and a piece of toast. At noon she usually eats an apple or an orange. After school she is famished and snacks on cookies, soda pop and ice cream. Frequently her evening meal consists of a pizza or milkshake and hamburger with her friends after school activities. When she eats dinner with her family she has a well-balanced meal, although she takes very small portions.

For the past two weeks Linda has felt queasy in the morning before breakfast and has noticed that she does not have as much energy as usual. She became worried when she missed her menstrual period and went to a teenage clinic for a pregnancy test. Her suspicions were confirmed and she learned that she was two months pregnant.

Her history and physical examination were unremarkable. Linda has been in good health and rarely misses school. A year ago she weighed 50 kg (110 lbs) and she has brought her weight down to 46 kg (101 lb); her height is 164 cm (65 in.). Her hemoglobin was 12 g per 100 ml, and there was no evidence of glucose or albumin in the urine. The nurse practitioner noted a concern about Linda's weight and the recent history of faddish diets. The nurse explored alternative future plans with Linda and learned that Linda opposes abortion. The nurse talked with Linda about the importance of a well-balanced diet and the relationship of nutrition to fetal development. She gave Linda pamphlets on nutrition and prenatal care and made an appointment for return to the clinic in two weeks.

During Linda's second visit to the clinic the nurse learned that Linda had not followed the recommended diet because she does not want to gain too much weight and lose her figure. The nurse is concerned that Linda's hostile attitude and ambivalence about the future are hindering her from considering her nutritional needs.

At this point Linda is uncertain about her plans for the future. She is contemplating either keeping the baby and getting her own apartment or else giving the baby up for adoption. She and her boyfriend still openly express affection for each other, but both are opposed to marriage now. His parents are unaware of the pregnancy. Linda's parents were upset to learn about the pregnancy, but they have told Linda that they will support her in whatever decision she makes. Linda's aunt who lives out of the state has offered her a place to stay until she has the baby.

Mr. and Mrs. B are particularly upset about the disruption of future school plans if Linda decides to keep the baby. Linda is hostile to any suggestions that her parents make as she feels that decisions regarding the baby are her own to make.

Linda missed several days of school when she felt nauseated. She has not told any of her friends that she is pregnant and is worried that they will find out. The nurse gave Linda some tips on how to cope with morning sickness and arranged for a follow-up visit. She was also given a prescription for vitamin and iron supplements.

Physiologic Correlations

1. Why is Linda medically, nutritionally, and psychologically at risk?
2. Describe the normal physiologic changes that should be expected in each of the following during the pregnancy: appetite; basal metabolism; gastrointestinal function; renal function; cardiovascular function; hormonal changes.
3. Why is Linda's recent weight loss and her underweight of some concern to the nurse practitioner?

Nutritional Assessment

4. Compare the Recommended Dietary Allowances for Linda prior to her pregnancy with those during pregnancy.
5. Based on the brief record of Linda's diet given in the case study, what are likely to be the most serious nutrient deficiencies?
6. What is likely to be the effect of Linda's caloric restriction on the ultimate utilization of protein?
7. What undesirable nutritional effects may arise from the emotional stress that Linda is undergoing?
8. How does Linda perceive her problems?

Planning the Diet

9. How much weight should Linda gain each trimester? What growth in tissues, including the fetus, account for these changes?
10. List the amounts of foods that Linda should include from each of the food groups.
11. Since Linda believes that milk is fattening and does not like it, what suggestions can you make for adequate nutrient replacement? Why is a calcium supplement less desirable?
12. Why is it important for Linda to take an iron supplement in addition to an adequate diet?
13. What justification is there for Linda to take a vitamin supplement?
14. Why is salt restriction not advisable?

Dietary Counseling

15. Linda is not likely to take very seriously a statement such as "You should eat these foods because they are good for you and the baby." What techniques and approaches do you need to use in counseling her about diet?
16. What assets does Linda have toward an effective dietary program?
17. Why should you be cautious about making firm statements regarding good nutrition leading to a successful outcome of pregnancy?
18. What dietary modifications will reduce the tendency to morning sickness?
19. Since Linda is so concerned about her weight, what approach can you use to help her understand the need for increased nutrient requirements?
20. The nurse has recommended that Linda attend prenatal classes that are being held for girls of her age. What might be appropriate objectives for such classes?

References for the Case Study

ABRAMS, B.: "Helping Pregnant Teenagers Eat Right," *Nursing '81*, 11:46–47, March 1981.

COMMITTEE ON ADOLESCENCE, AMERICAN ACADEMY OF PEDIATRICS: "Statement on Teenage Pregnancy," *Pediatrics*, 63: 795–97, 1979.

CORBETT, M. A., and BURST, H. V.: "Nutritional Intervention in Pregnancy," *J. Nurs. Midwife*, 28:23–29, July/August 1983.

GORMICAN, A., et al.: "Relationships of Maternal Weight Gain, Prepregnancy Weight, and Infant Birthweight," *J. Am. Diet. Assoc.*, 80:662–67, 1980.

JOHNSON, C. A., et al.: "A Teaching Intervention to Improve Breastfeeding Success," *J. Nutr. Ed.*, 16:19–22, 1984.

TRUSWELL, A. S., and DARNTON-HILL, I.: "Food Habits of Adolescents," *Nutr. Rev.*, 39:73–88, 1981.

References

1. Richmond, J., and Filner, B.: "Infant and Child Health: Needs and Strategies," in *Healthy People: The Surgeon General's Report on Health Promotion and Disease Prevention*. U.S. Department of Health, Education and Welfare, Washington, D.C., 1979, pp. 307–332.

2. Committee on Maternal Nutrition, Food and Nutrition Board: *Maternal Nutrition and the Course of Pregnancy. Summary Report*. National Research Council–National Academy of Sciences, Washington, D.C., 1970.

3. Hook, E. B.: "Dietary Cravings and Aversions During Pregnancy," *Am. J. Clin. Nutr.*, 31:1355–62, 1978.

4. Food and Nutrition Board: *Recommended Dietary Allowances*, 10th ed. National Research Council–National Academy of Sciences, Washington, D.C., 1989.

5. Naeye, R. L.: "Weight Gain and the Outcome of Pregnancy," *Am. J. Obstet. Gynecol.*, 135:3–9, 1979.

6. Review: "Maternal Weight Gain and the Outcome of Pregnancy," *Nutr. Rev.*, 37:318–21, 1979.

7. Brennan, R. E. et al.: "Assessment of Maternal Nutrition," *J. Am. Diet. Assoc.*, 75:152–54, 1979.

8. Stearns, G.: "Nutritional State of the Mother Prior to Conception," *JAMA*, 168:1655–59, 1958.

9. McGanity, W. J., et al.: "Vanderbilt Cooperative Study of Maternal and Infant Nutrition. XII. Effect of Reproductive Cycle on Nutritional Status and Requirements," *JAMA*, 168:2138–45, 1958.

10. Thomson, A. M., and Hytten, F. E.: "Nutrition in Pregnancy and Lacation," in *Nutrition: A Comprehensive Treatise*, Vol III. G. H. Beaton and E. W. McHenry, eds. Academic Press, New York, 1966, pp. 103–45.

11. Burke, B. S., et al.: "Nutrition Studies During Pregnancy," *Am. J. Obstet. Gynecol.*, 46:38–52, 1943.

12. Kennedy, E. T., et al.: "Evaluation of the Effect of WIC Supplemental Feeding on Birth Weight," *J. Am. Diet. Assoc.*, 80:220–27, 1982.

13. Iber, F. L.: "Fetal Alcohol Syndrome," *Nutr. Today*, 15(5):4–11, September/October 1980.

14. Beagle, W. S.: "Fetal Alcohol Syndrome: A Review," *J. Am. Diet. Assoc.*, 79:274–76, 1981.

15. Committee on Nutrition of the Mother and Preschool Child, Food and Nutrition Board: *Alternative Dietary Practices and Nutritional Abuses in Pregnancy*. National Research Council–National Academy of Sciences, Washington, D.C., 1982.

16. Expert Panel on Food Safety and Nutrition, Institute of Food Technologists: "Caffeine," *Contemp. Nutr.*, 9(5), May 1984.

17. Linn, S., et al.: "No Association Between Coffee Consumption and Adverse Outcomes of Pregnancy," *N. Engl. J. Med.*, 306:141–45, 1982.

18. Lackey, C. J.: "Pica During Pregnancy," *Contemp. Nutr.*, 8(11): November 1983.

19. Alton, I. R.: "Nutrition Services for Pregnant Adolescents within a Public High School," *J. Am. Diet. Assoc.*, 74:667–69, 1979.

20. Brennan, R. E., et al.: "Nutrient Intake of Low-Income Pregnant Women: Laboratory Analysis of Foods Consumed," *J. Am. Diet. Assoc.*, 83:546–50, 1983.

21. Moser, P. B., and Allen, D.: "Zinc Intakes of Lactating and Nonlactating Women: Analyzed vs. Calculated Values," *J. Am. Diet. Assoc.*, 84:42–46, 1984.

22. Orr, R. D., and Simmons, J. J.: "Nutritional Care in Pregnancy," *J. Am. Diet. Assoc.*, 75: 126–31, 131–36, 1979.

23. Thomas, M. R., and Kawamoto, J.: "Dietary Evaluation of Lactating Women with or without Vitamin and Mineral Supplementation," *J. Am. Diet. Assoc.*, 74: 669–72, 1979.

24. Shulman, P. K.: "Hyperemesis Gravidarum: An Approach to the Nutritional Aspects of Care," *J. Am. Diet. Assoc.*, 80: 577–78, 1982.

25. Roe, D.: "Nutrition and the Contraceptive Pill," in *Nutritional Disorders of American Women*, M. Winick, ed. John Wiley and Sons, New York 1977.

26. Hudiburgh, N. K., and Milner, A. N.: "Influence of Oral Contraceptives on Ascorbic Acid and Triglyceride Status," *J. Am. Diet. Assoc.*, 75: 19–22, 1979.

27. Review: "The Effect of Oral Contraceptives on Blood Vitamin A Level and the Role of Sex Hormones," *Nutr. Rev.*, 37:346–48, 1979.

28. Review: "The Vitamin B_6 Requirement in Oral Contraceptive Users," *Nutr. Rev.*, 37:344–45, 1979.

20

Nutrition During Infancy

Growth and Development

GROWTH is an increase in the size of the body or any parts of the body. It includes an increase in cell numbers and cell size. DEVELOPMENT entails the maturation of the body tissues, organs, and metabolic systems so that the intended functions can be performed.

The full-term infant enters the world able to function independently of the uterine environment in those physiologic aspects that are essential for survival—respiration, cardiovascular function, body temperature control, ingestion, digestion, absorption, and metabolism. During the first year the rate of growth and development will exceed that of any year in his later life. Each infant's physical growth and development are determined by genetically acquired characteristics, the prenatal quality of nutrition, and the nutritional adequacy of the postnatal diet.

CHANGING FEEDING PATTERNS AND CURRENT ISSUES

Infant feeding practices change as research identifies new and better ways. But they also change for environmental, cultural, and socioeconomic reasons. Sometimes the issues are emotionally charged—among pediatricians and nutritionists as well as among parents!

In the United States and other developed countries there has been a resurgence of interest in breast feeding, especially among educated women of middle and higher socioeconomic classes, and to a somewhat lesser extent among women of lower socioecomic status. For those who use artificial feeding, commercial formulas now account for about 90 per cent of all bottle feedings. In the developing countries, by contrast, breast feeding has been declining; yet, for a number of reasons, bottle feeding becomes a hazardous substitute.

With understanding of the adequacy of human milk for the infant and in consideration of the development of feeding behavior, the introduction of solid foods before the infant is 5 to 6 months old is now believed to be undesirable. There are, likewise, proponents of home-prepared rather than commercially produced baby foods. Parents often express concern about modified starches and additives in commercial foods.

Many mothers of infants are employed away from the home, sometimes because they wish to continue their careers, and often because they need to work in order to maintain a livelihood for themselves and their infants. What are the essential needs for maintaining nutrition and nurturance when some of the infant's care is delegated to others? Society has not yet provided fully satisfactory solutions.

The emphasis in recent years on the prevention of diseases has raised the question: Will modification of the infant's diet help reduce the risks or prevent chronic diseases? There are concerns, and indeed controversies, about the intake of energy, sugar, fat, cholesterol, and salt.

Intensive care units in hospitals are now able to dramatically reduce the mortality rate of low-birth-weight infants. These advances are implemented only at considerable financial cost, and sometimes much emotional turmoil on the part of the parents. There are two critical issues: What measures can be taken to reduce the incidence of low birth weight? (See Chapter 19.) How are the nutritional needs of the low-birth-weight infant best met?

Each of these issues will be considered in this chapter. Although some controversies persist, the health professional can help parents to make prudent choices for the well-being of their infants.

Body Size The infant loses some weight during the first week after delivery but has regained his birth weight at 7 to 10 days. Thereafter the full-term infant will gain 140 to 225 g (5 to 8 ounces) weekly during the first 4 or 5 months, thus doubling the birth weight. For the remainder of the year he or she will gain 110 to 140 g (4 to 5 ounces) each week, so that the weight is tripled by the time the infant is 10 to 12 months old. On his or her first birthday the infant will have achieved one sixth to one seventh of the adult weight.

The normal birth length of 50 to 55 cm (20 to 22 in.) increases by another 23 to 25 cm (9 to 10 in.) during the first year. With the increase in length the body proportions are also changing. The trunk becomes longer as do also the short arms and legs. The baby's head grows rapidly during fetal life and during the first year. By the end of the second year the head circumference is about two thirds of its final size.

Body Composition Weight gains consist of water, muscle and organ tissues, adipose tissue, and skeletal structures. At birth the infant's body consists of as much as 75 percent water, about 12 to 15 percent fat, and poorly developed muscles. By the end of the first year the water content has decreased to about 60 percent, the fat has increased to about 24 percent, and lean body mass has correspondingly increased. From birth onward girls have more adipose tissue than boys.

The skeleton contains a high percentage of water and cartilage at birth. During the first year the bones increase in length, width, and level of mineralization. The calcium content of the skeleton at birth is tripled by the end of the first year.

Cardiovascular-Respiratory Systems Infants have rapid heart (120 to 140 per minute) and respiratory (20 per minute) rates. At birth the hemoglobin level of the well-nourished infant is 17 to 20 g per dl. This provides a reserve for expansion of the blood circulation and adequate oxygen-carrying capacity to the growing tissues during the first 4 to 6 months. By 6 months of age the hemoglobin level has dropped to 11 to 12 g per dl or lower. The failure to anticipate this decline and to supply iron can lead rapidly to anemia.

Gastrointestinal System The full-term infant is able to digest protein, emulsified fats, and simple carbohydrates such as lactose. There is little secretion by the salivary glands until 2 to 3 months at which time the increased salivation becomes evident with drooling. Also, during the first few months the pancreatic amylases are not produced at levels for satisfactory digestion of complex carbohydrates.

Renal System The kidneys reach their full functional capacity by the end of the first year. During the first few months the glomerular filtration rate is somewhat lower, and therefore the excretion of a high concentration of solutes is more difficult. The healthy, full-term, growing infant rarely has problems of renal solute load, because the relatively high intakes of protein and minerals are used for tissue synthesis.

Young infants also excrete greater amounts of some amino acids, but the reabsorption of other amino acids such as phenlyalanine is high. Thus, 97 to 98 percent of phenylalanine may be reabsorbed even though blood levels are high, as in phenylketonuria, one of many genetic diseases.

Brain Development The brain develops rapidly in fetal life and during infancy and early childhood. By the age of 4 years the brain has reached 80 to 90 percent of its adult size. The increase in the number of brain cells is most rapid during fetal life and in the first 5 to 6 months after birth. Thereafter, the rate of cell division declines but continues into the second year. If malnutrition is unusually severe during pregnancy and during the first few months of life, as in the marasmic infant, the number of brain cells is greatly reduced. Once the critical period of cell division has passed, an adequate diet given subsequently cannot bring about an increase in cell numbers. It is difficult to separate the influences of malnutrition and of environmental deprivation on the ultimate outcome with respect to mental development.

Feeding Behavior The development of feeding behavior depends on maturation of the nervous system which controls muscular coordination. At birth the baby is able to coordinate sucking, swallowing, and breathing. The eyes cannot yet be focused, but by the ROOTING REFLEX the baby can find nourishment; that is, when the cheek and lips nearest the nipple are stroked the infant will turn toward the stimulus and seek the nipple and suckle.

For about 3 months the baby suckles rhythmically with an up and down movement of the tongue. If solid food is placed on the tongue at this age, the same tongue movements result in food being pushed out of the mouth (EXTRUSION REFLEX).

At 12 to 16 weeks the sucking pattern changes and the tongue moves back and forth instead of up and down. When food is placed on the tongue the baby is able to draw in the lower lip when the spoon is withdrawn, transfer the food to the back of the tongue and swallow it.

By 6 months of age the infant has better coordination of eyes and hands, grasps objects within reach, and puts them into the mouth. The baby also develops chewing movements and it is appropriate to give him or her zwieback or crackers.

Mother–infant bonding developed from the earliest days, whether by breast- or bottle-feeding, influences not only the establishment of desirable food behavior but is also important for the social, emotional, and psychologic values that develop throughout infancy and childhood.

Nutritional Assessment

Measurements Each infant is individual and serves as his or her own best control in the measurement of progress. Although it is useful to make comparisons with stated norms such as length and weight, it is also dangerous to expect every infant to conform exactly to such norms. No single criterion of physical status by itself is indicative of the quality of nutrition, but a series of measurements over a period of time are likely to be reliable indicators. (See also Chapter 23.)

Weight, length, head circumference, and skinfold thickness can be compared with standards for infants of a given age. (See Length and Weight Charts, Tables A-7, A-8, A-11, and A-12.) An infant that falls within the 25th and 75th percentile is within the range of most infants. If the baby falls within the 90th to the 95th percentile for weight and/or length, he or she exceeds all but 5 to 10 infants in each 100. Thus, weight at the 90th percentile should be monitored for the onset of obesity. Conversely, an infant that falls at the 5th to 10th percentile may be experiencing growth failure, and its causes should be sought.

Some important questions to ask in making an assessment are these:

From time to time do the infant's measurements fall within a percentile level, or are there deviations up or down? If there are deviations, what are the possible explanations—illness, inadequate or excessive feedings?

How does the infant's height and weight pattern compare with that of his parents and siblings? For example, infants of parents who are short and slender might be expected to fall at a lower percentile level, yet show steady progress at that lower level. A difference of two percentile levels between the infant and siblings merits some further study.

What is the relationship of weight and length? If they differ by two percentile levels, one should try to determine the causes for the difference.

Other criteria of satisfactory quality of nutrition are these:

Normal levels of hemoglobin and hematocrit for age
Steady rate of weight gain, but some weekly fluctuations to be expected
Healthy, smooth skin
Firm muscles with moderate amount of subcutaneous fat
Tooth eruption beginning at about 5 to 6 months; 6 to 12 teeth by end of first year
Normal elimination for type of feeding
Vigorous and happy; sleeps well
Absence of handicaps that interfere with feeding
Absence of metabolic errors that require a modified diet

Nutritional Status Many studies have shown that most infants in the United States receive an adequate diet of all nutrients and are well nourished. Second generations of immigrants to the United States have generally been taller than their parents. Also in developing countries the children of privileged families are taller than those who are deprived. This effect on stature is generally ascribed to better nutrition and better health, including immunization against common diseases.

Iron-deficiency anemia occurs in about 10 percent of infants from low socioeconomic groups and in about 1 percent in infants from families of higher socioeconomic status. Multiple births and premature infants are more susceptible to iron-deficiency anemia if they do not receive iron supplements within the first few months of life.[1]

Even in the United States there are occasional instances of failure to thrive, vitamin deficiencies such as scurvy or rickets, deficiencies in trace minerals such as zinc, and protein-calorie malnutrition. When such conditions are encountered, the underlying causes must be sought, for they may range from poverty to ignorance of the infant's needs to infant neglect to metabolic errors that have not been diagnosed.

Nutritional Requirements

The amount of human milk ingested by the healthy infant from a well-nourished mother has been used as the primary basis for the recommended allowances during the first 6 months.[2] In some instances the nutrient levels have been set higher for babies who are receiving formulas. For the second 6 months the al-

Table 20-1. **Comparison of Recommended Dietary Allowances for Normal Infants with Composition of Human Milk, Cow's Milk, and Milk-Based Formula***

| Nutrient | Dietary Allowances | | Human Milk per 1,000 ml† | Cow's Milk (Whole) per 1,000 ml | Milk-Based Formula per 1,000 ml |
	0–6 Months	6–12 Months			
Weight, kg	6	9			
lb	13	20			
Height, cm	60	71			
in	24	28			
Water, ml			897	894	875
Energy, kcal	kg×115	kg×105	718	620	670
Protein, g	kg×2.2	kg×2.0	10.6	33.4	15–16
Fat, g			44.9	33.9	33–37
Carbohydrate, g			70.6	47.3	70–72
Vitamin A, RE	375	375	656	315	340–500
IU	1,875	1,875	2,470	1,279	1,700–2,500
Vitamin D, μg	7.5	10		10‡	10
Vitamin E, mg TE	3	4	1.3–3.3	5.7	5.7–8.5
Ascorbic acid, mg	30	35	51	10	55
Thiamin, mg	0.3	0.4	0.14	0.39	0.4–0.7
Riboflavin, mg	0.4	0.5	0.37	1.65	0.6–1.0
Niacin, mg NE	5	6	2.0	0.85	7–9
Vitamin B-6, mg	0.3	0.6	0.11	0.43	0.3–0.4
Vitamin B-12, μg	0.3	0.5	0.46	3.63	1.5–2.0
Folacin, μg	25	35	51	51	50–100
Calcium, mg	400	600	328	1,208	550–600
Phosphorus, mg	300	500	144	945	440–460
Sodium, mg	120§	200§	141	498	250–390
Potassium, mg	500§	700§	523	1,544	620–1,000
Magnesium, mg	40	60	31	132	40–50
Iodine, μg	40	50	30–100		40–70
Iron, mg	6	10	0.3	0.5	1.4–12.5#
Zinc, mg	5	5	1.8	3.9	2.0–4.0

  * Food and Nutrition Board: *Recommended Dietary Allowances*, 9th ed. National Research Council–National Academy of Sciences, Washington, D.C., 1980.
  † One liter of human milk = 1.025 g; 1 liter of cow's milk = 1.017 g.
  ‡Assumes fortification of cow's milk with 10 μg vitamin D.
  § Allowances for sodium and potassium are ranges considered to be safe and adequate.
  # Values for formula not fortified and fortified with iron.

lowances are based on the consumption of a formula and a mixture of solid foods. The recommended allowances are listed in Table 20-1.

Energy The energy needs of the infant for the first 6 months range from 95 to 145 kcal per kg and for the second 6 months from 70 to 135 kcal per kg.[2] About half the energy expenditure is accounted for by the basal metabolism alone in order to regulate the temperature of the body with its high skin surface, and to maintain the high level of metabolic activities. During the first 4 to 5 months a normal rate of growth accounts for as much as one third of the total energy requirement. For the remainder of the year about a tenth of the energy requirement is for growth, while an increasing proportion is needed for activity. Babies who are active and who cry a lot have much higher energy requirements than those who are placid. The general well-being, rate of weight gain, and appetite give clues to the adequacy of the energy intake.

Protein The infant adds about 3.5 g protein daily to his or her body during the first 4 months and thereafter about 3.1 g per day for the rest of the year. This results not only in a net increase in body size but also in an increase of the percentage of body protein from 11 to 14.6.[2]

Human milk furnishes about 2 to 2.4 g protein per kg per day during the first month of life, but by the sixth month this has fallen to 1.5 g per kg per day. In the recommended allowances this lower level has been adjusted to 2.0 g per kg for the second 6 months in order to allow for the lesser efficiency of the protein in a mixed diet.

Carbohydrate There is no recommended allowance for carbohydrate for infants. Lactose accounts for about 38 to 40 percent of the calories in human milk. Since the lactose content in cow's milk is lower, lactose or another simple carbohydrate is added to commercial formulas. Sucrose, cane syrup, or dextrimaltose are commonly added to home-prepared formulas.

Fat About 45 to 50 percent of calories in human milk and in most formulas are provided by fat. Such a proportion helps meet the high energy requirements of the infant in an efficient way.

Human milk supplies from 6 to 9 percent of its calories as linoleate. A formula that furnishes 3 percent of calories as linoleic acid will meet the infant's needs.[2]

Low-fat formulas are contraindicated, since it is difficult to achieve sufficient caloric intake for satisfactory weight gain. Low-fat formulas will not furnish enough linoleic acid unless it is added to the formula. If the concentration of the formula is increased, there will be greater deamination of amino acids and thus a considerable increase in the renal solute load.

The desirable level of cholesterol intake is not known. Human milk contains significantly more cholesterol than commercial formulas made with vegetable oils. Cholesterol is required for the synthesis of bile salts, the development of the central nervous system, and the elaboration of enzymes that control the body's synthesis of cholesterol.[3] Two questions remain unanswered: Does restriction of cholesterol in the formula impair the synthetic processes? Does restriction of cholesterol in infancy and early life help reduce the incidence of atherosclerosis?

Water The normal daily turnover of water by the infant is about 15 percent of body weight. The water loss from the skin is large because of the greater surface area in relation to body weight. The ability of the kidneys of the young infant to concentrate urine is much less than that of older children or adults. Hence, to excrete a given amount of solute, chiefly urea and sodium chloride, a larger volume of fluid is required. The osmolar load of breast milk is well within the excretion capacity of the kidney, but more concentrated formulas could present an excessive osmolar load.

Infants require about 150 ml water per 100 kcal. This requirement is met by breast milk, and by formulas containing 5 to 10 percent sugar and enough water to give a concentration of 65 to 70 kcal per dl.

High environmental temperatures, vomiting, or diarrhea lead to greatly increased water losses that must be made up to prevent dehydration and electrolyte imbalance.

Minerals Iron is probably the mineral element that requires the most emphasis in infant feeding, especially for infants of lower socioeconomic groups. The iron stores of the healthy infant are adequate for 4 to 6 months after birth. The iron content of breast milk is low but about half that present is absorbed, whereas the rate of absorption from formulas is about 10 percent. An intake of 1 mg iron per kg per day beginning about the third month will maintain hemoglobin levels in normal infants. The recommended allowance of 6 and 10 mg, respectively, for the first and second half of the year is based on an average need of 1.5 mg per kg.[2]

The American Academy of Pediatrics recommends that iron supplementation (not more than 15 mg per day) should begin at 4 to 6 months for normal infants and at 2 months for preterm infants.[4]

The recommended allowance for calcium is based on about 60 mg calcium per kg body weight, the amount supplied to breast-fed infants.[2] Breast-fed infants retain about 50 to 60 percent of the total calcium intake, whereas bottle-fed infants retain 25 to 30 percent of a cow's milk formula. Since formulas contain a much higher proportion of calcium, the net retention is approximately the same. The calcium-to-phosphorus ratio during the first six months should be 1.3 to 1 in order to offset the tendency toward hypercalcemia that sometimes occurs with a high phosphorus intake.

The infant requires about 1.0 to 1.5 mEq sodium for daily growth, and losses from the skin and excretions are about 1 to 2 mEq daily. The total sodium needs are estimated to be 2 to 5 mEq (45 to 115 mg) daily.[5] The average daily intake of sodium ranges from 13 mEq (300 mg) at 2 months to as much as 60 mEq (1400) by the sixth month, especially if salt is added to solid foods.

The allowances for magnesium, zinc, and iodine, listed in Table 20-1, are adequately met by human milk or formulas. For safe and adequate intakes of electrolytes and some trace minerals and vitamins see table inside front cover. The safe level of fluoride intake is achieved when formulas are diluted with water that contains 1 ppm fluoride. Some pediatricians recommend fluoride supplementation for infants that are breastfed and those who live in areas in which the water fluoride content is low.

Vitamins Human milk from a healthy, well-nourished mother supplies sufficient levels of vitamins for the infant with the possible exception of vitamin D. Although some studies have indicated that a water-miscible form of vitamin D is present in human milk and will meet the infant's needs, a supplement is usually recommended. Formulas generally contain the 10 μg (400 IU) vitamin D recommended for the first year.[2]

The plasma vitamin E content of newborn infants is low but rises rapidly to normal levels by the end of the first month. The need for vitamin E is normally met by human and cow's milk. A vitamin E supplement may be required if formulas have an increased level of polyunsaturated fatty acids and are also fortified with iron. The presence of iron increases lipid peroxidation, reduces the available level of vitamin E, and leads to anemia, reticulocytosis, and thrombocytosis.[6] At birth an intramuscular injection of 0.5 to 1.0 mg phytylmenaquinone (vitamin K_1) is recommended. Thereafter intestinal synthesis of vitamin K is adequate to meet the infant's needs.

Human milk will meet the ascorbic acid needs of normal infants. Formula-fed infants require supplementation if the formula itself is not fortified. When increased amounts of protein are given, infants require additional amounts of ascorbic acid for the metabolism of tyrosine. Human milk is low in vitamin B-6, but the infant is born with a store of this vitamin that is adequate until other foods are added.

Breast Feeding

Resurgence of Interest Up to the early part of the twentieth century, an infant's survival depended primarily on the availability of human milk from the mother or a wet nurse. Safer milk supplies and increasing knowledge of ways to adapt cow's milk for infants led to widespread use of home-prepared formulas based on certified or pasteurized cow's milk or evaporated milk. By 1940 evaporated milk formulas accounted for the feedings of 6 of every 10 infants while in the hospital and of 8 of every 10 infants at 5 to 6 months of age.[7] Breast feeding continued to decline, while commercial formulas gradually began to replace evaporated milk formulas. By 1975 one of every four infants was breast fed and three of every four received a commercial formula[8].

During the late 1970s, there occurred a remarkable increase in breast feeding. By 1981, at 1 week of age, 56 percent of infants were breast fed, with commercial formulas accounting for the rest. This resurgence of interest in breast feeding can be explained by several factors: (1) better informed mothers regarding the advantages of breast feeding; (2) adaptation of routines in obstetric units to encourage breast feeding; (3) support given by the La Leche League to mothers; and (4) ecologic concerns of many people in the 1970s with emphasis on the "natural."[9]

Nutritional Characteristics of Human and Cow's Milk Human milk is the most balanced food for the infant. Human and cow's milk are similar in their energy value and in the amount of fat. Cow's milk contains substantially higher levels of most nutrients, but supplies less lactose, ascorbic acid, niacin, and vitamin A than does human milk. (See Table 20-1.)

Lactalbumin accounts for 60 percent of the protein in human milk, while in cow's milk only 15 percent of the protein is lactalbumin. The remaining protein in both milks is primarily casein. For the infant lactalbumin provides an amino acid pattern that most nearly approaches that of the body tissues. Some recent research has focused on the taurine content of human milk, and the possibility that taurine may be an essential amino acid for the infant.[10] Taurine is involved in the formation of bile salts that are essential for fat absorption, and may also be required for the development of the nervous system. However, there is no evidence that infants receiving formulas with little or no taurine have been adversely affected.

Newborn babies absorb about 95 to 98 percent of the fat from human milk but only about 80 percent of fat from a milk-based formula.[11] Human milk has a high lipase activity, and also a higher level of linoleic acid.

Cow's milk contains about three times as much ash as does human milk. Most of this is accounted for by higher contents of calcium, phosphorus, sodium, and potassium. The calcium-to-phosphorus ratio in cow's milk is about 1:1 and in human milk 2:1.

Human and cow's milk differ considerably in their vitamin contents. Human milk can furnish the ascorbic acid needs of the infant, but cow's milk cannot. Both milks provide satisfactory levels of other vitamins except vitamin D.

Other Advantages of Breast Feeding Human milk forms fine, flocculent curds in the stomach, thus enhancing digestion and leading to more rapid emptying of the stomach. Also, the solute content of human milk is lower than that of cow's milk and leads to less secretory load for the developing kidneys. However, today's commercial formulas produce a fine curd and have a solute load comparable to that of human milk.

For even a few weeks breast feeding confers advantages to the infant by reducing the likelihood of allergies and serious illnesses. The colostrum and mature milk confer immune properties that are low or missing in cow's milk.[11] Human milk contains about as many leukocytes as are found in blood. They bring about phagocytosis, and also secrete complement, lysozyme, and lactoferrin. Most classes of immunoglobulins (IgA, IgG, and IgM) are present. Lysozymes split bacterial walls, while lactoferrin retards growth of bacteria such as *Escherichia coli* and *Shigella*. The BIFIDUS factor in human milk increases the growth of lactobacilli and helps to convert lactose to lactic and acetic acids. With the consequent lowering of the pH of the intestinal tract, the growth of enteropathogenic organisms is reduced. Lipid factors (lipase and monoglyceride) have also been identified as antimicrobial agents.

In lower socioeconomic groups breast-fed infants have a lower mortality rate, probably because there is no problem of sanitation. On a practical basis breast feeding eliminates preparation of a formula; the feeding is immediately available at the proper temperature; and errors in formula dilution or home preparation of a formula are avoided.

Claims are often made for psychologic advantages of breast feeding. A bonding between mother and child is established; that is, the baby feels safe, warm, and protected and the mother has a sense of satisfaction and closeness to the baby. Yet it is difficult to prove that the formula-fed baby is in any way disadvantaged in this respect.

The cost of the additional foods needed to produce milk by the mother varies widely depending on the choices made. Breast feeding is likely to be more economical than feeding with commercial formulas. Generally, the cost of the additional food required by the mother for lactation compares with the cost of the now rarely used evaporated-milk formulas.

In the developing countries breast feeding can be lifesaving. Yet in many countries breast feeding is declining. This has come about because some mothers are working and are unable to feed their babies, while others have come to regard bottle feeding as a status symbol. Many people in these countries do not have sufficient income to purchase the amounts of formula that the infant requires. They resort to excessive dilution and the infant becomes malnourished. Water supplies are often contaminated and refrigeration is lacking. With the contamination of the formulas, the

Figure 20-1. Breast feeding provides the best nourishment for the baby. It also confers immunity against some infections during the early months of life. (Courtesy, Health Education Associates, Glenside, Pennsylvania, and Charles M. Cadwell, photographer.)

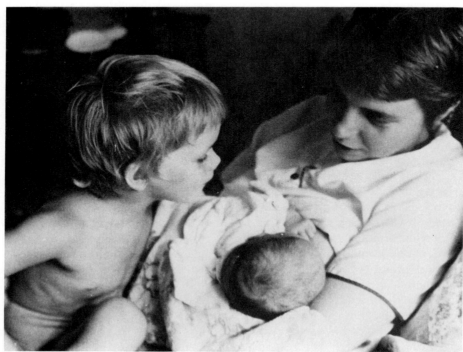

subsequent diarrhea leads to loss of nutrients, dehydration, acidosis, and a high mortality rate. (See Figure 20-1.)

Human Milk Production   The female breast consists of glandular tissue and fibrous, fatty connective tissue called the stroma. There are 15 to 20 lobes that converge on the nipple. Each of the lobes includes smaller units called lobules, which in turn contain the alveoli, the milk-secreting glands. Nutrients are supplied to the alveoli by the rich bed of capillaries in the connective tissue.

Lactation involves the synthesis of milk by the alveoli, the release of milk into the ducts, the collection of milk in the reservoirs underneath the areola (the pigmented area surrounding the nipple), and the ejection of milk through the nipple. During pregnancy the breasts enlarge, and there is a marked increase in the formation of alveoli. PROLACTIN is the primary hormone involved in milk production, although insulin, thyroid hormone, glucocorticoids and mineralocorticoids are also essential. Prolactin production by the anterior pituitary begins in pregnancy but its release is inhibited by high circulating levels of estrogen and progesterone. After birth prolactin secretion is stimulated by the sucking of the infant and milk production takes place in the alveoli.

The infant's sucking triggers nerve impulses to the hypothalamus, which stimulates the posterior pituitary to release OXYTOCIN, the primary hormone involved in milk ejection, also known as the LET-DOWN REFLEX. Oxytocin causes myoepithelial cells that surround the alveoli to contract, thus forcing milk into the lactiferous ducts and into the reservoirs beneath the areola, and ejection through the nipple.

Once lactation has become well established, the letdown reflex may be triggered by the cry of the infant and even the thought of the infant at feeding time. The reflex is strongly inhibited by emotional upsets, some drugs such as sedatives, and by alcohol—all of which may lead to lactation failure.

Women vary widely in their ability to produce milk. They are likely to be less successful with their first babies. But if the advantages of breast feeding are explained to them and they are given guidance regarding diet, exercise, freedom from stress, and care of the breasts during pregnancy, most women can successfully breast feed.

Initiation of Feeding   In order to foster breast feeding the mother and infant should not be separated during the first 24 hours after delivery. An important role of the nurse is to assist a new mother to achieve an effective feeding technique. With the mother reclining or comfortably seated, the infant is held in a semireclining position. When the baby's cheek nearest to the breast is touched, the infant will turn toward the breast to find the nipple. Too often an attempt is made to push the baby's other cheek, only to have the infant turn away.

The baby's mouth should grasp the breast around the areola, not just the nipple. If the nipple only is engaged, the baby will have to suck too hard to extract the milk, and becomes fatigued and frustrated. Also, the nipple becomes very sore.

At first the baby receives only a small amount (10 to 40 ml) of a clear yellowish secretion known as COLOSTRUM. This fluid supplies only small amounts of nutrients but furnishes important immune factors. Mature milk is produced in sufficient amounts after 4 to 5 days if the infant has been feeding satisfactorily. The initial loss of weight after delivery is generally regained by the end of the first week to 10 days.

The baby may get enough food by emptying one breast, but if the baby is still hungry he or she should be offered the other breast. At the next feeding the breast that was not emptied should be offered first.

When the baby stops sucking he or she should be held over the shoulder and patted on the back to release any air that may have been swallowed. Some babies burp best if they are laid across the knee, abdomen down, and patted. Some babies suckle so vigorously and swallow so much air that they require two or three burpings for each feeding.

Self-Demand Feeding   Healthy infants will establish, after a few weeks, schedules of their own that are reasonably regular from day to day if they are fed when they indicate that they are hungry.

The success of self-demand feeding depends upon the mother's ability to determine when the child is hungry. The infant who cries at intervals much shorter than 3 hours may be underfed, may have swallowed too much air at the previous feeding, or may be crying because of other discomforts.

The very young infant may require as many as 10 to 12 feedings at first but soon establishes a rhythm of feeding which falls into approximately 3- to 4-hour intervals. After the second month, the night feeding usually may be discontinued. By the end of the fourth or fifth month, the infant sleeps through the night and will no longer require a feeding around 10 P.M.

Adequacy of Feeding   About 150 to 165 ml human milk per kilogram body weight (2.5 ounces per pound) result in satisfactory weight gain. The baby is getting enough milk if he or she is satisfied at the end of a 15- to 20-minute feeding, falls asleep promptly and sleeps quietly for several hours thereafter, and makes satisfactory gains from week to week. The infant should be weighed once a week in the same amount of clothing each time. If the milk intake is inadequate one or more breast feedings may be replaced with a formula. At 5 to 6 months supplementary foods may be added.

During the first 5 or 6 months the breast-fed baby who is gaining at a normal rate receives all the nutrients needed with a few exceptions. These supplements are generally recommended:

Vitamin K is usually given parenterally shortly after birth
10 μg (400 IU) vitamin D as a water–miscible preparation, beginning a week to 10 days after birth [12]
Iron (not more than 15 mg) at 4 to 6 months; may be given as iron-fortified cereal or as iron drops [4]
Vitamin B-12 if the mother is a strict vegetarian

At 5 to 6 months baby foods are introduced and will gradually contribute increasing amounts of nutrients. (See page 290.)

Weaning When the supply of milk declines or breast feeding must be terminated for any reason, the baby is gradually weaned by offering a formula for a single feeding. After 4 to 5 days the baby is offered the bottle for the second feeding, and so on. When breast feeding has been successful for most of the year the baby can be weaned directly to cup feedings of formula.

Contraindications Breast feeding must be discontinued when (1) chronic illnesses are present in the mother, such as cardiac disease, tuberculosis, severe anemia, nephritis, and chronic fevers; (2) another pregnancy ensues; (3) it is necessary for the mother to return to employment outside the home; or (4) the infant is weak or unable to nurse because of cleft palate or harelip. Some places of employment are now providing day-care nurseries and in some of them it is possible for the woman to breast feed her baby.

If the mother has an acute infection it may be necessary to temporarily halt breast feeding. In such a situation the mother's breasts should be completely pumped at regular intervals so that the breast supply will not diminish.

A number of drugs are transmitted to the mother's milk and the baby may have adverse reactions to them. These include anticoagulants, some antibiotics, anticancer drugs, nicotine from heavy cigarette smoking, tranquilizers and sedatives, and "street" drugs. Occasionally breast milk can be contaminated by environmental pollutants such as DDT and PCBs. (See page 253.)

Bottle Feeding

Today's commercial formulas provide safe, easily digested, and nutritious alternatives for infants whose mothers are unable to breast feed or who, for some reason, are not convinced that they should do so. The choice is made by the mother and she should never be made to feel guilty in choosing to bottle feed the baby. Although much is made of mother–infant bonding with breast feeding, such interaction can also be fostered with breast feeding. Indeed, the father can also feed the baby and establish a close father–baby bond. Bottle feeding may free some mothers for additional time with other children. (See Figure 20-2.)

Although bottle feeding does not confer immune properties to the infant, this difference is probably not of major significance when formulas are used according to strict observance of rules of sanitation.

Figure 20-2. Infants are successfully fed by formulas when breast feeding is not possible. The baby should be held comfortably during the feeding. (Courtesy, Ross Laboratories, Columbus, Ohio.)

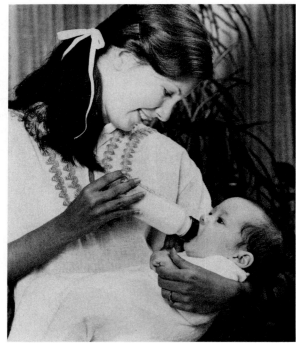

Regulation and Safety of Infant Formulas Under the Infant Formula Act of 1980 the Food and Drug Administration regulates the composition of all infant formulas under the category "Foods for Special Dietary Use." All infant formulas must contain at least the minimum levels of the essential nutrients, these levels having been established by a committee of the American Academy of Pediatrics.[13] The formulas must be produced to ensure safety and wholesomeness. Manufacturers must notify the FDA of any proposed changes in composition, and must keep records of production and distribution for 2 years. The FDA must be notified of any problems that arise.

Commercial formulas have enjoyed remarkable success. That these formulas have met the infant's needs has been documented over and over again. Indeed, the growth and development of formula-fed and breast-fed infants are comparable.

There have been, however, some rare adverse effects of formula feedings.[14] Thus, if a needed nutrient is missing from a formula there may be signs of deficiency if the formula is the sole source of food. Infants who were fed a milk-based formula with low levels of linoleic acid had skin lesions that disappeared when linoleic acid was added. One of the most frequently cited examples occurred during the early 1950s when infants fed a formula in which processing had destroyed the pyridoxine developed anemia, failure to thrive, vomiting, and occasionally convulsive seizures.

One of the most recent problems to arise with formula feeding has been a chloride deficiency observed in infants who were fed a soy-based formula as the sole source of nutrition.[15] The infants had a metabolic alkalosis characterized by vomiting, constipation, failure to thrive, and low blood levels of chloride, potassium, and sodium together with increased plasma bicarbonate and blood urea nitrogen. The addition of potassium chloride to the formula corrected the electrolyte imbalance.

The failure of commercial formulas is more often the result of improper use by the mother, that is, excessive dilution, too little dilution, contamination by polluted water, or holding at temperatures where bacteria thrive. These are major reasons why bottle feeding is discouraged in the developing countries.

Proprietary Premodified Formulas About 95 percent of formula-fed infants are now being given commercially prepared formulas. Some of these are available in dry form; some are concentrated, requiring dilution with water; some are ready-to-use to be measured into the bottle; and some are available in dispos-

able nursing bottles. Their cost is moderate to expensive; packaging in disposable bottles for each feeding increases the cost considerably.

Proprietary formulas are available not only for healthy babies but for a variety of conditions such as lactose intolerance, allergies, and inborn errors of metabolism. (See also pages 447/582/591.) The formulas for healthy infants are patterned on the composition of human milk. (See Table 20-1) They are homogenized and have a low curd tension. Nonfat dry milk is used for milk-based formulas. Typical adaptations of cow's milk include the following:

Protein content is lowered; the protein is treated to produce a fine, flocculent, easily digested curd.
Butterfat is removed, and vegetable oils, such as corn oil are substituted to increase the linoleic acid content.
The cholesterol content is usually low.
Lactose or other carbohydrate is added.
Calcium, phosphorus, and other mineral levels are lowered by dilution.
Vitamins A, D, E, and ascorbic acid are added to meet the infant's needs.
Iron may be added; iron-fortified formulas should be encouraged throughout the first year.

Home-Prepared Formulas A formula prepared in the home using evaporated milk, cane sugar, and ascorbic acid tablets is relatively inexpensive. Neither whole cow's milk nor skim milk is suitable for the first year. Although some savings can be effected by preparing the formula in the home and most babies thrive on them, the families that can most benefit from these savings are sometimes least able to understand the importance of proper measurements and sanitary preparation. An initial evaporated milk formula may include

8 ounces evaporated milk (1 ounce per pound)
16 ounces water (2 ounces per pound)
1½–2 tablespoons corn syrup or cane sugar

Honey is not recommended for infant formulas because its use has occasionally led to infant botulism.[16] As the baby grows the amount of evaporated milk is increased until by 4 to 6 months equal parts of milk and water (about 16 ounces of each) are being used. At that time solid foods are gradually being introduced, and no further increases in the amount of formula are required.

Sterilization of Formula. Terminal sterilization of the formula is preferred. The steps are as follows:

1. Pour measured amount of formula into thoroughly washed bottles.
2. Put nipples on bottles and test the flow of milk.
3. Cover loosely with nipple covers.
4. Place bottles on rack in sterilizer and add water to halfway level of bottles.
5. Cover sterilizer, bring water to boiling, and maintain boiling for 25 minutes.
6. Remove bottles as soon as they can be handled, and cool slightly.
7. Store in refrigerator.

Technique of Feeding The feeding is usually warmed to body temperature, but no adverse effects have been noted when it is given cold. As with breast feeding the baby should be held in a semireclining position. The baby should never be propped up and allowed to feed alone.

An overly large hole in the nipple leads to rapid taking of the formula and excessive swallowing of air, discomfort, and perhaps regurgitation. On the other hand, a very small hole in the nipple will necessitate too long a period of feeding. During the feeding the nipple should be filled with fluid, and not air, so that less air is swallowed. Even so, the infant will need to be "burped" one or more times as experience shows to be necessary.

The baby should not be expected to finish the entire amount of formula in the bottle at each feeding. The mother soon learns how much the baby will usually take at each feeding and can adjust the amounts of formula in the bottle. Any formula remaining at the end of each feeding must be discarded.

Supplements for Formula Feeding Proprietary formulas fortified with iron require no supplementation except for fluoride if the water supply is not fluoridated. Home-prepared formulas should be supplemented with 35 mg ascorbic acid within 2 weeks after birth. Synthetic ascorbic acid is preferable since young babies are sometimes allergic to citrus juices. This may be added to the formula or given with water. At 4 to 6 months iron-fortified cereal is given to meet the iron need. If the water is not fluoridated a fluoride supplement is indicated. When soy–milk formulas are used it is essential that a vitamin B-12 supplement be provided if the formula itself is not fortified.

Solid Foods

Rationale for Timing In the last quarter century most babies have been introduced to solid foods at an early age—sometimes within a few weeks after birth. It was believed that such foods would help the baby to sleep through the night although there is no evidence for this. Many also believed that the early introduction of solid foods would improve acceptance of a variety of foods. However, the sense of taste is not well developed until 3 or 4 months. Mothers were often prodded to early feeding by relatives and friends. Indeed, it was considered to be an accomplishment for the baby to be accepting solid foods!

Pediatricians and nutritionists now recommend that solids be introduced at about 6 months for breast-fed babies and at 4 to 6 months for formula-fed babies. This is more in accord with the time at which lessening of the extrusion reflex occurs and the increased ability to transfer food to the back of the mouth and to voluntarily swallow it. Moreover, fewer allergic reactions are likely when the mucosa of the intestinal tract is less permeable to foreign proteins. Each baby should be allowed to develop a feeding behavior according to his or her neuromuscular coordination.

Proprietary and Home-Prepared Baby Foods Commercially prepared baby foods are convenient, bacteriologically safe, moderate in cost, and available in considerable variety. Baby meats contain more protein than do soups and meat dinners. Desserts that contain sugar contribute to a liking for sweets. Manufacturers have eliminated sugar in some fruits and have reduced the amounts in desserts and fruits that are more acidic. Likewise, salt is no longer added.

Modified food starches have been added to dinners, high-meat dinners, fruits, and desserts in order to retain proper texture, consistency, and uniformity of ingredient distribution. In a study of 430 infants modified starches provided an average of only 2 percent of caloric intake and appeared to be well utilized. Only four of the infants in this study had a modified starch intake accounting for as much as 10 percent of total caloric intake.[17]

With a little expenditure of time and careful attention to sanitary handling of food, the mother can prepare satisfactory foods for the infant, usually at lower cost. Many of the foods prepared for the family can be used, but they should not be salted or sweetened. The mineral and vitamin content is more variable than that of commercial foods. If foods are cooked in a minimum amount of water, puréed or chopped as soon as cooked, and fed to the baby promptly, the nutrient retention should be good. Individual portions may be frozen in ice-cube trays, and stored in plastic bags kept in a freezer for several weeks.

Home-prepared beets, spinach, carrots, and broccoli are not recommended until the latter part of the first year, since they contain appreciable amounts of nitrates.[18] The relatively low acidity of the young infant's stomach favors the conversion of nitrates to nitrites. When absorbed, nitrites change hemoglobin to methemoglobin. This reduces the oxygen-carrying capacity of the blood. Although this is not a widespread problem, it is prudent to delay the introduction of these home-prepared vegetables. Commercially processed carrots, spinach, and broccoli do not present this problem.

Choices for Solid Foods By the end of the year the baby will be consuming 300 to 450 g (10 to 16 oz) of solid foods. Correspondingly, the amount of breast milk or formula ingested will decline to about three fourths of a liter. Formula, rather than fresh whole cow's milk, should be continued throughout the first year. Fresh whole cow's milk is low in iron and unless heated at a high temperature (as in evaporated milk) occasionally causes gastrointestinal bleeding. A typical sequence for adding solid foods is shown in Table 20-2.

Cereals. Iron-fortified rice cereal is preferred initially since it is less likely to produce allergic reactions than are wheat and oats. The dry cereal is mixed with some of the formula, initially using a semiliquid and, later, a more solid consistency.

Crisp toast, zwieback, and graham crackers may be given when teeth appear.

Table 20-2. Typical Sequence for Adding Solid Foods*

The amounts stated below for each age grouping are approximate, and will vary from one infant to another.

5 to 6 months if breast-fed; 4 to 6 months if formula-fed
 Dry, iron-fortified infant cereal—2 to 3 tablespoons
 Strained, unsweetened fruit—2 tablespoons
 Strained vegetable—2 tablespoons

6 to 7 months
 Dry infant cereal—¼ cup
 Fruits and vegetables—3 tablespoons each
 Start strained meat—2 tablespoons

7 to 8 months
 Fortified infant cereal—½ cup
 Mashed or chopped fruits and vegetables—¼ cup each
 Meat—3 tablespoons
 Add zwieback, toast, potatoes

8 to 12 months
 Cereal—½ cup
 Chopped fruits and vegetables—⅓ cup of each
 Meat—¼ cup; may be chopped or ground
 Add mashed cooked egg yolk, cottage cheese or other soft cheese,
  or mashed dried cooked beans or peas

*See page 294 for guidelines for introduction of new foods.

Fruits. Mashed ripe banana or mild-flavored cooked or canned puréed and later chopped fruits without added sugar—applesauce, pears, peaches, prunes—are accepted well. Orange, grapefruit, grape, and apple juices—all unsweetened—are initially diluted with water, given in very small amounts, and then given full strength.

Vegetables. Puréed carrots, peas, green beans, and squash are better accepted initially than are spinach, asparagus, or broccoli.

Protein-Rich Foods. Hard-cooked egg yolk should be mashed and mixed with a little formula, cereal, or vegetable. Only ½ teaspoon should be given initially lest there be an allergy to egg protein. Egg white is not given until the infant is a year old, and then it must be well cooked.

Strained, and later ground or chopped, beef, chicken, turkey, tuna fish, and other fish (with careful removal of all bones) are added by the seventh or eighth month. Cottage cheese or other soft cheese or mashed dried cooked beans may be substituted occasionally for the meat or egg.

Feeding Problems and Nutritional Issues

Regurgitation and Colic The small amounts of food regurgitated by many babies is no cause for concern. Vomiting is more serious and should receive the prompt attention of the pediatrician.

Some babies cry loudly and for long intervals following feeding. Usually they have swallowed excessive amounts of air and have been inadequately burped. However, some babies continue to cry even with burping and the parents become quite distraught. These colicky babies usually grow well; the parents need reassurance that they are progressing satisfactorily and will usually outgrow the colic within a few months. Colic sometimes occurs because the baby is overfed, is tired, or is cold.

Some breast-fed infants who become colicky may be allergic to their own mother's milk if the mother is drinking cow's milk. A recent study showed that many breast-fed infants no longer had colic when their mothers gave up cow's milk.[19]

Constipation Formula-fed infants usually have but one bowel movement daily, whereas breast-fed infants have two or three. Only when the stools are hard and dry and eliminated with difficulty does constipation exist. Prune juice or strained prunes given daily usually suffice to correct the constipation.

Diarrhea Infantile diarrhea may be caused by bacterial or viral infection or by injudicious ingestion of some foods. Other causes of diarrhea include allergy, lactose intolerance, and malabsorption syndromes such as cystic fibrosis and gluten enteropathy. An infant who is malnourished is more susceptible to diarrhea; diarrhea, in turn, can initiate or accentuate malnutrition.

Diarrhea is a serious problem that can be life threatening if it persists in an infant. The losses through the stool include fluid, base, sodium, potassium, and chloride. The consequences of these losses are dehydration, acidosis, fever, and reduction of kidney function. Vomiting causes loss of acid and a lowering of total body anions and cations. The younger the infant the more serious the problem.

If the diarrhea is mild and of short duration, the pediatrician may recommend that the mother give the infant an oral glucose–electrolyte solution available from the pharmacy. As soon as this solution is tolerated the infant is gradually introduced to a half-strength formula (10 kcal per ounce), and in stages to the full strength formula. The mother must receive precise instructions for the use of the glucose-electrolyte solution and for the formula, and must keep records of intake and losses.

When diarrhea is severe and vomiting precludes oral feeding, hospitalization becomes necessary. The infant is given glucose and electrolytes by intravenous feeding or may require hyperalimentation.

Many infants with moderate to severe diarrhea have a transient intolerance to lactose and sometimes to other carbohydrates. For these infants soy–isolate or casein hydrolysate formulas are sometimes used.* Convalescence may be prolonged and increases in concentration and in volume of formula must be made with caution.

Hazards of Overconcentrated Formulas Formulas are sometimes insufficiently diluted with water because of error, or because the mother mistakenly believes that the baby will be better nourished if the formula is more concentrated. Also, if skim milk is boiled, as was formerly recommended for infants with diarrhea, the solute concentration increases unless the water lost by evaporation is replaced. With the higher solute concentration the kidney requires additional water for the excretion of metabolic

---

* Isomil (Ross Laboratories, Columbus, Ohio), Mullsoy and NeoMullsoy (Syntex Laboratories, Inc., Palo Alto, California), and Nutramigen, Pregestimil, and ProSobee (Mead Johnson & Company, Evansville, Indiana).

wastes. Dehydration becomes increasingly severe, and, if not corrected, could lead to renal failure and coma.

Bottle Mouth Syndrome This condition of rampant dental caries affects especially the maxillary incisors (four upper anterior teeth). Infants who are allowed to use the bottle with milk or juice in it as a pacifier at bedtime, or who breast feed at night after 1 year, or who suck on a pacifier dipped in a sweetener are especially susceptible to the condition. The teeth are bathed with the liquid containing the fermentable carbohydrate and in severe cases may be destroyed.

Salt Intake Salt taste is a learned behavior. Babies will accept unsalted and salted foods equally well, and much of the salt added to infant foods seems to be a response to the mother's, and not the infant's, taste. Normal salt intakes exceed requirements by a wide margin. The healthy baby readily excretes the excess and seems to be able to adapt to a wide margin of intake. Based on animal research as well as epidemiologic studies, many clinicians are concerned that excessive salt intake could lead to hypertension in later life. A sodium intake that is within the safe and adequate range is a prudent measure to take. (See page 284.) Manufacturers of baby foods now omit salt in their products. Mothers, likewise, should prepare foods for the baby and their young children that contain no added salt.

Sugar Intake Breast-fed babies as well as most babies given commercial formulas ingest lactose, a sugar that is not very sweet. When home-prepared formulas are used, the sugar or corn syrup added to meet the caloric requirement should be used only until solid foods are added.

Infants do not need to be taught to like sweet foods. Three objections can be raised to the use of sugar in the infant diet: (1) the role in dental caries; (2) the contribution of energy without a corresponding contribution of other nutrients; (3) the initiation of a lifetime habit of overuse of sweet foods.

Some mothers who are concerned that cane sugar never be used will substitute raw sugar, brown sugar, or honey. All these condition the infant to sweet foods and supply only insignificant amounts of nutrients other than carbohydrate; also, honey sometimes poses the threat of botulism.

Obesity Some studies have shown that infants who remain in the 90th percentile of weight during the first year are more likely to become obese in later life than are infants whose weight remains within the 25th to 75th percentile. According to these studies, adipocytes increase at an abnormal rate until adolescence. Thereafter, the number of cells remains fixed throughout life, but the size of each cell increases enormously. When weight is lost the size of the cells decreases but the cells themselves remain intact. A recent study showed a close correlation between excessive weight gains at 6 weeks, 3 months, and 6 months, and overweight and obesity at 6 to 8 years.[20] More recently it has been suggested that the fat cell theory is speculative, and that fat infants will not necessarily remain fat.[21]

Infantile obesity must be approached individually.[22] It is not necessarily caused by bottle feeding instead of breast feeding, or the early introduction of solid foods. Nor is it caused by a mother's inability to heed the baby's satiety signals. Some mothers, however, may prod the baby to finish the bottle, thinking that the baby will be undernourished if the amounts recommended by the nutritionist or pediatrician are not consumed. Other mothers may give food to their babies whenever they cry to keep them quiet.

Babies who are inactive will have lower energy requirements, and their caloric intake needs to be monitored. Nonfat milk formulas should not be used in the first year. Any solid foods that are given should be rich in nutrients but restricted in the amounts of fat that they contain. The obese infant should be monitored for gains in height and weight, the objective being to allow the baby to "slim out" and to maintain a more moderate rate of gain. Inactivity in an infant is a tendency to be watched in the forthcoming years when the child needs special encouragement to activity.

Anemia Iron, folacin, and vitamin B-12 deficiency can cause anemia. Of these, iron deficiency is by far the most common. It is rare in breast-fed babies. The healthy, full-term infant is born with an iron store sufficient for hemoglobin synthesis up to 4 to 6 months. Thereafter, the infant should be given iron-fortified cereal or an iron-fortified formula. If anemia occurs it may persist into the second or third year and may interfere with growth and development.

Human milk and proprietary formulas supply sufficient folacin for the infant. Home-prepared formulas from evaporated milk are likely to contain little folacin because of the destruction during the sterilization of the formula. If such home-prepared formulas are used, a folacin supplement may be prescribed.

Vitamin B-12 deficiency has been observed in infants who were breast-fed by mothers who had long been strict vegetarians and who had therefore depleted their own stores of vitamin B-12.[23] Deficiency may also occur if a home-prepared soy formula is used without supplementation with vitamin B-12. Home-prepared soy formulas are likely to be deficient in other nutrients as well, and their use is not recommended.

Growth Failure Infants may fail to grow for a variety of reasons. In some there are errors of metabolism that must be treated with an appropriate modified formula. (See page 588.) Others have congenital heart conditions that require surgery before adequate feeding can take place. Infants who are small for gestational age are likely to experience a slow rate of growth and may never fully catch up.

Growth failure also occurs because of a poor physical and emotional environment in the home. The infant may be unwanted and thus fails to get nutritional or emotional support. Mothers may be burdened with poverty and may have many children that distract them. Some mothers may have failed as children to get the emotional support they needed. Other young mothers do not know how to interact with their infants; they don't hold them or talk to them but leave them untended in their cribs.

When physical and emotional support are severely lacking, the infant may progress to a marasmic state, including wasting, dehydration, and diarrhea. (See page 352.) Growth and development are resumed only when the infant is provided with adequate nutrition and also with emotional stimulation with holding and being cared for. In the severely depleted infant, it is essential to replace fluid and electrolyte losses by oral or intravenous solutions. At first half-strength formulas are used, and the concentration is gradually increased according to the infant's tolerance.

Allergy A special problem in infants and young children is milk sensitivity. From 1 to 3 percent of all children are sensitive to cow's milk. In many instances this may be associated with infection and emotional stress; in others genetic factors may be a cause. (See Galactose Disease and Lactose Intolerance, page 593.)

In milk sensitivity changing the form of the milk sometimes improves tolerance—that is, boiled, powdered, acidulated, or evaporated milk may be satisfactory when fresh cow's milk is not. Many children outgrow their sensitivity to milk by 1 or 2 years. At this age the child should be given small amounts of milk to determine tolerance.

In infants with true milk allergy the response to the ingestion of milk is immediate and may lead to colic, spitting up of the feeding, irritability, diarrhea, and respiratory disorders. In some infants a delayed reaction may occur hours to days following the ingestion of milk, and thus it becomes difficult to determine the cause.

Each of the common proteins in milk has been found to be allergenic, but alpha-lactoglobulin is the most common. Several hypoallergenic formulas are available with a casein hydrolysate, meat, or soybean often used as the protein source.* Eggs, citrus fruits, corn products, wheat, chicken, fish, and pork are relatively common allergens. These foods should be introduced, one at a time, during the second 6 months so that any allergic tendency can be determined.

COUNSELING THE MOTHER

Community Resources   The La Leche League International is a lay group that supports breast feeding.* It issues practical guidelines for the pregnant woman in preparation for breast feeding, and also for initiation of the new infant to the breast. Through local chapters new mothers can talk with other mothers to air their concerns and to receive advice.

To families who qualify on the basis of low income, the WIC program (see page 275) provides food supplements for infants who are at high nutritional risk, for example, low-birth-weight infants, those who fail to gain or who gain excessively, and those who are anemic. A typical food allowance for the infant includes iron-fortified formula, cereal high in iron, and fruit juice.

Infant Feeding   The nutritionist or nurse who counsels the pregnant woman should present the advantages of breast and formula feedings, but the choice should be freely made by the woman without any pressures whatsoever. If she chooses to breast feed, she needs guidance prior to delivery on diet and care of the breasts. The new mother nursing a baby for the first time sometimes needs guidance and encouragement from the nurse and directions for support of the breast and care of the nipples.

*La Leche League International, 9616 Minneapolis Avenue, Franklin Park, IL 60131.

* Nutramigen (Mead Johnson and Co., Evansville, Indiana); MBF (Meat-base formula) (Gerber Products Company, Fremont, Michigan); and Neomullsoy (Syntex Laboratories, Palo Alto, California).

If commercial formulas are selected, these points must be emphasized: reading of labels for proper dilution of formulas; sanitation of bottles into which formulas are placed; refrigeration of formula once it is mixed.

If formulas and baby foods are to be home prepared, detailed written and illustrated instructions should be provided. In addition the dietary counselor should demonstrate measurements, sanitation of utensils, and terminal sterilization of the formula.

Introduction of New Foods   These practical suggestions are intended to help the mother give the baby a smooth adjustment to new foods.

1. Hold the baby upright while feeding to facilitate swallowing and to enhance the baby's feeling of security.
2. Give very small amounts of any new food—teaspoonfuls or even less—at the beginning.
3. Introduce only one new food each week. Allow the infant to become familiar with that food before trying another. Watch for any allergic symptoms.
4. Use foods of smooth rather thin consistency at first. Gradually the consistency is made more solid as the infant learns how to use the tongue in propelling food to the back of the mouth. With a small spoon food is placed on the middle of the tongue, thereby facilitating swallowing.
5. Never force an infant to eat more of a food than he or she takes willingly.
6. If, after several trials, it is apparent that a baby has an acute dislike for a food, omit that item for a week or two and try it again. If the dislike persists it is better to forget about that food for a while and substitute another.
7. Gradually introduce variety from each group of foods. Babies, like older persons, tire of repetition of certain foods.
8. When the baby is able to chew, gradually substitute finely chopped foods for strained foods. Include some zwieback or dry toast.
9. Avoid showing in any way a dislike for a food that is being given.
10. During the first year avoid giving any foods that the baby cannot chew and that can cause choking and obstruction of the airway. These include nuts, popcorn, stringy foods, raisins, candies, round cylindrical foods such as hot dogs, or chunks of meat.[25]
11. Finally, recognize that the baby learns about food also by touching it. Sometimes the infant tries to feed himself or herself by hand. Later, when the baby tries to use a spoon but finds it frustrating to get food onto the spoon and into the mouth, hand feeding may again

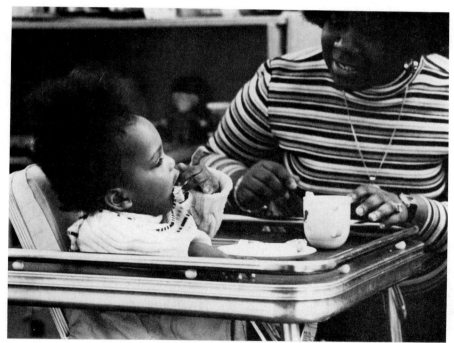

Figure 20-3. Infants also learn about foods by touching them. This infant begins to coordinate finger movements and also begins to assert some independence by picking up the food instead of letting her mother feed her. (Courtesy, Handicapped Children's Unit, St. Christopher's Hospital for Children, Philadelphia.)

be resorted to. The mother needs to exercise understanding, patience, and discretion in helping the baby get the feel of food and in feeding with the spoon. This is usually a messy time in the course of learning to self-feed. (See Figure 20-3.)

Nutrition for Low-Birth-Weight Infants

Remarkable progress has been made in recent years in the survival rate of low- and very-low-birth weight infants. This has become possible in hospital intensive care nurseries, where attention is focused on the maintenance of breathing, thermal support, fluid and electrolyte control, and nutritional adequacy. A report from one such unit indicated survival to range from 80 to 90 percent for infants who weighed 1,001 g or more and 48 percent for infants weighing 501 to 1000g.[26]

Definitions A low-birth-weight infant (LBW) is one whose weight at birth is 2,500 g (5½ pounds) or less. A very-low-birth-weight infant (VLBW) weighs 1,500 g or less.

Low-birth-weight infants born prematurely may have a weight appropriate for the gestational age (AGA). They have had satisfactory nutrition up to the time of birth and usually their growth and development is satisfactory.

Other low-birth-weight infants, whether premature or full term, may have a weight that is small for gestational age (SGA) or "light for date." These SGA infants are poorly nourished because of severe maternal malnutrition, insufficient placental transfer of nutrients, or genetic abnormalities. These infants grow and develop slowly, and some never fully catch up.

Developmental Problems The LBW infant is born with poorly developed muscle tissues, very little body fat, low stores of iron, and an inadequately mineralized skeleton. Because there is very little fat and practically no glycogen, the energy stores are minimal and hypoglycemia and starvation result unless calories are supplied early. The energy needs are high because the surface area is proportionately great and because the extremely small deposits of subcutaneous fat result in a higher rate of heat loss.

The infant of less than 34 weeks has poor sucking and swallowing reflexes. Absence of the peristaltic waves of the esophagus together with incomplete functioning of the esophageal sphincter is not uncommon. These deficiencies frequently lead to regurgitation and aspiration, with its attendant danger.

The capacity of the stomach is small and the emptying time is slow. Bile salt deficiency reduces the ability to digest and absorb fat and fat-soluble vitamins. Reduced disaccharidase activity is common. Lactose intolerance is often seen in the first weeks of life. Protein digestion is adequate, but casein curds can lead to LACTOBEZOAR, a concretion formed in the stomach.

Because the kidneys are immature, there is a reduced capacity to excrete wastes and consideration must be given to the concentration of nitrogenous constituents and electrolytes. When there is evidence of growth the renal solute load is reduced because of the use of nitrogen and minerals for tissue synthesis.

Nutritional Requirements The goal in nutritional care is to provide a level of nutrients that would allow the same rate of growth and development as would have been achieved in utero at full term. The exact needs are not known but advisable intakes are summarized in Table 20-3. The nutritional care protocol and guidelines used by Rickard and associates[26] were as follows:

Age to low weight, days	8
Weight loss, percent	10
Age to regain birth weight, days	14
Age to achieve full caloric intake, days	7
Age to achieve initial sustained weight gain, days	7
Energy intake, kcal/kg	
To low weight	
Enteral	80
Parenteral	60
During initial sustained gain (mean 19 g per day)	100
During gains of 20 g or more per day	
Enteral	120
Parenteral	90

Based on body weight the estimated requirements are as follows:

Fluid: 150 to 200 ml per kg
Energy: at 120 kcal per kg the LBW infant grows at about the same rate as in utero; that is, about 20g per day.
Protein: 3 to 5 g per kg

Minerals. Hypocalcemia and rickets are perplexing problems for LBW infants. Calcium supplementation is needed if preterm human milk is used, and if special formulas do not supply the advisable intakes. Hy-

ponatremia occurs if the sodium intake is not increased as the infant grows. From time to time the serum and urine sodium concentrations should be checked. LBW infants have stores of iron for only 2 to 3 months, at which time an iron supplement (2 mg per kg) is recommended. At this age the infant can usually take an iron-fortified standard formula.

Vitamins. Preterm infants have high requirements for folacin, ascorbic acid, vitamin B-12, vitamin D, and vitamin E. (See Table 20-3.) The intake of the infant is very small, so that neither preterm milk nor special formulas will meet the vitamin needs, and a multivitamin supplement is generally prescribed.

Preterm Milk Feeding Some low-birth-weigh infants can be breast-fed by their own mothers. LBW infants progress more rapidly with preterm milk because its composition is more suited to the infant's needs than is term milk.[27] If the infant is unable to suck, the mother can pump her breasts. Lactation failure by mothers of LBW infants is high.

The composition of preterm milk varies widely from one woman to another, and changes as lactation proceeds. Some studies have shown that preterm milk is higher in immune properties, total nitrogen, protein nitrogen, sodium, chloride, iron, cholesterol, phospholipids, and polyunsaturated fatty acids.[28,31] The caloric, calcium, potassium, and magnesium levels were found to be similar to those of full-term milk. Supplements of calcium are generally required. Little is known of the vitamin concentration of preterm milk, but supplements are generally advised.

Selection of Formula Considerable improvement in formulas available for feeding VLBW and LBW infants has been made within the past few years. Such formulas are subject to change as new studies are completed, and the most recent data available from the manufacturers should form the basis for selection for a given infant. Some of these formulas have been described as having the following characteristics[26,32]:*

Energy: 81 kcal per dl instead of 67 kcal per dl, as in standard formulas.
Protein: 2.5 to 3.0 g per 100 kcal; regular formulas supply 2.2 g per 100 kcal.
The whey-to-casein ratio is 60:40 and gives a better distribution of amino acids than that provided by

---

* Enfamil Premature with Whey (Mead Johnson Nutritional Division, Evansville, Indiana); Similac Special Care (Ross Laboratories, Columbus, Ohio); and "Preemie" SMA (Wyeth Laboratories, Philadelphia).

Table 20-3. Advisable Intakes for Low-Birth-Weight Infants*

	Infant's Weight			Infant's Weight
	800–120 g per 100 kcal	1,200–1,500 g per 100 kcal		800–1,500 g
Protein, g	3.1	2.7	Vitamin A, IU	500
Calcium, mg	160	140	Vitamin D, IU	600
Phosphorus, mg	108	95	Vitamin E, IU	30
Sodium, mEq	2.7	2.3	Vitamin K, μg	15
Potassium, mEq	1.9	1.8	Ascorbic acid, mg	60
Chloride, mEq	2.4	2.0	Thiamin, mg	0.2
Magnesium, mg	7.5	6.5	Riboflavin, mg	0.4
Zinc, mg	0.5		Niacin, mg equiv.	5.0
Copper, μg	60		Vitamin B-6, mg	0.4
Iodine, μg	5		Folacin, μg	60
Manganese, μg	5		Vitamin B-12, μg	1.5
			Biotin, μg	12
			Pantothenic acid, mg	2.0

* Adapted from Rickard, K. A., et al.: "Nutritional Outcome of 207 Very-Low-Birth-Weight Infants in an Intensive Care Unit," *J. Am. Diet. Assoc.*, **81**:677, 1982.

standard formulas with a whey to casein ratio of 18:82. Also, the high whey-to-casein ratio reduces the likelihood of formation of lactobezoar.

Fat: Some of the fat is provided by medium-chain triglycerides (MCT), which are more readily absorbed than are the longer-chain fatty acids. The proportion of polyunsaturated fatty acids, iron, and vitamin E is controlled to avoid hemolytic anemia.

Carbohydrate: The special formulas contain lower levels of lactose with the balance of carbohydrate being furnished by glucose polymers, which are readily digested and utilized.

Osmolality: To avoid excess solute load for the gastrointestinal tract and renal system, the osmolality of the special formulas is similar to that of human milk.

Minerals and vitamins: Variations from one formula to the next should be considered when determining the need for supplementation. Usually supplementation is advisable, since the volume of formula intake may be too low to supply desirable levels.

Method of Feeding Some older (34 weeks gestation or more) LBW infants are able to suck and are fed by nipple. If the infant tires too much, part of the feeding may be given by gavage. Enteral feeding is preferred for the VLBW infant if the clinical status is stable; that is, there is no abdominal distention, reflux, or diarrhea.[26] Intragastric feeding is preferable to transpyloric feeding because there are fewer complications. When enteral feeding is not feasible,

peripheral parenteral nutrition (glucose, electrolytes, vitamins, amino acids) is used. Total parenteral nutrition by central vein is an option when oral and enteral routes are impossible for extended periods of time.

Schedule of Feeding The feeding schedule for infants weighing less than 1,500 g but having no complications has been described by Rickard and associates[26,33]:

First day: Give 80 to 100 ml per kg of 10 percent glucose–electrolyte solution. Over the next few days, gradually increase the amount to 100 to 200 ml per kg.

Second day: Give about 3 ml per kg of a half-strength formula (12 kcal per ounce). Give feedings about every 2 hours for the smallest babies. At every other feeding, increase the amount of formula by 1 to 2 ml, provided that there are no adverse effects. Continue the intravenous solution to achieve 80 to 150 ml per kg total fluid intake.

Third day: Give full strength formula (24 kcal per ounce). Gradually increase the size of the feedings as on the second day. Continue the intravenous solution, gradually decreasing the amount as the amount of formula given increases.

Fourth day: If the enteral intake is less than 80 kcal per kg, increase the formula concentration, or add peripheral parenteral nutrition, or transpyloric feeding.

Seventh day: If enteral intake is less than 100 kcal per kg, consider the alternative options for day 4.

Infant from Birth to Six Months

After Mr. D completed college, Mr. and Mrs. D were married and moved to Maine, where he has taught history to junior high school students for the past five years. Mrs. D attended business school after completing high school and has been a legal secretary for the past 7 years.

Mr. and Mrs. D excitedly awaited the arrival of their first child. They were a bit nervous about caring for a new baby, since neither of them had had experience with infants. They attended prenatal and childbirth education classes which helped them to feel more at ease about becoming new parents.

Mrs. D had an uncomplicated pregnancy, labor, and delivery. At birth their son, Jon, weighed 2.7 kg (6 lb) and was 51 cm (20 in.) long. No congenital abnormalities were found. Mrs. D nursed him for the first time in the delivery room. While in the hospital she was able to have her baby with her as much as she wanted during the day. The nursing staff was helpful in answering her many questions related to feeding and child care.

Upon discharge from the hospital, 4-day-old Jon weighed 2.5 kg (5½ lb). Mrs. D became concerned about the adequacy of her milk supply, especially since the baby was small and fussy. Her worries were reinforced by the lack of support from others. Everyone remarked about Jon's small size. Mrs. D became very sensitive about the comments concerning her boy's size and to the suggestions about breast feeding and caring for her baby.

At his 2-week checkup, Jon weighed 2.6 kg (5 lb 13 oz). The pediatrician told the mother that Jon's weight gain was below the normal range expected for babies of his age. However, the baby had almost regained his birth weight and all clinical signs were normal. The pediatrician suggested that Mrs D supplement the evening feeding with Enfamil formula. He also suggested how to build up her milk supply, such as increasing the frequency of feedings, increasing fluid intake, eating a well-balanced diet, and getting adequate rest.

At his 6-week checkup, Jon weighed 3.4 kg (7 lb, 8 oz) and measured 54 cm (21 in.). Mrs. D was much more confident about breast feeding, and her milk supply was well established. Mrs. D asked about the safety of food additives in commercially prepared baby foods and questioned whether she should prepare her own baby food.

She was also bewildered by the differing advice she heard from people as to when solid foods should be introduced. The pediatrician advised that solids be introduced when Jon reaches 5 to 6 months of age. He also recommended that she attend nutrition class for new mothers on diet additions for infants.

Mrs. D started Jon on rice cereal fortified with iron at 5 months of age and then introduced fruits such as applesauce and bananas. He tolerated solids well and had little difficulty in learning to eat from a spoon. Vegetables were gradually added to the diet when he was 6 months old.

At the 6-month checkup Jon weighed 6.4 kg (14 lb) and had grown 4.5 cm (2 in.). He now has a double chin and looks chubby. Mrs. D now worries that Jon is becoming overweight. She has decided to wean him and wonders whether she should start him on skim milk or continue to use the formula.

Physiologic Correlations

1. What factors enter into a baby's size at birth?
2. In addition to height and weight, list other measurements and clinical signs that indicate normal growth and development.
3. How does the infant's body differ from that of the older child or adult in water content? fat content? surface area?
4. What are the nutritional implications of the differences in body composition?
5. According to the NCHS growth charts, Jon's length and weight fall between the fifth and tenth percentiles. The pediatrician is not concerned about this and explains to Mrs. D that Jon is "his own best control." What does he mean by this?

Nutritional Assessment

6. Jon's first feedings from the breast were small amounts of colostrum. What is colostrum?
7. What is the normal weekly rate of weight gain during the second 6 months?
8. List the Recommended Dietary Allowances for Jon for the first 6 months and for the second 6 months for energy, protein, vitamin D, ascorbic acid, calcium, and iron.
9. State two reasons why the energy requirements are so high.
10. What mineral requires particular attention in planning Jon's diet for the second 6 months? Why?
11. What factors may contribute to overfeeding of infants?

Planning the Diet

12. Which of the following constituents are higher in human milk when compared with whole cow's milk: casein; lactalbumin; fat; lactose; calcium; phosphorus; vitamin A; thiamin; riboflavin; niacin?

13. List the ways in which cow's milk is adjusted to simulate human milk in the preparation of commercial formulas.

14. Why is ascorbic acid initially given to Jon in synthetic form rather than as orange juice?

15. How would you go about introducing orange juice to Jon?

16. Why is the proprietary rice cereal better for Jon than a home-prepared cereal?

Dietary Counseling

17. What suggestions would you make for weaning Jon from the breast to the bottle and then to a cup?

18. List five suggestions that you could give to Jon's mother regarding the introduction of solid foods.

19. What factors will influence the amounts of food that Jon may eat?

20. Write a typical day's menu for Jon at 6 months. Include suggested times and amounts of foods.

References for the Case Study

AHN, C. H., and MACLEAN, W. C.: "Growth of the Exclusively Breast-fed Infant," *Am. J. Clin. Nutr.*, 33:183–92, 1980.

COOPER, A., and HEIRD, W. C.: "Nutritional Assessment of the Pediatric Patient Including the Low-birth-weight Infant," *Am. J. Clin. Nutr. (Suppl.)*, 35:1132–41, 1982.

FOMON, S. J., et al.: "Recommendations for Feeding Normal Infants," *Pediatrics*, 63:52–59, 1979.

HIMES, G. H.: "Infant Feeding Practices and Obesity," *J. Am. Diet. Assoc.*, 75:122–25, 1979.

MARLIN, D. W., et al.: "Infant Feeding Practices," *J. Am. Diet. Assoc.*, 77:668–76, 1980.

OWEN, A. L.: *Feeding Guide: A Nutritional Guide for the Maturing Infant.* Health Learning Systems, Inc., Bloomfield, N.J. Available from Mead Johnson Nutrition Division, Evansville, Indiana.

POPESCU, C. B.: *Breast or Bottle?* American Council on Science and Health, New York, 1983.

QUANDT, S. A.: "The Effect of Beikost on the Diet of Breast-fed Infants," *J. Am. Diet. Assoc.*, 84:47–51, 1984.

STAHL, M. D., and GUIDA, D. A.: "Slow Weight Gain in the Breast-fed Infant: Management Options," *Pediatr. Nurs.*, 10:117–20, March/April 1984.

YEUNG, D. L., et al.: "Infant Fatness and Feeding Practices: A Longitudinal Assessment," *J. Am. Diet. Assoc.*, 79:531–35, 1981.

References

1. Owen, G., and Lippman, G.: "Nutritional Status of Infants and Young Children: U.S.A," *Pediatr. Clin. North Am.*, 24:211–27, 1977.

2. Food and Nutrition Board: *Recommended Dietary Allowances*, 10th ed. National Research Council–National Academy of Sciences, Washington, D.C., 1989.

3. Jackson, R. L.: "Maternal and Infant Nutrition and Health in Later Life," *Nutr. Rev.*, 37:33–37, 1979.

4. Committee on Nutrition, American Academy of Pediatrics: "Iron Supplementation for Infants," *Pediatrics*, 58:765–67, 1976.

5. Filer, L. J.: "Salt in Infant Foods," *Nutr. Rev.*, 29:27–30, 1971.

6. Williams, M. L., et al.: "Role of Dietary Iron and Fat on Vitamin E Deficiency Anemia of Infancy," *N. Eng. J. Med.*, 292:887–90, 1975.

7. Committee on Nutrition, American Academy of Pediatrics: "The Promotion of Breast Feeding," *Pediatrics*, 69:654–61, 1982.

8. Martinez, G. A., et al.: "1981 Milk-Feeding Patterns in the United States during the First 12 Months of Life," *Pediatrics*, 71:166–70, 1983.

9. Review: "Adequacy of Lactation in Well-Nourished Mothers," *Nutr. Rev.*, 40:136–38, 1982.

10. Rassin, D. K., et al.: "Feeding the Low-Birth Weight Infant. II. Effects of Taurine and Cholesterol Supplementation on Amino Acids and Cholesterol," *Pediatrics*, 71:179–86, 1983.

11. Kabara, J. J.: "Lipids as Host-Resistance Factors in Human Milk," *Nutr. Rev.*, 38:65–73, 1980.

12. Fomon, S. J., et al.: "Recommendations for Feeding Normal Infants," *Pediatrics*, 63:52–59, 1979.

13. Committee on Nutrition, American Academy of Pediatrics: "Commentary on Breast Feeding and Infant Formulas, Including Proposed Standards for Formulas," *Nutr. Rev.*, 34:248–56, 1976.

14. Roy, S.: "Perspectives on Adverse Effects of Milks and Infant Formulas Used in Infant Feeding," *J. Am. Diet. Assoc.*, 82:373–77, 1983.

15. Linshaw, M. A., et al.: "Hypochloremic Alkalosis in Infants Associated with Soy Protein Formula," *J. Pediatr.*, 96: 635–40, 1980.

16. Arnon, S. S., et al.: "Honey and Other Risk Factors for Infant Botulism," *J. Pediatr.*, 94:331–36, 1979.

17. Filer, L. J., Jr.: "Modified Food Starches for Use in Infant Foods," *Nutr. Rev.*, 29:55–59, 1971.

18. Raab, C. A.: "The Nitrite Dilemma: Pink and Preserved?," *J. Nutr. Educ.*, 5:8–9, 1973.

19. Jacobsson, I., and Lindberg, T.: "Cow's Milk Proteins Cause Infantile Colic in Breast-Fed Infants: A Double-Blind Crossover Study," *Pediatrics*, 71:268–71, 1983.

20. Eid, E. E.: "Follow-up Study of Physical Growth of Children Who Had Excessive Weight Gain in First Six Months of Life," *Br. Med. J.*, 2:74–77, 1970.

21. Yeung, D. L., et al.: "Infant Fatness and Feeding Practices: A Longitudinal Assessment," *J. Am. Diet. Assoc.*, **79**:531–35, 1981.

22. Dubois, S., et al.: "An Examination of Factors Believed to be Associated with Infantile Obesity," *Am. J. Clin. Nutr.*, 37: 1997–2004, 1979.

23. Review: "Vitamin B-12 Deficiency in Breast-Fed Infant of a Strict Vegetarian (Clinical Nutrition Case)," *Nutr. Rev.*, **37**:142–44, 1979.

24. Lebenthal, E.: "Cow's Milk Protein Allergy," *Pediatr. Clin. North Am.*, **22**:827–33, 1975.

25. Lecos, C.: "Determining When a Food Poses a Hazard," *FDA Consumer*, **17**:25–28, 1983.

26. Rickard, K. A., et al.: "Nutritional Outcome of 207 Very-Low-Birth-Weight Infants in an Intensive Care Unit," *J. Am. Diet. Assoc.*, **81**:674–82, 1982.

27. Review: "Preterm Human Milk Improves the Growth of Preterm Infants," *Nutr. Rev.*, **41**:304–305, 1983.

28. Gross, S. J., et al.: "Nutritional Composition of Milk Produced by Mother's Delivery Preterm," *J. Pediatr.*, **96**:641–44, 1980.

29. Bitman, J., et al.: "Comparison of the Lipid Composition of Breast Milk from Mothers of Term and Preterm Infants," *Am. J. Clin. Nutr.*, **38**:300–12, 1983.

30. Review: "Differences between the Immunology of Term and Preterm Milk," *Nutr. Rev.*, **41**:237–38, 1983.

31. Review: "Biochemical Differences between Preterm and Term Milk," *Nutr. Rev.*, **41**:79–80, 1983.

32. Brady, M. S., et al.: "Formulas and Human Milk for Premature Infants: A Review and Update," *J. Am. Diet. Assoc.*, **81**:547–82, 1982.

33. Rickard, K., and Gresham, E.: "Nutritional Considerations for the Newborn Requiring Intensive Care," *J. Am. Diet. Assoc.*, **66**:592–600, 1975.

21

Nutrition for Children and Teenagers

Each person inherits a unique genetic pattern upon which the environment throughout life brings about modifications in physical, biochemical, mental, and emotional characteristics. The rate of growth and maturation and the activity of the child and teenager, rather than chronological age, are the more accurate predictors of nutritional needs. Desirable food behaviors for a lifetime have their beginnings in childhood and adolescence.

Growth and Development

Preschool and School Children Neither growth nor development occurs at a uniform rate. The rapid growth in overall size that occurred in fetal life and during infancy is followed by a long period of very gradual growth that accelerates again in the adolescent years. The three phases of cellular growth continue: rapid cell division; slowing of cell division but increase in cell size; and cessation of cell division with continuing protein synthesis and increase in cell size. These phases follow a chronologic schedule with the timing differing for the various organs and tissues of the body. For example, brain development is rapid during fetal life and infancy whereas sexual maturation takes place during the teen years.

During the second year the toddler increases in height by 10 to 12 cm (3.8 to 4.8 in.), and in the third year by 7 to 9 cm (2.7–3.5 in.). Half of the adult height is usually achieved by the age of 2½ to 3 years. After the third year, the annual gain in height averages 5 to 6 cm (2.0–2.3 in.) and occurs rather evenly throughout the childhood years. Wide variations in height occur depending upon the genetic potential and the living environment. For example, based on the NCHS standards (see Table A-13) the 5-year-old boy at the 95th percentile is about 15 cm (6 in.) taller than is the boy at the 5th percentile. By the time he is ten the difference is about 22 cm (8.9 in.). At each age

NUTRITIONAL ISSUES AND PROBLEMS

Parents voice continuing concerns about the foods that their children need and especially about ways to achieve desirable habits. Common problems that adversely affect the nutritional status of children and teenagers are preventable. These include obesity, underweight, growth failure, anemia, and dental caries.

The role of a prudent diet during the early years of life in the prevention of chronic conditions in adult life, including arteriosclerosis, hypertension, diseases of the heart, and cancer, is supported by many and disputed by others. What is a responsible position to take on such controversy in the feeding of children?

The use of additives in foods is looked upon with dismay by many parents. Especially this relates to the popular additive-free diet for the treatment of hyperactivity in preschool and school children. Controlled research has not supported the value of such a diet.

Other concerns of parents and health professionals include sugar (see page 78), salt (see page 143), "junk foods" (see page 239), "fast foods" (see page 239), "organic" and "natural" foods (see page 239), and vegetarian diets (see page 230).

throughout childhood boys are a little taller than girls.

The toddler gains about 2½ to 3 kg (5.5 to 6.5 pounds) in the second year and has approximately quadrupled the birth weight. Thereafter the gains are gradual throughout childhood and average about 1½ to 2 kg (3.3–4.4 pounds) per year. As with height, so there are wide differences in weight at a given age. For example, the 5-year-old boy at the 95th percentile will weigh 8 kg (17.6 pounds) more than the boy at the 5th percentile. (See Table A-13.) At 10 years the difference is about 21 kg (46 pounds). At each age throughout childhood boys weigh somewhat more than girls, until about 11 to 13 years when girls are somewhat heavier.

During the second year the somewhat chubby baby "slims out." The legs become longer, the muscle mass increases, and the bones become increasingly mineralized. The body water decreases gradually with the addition of adipose tissue and of minerals to the bones. The body protein content has increased from 14.6 percent at the end of the first year to the adult level of 18 to 19 percent of body weight by 4 years of age.[1] At a given age girls have a higher percentage of body fat than boys but less muscle tissue.

Adolescent Growth and Development The adolescent period covers almost a decade. It is characterized by rapid increase in height and weight, by hormonal changes, by sexual maturation, and by wide swings in emotions. The patterns of body water, lean body mass, bone, and fat show increasing differences between boys and girls. The skeleton has usually reached its full size in girls by the age of 17 years, and in boys at 20 years. The water content of the bones gradually diminishes as the mineralization increases. Provided that the diet remains good, bone mineralization continues for several years after the attainment of full size.

For a year or two before and during adolescence the growth rate accelerates and is second only to that of infancy. The growth spurt in girls occurs at approximately 11 to 14 years and in boys between 13 and 16 years. The annual peak rate for height and weight in girls averages about 9 cm (3.5 in.) and 8 to 9 kg (17.6–19.8 pounds), respectively. For boys the annual peak rate, reached about 2 years later, is 10 cm (3.8 in.) and 10 kg (22 pounds).

Along with the spurt in height of girls, development of the breasts and axillary and pubic hair takes place. Menarche occurs after the peak velocity in growth. With these changes in growth the fat content of the girl's body has increased from about 10 percent at 9 to 10 years to 20 to 24 percent at the beginning of menarche. The fat content of the girl's body at age 20 is about 1½ times that of boys.

By 18 to 20 years boys have achieved their full height, but small increases in stature are often observed during the next decade. At the end of the growth period boys will have 1½ times as much lean body mass as girls. At the beginning of the growth spurt sexual changes in boys appear: deepening of the voice; broadening of the shoulders; development of axillary, body, and pubic hair; and growth of the penis and testicles.

Nutritional Status of Children

Nutritional Assessment Health professionals should be trained to make accurate anthropometric measurements of children, to evaluate food intake, and to interpret biochemical and clinical data. (See Chapter 23 for methods of nutritional assessment.) Measurements on children are usually indicated at 6 months to yearly intervals, but oftener if there are abnormalities of growth and development. Some questions that the health professional might ask are these:

How do current measurements of height, weight, and skinfold compare with earlier measurements? If there have been shifts in the percentile channels, what are some reasons for such shifts? (See Tables A-7 through A-17.)

What is the relationship of height to weight? For example, suppose the height is at the 75th percentile and the weight at the 25th percentile, then it would appear that underweight is a problem. Or if the weight is at the 75th percentile and the height at the 25th percentile, then it seems that obesity is a problem. If height and weight are two or more percentiles apart, further study is needed to determine the cause and to initiate corrective measures.

What is the health status? Any infections? Any chronic diseases that affect growth and development? Any surgery?

Every mother, teacher, or nurse should be aware of the characteristics of the well-nourished child:

SENSE OF WELL-BEING: alert, interested in activities usual for the age; vigorous; happy
VITALITY: endurance during activity, quick recovery from fatigue; looks rested; does not fall asleep in school, sleeps well at night
WEIGHT: normal for height, age, and body build
POSTURE: erect; arms and legs straight; abdomen pulled in; chest out
TEETH: straight, without crowding in well-shaped jaw

GUMS: firm, pink; no signs of bleeding

SKIN: smooth, slightly moist; healthy glow; reddish-pink mucous membranes

EYES: clear, bright; no circles of fatigue around them

HAIR: lustrous; healthy scalp

MUSCLES: well developed; firm

NERVOUS CONTROL: good attention span for age; gets along well with others; does not cry easily; not irritable and restless

GASTROINTESTINAL FACTORS: good appetite; normal, regular elimination

(See also Table 23-1 for abnormal signs that result from faulty nutrition.)

Dietary Adequacy Numerous surveys of the diets of children have shown that the intakes of calcium, iron, ascorbic acid, and vitamin A are often below recommended allowances. The National Food Consumption Survey of 1977 identified the age groups that had average intakes of nutrients below the RDA.[2] It must be remembered, however, that average intakes conceal those persons who might have had intakes much lower or higher than the RDA. In this survey the averages that were significantly low were these:

Toddlers, 1 to 2 years: iron
Females, over 12 years: calcium, iron
Females, over 15 years: vitamin B-6

Surveys on the diets of children have shown that a direct correlation exists between the adequacy of the diet and the socioeconomic status. Based on the caloric level, the quality of the diet of children in poor families is generally good. The principal problem lies in an insufficient quality of food to meet the child's need. The diets of Hispanic and black children were often low in iron, ascorbic acid, and vitamin A.[3]

Nutritional Status Because the RDAs provide a margin of safety for most persons, a diet that fails to meet these standards cannot be interpreted as a decline in nutritional status. Indeed, national studies[3-5] have shown that children and teenagers, for the most part, have satisfactory nutritional status. Better economic conditions and access to assistance in nutrition programs have contributed substantially to improvement in recent years. Nonetheless, several nutritional problems persist to a varying degree and these should be addressed so that they can be prevented or corrected. These problems occur more frequently in the lower socioeconomic groups.

1. *Dental caries*: Begins in preschool years and continues throughout the growing years and into adulthood. It occurs in all economic groups and is so widespread that the child with no tooth decay is in a minority.

2. *Anemia*: That caused by iron deficiency is present in 5 to 10 percent of children in some groups and as high as 25 to 30 percent in other groups. Infants and toddlers are especially vulnerable, as are girls over 10 years of age. Anemia also occurs in some teenage boys.

3. *Obesity*: Occurs in about 10 to 20 percent of children and teenagers who have a greater likelihood of being obese as adults.

4. *Growth failure*: A significant number of children are underweight and undersized. (See Figure 21-1.) Such children usually tire easily, are irritable, and are susceptible to infections.

5. *Pregnancy*: Adolescent pregnancy poses a nutritional problem of considerable importance. (See Chapter 19.)

6. *Aberrations of food intake*: Include *anorexia ner-*

Figure 21-1. Growth retardation. The child on the right is 3 years younger than the child on the left. Not only is he better nourished and healthier than the other child, but his parents who are equally poor keep their child cleaner and better dressed. (UNICEF photo by Chavez.)

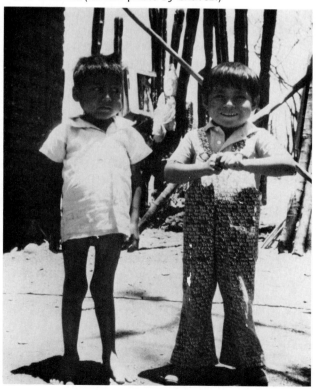

vosa and *bulimia*. These are serious nutritional and psychologic problems most often seen in adolescent girls. (See page 498).

These problems are preventable when nutritional assessment is made periodically throughout childhood and when intervention is made as soon as there are indications of abnormalities. (See pages 309–318.)

Dietary Allowances

Because the anabolic activities are considerable during the entire period of childhood, the nutritional requirements in proportion to body size are much higher than they will be in the adult years. Moreover, childhood and adolescence are times of considerable physical activity and hence the energy requirement is greater. The recommended dietary allowances are designed to support optimum growth and development. When using these allowances it is important to interpret them in terms of the child's size as well as with reference to chronologic age. (See table inside front cover.)

Energy At any given age the energy requirements will vary widely depending upon the level of growth and activity. A deficit of as little as 10 kcal per kg body weight can lead to growth failure and reduced nitrogen retention even though the protein intake is adequate.[6] Average energy requirements for each age category are listed in Table 21-1. Although the total energy requirements increase with age, the per kilogram allowances gradually decline.

Table 21-1. Recommended Energy and Protein Allowances for Children and Teenagers*

Age	Energy		Protein	
Years	Per day (kcal)	Per kg (kcal)	Per day (g)	Per kg (g)
Children				
1–3	1,300	100	16	1.2
4–6	1,800	90	24	1.2
7–10	2,000	71	28	1.0
Boys				
11–14	2,500	55	45	1.0
15–18	3,000	45	59	0.9
Girls				
11–14	2,200	49	46	1.0
15–18	2,200	40	44	0.8

*Calculations per kilogram body weight are based on mean weights for each age category. (See table inside front cover.)

Protein The protein allowances range from 1.8 g per kilogram at 1 to 3 years to the adult level of 0.8 g per kg by 18 years of age. (See Table 21-1.) From 10 to 15 percent of calories are normally derived from protein—a level that exceeds the recommended allowances.

Minerals The recommended calcium and phosphorus allowances are 800 mg for children from 1 to 10 years, and 1,200 mg for adolescents. The greatest retention of calcium and phosphorus precedes the period of rapid growth by 2 years or more, and liberal intakes of these minerals before the age of 10 are a distinct advantage. Children whose diets have been poor require a diet adequate in nutrients for as long as 6 months before they can equal the calcium and phosphorus retention of children on a good diet. Such a lag in retention can be a special hazard for the poorly nourished girl who becomes pregnant.

Adequacy of calcium intake is directly correlated with the intake of milk or milk foods. All nonmilk foods in the diet can be expected to yield only 200 mg calcium to young children, and 300 mg calcium to older children.

The data on magnesium requirements for children are limited. The allowances range from 150 mg for children at 1 to 3 years to 250 mg at 7 to 10 years. Boys from 11 to 18 years should receive daily allowances of 350 to 400 mg, and girls should receive 300 mg. One quart of milk furnishes about 120 mg magnesium, and dark green leafy vegetables are also good sources. Although many diets reasonably adequate in other nutrients fail to provide the recommended allowances for magnesium, symptoms of magnesium deficiency have not been demonstrated.

The safe and adequate intake of sodium ranges from 325 to 975 mg for toddlers and increases to 900 to 2,700 mg for teenagers. (See table on the inside front cover.) Children and teenagers consume more sodium than they need or that is desirable.

The recommended allowances for iron are 15 mg at 1 to 3 years, 10 mg at 4 to 10 years, and 18 mg at 11 to 18 years. To meet these allowances, careful choice of iron-rich foods is necessary, including a variety of meats, legumes, whole-grain or enriched breads and cereals, and green leafy vegetables, together with some fruits. The absorption of iron in vegetables and cereals improves when meat or a good source of ascorbic acid is eaten in the same meal. (See page 125.)

The allowance for zinc is 10 mg for preadolescent children and 15 mg for teenagers. Animal foods furnish higher levels of zinc than do vegetable foods.

The recommended allowance for iodine ranges

from 70 μg for toddlers to 150 μg at 11 years and throughout adult years. Iodized salt provides about 76 μg per g of salt.

The safe and adequate range of intake for fluoride is 0.5 to 1.5 mg for toddlers and increases to 1.5 to 2.5 mg for teenagers. A water supply that contains 1 ppm of fluoride will meet the need.

Copper, manganese, chromium, and selenium are other trace minerals for which safe and adequate intakes have been recommended. (See table inside front cover.) When diets supply recommended levels of other nutrients, these elements will also be supplied at satisfactory levels.

Vitamins The vitamin requirements of children have not been extensively studied. Throughout childhood and adolescence 10μg (400 IU) vitamin D should be provided—an allowance met by 1 quart of fortified milk. The vitamin A needs are related to body weight with the allowance increasing from 400 RE (2,000 IU) at 1 to 3 years to 1,000 RE (5,000 IU) for boys and 800 RE (4,000 IU) for girls. These allowances are easily met by including milk, margarine or butter, dark green or deep yellow vegetables and fruits, egg yolk, and liver. The vitamin E allowances ranging from 6 to 10 mg alpha-tocopherol equivalents are provide by vegetable oils, margarines, whole grains, legumes, nuts, and dark green leafy vegetables.

Ascorbic acid allowances range from 45 mg for 1-to-6-year-olds to 60 mg for 15- to 18-year-olds. Thiamin and niacin allowances are 0.5 and 6.6 mg, respectively, for each 1,000 kcal. The range of riboflavin allowance is from 0.8 to 1.2 mg for children, up to 1.8 mg for boys, and up to 1.3 mg for girls.

Vitamin B-6 allowances are based on 0.02 mg per g of expected protein intake as estimated from surveys of food consumption.[1] Thus, toddlers should receive 0.9 mg, per day, whereas teenage girls and boys need 1.4 to 2.0 mg.

Folacin allowances supply 8 to 10 μg per kilogram body weight. Green leafy vegetables, fruits, legumes, and liver supply generous amounts. Vitamin B-12 needs of 2.0 μg are readily met when the diet includes foods from animal origin.

Food Behavior

Food Habits and Development Food continues to be a major factor in the development of the whole person throughout the growing years. Food becomes a means of communication; it has cultural and social meanings; it is intimately associated with the emotions; and its acceptance or rejection is highly personal.

The environment in which the child lives determines the food behavior and the quality of nutrition. One way to study the influence of environmental factors on the nutritional status of preschool children is to consider the family as one ecosystem and the child as a second ecosystem.[7] The family has responsibility for the child's food, controls the child's access to the foods, and establishes the emotional climate. Interacting factors within the family include the family composition, income, general education, the stability of the family, the quality of housing, the attitudes toward food, parental knowledge of nutrition, attitudes toward child rearing—authoritarian or nonauthoritarian—and others.

The child is the second ecosystem. From the family ecosystem he or she draws on information, materials, and energy. The nutrient supply from the family ecosystem is processed by the child for his or her own physical development and nutritional status. Also from the family's system the child develops attitudes and values that determine food behavior.

Upon entering school the child acquires further information, attitudes and values from teachers, school food services, and peers. Although food behavior within a family, cultural, and community setting may have many similarities, the food behavior for each individual is unique corresponding to environmental exposure.

Good food habits have several characteristics. First, the pattern of diet permits the individual to achieve the maximum genetic potential for his or her physical and mental development. Second, the food habits are conducive to delaying or preventing the onset of degenerative diseases that are so prevalent in American society today. Third, the food habits are part of satisfying human relationships and contribute to social and personal enjoyment. The development of food habits is a continuous process in which each year builds on what has gone before. The responsibility of parents and all who work with children goes far beyond ensuring the ingestion of specified levels of nutrients. It requires the application of knowledge from the fields of human behavior and development, psychology, sociology, and anthropology.

Common Dietary Errors Studies of food habits of children have shown repeatedly that the foods requiring particular emphasis for the improvement of diets are milk, dark green leafy and deep yellow vegetables, and whole-grain or enriched breads and cereals. Among the food habits that contribute to these deficiencies are these:

POOR BREAKFAST OR NONE AT ALL: lack of appetite; getting up too late; no one to prepare breakfast; monotony of breakfast foods; no protein at breakfast, meaning that the distribution of good quality protein is poor even though the day's total may be satisfactory; too little fruit, meaning that ascorbic acid often is not obtained.

POOR LUNCHES: failure to participate in school lunch program; poor box lunches; spending lunch money for snacks or other items; unsatisfactory management of school lunch program with resultant poor menus, poor food preparation, excessive plate waste.

SNACKS: account for as much as one fourth of calories although some do not provide significant amounts of protein, minerals, and vitamins; may be eaten too close to mealtime, thus spoiling the appetite.

OVERUSE OF A FEW FOODS: some young children drink too much milk and eat a limited variety of foods. Teenagers may eat excessive amounts of fast foods and fail to get the nutrients not provided by those foods. (See page 239.)

SELF-IMPOSED DIETING, ESPECIALLY BY TEENAGE GIRLS: caloric restriction but no consideration given to protein, minerals, and vitamins.

IRREGULAR EATING HABITS: few meals with the family group; no adult supervision in eating; children often prepare own meals without guidance.

FOOD DISLIKES: little exposure to new foods; limited variety from day to day.

Diet for the Preschool Child

Food Selection Correlated with Behavioral Changes The nutritional requirements of the child cannot be satisfied apart from an understanding of behavioral changes that occur. Toddlers begin to show independence and to assert themselves. They are alert to the attitudes of others, and readily learn that they can use food as a weapon to gain attention. They mimic siblings and parents. They have a short attention span and are easily distracted from eating. Their response to food is often inconsistent.

Toddlers want to feed themselves and should be encouraged to do so. However, they have limited muscle coordination and their eating behavior can best be described as messy. Although they can use a spoon to pick up food, they may turn over the spoon upon bringing it to the mouth if they have not yet developed wrist coor-

dination. Eating with one's fingers is not only convenient for the toddler but is another way of learning about the texture of food.

If given the opportunity the toddler quickly learns to take advantage of parents through his or her food behavior. As the child enters the 3- to 5-year-old group the attention span is somewhat longer, and muscle coordination is much better although the child still has some problems from time to time in the handling of utensils. (See Figure 21-2.)

During the second year the appetite tapers off corresponding to the slower rate of growth. Beal[8] found that healthy, well-nourished girls reduced their milk intake as early as 6 months and returned to higher intakes at 2 to 3 years of age. Boys also reduced their milk intake at about 9 months, but started to increase their consumption between 1 and 2 years. An intake of 2 cups or less is not uncommon for a period of time. Some children's appetites improve by 5 years or earlier, but other children have poor appetites well into the school years.

Many mothers must be reassured that the child will remain well nourished provided that foods of high nu-

Figure 21-2. The young child gradually develops muscle coordination as he tries to feed himself. A word of encouragement now and then is helpful. (Courtesy, U.S. Department of Agriculture.)

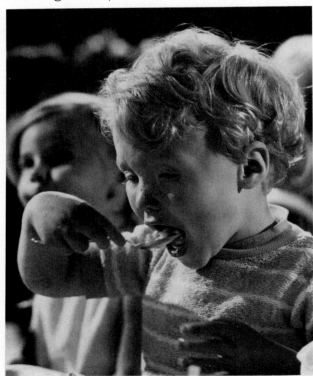

trient density are offered, and that feeding does not become an issue between mother and child. Some compensation for the reduced consumption of milk may be made by incorporating milk into foods such as simple puddings. The occasional use of flavorings such as molasses or cocoa may increase milk acceptance. Children are sometimes encouraged to drink milk if they are permitted to pour it for themselves from a small pitcher. Cottage cheese, yogurt, and mild American cheese are often well liked and help increase the calcium and protein intakes.

Because young children have a high taste sensitivity, it is generally believed that they prefer mildly flavored foods. However, a recent review disputes this, and points out that many studies indicate likes and dislikes for both mildly flavored and strongly flavored vegetables.[9] Plain foods are preferred to mixtures such as casserole dishes, creamed dishes, and stews; yet young children like macaroni and cheese, spaghetti with meat sauce, and pizza. Preschool children do not like extremes of food temperatures, and may seem to dawdle until the mashed potatoes are lukewarm or the ice cream is beginning to melt.

The feel of food is important to young children, and they enjoy foods that can be picked up with the fingers such as pieces of raw vegetables, small sandwiches, strips of cheese or meat, and narrow wedges of fruit. The ability to chew food should determine the textures that are given. Toddlers may be given chopped vegetables and ground meat, whereas the 3- to 5-year-old can manage diced vegetables and minced or bite-size pieces of tender meat. Foods that are stringy such as celery, sticky such as some mashed potatoes, or slippery such as custard are often disliked because the child is not familiar with the texture.

Food jags are not uncommon, especially between the ages of 2 and 4 years. The child may shun all but a few foods, such as milk or peanut butter-and-jelly sandwiches. Such occurrences do not last too long, if the parent does not show concern, and if the foods which constitute the child's preference at the moment are nutritious in general.

Preschool children are almost constantly active. Their interest is readily diverted from food. If they become overtired or excessively hungry, their appetites may lag a great deal.

Daily Food Allowances. A selection of a variety of foods from the milk, meat, vegetable–fruit, and bread–cereal groups provides a sound basis for the child's diet. Although intakes vary widely, the following amounts provide a guide:

2 cups low-fat milk, fortified with vitamin D
3–4 eggs per week
1–3 ounces chopped meat, fish, or poultry; or equivalent of cheese, legumes, or peanut butter
4 ounces orange juice or other source of ascorbic acid
2–4 tablespoons other fruit such as banana, peaches, pears, apple, apricot, prunes
2–4 tablespoons vegetables, including deep yellow and dark green leafy
1 potato
1 raw vegetable such as carrot sticks, cabbage slices, lettuce, tomato
⅓ to ⅔ cup enriched dry or cooked cereal
1–3 slices enriched or whole-grain bread

The three-meal pattern used for adult members of the family is appropriate for the child, but some snacks in midmorning and midafternoon are also necessary. Very active children become excessively fatigued and hungry if they are not fed between meals. Snacks should make a liberal contribution to the nutrient requirements. Some that are suitable for preschool children are

Fruit juices without sugar
Milk and milk beverages; yogurt, plain or with fruit
Cheese cubes, cottage cheese
Fruit of any kind
Raw vegetables: carrot sticks, celery sticks, cauliflower buds, green beans, rutabaga sticks, broccoli buds, zucchini slices, cherry tomatoes, green pepper slices
Molasses, oatmeal, or peanut butter cookies
Dry cereal from the box or with milk
NOTE: Children under 3 years should not be given nuts, popcorn, seeds, chunks of meat, or vegetable sticks since they may choke on them and aspirate the food items.

Establishing Good Food Habits   Suggestions have been made in the preceding chapter for the establishment of good food habits in the infant. In addition, the following considerations are conducive to the development of good food habits in the preschool child.

Meals should be served at regular hours in a pleasant environment. The child should be comfortably seated at a table. Deep dishes permit the child to get the food onto the fork or spoon with greater ease. A fork, such as a salad fork with blunt tines, and a small spoon can be handled comfortably. A small cup or glass should be only partially filled with liquid to minimize spilling; however, the coordination of eye, hand, and mouth is difficult and some spilling is to be expected.

Children enjoy colorful meals just as adults do. But, then, one may wonder why they prefer brown foods such as meat and peanut butter to the brightly colored green or yellow vegetables.[9] Thus, food preferences result from the interaction of many variables. The appetites of children vary from day to day, and like adults they react strongly to portions that are too large. It is much better to serve less than the child is likely to eat and to let him or her ask for more.

Even favorite foods should not be served too often. Breakfasts do not need to be stereotyped. A hamburger or sandwich and an orange cut in sections to be picked up with the fingers is just as satisfactory as a juice, cereal, and egg breakfast.

Fewer difficulties are likely to be encountered if new foods are given at the beginning of the meal when the child is hungry. A food is more likely to be accepted if it is given in a form that can be easily handled, that can be chewed, and if some favorite food is also included in the same meal. A taste or two is enough for any new food that is offered. Encouragement and praise are helpful, but favorite foods should not be used as a bribe or reward for taking the new food. Any new food should be offered at regular intervals until the child learns to accept it.

Whether the preschool child should eat with other members of the family or alone is a matter that individual parents must determine for the child's greatest good and the family's convenience. In most situations the young child should eat with the rest of the family because the interactions between family members are a part of normal development. If, however, the evening meal must be late, if the child becomes overexcited about the family doings, or if the child is expected to live up to a code of behavior beyond his or her young years, it is better that the child be allowed to eat before the rest of the family in a pleasant, quiet atmosphere with the parent nearby. Even so, an occasional meal with the family is a treat for the child and parent if tension can be avoided. Since children are great imitators, they enjoy doing just as the parents or the other children are doing.

The child may well learn early in life that he or she is expected to eat foods that are prepared, but this does not mean that nagging or bribery will accomplish anything. Children, like adults, enjoy attention, and they are quick to realize that food can be a powerful weapon for gaining such attention. A display of concern or the use of force in getting a child to drink milk or to take any other food can have nothing but unfavorable effects. When a child refuses to take a food, the unwanted item should be calmly removed without comment after a reasonable period of time. If the child is refusing to eat because this behavior attracts attention, the parent should make certain that the child receives a full share of affection and companionship at other than mealtimes. If this is done the child will lose interest in using food as a weapon.

Diet for the Schoolchild

Characteristics of Food Acceptance Elementary school children are usually better fed than preschool children or adolescents. Group acceptance is extremely important at this time, and the child needs to be able to keep up with classmates and to have a sense of accomplishment. When the child goes to school for the first time he or she makes acquaintance with food patterns that may be different from those at home. The child learns that certain foods are acceptable to the peer group, whereas other foods from a different cultural pattern may be looked upon with disdain; as a result he or she may be unwilling to accept these foods at home—good though they may be. On the other hand, within a group the child is willing to try foods with which he or she is unacquainted and would not try alone. (See Figure 21-3.)

Schoolchildren have relatively few dislikes for food except possibly for vegetables, which are usually not eaten in satisfactory amounts. By the time children reach 8 to 10 years of age the appetite is usually very

Figure 21-3. Young school boy with a good appetite eagerly awaits a familiar food. (Courtesy, Metropolitan Medical Center, Minneapolis.)

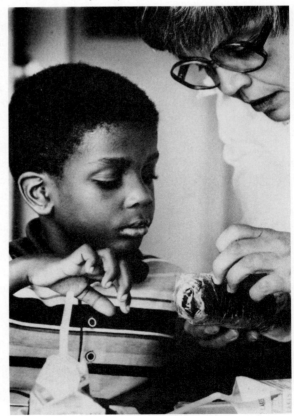

good. Feeding problems are more likely to result because parents are unduly concerned with behavior at mealtime which does not come up to adult standards. Most children of this age are in a hurry, and do not like to take time for meals. Breakfast, especially, is likely to be skipped.

Schoolchildren are subject to many stresses which affect the appetite. Communicable diseases occur often in this age group. They reduce the appetite on the one hand, but they increase body needs on the other. Schoolwork, class competition, and emotional stresses in getting along with many children may have adverse effects on appetite, as may also an unbalanced program of activity and rest.

Choice of Foods   Table 21-2 lists the kinds and amounts of foods which may be taken in a day by healthy schoolchildren. A number of other equally satisfactory patterns could be devised for different cultural groups. A diet for adults which places emphasis first on the inclusion of protein, minerals, and vitamins is also a good one for schoolchildren. The amount of milk given to children should be greater than that for the adult. Although no foods need to be forbidden to this age group, it is extremely important that high-carbohydrate and high-fat foods not be allowed to replace essential items of the diet.

Food Habits   The suggestions concerning good food habits for preschool children also apply to schoolchildren. A good school lunch program (see page 310) may introduce new foods in a setting where the child is anxious to conform to the group. The elementary teacher should integrate nutrition education with the total classroom experience so that good food habits are strengthened.

Since children are likely to be in a hurry, it is often wise to require that a certain time be spent at the table—say 15 or 20 minutes—so that the child will take time to eat. Children learn good manners by imitation of adults, and not by continuous correction at the table. During the elementary-school years, little can be gained by overemphasis of manners. In fact, the food intake may be adversely affected.

Diet for the Teenager

Adolescent Dietary Problems   Even boys and girls who have had an excellent pattern of food intake sometimes succumb to bizarre, unbalanced diets dur-

Table 21-2.   Foods to Meet Nutritional Needs of Elementary School Children and Teenagers

Food	6 to 10 Years	10 to 12 Years	12 to 16 Years
Milk, vitamin-D fortified	2–3 cups	3–4 cups	4 cups or more
Eggs	3–4 per week	3–4 per week	3–4 per week
Meat, poultry, fish	2–3 ounces (small serving)	3–4 ounces (average serving)	4 ounces
Dried beans, peas, or peanut butter	2 servings each week. If used as an alternative for meat, allow ½ cup cooked beans or peas or 2 tablespoons peanut butter for 1 ounce meat		
Potatoes, white or sweet (occasionally spaghetti macaroni, rice, noodles, etc.)	1 small or ⅓ cup	1 medium or ½ cup	1 large or ¾ cup
Other cooked vegetable (green leafy or deep yellow 3 to 4 times a week)	¼ cup	⅓ cup	½ cup or more
Raw vegetable (salad greens, cabbage, celery, carrots, etc.)	¼ cup	⅓ cup	½ cup
Vitamin C food (citrus fruit, tomato, cantaloupe, etc.)	1 medium orange or equivalent	1 medium orange or equivalent	1 large orange or equivalent
Other fruit	1 portion or more as: 1 apple, 1 banana, 1 peach, 1 pear, ½ cup cooked fruit		
Bread, enriched or whole grain	3 slices or more	3 slices or more	4–6 slices or more
Cereal, enriched or whole grain	½ cup	¾ cup	1 cup or more
Additional foods	Butter or margarine, desserts, etc., to satisfy energy needs.		

ing the adolescent years. Teenagers have many concerns about their development such as the size and shape of the body, sexual development, skin conditions, vitality, attractiveness, and approval by their peers. They feel independent and seek freedom to make their own decisions. It is a period when family conflict is likely to increase. The advice of teachers and coaches is often taken more seriously than that of parents.

The teenager is concerned about his or her weight. Most girls want to weigh less; they want smaller hips, smaller thighs, and smaller waists but larger busts. Most boys want to weigh more and they equate overweight with muscle development which is desirable. They want a larger upper torso and arms, an indication of strength.[10]

Stresses of various kinds have an adverse effect on nutrition. The incidence of tuberculosis is higher than it should be in adolescent years and in early adulthood and is believed to occur more frequently in those who have inadequate diets, especially with respect to protein and calcium. Teenage pregnancy can have serious effects on the girl who has a poor intake of essential nutrients. (See page 271.)

Emotional difficulties often stem from the feeling of social inadequacy or the pressures of schoolwork. Where there is conflict within the home because of the teenager's food choices, failure to accept responsibilities, the use of money, dating hours, and so on, the emotions not only determine the food intake but also modify nutrient utilization. For example, negative nitrogen and mineral balances have been observed when students were taking examinations or when young women were upset about a pregnancy.

Selection of Foods Because of their high energy requirements boys are more likely to meet their nutrient needs than are girls. Emphasis upon green leafy and deep yellow vegetables is necessary for both boys and girls. In addition girls need to increase their intake of milk and whole-grain or enriched breads and cereals. The list in Table 21-2 serves as a starting point for the planning of meals.

Snacks furnish about one fourth of the energy requirement of most adolescents. They should also furnish an equivalent amount of the day's allowance for protein, minerals, and vitamins. Thus, sandwiches, hamburgers, pizza, fruit, and milk are types of snacks to be encouraged. A recent study has shown that typical teenage snacks are better nutritionally than many people have believed them to be. For each 100 kcal supplied by the snacks there are substantial contribu-

tions of protein, calcium, iron, vitamin A, thiamin, riboflavin, and ascorbic acid.[11] (See Figure 21-4.)

The School Athlete The energy needs of the athlete increase during activity, and often range between 3,000 and 6,000 kcal—sometimes more. With this increased energy requirement there is also an increased need for thiamin, riboflavin, and niacin. The recommended allowances for protein will meet the needs for growth of adolescents, for tissue turnover, and for the development of muscles during athletic conditioning. The nutrient needs are easily met when the amounts of foods listed in Table 21-2 become the basis for food selection. Many high school youth are poorly informed about the nutritional requirements for physical activity and sometimes resort to faddish and even dangerous practices regarding food and fluid intake. Athletes sometimes have strong opinions about specific foods that will help them to win, and such preferences can be respected within the general bounds of good nutrition and fluid balance. There is no evidence, however, that wheat germ, honey, bee pollen, lecithin, protein supplements, brewer's yeast, sunflower seeds, vitamin E, ascorbic acid, or vitamin–mineral supplements have any special value in promoting endurance or skills.[12] (See Chapter 25.)

Community Resources

School Food Services The initial focus of the school lunch was to provide a market for food surpluses, with the feeding of children as a commendable outcome. The National School Lunch Act was passed in 1946 "to safeguard the health and well-being of the nation's children." Several laws, especially the Child Nutrition Act of 1966, have been enacted to expand the program to include school breakfasts and to provide cash assistance; donation of surplus food commodities; and technical assistance in the purchase and use of foods and in the management and equipment of the school lunchroom. The school lunch program has always been regarded as a laboratory for nutrition education.

To participate in the program a school must agree to operate the program on a nonprofit basis; provide free or reduced-price lunches for needy children; serve all children regardless of race, color, or national origin; and serve lunches that meet the requirements established by the Secretary of Agriculture. Children who are eligible for free or reduced-price meals must not be identified by placing them in separate lines, re-

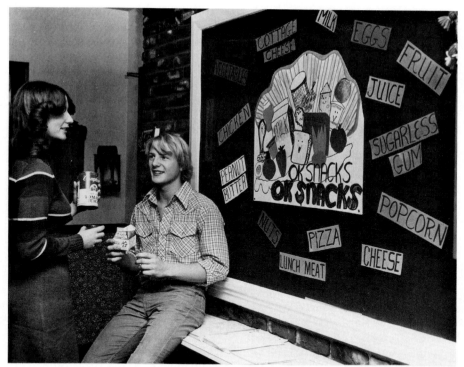

Figure 21-4. Well chosen snacks contribute an important share of nutrients toward the day's allowance. (Courtesy, Harry Broder and Marple-Newton School District, Newtown Square, Pennsylvania.)

quiring them to sit in places set apart, or requiring them to provide service as a reimbursement for the meal.

The type A pattern for preschool and schoolchildren includes milk, protein-rich food, vegetables and fruits, and whole-grain or enriched bread or an alternate.

Junior and senior high school students are eligible for the "offer vs. serve" pattern; that is, the five items of the type A pattern (milk, meat, vegetables, fruits, breads-cereals) are offered and the student may select three of these items. This option is intended to reduce plate waste by omitting foods that the student doesn't like. A study of free-choice lunches actually consumed by high school students showed that the nutritional values were as high as type A lunches actually eaten.[13] Intakes by girls of vitamins A and C and iron were marginal. Free-choice programs should be combined with an ongoing program of nutrition education.

A controversial issue for nutritionists and parents has been the introduction of fast foods into some school lunch programs. Proponents of such a program maintain that participation is much better than with the traditional type A lunch. When salads and citrus juices are provided with the usual fast-food items, the nutrient requirements of the type A lunch can be met. Opponents point out that the limited variety of foods can result in deficient intakes of some nutrients such as trace minerals, and that few choices will not help children to develop acceptance of a wide range of foods. (See page 239.)

School Breakfast Program. Breakfasts are planned to provide one fourth to one third of the recommended allowances. A breakfast includes: milk, fruit, bread or cereal, and when practicable, a serving of protein-rich food such as 1 egg, cheese, or 2 tablespoons peanut butter.

Additional foods to round out the breakfast and to satisfy the appetite may include foods of popular appeal such as doughnuts, potatoes, or bacon; sweeteners; butter or margarine.

WIC Program. The Special Supplemental Feeding Program for Women, Infants, and Children (WIC) provides food vouchers for children up to 5 years who are at risk from economically deprived families. Children at risk include those known to have inadequate diets, who are anemic, or who have deficient growth patterns. Food supplements that meet standards set

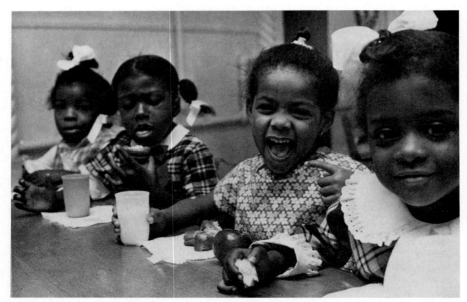

Figure 21-5. Preschool children in a day-care center are provided nutritious meals and snacks. The food service program is similar to that in the elementary and secondary schools. The Child Nutrition Program provides cash and USDA donated foods. (Courtesy, USDA)

by the U.S. Department of Agriculture include milk, eggs, fruit juices, and iron-fortified cereals. (See Figure 21-5.)

Nutritional Issues and Problems

Preventive Aspects of Children's Diets There is general agreement that a nutritionally adequate diet at suitable caloric levels to bring about desirable growth and development can prevent obesity, underweight, growth failure, dental caries, and anemia. Continuous monitoring of growth and nutritional status by health professionals and parents is essential to nip any incipient problems in the bud. Yet the incidence of these problems remains high. Some insight to the causes of these problems as well as some special cautions for prevention and treatment are discussed on the pages that follow.

Substance abuse—tobacco, alcohol, marihuana, amphetamines, cocaine, heroin, and others—has serious immediate and long-term consequences for teenagers. The physiologic and psychologic effects of these substances on the individual and the strategies for dealing with the problem are beyond the scope of this book. However, it is pertinent to point out that health professionals must be alert to the negative impact that substance abuse has on nutritional status. It is fairly obvious that money may be used to purchase the alcohol or drugs instead of food, resulting in inadequate

food intake. Some drugs interfere with appetite resulting in bizarre and inadequate food intakes. Hepatitis and other infections that often occur may further inhibit the appetite but also increase the nutrient requirements.

Of children 11 to 14 years of age it has been reported that 40 percent had one or more of the risk factors for arteriosclerosis: cigarette smoking, overweight, poor physical fitness, elevated serum cholesterol, hypertension, or diabetes.[14] Health professionals should screen children for the existence of such risk factors and should provide counseling to children and their parents on the appropriate modification of diet and lifestyle in an effort to eliminate these risk factors.

Controversy continues, however, about recommending that all children restrict the intake of fat, sugar, and salt in order to reduce the risk of chronic disease in later life. Many nutritionists recommend moderation in the intake of salt, sugar, and fat together with an increase in dietary fiber. More specifically, the intake of whole-grain breads and cereals, and fruits and vegetables—both raw and cooked—should be increased. Also, recommended amounts of milk that is lower in fat content (skim, 1 or 2 percent) and of lean meat for the various age groups should be provided. (See Table 21-2.) Such moderate changes have several benefits: (1) reduced levels of fat and sugar help control caloric intake so that desirable weight can be maintained; (2) reduced levels of fat and sugar leave more room for nutrient dense foods in the diet, thus improving the likelihood of nutritional adequacy; and (3) the moderation of diet in childhood increases the likelihood that degenerative changes can be delayed or prevented. (To reduce salt intake, see page 142; to reduce fat intake, see page 97.)

Obesity About 80 percent of youngsters who are obese remain so as adults. Because of the physiologic and psychologic disadvantages of obesity, prevention, by regulation of food intake and activity patterns in childhood, has important implications for the later years. The social and psychologic effects of obesity can be devastating to the child or teenager. The obese child is teased about his or her fatness, is excluded from many peer activities, and is made to feel unwanted. Peers may describe the obese child as fat, sloppy, lazy, dirty, or stupid.[15] Storz and Greene[16] found that adolescent girls, whether obese or within normal weight, more often described their appearance with negative adjectives (fat, hippy, skinny, unattractive, ugly) than with positive adjectives (slender, just right, pleasingly plump, attractive, beautiful). To cover up for loneliness and lack of social relationships or failure in everyday school activities, the child resorts to eating foods high in unneeded calories. Parents often complain that their teenagers eat too many "junk" foods or fast foods. (See page 239 for fuller discussion.)

Juvenile-onset obesity is characterized by an increased number and size of adipose cells. Once formed, the excess number of cells cannot be altered by dieting; only the size can be reduced. However, environmental factors are more likely to be important contributors to obesity.

Some children overeat because the pattern of overfeeding established in infancy is carried over into childhood. An abundance of rich, high-calorie foods is readily available and, together with relative inactivity, becomes part of the family pattern.

In one study, several factors accounted for greater food intake by obese boys than their nonobese brothers both at home and at school: mothers tended to serve the obese boys larger portions; obese boys left less food on their plates; and they purchased more food at school or obtained it from their nonobese peers. Activity patterns also differed in the two groups. Compared with control subjects, the obese boys were less active at home but equally active at school. However, when oxygen consumption was measured, energy expenditure in the obese boys was greater than that of the nonobese. Thus, increased energy intake was more important than differences in energy output in maintaining the obese state in these boys.[17] Other studies have shown that obese children do not eat any more food than normal weight children and, in fact, may eat less, but their energy expenditure is considerably less.[18] They avoid active sports, and when they do participate they manage to become involved as little as possible.

Treatment of obesity includes behavioral modification, social support, and physical activity. Young children progressed better when the parents played an active role, but 12- to 16-year olds lost more weight when they attended sessions without their mothers.[15] School programs for weight control often provide significant support. For the moderately obese behavioral modification may be sufficient to bring about weight loss without imposing a rigid dietary regimen. (See page 371.) For those who are very obese a diet together with behavioral modification is likely to be most successful.

For young, moderately obese children the goal should be to provide a normal rate of growth rather than to effect loss of weight. The emphasis is placed on a nutritionally adequate diet with restriction of nutrient-deficient foods. Physical activity such as cycling, walking, and hiking do not require peer competition and may be better accepted by the child.

The caloric intake for teenagers should be adjusted to bring about a loss of at least 1 pound, but not more than 2 pounds, weekly. Far too often teenagers adopt some crash diet that may be damaging to health; yet they find that the weight losses—often mostly water—are only temporary. For teenage girls a 1,200- to 1,500-kcal diet will usually lead to satisfactory weight loss. Because they are likely to be more active, teenage boys can lose satisfactorily on 1,500- to 1,800-kcal diets. (Low-calorie diets are described on pages 372–74.) Adolescents should include at least 3, preferably 4, cups of low fat milk in these diets.

Underweight With today's emphasis on slimness, often little attention is paid to the incidence of underweight. Children and teenagers who are underweight tire easily, are irritable and restless, and are less alert so that progress in school is likely to be slower. They are more susceptible to infections. Tuberculosis can occur in some underweight adolescents.

The causes for underweight, as for overweight, are many. Basically the intake of calories has been insufficient. The deficiency may have come about because of an underlying disease process that requires correction, lack of sufficient food owing to poverty, the parent's poor understanding of the child's nutritional needs, or an emotional climate within the home that precludes satisfactory food intake. Is the mother too tense about what the child eats, and does she convey this concern to the child? Do the parents force or coax the child to eat? Is the child too tired when meals are served? Does the child receive less attention than siblings? Are meals skipped? What are the snacking patterns?

The dietary counselor must determine the daily food intake and evaluate it in terms of the Daily Food Guide. The diet is improved qualitatively by the inclusion of foods that are in short supply from any of the food groups, and quantitatively by increasing the caloric intake. Any additions to the diet must be made gradually since noticeable increases in the amounts of food often discourage intake. After school and at bedtime nutritious snacks may be sufficient to increase the caloric intake so that weight gain occurs. Guidance of the child and parents toward the improvement of the environment is as important as are the essentials of diet itself.

Growth Failure A variety of conditions may lead to growth failure including hunger and famine resulting in protein-energy malnutrition (see page 351); malabsorption (see page 443); anorexia nervosa (see page 377); changes in metabolic requirements as in diabetes mellitus; poor physical and emotional environment in the home leading to child neglect or even physical abuse; and preoccupation with slimness as in a recently described syndrome, "fear of obesity."

Growth retardation was observed in a group of children, 9 to 17 years of age, mostly male, and was diagnosed as fear of obesity.[19] The children had poor eating habits, meals were often skipped, and the meals that were eaten had a low volume. The intakes ranged from "junk" foods to high fiber diets. The diets were low in calories, protein, minerals and vitamin D, although there was no evidence of iron deficiency or rickets. The subjects had short stature and were 5 to 23 percent below expected weights for heights. All the children had delayed bone growth and half had delayed puberty. With an adequate diet weight gain again took place, and a few months later growth in height occurred. The subjects differed from anorexia nervosa in a number of ways: they did not have a distorted body image; did not use laxatives and diuretics; did not compulsively exercise; and did not require psychotherapy to improve. However, it is believed that this syndrome, if untreated, could lead to anorexia.

The correction of growth failure requires treatment of any pathologic conditions, improvement of the environmental situation, psychologic intervention and

improvement of the diet. Gradual changes are made in food selection from the Daily Food Guide and toward increasing the caloric intake. The dietary counselor must assist the client and the parents to develop new attitudes, values and motivation.

Anemia Preschool children who have anemia are most likely to have been iron-deficient since infancy because they did not receive iron-fortified cereals or formula during the first year, and have continued to ingest an iron-poor diet. Some children drink excessive quantities of milk and eat only small amounts of iron-rich foods.[20] Still others live in geographic areas where there is a high incidence of intestinal parasites such as hookworm. The anemia often becomes evident when an infection further depletes the iron-poor reserves.

Although most teenagers do not have anemia, adolescence is a particularly vulnerable time, especially for girls. With well-chosen diets at calorie levels to maintain optimal weight for age, the iron intake is likely to be 10 to 12 mg per day—not the 18 mg of the RDA. For many girls such an intake may appear to be adequate, but may not provide the iron reserves needed when menstrual losses are high or when the body is stressed by illness or the additional demands of pregnancy. Unfortunately, many teenagers have particularly bizarre, inadequate diets that do not begin to meet the growth needs and that further deplete iron reserves.

The prevention of iron-deficiency anemia requires emphasis on the inclusion of meat or ascorbic acid at meals to enhance the absorption of nonheme sources of iron, and frequent selection of iron-rich foods such as liver and other organ meats, meat, enriched breads and cereals, dried fruits, legumes, and green leafy vegetables.

An existing iron-deficiency anemia cannot be effectively treated by diet alone, since it is impossible to achieve therapeutic levels of iron from foods alone. Iron supplements such as ferrous sulfate, gluconate, or fumarate are prescribed. Oral therapy is as effective as parenteral therapy. An initial intolerance occurs in some but it disappears with adjustment to the medication. It is helpful to take the salts after meals. Dietary counseling with emphasis on the factors for prevention is required.

Dental Caries The foundation for the development of sound teeth is provided to the fetus during pregnancy. Protein, calcium, phosphorus, vitamins A and D, and ascorbic acid are especially involved in tooth structure.

Dental caries is an infectious disease that occurs in

earliest childhood and persists throughout life. Bacteria, *Streptococcus mutans*, thrive in dental plaque that surrounds the teeth. The bacteria produce acids that destroy the tooth enamel and dentin. For their growth and multiplication the bacteria require carbohydrate, especially sugars such as sucrose. The destruction of tooth surfaces depends on the length of time that bacteria have access to sugar and the frequency of such access. Thus, small amounts of sugar consumed at frequent intervals are likely to be more harmful than a larger amount taken at a single time.

Several steps can be taken to reduce the incidence of dental caries:

1. Use water with a fluoride concentration of 1 ppm, since fluoride helps harden tooth structures and make them more resistant to bacterial action. If fluoridated water is not available, a supplement may be prescribed by the pediatrician. Fluoridated toothpaste and mouth wash also help to reduce the cariogenic effect.
2. Reduce the frequency of tooth contact with sticky and sweet foods.
3. Brush teeth after meals and after consuming a sticky, sweet snack; better still, avoid such a snack! At a minimum, rinse the mouth well with water after eating food.
4. Visit the dentist regularly for removal of dental plaque and for any needed repairs.

Hyperactivity *Learning disability, minimal brain function, attention deficit disorder, hyperactivity,* and *hyperkinesis* are among the terms used to describe related disorders variously estimated to occur in 3 to 10 percent of school-age children. The children have a number of behavioral problems: heightened level of activity; inappropriate activity; short attention span; rebelliousness; and sometimes violent behavior. The symptoms occur before age 7 but may not be diagnosed until school years when the child is found by teachers to be a behavior problem. Sometimes the behavior is caused by central nervous system injury as from lead poisoning or another toxic substance, infection, or prolonged oxygen deficit. More commonly, the etiology is unknown.

In 1973, Dr. Ben Feingold, an allergist, claimed that a diet free of food additives, especially artificial flavorings and colorings together with salicylate-containing foods such as tomatoes, cucumbers, and many fruits, was fully successful in about one half of children treated.[21] Another fourth of the children improved somewhat. Many parents of hyperactive children adopted the rigorous dietary regimen with enthusiasm and claimed that their children were helped.

Dr. Feingold's report was widely criticized because it did not follow acceptable scientific standards and controls. In response to the issues raised, The Nutrition Foundation organized a study to review Dr. Feingold's claims and other literature pertaining to the syndrome, and encouraged further research. After numerous carefully controlled studies and the literature review had been completed, a comprehensive report was issued in 1980.[22] In only a few instances did there appear to be any success with the diet—by no means the high success rate reported by Dr. Feingold. It has been suggested that the special attention that parents must give to the diet and the child may have some beneficial effects on behavior. In idiopathic hyperactivity, central nervous stimulants such as methylphenidate administered by an experienced clinician appear to be of more value.[21]

Some parents, despite research evidence that diet appears to be of only limited value, prefer to use the diet rather than use a medication. There is no evidence that the diet is harmful or nutritionally deficient. However, the dietary counselor should help parents evaluate the diet they are using to be certain that it provides all the nutritional essentials.

Some have claimed that a high sugar intake is a cause of hyperactivity.[23] Like the Feingold diet, the reports have been based on anecdotal observations rather than controlled, double-blind studies (neither the subject nor the observer, such as parent or teacher, know what treatment is being tested). To date there is little, if any, scientific support for claims that a high sugar intake adversely affects behavior or that elimination or lowering of the sugar intake will correct or prevent these problems.[24]

Lead Poisoning Young children often ingest nonfood substances (pica) such as dirt, crayons, paint chips, and plaster. According to the Second National Health and Nutrition Examination Survey (1976–80) 4 percent of all children aged 6 months to 5 years had elevated blood levels of lead. The incidence was five times as high in urban areas as in rural areas.[25] Children of black and Hispanic families with low incomes and living in old houses and apartments with flaking paint are particularly susceptible.

Anorexia, vomiting, weight loss, and increased restlessness have been found.[26] Excessive ingestion of lead severely affects the nervous system, the bone marrow, and the kidneys.[27] In young children the effect on the central nervous system leads to hyperactivity, impaired intellectual function, and in severe cases to coma, convulsions, and death. Lead interferes with the activity of several enzymes involved in hematopoiesis. The anemia resulting from lead toxicity and also from iron deficiency can be severe. Damage to the kidney leads to increased excretion of glucose, amino acids, and phosphates, and is also believed to interfere with the conversion of 25-$(OH)D_3$ to 1,25-$(OH)_2D_3$, the active form of vitamin D.[26,27]

The absorption of lead is 5 to 10 times as high in children as in adults. Lead also readily crosses the placental membranes so that the infant of a woman with lead intoxication is also subject to toxicity. Absorption of lead is significantly greater in children whose diets are deficient in calcium, iron, and zinc. Children living in poverty who are most likely to be malnourished are also those who are more likely to be exposed to lead hazard.

Chelation therapy (calcium disodium EDTA) is used effectively. Iron supplementation is generally indicated. The focus on the prevention of lead poisoning in children should be on the removal of lead paint in housing—a monumental task in many urban areas. Screening of children for lead toxicity is an essential public health measure. The nutritionally adequate diet required for growth and development is also important for reducing the absorption of lead and thus is protective against toxicity.

CASE STUDY 6

Preschool Girl with Obesity

Kathy T is a chunky 4-year-old who weighs 22 kg (48 lb) and is 103 cm (40½ in.) tall. She has a pale complexion and a docile disposition. She lives with her parents, a 6-year-old sister, Susan, a 2-year-old sister, Denise, and a 6-month-old brother, Kevin, in a rural town in the Midwest.

The T family's home is a modest one with a large yard that contains a vegetable garden. Kathy's father has seasonal employment at the implement dealership in town. Mrs. T's day is a busy one, with Denise and Kevin requiring much attention. Mrs. T is nursing Kevin and has started him on commercially prepared baby foods.

The T family lives on an income of $15,000 per year. About $275 is spent on food each month. Mrs. T tries hard to get the most for her money. In the tenth grade she had a unit on nutrition and she is eager to feed her family well. She gives the children plenty of milk. She often uses soups or casseroles with rice or macaroni as main dishes. Peas and corn are the only vegetables the family enjoys. Desserts such as cake or ice cream are usually served at the dinner meal. Mrs. T often uses candy and cookies to reward the children.

Both Kathy's parents and Susan are slender. Although Mr. and Mrs. T are a bit concerned about Kathy's weight, they are comfortable in believing that she is just passing through a stage and will eventually become slim like her sister. Since there are few children Kathy's age in the neighborhood, her parents decided to enroll her in the community Head Start program.

Before her enrollment in the Head Start program, Kathy had her required health screening completed. Abnormal findings included the identification of four carious teeth and a hemoglobin of 9.5 g per dl. When reviewing Kathy's growth pattern, the physician noted that at birth Kathy weighed 3.6 kg (7 lb, 14¾ oz) and was 56 cm (22 in.) long. Mrs. T reported that she had breast-fed Kathy and had started her on infant cereal at 2 months of age. By the end of the first year of life, Kathy was eating many table foods and drinking whole milk. She weighed 13.1 kg (28.8 lb) on her first birthday. At age 2 her weight was 17.3 kg (38.0 lb) and at age 3 it was 19.6 kg (43.1 lb). The physician recommended that Kathy's weight be watched; she prescribed vitamin supplements with iron.

In preparation for preschool, Kathy gets up at 7:00 A.M. Before she leaves she has a breakfast that usually includes a glass of whole milk, a bowl of presweetened cold cereal, and a piece of toast with jelly. Kathy arrives at school at 8:30. The children are offered a breakfast that includes a small glass of juice, a half pint of whole milk, an egg, and toast or a bowl of hot cereal. Kathy eats this breakfast with the other children.

Most of the morning is spent in free-play activities. When choosing her own interests, Kathy usually spends her time in the quiet story-telling corner. The teachers encourage her to become involved in large-muscle activities.

Lunch is served at 11:30 A.M. A typical meal includes a carton of whole milk, a hot dish such as macaroni and cheese, green beans, carrot and celery sticks, buttered bread, and chocolate pudding. Kathy eats well but usually takes only a taste of the hot vegetables. In the afternoon 1 hour of free play is followed by a 45-minute nap, after which a snack of juice and cookies is served.

Kathy comes home about 3:00 P.M., where she watches television until dinner time. Her mother usually gives her an afterschool snack such as a soft drink and a couple of cookies. Dinner is served about 5:30 P.M. Most evening meals consist of a casserole such as escalloped potatoes and ham or spaghetti and meat balls, peas or corn, bread and butter, gelatin dessert, a glass of whole milk, and cake, pie, ice cream, or pudding. The family watches television until bedtime and often has a snack of popcorn or potato chips.

Physiologic Correlations
1. What factors have been contributing to Kathy's obesity?
2. At what stage in life does the number of adipocytes increase sharply?
3. Compare Kathy's annual increase in weight with average rates of gain by children during the same time span.
4. What is a normal hemoglobin value for Kathy?
5. What factors in Kathy's history may contribute to the incidence of dental caries? Are there other factors that should be explored?

Nutritional Assessment
6. Using the Physical Growth NCHS Percentiles, locate Kathy's height and weight on the charts. How does she compare with other girls of her age?
7. Kathy's average daily energy intake is about 2,100 kcal. How does this compare with the recommended allowance for a girl of Kathy's age?
8. List the requirements per kilogram of body weight for a girl of Kathy's age for energy and for protein.
9. How much iron should Kathy obtain in her diet each day?
10. What dietary inadequacies might have contributed to Kathy's low hemoglobin level?

Planning the Diet
11. List the amounts of foods from each food group that would be appropriate for Kathy. Estimate the caloric value of these foods.
12. Prepare a list of snacks that would be suitable for Kathy after school and in the evening, giving attention to energy values and also to foods that are likely to reduce the incidence of dental caries.

Dietary Counseling
13. For each of the food groups in the Daily Food Guide, list some recommendations that will help Mrs. T to supply the foods needed for her family without exceeding her budget.
14. Determine whether the family income qualified them for Food Stamps. What referral is needed so that she can get them?
15. What suggestions can be made regarding Kathy's breakfast pattern?
16. Mrs. T is relieved that the physician has prescribed multivitamins and iron for Kathy, as she feels that this will take care of the nutritional problems. Explain fully why this sense of relief is not justified.

LASKY, P. A., and EICHELBERGER, K. M.: "Symposium on Obesity: Implications, Considerations, and Nursing Interventions of Obesity in Neonatal and Preschool Patients," *Nurs. Clin. North Am.*, **17**:199–205, June 1982.

MALLICK, M. J.: "Health Hazards of Obesity and Weight Control in Children: A Review of the Literature," *Am. J. Publ. Health*, **73**:78–82, 1983.

PHILLIPS, M. G.: "Nutrition Education for Preschoolers: The Head Start Experience," *Children Today*, **12**:20–24, July/August 1983.

References

1. Food and Nutrition Board: *Recommended Dietary Allowances*, 10th ed. National Research Council–National Academy of Sciences, Washington, D.C., 1989.
2. Pao, E. M.: "Nutrient Consumption Patterns of Individuals, 1977 and 1965," *Family Econ. Rev.*, Spring 1980, pp. 16–20.
3. Owen, G. M. et al.: "A Study of Nutritional Status of Preschool Children in the United States, 1968–70." *Pediatrics, (Suppl.)*, **53**:598–646, 1974.
4. *Ten-State Nutrition Survey 1968–1970*: Pub. No. (HSM) 72–8132, U.S. Department of Health, Education and Welfare, 1972.
5. Abraham, S. et al.: *Preliminary Findings of the First Health and Nutrition Examination Survey, United States, 1971–72. Anthropometic and Clinical Findings*: Pub. No. HRA 75–1229, U.S. Department of Health, Education and Welfare. 1975.
6. Macy, I. G., and Hunscher, H. A.: "Calories—A Limiting Factor in the Growth of Children," *J. Nutr*, **45**:189–99, 1951.
7. Sims, L. S., and Morris, P. M.: "Nutritional Status of Preschoolers: An Ecologic Perspective," *J. Am. Diet. Assoc.*, **64**:492–99, 1974.
8. Beal, V. A.: "Dietary Intake of Individuals Followed Through Infancy and Childhood," *Am. J. Publ. Health*, **51**:1107–17, 1961.
9. Hertzler, A. A.: "Children's Food Patterns—A Review: 1. Food Preferences and Feeding Problems," *J. Am. Diet. Assoc.*, **83**:551–60, 1983.
10. Huenemann, R. L. et al.: "A Longitudinal Study of Gross Body Composition and Body Conformation and Their Association with Food and Activity in a Teen-age Population. View of Teen-age Subjects on Body Conformation, Food and Activity," *Am. J. Clin. Nutr.*, **18**: 325–38, 1966.

11. Thomas, J. A., and Call, D. L.: "Eating Between Meals—A Nutrition Problem Among Teen-agers?" *Nutr. Rev.*, 31:137–39, 1973.

12. American Dietetic Association: "Statement on Nutrition and Physical Fitness," *J. Am. Diet. Assoc.*, 76: 437–43, 1980.

13. Jansen, G. R., and Harper, J. M.: "Nutrition vs. Waste in School Menus," *National Food Rev.*, Winter 1980, pp. 32–34.

14. Williams, C. L., et al.: "Primary Prevention of Chronic Disease Beginning in Childhood: The 'Know Your Body' Program: Design of Study," *Preventive Med.*, 6:344–57, 1977.

15. Brownell, K. D.: "The Psychology and Physiology of Obesity: Implications for Screening and Treatment," *J. Am. Diet. Assoc.*, 84:406–414, 1984.

16. Storz, N. S., and Greene, W. H.: "Body Weight, Body Image, and Perception of Fad Diets in Adolescent Girls," *J. Nutr. Educ.*, 15:15–18, 1983.

17. Waxman, M., and Stunkard, A. J.: "Caloric Intake and Expenditure of Obese Boys," *J. Pediatr.*, 96:187–93, 1980.

18. Huenemann, R. L. "Food Habits of Obese and Non-Obese Adolescents," *Postgrad. Med.*, 51:99–105, May 1972.

19. Pugliese, H. T., et al.: "Fear of Obesity: A Cause of Short Stature and Delayed Puberty," *N. Engl. J. Med.*, 309:513–18, 1983.

20. Dallman, P. R., et al.: "Iron Deficiency in Infancy and Childhood," *Am. J. Clin. Nutr.*, 33:86–118, 1980.

21. Lipton, M. A., and Mayo, J. P.: "Diet and Hyperkinesis—An Update," *J. Am. Diet. Assoc.*, 83:132–34, 1983.

22. National Advisory Committee on Hyperkinesis and Food Additives: *Final Report to the Nutrition Foundation*. The Nutrition Foundation Office of Education and Public Affairs, Washington, D.C., 1980.

23. Prinz, R. J., et al.: "Dietary Correlates of Hyperactive Behavior in Children," *J. Consult. Clin. Psychol.*, 48: 760–69, 1980.

24. Rumsey, J. M., and Rapoport, J. L. in *Nutrition and the Brain*, Vol. 6, R. J. Wurtman and J. J. Wurtman, eds. Raven Press, New York, 1983, pp. 135–36.

25. "Update: Childhood Lead Poisoning," *J. Am. Diet. Assoc.*, 80:592–94, 1982.

26. Review: "Clinical Nutrition Case: Metabolism of Vitamin D in Lead Poisoning," *Nutr. Rev.*, 39:372–73, 1981.

27. Mahaffey, K. R.: "Nutritional Factors in Lead Poisoning," *Nutr. Rev.*, 39:353–62, 1981.

22

Nutrition for Older Adults

The goal of nutritional care for the vast majority of persons in the later years of life is to help achieve healthful, purposeful, and independent living. A much smaller segment of the population requires coordinated health and social services including nutritional rehabilitation because they have suffered illness, physical disability, socioeconomic deprivation, or other handicap.

Who Are the Elderly?

Demographic Profile   What is meant by "old"? Chronologic age cannot be used to define physical and mental abilities. To be eligible for programs under the Older Americans Act (see page 325), the client must be at least 60 years of age. To qualify for Social Security and Medicare the individual must be 65 years, with some increase in age eligibility being contemplated by legislators. Retirement from one's occupation may come as early as the late 50s or as late as the 70s. Some people are "old" in their middle years,

and others are "old" only when they reach their 90s or beyond.

The "graying of America" describes the increasing ratio of older persons in the population. About one person in nine in the United States is 65 years or older, which accounts for approximately 27 million people. About one third of this elderly population is 75 years and over. Today at birth the white male has a life expectancy of almost 72 years and the white female of 77 years. The life expectancy for blacks is about 5 years less. Most of the increase in life expectancy since the early years of this century has resulted from greatly reduced infant mortality and not from the lengthening of the life span in the later years.

Upon reaching age 65, men can expect to live about 14 years longer and women 18 years. For every 100 men over 65 years there are 146 women. There are five times as many widows as there are widowers. One third of older women live alone, but most men over 65 years are living with their wives. Thus the problems of aging are much more acute for women,

CONCERNS RELATED TO NUTRITIONAL CARE

Although older adults have essentially the same human needs as do younger adults, many circumstances in their lives lead to a number of concerns.

Negative stereotypes exist not only in the general population, but are also held by health workers whose services are provided largely to a small percentage of the aging population.

More and more older people live alone, often in homes too large for them, and that they are unable to maintain because of physical or financial limitations.

Many older persons do not understand what their nutritional needs are or how to meet them. Others are unable to shop for food or to prepare it.

Some older people are especially susceptible to the exaggerated claims that certain foods or supplements will sustain health and vigor, prevent disease, or lengthen life.

With advancing years, especially after age 75, more people are frail, have one or more chronic diseases, and are physically disabled. They may need many kinds of services, including comprehensive arrangements for nutritional care.

By a physician's prescription or by self-medication many elderly are taking a variety of drugs. These can compromise good nutrition, but in certain situations food can also interfere with the effectiveness of the medications.

since they live longer, more frequently live alone and are isolated, and have lower incomes.

Low income and lack of education are more characteristic of blacks and Spanish Americans. Although most older persons are healthy, the average per capita expenditure for health care for the over-65-year group is about three times as high as that for the 19- to 64-year group. Although persons over 65 years account for about 11 per cent of the population, they utilize about one third of the nation's hospital beds.

Stereotypes and Realities Some unfortunate stereotypes about older persons exist in all segments of our society: that they are set in their ways, lonely, sick, poor, handicapped, no longer able to contribute to society, senile, living in nursing homes, and so on. Although some of these characteristics apply to millions of older persons, they are not descriptive of most older persons. The elderly who have lived 60, 70, or 80 years have been molded by their heredity, health, family, education, occupation, and numerous social, economic, and cultural factors. With the passage of time they have become increasingly complex individuals, and they make up a highly heterogeneous population.

Older adults fall into three subgroupings: those in middle age are likely to be at the peak of their careers and the fulfillment of their hopes, but are beginning to think about retirement; those for whom retirement has become a fact rightfully should be able to live up to high expectations; those in old age experience a decline with increasing dependency based upon state of health, economics, and social change.

Most older Americans have had a good marriage and family life, have financial security, and live comfortably. They live independently in their own homes, some live with their children, relatives, or friends, and only about 5 percent are confined to nursing homes. These older adults have learned to cope with many changes that occur in the later years: retirement, reduced income, death of loved ones, physiologic and pathologic changes, and so on. They lead productive lives by engaging in volunteer activities in the community, by working part time and sometimes full time, and by contributing to family welfare. They are physically active and enjoy life. They manage their own resources for healthful living, for pursuit of hobbies, and for travel. They have a strong sense of personal worth and spiritual values. In every sense they are a part of the community in which they live and not apart from it. They are a valuable source of experience, skills, and talents.

Physiologic and Biochemical Changes

The Aging Process AGING is a continuous process that begins with conception and ends with death. The Greek word for *old man* is *geron* and that for *treatise* is *logos*; therefore, the term GERONTOLOGY refers to the science that deals with the physiologic, psychologic, and socioeconomic aspects of aging. The suffix *-iatrics* means *the treatment of*; thus, GERIATRICS is the specialty in medicine concerned with the prevention and treatment of disease in older persons.

Each species appears to have a built-in limitation of the life span. Moreover, within the organism each cell type has a given life span. Some cells, such as those of the gastrointestinal mucosa have a very short life span—about 2 to 3 days. By the age of 2 the individual has a full complement of brain cells that will serve him or her throughout life. Some cells continue to divide and reproduce throughout life—for example, cells of the gastrointestinal mucosa, skin, and hair, while others appear to be programmed to divide a specific number of times and then cease reproducing—such as muscle and nerve cells.

With time there is a decline in the number of functioning cells of various organs so that performance is reduced. Two quite different examples illustrate the problem: A reduction in the number of taste buds reduces taste acuity and may modify the acceptance of food; a reduction in the number of functioning nephrons reduces glomerular filtration and renal blood flow so that wastes are less efficiently removed.

Theories of Aging The causes of cell aging are not known. On a molecular basis aging is the result of changes in cell metabolism or of cell death. Both genetic and environmental factors determine the rate of aging. No single theory of aging is generally accepted. Among the theories that have been set forth are the following[1-3]:

1. Modification of biologic information: The nuclear DNA may be damaged faster than it can be repaired, or there might be a defect in the repair mechanism. Alteration in the DNA can lead to transcription of faulty information to mRNA. Errors in the RNA assembly of amino acids lead to faulty protein synthesis so that enzymes required for normal cellular function are not produced.

2. Programmed life span or biologic time clock: Cells may be programmed to divide and replicate a given number of times, after which they lose their capacity to replicate. By genetic coding in the brain according to a precise timetable, signals are

sent by neural and hormonal stimulation or inhibition to organs and peripheral tissues. Thus, the "self-destruct" mechanism of the cells is ordered.

3. Wear and tear: Cells are subjected to insults and injuries by mechanical and thermal alterations, ionizing radiations, and uncontrolled chemical reactions. Highly reactive free radicals can react with polyunsaturated fatty acids to form peroxidation products that disrupt the cell membrane; that produce disintegration of the mitochondria (the cell's energy powerhouse) so that the ability to bring about electron transport and phosphorylation is reduced; or that release lysosomes (the "suicide bags" within the cells) so that cell death occurs. Some research indicates that vitamin E, selenium, and ascorbic acid may play a role in reducing the peroxidation reactions.

4. Crosslinkage: Because collagen accounts for about 40 percent of all protein in the body, there is a great interest in studying the changes that occur in it with advancing years. With aging there appears to be an increased number of hydrogen and ester bonds forming crosslinks between molecules of the collagen fiber. As the number of crosslinks increases, the collagen is immobilized. With the increasing rigidity of collagen, the skin, blood vessels, and respiratory system lose their elasticity, and the joints become stiff.

5. Immunologic changes: Immunologic function declines with age. On the one hand, the antibody synthesis may be defective so that the body's ability to counteract damaging substances is reduced. On the other hand, an increased response to endogenous antigens (autoimmune reactions) leads to increased destruction of normal body cells.

Body Composition   With aging a progressive decline in the water content and lean body mass is accompanied by an increasing proportion of body fat. By 80 years it is estimated that half the muscle cells remain. Specific functioning cells are replaced in part by nonspecific fat and connective tissue. The increase in the proportion of body fat occurs even though the weight remains unchanged.[4]

The changes in connective tissue, which is so abundant in the human body, are of especial significance. Collagen is one of the fibrous materials found in tendons, ligaments, skin, and blood vessels. With aging the amount of collagen increases and it becomes more rigid; the skin loses its flexibility, the joints creak, and the back becomes bent.

Function of the Gastrointestinal Tract   The senses of taste and smell are less acute in later years so that some of the pleasure derived from food is lost. Less saliva is secreted so that swallowing becomes more difficult. Because of tooth decay and periodontal disease more than half of persons over 70 years have lost some or all of their teeth. Many have ill-fitting dentures or none at all so that chewing is difficult. Consequently, these persons eat more soft, carbohydrate-rich foods that fail to provide adequate intakes of protein, minerals, and vitamins.

Digestion in later years is affected in a number of ways. Annoying delay of esophageal emptying occurs in many older persons. Hiatus hernia leads to increased complaints of heartburn and intolerance to foods. A reduction of the tonus of the musculature of the stomach, small intestine, and colon leads to less motility so that the likelihood of abdominal distention from certain foods is greater, as is also the prevalence of constipation. The volume, acidity, and pepsin content of the gastric juice is sometimes reduced. In turn there is interference with the absorption of calcium, iron, zinc, and vitamin B-12.

Fats are often poorly tolerated because they further retard gastric emptying, because the pancreatic production of lipase is inadequate for satisfactory hydrolysis and because chronic biliary impairment may reduce the production of bile or interfere with the flow of bile to the small intestine.

Cardiovascular and Renal Function   The progressive accumulation of atheromatous plaques leads to narrowing of the lumen of the blood vessels and loss of elasticity. There is a decline in cardiac output, an increased resistance to the flow of blood, and a lessened capacity to respond to extra work. As the rate of blood flow is reduced the digestion, absorption, and distribution of nutrients is retarded. A reduced blood flow together with a smaller number of functioning nephrons lessens the glomerular filtration and the tubular reabsorption so that the excretion of wastes and sometimes the return of nutrients to the circulation is less efficient.

Metabolism   From age 25 years the basal metabolism decreases about 2 percent for each decade owing to the increasing proportion of body fat and the lesser muscle tension. The decline in basal metabolism is less in persons who remain healthy and pursue vigorous activity in their later years. The ability to maintain normal body temperature is also lessened, and hypothermia in the elderly can be especially dangerous.

Carbohydrate Metabolism. Usually the fasting blood sugar is normal. Likewise, the absorption of carbohydrate is not impaired. However, when a carbohydrate load is presented, as in the glucose tolerance test, the blood sugar remains elevated for a longer period of time than it does in younger persons. Following exercise, the levels of blood lactic acid and pyruvic acid are often above normal limits.

Fat Metabolism. With increasing age the blood cholesterol and blood triglyceride levels gradually increase. The kind and amount of fat and carbohydrate in the diet, the degree of overweight, the stresses of life, and many other factors are believed to be responsible for these changes.

Factors Influencing Food Habits

The food habits of the elderly are the result of the lifetime influences of cultural, social, economic, and psychological factors. The individual who has had poor food habits throughout life is not likely to be in as good health as the one who has enjoyed the benefits of a good diet. Good diet in later years cannot completely make up for the years of inadequacy or correct irreversible changes. Furthermore, an older individual is not likely to change his or her whole pattern of eating. Nevertheless, even the individual with poor food habits who is in a poor state of nutrition can benefit greatly from the application of the principles of good nutrition.

Socioeconomic Factors Insufficient income is probably the chief factor limiting dietary adequacy. About one sixth of persons over 65 years of age in 1980 were below the Bureau of Census Poverty Index.[5] Poverty is twice as prevalent in women as in men. Four of every ten blacks and three of every 10 Hispanics have incomes below the poverty level.

Many persons must rely solely on Social Security income. Others have pensions and some savings, but fixed incomes make it increasingly difficult to meet ever-increasing costs for the essentials of life. Although Medicare and Medicaid provide substantial benefits for health care, the costs of medications and catastrophic illness can use up life savings and reduce the available income.

Housing is a major problem for many older persons. Most older people continue to live in their own homes but find it increasingly difficult to pay the exorbitant charges for fuel and other utilities as well as the ever-increasing real estate taxes. Those who live in apartments are often unable to afford higher rents, so they are forced to move to less desirable places. Many live in neighborhoods where they are afraid to walk on the streets because they might be robbed or physically assaulted. Living in a single room with no facilities for food preparation is the lot of many elderly.

Transportation to shopping facilities, physician, dentist, and churches is a serious problem for many older people. Some cannot afford to drive an automobile and others have lost the ability to drive safely. Even those who live near public transportation find it difficult to manage bags of groceries while boarding or getting off vehicles. Nearby independent food stores offer convenience but the food costs are likely to be higher.

Shopping itself can be a problem. With thousands of items in supermarkets, the shopper finds it more difficult to make economical, nutritious choices. Failing vision means that one cannot read the fine print on labels or compare costs of various brands.

Psychologic Factors Loneliness and social isolation powerfully affect food intake. Upon retirement some elderly persons lose their sense of worth, since they are no longer consulted for advice or see their former co-workers. Some older adults have lost their loved ones, live far away from their children, or are neglected by their relatives. They often have little desire to prepare meals and may eat only those foods that are conveniently available. Others eat compulsively to assuage their feelings of loneliness, depression, and despair. Erratic eating habits in turn perpetuate the mental depression.

Food Misinformation and Faddism Older adults are justified in their hopes that a nutritionally balanced diet throughout life will improve health and prolong life. However, the present generation of elderly have had less education than the younger generations, and they may be more influenced by exaggerated claims for health foods and supplements. Advertising for these products usually extols the values they have in correcting deficiencies and removing symptoms. The individual makes a self-diagnosis based on a graphic description of symptoms and buys the product to alleviate these symptoms, real or imagined. Although the product is likely to be safe, it is often not needed and the money spent could better be used for a good diet. More important, by self-diagnosis one may wait too long before seeking medical advice. Among the exaggerated claims being made for special products are these:

Typical diets do not furnish sufficient amounts of trace minerals and a supplement should be taken daily. (NOTE: a diet consisting mostly of *highly processed* foods could indeed be lacking some trace minerals.)
Vitamin E will prolong life and prevent heart attacks.
Garlic and parsley reduce blood pressure.
Lecithin supplements will prevent or treat heart disease.

The elderly also hold a variety of erroneous beliefs about foods that are normal constituents of the diet. Among these are:

Older people do not need milk. It is expensive, and also causes flatulence and constipation.
Fruits are too "acid."
Raw vegetables and whole-grain breads and cereals irritate the lining of the stomach and intestines and cause diarrhea.
Pork causes high blood pressure. (NOTE: persons using antihypertensive drugs are sometimes advised by their physicians not to eat pork. They should avoid salted meats such as bacon, salt pork, and ham, but there is no reason to restrict fresh pork.)
Honey and vinegar reduce the symptoms of arthritis.

Dietary Management

Nutritional Status The principles and techniques for assessing nutritional status are described in Chapter 23. Unfortunately many of the widely used measurements are of limited value for use with the elderly inasmuch as the available standards are not applicable to the older population. A single measure of body weight is a poor indicator of nutritional status in most elderly persons. However, health professionals should be encouraged to follow body weight on a continuing basis, since loss of body weight may be an indicator of loss of appetite or of illness, while a sudden gain in body weight could occur because of fluid retention. One of the more reliable indicators of malnutrition is a reduced level of serum albumin. This can result from a diet inadequate in protein over a long period of time or from some fault in the synthesis of albumin. The state of malnutrition is usually fairly well advanced by the time the serum albumin levels are lowered.

Many studies on nutritional status have been carried out on selected population groups such as the elderly in nursing homes, or on those with low incomes. Such studies are useful for identifying the nutritional problems of these particular groups, but they are hardly representative of the needs of all older Americans. In general, surveys have shown that blacks and Spanish Americans are most likely to have deficient diets and to show evidence of biochemical deficiency.

Low income and lack of education are important contributing factors.

Obesity is a frequent finding in those under 75 years; it is less common in persons over 75 years. In the later years a moderate level of overweight—10 to 20 percent above standards for height, weight, and body frame—is desirable.

On the basis of nutrient intakes per 1,000 kcal, most studies show that the quality of the diet of the elderly is generally good. However, significant numbers fail to eat enough food, so that the total nutrient intakes do not meet the recommended allowances. The 1971 HANES survey showed that 56 percent of persons 60 years or older had diets inadequate in calcium, iron, vitamin A, and vitamin C.[5] According to the Household Food Consumption Survey,[6] calcium and vitamin B-6 intakes were most significantly below recommended allowances for women.

Of the dietary inadequacies, that of calcium is probably most serious since it is one of several risk factors for osteoporosis. (See page 326.) Seventy-five percent of all women over 35 years of age ingest only three fourths or less of the RDA for calcium.[7] The average intake by men over 65 is 600 mg and by women over 65 is 480 mg.[8] Vitamin D deficiency in the elderly is not common, but it can occur if the individual does not drink vitamin D milk and also has limited exposure to sunlight.

Most elderly meet their 10-mg dietary allowance for iron.[9] Nonetheless, hypochromic microcytic anemia characteristic of iron deficiency is surprisingly common in older persons. In women especially this could reflect a lifelong inadequacy of iron intake or a diet with a low bioavailability of iron. Many elderly reduce their consumption of meat which is a good source of heme iron, and which also improves the bioavailability of iron from plant sources. In anemia it is important to rule out any small, often undetected, losses of blood from the gastrointestinal tract.

The elderly are often concerned that they may have a zinc deficiency, largely because of the emphasis given by advertisers of zinc supplements. A recent survey showed that the elderly with a mean age of 71 to 75 years ingested only half the RDA for zinc.[10] The elderly showed a lower hair concentration of zinc and lower taste acuity. However, the authors caution that there is currently no precise definition of low zinc status, nor is the frequency of zinc deficiency known.

Most elderly consume less than the RDA for folacin and magnesium, but there is no evidence of a high level of biochemical deficiency for these nutrients.[11] The present RDA levels may be higher than needed. Diets also are often low in vitamins A and C.

But a high percentage of the elderly are using vitamin supplements, often to excess.

Dietary Allowances   Only limited data on nutritional requirements of the elderly are available.[4] The RDA for the nutrients are set for all healthy persons over 51 years and, except for iron, are the same as those for adults 23 to 50 years of age. It is to be expected that the nutritional requirements of healthy vigorous persons in their 60s will differ from those in their late 70s and 80s who are likely to be more sedentary and perhaps less healthy. Also, individual adjustments are necessary according to existing nutritional status, infections, interference with digestion and absorption, deficiencies of cardiovascular and renal function, and the use of medications.

Energy.   The mean requirement for men 51 years and over is 2,300 kcal. For women of 51 years and over the mean energy requirement is 1,900 kcal. For persons over 75 years the requirement is likely to be lower. For any given individual the actual caloric requirement varies by as much as ± 20 percent.

Protein.   Some studies indicate that the elderly require more protein than do younger adults in order to maintain nitrogen balance, while others have suggested lower intakes of protein. Gersovitz and co-workers[12] found that healthy subjects (70 to 99 years) were in negative balance when they were fed egg protein at the RDA level (0.8 g per kg). They recommend a protein intake higher than the RDA for persons over 70 years of age.

The likelihood of negative nitrogen balance is greater when the energy intake as well as the protein intake is reduced. Generally, an allowance of 12 percent of calories from protein will permit a satisfactory intake.

Fat and Carbohydrate.   The fat intake should be restricted to 30 to 35 percent of calories, with preference given to sources of fat that are high in polyunsaturated fatty acids. Thus, the carbohydrate level of the diet will range from 53 to 58 percent of the calories.

Fiber.   A liberal intake of dietary fiber is recommended, since it helps maintain normal peristaltic activity of the lower bowel, and may reduce the formation of diverticula. (See page 76.)

Minerals.   The mineral requirements of the elderly are not known, but the RDA are believed to be satis-

factory for most persons. However, because bone loss is so persistent in later years a calcium intake of 1,000 to 1,500 mg may be preferable to the 800-mg level of the RDA.

Sodium intake requires particular attention, since many elderly have hypertension and are taking antihypertensive medications. Such persons are usually cautioned to reduce their intake of sodium. The minimum requirement for sodium is 500 mg, which accounts for one sixth of the sodium most adults generally ingest.

The minimum requirement for potassium by adults is 2,000 mg. Persons taking diuretics have increased excretion of potassium and need to increase their potassium intake.

Vitamins.   Whether the elderly require higher or lower levels of vitamins than younger adults is not known. Generally, they will be well nourished if their diets supply the RDA set for younger adults. In some circumstances, such as infections, surgery, and malabsorption disorders, supplements are indicated.

Meal Plans   Since the caloric requirement for older persons is lower than that for younger adults, the diet must be one of higher nutrient density. Especially for women, there is little margin remaining for foods high in sugar and fat that are nutrient poor but that also can lead to weight gain and obesity. The basic diet outlined for adults on page 38 serves as a foundation for the diet after 50 years. It furnishes about 1,200 kcal and most of the nutrients at recommended levels. The levels of folacin, vitamin B-6, magnesium, and zinc do not meet the recommended levels. Thus, in the selection of foods to add to the basic diet, particular emphasis should be given to good sources of these nutrients.

Daily meal patterns followed in earlier years are satisfactory for older persons. Breakfast is often the best meal of the day and it should be planned to contribute a significant proportion of the day's nutrients. Some prefer to have the heavier meal at noon rather than at night. Others enjoy a midafternoon snack.

A wide variety of frozen dinners and breakfasts are available in most markets. Most are labeled with nutritional information and provide satisfactory levels of nutrients. Although these meals are more expensive than comparable meals prepared in the home, they provide an alternative for those who have little inclination or limited physical ability to prepare meals from scratch. A serving of fruit or salad and a glass of milk should be included with these meals.

People who live alone miss the social interaction

that takes place at mealtime. They must be encouraged to develop regular meal patterns and to prepare foods they enjoy. One elderly woman who lives alone likes to share Sunday morning breakfast with a friend who also lives alone. She sets her table by a window where they can see the garden and watch the activities of the birds. During the week she and two women who also live alone take turns having lunch together in each others' homes.

Community Resources for Nutrition

Senior Centers The intention of the revised Older Americans Act (1978) is to provide essential services to older Americans so that they can remain in their homes rather than being forced into more expensive institutional facilities. This act provides funding for meals and supporting social services that are provided in senior centers or to persons who are homebound. Although all persons over 60 years are eligible for the programs, priority is given to those who have low income, physical limitations, live alone, and are over 75 years.

A noon meal that furnishes at least one third of the recommended dietary allowances is served at community centers at least 5 days a week. (See Figure 22-1.) Modified diets are furnished according to need. Some centers also serve breakfasts or afternoon snacks. The supporting services may include information and referral; outreach activities; health screening; health and nutrition education; diet counseling; transportation to centers, shopping, and physician's offices; legal aid; crafts and recreational activities and so on.

Many programs for the aging are now providing day care for elderly who cannot remain alone in their homes while other family members are away. Usually the facilities for these persons are separate from those who attend the senior centers. Because these individuals are more infirm and have a variety of health problems, some supervision by a nurse is indicated. The nurse makes an evaluation of the individual's state of health and works under the direction of the physician in administering medications or other therapy. Close attention to intake of food is important. Many of these elderly become more alert and cooperative as their nutrition improves.

Home-Delivered Meals Through funding under Title III-C of the Older Americans Act, home-delivered meals are available to the elderly who cannot come to the senior centers. Some of the programs deliver a noon meal 5 days per week, while others

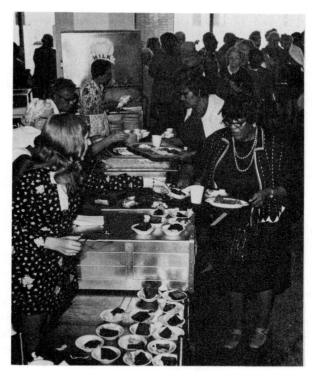

Figure 22-1. Through the Older Americans Act and by state and community support a noon meal and a spectrum of social services are available in senior centers five days a week. (Courtesy, *Aging Magazine.* October 1975, Administration on Aging, Department of Health, Education, and Welfare, Washington, D.C.)

provide two meals daily for 5 to 7 days. Nutrition counseling is an important part of this program.

Meals-on-Wheels is a voluntary program sponsored by civic or religious organizations. Meals are delivered to ill and disabled persons of any age who have no one to prepare food for them. Usually the program provides a noon meal and a sack lunch for the evening meal 5 days a week. Each recipient pays for the cost of the food, but the meals are packed and delivered by volunteers. For those who are unable to pay the full cost of the food, a sliding scale of payment can usually be arranged.

Food Stamps Many older Americans are unaware that they may be eligible to receive food stamps, while others refuse to accept stamps because they prefer not to accept what they consider charity. Dietary counselors should encourage eligible individuals to use the stamps, thereby increasing the likelihood of an adequate diet.

Nutrition-Related Health Problems

About one person in five over 65 years of age identifies some serious health problems. Some of these problems are the consequence of poor nutrition throughout life. Others are not caused by faulty nutrition but may have profound effects on nutritional status because they affect appetite and the ability to digest, absorb, and metabolize nutrients or because of limited physical powers that affect the ability to obtain an adequate diet.

Osteoporosis

Osteoporosis is a major cause of disability in the elderly. This age-related disorder is characterized by a decrease in total bone mass without a change in chemical composition. It occurs when the rate of bone resorption exceeds the rate of formation. The reduction in the number of cells results in a decrease in the thickness of the cortex, a thinning of the trabeculae, and an increased porosity of bone. Consequently, fractures of the vertebrae, femur, and radius occur with greater frequency, often in spite of little or no trauma.

Probably 90 percent of all fractures are caused by osteoporosis. The rate of femoral fractures alone doubles for each decade after age 50, at an annual cost of about $1 billion in the United States.[13] Three to four of every 10 women over age 65 suffer fractures.[14] Osteoporosis occurs four times as frequently in women as in men. The longer women live beyond the menopause, the greater the likelihood of fracture. Thin women of small stature are more susceptible than those of larger body frame. The incidence is higher in whites than in blacks and in Caucasians from northern Europe than in those from the Mediterranean area.

Etiology   After the age of 30 to 35 the annual rate of bone loss is 0.5 percent in both men and women. This rate increases to at least 1 percent annually for 10 years or more after the menopause.[15] The etiology of osteoporosis is multifactorial and includes the following age-related changes:

Decreased estrogen production associated with the menopause
Long-time low intake of calcium[15,16]
Decreased absorption of calcium
Reduced circulating level of calcitriol (vitamin D hormone)[17,18]
Increased urinary loss of calcium
Increased urinary excretion of hydroxyproline, representing collagen breakdown
Reduced physical activity, with calcium losses in immobilization dramatic[19]

There is no consistent alteration in the levels of plasma calcium, phosphorus, and alkaline phosphatase.[20] Although the role of dietary factors is not clear, calcium deficiency must be considered a possible risk factor. Those who chronically have low intakes of calcium appear to have a higher risk of osteoporosis than those who have developed maximum bone mass because of a lifelong higher intake of calcium.[21] But not all persons with low calcium intake develop osteoporosis.

An increased intake of phosphorus through the use of many processed foods and soft drinks to which phosphorus compounds have been added has been suggested as a possible factor leading to negative calcium balance. However, it has not been demonstrated in humans that wide variations in phosphorus intake and in the calcium-to-phosphorus ratio lead to negative calcium balance.[8] If soft drinks are consumed in place of milk, the calcium intake would be substantially reduced.

High intakes of alcohol, caffeine, protein, and/or fiber can increase calcium loss, but the clinical significance of these effects when ordinary mixed diets are consumed is not known.[22]

Clinical Characteristics   Low back pain that is sometimes severe, kyphosis of the dorsal spine, and skeletal fractures are the primary symptoms of osteoporosis. Loss of height—sometimes several inches—follows collapse of the vertebrae.

Treatment   Just as the causes of osteoporosis are poorly defined, so there is also much controversy about the treatment. Low-dose cyclic estrogen–progestagen therapy together with a daily 500-mg supplement of calcium over a 3-year period was found effective in reversing mineral loss from bone in a group of Danish women. Those who received the hormone therapy plus calcium had an annual bone accretion of 1.3 percent, while women who received only the calcium supplement and a placebo experienced an annual mineral loss of 1.9 percent.[14] However, the use of estrogens following the menopause has been associated with an abnormal incidence of cancer of the uterine endometrium. The estrogen–progestagen combination is believed to reduce this risk. Thus, in using hormone therapy one must consider whether improvement in bone mineralization and prevention of fractures outweighs the possible risk of cancer.

From a nutritional point of view, an intake of 1,000 to 2,000 mg calcium slows the rate of calcium loss.[8,15,16,19] Since the average calcium intake by elderly women is about 500 mg, the addition of 3 to 4 cups of milk would raise the intake to 1,500 mg or so. Those who are not likely to consume this level of milk may use supplements of calcium gluconate, calcium carbonate, or calcium lactate.

A liberal intake of calcium accompanied with physical activity may arrest the deterioration of bone mass. Exercise that involves weight-bearing movement, as in walking or running, is helpful, but calisthenic-type exercises are not effective.[19] According to Raisz,[15] there have been no controlled clinical trials to demonstrate the effectiveness of parathormone, growth hormone, calcitonin, or vitamin D metabolite.

Prevention The only rational approach to osteoporosis is prevention. But just as the etiology and treatment are confusing, there are no clear-cut guides to prevention. If women can enter the sixth decade of life with a well-fortified bone mass, the severity of bone loss can be ameliorated. This suggests that women especially must ingest liberal levels of calcium throughout their lives—1,000 to 1,200 mg being preferable to the 800 mg recommended by the RDA.

Persons living in areas where the naturally occurring fluoride in water is high have a remarkably lower incidence of hip fractures. Based on data from the National Health Interview Survey (1973–77) Madens and co-workers found that fluoride levels of 0.7 ppm (the level recommended for protection against dental caries) was not protective.[23] Further research is required to determine the fluoride level that is protective without being toxic.

Other Health Problems

The incidence of chronic diseases such as arthritis, diabetes mellitus, and those of the gastrointestinal tract, and the cardiovascular and renal systems increases with age. The dietary management of these conditions is discussed in Part III of this book. Some problems associated with these conditions that health professionals might encounter in working with any group of older persons are described briefly below.

Arthritis afflicts a significant number of older persons who may need assistance in shopping for food and preparing it. Health professionals need to be aware of the many false claims for treatment and cure by a special diet or some device. A diet that meets nutritional requirements contributes to a sense of well-being, although it is not likely to modify the arthritic process. Those persons who are obese will experience some improvement by losing weight, thereby reducing the load on weight-bearing joints. (See Chapter 37.)

Periodontal disease is highly prevalent after age 35. It is characterized by a loss of bone mass in the jaw followed by loosening of the teeth and their eventual loss. With the continuing bone loss, dentures will fit poorly, so that chewing becomes difficult. Marked improvement in nutritional status is often possible when appropriate dental care is given. The following list includes foods that are appropriate when chewing is difficult:

Milk as a beverage
Cottage cheese; American cheese in sauces or casserole dishes
Eggs, soft cooked, scrambled, poached
Tender meat, or poultry, finely minced or ground; flaked fish; finely diced meat in sauces often taken more readily
Soft raw fruits as banana, berries; canned or cooked fruits; fruit juices
Soft-cooked vegetables, diced, chopped, or mashed. Raw vegetables such as tomatoes can often be eaten if finely chopped—skin and seeds removed
Cooked and dry cereals with milk
Bread, crackers, and toast with hot or cold milk
Desserts: diced cake with fruit sauce; fruit whips; gelatin; ice cream and ices; puddings; pie, if crust is tender and cut up

Occasional social drinking of alcoholic beverages is not considered harmful to the elderly; it may even be beneficial. Alcohol addiction, on the other hand, is a serious problem that afflicts a million or so older Americans. It is particularly damaging when money available for the purchase of food is spent instead for alcoholic beverages. Excessive use of alcohol can lead to mental confusion, and may interfere with the metabolism of some medications. (See Chapter 27.)

Constipation in older persons results in part from reduced tonus of the lower intestine. However, the most important contributing factors can be controlled by the individual: ingesting 1,200 to 2,000 ml fluid daily; increasing fiber intake by including generous amounts of fruits, vegetables, and whole-grain breads and cereals; and regular habits of elimination.

Sodium restriction is recommended for many older persons, especially those who are taking antihypertensive medications. (See also Chapter 39.) The moderate restriction that is usually indicated does not need to result in loss of food palatability, and requires only some rather common sense changes:

1. Remove salt shaker from the table. (Alternatively, women can place clear tape over most of the holes if their spouse insists on using salt.)
2. Avoid obviously salty foods such as pickles, relishes, meat sauces, salted meats and fish, snacks such as potato chips and pretzels.
3. Use ½ to ¾ as much salt as specified in recipes for preparing meats and vegetables.
4. Make cakes, cookies, and desserts from scratch and omit salt.
5. Learn to use herbs, spices, lemon juice, and other substitute flavorings.

Potassium loss is increased with the use of many diuretics. Meats, fruits, and vegetables are good sources of potassium; a varied diet including these foods will meet the needs of most persons.

Medications

With increasing health problems in later years there is also an increasing use of medications, either according to a physician's prescription or through use of over-the-counter preparations. In fact, expenditures for drugs by those with a limited income may restrict the money available for food. Some drugs affect nutritional status because of change in appetite and sense of taste, nausea, vomiting, and interference with absorption and excretion. (See Chapter 27 and Appendix B.)

Nutrition for Clients in Nursing Homes

The Nursing Home Population About 1 of 20 persons over 65 years of age lives in a nursing home and will remain there for the rest of his or her life. Most of these clients are women, and almost half are childless. The average age is 81 years. As in any aging population, they present a wide spectrum of problems that may include limited mobility, poor vision, loss of hearing, altered behavior, loss of socialization skills, slowed reaction time, food idiosyncrasies, ill-fitting or absent dentures, inability to feed self, malnutrition, and chronic disease.

Some Behavior Problems Weiner[24] described four categories of pathologic–psychologic reactions in aging persons in nursing homes; anxiety, depression, suspicion, and confusion. In some individuals all of these may be present to a varying degree or they may appear one after the other. Each type of reaction requires specific measures in feeding.

The anxious person requires assurance that everything is all right. This individual worries about the effects that foods may have on bowel function and often asks questions about which foods are constipating. Worry about food may increase gastrointestinal motility, so that the person has cramps or may reduce motility so that he or she becomes distended. The anxious person needs to be comforted, to have someone around, to be made to feel secure, and to be given special consideration by being served favorite foods as often as possible.

The depressed individual feels that his or her situation is hopeless and has a conscious or unconscious desire to die. Reassurance only frightens the person more and he or she will continue to demand more and more of it until there seems to be no end to the demands. Such individuals need external control and should be told firmly exactly what they must do, that they must eat, that they will be taken care of, and that they will be helped to eat what they need for their nourishment. Sometimes spoon feeding is needed to get them started. It is not advisable for these individuals to choose their own menu.

The suspicious person is afraid of being hurt and often suspects that the food is poisoned. Such persons feel that they must constantly be on watch lest something happen to their security. Efforts to reassure them to the contrary only increase their suspicions. Matter-of-factly they should be told that there is nothing wrong with the food, but it may be necessary for the attendant to taste the food in their presence to show that it is not poisoned. The suspicious person, unlike the depressed person, must not be forced to eat. He or she should be allowed to eat or not to eat what is presented.

The confused person has usually had some brain damage as in a stroke, from diabetic or hepatic coma, or from head injury. Such persons do not know what is happening around them and often become anxious, depressed, or suspicious. They may not know where they are and, regardless of what they are told, they believe themselves to be in their own home as adults or in their childhood home. They need help in understanding what is going on around them. With respect to feeding, they need to be told that it is mealtime, what meal it is, and what foods are on the tray. When a favorite food is served, it is a good idea to specially identify it.

Meeting Nutritional Needs The condition that necessitates admission to a nursing home is also likely to be one that contributes to malnutrition. Each new admission should be evaluated for nutritional status and a care plan developed for maintaining or improving nutritional health. A dietary history helps establish past food intakes and food preferences. Body weight should be determined weekly, if possible, and any changes should be evaluated for needed therapy. Monitoring the daily food intake helps determine not only how well the client is eating but also what foods are liked and disliked.

Meal planning should follow the principles applicable to any population. (See Chapter 14.) A selective menu emphasizes to clients that they can still make some choices in their lives and usually helps improve food intake. Portions should be adjusted to each individual's appetite, since overly large portions often discourage eating. Group dining is preferred except when behavior or physical limitations make this impossible.

The main meal in many nursing homes is usually served at noon. To accommodate employee schedules, the evening meal is often served early (4 to 5 P.M.), resulting in a long interval between supper and breakfast. If such scheduling is unavoidable, an evening snack such as pudding, milk and cookies, or fruit should be provided.

Some clients who are malnourished and who have poor appetites may require supplementary feedings that supply protein, energy, minerals, and vitamins. Several proprietary supplements are convenient, palatable, and especially useful as an evening feeding. As nutritional status improves, so the alertness and general sense of well-being usually improves.

Although clients suffer a variety of chronic diseases, strict dietary regimens are rarely warranted.[25] Too much emphasis on a modified diet often leads to frustration and rebellion. Indeed, such enforcement may make it seem that one of life's last pleasures has been taken away. Although many clients require moderate sodium restriction, there is little justification for preparing all foods without any added salt—a practice followed in too many nursing homes. (See page 142.) Unless obesity is severely aggravating a condition such as arthritic joints, attempts at weight loss probably are not indicated.

DIETARY COUNSELING

With increasing age the problems of meal management become greater. The dietary counselor must consider the individual's income, the facilities for food preparation, the physical ability to shop for food and prepare it, the social and cul-

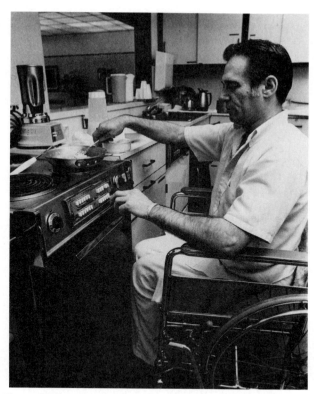

Figure 22-2. Older man who wants to be independent learns how to prepare his meals before his discharge from the hospital. (Courtesy, Metropolitan Medical Center, Minneapolis and Jeffrey Grosscup, photographer.)

tural background, and the individual attitudes toward food together with the motivation for obtaining an adequate diet. The counselor must be especially alert to the food beliefs held by the client and to the possibility that medications might interfere with food utilization.

Most older adults are anxious to improve their diets, but they also need assurance that some of their present practices have merit. They need assistance in planning simple meals that not only meet their nutritional requirements but are satisfying; advice concerning the best food buys for the money; information on the interpretation of labels; recipes suitable for one or two people; and suggestions for simple food preparation. (See Figure 22-2.)

The Daily Food Guide can be adapted to various cultural patterns. Special emphasis should be given to the inclusion of milk daily, except for those occasional persons who have lactose intolerance; of good sources of fiber including some fresh fruits and raw vegetables as well as whole-grain breads and cereals; and at least 1,200 to 1,800 ml water daily. Some salt restriction is desirable for most older persons. They need information not only on foods that contain much salt, but also on ways to reduce the use of salt in food preparation.

The elderly who live alone need encouragement to take time to prepare attractive meals and to make mealtime enjoyable. The following suggestions may help.

1. Serve colorful foods attractively on a tray if eating alone. Invite relatives or friends to share a meal from time to time.
2. Eat leisurely in pleasant surroundings; for example, by a window with a good view.
3. Include essential foods first. Sweets and fats should be moderately restricted. Use fresh fruits for dessert, with a calorie-rich dessert included occasionally as a special treat.
4. Adjust food selection to individual tolerance. For some this might indicate that one or more strongly flavored vegetables are not included, whereas others find fatty foods, fried foods, gravies, pastries, and rich cakes give discomfort. No foods need arbitrarily be omitted for all elderly just because a few have a poor tolerance.
5. Avoid coffee, tea, and cola beverages late in the day if insomnia is a problem.

CASE STUDY 7

Elderly Man with Depression

Mr. H age 76, is a retired barber who has lived in Charlestown, West Virginia all his life. He is proud of his Pennsylvania Dutch heritage. Several years ago he had to retire because of osteoarthritis in his upper spine. His present income consists of checks from Social Security and interest from a sizeable savings account.

Since his wife's sudden death 2 years ago Mr. H has been lonely and depressed. The H's had been married for 54 years and were very close. They had no children, and he has only one living relative, a brother who lives in Kansas. During the past year Mr. H has lost 4.5 kg (10 lb), and he looks thin, haggard, and unkempt. He is 173 cm (68 in.) tall and weighs 61 kg (134 lb). He has become withdrawn, smokes excessively, and is very fidgety. He no longer attends church or participates in the V.F.W. post where he had been active for years. He has refused many dinner invitations and rarely sees friends.

Mr. H lives alone in a two-bedroom ranch house which is filled with memorabilia. His day begins at 5:00 A.M., and he spends most of the day in his den watching television or listening to the radio. There are many filled ash trays in the room and a number of unopened pieces of mail. The days are long for Mr. H, and boredom is a problem. He has no hobbies or outside interests, and because of cataracts he has difficulty reading. After watching the late-late show on television he often falls asleep in his recliner in the den.

Mrs. H had done all the cooking and housekeeping tasks; as a result, Mr. H had never learned to cook. He does not use the kitchen, and he takes his laundry to a commercial firm, although there is a washer and dryer in the basement. In the refrigerator there is a can of juice, a jar of jam, some butter, and a loaf of bread.

Mr. H eats most of his meals in local restaurants. The menu selection is limited because he has a poor tolerance for fried foods. He tires of the menus and often skips meals. For breakfast he usually has only a cup of coffee and sometimes a piece of bread with butter and jam. When he doesn't go out at noon he may heat a can of soup and eat some more bread. He thinks he does not need much food because of his age. His diet is relatively high in carbohydrates and low in protein, minerals, and vitamins. His average caloric intake was found to be about 1,450 kcal.

Mr. H has made frequent visits to his family physician for minor somatic complaints since his wife's death. His physician expressed concern about Mr. H's ongoing depression and referred him to a psychiatrist. He also encouraged him to get involved in the local senior citizen's center, which had many activities in which he might become involved.

The psychiatrist placed Mr. H on tricyclic antidepressant therapy. After an unsuccessful trial with tricyclics, Mr. H was placed on Nardil (phenelzine sulfate) a monoamine oxidase inhibitor (MAO).

Pathophysiologic Correlations

1. State three changes in physiologic function that are characteristic of the aging process.
2. Mr. H says he does not like meat as much as he did a few years ago. What physiologic basis might there be for this change?
3. What factors might account for Mr. H's inability to tolerate fried foods?
4. What hormonal changes occur during aging? How do these changes affect nutrition?
5. What is the biochemical action of monoamine oxidase inhibitors?

Nutritional Assessment

6. List some physiologic, psychologic, and social factors that might have contributed to Mr. H's eating habits.
7. Since Mr. H's protein intake is inadequate, what other nutrients are also likely to be lacking in his diet?
8. Ten years ago Mr. H lost all of his teeth because of severe periodontal disease. What nutrient deficiencies might contribute to this inadequacy?
9. What is the relationship, if any, between periodontal disease and osteoporosis?
10. Although Mr. H has dentures he usually does not wear them because they do not fit well. Is it possible for Mr. H to have an adequate dietary intake if he doesn't use his dentures?

Planning the Diet

11. Outline the points you need to consider in planning for Mr. H's nutritional care.
12. Explain the importance of calcium in the diet of the elderly.
13. What foods are contraindicated for persons who are taking MAO inhibitors? Why? (See page 248.)
14. Suggest some practical ways for increasing protein intake that might be acceptable to Mr. H.

Dietary Counseling

15. Mr. H drinks very little milk. He feels that at his age he doesn't need milk, and he believes milk is constipating. How would you respond to these misconceptions?
16. The physician told Mr. H that attention to his diet was all that was needed to correct constipation. What specific changes are required?
17. On a late night radio program Mr. H heard that vitamin E is a "miracle" vitamin that delays aging. Is there any evidence to support this claim?
18. What suggestions can you offer for foods requiring little or no preparation that Mr. H could keep on hand so that he could eat a more substantial breakfast at home?
19. Mr. H would rather eat out than shop for groceries. What are some factors that make it difficult for older persons to shop for groceries?
20. Mr. and Mrs. H took great pride in their beautiful flower garden, especially their roses. Suggest some ways in which Mr. H's talents might be used to encourage him to become more active socially. What benefits would you expect this involvement to have? Could there be any nutritional benefits? Explain.

References for the Case Study

Axelson, M. L., and Penfield, M. P.: "Food- and Nutrition-Related Attitudes of Elderly Persons Living Alone," J. Nutr. Educ., 15:23–27, 1983.

Korcok, M.: "Add Exercise to Calcium in Osteoporosis Prevention," JAMA, 247:1106, 1982.

Luros, E.: "A Rational Approach to Geriatric Nutrition," Diet. Currents, 8 (6):November/December 1981.

Posner, B. M.: "Nutrition Education for Older Americans: National Policy Recommendations," J. Am. Diet. Assoc., 80:455–58, 1982.

Weiner, M. F.: "A Practical Approach to Encouraging Geriatric Patients to Eat," J. Am. Diet. Assoc., 55:384–86, 1969.

References

1. Marx, J. L.: "Aging Research. I. Cellular Theories of Senescence," Science, 186:1105–07, 1974.
2. Timiras, P. S.: "Biological Perspectives on Aging," Am. Scientist, 66:605–13, 1978.
3. Hayflick, L.: "Current Theories of Biological Aging," Fed. Proc., 34:9–13, 1975.
4. Munro, H. N.: "Major Gaps in Nutrient Allowances: The Status of the Elderly," J. Am. Diet. Assoc., 76:137–41, 1980.
5. Weimer, J. P.: "The Nutritional Status of the Elderly," Natl. Food Rev., 19:7–10, Summer 1982.
6. Pao, E. M.: "Nutrient Consumption Patterns of Individuals, 1977 and 1965," Family Econ. Rev., Spring 1980, pp. 16–20.
7. Abraham, S., et al.: Dietary Intake Findings, United States, 1976–1980, National Center for Health Statistics, U.S. Department of Health and Human Services, 1982.
8. Heaney, R. P., et al.: "Calcium Nutrition and Bone Health in the Elderly," Am. J. Clin. Nutr., 36:986–1013, 1982.
9. Lynch, S. R., et al.: "Iron Status of Elderly Americans," Am. J. Clin. Nutr. (Suppl.), 36:1032–45, 1982.
10. Hutton, C. W., and Hayes-Davis, R. B.: "Assessment of the Zinc Nutritional Status of Selected Elderly Subjects," J. Am. Diet. Assoc., 82:148–53, 1983.
11. Rosenberg, I. H., et al.: "Folate Nutrition in the Elderly," Am. J. Clin. Nutr. (Suppl.), 36:1060–66, 1982.
12. Gersovitz, M., et al.: "Human Protein Requirements: Assessment of the Adequacy of the Current Recommended Dietary Allowances for Dietary Protein in Elderly Men and Women," Am. J. Clin. Nutr., 35:6–14, 1982.

13. Gallagher, J. C., et al.: "Epidemiology of Fractures of the Proximal Femur in Rochester, Minnesota," *Clin. Orthop.*, **150**:163–71, 1980.
14. Review: "Hormones, Nutrients and Postmenopausal Bone Loss," *Nutr. Rev.*, **40**:13–15, 1982.
15. Raisz, L. G.: "Osteoporosis. Review," *J. Am. Geriatr. Soc.*, **30**:127–38, 1982.
16. Spenser, H. et al.: "Factors Contributing to Calcium Loss in Aging," *Am. J. Clin. Nutr.*, **36**:776–87, 1982.
17. De Luca, H. F.: "The Vitamin D System: A View from Basic Science to the Clinic," *Clin. Biochem.*, **14**:213–22, 1981.
18. Slovik, D. M., et al.: "Deficient Production of 1,25 Dihydroxy Vitamin D in Elderly Osteoporosis Patients," *N. Engl. J. Med.*, **305**:372–74, 1981.
19. Korcok, M.: "Add Exercise to Calcium in Osteoporosis Prevention," *JAMA*, **247**:1106, 1982.
20. Review: "Osteoporosis and Calcium Balance," *Nutr. Rev.*, **41**:83–85, 1983.
21. Matkovic, V., et al.: "Bone Status and Fracture Rates in Two Regions of Yugoslavia," *Am. J. Clin. Nutr.*, **32**:540–49, 1979.
22. Heaney, R. P., and Recker, R. R.: "Effects of Nitrogen, Phosphorus, and Caffeine on Calcium Balance in Women," *J. Lab. Clin. Med.*, **99**: 46–55, 1982.
23. Madans, J., et al.: "The Relation Between Hip Fracture and Water Fluoridation: An Analysis of National Data," *Am. J. Publ. Health*, **73**:296–98, 1983.
24. Weiner, M. F.: "A Practical Approach to Encouraging Geriatric Patients to Eat," *J. Am. Diet. Assoc.*, **55**: 384–86, 1969.
25. Luros, E.: "A Rational Approach to Geriatric Nutrition," *Diet. Currents*, **8**(6):November/December 1981.

23

Nutritional Assessment and Dietary Counseling

Assessment of Nutritional Status

NUTRITIONAL ASSESSMENT is the process whereby the state of nutritional health of an individual, or group of individuals, is determined. It includes anthropometric, clinical, biochemical, and dietary data. The conclusions reached through nutritional assessment become the basis for the development of intervention programs in the community, and for the planning and implementation of nutritional care for individuals.

NUTRITIONAL STATUS refers to the health of an individual as it is affected by the intake and utilization of nutrients. Nutritional health can be described at several levels. *Normal nutrition* implies a sufficiency of nutrients and energy intake—neither deficiency nor excess—that affords the highest level of wellness. *Malnutrition* includes deficiency or excess of one or more nutrients and/or calories. At one extreme are the manifestations of severe nutritional deficiency in which the sequence has consisted of tissue depletion followed by measurable biochemical alterations and finally by clinical signs. At the other extreme are the signs related to excessive intake of one or more nutrients. A given individual, however, may show signs of deficiency and excess at the same time. For example, an obese person sometimes has an inadequate intake of some nutrients despite an excessive caloric intake.

Procedures commonly used in nutritional assessment are described in the sections that follow. The assessment ranges from the application of rapid screening techniques to a given population in a community or newly admitted patients in a hospital to very comprehensive studies on patients who require aggressive intervention for the correction of nutritional deficiencies. The assessment of the hospitalized patient is further described in Chapter 26.

Anthropometric Measurements

ANTHROPOMETRY deals with comparative measurements of the body. These measurements permit estimations of body fat, muscle tissue, and bone. They may include height, weight, head, arm, and chest circumference, skinfold, bony widths measured with calipers, x-ray measurements of hand and wrist to show bone development, and films of the hip to measure body fat.

Body Composition Body weight is a composite of body water, lean tissue, adipose tissue, and bone. The average percentage of fat in healthy, nonobese women is 24, and that for men is 17. Correspondingly, the percentage of body water and lean mass differ in men and women. The proportions of water, lean mass, and fat also change with age and are modified by diet and exercise. A person with a sedentary lifestyle may have a high proportion of fat, while an athlete of the same height and weight has a highly developed musculature and much less body fat. Or, for a given individual with a change in activity, a shift in the proportion of fat and lean mass can occur without change in body weight. An elderly person, even though she is active, will have a higher percentage of body fat than the young individual with the same level of activity.

Research Techniques for Measuring Body Composition. In research laboratories a number of techniques are used to measure body composition. UNDERWATER WEIGHING (densitometry) applies the Archimedean principle of water displacement by the fully submerged individual. The specific gravity is determined by dividing the body weight by the body volume. Tables have been developed that show the percentage of body fat for a given specific gravity. A body specific gravity of 1.048 is equivalent to 25 per cent body fat; a specific gravity of 1.002 is equal to a fat content of 49.3 percent.[1]

MULTIPLE ISOTOPE DILUTION (total and extracellular body water) is based on the principle that certain substances distribute themselves evenly within specified fluid compartments. After time has been allowed for this distribution to take place, a blood sample can be analyzed for the concentration of the substance. Deuterium oxide, radioactive tritium oxide, and antipyrine distribute evenly throughout all body compartments and are used to determine total body water. Inulin is distributed only in the extracellular fluid compartments and can be used to differentiate between the intracellular and extracellular compartments.

TOTAL BODY POTASSIUM applies the concept that body cells contain a constant amount of potassium and that its measurement is therefore an indicator of lean body mass. The body potassium can be measured by injecting radioisotope ^{42}K, allowing time for its equilibration within the cells, and then withdrawing samples for analysis. Another technique involves the measurement of the naturally occurring ^{40}K in the body with a low-level whole-body scintillation counter. Since ^{40}K accounts for 0.012 percent of naturally occurring potassium, the total body potassium can be calculated.

Weight Serial measurements of weight help establish the pattern of growth during childhood. For healthy adults, increase in body weight usually, but not always, indicates an increase in body fatness. In some pathologic conditions such as diseases of the heart, kidney, or liver, a rather sudden increase in body weight is an indication of fluid retention. A decrease in body weight of an adult or a child often accompanies a disease process in which there is a reduction of appetite, a defect in absorption or utilization, or an increase in metabolism. In each of these instances, the cause must be determined.

Lever balances with weights that cannot be removed should be used. The scale should be checked from time to time for accuracy. Bathroom scales, while useful in the home, are not sufficiently accurate for clinical purposes. The individual should be weighed at the same time of the day, preferably before breakfast and after voiding.

Height and Length Although height is genetically determined, socioeconomic deprivation during the period of growth is a leading cause of failure to reach genetic potential. Standing height is preferably measured against a fixed scale attached to a wall. The client is told to stand erect with feet together and heels back against the wall and eyes looking straight ahead.

Under 2 years of age recumbent length (crown to heel) is measured by means of a specially designed board or table with a fixed headboard and a moveable footboard. Two people are needed to position the child and to make the measurement. The measurement is made to the nearest centimeter or fourth of an inch. For young children the recumbent length is 1 to 2 cm greater than that for standing height. For children over 3 years of age the sitting height is sometimes determined.

Height-Weight Standards for Adults The Metropolitan Life Insurance Company revised height-weight tables published in 1983 and the percentile weight distribution based on HANES data, 1971 to 1974, may be used to determine the weight status of adults. (See Tables A-16 through A-18.)

For these standards body frame is an important consideration for determining the weight range that is appropriate for a given individual. Wrist circumference and elbow breadth are two measurements commonly employed for determining body frame as small, medium, or large. (See Appendix Table A-15.)

Desirable weight is a highly individual matter and is best determined in association with other factors of health and well-being. In the clinical setting it is more relevant to compare the usual weight and the current weight, using the following calculation:

$$\text{Percentage of usual body weight} = \frac{\text{actual weight}}{\text{usual weight}} \times 100$$

If this percentage is 90 or less, aggressive nutritional support may be indicated.

Height-Weight Standards for Children The National Center for Health Statistics (NCHS) has published growth data for boys and girls from birth to 36 months and from 2 to 18 years. (See Tables A-7 through A-14.) A single value plotted on a chart indicates where a child ranks in relationship to other children of the same age and sex in the United States. The child who falls within the 25th and 75th percentiles is within normal limits. A single weight above or below these limits is not significant, but if values fall consistently below or above these limits the child should be monitored more closely to determine the pattern of growth. Children who fall above the 95th or below the 5th percentile should be given top priority for further assessment.

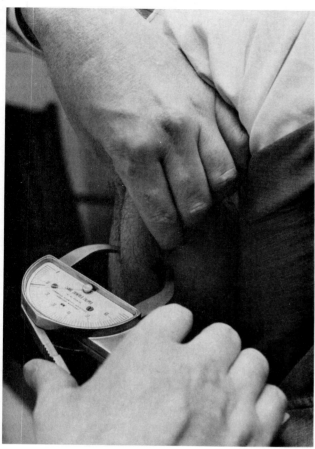

Figure 23-1. The caliper is applied at the skinfold of the upper back arm exactly midpoint between the acromion and olecranon processes. (Courtesy, *Roche Medical Image,* Hoffmann La Roche, Inc.)

Skinfold Measurements About 50 percent of the body's adipose tissue is located in the subcutaneous layer. Therefore, measurements of skinfold thickness can be made to determine the approximate fat stores in the body. The triceps, biceps, subscapular, abdominal, hip, pectoral, and calf areas have been studied. To reduce errors, practice in taking the measurements is needed to develop the needed skill. The same arm or the same side of the body should be used for initial and subsequent measurements. Also, the same type of caliper should be used each time. Measurements that involve more than one skinfold area are more reliable than a single measurement.

The following procedure is used for making a triceps skinfold (TSF) measurement. (See Figure 23-1.)

1. Locate the midpoint on the back of the upper arm as follows:
   a. The client holds the arm at a 90° angle across the chest.
   b. With a tape the technician measures the distance from the acromion process (the bony eminence at the shoulder) to the olecranon process (the lateral eminence at the elbow) and marks the midpoint.
2. Let the arm hang loosely. With the thumb and forefinger grasp the fold of skin and subcutaneous tissue directly in line with the olecranon process and about 1 cm above the midpoint mark. Pull the fold away from the underlying muscle tissue.
3. Place caliper* over the fold at the midpoint mark and exert pressure at 10 g per mm². Read after 2 to 3 seconds.
4. Repeat the measurement twice. Average the readings.
5. Compare with standard table of triceps measurements. (See Table A-19.)

The subscapular skinfold (SSS) is measured as follows:

1. The client is standing and with arms hanging relaxed at the side.
2. Locate the subscapular site exactly 1 cm below the tip of the right scapula.
3. With the thumb and forefinger of the left hand grasp the skinfold and subcutaneous tissue about 1 cm above the site. Pull the fold away from the subcutaneous muscle.
4. Apply the caliper jaws about a centimeter below the fingers. The jaws should be on a downward and lateral axis.
5. Read the measurement to the nearest millimeter. Repeat the measurement twice. Take an average of the readings and compare with the standards in Table A-20.

The sum of triceps and subscapular skinfolds (SOS) gives a somewhat more reliable measure of body fatness than either measurement alone. (See Appendix Table A-21.) Skinfold measurements may vary in racial and ethnic groups, but little is known of these variations. A measurement at or below the 10th percentile indicates depletion of fat and nonprotein caloric reserves, while one at or above the 90th percentile indicates excessive body fat. At either of these extremes further evaluation of nutritional status is indicated.

Arm and Muscle Circumference At the midpoint that was located for the triceps skinfold, the circumference of the arm (MAC) can be measured to 0.1 cm with a flexible, nonstretchable tape or an insertion type tape. The tape must be in complete contact with the skin surface without compressing the underlying fat. With data from the MAC and TSF a calculation

---

* Lange Skinfold Calipers, Cambridge Scientific Industries, Cambridge, Md. 21613.

can be made for the midarm muscle circumference (MAMC) as follows:

$$\text{MAMC}_{cm} = \text{MAC}_{cm} - (0.314 \times \text{TSF}_{mm})$$

Standards for the midarm circumference and the midarm muscle circumference are listed in Table A-22.

The calculation for the midarm muscle circumference provides an estimation of the somatic protein (skeletal muscle) in the body. It is only an approximation of muscle size, since it does not take into account bone size. In cachectic individuals the bone is a larger proportion of the arm size. Measurements that fall below the 5th percentile are evidence of depletion, while those at the 10th percentile indicate marginal depletion.

Clinical Findings

Sequence of Onset of Symptoms Detectable clinical signs of nutritional deficiency result from the following sequence of events: (1) an inadequate supply of one or more nutrients, whether through an inadequate diet or a failure of utilization, (2) gradual tissue depletion, followed by (3) changes in blood levels of nutrients or metabolites, and leading to (4) symptoms characteristic of the deficiency.

Interpretation In a physical examination a physician may complete a head-to-toe examination, but in many nutritional studies a selective list of observations is sufficient. (See Figure 23-2.) Table 23-1 lists signs that are useful in making a nutritional assessment. The principal nutrients that may be lacking are also listed. For a full description of deficiency for a given nutrient the reader is urged to review the discussion in the chapters pertaining to the nutrients, especially Chapters 5, 9, 11, 12, and 13.

Nurses, nutritionists, and teachers who are observant of the children or adults with whom they work can detect many physical and behavioral signs, such as those listed in Table 23-1, that are suggestive of impaired nutritional health. While these observations should not be equated with a specific diagnosis, they are useful in identifying other studies that need to be made and for referring the individual to a physician for further study and for appropriate intervention measures.

Classic deficiency diseases such as scurvy, pellagra, and rickets are rare in the United States. It is more difficult to arrive at a certain diagnosis when the defi-

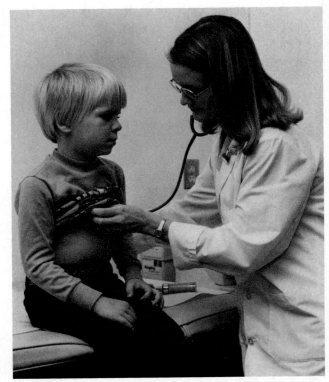

Figure 23-2. The physical examination is an important part of the assessment for nutritional status. (Courtesy, Diabetes Education Center, Minneapolis.)

ciency is moderate. Many of the clinical signs are nonspecific for nutritional deficiency and are the result of a variety of circumstances. For example, a student may complain of inability to concentrate, of irritability, and of always feeling tired. Such symptoms are characteristic of moderate thiamin deficiency, but they are equally likely to be caused by failure to get enough sleep or may result from some pathologic change unrelated to nutrition.

Nutritional deficiencies usually result from lack of several nutrients, although the lack of one may seem to predominate. Thus, the child who has a large pot belly and swollen legs characteristic of protein deficiency in kwashiorkor may show signs of pallor suggesting a lack of iron or vitamin B-12 as well as changes in the eyes suggestive of vitamin A deficiency.

In addition to the signs descriptive of primary nutrient deficiencies, the nutritionist and nurse must be especially alert to client's complaints of abnormalities of ingestion or digestion of food such as nausea, fear of eating certain foods, and changes in bowel habits—especially persistent diarrhea. Drug addiction and alcoholism are important contributors to malnutrition.

Table 23-1. Clinical Signs That May Be Associated with Nutrient Deficiency*

Abnormal Signs	Some Possible Nutrient Lacks
Attendance	
Frequent absence from school or work	
Growth failure (children)	
Failure to increase in stature or weight	Energy, protein, zinc
Behavior	
Easily fatigued; listless; apathetic; depressed; nervous; irritable; inability to concentrate; complaints of insomnia; poor work capacity	Multiple deficiencies including energy, protein, B complex
Skin	
Dry, flaky, rough	Vitamin A, essential fatty acids
Bed sores, poor wound healing, edematous	Protein, vitamin C
Excessive bruising	Vitamin K
Keratinization	Vitamin A
Pinpoint, purplish hemorrhagic spots	Ascorbic acid
Symmetrical dermatitis	Niacin
Hair	
Thin, sparse, dry, lusterless, easily plucked out, change in pigments with distinct bands	Protein, energy
Face	
Pale	Iron, vitamin B-6, B-12, folacin
Scaling around nose	Riboflavin, niacin, vitamin B-6
Swollen (edema)	Protein
Eyes	
Pale	Iron
Dry and scaly at corners	Riboflavin, vitamin B-6
Sensitive to bright light, itching	Riboflavin
Increased vascularity	Riboflavin, niacin, vitamin B-6
Nightblindness, Bitot's spots, soft cornea, xerophthalmia	Vitamin A
Lips	
Fissuring at corners	Iron, riboflavin, niacin, vitamin B-6
Swollen, puffy	Riboflavin, niacin
Tongue	
Pale	Iron, vitamin B-12, folacin
Swollen	Niacin, vitamin B-12, folacin
Raw, scarlet red	Niacin
Magenta red	Riboflavin
Atrophy of papillae	Iron, B complex
Teeth	
Mottled enamel	*Excess* fluoride
Caries	*Excess* sugar; poor dental hygiene
Gums	
Spongy, swollen, bleeding	Ascorbic acid
Nails	
Brittle, ridged, spoon shaped, pale nail beds	Iron
Glands	
Enlarged thyroid	Iodine
Muscles	
Wasted	Protein, energy
Sore, painful	Ascorbic acid, potassium
Weak	Ascorbic acid, potassium, magnesium
Skeletal	
Poor posture, delayed closing of fontanelles (infant), knock knees, bowed legs, beading of ribs, enlarged joints	Vitamin D, calcium
Fleeting joint pains	Ascorbic acid

Table 23-1 (cont.)

Abnormal Signs	Some Possible Nutrient Lacks
Gastrointestinal system	
Anorexia	B-complex
Enlarged liver with fatty infiltration	Protein
Cardiovascular system	
Hypertension	*Excess* calories, sodium
Dyspnea	Iron, thiamin, vitamin B-12
Arrhythmia	Potassium
Neurologic System	
Mental confusion	Thiamin, niacin
Loss of knee and ankle joints, calf tenderness	Thiamin
Muscle tremor	Magnesium
Motor weakness, peripheral neuritis	Thiamin, niacin, vitamin B-12, pantothenic acid
Convulsive seizures (infant)	Vitamin B-6
Burning sensation of feet	Pantothenic acid

* Sources of data:
Expert Committee on Medical Assessment of Nutritional Status. Tech. Rep. Series, No. 258, World Health Organization, Geneva, 1963, pp. 57–58.
Preliminary Findings of the First Health and Nutrition Examination Survey, 1971–71. Anthropometric and Clinical Findings. U.S. Department of Health, Education and Welfare, Pub. No. (HRA) 75-1229.
Letsou, A. P., et al.: *A Guide to Nutritional Care.* Nutritional Division, Mead Johnson, Evansville, Indiana.

The influence of many pathologic conditions on nutritional status are described in Part III of this book.

Laboratory Studies

Scope and Purposes With some biochemical tests deficiencies or excesses can be detected before symptoms are apparent, thus making it possible to institute nutritional corrections early. Some biochemical determinations also help to confirm clinical and dietary data so that a diagnosis can be made and nutritional care can be planned and implemented. Other biochemical studies do not necessarily give a clue to nutritional status, but the findings may be significant for the initiation of appropriate therapeutic diets.

Whole blood, blood serum, blood plasma, urine, feces, hair, and biopsy of liver and bone are among the materials used for biochemical studies. Analyses may be made for *nutrient levels* such as glucose, lipids, amino acids, vitamins, and minerals, for concentrations of *metabolic products* such as serum proteins, hemoglobin, and enzymes, or for *excretory substances* such as urea, creatinine, vitamins, and intermediary metabolites. (See Figure 23-3.)

Hemoglobin, hematocrit, and white cell counts are routinely measured in nutrition surveys, hospitals, and outpatient facilities. The visceral protein status can be measured by determinations of serum albumin, serum transferrin, and total lymphocyte count. The immune response is another measure of the body's visceral protein reserves. (See page 471.) Studies on the apparent nitrogen balance and on creatinine excretion require accurate 24-hour collection of urine, and are therefore performed primarily on hospital patients suspected of undernutrition. The significance of these measurements is discussed in Chapter 26. Blood levels of minerals and vitamins and urinary excretions of vitamins and their metabolites are measured less often.

Interpretation Normal values for various blood and urine constituents are listed in Tables A-27 and A-28. The interpretation of biochemical data requires an understanding of the metabolic pathways of the constituent being tested and of the factors that influence the levels of this constituent in the body. For example: time of day when sample was taken; whether the sample is obtained fasting or following a meal; age, sex, and body weight; the present dietary intake; interactions of nutrients—especially if there is a nutrient imbalance; effect of medications—steroids, antibiotics, and others.

The methods for some determinations vary from laboratory to laboratory. Thus, it is important to interpret the results according to standards set up by the laboratory. To complicate the interpretation further,

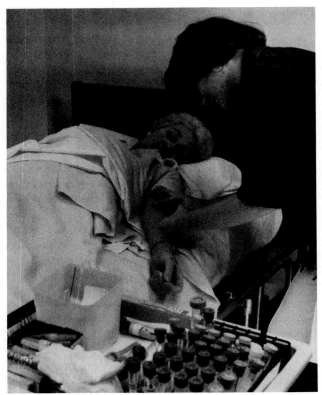

Figure 23-3. Blood studies are useful for assessment of nutritional status as well as for purposes of diagnosis and therapy. (Courtesy, University of Minnesota Health Sciences Center, Minneapolis.)

there is controversy on the values to be accepted as normal. For example, some clinicians make a diagnosis of anemia if the hemoglobin level is less than 12 g per dl, while others use 10 g per dl as the cutoff point for a normal value. Another example relates to changing interpretation with new evidence from research. Thus, the acceptable range for blood cholesterol is lower than it was a decade or two ago.

The measured constituents may deviate from normal values because of inappropriate nutrient intake, faulty absorption, alterations in intermediary metabolism, increased destruction of specific components, defective waste elimination, or a combination of two or more of these. Some findings may reflect current nutrient intake, whereas others are the result of long-term effects.

Various homeostatic mechanisms maintain normal levels in the blood at the expense of tissue and storage forms, or by reducing the excretion of a given substance. Only when dietary and tissue sources no longer suffice to replenish the blood constituents, or when there is interference with release from the stores, will the blood levels fall.

Several examples illustrate some problems of interpretation. A normal value for total serum protein does not always rule out protein deficiency. A fractionation of the serum proteins might indicate hypoalbuminemia together with elevated globulin fractions. The serum albumin concentration is not a sensitive indicator of early protein deficiency, since it is reduced only when the tissues have been severely depleted. When the serum albumin is reduced, there remains the question of etiology: Was there extreme dietary lack of protein over a prolonged period? Is there a defect in the formation of albumin by the liver? Are there large daily losses in exudates as in burns, or urine as in nephrosis?

Biochemical findings do not always correlate with dietary findings. For example, suppose the hemoglobin and hematocrit levels were found to be normal, but the diet study indicated that the iron intake did not meet the recommended allowances. How shall this be interpreted? On one hand, the iron allowances include a margin of safety for most people and it may be that in the given instance the need for iron was less than the allowances so that the hemoglobin level was normal. But there is another consideration: because of homeostatic mechanisms, the hemoglobin level might be normal but tissue reserves are depleted. Thus, values for serum iron and for transferrin saturation might be sought to define the body's iron reserves.

Dietary Assessment

Scope and Purposes   Dietary assessment is an important part of nutritional assessment, but it cannot be used alone to make a diagnosis of nutritional health. It is an aid in the interpretation of anthropometric, clinical, and laboratory findings and provides a foundation for dietary counseling. However, obtaining accurate information on food intake and the interpretation of that information have been problems for many years. Rapid cost-effective screening may be conducted by trained paraprofessionals to identify persons at risk, as in a community nutrition program. A comprehensive assessment requires much more time, is more expensive, and in the clinic/hospital setting is reserved for those persons at risk and who require intensive nutritional rehabilitation. Dietary assessment is also an important aspect of surveys of nutritional status of population groups. The methods used in these instances must be appropriate for the purposes intended.

Twenty-Four-Hour Recall   This is probably the most widely used method on which subsequent dietary counseling is based. It may require from 15 to 20 minutes to as much as an hour of the interviewer's time. The client recalls food intake for the preceding 24 hours by interview or by completing a questionnaire. He or she recalls what was eaten, how much food was eaten, how the food was prepared, and when it was eaten. Food models, cups, glasses, and bowls of various sizes and a ruler help clients to estimate portion sizes.

By itself, the 24-hour recall is not a reliable indicator of food intake.[2-5] If it is used together with a food frequency list as a crosscheck, or if it is used randomly when the client has a follow-up counseling session, the 24-hour recall is a useful tool.

Among the disadvantages of the 24-hour recall are these: some people find it difficult to remember everything they ate on the preceding day, especially if their eating patterns are irregular; estimating portion sizes is likely to be variable; the recalled day may not be typical of the usual intake; or the person may not be entirely truthful, citing what he or she wants the interviewer to think he or she ate.

Food Frequency This consists in asking the client (by interview or by a checkoff list) how often (daily, weekly, monthly) specific foods are eaten. The frequency list may include a few broad groupings of foods or more than a hundred foods common to the geographic region. Detailed lists are especially useful in the diagnosis of allergies. Some lists are restricted to certain categories of particular concern such as fat-rich foods, sugars, sweets, and desserts, or foods high in salt. When an estimation of calories and nutrients is to be made it is also essential to record the amounts of foods that are customarily eaten.

To determine the adequacy of diets Strohmeyer and associates have described a simplified scoring approach that is based on the four food groups.[6] Using a dietary intake form clients circle the size of portions that are consumed from each group and the number of times per week that these foods are eaten. Clients are also encouraged to compute their own scores. These nutritionists found the correlation of the scores with a nutrient analysis based on a weighed food diary was good; that is, when scores were low, the nutrient analysis also showed the diets to be lacking in some nutrients. The clients were able to complete the form in 4 to 7 minutes. Their active participation provided a positive approach to further counseling.

Food Diary Persons are sometimes asked to keep a food diary for several days. Generally it has been recommended that a 3-day record be taken on midweek days. A recent study has found that a 4-day record beginning on Friday and continuing through Monday was more indicative of food intake.[7]

When the record is carefully kept, as by a mother for her child or by an adult who is motivated to effect improvement in his or her diet, much useful information on food habits is made available. But this method too has its disadvantages. People who are illiterate obviously cannot keep the record. Other persons modify their diets during the record-keeping period to simplify the recording; still others are unable to estimate food portions accurately; and for many it is burdensome to keep the record.

Observation of Food Eaten For patients at risk nurses and dietetic technicians should observe the kinds and amounts of foods that are served and also any food remaining at the end of the meal. On menu lists some patients are capable of providing reliable records—a useful exercise for dietary counseling. Such observations are essential when an estimate is to be made of energy intake and nutrients, and also for a nitrogen balance study. (See page 391.)

Weighed Intake This method consists of weighing, on a gram scale, the amount of food served, and the amount of food not eaten. The procedure is used primarily for research on food consumption and for controlled diets used for the study of nutritional requirements.

Diet History As the term implies, the diet history is a record of dietary practices of the individual over a period of time. The food intake by recall, frequency, or diary is a part of the diet history. Information is also included on the socioeconomic environment and the medical history. Much of this information is available in medical or health records and no client should be subjected to a second questioning on these items. A form for making a nutritional assessment and completing a dietary history is presented in Appendix C.

Dietary Evaluation Once the data have been assembled, what methods can be used for dietary evaluation?

Food Groups and Dietary Inspection. Typical diet patterns according to 24-hour recall or food diary can be checked against the food groups to determine whether the amounts eaten from each group are equal to the amounts recommended. This is a rapid but rather crude evaluation technique. It is most useful when the client eats a wide variety of food from each group rather than a limited choice. It is also more useful when it is used randomly for follow-up counseling sessions.

Dietitians who are conversant with the nutritive values of various foods can often make important evaluations by review of the food intake. For example, a diet that supplies little or no milk suggests that the intake of calcium and riboflavin, and possibly protein, are likely to be inadequate. A diet that includes no animal foods is one that lacks vitamin B-12, and so on.

Calculation of Nutritive Values. The exchange lists for meal planning provide a rapid method for estimating calories, protein, fat, and carbohydrate. (See Table A-4.) For foods not included in the exchange lists, information on nutritive values is obtained from a table of food composition. (See Table A-1).

Heretofore, detailed calculations for many nutrients have been time consuming and have been restricted to surveys of nutritional status in populations and to research pertaining to nutritional requirements. Only rarely have such detailed calculations been used as a basis for dietary assessment of a client and as a basis for dietary counseling. Today many dietitians have access to computers and are able to obtain information on the nutrient intakes of their clients. However, some computer data bases are more complete than others, and there remains a need for "reliable, valid computerized analysis systems."[8] (See Chapter 44.)

The limitations of calculations must also be recognized. Portion sizes must be carefully determined if the calculations are to be meaningful. Also, food composition varies widely, depending on variety, environmental conditions in production, and methods of food preparation. There is also considerable variability in the availability of nutrients to the body, depending on food source, the mixture of foods that is ingested, and the environment within the gastrointestinal tract.

After calculations have been completed, comparisons are often made with the recommended dietary allowances for the age and sex category of the individual. When such comparisons reveal intakes below the RDA, they cannot be interpreted as indicating nutritional deficiency. It must be remembered that the RDA furnish a substantial margin of safety for most individuals. A diet that supplies less than two thirds of the RDA is rated as one that increases the risk of nutrient deficiency.

Food Analysis Food analysis is used for some metabolic studies. All food to be eaten is weighed. Dupli-cate samples of each food are weighed for analysis in a laboratory for energy and nutrient content.

Dietary Counseling

Dietary counseling is the process whereby people are helped to deal with their dietary and nutritional problems. (See Figure 23-4.) The goal of the counseling is to bring about a desirable change in food behavior. In the process the principles of food and nutritional sciences are translated into practices that are appropriate and acceptable to the client.

Clients and Counselors

Clients Nurses and dietitians often think of counseling in terms of patients who require modified diets. To be sure, such counseling is essential to nutritional care of the patient, but it is a limited view. Many healthy people will have an enhanced sense of well-being if their diets are improved. With today's emphasis on prevention of disease, most people can be helped to reduce the risk of some illness by appropriate dietary counseling. Thus, the client might be a

Figure 23-4. Dietary counseling is effective when the counselor assists the client in setting realistic goals and provides the necessary guidance, including information regarding menu planning, food purchasing, food preparation, and available community resources. (Courtesy of Upjohn Health Care Services, Inc.)

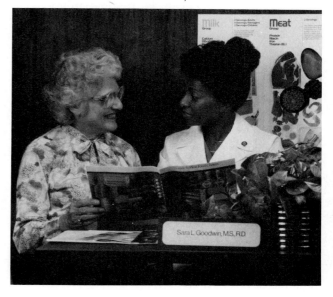

child in school who is becoming obese; a mother enrolled in a WIC program; an elderly person participating in a congregate feeding program; a homemaker receiving food stamps, and so on. It could be someone who receives such counseling as part of the program of a health maintenance organization, or an executive in a corporation that provides surveillance of the health of its employees. Some clients are counseled toward better behavior patterns, whereas others can receive assurance that their present diets are indeed satisfactory.

Client Responsibility Each person is responsible for his or her own health. Thus, the individual must be an active participant throughout the counseling process. In many instances members of the family must be involved. For a very young child the parent, of course, is the principal participant in the counseling process. For the child old enough to take some responsibility for his or her nutritional health, the counseling involves the child, with the parent as an observing supporter whose actions will help the child to implement the needed changes. The spouse of a client provides support and willingness to help in the change process. But only the client can effect the modification of behavior, so it is essential that he or she be directly involved.

Counselors The dietitian is the professional person who by education and experience is best qualified to provide dietary counseling. But in the absence of a dietitian, a nurse often provides dietary counseling to clients, for example, in a school, or in the home, or in an extended care facility. Other members of the health team are often involved. In some situations the client may be referred to a social worker to help solve some financial problem that requires welfare assistance, or to arrange for supportive services such as home-delivered meals, homemaker services, and transportation. Modified diets are usually prescribed by a physician who should also assume responsibility for discussing the reasons for such a prescription with the patient.

Attributes of a Successful Counselor Needless to say, thorough knowledge of the sciences of food and nutrition and of their practical applications are prerequisite to satisfactory counseling. One can scarcely advise on low-cost diets if one is not familiar with food costs and budgeting. Nor can one advise on food substitutions without being able to make comparisons of nutritive values. If one does not have an understanding of the basic principles of food preparation,

there is little likelihood that sound directions can be given to the client. Equally important is an understanding of factors that influence food behavior and of techniques that can be used to help the client arrive at decisions to make the necessary change. (See also guidelines on page 343.)

Steps in the Counseling Process

Each step leads to the next:

Assessment→Planning→
Implementation→Evaluation

Assessment This is a process of gathering and evaluating data as a means of improving the client's nutritional practices. It describes the client with respect to nutritional status, food behavior, and environment. It includes the social, medical, and dietary history. (See page 340.) Each assessment must arrive at a conclusion upon which the plan is developed.

Planning Based on the assessment (1) reasonable objectives are set toward which the client is willing to work; (2) ways are described to achieve the stated objectives; and (3) a plan is devised for evaluation of the results. A satisfactory plan applies the principles of food and nutrition sciences within the context of the client's social, economic, psychological, and physical environment. The plan is the blueprint for action.

Implementation Understanding and attitude are basic to putting a plan into action. Implementation means that the client is able, independently, to plan his or her own menus, to prepare foods appropriate to the needed changes (or to supervise such preparation), and to consume the needed amounts of food. It includes the client's selection of food in the marketplace with respect to cost, information on labels, and so on. It means that the client applies each day those modifications of food behavior to which he or she is committed.

Evaluation The progress of a client toward achieving personal goals should be evaluated from time to time by the client and the counselor. The evaluation confirms the degree of success by the client. Did the client understand the plan that was set? Was he or she motivated to make the needed changes? What support systems were available to the client? How consistently was the plan followed? Were the counselor's techniques appropriate for the client?

Each evaluation becomes, in effect, a reassessment

or addition to the initial assessment. This may lead to revision of the plan, if needed, and then to changes in implementation. Sometimes the evaluation may show that an individual cannot be helped or does not want to be helped; this too should be recognized.

Some Counseling Guidelines

1. Review the medical record. Before meeting with the client, abstract from the record all pertinent information on family, socioeconomic status, anthropometric measurements, symptoms and complaints, laboratory studies and so on.

2. Provide for a comfortable setting. Pleasant, quiet surroundings are conducive to a positive outcome. During the session the client should have the undivided attention of the counselor. Clients should not be distracted by noise or interruption of the counselor by other professionals or by telephone calls.

3. Set a time for the counseling session in advance. For a patient in the hospital the counseling should take place before the day of discharge. For clinic patients who have appointments with several professionals, it is important that they be scheduled for the same day and with no long waits between these appointments. Be aware of the attention span of the client. Especially for those who are ill in the hospital it may be better to schedule several short sessions. Generally, not more than an hour is scheduled for the initial session, with 15 minutes to one half hour being sufficient for follow-up sessions.

4. Introduce yourself to the client. Give your title as well as your name. Address the client by name. Explain the purpose of the session. Let the client know that you are there to help.

5. Listen effectively. Maintain eye-to-eye contact while the client is talking. Allow ample time for the client to voice any problems and complaints. When the client stops talking, give him or her a moment to go on, or perhaps prompt the client by saying "Yes, I understand. Go on." Interrupt only when there is a point that needs clarification or if the conversation becomes irrelevant. What does the client say first? How intense are the feelings expressed? Do the words mask true feelings? Note the tone of voice as well as the attitudes and facial expressions. As the counselor you should avoid facial expressions or comments that suggest criticism of what is being said or that might imply that you are getting impatient.

6. Ask open-ended questions that are nondirective.

For example, the question, "What kind of cereal do you eat for breakfast?" suggests to the client that he or she should have eaten breakfast and that it should have included cereal. It is better to say, "Tell me when you first ate yesterday." Then, "What did you eat?" and "How much did you eat?" and "How was it prepared?"

7. When eliciting information respond in a noncommittal way. Do not express approval or disapproval until all the data gathering is completed. For example, if a client tells you he has orange juice every day for breakfast, your approval at that point could lead him to describe a fictional intake of other foods to gain further approval. It might be better to say, "Show me which size glass you usually use for your juice. . . . Go on."

8. Use nontechnical terminology. Avoid using medical terms or abbreviations. But almost every client will have heard someone using words that he or she does not understand. You should be prepared to explain such terms when the client asks about them.

9. Set realistic objectives. Some of these will be for immediate action, while others are long range. What is the client's concept of his or her problems? How does the client feel about them? What ability does the client have to solve them? Making a list of the problems helps set up some priorities. People often feel overwhelmed by many problems and are unable to make progress in solving them. A small problem that seems important to the individual and toward which some success can be anticipated should be singled out for attention. Then, with time, other problems can be attacked. For example, learning to cook an inexpensive one-dish meal may be a genuine accomplishment for an unskilled homemaker. Or increasing the caloric intake by 200 each day for a period of time might be a good beginning for one who needs to gain weight, whereas a larger goal—500 to 1,000 kcal a day—would be too difficult.

10. Prepare an individualized written dietary plan. This plan is developed with the client—not imposed by the counselor. Something good can be found in every dietary pattern, and at this point it is appropriate to commend the client for those aspects of the diet that he should continue to use. Any change in diet represents a threat to one's way of life. Negative critical attitudes toward current practices are rarely helpful. The plan includes a listing of the objectives to which the client is committed as well as the meal plan itself. In

addition the plan may be supplemented with printed food lists, guidelines for preparation of food, and markets where special foods and supplements may be purchased if they are not available in the usual market used by the client. The uses of any printed materials must be fully explained.

11. Provide opportunity for feedback. For example, from a list of foods or a menu card, a client might show what food selection she could make to conform to her diet plan. The patient in the hospital can learn to relate menu items to the exchange list or might use food models to set up a sample meal. Give the client opportunity to ask questions.

12. Bring the counseling session to a close. If follow-up is needed, schedule a time for the next appointment. Tell the client how to obtain answers to questions that may arise after he or she gets home.

Problems and Review

1. *Key words*: anthropometry; assessment; dietary counseling; dietary history; evaluation; food diary; food behavior; food frequency; nutritional status; skinfold measurement; 24-hour recall.
2. List some physical and behavioral signs that might suggest to a teacher that a child should be further assessed for nutritional status.
3. *Problem*. Develop a list of five foods commonly used from each of the food groups. Then interview a classmate to determine the frequency with which he or she consumes these foods. Determine the amounts of food consumed. What are the advantages of this approach? What limitations did you encounter?
4. Based on a dietary history, including a 3-day food record, it was determined that the diet furnished the recommended allowances for protein, calories, and ascor-

bic acid. All of the B-complex vitamins and iron fell within 70 to 90 percent of the allowances. What evaluation would you make of such information? Explain fully.

5. *Problem*. Obtain a diet history from a classmate using the form in Appendix C.
   a. Compare the 24-hour intake of food with the recommended amounts in the Daily Food Guide.
   b. Which nutrients are likely to be adequate? Which nutrients require more emphasis?
   c. Using the exchange lists in Table A-4, calculate the protein, fat, carbohydrate, and caloric intake of the 24-hour food intake. For foods not covered in the exchange lists, look up values in Table A-1.

References

1. Rathbun, E. N., and Pace, N.: "Studies on Body Composition. I. The Determination of Total Body Fat by Means of the Body Specific Gravity," *J. Biol. Chem.*, **158**:667–76, 1945.
2. Alford, H., and Ekvall, S.: "Variability of Dietary Assessment Values among Nutrition Students," *J. Am. Diet. Assoc.*, **84**:71–74, 1984.
3. Beaton, G. H., et al.: "Sources of Variance in 24-hour Dietary Recall Data: Implications for Nutrition Study Design and Interpretation. Carbohydrate Sources, Vitamins, and Minerals," *Am. J. Clin. Nutr.*, **39**:986–95, 1983.
4. Carter, R. L., et al.: "Reliability and Validity of the 24-hour Recall," *J. Am. Diet. Assoc.*, **79**:542–47, 1981.
5. Todd, K. S., et al.: "Food Intake Measurement: Problems and Approaches," *Am. J. Clin. Nutr.*, **37**:139–46, 1983.
6. Strohmeyer, S. L., et al.: "A Rapid Dietary Screening Device for Clinics," *J. Am. Diet. Assoc.*, **84**:428–32, 1984.
7. St. Jeor, S. T., et al.: "Variability on Nutrient Intake in a 28-day Period," *J. Am. Diet. Assoc.*, **83**:155–62, 1983.
8. Hoover, L. W.: "Computerized Nutrient Data Bases. 1. Comparison of Nutrient Analysis Systems," *J. Am. Diet. Assoc.*, **82**:501–505, 1983.

24

Nutritional Problems and Programs in the Community

Focus on Public Health Nutrition

The term PUBLIC HEALTH NUTRITION is generally understood to be concerned with those problems of nutrition that affect large numbers and that can be solved most effectively through group action. The term COMMUNITY may be used to refer to any group of people; it might be, for example, a small, closely knit group such as the student community, or the low-income area of a city, or an entire city or a nation.

Physicians, nurses, dietitians, nutritionists, social workers, home economists, and teachers must be informed citizens regarding nutrition concerns of the local community, the state, the nation, and even the world. They have a responsibility to assume leadership in identifying nutritional problems and in finding solutions to these problems. The solutions might result in direct services to clients, in expanded programs of nutrition education, in agency activities to develop new programs, and in taking a position on proposed legislation that affects the nutritional well-being of the population.

Malnutrition— A Worldwide Concern

Scope of Malnutrition

Incidence and Nature of Malnutrition Malnutrition is an inclusive term that involves the lack, imbalance, or excess of one or more of some 50 or so nu-

---

ISSUES PERTAINING TO PUBLIC HEALTH NUTRITION

—Malnutrition exists to some degree in the United States and other affluent nations but assumes epidemic proportions in more than 100 developing countries. What are the principal problems in the United States? In the developing countries? Which segments of the population are most vulnerable?

—The purpose of a national food and nutrition policy is to assure a nutritionally adequate, satisfying diet at reasonable cost to all people of the nation. Who decides what such a policy should be? What recommendations have been made for the components of such a policy in the United States? What elements in the development of such a policy are likely to be controversial?

—Protein-energy malnutrition is a major problem for the children of the developing coun-

tries. What are the factors in the host–agent–environment triad that interact in its causation? What four measures have been proposed for its prevention and treatment by the United Nations Children's Fund?

—Lifestyles are rapidly changing in the developing nations. What are some of these changes that adversely affect nutrition?

—Rapid population increase is viewed by many as leading to a losing battle to feed the world's people. In addition to measures for controlling population growth, primary emphasis is placed on improving the production of cereal grains. What major hindrances exist in the developing countries for achieving adequate grain production? What are some realistic ways to make up for some of the nutritional deficiencies of the cereal grains?

---

trients that are required by the body. The classic nutritional deficiencies are rarely encountered in the United States and Western Europe. Occasionally beriberi is seen in severe alcoholics. Marasmus, a severe form of protein-calorie malnutrition, is not unknown in the United States but is almost always traceable to child neglect. Iatrogenic malnutrition in hospital patients has also been described. (See page 393.)

Nutritional deficiencies and excesses are important problems in the United States, but there is no reliable estimate of their incidence. Obesity and dental caries assume epidemic proportions in the population. Iron-deficiency anemia occurs in significant numbers of preschool children, teenage girls, women during the child-bearing years, and the elderly. Osteoporosis is a widespread problem in older women. About 550,000 Americans die annually from heart attacks, 170,000 from strokes, and 440,000 from cancer. Multiple factors are involved in the etiology of these diseases, of which diet is one. Excessive intakes of calories and fat are primary dietary targets.

An estimate of the Food and Agriculture Organization of the United Nations indicates that one quarter of the people in the developing countries are undernourished. (See Table 24-1.) More than three fourths of the world's undernourished live in the Far East. Children are most severely affected. The incidence of the principal problems is estimated as follows[1]:

Low birth weight: 22 million births annually are below 2,500 g
Anemia: 260 million women of child-bearing age; 200 million preschool children
Xerophthalmia and blindness: 250 million in developing countries go blind each year
Endemic goiter: 200 million
Protein-energy malnutrition, children up to age 4 years: 9.4 million severe cases and 98 million mild cases.[2] (See Figure 24-1.)

Nutritional Deficiencies The nutritional deficiencies arising from lack of specific nutrients, the nutritional problems encountered at various stages of the life cycle, and the effects of disease upon nutrition are discussed in detail in appropriate chapters of this text. Table 24-2 summarizes the principal nutritional deficiencies on the world scene today and includes a cross-reference to the chapters within this text where a fuller description is available.

In the initial stages of development a deficiency is so mild that physical signs are absent and biochemical methods generally cannot detect the slight changes. As tissue depletion continues the biochemical changes can be measured in body fluids and tissues. With further depletion the physical signs become apparent until finally the full-blown signs of the predominating classic deficiency can be recognized.

Nutritional deficiencies rarely occur singly inasmuch as an inadequacy of food almost always reduces the intake of more than one nutrient. Moreover, the metabolic interdependence of nutrients means that a lack of one will interfere with the proper utilization of another, many examples of which have been cited in Chapters 5 through 13.

Primary nutritional deficiencies are those that are caused by inadequate or imbalanced intake of food. These conditions are the result of many environmental factors, some of which are discussed more fully on page 349.

Secondary deficiencies are those that result from some fault in digestion, absorption, and metabolism so that tissue needs are not met even though the ingested diet would be adequate in normal circumstances. Thus, the restoration and maintenance of good nutrition are important concerns in clinical nutrition.

Classic deficiency diseases are diagnosed relatively easily because the physical and biochemical findings are prominent and specific. Nevertheless, the diagnosis of even these may be missed when the disease is seldom seen by clinicians, as is the case in the United States.

Economic Cost of Malnutrition The maintenance of health and the treatment of disease are important not only for humanitarian reasons but also in eco-

Table 24-1. Estimates of Undernutrition in Developing Countries*

	Latin America	Africa	Near East	Far East
Population, millions	317	320	192	1,090
Number undernourished, millions	41	72	19	303
Percentage undernourished	13	23	10	28
Daily caloric deficit, billions	30	52	15	214

* Data from *UNICEF News*, Issue 113, 1982, p. 9.

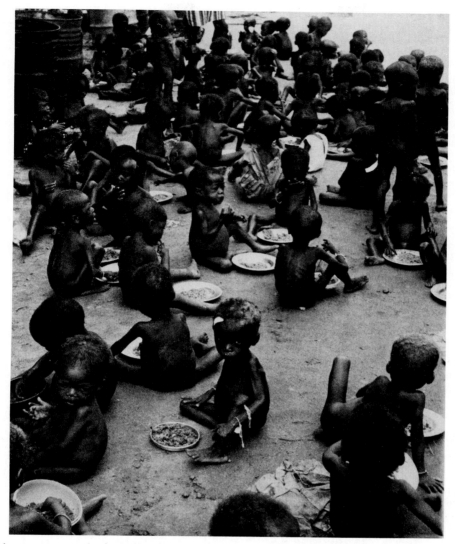

Figure 24-1. Children are among the first victims of food scarcity. Here some children are being fed a mixture of stockfish and beans from an improvised kitchen in a Niger clinic. Note the emaciation and pot bellies in some of the children. (UNICEF photo by Poul Larsen.)

nomic terms. What is good nutrition really worth? Can a preventive program in nutrition be economically justified? The answers are not easy to obtain. Health care costs in the United States during 1983 were estimated to be $355 billion, representing 10.7 percent of the gross national product. These costs continue to escalate at a rapid rate. According to testimony given by Dr. George Briggs at 1972 hearings before the Senate Select Committee on Nutrition and Human Needs, poor dietary habits may account for as much as one third of the total health care bill.[3]

In the developing countries child wastage due to malnutrition has been singled out as being especially restrictive in an economic sense. Children comprise up to half of the population in many developing countries, but most of them will never reach maturity. The costs involved in their short lives include extra food consumed by the mother during pregnancy, the costs of childbirth, the food, clothing, and shelter consumed by the child while living, and even the costs of burial. These malnourished children are consumers without ever reaching the status of producers and their own brief existence has usually been miserable.

When malnourished children survive to adulthood their stunted growth, retarded mental development, lessened ability to learn, reduced work efficiency, and physical defects including blindness are among the handicaps that beset them.

Table 24-2. Summary of Diseases of Malnutrition

Principal Disease Conditions	Nutrient Imbalances
Deficiencies	
Underweight	Calorie deficit (Chapter 25)
Protein-calorie malnutrition	
Kwashiorkor	Principally protein lack (page 352)
Marasmus	Calorie-protein lack (page 352)
Dental caries	Calcium, phosphorus, fluorine, vitamins A and D (Chapters 9, 11)
Anemia, microcytic, hypochromic	Iron (Chapter 9)
Macrocytic in infancy, pregnancy, malabsorption	Folacin (Chapter 13)
Pernicious (absorptive defect)	Vitamin B-12 (Chapter 13)
Goiter, endemic	Iodine (Chapter 9)
Osteoporosis	Possibly calcium, vitamin D; endocrine factors (Chapter 22)
Osteomalacia	Vitamin D, calcium, phosphorus (Chapter 11)
Scurvy; hemorrhagic tendency; inflamed gums; loose teeth	Ascorbic acid (Chapter 12)
Beriberi; polyneuritis, circulatory failure; emaciation; edema	Thiamin (Chapter 13)
Pellagra; glossitis; dermatitis; diarrhea; nervous degeneration; dementia	Niacin (Chapter 13)
Cheilosis; scaling of skin; cracking of lips; light sensitivity; increased vascularization of eyes	Riboflavin (Chapter 13)
Growth failure, anemia, convulsions in infants	Vitamin B-6 (Chapter 13)
Night blindness; keratomalacia; xerophthalmia; blindness	Vitamin A (Chapter 11)
Rickets; bone deformities	Vitamin D (Chapter 11)
Hemorrhagic tendency in infants	Vitamin K (Chapter 11)
Excesses	
Obesity	Calorie excess (Chapter 25)
Toxicity; changes in skin, hair, bones, liver	Vitamin A excess (Chapter 11)
Hypercalcemia, calcification of soft tissues	Vitamin D excess (Chapter 11)
Dental caries	Sticky sugars (Chapter 6)
Atherosclerosis; cardiovascular and cerebrovascular disease*	Too much saturated fat, cholesterol; ?simple sugars (Chapter 38)
Hypertension*	Calorie excess; ?too much salt (Chapter 39)
Diverticulosis; irritable colon*	Excessively refined diets (Chapter 30)
Cancer of the colon*	?Excessively refined diets; ?excess of fat leading to excess metabolites of sterols and bile acids (Chapter 35)

*In these diseases diet is only one of a number of risk factors that must be considered; more research is needed to fully establish the role of diet.

Factors Contributing to Malnutrition

The causes of malnutrition are complex. They include conditions that preexist within the individual—the *host*, the quality of the *environment*, and the specific *agents* that provoke the problem. Each element of this triad interacts with others. For example, many people in the United States suffer from some degree of malnutrition but the food supply, water, and waste disposal meet high standards of sanitation and safety so that health remains relatively good. On the other hand, people in some developing countries suffer the same degree of undernutrition but are exposed to grossly contaminated food and water so that life-threatening illness results. (See Figure 24-2.)

Susceptibility of Individuals   Within a given environment some individuals are more susceptible than others to malnutrition. Normal adults can usually survive moderate nutritional deficits rather well. Among the vulnerable groups are these:

1. Infants and preschool children: their nutritional requirements are high during rapid growth. When nutrients are not available for a given stage of development, the physical or mental rehabilitation may be delayed or may be unattainable.
2. Pregnant women: inadequate diets compromise the development of the fetus as well as the mother's own nutritional status and her freedom from the complications of pregnancy.
3. The elderly: malnutrition results from chronic ill health and long-standing nutritional deficiency; endocrine imbalances; inability to chew; physical handicaps that prevent adequate shopping or food preparation; loneliness and lack of interest in eating; and misconceptions concerning diet.

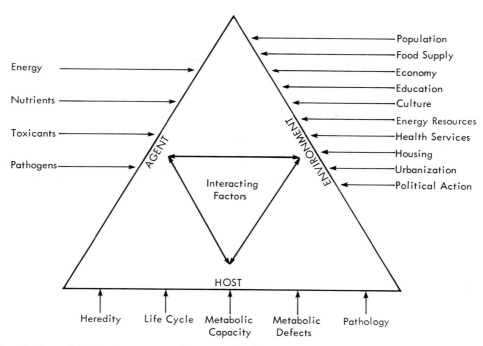

Figure 24-2. Many factors of the host-agent-environment triad interact to determine the quality of nutrition.

4. The sick: poor appetites; psychiatric disorders that prevent eating; infections; fevers and metabolic disorders that increase nutritional requirements; allergy; blood losses; injuries; gastrointestinal disorders that lead to fear of eating; diarrhea; malabsorption; and so on.

The vulnerability of these groups to malnutrition is considered when priorities are assigned to food assistance and to educational programs.

Environmental Factors that Favor Malnutrition In the United States and throughout the world poverty and ignorance are leading causes of malnutrition. Lack of available food is a principal cause of malnutrition in the underdeveloped and the developing countries of the world, but not in North America, Europe, and Oceania.

Poverty. In the United States approximately 34 million people are living at or below the poverty level.[4] They are to be found in the slums of the cities and in rural areas as well. Minority groups including blacks, Puerto Ricans, Spanish Americans, American Indians, and many people living in Appalachian regions constitute important segments of the poor population. The plight of no group in the United States is less favorable than that of the migrant farm workers who have few if any roots in a community and who often do not have the services of agencies that can provide assistance.

Two billion people live in about 100 poor underdeveloped nations of the world. Two thirds of these people live in Asia. Their per-capita income ranges from moderate to extreme poverty. In 1981 the per-capita income in the richest countries was about 220 times what it was in the poorest country. This gap will widen unless population growth is slowed and economic development is increased.[5]

Poverty means too few dollars to spend for food; competition between food and other necessities of life as well as things that give personal satisfaction for the available income; lack of food storage and preparation facilities; inability to purchase foods under the most favorable price conditions; and crowded, often unsanitary housing. Poverty results in a vicious cycle: poverty→inadequate diet→undernutrition→illness→inability to work→poverty.

Population Growth. The population of the world in 1984 was estimated to be 4.76 billion.[5] It is increasing by 80 to 90 million per year (about 10,000 every hour of every day!). By the end of this century about 6.1 billion persons will share the earth's resources—but not equally.

One half the world's people live in the Far East, but only one fourth of the world's food supply is produced there. If the entire world food supply could be evenly distributed, it would just about meet the energy needs of today's population. By the end of the century food production will need to increase by more than one fourth to meet the present-day inadequate levels. Any improvement in nutritional status would require far greater improvement in food production.

Population control is a possible answer to meeting world food needs. In recent years there has been some reduction in the rate of population increase. But population control involves religious, political, economic, and personal values. In countries where infant and child mortality is high, birth control may not seem realistic to a couple that wants survivors who can care for them in their old age.

Inadequate Supply of Food. Within a 40-year time span world grain production increased from 631 million metric tons in 1950 to 1620 million metric tons in 1981.[6] This remarkable increase was accounted for primarily by a doubling of the yield per acre of land. During this same period population increased at a rapid rate so that the grain available per person had improved at a somewhat slower rate (251 kg grain per person in 1950 to 365 kg per person in 1981). Although this increase in grain production was dramatic, it did not occur evenly throughout the world.

Since 1972–73 there has been a deepening food crisis throughout the world. Natural disasters such as the floods in Bangladesh and India, the severe droughts for several years in the Sahel, Africa, and political upheaval as in Campuchea have severely curtailed food production, leading to starvation for millions of people. The tragedy of famine in several countries of Africa is causing millions of deaths. The continuing drought greatly reduces the amount of grain that can be produced. Moreover, economic and political factors as well as severe problems of food distribution further complicate the problem.

In affluent countries people are demanding more and more animal foods, especially meat, and thus excessive amounts of grain must be fed to animals rather than being used directly for human food. As the economy of developing nations improves, the consumption of animal foods by its people increases. Yet, there is a finite limit to the acreage available for agriculture, for water resources, and for pesticides and fertilizers.

Tremendous increases in oil prices have made it impossible for farmers in developing countries to adopt modern methods of agriculture that depend on energy resources, or to purchase fertilizers that are dependent upon oil for their production. Food spoilage is excessively high because of lack of processing, storage, and distribution facilities. Where agriculture is most primitive the diets are almost always at the subsistence level. Thus, there is no food left over for an emergency. In the developing countries governments are usually unable to finance the irrigation programs needed for crops, the industrial plants for food processing and storage, and the roads for food distribution.

Urbanization. Jelliffe[7] described the flood of rural dwellers to the cities that is now occurring throughout the entire world as "disurbanization" because the influx is too rapid to accommodate people in terms of employment, housing, food, and services. The shanty towns and ghettos provide surroundings that are often worse than the rural areas left behind. Because they need cash to purchase food, people find themselves with diets that are more meager than their rural fare.

Infants and children suffer most from this trend. Infants are often weaned early, partly because the mother seeks employment and partly because she is trying to emulate the women of the Western world who do not breast feed their babies. Unfortunately, the substitute feedings for the baby are insufficient in quantity, often poor in quality, and likely to be grossly contaminated with bacteria.

Cultural Factors. Malnutrition sometimes results because people refuse to eat foods prohibited by religious beliefs or taboos and superstitions, those that lack prestige value, and those that are unfamiliar.

The taking of life is prohibited by some religions and no flesh foods may be eaten. This restriction excludes even eggs and milk for some. The prohibition against the taking of life may also mean that pesticides will not be used against rodents, thus resulting in high food losses in some countries. In India the sacred cows still compete seriously for the food supply of humans.

Social customs, taboos, and superstitions interfere with adequate food intake, especially by vulnerable groups. In some of the developing countries the father and other men in the family eat first and are given the choicest share of food. When food is scarce, women and children may get less than they need. Many primitive people believe that foods are endowed with specific qualities that can influence the personality of the unborn child or that can mark him or her physically. Thus, animal foods in particular may be taboo for pregnant and lactating women.

To be accepted food must be familiar. People to whom rice is the staple do not quickly change to a diet consisting principally of wheat. Even a change in a familiar food will reduce its acceptability. The new high-yielding varieties of rice and corn are less well liked by the people who use them because they are slightly different in color and texture and have somewhat different cooking qualities.

Plentiful foods may be ignored because they lack status value even though they are of excellent nutritive quality, whereas other foods of more marginal value may be selected because of their prestige value. Poor people often resent gifts of food that are classified as surplus. In the developing countries spices, fats, oils, sweets, tea, coffee, and cola beverages are often purchased because they are equated with a higher standard of living.

Lack of Education. People of all income classes and at all educational levels lack knowledge regarding the essentials of an adequate diet. Those who are ignorant concerning nutrition are particularly susceptible to food faddism, superstition, and nutritional quackery.

A limited education exacts a particularly severe toll from those who are also poor. It is, for many of them, the cause of their poverty inasmuch as people with minimal education and technical skills are unable to secure employment to earn a satisfactory living wage. Somehow, the poor must use each dollar more carefully but they have too little consumer information to help them. Moreover, inasmuch as the amount and quality of food available to them are limited, they need to employ the best techniques in food preparation to preserve nutritive values—but they lack the facilities and skills to do so.

Misinformation and Faddism. A fad is a fashion of the moment—here today, gone tomorrow. Fads sometimes disappear, only to reappear some years later in a new form. Persons of all ages fall prey to exaggerated claims: the teenage girl or woman looking for a quick way to lose some weight; the teenage boy seeking athletic prowess; the elderly person hoping for some panacea for impaired health. In each instance lack of education in nutrition, the influence of peers, and the pressures of advertising may have been influential.

Certain code words are widely used by food faddists and quacks to characterize foods, supplements, and devices. The "good" words include *health food, prevent, cure, pep and energy, organic, natural, herbal, fiber, supplement* (vitamin, mineral, protein), *vegetarian*, and many others. The "bad" words include *additive, chemical, devitalized, pesticide, preservative, processed, synthetic.* With a liberal use of "good" and "bad" words, the faddist develops a rationale for a given product or practice that manages to sway the uninformed consumer. In addition to claims for health maintenance, the faddist makes exaggerated and untrue statements regarding the prevention and cure of numerous diseases and conditions: arthritis, cancer, diabetes, hypoglycemia, hyperactivity, obesity, retardation of aging, maintenance of sexual virility, skin disorders, and so on.

Many fads and myths related to food are probably harmless. But if a consumer adopts a particular food, diet, supplement, or device as a treatment for disease without consulting a physician, the harm can be serious indeed. A second danger of food faddism is economic. About $1.5 billion is spent annually for "natural," "organic," and "health foods." Such foods are neither more nor less nutritious than their counterparts available in supermarkets, but they are usually much more expensive. For persons with limited income the additional expenditure for such foods could mean the elimination of other needed foods.

Protein-Energy Malnutrition

Forms of PEM CHRONIC MILD PROTEIN-ENERGY MALNUTRITION affects up to 50 percent of all children in the developing countries. The symptoms are nonspecific, with the chief characteristic being growth retardation or growth failure. Often the deficit is not detected unless the age of the child is known since the height and weight may be proportionate. A comparison of the child's height with standards for age is useful in determining whether growth is impaired. Children with mild deficiency often progress to severe deficiency when an infection or diarrhea is present. This progression is further hastened if the mother feeds a limited diet to the sick child.

KWASHIORKOR and MARASMUS are two facets of the same disease. The similarities and differences between the two are summarized in Table 24-3. Kwashiorkor is the severe form of protein deficiency occurring after 12 months of age, and characterized by marked edema, skin and hair changes, enlarged liver, and reduced levels of serum albumin, digestive enzymes, and lowered immune systems response.

Marasmus usually occurs during the second half of the first year. Its dominant characteristic is emaciation demonstrated by severe loss of subcutaneous tissue and muscle atrophy. Biochemical changes are less severe than in kwashiorkor, indicating adaptation to a lower level of existence for the body systems. (See Figure 24-3.)

Mixed PEM presents symptoms of kwashiorkor and marasmus. For example, when the marasmic child

Table 24-3. Protein-Energy Malnutrition: Kwashiorkor and Marasmus

Kwashiorkor	Marasmus
Principal nutritional deficit	
Protein	Calories, protein
Age of onset	
18 months to 3 years	6–12 months
Clinical findings	
Edema, pot belly, often swollen legs	No edema
Mild to moderate growth retardation; weight loss may be masked by edema	Weight loss of 40 percent or more
Subcutaneous fat normal to slightly lower	Severe growth failure; emaciation
Slight muscle atrophy	Severe loss of subcutaneous tissue
Round face with edema	Severe muscle atrophy
Dry, flaky, peeling, pigmented skin; sometimes ulcerated	Wrinkled face like a little old man; head often appears large
Thin, dry, easily plucked hair with pigmented bands ("flag sign")	Skin changes rare
Enlarged liver with fatty infiltration	Hair changes are common
Xerophthalmia leading to blindness	Liver normal or mildly enlarged; no fatty infiltration
Frequent anemia	Frequent anemia
Frequent infections; diarrhea	Frequent infections; diarrhea
Profound apathy, irritable, whimpers, sits where placed	Often appears bright eyed and alert; minimum activity
Biochemical changes	
Low serum albumin	Serum albumin normal or nearly so
Low serum transferrin	Serum transferrin low to normal
Low immune system response	Normal immune system response
Enzyme deficiency—amylase, lipase, trypsin	Normal enzyme activity
Some potassium deficit	Potassium deficit severe
Response to treatment	
Fairly rapid recovery; sudden death sometimes occurs	Long period of recovery

encounters an infection, the ability to maintain a level of homeostasis with respect to visceral proteins is lost and there is rapid decline in the serum albumin. Edema and decline in immune response follow. The condition is life threatening.

Iatrogenic PEM has been described as a too common finding in hospitalized patients, especially those under severe stress of surgery or injury, and accompanied by a deficient supply of nutrients by enteral or intravenous routes. (See page 393.)

Etiology Dr. Cicely Williams, a pediatrician, in the 1930s observed a syndrome in infants and children in Ghana which was called kwashiorkor. This is "the disease the deposed baby gets when the next one is born."[8] In the developing countries babies are usually breast fed for 18 to 24 months, and sometimes longer. Upon the birth of another child, the older child is deposed from the breast and subsists largely on a high-carbohydrate low-protein diet provided by the staple foods of the country. The symptoms become apparent about 3 to 4 months after the child has been weaned and have their highest incidence between 2 and 5 years of age. Not only is the child deprived of the mother's milk but he is also left to fend for himself.

In Africa the staples to which the child is weaned are cassava, plantain, and millet; in Central America and South America they are corn and beans; and in Asia, rice and some legumes. These foods do not provide sufficient amino acids for the rapid growth needs of the infant.

Marasmus occurs because (1) the mother's supply of breast milk is inadequate to meet the infant's nutritional needs, (2) breast feeding is not supplemented with other foods at the age of 5 to 6 months, or (3) inadequate, unsanitary formulas have been substituted for breast feeding. Because formulas are expensive, they may be diluted excessively so that they provide neither the calories nor the protein the infant needs.

Synergism Between Malnutrition and Infection When a diet is nutritionally inadequate but the sanitation is good and infections are minimal, the onset of deficiency symptoms is gradual. Likewise, when a well-nourished child succumbs to an infection, the period of illness is usually short, the residual effects are few, and the mortality rate is low. Conversely, the coexistence of malnutrition and infection vastly increases the severity of both; that is, a synergism exists between the two. (See Figure 24-4.) The child with

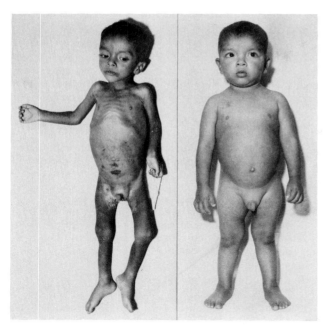

Figure 24-3. Severe protein-calorie malnutrition. Two-year-old child 2 weeks after admission and 10 weeks after treatment with INCAPARINA. (Courtesy, Institute of Central America and Panama, and the *Journal of the American Dietetic Association*.)

prekwashiorkor rapidly advances to kwashiorkor if gastroenteritis, measles, or some other infection is also present. Infections that are ordinarily mild become so severe in the malnourished that the resulting death rate is high. In some countries the mortality from measles is 400 times greater than in the United States—not because of increase in virulence but because of coexisting malnutrition.

Mental Development   One of the most serious consequences of PEM could be the arrest of mental development. Teachers have long observed that children who came to school without breakfast were irritable, nervous, had a short attention span, and were unable to concentrate on the tasks set before them. Such behavior is greatly accentuated in chronic undernutrition. The apathy, lack of curiosity, and reduced activity of the child with kwashiorkor greatly reduces the learning that can take place during this period of life when the normal rate of learning is nothing short of fantastic. Malnutrition is not an isolated occurrence but is generally associated with adverse environmental conditions such as parental ignorance, poverty, poor housing, crowding, and social isolation. These environmental factors, superimposed upon the malnutrition, can delay behavioral and intellectual development for months or even years. The longer the pe-

riod of delay, the greater is the likelihood that full development will not occur.

Since the most rapid brain growth occurs during the third trimester of pregnancy and during the infant's first year, it might be expected that permanent damage might occur if there is severe undernutrition at this time. Malnourished children have smaller head circumferences. Also, analyses of brain tissues of children that died of marasmus showed lower brain weight and fewer brain cells than in brain tissues of healthy children who died in accidents.[9] Thus, it might be inferred that such reduction in brain development could result in permanent mental retardation. To what extent such damage can be corrected by vigorous nutritional rehabilitation is not known. Some studies have shown that severely malnourished children were able in their school years to catch up to their normal peers.[10]

Prevention and Treatment of PEM   Four key elements for the prevention of infant deaths in the developing countries were described in the 1982 report of State of the World's Children.[11]

1. Keep a growth chart in the home. Most mothers of malnourished children don't know that anything is wrong. A growth chart together with regular weighing of the child helps make malnutrition visible and reduces the incidence of serious disease.
2. Use oral rehydration. About 5 million children die each year from dehydration caused by diarrhea. Most of these children can be saved by a mixture of sugar, salt, and water given orally in the home or the clinic. The inexpensive packets should be promoted by nations throughout their health systems,

Figure 24-4. The prognosis in malnutrition or infection occurring independently is good if appropriate therapy is instituted promptly. When malnutrition and infection interact, the severity of both is greatly increased and the prognosis is guarded.

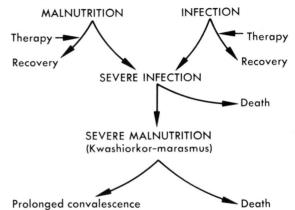

educational channels, mass media, industry, labor, and religious groups.

3. Promote breast feeding aggressively. This could save up to a million lives a year. In developing countries bottle feeding using powdered milk, often diluted with polluted water, and given in unsanitary bottles takes many lives.

4. Immunize infants and children. Immunizable diseases take about 5 million lives a year. Protection against these diseases costs about $5 per year.

On a continuing basis one of the best ways to improve the nutrition of the toddler is to improve the food supply of the entire family, since this helps ensure that the child will receive his needed share. Achieving such a goal involves improvement of the locally available food supplies, income, and education. Food mixtures that contain sufficient quantities of essential amino acids to meet the growth needs of children have been developed in a number of countries. (See page 361.)

When electrolyte imbalance and dehydration are present, the initial therapy must be directed to restoration of fluid–electrolyte balance. In severe malnutrition a deficit of potassium is likely to be present. This deficit could lead to cardiac failure if feeding is too vigorous at the beginning of therapy. Once rehydration has been accomplished a half-strength formula of skim milk is fed (providing that breast feeding is not possible), with gradual increases to a whole-milk formula that furnishes 125 to 150 kcal and 3 to 4 g protein per kg.

Anemia and vitamin A deficiency become more apparent as growth resumes and blood volume increases. These complications can be prevented by using formulas that are fortified with vitamins A and D, and with iron and folacin. A single injection of 100,000 IU water miscible vitamin A may be given instead of the daily supplementation of the formula.

Community Nutrition Services for Prevention and Intervention

National Food and Nutrition Policy

The objective of a national nutrition policy is to promote wellness or nutritional health. In 1974 the Nutrition Consortium (American Institute of Nutrition, American Society for Clinical Nutrition, The American Dietetic Association, and The Institute of Food Technology) published the following goals for a national nutrition policy*:

1. assure an adequate wholesome food supply at a reasonable cost to meet the needs of all segments of the population, this supply being available at a level consistent with the affordable life style of the era;
2. maintain food resources sufficient to meet emergency needs and to fulfill a responsible role as a nation in meeting world food needs;
3. develop a level of sound public knowledge and responsible understanding of nutrition and foods that will promote maximal nutritional health;
4. maintain a system of quality and safety control that justifies public confidence in its food supply;
5. support research and education in foods and nutrition with adequate resources and reasoned priorities to solve important current problems and to permit exploratory basic research.

To attain these goals, it is essential to:

1. maintain surveillance of the nutritional status of the population and determine the nature of nutritional problems observed;
2. develop programs within the health care system that will prevent and rectify nutritional problems;
3. assist the health professions in coordinated efforts to improve the nutritional status of the population through the life cycle;
4. develop programs for nutrition education for both health professionals and the general public;
5. identify areas in which nutrition knowledge is inadequate and foster research to provide this knowledge;
6. assemble information on the food supply, including food protection and distribution, and provide nutritional input in the regulation of foreign agricultural trade;
7. determine the nutrient composition of foods and promote and monitor food quality and safety;
8. cooperate with other nations and international agencies in developing measures for solving the world food and nutrition problems."*

In 1980 the National Nutrition Consortium reaffirmed the recommendations for a national nutrition policy, and also stated: "It endorses the principle of dietary guidelines which emphasize weight control, and stress moderation in the use of alcohol, fat, sugar, and salt."† During the past decade many nations have adopted guidelines that are similar to the recommendations of the several guidelines published in the United States. (See pages 29 to 32.) While endorsing the principle of dietary guidelines, the Consor-

---

* The National Nutrition Consortium, Inc: "Guidelines for a National Nutrition Policy," *Nutr. Rev.*, 32:153–57, 1974.
† National Nutrition Consortium: "Guidelines for a National Nutrition Policy," *Nutr. Rev.*, 38:96–98, 1980.

tium has cautioned that diet is only one of many factors that must be controlled if the incidence of chronic diseases is to be reduced. A national food and nutrition policy must evolve with new findings in research and in clinical experience.

At the governmental level the U.S. Department of Agriculture has stated the food and nutrition policy is "to ensure that there will continue to be an adequate, safe, palatable, nutritionally balanced, and reasonably priced food supply, equitably available to all Americans."* Before the 1970s the government programs in the agricultural sector dealt primarily with the needs of farmers. But the nation's economy and inflation, the world's inability to meet the expanding needs for food, the interdependence of nations, and even the changing perceptions of dietary needs required a reorientation of policy. Thus, the Food and Agriculture Act of 1977 was a response to the needs of consumers as well as farmers. The 1977 act provides for expansion of human nutrition research. It provides for the first federally mandated program of nutrition education for children. Another consideration

is that "nutritional goals may require changes in the types of commodities at the farm level and thus change the emphasis of government programs for producers, marketing promotion, regulation, and research."† Other important provisions of this act are the food assistance programs. (See Table 24-4.)

Nutrition Education

Scope of Educational Programs Education means change in behavior. It moves the individual from lack of interest and ignorance to increasing appreciation and knowledge and finally to action. Nutrition education offers a great opportunity to individuals to learn about the essentials of nutrition for health and to take steps to improve the quality of their diets and thus their well-being.

Nutrition education must continue throughout the individual's life in order to accommodate for developments in nutrition science and for changing economic

---

* *Food and Nutrition for the 1980's: Moving Ahead.* U.S. Department of Agriculture, Washington, D.C., April 1979, p. iii.

† *Agricultural-Food Policy Review*, Economics, Statistics, and Cooperative Services, U.S. Department of Agriculture, Washington, D.C., February 1980, p. 81.

Table 24-4. Some Examples of Federally Sponsored Nutrition Programs

Administered by the Food and Nutrition Service, U.S. Department of Agriculture	
National School Lunch Program	Cash and food subsidies to school programs; reduced and free meals for the poor. See page 310.
School Breakfast Program	Especially for low-income areas. See page 311.
Special Milk Program	Reimbursement for milk served to children.
Summer Food Service Program	Assistance to public and nonprofit institutions operating recreational programs in low-income areas.
Food Stamp Program	See page 358.
Supplemental Food Program for Women, Infants, and Children (WIC)	Food supplements to supply nutrients low in diets of high-risk persons. See page 275.
National Education Training Program	Education in schools see page 356.
Administered by Cooperative Extension Service, U.S. Department of Agriculture	
Expanded Food and Nutrition Education Program (EFNEP)	See page 359.
Administered by the U.S. Department of Health and Human Services	
Nutrition programs for the elderly Congregate meals Home-delivered meals Nutrition education	See page 325.
Early and Periodic Screening, Diagnosis, and Treatment	Preventive medical care for persons under 21 who are Medicaid beneficiaries.
Maternity and Infant Care Projects (MIC, M&I)	Multidisciplinary prenatal care to high-risk women, and to high-risk infants. See page 275.
Children and Youth Projects (C&Y)	Comprehensive health care to preschool and school children in low-income areas.
Head Start	Multiple health services to children 3 years to school age in low-income areas.

circumstances, health requirements, and the new food products appearing in the nation's markets. This requires a greatly expanded use of the mass media, and the involvement of governmental and private agencies and universities, as well as the food industries.

Dietary counseling, described in Chapter 23, is an example of education in nutrition on a one-to-one basis and is designed to bring about desired changes in food behavior as identified by nutritional assessment. Educational activities at the community level are available at health centers, maternal and child-care centers, day-care centers, programs for the elderly, youth organizations, women's clubs, and special purpose programs such as those for alcoholism, drug abuse, and the handicapped.

In 1977 an amendment to the Child Nutrition Act provided funding to state educational agencies to develop and implement nutrition education for all children of school age. This program, popularly referred to as NET (Nutrition Education and Training Program), has led to the development of curricula and educational materials, the training of school food service personnel in nutrition and management, and the instruction of classroom teachers.

Leaders in business and industry have recognized that health maintenance and disease prevention by employees is cost effective. In recent years many organizations have introduced programs to employees on smoking cessation, stress management, hypertension, drug and alcohol abuse, weight management, exercise, and nutrition. For example, a nutrition education program can be conducted during a lunch hour or after work, allowing about one hour weekly for 8 to 10 weeks. Some topics covered are mineral and vitamin supplements, dietary fiber, carbohydrate, protein, and fat needs, food labeling, and food for sport.[12] Nutrition education is coordinated with the cafeteria and vending services; for instance, caloric information is provided for foods to assist employees in selecting foods that will control weight.

Concepts for Food and Nutrition Education A concept is "an idea around which the content of nutrition education curricula can be built."* Concepts have been developed by the Interagency Committee on Nutrition Education, U.S. Department of Agriculture in 1964, and by the White House Conference on Food, Nutrition and Health in 1969.[13,14] These and other concepts were used to develop an updated set of concepts by a committee of the Society for Nutrition Education. They are as follows†:

1. Nutrition

Nutrition is the process by which food is selected and becomes part of the human body.

2. Food and Its Handling

   A. Food contains nutrients that work together and interact with body chemicals to serve the needs of the body.
   B. No one food, by itself, contains all the nutrients in the appropriate amounts and combinations needed for optimal growth and health.
   C. Many different combinations of food can provide the needed nutrients in appropriate amounts.
   D. Food contains important nonnutritive components, such as dietary fiber, which are needed for healthy functioning of the body.
   E. Toxicants, additives, contaminants, and other nonnutritive factors in food affect its safety and quality.
   F. The way food is grown, processed, stored, and prepared for eating influences the amount of nutrients in the food and its safety, appearance, taste, cost, and waste.
   G. Food requires varying amounts of energy and other resources to produce, process, package, and deliver it to the consumer.

3. Nutrients and Dietary Components

   A. Nutrients in the food that we eat enable us to live, to grow, to keep healthy and well, and to be active.
   B. Each nutrient—carbohydrates, protein, fats, vitamins, minerals, and water—has specific functions in the body.
   C. Nutrients must be obtained from outside the body on a regular basis because the body cannot produce them in sufficient amounts.
   D. Most healthy people can obtain all the nutrients, in the amounts needed, from a variety of foods.
   E. Nutrients are distributed to and used by all parts of the body.
   F. Nutrient interactions may affect the amounts needed and their functioning.
   G. The body stores some nutrients and withdraws them for use as needed.
   H. Nutrients are found in varying amounts, proportions, and combinations in the plant and animal sources which serve as food.
   I. Ongoing scientific research determines nutrients, their functions, and the amounts needed.
   J. Both dietary excesses and nutrient deficiencies affect health.
   K. Optimum intakes of nutrients and dietary components have both upper and lower limits.

---

* "SNE Concepts for Food and Nutrition Education," *J. Nutr. Educ.*, **14:**1, 1982.

† "SNE Concepts for Food and Nutrition Education," *J. Nutr. Educ.*, **14:**1–2, 1982.

L. All persons throughout life have need for the same nutrients, but the amounts of nutrients needed are influenced by age, sex, size, activity, specific activity, specific conditions of growth, state of health, pregnancy, lactation, and environmental stress.

4. Nutrition and Physical Activity

A. Balancing energy intake and energy expenditure is important for achieving and maintaining desirable body weight.
B. There is a synergistic relationship between nutrition and physical activity which affects health and well-being.

5. Food Selection

A. Food, that is, what people consider edible, is culturally defined.
B. Physiological, cultural, social, economic, psychological, and geographical factors influence food selection.
C. Knowledge, attitudes, and beliefs about food and nutrition affect food selection.
D. Food availability and merchandising influence food choices.

6. National and International Food Policy

A. Food plays an important role in the physical, psychological, and economic health of a society.
B. Food production, distribution, and merchandising systems have economic, social, political, and ecological consequences.
C. Effective utilization of individual and community resources is beneficial for the economic and nutritional well-being of the individual, family, and society.
D. The availability of food and maintenance of nutritional well-being is a matter of public policy.
E. Knowledge of food and nutrition combined with social consciousness enables citizens to understand and participate in the development and adoption of public policy affecting the nutritional well-being of societies.

From these concepts, the educator selects those around which the content of a given curriculum is built. The next step in the development of the teaching plan is to identify the objectives—that is, to determine exactly what learning is to take place. Then methods for implementing these objectives that are appropriate for the learners are incorporated into the teaching plan.

Nutritional Services

Nature of Services In the hospital or clinic the nurse and dietitian give direct service to the individual. Nutrition services of the community are also provided on an individual basis, especially at the city-county level. For example, such direct services are given by a public health nurse, a nutritionist, a home-maker from a welfare agency, or a volunteer who delivers a hot meal to an aged person.

Community programs in nutrition seek to improve nutrition through research, education, improvement of the food supply, and feeding. A complex network of agencies exists at the local, state, and national level for providing nutrition services to the people at all stages of the life cycle. Health workers must know what public and private resources exist in the community so that they are able to make appropriate referrals for assistance. The following activities are representative of those included in nutrition programs.

1. Define the place of nutrition in program areas.
   a. Conduct surveys of the community needs in cooperation with universities and other health agencies.
2. Provide materials on nutrition information.
   a. Analyze and interpret findings of science.
   b. Prepare leaflets on topics such as: weight control; meal planning; infant feeding; food misinformation; diet patterns for various cultural groups; teenagers; senior citizens.
   c. Prepare diet manuals, food value charts, exhibits, newspaper, magazine, radio, and television releases.
3. Provide consultant service to agencies and institutions: child care, nursing homes, small hospitals, mental hospitals, homes for the elderly.
   a. Planning food service facilities.
   b. Personnel training; budgeting; menu planning; purchasing; sanitation; preparation and service of food; therapeutic diets.
4. Work with schools: elementary, secondary, college, medical, nursing, allied health.
   a. Assist in developing programs in nutrition education.
   b. Conduct workshops for school faculty.
   c. Assist in training programs for school food service personnel; help to interpret educational value of school meals.
5. Cooperate with other health groups in rehabilitation and in chronic disease programs.
   a. Preparation of materials for professional and lay instruction.
   b. Conduct workshops for staff education of nurses, nutritionists, physicians, social workers, and other health professionals.
6. Work with clients individually or in groups in clinics, health centers, or by home visits.
7. Coordinate individual and group activities with social and welfare agencies.

8. Assist in programs of research with college departments of food and nutrition, medical schools, departments of health, private and federal agencies.

Helping People with Low Income

Characteristics of the Poor The poor are often thought of as a single group that can be described in terms of a "culture of poverty." Although certain characteristics of behavior are enforced upon them by reason of poverty, it is a serious error to regard the poor as a homogeneous group.[15]

Variations in Environment and Culture. Poor people living in Appalachia, the Mexican Americans of the Southwest, the Puerto Ricans, the American Indians, the black people in city ghettos, and many people in cities and in rural areas have one thing in common—lack of sufficient income to meet their basic needs. Their cultures, however, have little in common. Moreover, within each of these groups, individuals and families differ from one another in their values, aspirations, and style of living just as people of the more affluent society differ from one another. Some poor people come from families that have been poor for generations and have never known any other way of life; other people are poor because of changed circumstances brought about by unemployment, inflation, and health costs. Some of the poor have a fair level of education, whereas others are illiterate. Some homemakers are good managers and do a remarkable job in keeping the family together, whereas others lack even the simplest skills in homemaking and in child care. Some constantly strive for a better way of life, whereas others regard their present status as permanent and they can do little about it.

The Limitations of Poverty. A limited income restricts most poor people to living in declining neighborhoods with deteriorating houses, inadequate sanitation, crowding, and lack of privacy. There is a constant fear of eviction because of loss of income and failure to pay the rent.

Some of the poor are isolated from society. They move about from place to place—usually not by choice but by necessity—and therefore establish no roots in the community. Their participation in community activities is minimal and their contact with the outside world through newspapers and magazines is small. This isolation encourages suspicion of the motives of those who may try to help them; it also means that they are poorly equipped to cope with emergencies because they do not know what resources are available to them.

The poor must live from day to day and are unable to plan ahead. The future is uncertain, they are fatalistic about what is to come, and setting goals for the future seems pointless.

Lacking education, the poor may not be able to make the best use of the little money they have. They are often at the mercy of credit schemes that, over a period of time, exact large interest payments.

Most poor people have known little success. They feel that people look down on them and have little concern for them. They will often place more confidence in the advice of a neighbor, a faith healer, or a practitioner of folk medicine—all of whom are attuned to their way of living.

Social problems are not unique to the poor but they are likely to be more frequent. Many of the families have only one parent, usually the mother. Men in many households are unable to fulfill their roles as providers; they leave their homes so that their families can qualify for public assistance.

Better Nutrition for the Poor Adequate income is basic to an adequate diet. Before you can tell people what foods they require and how to prepare them, there must be food in the home to prepare or money with which to purchase it. During the 1970s, in response to the demonstrated food needs of the poor, there was rapid expansion of federal feeding programs. The cost of these programs in 1983 was about $19 billion. Of those who received food aid, 7 of 10 were white, 60 percent were under 15 years or over 65 years, and many were infirm. Others worked for low wages or had been laid off and could not find employment.[16]

Food Stamp Program. The Food Stamp Act, passed in 1964, is intended to increase the food purchasing power of the poor. It is the single largest source of food aid, and in 1983 benefited more than 21 million persons.

The stamps are issued to families and single persons who have an income of 130 percent or less of the federal poverty guideline. They may be used instead of money to purchase food and to buy seeds or plants for producing food. The elderly may use the stamps for their contribution to the congregate meal programs. Consumer education along with the distribution of food stamps is needed in order to realize maximum nutritional benefits.

Expanded Food and Nutrition Education Program. This program was started in 1968 to help low-income families improve their diets. The families are taught why they need a balanced diet; how to purchase nutritious foods; how to prepare and serve tasty meals; how to store food and keep it safe; how to use food stamps; how to keep a home garden whenever possible; and what resources and programs are available to them.

Program aides who will serve the families are given intensive training by home economists and nutritionists in the Cooperative Extension Service of the U.S. Department of Agriculture. The aides are mature, nonprofessional women usually selected from the community in which they will serve. These women are usually aware of the problems of the families with whom they work. Their assistance is less likely to be viewed with suspicion than is that of a helper who comes from a middle-class environment with different standards and values, and with little understanding of what it means to be poor.

International Agencies for Nutrition

Food and Agriculture Organization   The Food and Agriculture Organization of the United Nations (FAO) was founded in Quebec, Canada, in October 1945 the aims being:

To help the nations raise the standard of living;
To improve the nutrition of the people of all countries;
To increase the efficiency of farming, forestry, and fisheries;
To better the condition of rural people;
And, through these means, to widen the opportunity of all people for productive work.*

The headquarters office of FAO is in Rome where the work of the organization is supervised by a director-general. FAO maintains an intelligence service which gathers, analyzes, and distributes information on which action can be based, and advises governments on actions to take.

Technical assistance is provided in agriculture, economics, fisheries, forestry, and nutrition to member countries. The diversified projects have included development of food storage, processing, and marketing facilities; land reclamation through irrigation and drainage; control of animal diseases; development of grains of higher nutritive value; increased yields of

crops and greater resistance to disease; inland fish culture in ponds and rice fields; establishment of home economics programs in colleges; school feeding; and many others.

World Health Organization   The World Health Organization (WHO) was created in 1948 and is administered by a director-general with headquarters in Geneva, Switzerland, and with six regional offices, one of which is in Washington, D.C.

WHO is "the directing and coordinating authority for international health work." It is governed by two principles defined in its constitution:

UNIVERSALITY: The health of all peoples is fundamental to the achievement of peace and security. The enjoyment of the highest attainable standard of health is one of the fundamental rights of every human being without distinction of race, religion, political belief, economic or social condition.
CONCEPT OF HEALTH: Health is a state of complete physical, mental and social well-being and not merely the absence of disease or infirmity.†

The assistance that WHO renders to government includes:

strengthening national health services; establishing and maintaining epidemiological and statistical services; controlling epidemic and endemic diseases; maternal and child health; promotion of mental health to foster harmonious human relations; improvement of sanitation and of preventive and curative medical services.†

United Nations Children's Fund   To children in different countries UNICEF means different things. It may mean an injection to cure them of yaws, a crippling disease, or vaccination to protect against measles, or a massive dose of vitamin A to prevent blindness, or provision for a safe water supply, or food to stave off starvation as a result of drought, floods, and civil war.

Organized in 1947, UNICEF continued the emergency feeding in war-devastated countries of Europe, with emphasis upon protein-rich foods, especially milk. Now, in developing countries all over the world, programs are directed to infants, children, and pregnant and lactating women. Although UNICEF continues to provide emergency relief, most of its funds are now diverted to long-range programs, for it is realized that countries must be able to solve their own nutritional problems.

* *Food and Agriculture Organization—What It Is—What It Does—How It Works.* Leaflet, Food and Agriculture Organization, Rome, 1956.

† *World Health Organization—What Is It—What It Does—How It Works.* Leaflet, World Health Organization, Geneva, 1956.

United States Responsibility in World Nutrition
Each nation justifies its participation in programs to solve world nutrition problems on the basis of economic and political concerns as well as humanitarian considerations. Public Law 480, the Food for Peace Program, was adopted by Congress in 1954 as a means of using agricultural surpluses for feeding the world's needy people. The program is administered by the Agency for International Development (AID) in the Department of State.

Four aims of PL 480 have been identified: "It provides humanitarian assistance; expands international trade and develops markets for U.S. agricultural commodities; supports economic growth within the developing countries; and promotes the foreign policy of the United States."* Under this act the U.S. government provides low interest loans with long repayment terms to developing countries to enable them to purchase U.S. agricultural commodities. These concessions help to promote economic growth within the recipient countries. PL 480 also provides food donations through CARE, Catholic Relief Services, the United Nations World Food Program, and other relief agencies. In addition, the United States maintains a 4-million-ton Food Security Wheat Reserve to meet the urgent needs of developing countries.[17]

Increasing the World Food Supply

Priorities   The caloric deficit in the developing countries is enormous. (See Table 24-2.) People who are poor and for whom the food supply is scarce are in need of (1) sufficient calories to sustain life and (2) protein of adequate quality and amount. The food must be culturally acceptable and must have taste, odor, and texture properties that provide palatability. The foods must be locally available, easily transported, stable for long periods without spoilage in the absence of refrigeration, and low in cost.

Important enterprises of AID and foundations such as the Ford and Rockefeller Foundations have included the development of better agricultural practices, improved strains of plants, and protein mixtures of high nutritive value.

Potential Sources of Food   Cereal grains are the principal source of food for the world's people and will undoubtedly continue to rank first throughout the world. Agricultural scientists have brought about the so-called "green revolution." In many less developed countries high yields of cereals are being achieved by using improved strains of rice, wheat,

and corn, and by emphasizing modern agricultural practices including fertilizers and equipment.

Improved Cereal Quality.   Cereal grains are deficient in one or more of the essential amino acids and thus do not meet the needs for rapid synthesis of proteins required for growth. (See page 58.) An outstanding example of an improved cereal grain is opaque-2 corn, a hybrid variety that has been developed in which the lysine and tryptophan content of the endosperm is 50 per cent higher than in regular varieties. Also, the leucine content is lower so that the balance with isoleucine is improved. This development is of considerable significance to Central American, Latin American, and some African nations where corn is a staple food. In 1973 two varieties of high-lysine sorghum were developed. Eventually, this will be of benefit in arid regions of Asia and Africa where sorghum is a staple food.

Triticale is a man-made grain, combining the properties of wheat and rye. It contains a higher quality of protein than other grains, and it is more resistant to drought and cold than is wheat.

Amino Acid Supplementation.   To improve the protein quality of wheat requires additional lysine; rice needs lysine and threonine; legumes require methionine; and corn requires tryptophan and lysine. Although some amino acid supplementation is technically and economically feasible, nutrition scientists have been cautious about recommending it because an excess of certain amino acids can create an increased need for the next most limiting amino acid. Amino acid imbalances in low-protein diets can result in growth failure and other metabolic problems.

Other Plant Sources.   Legumes, including chick peas, peanuts, and many varieties of beans, are important sources of protein and calories in Central America, Africa, and India. Soybeans contain protein of superior quality and probably have not been utilized for human food as much as they might be. Cottonseed is a useful source of protein when the toxic pigment, gossypol, is removed.

Fish.   Seafoods are an important source of high-quality protein. However, since 1970 there has been a steady decline in the catch of fish. Much competition exists today between nations concerning fishing rights. Another serious problem is the pollution of the seas by oil, and agricultural, industrial, and municipal wastes. Polluted waters may kill fish, interfere with their reproduction, or render fish unfit to eat, for example, the mercury poisoning that has been traced to fish in isolated instances in Japan.

*Langan, K., et al.: "Food Aid: Help for Hungry Nations," *Natl. Food Rev.*, 24:15–18, Fall 1983.

Fish protein concentrate is a low-fat, bland powder produced from whole fish. It contains in excess of 80 percent protein, but problems of production and palatability have prevented wide use of this product.

Food Mixtures. Many food mixtures that apply the principle of the supplementary value of the proteins of various foods have been developed, particularly for the relief of protein-calorie malnutrition in children. These mixtures do not yet account for a sizable proportion of the world's protein needs. Among the mixtures that have been shown to be nutritionally satisfactory, economically feasible, and acceptable to the consumers are these:

C.S.M.: corn, soy, milk blend; developed for use in U.S. AID programs

INCAPARINA: the first mixture to be developed; cottonseed and corn flours, vitamins, minerals, and torula yeast; protein efficiency equal to milk; 26 percent protein; Central America.

BAL AHAR: a farinalike blend of bulgur wheat, peanut flour, nonfat dry milk, vitamins, minerals; 22 per cent protein; India.

GOLDEN ELBOW MACARONI (*General Foods*): corn, soy, and wheat flours; calcium carbonate, calcium phosphate, iron, B vitamins; 20 percent protein; Brazil.

LECHE ALIM: A cereal food of toasted wheat flour, fish protein concentrate, sunflower meal, skim milk powder; 27 percent protein; Chile.

PUMA (*Monsanto*); SACI (*Coca-Cola*); and VITASOY (*Lo*): beverages containing vegetable protein, sugar, vitamins; compete with soft drinks in price and are well accepted; 2.5 to 3 percent protein; Brazil, Guiana, Hong Kong.

Food for the Future. Leaves of plants such as alfalfa and single-celled plants, including yeasts, fungi, and algae, may become important sources of food in the more distant future. The techniques for producing them at low cost are not yet known, and major problems remain in developing products that are aesthetically acceptable. The high nucleic acid content leads to increased uric acid production and subsequent problems of excretion.

CASE STUDY 8

A Teenage Mother Needs Assistance in Meal Management

Eighteen-year-old Tania is the single parent of a 12-month-old daughter, Carrie. They live in a scantily furnished one-room apartment with limited kitchen facilities. The compact refrigerator has freezer space only for ice cube trays.

Tania works 4 hours daily, Monday through Friday, as a waitress in a local cafeteria. She receives her lunch at the cafeteria. While Tania is at work, Carrie is in a day care center, where she receives a morning snack and lunch.

Because of her low income, Tania qualifies for food stamps. She also receives vouchers for designated supplemental food for Carrie through the WIC program at the Health Department clinic where she received her prenatal care. Tania still finds it difficult to keep within a limited food budget. Since she has no convenient transportation of her own, Tania shops at the small neighborhood grocery store, where foods are more expensive. Also the meat and produce selections are minimal.

Tania is weaning Carrie from a bottle to a cup and serves her mostly table foods. The baby enjoys fruit juice in a bottle at bedtime and often falls asleep with her bottle in her crib.

Questions for Case Study

1. What are the criteria for participation in the WIC supplemental food program?
2. What foods are provided through the WIC program?
3. Tania told the nurse that on her way home she buys some food for their supper, such as hot dogs, potato salad, and cinnamon buns. How would you evaluate these choices?
4. What are some inexpensive ways to meet Tania's and Carrie's protein needs?
5. When using table foods for Carrie, what are some recommendations that could be made to Tania for their selection and preparation?
6. The nutritionist in the WIC program referred Tania to the local Cooperative Extension Service for assistance from a nutrition program aide. What kinds of assistance is a program aide prepared to give in Tania's home?
7. Tania is advised to refrain from giving Carrie the bottle of juice at bedtime. What are the reasons for this advice?
8. Since Tania had little experience in selecting a nutritious diet, what assistance might the nutrition program aide give in food selection on a limited budget?
9. With limited kitchen facilities, what are some practical guides that could be demonstrated to Tania in her home for easy-to-prepare meals?

References for the Case Study

PAREDES-ROJAS, R. R., and SOLOMONS, H. C.: "Food for Thought: Impact of a Supplemental Nutritional Program on Low-Income Preschool Children," *Pediatr. Nurs.*, 8:315–17, 1982.

UNITED STATES DEPARTMENT OF AGRICULTURE BULLETINS:
Family Food Budgeting for Good Meals and Nutrition
Food: The Hassle-Free Guide to a Better Diet, 1979.
Food for Families with Young Children
Money Saving Main Dishes
Making Food Dollars Count: Nutritious Meals at Low Cost

WATSON, M. L.: "The Relationship between Dietary Factors and Dental Caries," *J. School Health*, 52:39–41, 1982.

References

1. Goodloe, C.: "Nutrition, World Hunger, and the Demand for Food," *Natl. Food Rev.*, 24:12–15, 1983.
2. "Food and Nutrition: the Facts," *UNICEF News*, Fall Issue 113:9, 1982.
3. Briggs, G. M., cited by Frankle, R. T., and Owen, A. Y.: *Nutrition in the Community.* The C. V. Mosby Company, St. Louis, 1976, p. 12.
4. Census data 1984, *Philadelphia Inquirer*, May 20, 1984, p. 3 F.
5. Salas, R. M.: *State of World Population Report 1984.* U.N. Fund for Population Activities.
6. FAO source, cited by S. H. Wittwer: "Nutrition, Agriculture and World Health," *Food and Nutr. News*, 55(1):January/February 1983.
7. Jelliffe, D. B., and Jelliffe, E. F. P.: "The Urban Avalanche and Child Nutrition," *J. Am. Diet. Assoc.*, 57:111–18, 1970.
8. Williams, C. D.: "Kwashiorkor. A Nutritional Disease Associated with a Maize Diet," *Lancet*, November 16, 1935, p. 1151; reprinted in *Nutr. Rev.*, 31:350–51, 1973.
9. Winick, M., and Ross, P.: "The Effect of Severe Early Malnutrition on Cellular Growth of the Brain," *Pediatr. Res.*, 3:181–84, 1969.
10. "Energy-Protein Malnutrition and Behavior," *Nutr. Rev.*, 38:164–67, 1980.
11. "UNICEF Launches 1982 State of the World's Children Report," *UNICEF News*, Issue 114:34, 1982.
12. Murphy, C.: "Nutrition Education at the Worksite," *Nutr. News (Natl. Dairy Council)*, 46(4):December 1983.
13. Hill, M. M.: "I. C. N. E. Formulates Some Basic Concepts in Nutrition," *Nutr. Program News*, September–October 1964, U.S. Department of Agriculture, Washington, D.C.
14. "Conceptual Framework for Nutrition Education in the Schools," *White House Conference on Food, Nutrition and Health*—Final Report, p. 151, Government Printing Office, Washington, D.C., 1970.
15. Shoemaker, L.: *Parent and Family Life Education for Low-Income Families.* Children's Bureau Pub. 434-1965. U.S. Department of Health, Education and Welfare, Washington, D.C., 1965.
16. Gershoff, S. N.: "If There Is One Hungry Person . . . ," *Tufts University Diet and Nutrition Letter*, 2(1):7–8, March 1984.
17. Langan, K., et al.: "Food Aid: Help for Hungry Nations," *Natl. Food Rev.*, 24:15–18, Fall 1983.

25

Physical Fitness, Exercise, and Weight Control
Calorie-Restricted Diets

Physical Fitness

More and more Americans are realizing the importance of exercise as part of an overall program for a more healthy lifestyle. Many beginners may not realize the full benefit of exercise without specific guidance regarding the type, duration, intensity, and frequency of exercise that is most appropriate for them. Whether the goal is increased energy expenditure for weight control, improved cardiovascular fitness, or athletic training, the advantages of a program prescribed to meet the needs of the individual should not be overlooked. Such programs are likely to be associated with a lower attrition rate and fewer injuries.

The details of exercise physiology and exercise prescription are beyond the scope of this text. However, the essential components of exercise programs are described in the sections that follow.

Preexercise Assessment An evaluation of the individual's exercise capabilities is desirable before planning an exercise program. Especially for sedentary persons and those over 35 years of age a physical examination by a physician is highly recommended. Examination of the cardiovascular and musculoskeletal systems in particular, measurement of blood pressure, determination of serum cholesterol and triglycerides, and a cardiac stress test are usually included. On the basis of the assessment, an individualized exercise program can be prescribed. Specific directions are provided regarding the type, intensity, duration, and frequency of exercise.

Type of Exercise Aerobic exercise is required for improvement of cardiovascular fitness. Examples of aerobic activities are those that use large muscle groups, that can be maintained continuously, and that are rhythmic, such as walking briskly, bicycling, jogging, running, and swimming. The type of exercise planned into the program should be enjoyable in order to encourage compliance.

Intensity of Exercise The exercise program should begin with low-intensity exercise tailored to the individual, with consideration given to the usual type and amount of physical activity, degree of fitness, and physical limitations. The level of exercise that is sufficient to condition the muscles and cardiovascular system, thereby improving physical fitness, is called the *target zone*. This corresponds to a heart rate that is 70 to 85 percent of the maximal attainable heart rate. The maximal attainable heart rate and the target zone for each individual can be determined by means of an exercise stress test, but in common practice age-adjusted averages are used for both. The value for maximal attainable heart rate is roughly 220 beats per minute minus one's age; the target zone is 70 to 85 percent of this. For example, the maximum heart rate for an average 25-year-old is 200 beats per minute and the target zone is 140 to 170 beats per minute, whereas the maximal attainable heart rate in a 55-year-old is 165 beats per minute and the target zone is 115 to 140 beats per minute.[1] (See Table 25-1.)

Since the pulse rate is usually the same as the number of heart beats per minute, the pulse rate can be used to determine whether one is in the target zone. The pulse rate is counted for 6 seconds immediately after 3 to 5 minutes of exercise, and the result multiplied by 10 to obtain the rate for one minute. If the pulse rate is less than the target zone, more strenuous exercise is needed. The intensity of exercise should progress to the target zone over several weeks.

The intensity of exercise is expressed in terms of

Table 25-1. Maximal Attainable Heart Rate and Target Zones*

Age (years)	Maximal Attainable Heart Rate (beats per minute)	Target Zone (70 to 85 percent of maximum)
25	200	140–170
30	194	136–165
35	188	132–160
40	182	128–155
45	176	124–150
50	171	119–145
55	165	115–140
60	159	111–135
65	153	107–130

* Adapted from Zohman, L. R.: *Beyond Diet. Exercise Your Way to Fitness and Heart Health*, CPC International, Englewood Cliffs, N.J. 1974.

metabolic equivalents (mets) or kilocalories (kcal). *Mets* refer to the oxygen consumption required to perform any activity and are expressed as multiples of the resting energy expenditure. One met equals 3.5 ml oxygen consumed per kg per minute and represents the resting energy expenditure; 2 mets equal twice the resting energy expenditure, and so on. Examples of the energy cost of walking or cycling at various speeds are shown in Table 25-2. Activities with an energy cost of 5 to 6 mets, or 6 to 7 kcal per minute, are beneficial in improving fitness.[1]

After several weeks of regular exercise, some improvement in the physical fitness level should occur; the exercise becomes easier, and the intensity must be increased in order for further progress to take place. Once physical fitness is attained, the exercise program must be continued to maintain the level of fitness.

Duration of Exercise The exercise period is usually divided into three phases:

1. *Warmup period*: A period of 5 to 10 minutes of warmup protects the cardiorespiratory system from sudden stress and prevents muscular strain. It includes stretching exercises after which the activity of choice is begun at a slow pace. During this period the heart rate should be below the target zone.
2. *Stimulus phase*: This phase initially includes 15 to 20 minutes of exercise during which the heart rate is in the target zone. After fitness is attained, this period may be extended to 20 to 60 minutes.
3. *Cooldown period*: This phase consists of 5 to 10 minutes of exercise at lower intensity before stopping. The heart rate should be below the target zone. The cooldown period is necessary because abrupt cessation of intense activity traps blood in the muscles, resulting in inadequate supply to the brain, heart, and intestines, and may be accompanied by symptoms of dizziness, arrhythmias, nausea, and so on.

Table 25-2. Energy Cost of Walking and Cycling at Various Rates

Activity	Energy (kcal/minute)	Cost (mets)	Comment
Strolling, at 1 mph	2.0–2.5	1.5–2.0	Not sufficiently strenuous to promote
Walking, at 2 mph	2.5–4.0	2.0–3.0	endurance unless capacity is very low.
Walking, at 3 mph Cycling, at 6 mph	4.0–5.0	3.0–4.0	Adequate if capacity is very low
Walking, at 3.5 mph Cycling, at 8 mph	5.0–6.0	4.0–5.0	Good dynamic aerobic exercise
Walking, at 4.0 mph Cycling, at 10 mph	6.0–7.0	5.0–6.0	Dynamic, aerobic, and beneficial
Walking, at 5 mph Cycling, at 11 mph	7.0–8.0	6.0–7.0	Same as above
Jogging, 5 mph Cycling, 12 mph	8.0–10.0	7.0–8.0	Same as above, plus builds endurance
Running, 5.5 mph Cycling, 13 mph	10.0–11.0	8.0–9.0	Excellent conditioner
Running, 6.0 mph	11.0–12.0	10	Same as above

* Adapted from Zohman, L. R.: *Beyond Diet. Exercise Your Way to Fitness and Heart Health*, CPC International, Englewood Cliffs, N.J., 1974.

Frequency of Exercise For developing and maintaining physical fitness, aerobic exercise must be done 3 to 5 times per week with no more than 2 days between workouts. For persons with a low level of fitness more frequent sessions of short duration are needed. Once fitness is attained, more frequent workouts have no additional benefit.

Nutrition for Athletes

High-school and college-age youth often participate in competitive sports. Many of them are poorly informed about appropriate diets and resort to faddish and even dangerous practices regarding food and fluid intake.

Nutritional Requirements The nutrient levels set forth in the Recommended Dietary Allowances are satisfactory for planning the diet for athletes. The athlete's primary increased need is in the caloric intake which ranges from 3,000 to 6,000 kcal, and occasionally more. In proportion to the caloric intake, the need for thiamin, riboflavin, and niacin is increased. (See pages 179, 182, and 185.) These needs are more than met by the increased amounts of foods consumed from nutrient-rich food groups. There is no evidence that supplemental vitamins will improve athletic performance.

Some evidence indicates that iron status is less than optimal in both male and female athletes. The iron depletion is associated with low levels of plasma ferritin and transferrin saturation, but the hemoglobin level is normal. Elevated serum lactate levels following exercise with subsequent muscle fatigue occur and improve with correction of the iron depletion with heme iron.[2]

Protein. The recommended allowances for protein will meet the needs for growth of adolescents, for tissue turnover, and for development of muscles during athletic conditioning. A high protein intake does not increase the efficiency of muscle performance. Intakes exceeding 1g per kg are actually commonplace since food selections for a palatable diet are likely to include more protein-rich foods as the caloric requirement increases.

Fluid Needs. Fluid losses during prolonged, vigorous activity may account for up to 4 liters per hour. Dehydration reduces performance, and, if extreme, can be life threatening. About 2 hours before the event the athlete should consume about 500 ml water,

and 10 to 15 minutes before the competition another 500 ml water. During the competition it is better to ingest small amounts (100 to 200 ml) of chilled liquid every 10 to 15 minutes rather than a large amount at one time. Fluid consumed before and during the competition will not fully restore fluid balance, and the athlete should continue to drink water for the next 24 to 36 hours until his or her initial weight is restored.[3]

Electrolytes. Profuse sweating increases the losses of sodium, potassium, and chloride. Ordinary mixed diets furnish generous amounts of these electrolytes and replacement is not necessary during a competition. After the competition, any deficits can be corrected by consuming foods whose content is high in sodium chloride and potassium.[4] When fluid losses in excess of 4 liters per hour are anticipated, the team physician may recommend some electrolyte replacement during the competition.

Weight Control During the period when muscles are being developed some weight gain is experienced. A shift from fatty tissue to lean tissue also occurs. After seasonal activity in sports athletes need to reduce their caloric intake or substitute other activities of equal energy output, so that weight remains at desirable levels.

Athletes who must meet specific weight requirements, as for wrestling, should achieve the necessary weight loss by losing fat, not water. A nutritionally adequate low-calorie diet and the maintenance of physical activity over a period of time will accomplish such weight loss. Starvation and dehydration reduce effective performance and are dangerous.

Carbohydrate Loading The ability to sustain peak performance over an extended period of time (as in a marathon race) is influenced by the availability of muscle glycogen. To build up glycogen stores, two phases of preparation are recommended: First, about a week before the competition, the athlete exercises vigorously to deplete glycogen stores and consumes a diet high in protein and fat and restricted to about 100 g carbohydrate. Second, after 2 to 3 days of the glycogen-depleting phase, a diet low in fat, moderate in protein, and high in carbohydrate (250 to 500 g) is consumed for 3 to 4 days. Complex carbohydrates that also furnish minerals and vitamins are preferred to simple sugars.[5]

Carbohydrate loading is not recommended for short-term competition, since it can lead to a feeling of heaviness that is a disadvantage in high-intensity competition. Occasional adverse effects of carbohydrate loading including myoglobinuria, chest pains, and change in the electrocardiogram have been observed when glycogen loading has been used persistently. Carbohydrate loading is not advised for athletes in early adolescence and should be used no more than two or three times a year by high school- and college-age athletes.[3]

Pregame Meal Exercise immediately after a meal could lead to nausea, vomiting, distention, and cramping. In addition the blood flow is diverted to the gastrointestinal tract and not to the working muscles. A rapidly digested meal low in fat, moderately low in protein, and high in complex carbohydrate should be eaten 3 to 5 hours before the competition. It may include some lean meat, fish, or poultry, vegetables, fruits, bread, and 250 to 500 ml beverage. Contrary to popular opinion, there is no evidence that milk needs to be omitted. Because of their diuretic effects, coffee, tea, beer, and caffeine-containing soft drinks should be avoided. Athletes sometimes have strong opinions about specific foods that will help them win; such preferences should be respected within the general bounds of good nutrition and fluid balance. Nutritionally complete liquid meals can be fed much closer to the event because of their rapid gastric emptying time. They aid in hydration and help avoid the pregame nausea experienced by some athletes.

Ergogenic Properties Substances that increase the ability to work are ERGOGENIC AIDS. There is no evidence that wheat germ, honey, bee pollen, lecithin, protein supplements, gelatin, brewer's yeast, sunflower seeds, vitamin E, ascorbic acid, or vitamin-mineral supplements have any special value in promoting endurance or skills.[3]

Importance of Weight Control

The problem of overweight is one of great frustration for many North Americans. Relative affluence, abundance of a wide variety of foods, and lack of physical activity are a few of the factors that contribute to excessive calorie intake for many. Numerous weight reduction regimens have been described; yet the long-term success rate with all of these is limited. Because of the difficulty in achieving and maintaining appropriate weight once obesity is established, emphasis must be on prevention of over-weight beginning early in life. Several approaches to weight control are de-scribed in this chapter. None of these is appropriate for all patients; nevertheless, each has advantages for certain patients.

Hazards of Obesity The health consequences of obesity have been studied both retrospectively and prospectively. Life insurance statistics provide retrospective data suggesting that life expectancy is shorter in individuals who weigh more than the average of the population being studied, especially among those who are overweight at younger ages.[6]

In morbidly obese men, the mortality is markedly higher than that of the U.S. male population as a whole. A longitudinal study of 200 morbidly obese men revealed a 12-fold excess mortality rate in 25- to 34-year-olds and a sixfold increase in 35- to 44-year olds. The most common cause of death in these men was cardiovascular disease; the incidence was 30 percent higher than that of U.S. males in general. Obesity appeared to favor the development of degenerative diseases at an earlier age, with more rapid progression to clinical events.[7]

Prospective studies have shown that obesity correlates with increased incidence of hypertension, impaired glucose tolerance, increased plasma insulin levels, gallbladder disease, elevated serum lipid levels, with the exception of HDL-cholesterol, and hyperuricemia. Correction of the obesity is associated with improvement in these parameters.[8] The obese are at increased risk for cardiovascular disease. The Framingham Heart Study showed that obesity is a significant independent predictor of cardiovascular disease.[6,9] Data from both the Framingham Study and the Manitoba Study indicated that morbidity and mortality from cardiovascular disease increase with the duration of overweight.[6]

Obesity entails a respiratory cost in normal persons by increased work of breathing, a decrease in lung volume, and pulmonary hypertension. In any person with chronic pulmonary disorders such as emphysema and asthma obesity greatly increases the respiratory stress. The hazards of surgery and of pregnancy and childbirth are multiplied in the presence of excessive adipose tissue.

Overweight is a physical handicap as well as a primary health hazard. Obese people are more uncomfortable during warm weather because the thick layers of fat serve as an insulator. More effort must be expended to do a given amount of work because of the increase in body mass. Because of their lessened agility, obese people are more susceptible to accidents. Fatigue, backache, and foot troubles are common complaints of the obese.

Obesity and Faddism For a significant portion of the American population, weight control is a perplexing problem. For many, constant vigilance is necessary to prevent gain of unwanted pounds and for maintenance of the slim physique so highly valued in the American culture. This cultural attitude toward slimness is evident everywhere—television and magazine ads for reducing aids such as low-calorie formula diets, appetite suppressants, and special clothing designed to promote quick weight loss; use of slim models in advertising everything from clothing to work tools; book clubs and bookstores with their abundance of books on reducing diets—such books are frequently best sellers; women's magazines—practically every month one of these has a new weight-loss diet; drugstores and supermarkets which feature a wide variety of reducing candies, "dietetic" and "low-calorie" items. Especially among American women emphasis on slimness contrasts sharply with that of other cultures, southern Europe, for example, where women generally weigh more than their American counterparts.

Evaluation of Weight Status and Body Composition

Ideal or Desirable Weight Reference is often made to "ideal" or "desirable" weight. The term "ideal" body weight was used in the first Metropolitan Life Insurance Company weight tables, published in 1942, to express the concept of normal weight, which was defined as the weight associated with the least mortality.[10] It represented the average weight for each inch of height at age 30 for males and at age 25 for females. Persons with the lightest weights at each height were arbitrarily designated as having a small frame, those in the upper weight ranges as large frame, and those in between the lower and upper ranges as medium frame. The tables were intended to encourage persons to keep their weight below the average for their height. Before the development of the tables, maintenance of average weight for height was believed to be optimal for health, and it was considered normal to gain weight as one progressed from young adulthood to middle age and beyond.

The Metropolitan Life weight tables were revised in 1959. In these tables the term "desirable" weight was used to indicate weights associated with the least mortality.[6] The new tables were based on pooled data from 26 life insurance companies in the United States and Canada, representing nearly 5 million insured persons, from 1935 to 1954. Average weights for each

inch of height were compiled for men and women 25 years and older. As in the earlier table, ranges of weight were given for small, medium, and large frames, but the criteria for determining frame size were not specified.

The 1983 revision of the tables was based on weight data associated with the lowest mortality in some 4 million insured adults in the United States and Canada from 1954 to 1972. The terms "ideal body weight" and "desirable" body weight were not used in the 1983 revision because of the confusion resulting from the use of these terms.

The 1983 tables assumed indoor clothing weighing 5 pounds for men and 3 pounds for women, and a one inch heel height for both men and women. Instructions for determining frame size using elbow breadth were included inasmuch as the National Health and Nutrition Examination Survey, 1971–74 (NHANES I) data had indicated that elbow breadth is useful in determining frame size. However, no physical measurements of elbow breadth were taken for subjects represented in the Metropolitan Life tables. The tables assume that the population is distributed so that one half has a "medium" frame, one fourth, a "small" frame, and one fourth, a "large" frame.[10]

The Metropolitan Life tables are often used as a reference in evaluating weights of individuals. Nevertheless, several considerations pertaining to data collection should be kept in mind when using the tables:

1. The tables are based on data obtained more than a decade ago from a large group of insured, presumably healthy persons and are not representative of the population as a whole. Persons with diseases such as diabetes mellitus, heart disease, or cancer were excluded.
2. Although the weights listed in the tables are those associated with the least mortality over time, the weights were obtained when individuals applied for insurance, and the average length of follow-up was less than 7 years.[6]
3. Standardized technique was not used in obtaining weights used in the tables. Insurance applicants were weighed by many different physicians and nurses using various kinds of weighing apparatus; in all likelihood many of the machines were not calibrated. The type of clothing, the time of day, the season, and whether the subject was in a fasting or postabsorptive state when weighed were not reported.
4. Although 90 percent of subjects were actually weighed, the percentage of heights that were actually measured is not given. Some evidence indi-

cates that self-reported heights and weights tend to be inaccurate.[11,12]

5. The tables are based on data from persons 25 to 59 years of age. Applicability of the tables to older adults has been questioned.[13]

6. Finally, the average adult experiences a lifetime loss of height of approximately 1 inch in males and 2 inches in females. Concern has been expressed regarding the appropriateness of the tables for these persons.[13]

Average Weights The National Center for Health Statistics obtained weights and heights and other health indicators from some 13,645 persons who participated in the National Health and Nutrition Examination Survey of 1971–74.[14] Although the sample size was considerably smaller than that represented by the Metropolitan Life tables, the NHANES I data were based on a national probability sample and are representative of the civilian noninstitutionalized population aged 18 to 74 in the United States. Cross-sectional data were used—that is, subjects were weighed only once for the survey; follow-up over time was not done. The tables represent average weights for height, age, and sex of the population. (See Tables A-17, A-18.) Standardized techniques were used in weighing and measuring all participants. Calibrated scales were used. Subjects wore disposable paper examination gowns and foam rubber slippers. The total weight of clothing ranged from 0.20 to 0.62 pounds and is included in the weights shown in the tables. However, weights were obtained at various times of the day in different seasons, and subjects may have been in the fasting or fed state.

Average weights of the population are generally greater than the weights associated with the least mortality in insured persons. The latter are 10 to 20 pounds below the average weight in men and up to 5 pounds below average weight in women.[10] Average weight tends to increase with height and with age in both men and women. In men, average weights increase rapidly until 25 to 34 years and peak at 35 to 44 years for those whose height is 68 inches or more, and at 45 to 54 years for those less than 68 inches. Women tend to increase weight rapidly until 35 to 44 years of age. The rate of gain slows in the next decade, peaks at 55 to 64 years, and declines thereafter.[14]

Reference Weights The best weight for a given individual's age, height, bone structure, and muscular development is unknown. Height–weight tables provide a rough guide for estimating weight, but clinical judgment must be used in applying the information,

since the tables do not provide information on body composition.

Generally speaking, a deviation of not more than 10 percent above or below that listed for a given height and frame size is considered acceptable by many practitioners. Persons who are 10 to 20 percent above the reference weight are described as OVERWEIGHT. OBESITY refers to an excess of body fat as determined by measurement of triceps and subscapular skinfolds. However, some clinicians consider persons whose weight is 20 to 40 percent above the reference weight to be *mildly obese*, those 40 to 100 percent over the reference weight as *moderately obese*, and those 100 percent or more overweight as *severely* or *morbidly obese*.

Others use the *body mass index* (see inside back cover) as an indicator of obesity as it correlates highly with weight. Values between 24 and 27 in women or 25 to 27 in men indicate overweight; those over 27 indicate obesity.[15]

Body Composition The concern in prevention and management of obesity is not the overweight per se, but the excessive amount of adipose tissue that accompanies the extra weight. Some persons have an excess of body fat, although body weight falls within an acceptable range according to height–weight tables. These persons are obese, according to NHANES criteria. Others, such as football players, are overweight by the usual height–weight standards, yet have well-developed musculature and are not overfat. Still others are overweight due to fluid accumulation occurring in certain illnesses.

Body fatness can be measured by determining the thickness of subcutaneous tissues at designated body locations by means of calipers. (See Chapter 23 for a description of tests used to determine body composition.) The subscapular skinfold provides a better indication of fatness than does the triceps skinfold; nevertheless, the triceps skinfold is frequently used since it is conveniently measured.

For accuracy in classifying individuals as overweight or obese, determination of *both* body weight and skinfold thickness is needed. Persons above either the 85th or 95th percentile in both are classified as obese.[16]

Estimation of Weight Loss Adipose tissue in adults consists of about 75 percent fat, 23 percent water, and small amounts of protein and mineral salts.[17] Each kilogram of adipose tissue represents 7,700 kcal (1 pound = 3,500 kcal). An individual who consumes 100 kcal in excess daily ingests an excess of 3,000 kcal by the end of 1 month. Theoretically, this would result in a weight gain of 0.4 kg monthly, or 4.8 kg (about 10 lb) in a year. The weight gain from consistently overeating by this amount over a 5- to 10-year period would be considerable. It requires about 2 teaspoons of butter, or two 1-inch squares of fudge, or an oatmeal cookie to supply the additional 100 kcal each day.

Conversely, the loss of 1 kg of adipose tissue means that the diet would be deficient by 7,700 kcal for the total time period of the weight loss. A young woman requiring 2,000 kcal a day to meet her energy needs who consumes a diet that supplies only 1,200 kcal has a weekly deficit of 5,600 kcal, and the predicted adipose tissue loss would be 5600 ÷ 7,700 or 0.7 kg (1.6 pounds).

Weight loss does not always follow the predicted straight line for several reasons:

1. The type of diet may influence losses—on very-low-carbohydrate diets rapid weight loss occurs initially, due principally to losses of sodium, potassium, and water; on more conventional diets, such losses are less conspicuous.
2. As weight loss continues, the basal metabolic rate per unit of active tissue mass declines, resulting in a slower rate of weight loss.
3. The energy cost of activity decreases as a function of lower body weight. Furthermore, subjects tend to decrease overall activity in response to reduced caloric intakes.
4. Adherence to the diet may change over time.

The composition of the tissue losses is influenced by the dietary regimen. Losses of protein, fat, and water are greatest during total fasting; protein and fat losses are similar on isocaloric ketogenic (high fat) diets and mixed diets. Greater water losses on a ketogenic compared to a mixed diet give the appearance of a more rapid weight loss. Introduction of carbohydrate following use of total fast or a ketogenic diet is associated with a temporary weight gain due to fluid retention.

Obesity

Incidence The incidence of overweight and obesity among adults in the United States is high. The HANES data indicated that 19 percent of men and 28 percent of women are obese, if the 85th percentile is used as a cutting point.[18] (See Table 25-3.) Based on triceps and subscapular skinfolds, 3 percent of men and 5 to 6 percent of women are severely obese, using the 95th percentile as a criterion.[18]

Table 25-3. Overweight and Obesity Among Adults in the United States*

	Males		Females	
	Millions	Percent	Millions	Percent
Overweight, not obese	6.0	10.5	5.1	8.0
Obese, not overweight	3.8	6.6	3.9	6.1
Overweight and obese	7.3	12.7	13.8	21.5

* 85th percentile was used as cutting point.

† Adapted from Abraham, S., et al.: *Obese and Overweight Adults in the United States.* National Center for Health Statistics, Hyattsville, Md., 1983. DHHS Pub. (PHS) 83–1680. Vital and Health Statistics. Series II (230): 1–93, 1983.

Causes Obesity is invariably caused by an intake of calories beyond the body's need for energy. Theoretically, it can easily be corrected by bringing the energy intake and expenditure into balance; practically speaking, however, this is not easily accomplished. The reasons for an existing imbalance are many and complex, and some understanding of the problems of the individual must be gained before therapy can be effectively instituted. A thorough physical examination, a dietary history, and an investigation of habits relating to activity, rest, and family and social relationships are indicated.

Food Habits. Eating too much becomes a habit for many people. Sometimes this is the result of ignorance of the calorie value of food. The amounts of food are not necessarily excessive, but it is the extra foods, beyond the calorie need, that account for the gradual increase in weight, for example, the extra pats of butter, the spoonful of jelly, the second roll, the preference for a rich dessert, or the TV snack. Eating too much may result from having to maintain social relationships including rich party foods in addition to usual mealtime eating. Excessive amounts of carbohydrate-rich foods are sometimes eaten because they are cheaper than lower-calorie fruits and vegetables.

Activity Patterns. Many persons continue to gain weight throughout life because they fail to adjust their appetites to reduced energy needs. The many labor-saving devices in homes and in industry reduce the energy requirement. Most people enjoy sports as spectators rather than as participants. Riding rather than walking to school or work is common practice even for short distances. Other circumstances may further reduce the energy needs: (1) basal metabolism is gradually decreased from year to year (see Chapter 8); (2) changes in occupation may result in reduced activity;

(3) the middle years of life sometimes bring about a repose and consequent reduction of muscle tension; (4) periods of quiet relaxation and sleep may be increased; and (5) disabling illness such as arthritis or cardiac disease may reduce markedly the need for calories.

Psychologic Factors. For the individual who is bored, lonely, discontented, or depressed, eating can be a solace. Food often becomes the focal point of the day for those with little else to do or who are not motivated to seek another outlet for their problems.

Genetic Influences. Several investigators have shown that there is a high correlation between obesity in parents and their children. Data from the Ten-State Nutrition Survey indicate that triceps skinfold is greater in children whose parents are obese than in children of lean parents. By age 17, children of two obese parents are three times as fat as children of two lean parents.[19] Mayer noted that if both parents are of normal weight, only 7 percent of children will be obese; if one parent is obese, the incidence in children is 40 percent, and it climbs to 80 percent if both parents are obese.[20] Mayer's observations led him to conclude that food habits alone do not explain these differences; furthermore, he found a correlation between obesity and body build. The *endomorphic* or round, soft individual gains weight readily, whereas the *ectomorphic* or slender, wiry person rarely becomes overweight. This does not mean that obesity is inevitable for the endomorph, but it does mean that constant vigilance is required to avoid it.

Metabolic Abnormalities. Only a small percentage of obese cases can be attributed to endocrine disorders. A deficiency of the thyroid gland can reduce the basal metabolism, but overweight from this cause can be prevented if the diet is sufficiently restricted in calories.

A number of biochemical parameters are altered in obesity. These include abnormal glucose tolerance and elevations in fasting levels of plasma glucose, insulin, glucagon, free fatty acids, triglycerides, cholesterol, and uric acid. These tend to revert to normal as the individual loses weight.

Types of Obesity Based on anatomical characteristics of adipose tissue two types of obesity have been described.[21] *Hyperplasia*, characterized by an increased *number* of fat cells, as much as three to five times normal, occurs in childhood. Fat cells may or

may not be enlarged. In adult-onset obesity, the cells are greatly *enlarged*, or *hypertrophied*. The number of fat cells may be normal or increased. Fat distribution is likely to be centralized in this type, whereas the extremities are involved in the hyperplastic type.

Formerly it was believed that fat cell number increased early in life and in adolescence but stabilized thereafter. Weight gain or loss was thought to be characterized by changes in cell size but not in cell number. It is now known that after excessive energy intake for prolonged periods, cell number in adults can increase, perhaps stimulated when fat cells reach a maximum size. Similarly, after extensive weight reduction, the size of fat cells may decrease below detectable limits.

Conceivably the adult-onset type of obesity might have a better prognosis for achieving normal weight than the hyperplastic type would, due to the latter's greatly increased number of fat cells and the biologic tendency to keep them filled. Such persons may experience persistent symptoms of hunger similar to those seen in normal-weight persons in starvation.[22] However, some research suggests that the type of adipose tissue obesity is not a predictor of success in maintaining weight loss.[23] The activity of lipoprotein lipase increases during weight reduction, and the resultant increase in uptake of fatty acids may have a role in excess energy storage in the cell.[22] The risk of medical complications is thought to be related to the size of the fat cells; thus, decreasing the cells to normal size by weight reduction may lower risk.[22]

Classification of obesity on the basis of fat cell characteristics is not yet feasible in the clinical setting because the techniques for fat cell biopsy are not generally available. However, valuable clues can be obtained from the history of onset, biochemical alterations, and type of fat distribution.

Prevention of Obesity

Identifying Those Who Are Likely to Become Obese The most vigorous efforts to prevent obesity should be directed to those individuals who are most susceptible, namely, children of obese parents and children who have stocky frames. Certain periods of life are also likely to bring about obesity. Men of normal weight often begin to gain weight in the 20s and early 30s and women are more likely to gain in the mid-30s and 40s.[14] Following pregnancy weight gain is common. If these trends are recognized, the individual can elect to reduce caloric intake, or increase exercise, or both.

Education for Prevention The best hope for the prevention of obesity is through greatly expanded programs of nutrition education directed particularly to schoolchildren, teenagers, and mothers. The pattern for obesity is often set in infancy when the mother overfeeds the baby in the erroneous belief that a "fat baby is a healthy baby." Sometimes overeating becomes a habit with a child after an illness because the mother keeps urging food upon the child through her concern for his or her state of nutrition. During adolescent years food is often used to submerge the many problems that face the boy and girl. By recognizing these trends, the mother can do much to redirect the food habits. The education of the mother in terms of weight control for her family and the education of the child in the elementary and secondary school can be effective.

Increased Activity. In these times of affluence, mechanization, and automation many individuals become overweight because of lack of exercise. A pattern of activity is best taught during childhood and must also be emphasized during the school years. Too often competitive sports exclude the child who most needs the exercise. Physical education should be directed to those activities that are likely to carry over into adult life.

Treatment of Obesity

The essential components of treatment include behavior modification, calorie restriction, nutrition education, and exercise. Two criteria must be satisfied if the treatment is to be considered successful: (1) weight loss must be such that desirable weight according to body frame and state of health is achieved; and (2) the desired weight must be maintained.

Assessment of the Patient The treatment of obesity is a frustrating problem to the physician, nutritionist, and nurse because failures are so frequent. To a patient a failure can be demoralizing. Therefore, it is important that each patient be evaluated in terms of his or her medical and dietary history and emotional stability. Screening clients before beginning treatment identifies those who are highly motivated to lose weight and who have the social support and coping strategies needed to succeed. Weight reduction should be guided by a physician, since the physiologic and psychologic stresses of weight loss are not well tolerated by all. Brownell[22] emphasized the importance of social support for the individual determined to lose weight. Involvement of the spouse or other family members, fellow workers, or peers at school may all have a very positive influence in the treatment of obesity.

Some persons lose weight satisfactorily when shown how to keep the calorie intake within prescribed limits; others benefit from group methods or behavior modification; for others, a program designed to promote rapid weight loss initially is an important motivating factor.

Behavior Modification This is based on the premise that excessive food intake is a learned response that can be changed. By means of this concept the individual learns to focus attention on the environmental factors that influence his or her food intake and gradually to modify these so that a change in eating habits and subsequent weight loss occurs.

Initially the client is asked to keep a detailed record of food intake and activity patterns. From this, the client and counselor identify problem areas and outline strategies to overcome them. Emphasis is on changing eating patterns rather than on caloric intake or pounds lost. For example, if the problem is too much unstructured eating, such as frequent snacking while watching television, knitting or other activities might be recommended as a diversion. Some techniques that have been used successfully to control food intake include (1) eating only at specified times and places; (2) learning to eat more slowly; (3) omitting other activities, such as reading or watching television while eating; (4) using smaller plates and placing portions directly on the plate rather than serving family style; (5) use of a reward system; and so on. Individualized stepwise behavioral changes are sought.

The behavioral approach to weight control involves detailed record keeping by the client; thus, it is not suitable for all. Not all such programs include nutrition education in the essentials of a well-balanced diet. Subjects may thus lose weight initially by eliminating excessive eating, yet fail to improve their nutritional habits.

The long-term efficacy of behavior modification for weight control is not known. Some studies have indicated that attrition is lower for behavior modification programs than for other approaches. Nevertheless, for most subjects, weight loss by the end of the program is modest, 5 to 15 pounds, and only a small percentage of subjects achieve substantial weight loss after termination of the program.[22] At 1 year follow-up, patients treated by behavior modification tend to have less weight gain than do others.

Self-help Groups Some persons find that group support, such as that provided by TOPS or Weight Watchers, is a valuable aid in helping them continue a weight-reduction program. Most of these groups require the individual to weigh in at a weekly meeting; some charge a small fee. These groups are most effective for persons who need to lose only a modest amount of weight, and the attrition rate is relatively high after a few months. Weight losses of those who remain are modest, and there is no evidence that the weight losses are maintained.

Calorie-Restricted Diets Many widely accepted nutritionally sound diets are available and are designed to bring about steady weight loss, to establish good food habits, and to promote a sense of well-being. Such diets must be palatable, must fit into the framework of family food habits, and must not require additional expense or long preparation time. Basic considerations in planning weight-reduction diets include the following:

Energy. A diet that provides 800 to 1,000 kcal below the daily requirement leads to a loss of 3 to 4 kg (6 to 8 pounds) monthly. This gradual loss does not result in severe hunger, nervous exhaustion, and weakness that often accompany drastic reduction regimens. For most men 1,400 to 1,600 kcal is a satisfactory level, and for women 1,200 to 1,400 kcal are indicated. Diets that supply 1,000 kcal or less are rarely necessary except for individuals who are bedfast. In many elderly persons satisfactory weight loss is achieved only when energy intake is limited to 1,000 to 1,200 kcal; this is because of their reduced basal metabolism and reduced physical activity.

Protein. Although 0.8 g protein per kg desirable body weight is sufficient, an allowance of 1.5 g per kg improves the satiety value of the diet. Most dietary plans can include 70 to 100 g protein daily.

Fat and Carbohydrate. Many diets drastically restrict the fat intake and allow a moderate carbohydrate intake. (See the 1,000-kcal diet in Table 25-4.) Some patients prefer a more liberal fat intake and a reduced carbohydrate level, as in the high-protein moderate-fat 1,500 kcal diet. (See Table 25-4.)

Minerals and Vitamins. A multivitamin preparation, iron salts, and possibly calcium are indicated for diets containing 1,000 kcal or less. Calorie-restricted diets for obese children must be planned with the increased mineral and vitamin requirements in mind.

Table 25-4.   Food Allowances for Calorie-Restricted Diets

	Normal Protein, Moderate Carbohydrate, Low to Moderate Fat			High Protein, Low Carbohydrate, Moderate Fat
	1,000 kcal (exchanges)*	1,200 kcal (exchanges)	1,500 kcal (exchanges)	1,500 kcal (exchanges)
Starch/bread	2	3	5	2
Meat				
Lean	—	—	—	4
Medium fat	5	5	6	5
Vegetables	1	1	2	2
Freelist	As desired	As desired	As desired	As desired
Fruit	3	3	3	2
Milk, skim	3	—	—	—
Low fat	—	3	3	3
Fat	1	1	2	5
Nutritive value				
Carbohydrate, g	116	131	166	106
Protein, g	67	70	85	97
Fat, g	30	45	55	77
Energy, kcal	1,002	1,209	1,499	1,505

* See Table A-4 for Exchange Lists.

For these reasons the diets used for them are usually less restricted.

Daily Meal Patterns The diets in Table 25-4 have been calculated with the food exchange lists. (See Table A-4.) The vitamin and mineral values in most instances equal or exceed the RDA; the levels of some trace minerals such as zinc, copper, and others may be marginal.

These diets include 3 cups of milk, thus enhancing the calcium intake, and also providing a convenient bedtime snack, if desired. Some adults will prefer 2 cups of milk and more meat. This can be arranged by substituting one medium-fat meat exchange for 1 cup of skim milk. The caloric exchange for 1 cup of 2 percent milk would be one medium-fat and one low-fat meat exchange, thus giving a higher protein intake.

A great deal of flexibility in food choices is possible with the exchange lists. One important consideration is the satiety value of the diet. Inasmuch as proteins and fats remain in the stomach longer, the protein and fat allowance should be divided approximately equally between the three meals. Some plans permit six meals a day instead of three; in these, some protein should be provided at each feeding.

Foods to Restrict or Avoid. The individual who learns to select foods in appropriate amounts from the exchange lists does not require specific lists of foods to avoid. For some persons, however, it may help create calorie consciousness if listings of concentrated foods are provided. Part of the success of a reducing diet depends upon learning to be content with smaller portions of food and less concentrated foods. Some of the foods in the following list are permitted in specified amounts in the exchange lists, but others are best avoided altogether.

HIGH-FAT FOODS: butter, margarine, cheese, chocolate, cream, ice cream, fat meat, fatty fish, or fish canned in oil, fried foods of any kind such as doughnuts and potato chips, gravies, nuts, oil, pastries, and salad dressing

---

Sample Meal Patterns

	Normal Protein, Moderate Carbohydrate, Moderate Fat (1,500 kcal)	High Protein Low Carbohydrate, Moderate Fat (1,500 kcal)
BREAKFAST		
Unsweetened citrus fruit	1 exchange	1 exchange
Eggs	1	2
Bread	2 slices	1 slice
Butter or margarine	1 teaspoon	1 teaspoon
Milk, 2 percent fat	1 cup	1 cup
Coffee or tea		
LUNCH		
Meat, poultry, or fish	2 oz, medium-fat	4 oz, lean
Vegetable, raw or cooked	1 exchange	1 exchange
Bread	1 slice	None
Butter or margarine	1 teaspoon	2 teaspoons
Unsweetened fruit	1 exchange	1 exchange
Milk, 2 percent fat	1 cup	1 cup
DINNER		
Meat, poultry, or fish	3 oz, medium-fat	3 oz, medium-fat
Starch/bread	2 exchanges	1 exchange
Vegetable	1 exchange	1 exchange
FREE LIST		
Fruit	1 exchange	—
Milk, 2 percent fat	1 cup	1 cup
Fat	—	2 exchanges
Coffee or tea, if desired		

HIGH-CARBOHYDRATE FOODS: breads of any kind, candy, cake, cookies, corn, cereal products such as macaroni, noodles, spaghetti, pancakes, waffles, sweetened or dried fruits, legumes such as lima beans, navy beans, dried peas, potatoes, sweet potatoes, honey, molasses, sugar, syrup, rich puddings, sweets

BEVERAGES: all fountain drinks, including malted milks and chocolate, carbonated beverages of all kinds, rich sundaes, alcoholic drinks, sweetened drink mixes

Other Dietary Regimens Commercial low-calorie meal substitutes, as *formulas* in liquid or powder form, cookies, and combination dishes are popular. Generally, they are nutritionally adequate and possess the advantages of convenience and strict calorie control. Some persons find them useful initially while they are learning the essentials of dietary planning. Others substitute these preparations for one meal a day.

The principal disadvantages of the formula diets are these: (1) they do not retrain the individual to a new pattern of food habits that must be followed once the weight is lost; (2) they are monotonous if used for a long period of time; and (3) they may be constipating for some patients, whereas others occasionally experience diarrhea.

Starvation. Total starvation for weeks or months has been used in treatment of persons who fail to achieve weight loss by conventional methods. Prolonged fasting requires hospitalization to monitor for side effects that include postural hypotension, acidosis, transient liver and kidney impairment, and hyperuricemia. Rapid weight loss is accompanied by substantial loss of lean body mass in addition to adipose tissue loss. Subjects who are overweight, but not obese, tend to have greater losses of body weight and nitrogen during fasting than do the obese. The large losses of lean body mass that occur in these subjects concern many workers, and some have suggested that total fasting for weight reduction be used only for very obese persons.

One group has shown that during caloric restriction cumulative nitrogen balance is highly correlated with the serum insulin concentration. This, in turn, is related to total body fat mass. Thus, the hyperinsulinism of obese subjects with greater fat stores helps preserve protein homeostasis. In overweight subjects without massive fat stores, the lower serum insulin concentration may not be sufficient to prevent protein catabolism nor to stimulate protein synthesis enough to offset losses of lean tissue.[24] Theoretically, protein supplementation would replace some of the nitrogen losses in these subjects. Unfortunately, most subjects

who fast tend to rapidly regain the lost weight when the fast is discontinued because they have not been educated to adopt a new pattern of eating habits.

Protein-Sparing Modified Fast. Decreased losses of body protein have been reported with use of the protein-sparing modified fast which provides approximately 400 kcal per day and consists of 1.5 g of high-quality protein per kg of desirable body weight. No other calorie sources are permitted. Vitamin and mineral supplements are needed. About 2 g potassium and 5 g sodium chloride are used to prevent orthostatic hypotension. Modifications of this regimen permit a small amount of carbohydrate in the diet. Nitrogen metabolism is not significantly different on the latter diet compared to the hypocaloric protein diet, but sodium depletion is less, thus lessening the possibility of orthostatic hypotension. These programs require careful medical supervision, but not hospitalization. The long-term results in maintaining weight loss do not appear to be any more promising than with other approaches for the majority of persons; nevertheless, some individuals will find this approach to be highly effective.

Very-Low-Calorie Liquid Diets. During the 1970s use of very-low-calorie (less than 800 kcal) liquid formula diets was popular. Rapid weight loss occurred when the formulas were used as the sole source of calories. Most were composed of poor-quality protein and were deficient in several minerals. Unfortunately, a number of deaths were reported with use of the formulas. Subsequently, low-calorie liquid formulas composed of 35 to 70 g high-quality protein, 30 to 45 g carbohydrate, and supplemented with vitamins and minerals were developed. Various groups have found these diets safe when used for limited periods in patients who have been carefully screened and who are closely monitored throughout the diet. Supplementary vitamins and minerals are customarily given.[25]

Ketogenic Diets. Periodically, low-carbohydrate ketogenic diets are publicized as an aid to rapid weight reduction. Advocates of these diets claim that one need not be concerned about calorie intake as long as carbohydrate is sharply restricted or even eliminated from the diet and that the diet will produce more rapid weight loss than more conventional calorie-restricted diets. There is no scientific evidence that this type of diet is any more effective than better balanced diets in promoting weight reduction. Weight loss is attributed to a decrease in calorie intake as a result of the high satiety value of the diet, and to increased urinary excretion of water and sodium. Potential adverse effects include elevations in serum lipids, increased blood uric acid levels, postural hypotension, and fatigue. The effects of long-term ketosis are not known. The practicality of such diets for long-term weight reduction is questionable inasmuch as most subjects are unable to persevere in the regimen for long periods.

Exercise and Weight Loss   Moderate exercise on a consistent daily basis is an important aid in weight loss and should be a required component of any weight reduction program. The goals are to increase energy expenditure and to improve physical fitness. The exercise program should be planned in accordance with the guidelines discussed on page 363. (See Figure 25-1.) Contrary to popular opinion, moderate exercise does not lead to increased appetite; conversely, a diminution of activity does not lead to a corresponding decrease in appetite. On the other hand, passive exercise devices, such as mechanical vibrators and spot reducers, are ineffective methods of achieving loss of body fat. Some beneficial effects of regular sustained exercise include increased work capacity and cardiovascular efficiency, reduction in total fat stores, increased HDL-cholesterol, and improved muscle tone. Strenuous activity is accompanied by an increase in the metabolic rate for up to 24 hours; thus, expenditure of calories continues after the exercise is stopped. The attrition rate in exercise programs is as high as 50 percent.[22] Thus, it is important that the exercise program be enjoyable and easily incorporated into one's lifestyle.

Role of Hormones and Drugs   Most overweight persons have no deficiency of endocrine secretions and should not be led to believe that they have glandular disturbances, nor should they be exposed to the increased nervousness and irritability that result from such medication. Thyroid hormone is sometimes prescribed; however, it promotes loss of lean body mass rather than adipose tissue.

Anorexigenic drugs, such as amphetamines, are often used to suppress the appetite. These drugs are only temporarily effective, however, and require an ever-increasing dosage for sustained weight loss. They may produce insomnia, excitability, dryness of the mouth, gastrointestinal disturbances, and other toxic manifestations. For some patients they are a crutch and for others they have no effect on decreasing the appetite.

Figure 25-1.   Exercise such as bicycling is not only enjoyable but it also increases energy expenditure, thereby helping maintain normal weight. (Courtesy, National Association Plans, Inc. Philadelphia.)

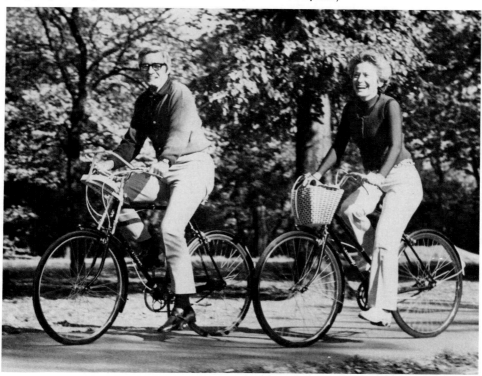

Human growth hormone offers theoretical advantages over other drugs, since it mobilizes fatty acids and decreases fat stores without enhancing nitrogen loss; however, inadequate supply and cost factors limit its potential use. Most drugs are of limited value in the treatment of obesity and should be used with great care because of the possibility of dependence and abuse.

DIETARY COUNSELING

Success in weight reduction is dependent on effective motivation and suitable knowledge.

Motivation and Psychologic Support   A diet prescription is worthless unless the client has some motivation for losing weight, such as the maintenance or recovery of health. The client must have the capacity for self-discipline, patience, and perseverance.

Although the motivation must come from within the client, the physician, nurse, and dietitian can be of immeasurable help toward initiating this motivation, and subsequently by providing encouragement and guidance at frequent follow-up visits. The client needs to understand that a calorie intake in excess of needs is the cause of overweight and that weight loss is accomplished only when the calorie intake is reduced below the client's needs. But this explanation is not enough. The client also needs to gain insight into the reasons he or she is overeating, and to work at correcting these.

Counseling and Group Sessions   Individual counseling is essential to determine the goals that are realistic for the client and to initiate a dietary regimen that is appropriate for the client's food habits and patterns of living. (See also Chapters 23 and 26.)

Group sessions are effective in that people compare their progress, share their problems in adhering to diets, and exchange ways to vary their diets. When groups are formed it is important that professional guidance be available from a physician, dietitian, or nurse. Each individual joining such a group should first be evaluated by the physician to determine his or her fitness for weight reduction.

Essential Knowledge   The dieter needs to understand that weight loss is accompanied by a reduction in the metabolic rate. This may explain the decreased rate of weight loss with time that many persons experience in spite of careful adherence to a calorie restricted diet. Further calorie restriction or increased energy expenditure will be required to continue weight loss. The importance of moderate regular exercise as an essential part of any weight reduction program should be pointed out to clients.

Most people are quite ignorant of the calorie values of foods. Each of the food exchange lists (Table A-4) provides a variety of foods that have approximately equal calorie values, and their consistent use helps to develop awareness of nutritive values. Many other tables of calorie values of foods are also available. Keeping a record of the daily calorie intake is useful, at least for a period of time. However, it is important that clear distinctions be made between the calorie values of foods that also supply protein, minerals, and vitamins and those foods that are principally carbohydrate and fat.

Portion control, taught by means of measuring cups, spoons, food models, or actual foods, is essential. Although a given diet is planned for a specific calorie level, it must be expected that the daily calorie intake may vary by as much as 200 to 300 kcal because of variations in food composition as well as in the precision of measurements.

Few dietetic foods are necessary. When fresh fruits are expensive or unavailable, water-packed canned fruits may be used. Artificial sweetening may be used if desired. Many low-calorie beverages currently available provide negligible calories.

Some clients ask about including cocktails and wine in their diets. If the physician permits these beverages, the client needs to know that each gram of alcohol supplies 7 kcal and that the calorie value of the beverage must be taken into consideration. A glass of dry table wine provides fewer calories than a cocktail. Usually an alcoholic beverage is restricted to one serving daily. (See Table A-1 for caloric values of alcoholic beverages.)

A single dinner in a restaurant can nullify careful adherence given to a diet for several days. Usually it is possible to select a clear soup, broiled or roasted meat without sauces, vegetables without sauces, and salad without dressing. Meat portions are likely to be larger than those allowed and the dieter will need to restrict intake to that allowed. The diet will not be exceeded too much if one foregoes the rolls, butter, and dessert. Many restaurants have menu selections suitable for dieters. For every dieter there are occasions when the limitations of the diet are exceeded, and such breaks in the dieting pattern should be anticipated. Each day gives an opportunity to begin again toward the goal of desired weight. Nevertheless, the person who has many social engagements will find it difficult to make the progress he or she would like to make. Occasionally, when one knows that the social event will make it difficult to keep within dietary restrictions, the intake at the preceding meal can be kept especially light. Most hostesses are very understanding about a guest who is on a diet and is therefore restricting the size of portions or letting some of the foods pass by without partaking of them.

Maintenance of Weight To lose weight is not easy; to maintain the desirable level of weight is even more difficult. The calorie-restricted diet planned with regard for the client's pattern of living also provides the basis for building a maintenance diet. The client must learn that a change in food habits is essential not only for losing weight but to maintain desirable weight. Thus, additions of foods should be made judiciously until weight is being kept constant at the desired level. It is important for the client to weigh himself or herself at weekly intervals or so in order to be sure that the foods added are in appropriate amounts.

If foods added for maintenance are also selected from the Daily Food Guide, the quality of the diet with respect to protein, minerals, and vitamins is thereby enhanced. On the other hand, the additions of concentrated high-calorie foods may be more difficult to control in amounts suitable for maintenance. For example, the sedentary person of middle age must continue to forego rich desserts and sweets except on rare occasions.

Eating Disorders

Just as psychologic factors have been noted as contributing to overeating, so they may contribute to eating too little food. Some patients with mental illness reject food to such an extent that severe weight loss results.

Anorexia Nervosa This psychiatric disorder is seen primarily in females with onset usually occurring in early adolescence. Most patients are from middle- and upper-class families. Epidemiological studies suggest an increased incidence of the disorder in recent years.[26] It is characterized by extreme weight loss, even to the point of emaciation, as a consequence of refusal to eat. Some authorities specify a weight loss of at least 25 percent for the diagnosis of anorexia nervosa.[27] Mortality rates in hospitalized patients range from 5 to 20 percent in various series. The individual often has a history of being "chubby" as a youngster. An over-riding desire to lose weight leads to self-imposed starvation, bizarre food habits, self-induced vomiting, hyperactivity, laxative abuse, and so on as means of preventing weight gain. The individual usually is able to carry on normal school and social activities while denying hunger and fatigue. Amenorrhea,

constipation, cold intolerance, hypotension, and bradycardia are characteristic findings. Visceral protein levels are adequate and cellular immunity is generally maintained. Anemia is not a common feature; serum iron and folate levels are normal. Hypercarotenemia is common. Plasma zinc, copper, and total iron-binding capacity are reduced.[28] The clinical signs and symptoms are reversible with weight gain.

Treatment. Every effort is made to avoid hospitalization; however, for some individuals, short-term intervention as tube feeding or total parenteral feeding is needed to prevent death by starvation. Ultimately, individual and family psychotherapy is needed to resolve the basic conflict. Various approaches are used to encourage resumption of normal eating patterns. Behavior modification is used in conjunction with other therapies. The initial goal is to prevent further weight loss and to establish regular eating patterns. The diet is planned to meet basal energy requirements with small weekly increments in calories until the desired weight is reached. In one setting weekly meetings between the patient and the dietitian are held in order to reinforce the importance of increasing calorie intake until the goal weight is reached.[29] Gradual changes in eating patterns and weight gain are sought. Once the goal weight is reached a plan for weight maintenance is formulated. Continued support and follow-up from the dietitian are essential. Another approach uses a contract between patient and therapist, in which privileges accorded the patient depend on achievement of a predetermined weight gain each day. Failure to gain the expected amount of weight results in suspension of privileges and use of supplemental feedings or tube feedings until the desired weight gain is reached.[30]

Bulimia This eating disorder is characterized by episodes of binge eating, or rapid intake of large amounts of high calorie food. When binge eating is accompanied by self-induced vomiting the term *bulimarexia* is used.[31]

The typical bulimic individual is in his or her late teens or early 20s. Most begin binging in order to lose weight, and the repeated episodes become habitual. A typical pattern involves binge eating several times daily for a few days. Large amounts of high calorie sweets or starchy foods are rapidly eaten, followed by self-induced vomiting, and laxative or diuretic abuse. A history of substance abuse (alcohol or drugs) is common. Both individual and group therapy are used. Individual nutrition counseling is also offered. Patients fear they will gain weight if they stop purging. By actively participating with the dietitian in planning the diet to meet their energy and nutrient needs, patients retain control and satisfactory intake is more likely. Bulimic individuals usually do not become severely malnourished. Unless the individual is more than 15 percent under his or her appropriate weight, a weight-maintenance diet is planned, and patients are taught to use the food exchange lists in selecting meals. Counting calories is discouraged, however. This approach permits the patient to discuss any nutritional concerns in detail, provides a source of reliable nutrition information, assures the patient of the dietitian's interest and support, and permits time spent with other counselors to focus on issues other than food.[32]

Underweight

Casual observation of most segments of society in the United States and Canada reveals that undernutrition and protein deficiency are not major problems in North America; in fact, quite the opposite appears to be true—overnutrition appears to be much more common than undernutrition. Nevertheless, persons affected by these conditions, especially the poor and elderly, enjoy less than optimal health because of fatigue, weight loss, and lowered resistance to infection.

To some extent, undernutrition and protein deficiency go hand in hand; those who are visibly undernourished are often found to be deficient in protein. On the other hand, some persons who do not appear to be undernourished, are, in fact, deficient in protein. With the availability of various types of nutritional support, both conditions are potentially reversible.

Causes Failure to ingest sufficient calories to meet the energy requirement results in underweight. Not infrequently this occurs in people who are very active, tense, and nervous, and who obtain too little rest. Sometimes irregular habits of eating and poor selection of foods are responsible for an inadequate calorie intake. Smokers generally weigh less than nonsmokers, and may make up a significant proportion of those at the low end of weight for height tables. Mortality is increased in persons weighing 15 percent or more below average.[6] The Framingham Heart Study indicated that this was in part due to cigarette smoking with its associated risks for mortality.[33]

Underweight also occurs in many pathologic conditions such as fevers in which the appetite is poor and the energy requirements are increased; gastrointesti-

nal disturbances characterized by nausea, vomiting, and diarrhea; cancer; and hyperthyroidism in which the metabolic rate is greatly accelerated. These will be discussed in Part III.

Changes in Body Tissue Compartments The extent of changes in body tissue compartments depends somewhat on the severity of the nutritional deprivation. In moderate undernutrition, losses occur primarily in visceral protein and muscle cell mass, while body fat is not affected. In severe undernutrition significant losses of both muscle cell mass and body fat occur. Prediction of the extent of changes in body tissue compartments can be made from knowledge of anthropometric measures and laboratory determinations of protein status, as discussed in Chapter 23.

Modifications of the Diet Before weight gain can be effected, the direct cause for the inadequate caloric intake must be sought. As in obesity, these causes in relation to the individual must be removed and a high calorie diet provided.

Energy. Approximately 500 kcal in excess of the daily needs will result in a weekly gain of about 0.5 kg (1 pound). For moderately active individuals diets containing 3,000 to 3,500 kcal will bring about effective weight gain. Somewhat higher levels are required when fever is high, or gastrointestinal disturbances are interfering with absorption, or metabolism is greatly increased.

Protein. A daily intake of 100 g protein or more is usually desirable, since body protein as well as body fat must be replaced.

Minerals and Vitamins. If the quality of the diet resulting in weight loss was poor, considerable body deficits of minerals and vitamins may likewise have occurred. Usually the high-calorie diet will provide liberal levels of all these nutrients. When supplements are prescribed, it is important that the patient understand that they are in no way a substitute for the calories and protein provided by food.

Planning the Daily Diet A patient cannot always adjust immediately to a higher caloric intake. It is better to begin with the patient's present intake and to improve the diet both qualitatively and quantitatively day by day until the desired caloric level is reached. Nothing is more conducive to loss of appetite than the appearance of an overloaded tray of food.

The caloric intake may be increased by using additional amounts of foods from the Daily Food Guide, thus increasing the intake of protein, minerals, and vitamins. For example, 500 kcal might be added to the patient's present intake as follows:

> 1 glass milk, 1 soft cooked egg, ½ cup ice cream, 2 oatmeal cookies or
> 1 glass milk, ½ cup cottage cheese, 5 saltines, ½ cup canned peaches

The judicious use of cream, butter, jelly or jam, and sugars will quickly increase the caloric level, but excessive use may provoke nausea and loss of appetite.

Some patients make better progress if given small, frequent feedings; but for many patients midmorning and midafternoon feedings have been found to interfere with the appetite for the following meal. Bedtime snacks, however, may be planned to provide 300 to 800 kcal, thus making it possible to follow a normal pattern for the three meals.

The following list of foods illustrates one way in which the Daily Food Guide may be adapted to a

high-calorie level. The meal patterns outlined for the high-protein diet (page 479) suggest suitable arrangements of these foods.

> 3 to 4 cups milk
> 5 to 7 ounces meat, fish, poultry, or cheese
> 1 egg
> 4 servings vegetables including:
>   1 serving green or yellow vegetable
>   2 servings white or sweet potato, corn, or beans
>   1 serving other vegetable
> 2 to 3 servings fruit, including one citrus fruit
> 1 serving whole-grain or enriched cereal
> 3 to 6 slices whole-grain or enriched bread
> 4 tablespoons or more butter or margarine
> High-calorie foods to complete the caloric requirement: cereals such as macaroni, rice, noodles, spaghetti; honey, molasses, syrups; hard candies; glucose; salad dressings; cakes, cookies, and pastry in moderation; ice cream, puddings, sauces

CASE STUDY 9
Obese Adolescent Female

Jody, age 17, is a freshman at City Community College, where she is majoring in business. After classes she works in a fast-food restaurant.

During summer vacation she had lost 20 pounds while on a well-known liquid formula diet. However, she has regained 15 pounds since the school term began. She is 165 cm (65 in) tall, medium in build, and currently weights 71 kg (156 lb).

Jody has been overweight since childhood. As a teenager she has tried numerous fad diets. She usually loses about 10 pounds but then regains the weight within a few months. She tends to binge on high-calorie foods when feeling nervous or lonely. On occasion, she has used laxatives after binging to avoid gaining weight. She has also been taking an over-the-counter appetite suppressant containing phenylpropanolamine daily during the past year.

One evening a forum was held on campus concerning "Eating Disorders." After the meeting, Jody talked with the speaker and expressed frustration regarding her difficulty maintaining weight loss and a fear of becoming bulimic. The speaker referred her to the Health Service nurse on campus who coordinates a weight-loss group for students.

Pathophysiologic Correlations
1. List several factors that may account for Jody's obesity.
2. What are some of the health consequences of obesity?
3. What type of adipose tissue cellularity is Jody likely to have?
4. Describe two common theories of obesity.
5. What are some psychological effects of obesity?
6. In what ways is Jody like the typical bulimic individual?

Nutritional Assessment
7. How do Jody's height and weight compare with the average for her age? (NOTE: Use the NCHS charts in the Appendix, Table A-9.)
8. What is an appropriate weight for Jody?
9. What factors have contributed to Jody's weight gain?
10. About how many calories does Jody need daily?
11. Why did the fad diets that Jody tried produce only a temporary weight loss?
12. What further information about Jody should you obtain in your assessment?
13. What is the likelihood that Jody can achieve and maintain average or slightly less than average weight?
14. How long should Jody expect to restrict calorie intake before she reaches a weight appropriate for her?

15. Is there any danger in taking appetite suppressants such as the one Jody uses?
16. What precautions should be taken in using liquid formula diets?

Planning the Diet

17. What are the components of a weight control program for Jody?
18. For each component of the program, list examples of two or three specific tips appropriate for teenagers.
19. What are some reasons that the usual advice to "decrease food intake and increase energy output" does not seem to be effective with teenagers?

20. What types of activities might be appropriate as part of an exercise program for Jody?
21. Outline the objectives in planning Jody's diet.
22. List some problems you foresee in planning Jody's diet.

Dietary Counseling

23. Outline the points you would emphasize in counseling Jody about her diet.
24. In addition to the dietary practices, what other recommendations should be made to Jody?
25. In what ways does exercise prevent obesity?
26. What problems might be anticipated by Jody in following the dietary recommendations?

References for the Case Study

CECERE, M. C.: "PIP (Positive Image Program): A Group Approach for Obese Adolescents," *Nurs. Clin. North Am.*, **18**:249–56, June 1983.

HOERR, S. L.: "Exercise: An Alternative to Fad Diets for Adolescent Girls," *Physician Sports Med.*, **12**:76–83, February 1984.

LANGFORD, R. W.: "Teenagers and Obesity," *Am. J. Nurs.*, **81**:556–59, 1981.

POTTS, N. L.: "Eating Disorders: The Secret Patient," *Am. J. Nurs.*, **84**:32–33, 1984.

WHITE, J. H.: "An Overview of Obesity: Its Significance to Nursing," *Nurs. Clin. North Am.*, **17**:191–98, June 1982.

WHITE, J. H., and SCHROEDER, M. A.: "Nursing Assessment," *Am. J. Nurs.*, **81**:550–52, 1981.

References

1. Zohman, L. R.: *Beyond Diet. Exercise Your Way to Fitness and Heart Health.* CPC International, Englewood Cliffs, N.J., 1974.
2. Smith, N. J.: "Nutrition and the Athlete," *Orthop. Clin. North Am.*, **14**:387–96, 1983.
3. American Dietetic Association: "Statement on Nutrition and Physical Fitness," *J. Am. Diet. Assoc.*, **76**:437–43, 1980.
4. Bergstrom, J., and Hultman, E.: "Nutrition for Maximal Sports Performance," *JAMA*, **221**:999–1006, 1972.
5. Forgac, N. T.: "Carbohydrate Loading: A Review," *J. Am. Diet Assoc.*, **75**:42–45, 1979.
6. Simoupoulos, A. P., and Van Itallie, T. B.: "Body Weight, Health, and Longevity," *Ann. Intern. Med.*, **100**:285–95, 1984.
7. Drenick, E. J., et al: "Excessive Mortality and Causes of Death in Morbidly Obese Men," *JAMA*, **243**:443–45, 1980.
8. Van Itallie, T. B.: "Obesity: Adverse Effects on Health and Longevity," *Am. J. Clin. Nutr.*, **32**:2723–33, 1979.
9. Hubert, H. B., et al.: "Obesity as an Independent Risk Factor for Cardiovascular Disease: A 26 Year Follow up of Participants in the Framingham Heart Study," *Circulation*, **67**:968–77, 1983.
10. "1983 Metropolitan Height and Weight Tables," *Stat. Bull. Met. Life Found.*, **64**:3–9, January–June, 1983.
11. Pirie, P., et al.: "Distortion in Self-Reported Height and Weight Data," *J. Am. Diet. Assoc.*, **78**:601–606, 1981.
12. Palta, M., et al.: "Comparison of Self-Reported and Measured Height and Weight," *Am. J. Epidemiol.*, **115**:223–30, 1982.
13. Russell, R. M., et al.: "Reference Weights. Practical Considerations," *Am. J. Med.*, **76**:767–69, 1984.
14. National Center for Health Statistics: *Weight by Height and Age for Adults 18–74 Years: United States, 1971–74.* National Center for Health Statistics, Rockville, Md., 1979. Data from the National Health Survey No. 208. DHEW Publ. (PHS) 79-1656. Vital and Health Statistics. Series 11. **208**:1–56, 1979.
15. Bray, G. A.: "Definition, Measurement, and Classification of the Syndromes of Obesity," *Int. J. Obesity*, **2**:1–14, 1978.
16. Frisancho, A. R.: "New Standards of Weight and Body Composition by Frame Size and Height for Assessment of Nutritional Status of Adults and the Elderly," *Am. J. Clin. Nutr.*, **40**:808–19, 1984.
17. Baker, G. L.: "Human Adipose Tissue Composition and Age." *Am. J. Clin. Nutr.*, **22**:829–35, 1969.
18. Abraham, S., et al.: *Obese and Overweight Adults in the United States.* National Center for Health Statistics, Hyattsville, Md., 1983. DHHS Publ. (PHS) 83-1680. Vital and Health Statistics. Series 11. **230**:1–93, 1983.
19. Garn, S. M., and Clark, D. C.: "Trends in Fatness and the Origins of Obesity," *Pediatrics*, **57**:443–56, 1976.
20. Mayer, J.: "Obesity: Causes and Treatment," *Am. J. Nurs.*, **59**:1732–36, 1959.
21. Hirsch, J., and Knittle, J. L.: "Cellularity of Obese and Non-Obese Adipose Tissue," *Fed. Proc.*, **29**:1516–21, 1970.
22. Brownell, K. D.: "The Psychology and Physiology of Obesity: Implications for Screening and Treatment," *J. Am. Diet Assoc.*, **84**:406–14, 1984.

23. Strain, G. W., et al.: "Do Fat Cell Morphometrics Predict Weight Loss Maintenance?" *Int. J. Obesity*, 8:53–59, 1984.

24. Merritt, R. J., et al.: "Consequence of Modified Fasting in Obese Pediatric and Adolescent Patients. I. Protein-Sparing Modified Fast," *J. Pediatr.*, 96:13–19, 1980.

25. Wadden, T. A., et al.: "Very Low Calorie Diets: Their Efficacy, Safety, and Future," *Ann. Intern. Med.*, 99:675–84, 1983.

26. Golden, N., and Sacker, I. M.: "An Overview of the Etiology, Diagnosis, and Management of Anorexia Nervosa," *Clin. Pediatr.*, 23:209–14, 1984.

27. Feighner, J. P., et al.: "Diagnostic Criteria for Use in Psychiatric Research," *Arch. Gen. Psychiatry*, 26:57–63, 1972.

28. Casper, R. C., et al.: "An Evaluation of Trace Metals, Vitamins, and Taste Function in Anorexia Nervosa," *Am. J. Clin. Nutr.*, 33:1801–8, 1980.

29. Huse, D. M., and Lucas, A. R.: "Dietary Management of Anorexia Nervosa," *J. Am. Diet Assoc.*, 83:687–89, 1983.

30. Sanger, E., and Cassino, T.: "Eating Disorders. Avoiding the Power Struggle," *Am. J. Nurs.*, 84:31–33, 1984.

31. Harris, R. T.: "Bulimarexia and Related Serious Eating Disorders with Medical Complications," *Ann. Intern. Med.*, 99:800–807, 1983.

32. Willard, S. G., et al.: "Nutritional Counseling as an Adjunct to Psychotherapy in Bulimia Treatment," *Psychosomatics*, 24:545–47, 1983.

33. Garrison, R. J., et al.: "Cigarette Smoking as a Cofounder of the Relationship Between Relative Weight and Long-Term Mortality: The Framingham Heart Study," *JAMA*, 249:2199–2203, 1983.

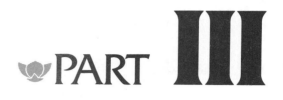

PART III

Therapeutic Nutrition

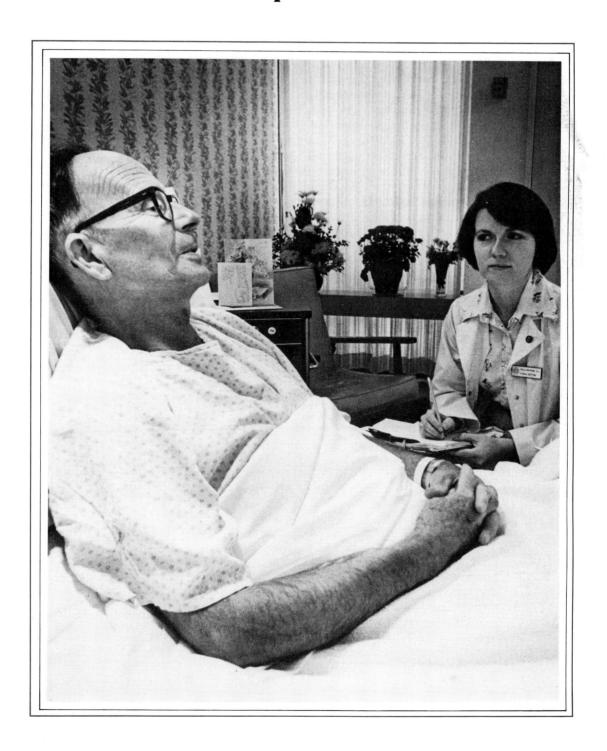

In Part III you will discover how nutrition principles can be applied to therapeutic interventions for individuals experiencing illness. Today, our nutritional interventions can be based upon a rapidly increasing knowledge base as hundreds of millions of dollars are allocated to the study of the role of diet in the prevention and treatment of disease.

Nutritional therapy in the form of a normal diet, or perhaps a diet modified slightly in texture, is supportive and restorative for many patients. For some others, dietary modification is the primary route of therapy as in weight correction, diabetes mellitus, and inborn errors of metabolism. For still others a highly sophisticated, life saving nutritional therapy by enteral and parenteral routes has become possible because of clinical research by physicians and nutritionists, and technologic developments by pharmacologists, biological scientists, and food scientists.

Nutritional therapy must also take into account any medications that are being used by the client. Some medications can interfere with the absorption and metabolism of nutrients. In turn, some nutrients and foods can interfere with or enhance the effectiveness of drug therapy. The timing of meals and medications as well as the inclusion or exclusion of specific foods are often critical to the maintenance of good nutritional status and effective medication.

In the hospital or nursing home patients expect to receive meals tailored to their particular needs. Dietitians and nurses find that meeting the nutritional needs of patients with widely varying nutritional requirements and individual food preferences and who often have persnickety appetites because of illness is an ongoing challenge to which they must respond. The number of days that patients remain in a hospital has been reduced through effective medical, surgical, and nutritional intervention. However, if relapse following discharge and subsequent readmission to the hospital are to be avoided, home health services including meals, when needed, and dietary counseling must receive far greater emphasis in health planning and implementation.

26

Comprehensive Nutritional Services for Patients

Introduction to Therapeutic Nutrition

Sooner or later most individuals will experience an acute or chronic condition that requires hospitalization. To the uninitiated, hospitals can be very frightening places. Food often is the only aspect of the daily routine that is familiar to hospitalized patients; if the usual food intake is not permitted because of the need for a therapeutic diet, food may become a source of apprehension. Regardless of the diagnosis or the type of diet prescribed, the satisfactory intake of food by the patient is essential for maintenance of tissue structures and body functions so that recovery from illness is not impeded. Inadequate intake of the proper nutrients, or impaired ability to digest, absorb, or metabolize foods leads to nutritional deficiency. This lowers the body's resistance and may initiate or aggravate diseases of nonnutritional origin. Illnesses such as infections, injuries, and metabolic disturbances lead to deficiencies even in previously well-nourished persons because of failure to ingest sufficient food or because the disease process greatly increases nutritional needs. Thus, a vicious cycle of disease, malnutrition, and prolonged convalescence ensues.

The principles of good nutrition have been discussed in Part I of this text. Practical application of these principles and adaptation of the normal diet for all age categories was the objective of Part II. Modification of the diet to the needs of individuals with some pathologic conditions is the objective of Part III. This introductory chapter in therapeutic nutrition presents an overview of some of the factors that may have a bearing on the nutritional status of hospitalized persons and the role of the health care team in meeting their nutritional needs. Much concern has been expressed about the prevalence of malnutrition in hospitalized patients and on the role of the health care team in assessing, preventing, and treating hospital malnutrition. Nutritional assessment has been de-scribed in Chapter 23. Further techniques for assessing nutritional status of hospitalized patients are described in detail in this chapter. Also described are the importance of nutrition in comprehensive health care and some ways in which nutritional services are provided for persons with health problems of a temporary or chronic nature that do not require hospitalization.

Purposes of Modified Diets   Most patients do not require dietary modification. Good nutritional care for them consists of supplying a normal diet that furnishes their nutritional, psychologic, and esthetic needs and taking measures to enable them to consume it. On the other hand, modified diets are the principal therapeutic agents in some metabolic diseases such as type II (non-insulin-dependent) diabetes mellitus. In other instances diet therapy supports the overall therapeutic program; for example, a sodium-restricted diet may be prescribed in addition to diuretics for some patients with hypertension. Modified diets are also used as preventive measures. One example of this is the fat-modified diet prescribed for individuals with elevated blood lipids who are at increased risk for ischemic (coronary) heart disease. For some conditions in which diet therapy formerly played a major role, drug therapy is now a more effective means of controlling symptoms. Use of cimetidine in peptic ulcer or allopurinol in gout has largely superseded the need for bland and purine-restricted diets in patients receiving these medications. Nevertheless, these diets are still used in some circumstances.

Team Approach to Nutritional Care   Meeting the patient's nutritional needs involves the coordination of several hospital departments. The core team is composed of the physician, nurse, and dietitian. With the advent of parenteral feeding formulas, the role of the clinical pharmacist is becoming increasingly recognized. At times, other health professionals, such as the social worker or physical therapist become directly involved. The relationships of each of these team members to one another and to the patient might be depicted as shown in Figure 26-1. The focus, of course, is on the patient who must actively participate, insofar as possible, in his or her health care. The physician prescribes the diet and should also give the patient some information concerning the reasons that a modified diet has been ordered. The dietitian is the specialist who translates the physician's written order into practicality in terms of foods or nutritional products or formulas. The dietitian assesses and evaluates the patient's nutritional status; formulates nutritional care plans; designs meal patterns individualized according to the patient's food habits and modified according to the therapeutic need; recommends appropriate proprietary formulas for enteral feeding; counsels the patient and family regarding any dietary modifications needed; and advises on nutritional effects of drug therapy. The dietary staff is also responsible for the preparation and service of food to the patient, and evaluation of the patient's response to the diet.

The nurse is the member of the health team who has the most constant and intimate association with the patient, and the direct services she or he gives to the patient differ from those of the physician and the dietitian. Through the nursing process the nurse identifies potential or actual patient problems related to nutrition and develops a care plan specifying the nursing interventions needed to achieve the desired patient outcomes. Some specific means by which nursing personnel assist in nutritional care include the following:

1. Maintaining lines of communication with the physician and dietitian regarding the patient's dietary needs:
   a. Obtaining a diet prescription if there is none, and arranging for food service to the patient
   b. Providing the dietitian and physician with information regarding the patient's response to the diet
   c. Serving as liaison between the patient and the physician and dietitian
2. Assisting the patient at mealtimes:
   a. Providing a pleasant environment conducive to eating
   b. Preparing the patient for the meal
   c. Giving assistance to the patient as needed, including feeding
   d. Helping the handicapped to adjust to self-feeding
   e. Giving encouragement and support to the patient
3. Interpreting the diet to the patient:
   a. Explaining the reasons for a modified diet and what may be expected of the diet
   b. Answering questions about the diet
4. Observing, recording, and reporting the patient's response to diet:
   a. Eliciting information regarding food habits, likes and dislikes, and attitudes toward diet
   b. Noting adequacy of food intake
   c. Reporting patient's response to dietitian and physician
5. Planning for home care:
   a. Identifying needs for outside assistance
   b. Arranging for counseling regarding home diet with member of family as well as patient

Factors to Consider in the Study of Diet Therapy
In order to function effectively in the provision of nutritional care, students of nursing and dietetics must have an understanding of (1) acute and chronic conditions which require a change in diet; (2) the rationale for dietary changes, characteristics of the diet, its beneficial and possible adverse effects, nutritional limitations of the various modified diets, and indications and contraindications for use; (3) ways in which drug therapy may influence food intake or utilization; and (4) the patient's tolerance for food.

A correctly planned diet is successful only if it is eaten. The dietitian and nurse must be able to apply the principles pertaining to the preparation and ser-

Figure 26-1. The central or "star" member of the team is the patient. The lines connecting the points of the star illustrate the lines of communication among all members of the team.

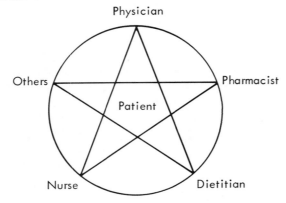

vice of appealing, palatable, and nutritious food. They must have the necessary understanding of the psychologic and emotional factors influencing food acceptance.

Patient care includes planning for full rehabilitation. For some patients a modified diet may be required for weeks, months, or even a lifetime; for others, guidance may be desirable in the improvement of a normal diet. Such planning necessitates consideration of social, religious, and cultural patterns, availability of foods, cost of food, suitable methods of food preparation, and so on.

The hospital or regional diet manual is used as the basis for planning modified diets. The American Dietetic Association has compiled a handbook in which the scientific basis for dietary modification in treatment of disease, dietetic terminology, and contents of various diets are listed.[1]

Effect of Illness on Food Acceptance and Utilization

The physiologic, psychologic, and emotional factors governing food acceptance have been discussed in Chapter 15. Likewise, a number of cultural food patterns have been presented in Chapter 16. Illness may modify or accentuate the influence of any of these factors.

The Stress of Illness The sick person has many fears: those relating to the outcome of the illness itself, economic concerns for self and family, emotional adjustments to having to depend on others during the illness, and anxiety about loss of love and self-esteem. The sick person may express fears in a number of ways: by being angry, self-conscious, talkative or reticent, uneasy, depressed, indifferent, impatient, hostile, apologetic for failure, or resentful.

When hospitalization becomes necessary, the sick person experiences additional stress. Some patients adjust easily to a hospital routine, but for others it is difficult. The patient is subjected to seemingly endless questions, physical examinations, laboratory tests, and ministrations of therapy by a parade of specialists and auxiliary workers who, too often, do not explain what is happening, thus causing much needless anxiety. On the other hand, the patient often experiences long delays when he or she requires attention to personal needs. Especially if primary care nursing is not provided, patients may feel that there is no specific person who has the primary concern and responsibility for his or her care. The loss of privacy is an especial embarrassment and even shock to an elderly individual who has never before been in a hospital. Likewise the loss of independence to eat when and what one wishes, to get out of bed or not, to come and go as one wishes, and so on, can be frustrating. Each member of the health care team should be concerned that the patient is treated with dignity and that his or her rights are observed. The American Hospital Association has prepared a bill of rights for patients in the interest of better patient care.[2]

Illness Modifies Food Acceptance Hospitalization itself may influence food acceptance. When the patient most needs the comfort and companionship of family and friends, he or she is relegated to eating alone. Perhaps the meal hours are different from those to which the patient is accustomed; the foods appearing on the tray may be unlike those usually eaten with respect to choice, or flavoring, or portion size; a single food that the patient strongly dislikes may be so upsetting that he or she is unable to eat anything served with it; managing a tray and the utensils for eating may be awkward when one is in bed; the patient may perceive expressed needs as being minimized or brushed aside. Some patients, under stress, use diet as a means of gaining attention from hospital personnel and later from family members. They may insist on meticulous attention to the minutest of details, in order to be noticed.

The disease process itself may have a profound effect on food acceptance. Some foods may produce marked anorexia, others may be distending, and still others may be irritants to the gastrointestinal tract. Food preferences may revert to those of earlier years. These may be bland foods of childhood, but they might be the special dishes associated with one's ethnic origin.

Modified Diets Impose Additional Problems When a patient is confronted with the need for a therapeutic diet, he or she may respond with comments such as these: "I just can't get it down." "This food is tasteless." "I can't afford such food when I go home." "Who is going to prepare my food at home?" "I can't buy these foods at work." Remarks such as these may indicate unwillingness to accept change; anger at those associated with the diet—nurse, dietitian, physician, or even mother or spouse who has nagged about the food habits at home; fears of having to eat disliked foods; of having to forego favorite foods; of loss of social status and self-esteem; or the feeling that diet is, in some way, a punishment.

The nurse and dietitian must try to allay the patient's fears by empathetic understanding and by providing help in budgeting, arrangements for food preparation, suggestions for making the diet more palatable, and other useful advice.

Nutritional Stress Emotional stress such as the taking of examinations leads to increased losses of nitrogen and calcium. In fact, persons under such stress may achieve balances only with considerable difficulty. One may reasonably assume that the anxiety concerning illness may also accentuate such losses.

Immobilization is also a stressful situation in which nitrogen and calcium excretions are elevated. In long-term illness, immobilization may be responsible for serious demineralization of bones.

Any trauma to the body such as bone fracture, wound injury, or infection increases the losses of nitrogen and various electrolytes. The secretion of several hormones is often increased, thereby elevating the needs for vitamins required to carry on metabolic processes.

Interpersonal Relationship with the Patient

The Needs of the Patient Each patient has physical, psychologic, social, and spiritual needs. The pathophysiologic aspects of illness are the immediate reasons for care by the health team, but other needs must not be overlooked. Each member of the health team has a unique contribution to make in providing for these needs. Some examples relating to nutritional care follow.

1. Each person wants to be treated as an individual. He or she has specific needs and values that are unique for him or her, and care should be personalized rather than making the patient fit into a general mold.
   Listening. Those who care for the patient must learn to listen carefully—not only to the words themselves but also to their tone and inflection. By taking time to listen, one may be made aware of a legitimate complaint about something wrong with the meals a patient receives—for example, cold coffee, an egg not cooked to his or her liking, or a vegetable the patient thoroughly dislikes. Such details are relatively easy to correct, and the patient is thereby made quite comfortable and satisfied. The seemingly casual conversation

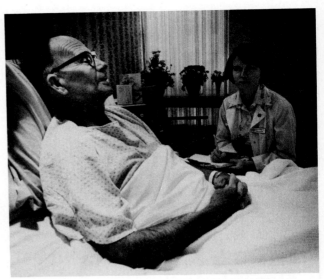

Figure 26-2.   The dietitian interviews the patient in a relaxed environment. She is nonjudgmental as she listens to him, and she skillfully elicits information by interjecting a question now and then. (Courtesy, Metropolitan Medical Center, Minneapolis.)

with the patient may bring to light that the past diet has been inadequate for a long period of time because of lack of teeth, poor health, inadequate income, or the inability to prepare food. Permitting the patient to talk about other things as well as the diet will often reveal that the problems encountered in food acceptance are actually a byproduct of the deep anxieties caused by other problems; through understanding, the patient can often be helped. (See Figure 26-2.)

2. Each person has a right to know what should be expected from the health team and what is expected of the patient. If a modified diet is prescribed, the patient should be given some understanding of the reasons for it and what he or she may expect by way of needed change in food habits. Reassurance with respect to the diet is essential, but it must be realistic in terms of the difficulties of adjustment to it and its legitimate role in the total therapeutic program. To illustrate, appropriate diets for obesity and diabetes are basic to treatment, but some patients may find the adjustment to the restrictions extremely difficult; to minimize the problems involved is to invite failure. A fat-restricted diet may be helpful to the patient with gallstones, but it should never be held as a guarantee that surgery would not be required at a later time. Likewise, a patient with cardiovascular disease may benefit from a fat-modified diet but

might eventually develop more serious cardiovascular disease regardless of the diet.

3. Each patient should be helped to participate in his or her own care. A selective menu can be a useful tool to help in making good choices for a normal as well as a modified diet. If dietary counseling is begun early, each meal helps the patient to learn what changes will be needed in the diet when the patient goes home. A patient who has a physical handicap should be helped to feed himself or herself as much as is possible, thereby increasing independence.

4. Each person expects that his or her behavior during illness will be accepted as part of the illness. The modification of food acceptance during illness as described on page 387 is an important expression of the change in behavior.

5. Each person expects to be treated with kindness, thoughtfulness, and firmness. The work of the dietitians, nurses, or homemakers is often more successful if they can place themselves in the patient's role, although they must guard against overidentification; if they become too close to the patient, they may accept his or her reactions as being always so reasonable that they are unable to do anything about changing them.

Recognition of Attitudes. How does the nurse or dietitian feel about the patient who does not eat the food, who eats too much, or who complains about the food a great deal? When the patient expresses resentment or hostility toward nurses or dietitians, do they realize that this may be against the dietary restrictions and not against them as individuals? It is important that they recognize their own attitudes toward the patient, lest they give the impression that they are pitying, superior, intolerant, resentful, or critical of him or her. Moreover, they must avoid an expression of any negative attitudes they may have toward food.

Nutritional Assessment of the Hospitalized Patient

All patients have the right to expect assessment of their nutritional status as a routine part of their care while they are hospitalized. Obviously, not all are malnourished, thus, the extent of the evaluation will vary from one individual to another. Preliminary screening will identify those who are at increased risk for malnutrition. (See Table 26-1.) For these individuals more detailed assessment is required in order to define the extent of the nutritional problem and plan

Table 26-1. **Some Factors That Increase Risk for Hospital Malnutrition**

1. Abnormal weight patterns
   a. Children—weight for height outside the normal range
   b. Adults—≥ 20 percent above or > 10 percent below desirable weight
   c. Significant unintentional recent weight loss (> 10 percent in 6 months)
2. Any condition characterized by insufficient intake of energy and nutrients
   a. Impaired ability to chew, swallow, taste, or smell food
   b. Diets with multiple restrictions in types of food and/or levels of nutrients; for example, clear liquid; extremely low-protein diets
   c. "Nothing by mouth" or use of intravenous feedings for more than a few days
   d. Chronic disease such as cancer or ulcerative colitis that influences appetite or ability to digest or absorb food
3. Increased nutritional needs
   a. Pregnancy, malabsorption, diarrhea, postoperative states, fever, sepsis, burns
   b. Continued external losses of bodily constituents; open, draining wounds; chronic hemorrhage; chronic dialysis
4. Drug therapy that interferes with nutrient utilization
5. Conditions characterized by abnormal levels of hemoglobin, hematocrit, lymphocytes, albumin, transferrin, cholesterol, blood urea nitrogen, etc.

and implement appropriate nutritional support. The particular techniques used in screening and in further assessment will depend upon the patient population and the resources and personnel available.

A number of anthropometric measurements, biochemical studies, clinical findings, and the dietary history are evaluated. These were discussed in Chapter 23. However, for patients at increased risk for protein-energy malnutrition, additional information is needed. Determinations of energy stores, lean body mass, visceral protein status, and immune competency are of particular interest to clinicians. It should be noted that few patients will have a completely normal profile of anthropometric, biochemical, and immune factors; however, the patient who is moderately or severely depleted in several of these parameters is likely to benefit from nutritional support. The validity of these measurements has been questioned by some on the grounds that they do not reflect changes in body composition[3,4] and do not accurately predict nutritional risk for individuals,[5] as opposed to groups of patients. Nevertheless, the techniques will continue to be important because of ease of use, convenience, and low cost. It must also be remembered that deficiencies of vitamins and minerals, especially trace minerals, are likely in patients whose protein or energy stores are depleted. Some indexes of nutritional status are listed inside the back cover of this text.[6-9]

Initial Screening Preliminary information obtained from the medical record and dietary history is useful in determining those patients likely to have nutritional problems that require intervention. (See Table 26-1.) Some rely on these two sources; others add various anthropometric, biochemical, and immunologic determinations, some of which are described in the sections that follow. One group has reported that serum albumin and total lymphocyte determinations are as useful as more detailed methods in identifying those at risk for nutritional complications.[10] If the initial evaluation suggests malnutrition, more extensive evaluation is needed.

Anthropometric Measurements

Skinfold, Arm Circumference, and Arm Muscle Circumference In the clinical setting, anthropometric measurements are used to estimate energy reserves and skeletal muscle protein reserves. Triceps and subscapular skinfolds, arm circumference, and arm muscle circumference measurements are frequently used. Techniques for taking the measurements have been described in Chapter 23. Some evidence suggests that arm muscle area and arm fat area, calculated from arm circumference and triceps skinfold, respectively, provide a better estimate of age-related tissue changes occurring in groups over time.[11] Data from the National Health and Nutrition Examination Survey, 1971–74, (NHANES I) indicated that anthropometric measurements may change significantly over a decade. Thus, it is important to consider age when anthropometric measurements are used in nutritional assessment. In men, arm circumference, arm muscle area, sum of skinfold thicknesses, and arm fat area increase with age up to 35 to 44 years, and then steadily decrease. Triceps skinfold shows no consistent trend with increasing age. In women, all these parameters tend to increase with age until 45 to 64 years, and thereafter stabilize or decrease.[11,12] Age- and sex-specific percentiles for several anthropometric measurements based on NHANES I data are shown in Tables A-19 through A-24.[11,12] Arm anthropometry nomograms for use in nutrition assessment are shown in Tables A-25 and A-26.[13]

Several considerations must be kept in mind when using anthropometric measures in nutritional assessment. Standardization of technique is important. Some practice in taking the measurements is required in order to develop the skill needed to minimize the margin of error. The same type of calipers should be used for initial and subsequent measurements. Care must be taken to see that arm measurements are made at the midpoint of the upper arm. Regardless of whether the right or left arm is used initially, subsequent measurements should be made on the same arm, with the patient in the same position. (See page 335.)

Anthropometric measurements do not reflect acute changes in body composition occurring in individual patients over short periods of time. Serial measurements, over time, are needed to evaluate changes occurring in tissue. Ideally, these should be made by the same person.

Assessment of Body Weight Determination of height and weight provides an indirect estimate of fat stores, assuming the patient is not edematous. Body build should be taken into account when estimating appropriate weight for height. Techniques used to determine body build, or frame size, include measurements of elbow breadth and wrist circumference. (See Table A-15.)

Height–Weight Tables. The Metropolitan Life Insurance Tables are widely used as a reference.[14] (See Table A-16). The tables indicate weights for given heights and frame sizes for men and women, ages 25 to 59 years. Weights and heights are given for individuals in indoor clothing and wearing shoes with 1-inch heels. Body frame size is based on elbow breadth and is distributed so that one fourth are designated as "small" frame, one half as "medium" frame, and the remaining one-fourth as "large" frame. Limitations of these tables were discussed in Chapter 25. (See page 367.)

Weight for height by population percentiles based on NHANES I data are shown in Tables A-7 to A-14 for infants and children, and Tables A-17 and A-18 for adults.[15,16]

For the hospitalized patient, evaluation of weight change often provides more useful information than comparison of the patient's weight to standard height–weight tables.

Percentage Usual Body Weight. A commonly used index compares the current weight with the patient's usual weight:

$$\text{Percentage usual body weight} = \frac{\text{current weight}}{\text{usual weight}} \times 100$$

Provided that the reported usual weight is accurate, a rough estimate of the degree of calorie malnutrition can be made. (See inside back cover.)

Recent Weight Change. Evaluation of weight change over time is useful in assessing risk for malnutrition (see formula on inside back cover). Weight loss of 5 percent in 1 month or 10 percent over 6 months is significant. Losses greater than these represent severe weight loss.[7]

Biochemical Studies

Lean Body Mass Urinary creatinine excretion is sometimes used as an index of lean body mass. Creatinine is derived from the breakdown of creatine, a substance found predominantly in muscle. Thus, creatinine excretion reflects the level of total body creatine and, therefore, skeletal muscle mass. In wasting disease, muscle mass is depleted and creatinine excretion is less than normal. Acceptable values for creatinine excretion range from 20 to 26 mg/kg body weight per 24 hours in men and 14 to 22 mg/kg body weight per 24 hours in women.[9]

Another measure of lean body mass is the creatinine–height index (CHI). This compares the patient's 24-hour creatinine excretion with that expected of a healthy adult of the same sex and height. The expected 24-hour creatinine excretion represents the mean creatinine excretion for healthy young adults of "ideal" weight (based on the 1959 Metropolitan Life Insurance standards). In these individuals, the creatinine coefficients are 23 and 18 mg/kg ideal weight for men and women, respectively (see inside back cover).[17] The ratio of the patient's creatinine excretion to the expected, or "ideal", is expressed in per cent. Values less than 80 percent are considered to represent moderate depletion of skeletal muscle mass.[6] Complete 24-hour urine collection and normal renal function are required for accurate test results.

In many clinical settings use of the creatinine–height index is not a practical means of assessing muscle mass because accurate 24-hour urinary collections are nearly impossible to obtain. The definition of "ideal" body weight is questionable. (See Chapter 25.) Furthermore, the "ideal" is based on creatinine excretion in young adults. Creatinine excretion decreases with age; thus, the creatinine–height index is not applicable to the elderly.[18]

Visceral Protein Status Direct measurement of visceral protein status is not feasible at present; thus, indirect measurements of serum transport protein concentrations are used to identify patients at nutritional risk. Albumin, transferrin, prealbumin, and retinol-binding protein levels have been measured.

Albumin. The serum albumin concentration is the most frequently assayed transport protein. Depression of the serum albumin concentration is associated with kwashiorkor in populations with deficient protein intake. However, many other factors besides deficient intake affect the serum albumin concentration. Included are stress, infections, absorptive defects, overhydration, inadequate synthesis occurring in severe liver disease, excessive losses in nephrotic syndrome or burns, and cancer, among others. Because of its relatively long half-life (18 to 20 days), albumin is not a useful indicator of early protein depletion, nor does it respond quickly to increases in dietary protein intake. Nevertheless, depletion of serum albumin level is associated with decreased resistance to infection, impaired wound healing, increased length of hospital stay, and increased morbidity and mortality.[6,19] Serum concentrations indicative of depletion are shown inside the back cover.

Transferrin. This is a more sensitive indicator of visceral protein status because it has a shorter half-life than albumin and will, therefore, indicate protein deficiency more rapidly. Decreased serum concentrations occur in stress, inflammation, liver disease, trauma, and so on. Transferrin is measured directly or is calculated from knowledge of the total iron-binding capacity (TIBC). The equation used to calculate transferrin from TIBC varies from one laboratory to another, depending on the specific test procedure used. Transferrin values associated with depletion are shown inside the back cover.

Other Transport Proteins. Prealbumin and retinol-binding proteins both have a short half-life, 2 to 3 days for prealbumin, and 8 to 10 hours for retinol-binding protein (RBP). For this reason both are of potential value in assessing acute changes in protein status. However, both are sensitive to stress, inflammation, surgical trauma, and liver disease and are rapidly depleted in these situations. Thus, low values do not necessarily indicate nutritional depletion. Furthermore, the tests are not available in many clinical settings. Normal values are shown inside the back cover.

Nitrogen Balance A rough estimate of nitrogen balance can be made from nitrogen intake and urinary urea nitrogen excretion. The latter accounts for about 80 percent of the nitrogen excreted from the body. Nitrogen losses are subtracted from nitrogen intake. Total nitrogen loss is estimated by adding a constant factor of 4 to urinary urea nitrogen to account for nonurea nitrogen losses. (See inside back cover.) Nitrogen balance is dependent on protein and energy intake. The balance data are of limited value in the initial assessment of protein depletion because such patients tend to conserve nitrogen more efficiently than better nourished individuals. Nitrogen excretion tends to increase as the severity of nitrogen depletion increases, however.

Vitamins and Minerals It is important to recognize that malnutrition in hospitalized patients is not limited to depletion of energy and protein reserves. Vitamin and mineral deficiencies may also occur. In one large study about 30 percent of hospitalized patients were found to have biochemical evidence of marginal or deficient status of thiamin, riboflavin, and vitamin C.[20] Individuals whose vitamin nutriture is marginal are at increased risk for deficiencies of these vitamins in infectious and catabolic diseases. Requirements for water-soluble vitamins, in particular, are increased in disease. Vitamin status is assayed by clinical observations, determination of blood levels, or by enzyme assays. Plasma levels reflect recent dietary intake, whereas intracellular levels are a better index of whole-body status.

Recent mineral intake is evaluated by measurement of both blood and urine levels. A fall in blood levels and a low urinary excretion are generally suggestive of an inadequate intake. Blood levels of trace minerals may shift in acute infections. For example, plasma zinc falls while plasma copper increases. Urinary excretion of zinc is increased in a number of catabolic conditions.

Other Biochemical Studies Other routine tests useful in assessing nutritional status of the hospitalized patient include serum urea nitrogen, blood glucose, alkaline phosphatase, prothrombin time, hematocrit, hemoglobin, mean corpuscular volume, mean corpuscular hemoglobin concentration, total iron-binding capacity, serum ferritin, percentage transferrin saturation, serum cholesterol, and serum triglycerides. Normal ranges for these tests are shown in Tables 9-6 and A-27.

Immune Competency

Cell-mediated immunity is an important host defense mechanism for resistance to infection. Morbidity and mortality from infections are increased when cellular immunity is depressed. One indicator of immune status is the *total lymphocyte count*. A value of less than 1,500 per mm^3 is associated with mild depletion. (See inside back cover.)

Delayed hypersensitivity skin tests using intradermal injections of recall antigens such as candida, streptokinase-streptodornase (SK-SD), and mumps are another means of evaluating immune function. The criteria for a positive response vary from one institution to another. A normal response is defined by some as a positive response to one or more antigens; others require a positive response to two or more antigens. Some consider the size of the response rather than the number of positive responses when differentiating normal from anergy. Both 5 mm and 10 mm have been used as cutoff points. Skin test responses are evaluated at 24 hours, 48 hours, or both, in various centers.

The term ANERGY refers to the failure to respond to any antigen, and indicates increased risk for sepsis. *Relative anergy* describes a response intermediate between anergy and normal and may refer to the number of positive responses or the size of the response to antigens. Patients in whom the total lymphocyte count and serum transport protein levels are low are likely to have abnormal responses to delayed hypersensitivity skin tests. The skin test responses are depressed in stress; in various benign infectious, inflammatory, and metabolic diseases; malignancy; certain drug therapies, such as steroids, immunosuppressants, chemotherapeutic agents, and cimetidine; general anesthesia; surgery; trauma; and burns.[21]

Follow-up Assessment If the initial assessment has indicated that nutritional support is needed, periodic follow-up is done to evaluate the effectiveness of nutritional therapy. One group recommends the following schedule: body weight, three times weekly; total lymphocyte count, weekly; albumin and transferrin, every 10 to 14 days; cell-mediated immunity, anthropometrics, and creatinine height index, every 21 to 30 days.[22]

Limitations of Nutritional Assessment The following points should be kept in mind concerning the various parameters used to assess nutritional status:

1. No one test is an accurate predictor of increased risk for nutritional complications. The best combination of tests is not known. Conflicting reports in the literature seem to suggest that the particular patient population, the number of patients studied, and the severity of stress may all influence the usefulness of certain tests as predictors.

2. Few patients have a completely normal profile when a number of parameters are assessed. In one study of surgical patients, only 3 percent had no abnormal measures. About one third of patients had three or more abnormal measurements of nutritional and immunologic status.[23]

3. Although some tests are useful in predicting increased risk of nutritional complications in groups of patients, the applicability of the data to individuals is meaningful only when associated with functional consequences. The measurements associated with functional consequences are recent weight loss of more than 10 percent, serum albumin less than 3.0 g per dl, weight and height less than 85 percent of standard, and anergy.[24]

4. In general, anthropometric data are not useful predictors of increased risk. Nevertheless, many malnourished patients have abnormal anthropometric measurements. Depressed levels of serum albumin and transferrin and the presence of anergy are all associated with increased morbidity and mortality.

Classification of Hospital Malnutrition Based on the information obtained from anthropometric, biochemical, and immune status determinations, three types of malnutrition have been described:

1. Marasmus, or protein-calorie malnutrition, is associated with depletion of energy reserves and lean body mass. Significant depletion of triceps skinfold, arm circumference, arm muscle circumference, and creatinine-height index is seen. Depression of visceral protein may occur, but is less pronounced. The patient has a wasted appearance.

2. Hypoalbuminemic malnutrition (kwashiorkor or protein malnutrition) is characterized by depressed serum albumin and transferrin levels and impaired cellular immunity. Patients often appear to have adequate energy stores.

3. A combination state is characterized by acute visceral protein depletion superimposed on protein-calorie malnutrition.

Nutritional Intervention

Assessment of Energy Needs The basal metabolic rate (BMR) of the hospitalized patient may be affected by a number of factors. For example, fever increases the BMR substantially while severe undernutrition lowers it. (See Chapter 8 for a discussion of other factors that influence the BMR.) Determination of the BMR is not done in the clinical setting. Instead, estimation of energy needs is based on the *resting metabolic expenditure* (RME), sometimes also called the resting or *basal energy expenditure* (BEE). The resting metabolic expenditure is assumed to be 10 percent greater than the basal metabolic rate, and is defined as the energy expenditure under normal conditions while at rest. (See page 104.)

Resting metabolic expenditure is measured by continuous expired air analysis in some centers. Where this technique is not available, the Harris–Benedict equations are used to predict basal energy expenditure.[25] These equations were derived in 1919 from the results of indirect calorimetry. Values obtained by measuring RME agree fairly closely with the predicted values for BEE in healthy subjects.[8] However, studies of malnourished general surgical or ventilator-dependent patients, or those with cancer, have shown that the predicted energy expenditure significantly underestimates the measured energy expenditure.[26] Total energy expenditure is estimated by adding the energy cost of activity and injury to the RME. The activity factor is increased 20 percent over the RME for patients confined to bed, and by 30 percent for ambulatory patients. The injury factor varies from 10 to 100 percent above the RME depending on the severity of the stress.[8] The formulas for predicting BEE are shown inside the back cover of this text. Nomograms for predicting resting energy expenditure in hospitalized patients have also been developed.[27]

Assessment of Protein Needs The requirement for protein in the hospitalized patient is influenced by the nutritional status before the illness or injury, the severity of stress, and the extent of nitrogen losses.

The previously well-nourished individual can usually tolerate a few days of inadequate protein intake. The adaptive response of the body in such situations is to utilize protein more efficiently and to decrease metabolic expenditure. On the other hand, the individual with serious illness or injury may be unable or unwilling to ingest sufficient calories and protein. A state of semistarvation added to the stress of the illness or injury may result in extensive nitrogen losses. Severely undernourished patients show less nitrogen loss than do those who were previously well nourished simply because their protein reserves are already depleted.

The nitrogen losses that accompany stress are inevitable. Increasing the protein intake will not prevent negative nitrogen balance from occurring during the peak catabolic period after severe stress (5 to 10 days post injury); however, it can improve nitrogen balance.

If nitrogen losses are known, the protein requirement is based on measured urinary losses, with correction for integumental and fecal losses. When urinary nitrogen losses are not measured, the protein requirement can be estimated by determining the energy requirement, and providing a calorie-to-nitrogen ratio of 150 : 1 during stress.[8] In severe stress the ratio may range from 100 : 1 to 150 : 1. During convalescence, adjustments in energy and protein intake are based on periodic 24-hour urinary urea nitrogen excretion. The protein requirement may decrease, although it is customary to maintain a calorie to nitrogen ratio of 150 : 1. Alternatively, monitoring of weight status is used to judge the adequacy of energy and protein intakes.

Documentation of Nutritional Care

Kardex Care Plans Many nursing and dietetic departments use a Kardex system for rapid access to important patient information and care plans. Some organize the same information into a notebook instead of a Kardex. The Kardex information is obtained from both the medical record and the patient. The amount of detail varies, but generally includes the diagnosis, allergies, scheduled tests or procedures, medications, and diet order.

The nursing kardex also includes the nursing diagnoses and interventions. For the sake of brevity, only the problem and etiology components of the nursing diagnosis are usually included in the Kardex. The signs and symptoms that make up the data base for the nursing diagnosis are not usually listed.[28]

The dietetic department Kardex lists specific information such as height, weight, pertinent laboratory values and medications, individual food preferences, food allergies, diet history, meal patterns for calculated diets, schedule for between meal feedings, nutrition assessment data, the nutrition care plan, and record of nutritional counseling. The dietitian is responsible for developing the nutritional care plan for each patient. The care plan includes (1) an assessment of the adequacy of the patient's usual dietary intake; (2) any nutritional problems and (3) plans for resolving these; (4) objectives for patient education, stated in terms of patient outcomes; (5) progress notes; (6) evaluation of nutritional care; and (7) readiness for discharge.

The Medical Record The medical record is the primary instrument for communication among those di-

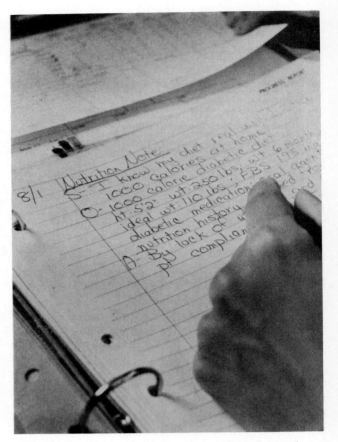

Figure 26-3. Entries into the medical record often make use of the SOAP format. Subjective and objective data are entered, as well as assessment of the problem, and the plans for resolving the problem. The chart should include progress notes concerning the patient's acceptance of his diet and any nutritional notes concerning the patient's acceptance of his diet and any nutritional deficiencies that may be present. Sometimes the intake of specific nutrients is calculated and charted. (Courtesy, Metropolitan Medical Center, Minneapolis.)

rectly concerned with the care of the patient; therefore, it should contain ongoing documentation of all aspects of health care provided to the patient, including nutrition. Many institutions use the "problem-oriented" approach. The record is organized according to the patient's key problems. This approach permits ready access to the problem of interest and knowledge of its current status by each member of the health care team. Entries into the record by team members are identified according to the problem and are organized so as to distinguish *subjective* and *objective* information, *assessment* data, and *plans* for resolution of the problem (SOAP format). (See Figure 26-3.) Nursing diagnoses are also recorded in the SOAP format.

Feeding the Patient

Environment for Meals   Time and effort directed toward creating an atmosphere conducive to the enjoyment of food are well spent. Such an environment implies that the surrounding areas are orderly and clean; that ventilation is good; and that distracting activities such as treatment of patients and doctors' rounds are not occurring at mealtime except as emergencies may arise.

Patients who are ambulatory enjoy eating with others. In some hospitals a dining room is provided for patients, and in others food service may be easily arranged at small tables set up in the patients' lounge.

Readiness of the Patient   The patient should be ready for the meal whether in bed or ambulatory. This may entail mouth care, the washing of the hands, and the positioning of the patient so that eating can take place in comfort. If tests or treatment unavoidably delay a meal, arrangements must be made to hold trays so that the food can be fresh and appetizing when the patient is ready to eat.

The Patient's Tray   The appearance of the tray is of the utmost importance since the patient's consumption of the food presented is the goal to be achieved. Foods should provide variety in color, textures, and flavors for appeal to the senses, should be attractively arranged on the tray, and should be served at the proper temperature. The tray should be of appropriate size for the food being served. China, glassware, and flatware should be spotless.

Assistance in Feeding   Some patients may require assistance in the cutting of meat or other dense foods, the pouring of a beverage, or the buttering of a piece of toast. Very ill or infirm patients must be fed. Ideally, the nurse should sit while feeding the patient so as to be at ease and avoid undue haste. Food will be enjoyed more if it can be eaten with reasonable leisure and if there is some conversation. Obviously, the nurse responsible for feeding several patients will make arrangements to delay tray service or to keep foods hot for those who must await their turn. (See Figure 26-4.)

Comprehensive Care Services

Concepts of Comprehensive Care   The provision of all necessary health services so that the patient can maintain or be restored to independent living is implied in the term *comprehensive care*. The components of comprehensive health care include screen-

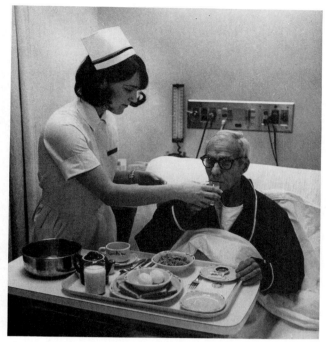

Figure 26-4.   Some patients require assistance at meals because they are too weak to feed themselves, while others need encouragement to eat. (Courtesy, Yale-New Haven Medical Center.)

ing, assessment, intervention, and follow-up. Careful evaluation and reevaluation of the client's physical, psychologic, economic, and social needs are required so that referral is made to the appropriate personnel for essential services. (See Figure 26-5.) The services may be provided on an inpatient basis, including hospital care for the acutely ill, a minimum-care facility within a hospital, or convalescent care in a nursing home. Care may be furnished through an outpatient clinic, utilizing a single service in a physician's office or multiple services provided by a clinic or health center. Home care, of course, implies services provided in the home, and can range from a single service such as nursing to coordinated services by many disciplines that could include medical, nursing, dental, dietetic, social, occupational therapy, physical therapy, and others.

Many home-care programs are now available, some of which are sponsored by the hospital whereas others are operated by for-profit organizations that work cooperatively with the hospital; still others are directed by a public or voluntary health agency. Such services require the assistance of a variety of technicians so that the services of the professional nurse, nutritionist, and others may be most effectively used.

Home parenteral nutrition is an example of one of the newer programs that require periodic monitoring

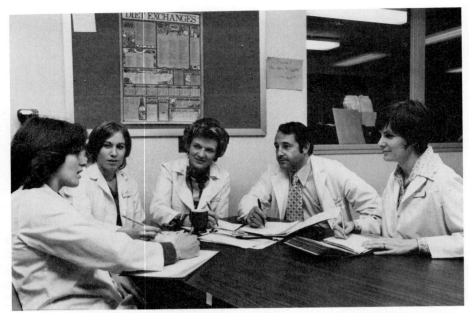

Figure 26-5. An important part of patient care involves adequate planning for the patient's discharge. here the social worker shares information with the occupational therapist, nurse, physician, and dietitian. (Courtesy, University of Minnesota Health Sciences Center, Minneapolis.)

by health team members. Family members are increasingly assuming responsibility for care of relatives who have serious health problems or who are terminally ill from cancer. The programs permit the patient to spend his or her last weeks or months among loved ones in a more comfortable environment.

Nutritional care is an essential and dynamic component of comprehensive health care. In fact, the ability to deliver the needed nutritional services and the quality of nutrition that the patient can maintain are often the decisive factors in restoring health, or in maintaining it. A brief discussion of some elements of home care follows.

Home-Delivered Meals Many individuals or couples with physical limitations can remain in their own homes rather than be institutionalized if they have access to home-delivered meals available from many senior centers or through the Voluntary Meals-on-Wheels program. (See page 325.) Others who are temporarily disabled by illness but who are ambulatory and can feed themselves may find it possible to return to their homes at an earlier time if they can procure their meals.

Homemaker Services The purpose of this service is to maintain the family in a healthful setting when no one in the family can fulfill the homemaking function. For example, the mother may be ill or convalescing from physical or mental illness; an aging person or couple is unable to perform the necessary tasks in the home, but could remain at home at less expense with homemaker assistance; death of the mother in a home with young children presents a major problem to the working father unless relatives help out or homemaker service is available.

The duties of the homemaker may include light housekeeping, meal preparation, marketing, laundry, and escort services to medical facilities. In some instances the homemaker also provides personal care such as bathing and grooming as supportive assistance.

A home health aide provides personal care to the client as supportive assistance and also as part of a medical care plan. She also assumes the general duties of homemaking listed previously. Generally she is employed by a nursing agency that is responsible for the supervision of the medical care plan. These services may be reimbursable through present regulations of Medicare when the medical care plan follows a period of hospitalization.

Nursing Homes The trend toward care of the elderly in institutional settings instead of the home is reflected by the substantial increase in the numbers of both nursing homes and residents in these homes during the 1970s. From 1969 to 1980 the number of nursing and related care homes in the United States with 25 or more beds increased by 27 percent; the number of residents increased by 75 percent.[29] Nearly 1.5 million persons reside in these homes. Although this represents a small percentage of the elderly, the numbers are expected to grow as the proportion of the population over age 65 increases.

Unfortunately, the medical, nursing, and nutritional care of residents in some nursing homes is less than optimal. Many physicians do not provide care to nursing home patients. State and federal regulations for long-term care facilities are more stringent than those for acute care facilities, yet reimbursement for services is substantially less. Under current Medicare guidelines, reimbursement for physician visits to skilled nursing homes is limited to one visit every 30 days; for intermediate care facilities one visit every 90 days is reimbursed. Nursing staff shortages are chronic in some areas, and a dietitian is available for consultation only a few hours a month in most nursing homes. In these situations, an ongoing record of the nursing diagnoses and nursing interventions can greatly facilitate patient care.

A common nursing diagnosis in many facilities is likely to be "alteration in nutrition." Many elderly persons have one or more chronic health problems that may affect nutritional status—diabetes mellitus, hypertension, diverticulosis, arthritis, stroke, constipation—to name a few. Poorly fitting dentures may limit the foods that can be eaten. Often the elderly seem to have lost interest in eating, owing in part to physiologic changes, and also to lack of socialization. Food intake is often remarkably improved if residents have a choice in menu selection, if therapeutic diet modifications are kept to a minimum, and if meals are taken in a common dining room with other residents rather than in the isolation of one's room. Company at mealtimes and assistance with eating are as important for some as what they are eating. Health care providers need to be alert to these needs, and to recognize that refusal to eat or complaints about the meals are sometimes means to gain attention. On the other hand, meals should be attractively served, at the proper temperature, and seasoned appropriately, with sufficient time allowed to enjoy the meals (see page 395).

Some guidelines for assessing and meeting the nutritional needs of the elderly in nursing homes were presented in Chapter 22.

Physical Handicaps, Rehabilitation, and Nutrition

Physical Handicaps Millions of Americans have physical handicaps that restrict their ability to care for themselves and to work. Physical disabilities cover a wide range: the individual who has lost a hand or an arm, or who is hemiplegic and has the use of only one arm; arthritics with stiff, swollen, painful joints and who have a limited range of motion; those with cerebral palsy, Parkinson's disease, or multiple sclerosis and for whom uncoordinated movements are a constant trial; those bound to a wheelchair; the blind; those who have limited cardiac and respiratory reserves such as patients with cardiac disease or emphysema; and many others.

Nutrition of the Physically Handicapped Adequate nutrition is essential in restoring a patient to his or her potential capacity for independence, yet the handicap itself may be the principal factor that favors malnutrition even though the supply of food is plentiful. The use of only one arm, or stiff, painful joints, or incoordinated movements present tremendous difficulties in feeding oneself and may limit the performance of simple kitchen tasks such as opening packages, cutting foods, peeling vegetables, and using appliances.

The energy balance is an important consideration. Some handicapped individuals have an increased energy requirement because they must exert a tremendous effort to complete tasks. The increased requirement, on the one hand, and the difficulties experienced in eating, on the other hand, lead to excessive weight loss and to tissue depletion. Other individuals confined to wheelchairs and who exert little effort may become obese and require a diet restricted in calories. (See Chapter 25.)

Good protein nutrition is essential for restoration of body tissues, to reduce the incidence of infection, and to maintain the integrity of the skin. For immobilized individuals decubitus ulcers are a frequent problem. During the early stages of immobilization the nitrogen losses from the body greatly exceed the intake. The accelerated catabolism of protein tissues appears to run a time sequence that is not wholly reversed in the early stages even though a high-protein diet may be used. Nevertheless, the replacement of these losses requires a high-protein diet over an extended period of time. (See Chapter 33.)

Excessive losses of calcium from the bones may lead to urinary calculi. A liberal fluid intake is essential to facilitate the excretion of calcium, and some restriction of the calcium intake is often prescribed. (See Chapter 40.)

Constipation is a frequent complication of those who are immobilized. Its prevention or correction requires a liberal intake of fluids, a diet containing sufficient bulk, and regular habits of elimination. (See Chapter 30 for further details.)

The Nature of Rehabilitation   Rehabilitation is the return of a handicapped individual to his or her maximum potential—to what the person will be able to do in the future. It is an individualized process in which therapy is designed specifically in terms of the patient's handicap, psychologic problems, family situation, and economic circumstances. It is individualized in that each patient's progress is measured against that person's own possibilities, not against some normal standard.

Rehabilitation may occur in a rehabilitation center, in a school for handicapped children, or in the home. The economic consideration is important inasmuch as rehabilitation is costly in terms of weeks or months in a rehabilitation center and the involvement of many specialists in the process. In addition, when the homemaker is handicapped, additional costs for a substitute in the home are likely to be appreciable.

The handicapped individual experiences helplessness, defeat, frustration, and even neglect. To surmount these difficulties becomes a constant uphill battle. Rehabilitation itself is usually slow, sometimes painful, and fatiguing both physically and emotionally. The patient needs the support of every member of the rehabilitation team.

The Rehabilitation Team.   The skills and techniques in physical medicine, physical therapy, occupational therapy, nursing, home economics, nutrition, social work, and psychology are utilized in rehabilitation. The patient is not only the focus of these specialized skills but part of the team and a participant in the plans for his or her restoration—as are members of the family. Each member of the team contributes skills in a way that complements but does not overlap or duplicate the efforts of another. The nurse is usually the coordinator of these services in the rehabilitation center.

Self-help Devices for Eating   Numerous devices for daily activities have been designed at the Institute of Rehabilitation Medicine of the New York University Medical Center. In addition, publications such as the *Mealtime Manual for People with Disabilities and the Aging* are valuable.[30] Many of the devices can be made in the home, and others are available at moderate costs. A few of the devices that are helpful to those who have only one arm or who have difficulty in holding articles or bringing food to the mouth are described in the following. (See Figure 26-6.)

Jointed Handles for Spoons and Forks.   When the motions of the arm and wrist are restricted, the joints of the utensil permit an angle that can approach the mouth.

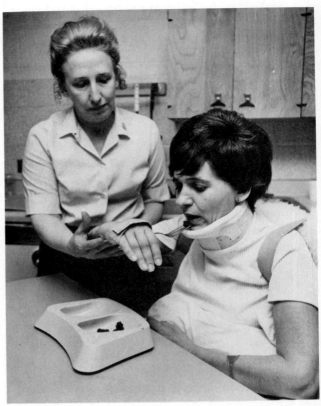

Figure 26-6.   This patient is learning to use a universal cuff to become independent in self-feeding activities. A bowl with suction cups adheres to the table and prevents slipping. This will be used to make learning less difficult and will be replaced with regular utensils when the skill is perfected. (Courtesy, Allied Services for the Handicapped, Inc., Scranton, Pennsylvania.)

Knife for Cutting.   A knife needs a firm support, and cutting is difficult for persons with the use of only one arm. A cuff fitted over the hand permits the knife to be held firmly. A serrated edge is better than one with a smooth edge.

Plate Guards.   These are placed at the edge of the plate; they keep food from spilling and provide a surface against which food can be pushed. A deep dish with straight sides is also helpful. The plate can be kept from sliding by placing it in a support constructed to hold it, or by setting it on a sponge.

Buttering Bread.   A right-angle ledge affixed to the corner of the breadboard will hold a piece of bread in place while it is being buttered.

Drinking Glass and Tube.   A drinking glass can be fitted with a holder that has a wide handle easily grasped by the hand. If it is difficult to bring the glass to the mouth, a wooden block into which a hole has been cut to hold a standard-size glass will hold the glass firmly on the table. A piece of plastic tubing bent at an angle for approach to the mouth can be used. To keep the plastic tube from slipping, a bulldog clip can be fastened to the edge of the glass and the tubing can be placed through the hole of the handle of the clip.

Aids in Food Preparation Homemaking is the single most frequent occupation of the physically handicapped. The rehabilitation of the homemaker in terms of food preparation skills and in overall homemaking activities benefits the entire family. Home economists, occupational therapists, and dietitians have specialized skills by which they are able to help the homemaker in simplification of procedures in food preparation and in more convenient kitchen arrangements.

The handicapped homemaker will find that each task requires a longer time to complete. As much food preparation should be completed in advance as possible so that there are few last-minute tasks. Arthritics fatigue easily and they should not attempt tasks that cannot be interrupted for a rest period. For many homemakers a list of things to be done is helpful.

Electric mixers, blenders, wedge-shape jar openers, electric can openers, long-handled tongs to reach packages and equipment out of reach, turntables in cupboards to hold supplies, sliding racks, magnetized equipment holders, and carts on wheels are among the pieces of equipment that facilitate work for the handicapped homemaker.

The person who has the use of only one arm needs firm support for devices. For example, a board with two stainless steel nails serves as a holder for vegetables to be peeled. A sponge underneath a bowl helps to keep it from sliding. Boxes can be held firmly between the knees and a scissors can be used with one hand to cut off tops.

For those who will be confined to a wheelchair indefinitely or who must sit while working, a redesign of the kitchen is essential. Counter surfaces need to be lowered so that work can be done while sitting. Knee-hole spaces are needed so that the chair or wheelchair can be partially underneath the work surface. Equipment and storage shelves must be within reach.

Nutrition for the Mentally Ill

The relationship of nutrition to mental disorders has intrigued some researchers for years—since the discovery early in the century that a substantial number of patients in mental hospitals suffered from pellagra-associated dementia which could be corrected with niacin. Out of this interest has grown the field of *orthomolecular psychiatry*, which advocates use of pharmacologic doses of vitamins as an adjunct to traditional therapy in treatment of mental disorders. Megadoses of niacin along with other B vitamins, ascorbic acid, and certain minerals and specific drug therapy have been advocated for use in treatment of schizophrenia. However, controlled studies have failed to show significant clinical improvement with this treatment in schizophrenia. Most traditional psychiatrists reject the hypothesis that megavitamins have therapeutic value in treatment of mental disorders.

An association between schizophrenia and celiac disease has been proposed based on the increased probability of celiac disease in schizophrenics and of schizophrenia in patients with celiac disease. Schizophrenic patients treated with a milk- and cereal-free diet have reportedly shown improvement of symptoms which was reversed when gluten was added to the diet.[31,32] Further controlled studies are needed to test this hypothesis.

Although a therapeutic role for specific dietary factors has not been clearly established in psychiatric disorders, diet is nevertheless an important part of the total program of rehabilitation for the psychiatric patient. Aside from its nutritional necessity, food provides basic security and pleasurable satisfaction. The patient needs to feel that someone is genuinely concerned about his or her welfare and cares for him or her. The dietitian and nurse—through the care shown in meal planning, preparation, and service, and through their expressions of interest to the individual—are participants in the therapy.

Planning a nutritionally adequate diet is obviously not enough. The service of food that is attractive to the eye, tempting in aroma, and satisfying to the palate is just as important in the psychiatric hospital as in any other feeding situation. The mentally ill may express marked irritability when given foods they dislike. Food service in a cafeteria permits the patient to exercise some choice in food selection, and thus helps to eliminate some of the irritations. On the other hand, staff-shared family-style meal service is favored by some and permits opportunity for closer rapport between staff and patients.

Patients react favorably and are less destructive when an attractive dining environment is provided. A well-planned dining room with a cheerful color scheme, curtains or draperies at the windows, small attractive tables, and suitable background music is conducive to food acceptance and contributes to the therapy of the patient. Attention to birthdays, holidays, and other special events provides additional evidence that the patient is cared for.

Psychiatric patients frequently eat inadequate or excessive amounts of food. A regular schedule of weighing of patients—about once a month—will help detect such changes, and correction can be started before marked weight change has occurred. Marked weight gain is not uncommon. It would seem easy to control this in a hospital by providing a diet designed for weight maintenance. However, the privileges of food purchases from a canteen and food gifts from relatives and friends must be taken into consideration. Patients are often known to eat food left by other patients.

Refusal to eat is a problem presented by other psychiatric patients. The nurse or attendant should note any patient who refuses more than half of a meal. A 4- or 5-day simple checklist helps identify whether the refusal follows a pattern with respect to a particular food or meal. Refusal of food sometimes denotes an underlying physical illness about which the patient who is withdrawn or mute does not complain. Those who need to gain weight may require close supervision in taking small, frequent feedings; some may be helped if butter is spread on the bread, milk and sugar are put on the cereal, the milk container is opened, the meat is cut, and so on; sincere words of encouragement should be offered when progress is made. Tube feeding (see Chapter 28) may be resorted to when all attempts to achieve satisfactory intake of food fail.

Feeding the mentally retarded presents many problems that may be especially acute in the child. The management of the diet for these patients is discussed in Chapter 43.

CASE STUDY 10

Elderly Man with Cerebrovascular Accident

Mr. P, age 84, is a retired land developer who lives in a two-story home in Arizona. He never married and has no close living relatives. He is well known in the community for his support of the arts and commerce. He takes pleasure in playing the violin and traveling. He belongs to the country club and enjoys golfing.

Mr. P, a man of moderate build, is 170 cm (67 in.) tall, and weighs 67 kg (147 lb). He is in good physical condition. Mr. P is very independent and still drives his automobile. He does his own cooking and appreciates fine wines. Occasionally he eats with friends in restaurants. A housekeeper comes in once a week to do the cleaning and grocery shopping.

When Mr. P awakened one morning he was unable to move the left side of his body. He fell to the floor when getting out of bed but managed to crawl to the telephone to call his neighbor. The neighbor recognized Mr. P's voice but could not understand what he was saying. She called the ambulance and the paramedics rushed Mr. P to the hospital.

Subsequent neurologic findings indicated a partial thrombosis of the right middle cerebral artery. Mr. P displayed general disorientation, left hemiplegia, left hemianopsia, and dysphagia. The muscles in his left arm and leg were completely flaccid.

Initially Mr. P was fed intravenously. As his diet was advanced to clear liquids he coughed frequently during feedings. The nurse noticed that Mr. P ate only those foods on the right side of his tray. Because of dysphagia and persisting disorientation at mealtimes, he was referred to the dysphagia team. The nutritionist on the team planned a diet to meet prescribed consistency and nutritional needs. During his hospital stay his diet was progressed to a mechanical soft diet.

Pathophysiologic Correlations
1. What is meant by "cerebrovascular accident" (CVA)?
2. What was the probable cause of the cerebral artery thrombosis Mr. P suffered?
3. Identify some of the nursing diagnoses that might apply in Mr. P's case.
4. What is the probable reason that Mr. P eats only the foods on the right side of his tray? Suggest a solution.

Nutritional Assessment
5. List some ways in which body composition and function change with aging.
6. Intakes of several nutrients are likely to be less than desirable in the elderly. List these nutrients and some possible reasons for the reduced intake.
7. How might iron status be assessed in the elderly?
8. What factors contribute to negative nitrogen balance in elderly persons in spite of adequate protein intakes?

9. What factors contributed to the alteration in nutrition experienced by Mr. P?
10. What was likely to be the primary feeding difficulty?
11. List the nutritional problems of particular concern when a patient is confined to a wheelchair.
12. Identify the feeding problems that must be resolved in patients such as Mr. P.

Planning the Diet

13. What types of foods could Mr. P handle best? Give examples.
14. State the rationale for a mechanical soft diet.
15. The first dinner tray delivered to Mr. P after he was placed on the mechanical soft diet contained ground meat. At first he thought this was an error, but when he was assured that the menu was correct he protested vehemently and refused to eat anything on his tray. How would you handle this situation?
16. Indicate the appropriate nursing interventions for the alteration in nutrition experienced by Mr. P.
17. What are the expected outcomes of the nursing interventions?
18. How would you go about teaching Mr. P to eat with his left hand?

19. Mr. P is so embarrassed by his drooling and messy eating that he refuses to eat in front of anyone. He does not even want the nurse present. Yet if left alone in his private room he hardly touches his food. What would you recommend?

Dietary Counseling

The nurse specialist in rehabilitation consulted with the staff of the extended care facility at the time of Mr. P's transfer. A consultant dietitian gave continuing assistance of dietary management.

20. Because of the difficulty of managing dishes and flatware with one hand, several feeding devices were suggested for Mr. P's use. List some possibilities.
21. List the steps you would emphasize in teaching Mr. P to swallow foods and liquids.
22. Mr P has problems with constipation. What are some dietary adjustments that can be made to alleviate this?
23. Mr. P's appetite is poor. What suggestions can you give to improve his food intake?
24. Mr. P's friends bring food to him three or four times a week. What suggestions can you give for the best food gifts? Give your reasons.

References for the Case Study

CALLAHAN, M. E.: "Caring for A Stroke Patient Like Me," *Nursing*, '84, **14**:65–67, May 1984.

KADAS, N.: "The Dysphagic Patient: Everyday Really Counts," *R.N.*, **46**:38–41, November 1983.

KAVCHAK-KEYES, M. A.: "Comeback From Disaster: Helping the Stroke Patient Learn to Help Himself," *Nursing*, '84, **9**:32–35, January 1979.

TILTON, C. N., and MALOOF, M.: "Diagnosing the Problems in Stroke," *Am. J. Nurs.*, **82**:596–601, 1982.

WILLIAMS, H., et al.: "Treating Dysphagia," *J. Gerontol. Nurs.*, **9**:638–39ff, 1983.

References

1. American Dietetic Association: *Handbook of Clinical Dietetics*, Yale University Press, New Haven, Conn., 1981.
2. American Hospital Association: "Statement on a Patient's Bill of Rights," *Hospitals*, **47**:41, February 16, 1973.
3. Forse, R. A., and Shizgal, H. M.: "The Assessment of Malnutrition," *Surgery*, **88**:17–24, 1980.
4. Michel, L., et al.: "Nutritional Support of Hospitalized Patients," *N. Engl. J. Med.*, **304**:1147–52, 1981.
5. Buzby, G. P., et al.: "Prognostic Nutritional Index in Gastrointestinal Surgery," *Am. J. Surg.*, **139**:160–67, 1980.
6. Grant, J. P., et al.: "Current Techniques of Nutritional Assessment," *Surg. Clin. North Am.*, **61**:437–63, 1981.
7. Blackburn, G. L., and Harvey, K. B.: "Nutritional Assessment as a Routine in Clinical Medicine," *Postgrad. Med.*, **71**:46–55ff, May 1982.
8. Long, C., et al.: "Metabolic Response to Injury and Illness: Estimation of Energy and Protein Needs from Indirect Calorimetry and Nitrogen Balance," *J.P.E.N.*, **3**:452–56, 1979.
9. Simko, M. D., et al.: *Nutrition Assessment*, Aspen Systems Corporation, Rockville, Md., 1984.
10. Seltzer, M. H., et al.: "Instant Nutritional Assessment," *J.P.E.N.*, **3**:157–59, 1979.
11. Frisancho, A. R.: "New Norms of Upper Limb Fat and Muscle Areas for Assessment of Nutritional Status," *Am. J. Clin. Nutr.*, **34**:2540–45, 1981.
12. Bishop, C. W.: "Reference Values for Arm Muscle Area, Arm Fat Area, Subscapular Skinfold Thickness, and Sum of Skinfold Thickness for American Adults," *J.P.E.N.*, **8**:515–22, 1984.
13. Gurney, J. M., and Jellife, D. B.: "Arm Anthropometry in Nutritional Assessment: Nomogram for Rapid Calculation of Muscle Circumference and Cross-Sectional Muscle and Fat Areas," *Am. J. Clin. Nutr.*, **26**:912–15, 1973.
14. Metropolitan Life Insurance Company: "1983 Metropolitan Height and Weight Tables," *Stat. Bull. Metrop. Life Found.*, **64**:3–9, January–June, 1983.
15. National Center for Health Statistics: "NCHS Growth

Charts, 1976," *Monthly Vital Statistics Report*, Vol 25, No. 3, supp. (HRA) 76-1120. Health Resources Administration, Rockville, Maryland, June 1976. (Charts prepared by Ross Laboratories, Columbus, Ohio.)

16. Sidney, A., et al.: "Weight by Height and Age for Adults 18–74 Years, United States, 1971–74," *Vital and Health Statistics*. Series 11. No. 28 DHEW Pub. No. (PHS) 79-1656. National Health Survey, Rockville, Md., 1979.

17. Blackburn, G. L., et al.: "Nutritional and Metabolic Assessment of the Hospitalized Patient," *J.P.E.N.*, 1:11–22, 1977.

18. Mitchell, C. O., and Lipschitz, D. A.: "The Effect of Age and Sex on the Routinely Used Measurements to Assess the Nutritional Status of Hospitalized Patients," *Am. J. Clin. Nutr.*, 36:340–49, 1982.

19. Anderson, C. F., and Wochos, D. N.: "The Utility of Serum Albumin Values in The Nutritional Assessment of Hospitalized Patients," *Mayo Clin. Proc.*, 57:181–84, 1982.

20. Lemoine, A., et al.: "Vitamin B_1, B_2, and C Status in Hospital Inpatients," *Am. J. Clin. Nutr.*, 33:2595–2600, 1980.

21. Twomey, P., et al.: "Utility of Skin Testing in Nutritional Assessment: A Critical Review," *J.P.E.N.*, 6:55–58, 1982.

22. Blackburn, G. L., and Thornton, P. A.: "Nutritional Assessment of the Hospitalized Patient," *Med. Clin. North Am.*, 63:1103–15, 1979.

23. Mullen, J. L., et al.: "Implications of Malnutrition in the Surgical Patient," *Arch. Surg.*, 114:121–25, 1979.

24. Bistrian, B.: "Anthropometric Norms Used in Assessment of Hospitalized Patients," *Am. J. Clin. Nutr.*, 33:2211–14, 1980.

25. Harris, J. A., and Benedict, F. G.: *A Biometric Study of Basal Metabolism in Man*, Carnegie Institution of Washington. Pub. No. (279) 189–90, Washington, 1919.

26. Roza, A. M., and Shizgal, H. M.: "The Harris Benedict Equation Re-evaluated: Resting Energy Requirements and the Body Cell Mass," *Am. J. Clin. Nutr.*, 40:168–82, 1984.

27. Rainey-McDonald, C. G., et al.: "Nomograms for Predicting Resting Energy Expenditure of Hospitalized Patients," *J.P.E.N.*, 6:59–60, 1982.

28. Gordon, M.: *Nursing Diagnosis. Process and Application*, McGraw-Hill Book Company, New York, 1982.

29. Strahan, G. W.: "Trends in Nursing and Related Care Homes and Hospitals, United States, Selected Years 1969–80," *Vital and Health Statistics*. Series 14. No. 30 DHHS Pub. No. (PHS) 84-1825. Public Health Service, Washington, D.C. U.S. Government Printing Office, March 1984.

30. Klinger, J. L., et al.: *Mealtime Manual for People with Disabilities and the Aging*, Campbell Soup Company, Camden, N.J., 1978.

31. Singh, M. M., and Kay, S. R.: "Wheat Gluten as a Pathogenic Factor in Schizophrenia," *Science*, 191:401–2, 1976.

32. Dohan, F. C., et al.: "Relapsed Schizophrenics: More Rapid Improvement on a Milk- and Cereal-free Diet," *Br. J. Psychiatry*, 115:595–96, 1969.

27

Food, Nutrient, and Drug Interactions

Drug therapy plays an important role in the management of many acute and chronic diseases. In recent years clinicians have developed a greater awareness of the potential effects of drug therapy on nutritional status and, conversely, of the influence of nutrition on drug effectiveness. Nevertheless, knowledge of drug–nutrient interactions is still in its infancy, and much more research is urgently needed. Animal studies have elucidated many potential drug–nutrient interactions, but the applicability of many of these studies to humans is uncertain.

Drug therapy may influence nutrient intake, absorption, metabolism, or excretion; likewise foods or their components may affect the absorption, metabolism, and excretion of drugs. This chapter presents a brief overview of these potential interactions with representative examples using commonly prescribed drugs. A description of ways in which selected drugs influence nutritional status is shown in Appendix B.

The potential for diet–drug interactions is greatest in those on long-term drug therapy, the malnourished, those with chronic diseases, children, and the elderly. Especially among the elderly in whom chronic disease states, physiologic changes associated with aging, inadequate food intake, multiple drug therapies, and poor drug compliance, or medication errors are likely, is close monitoring of the effects of drug therapy needed. Health care professionals responsible for the nutritional care of all these groups of patients must be aware of potential drug–nutrient interactions. Nutritional assessment should include a review of all medications and the type of diet the patient is receiving. Plans for educating the patient regarding appropriate timing of drugs in relationship to meals and any dietary modifications needed because of drug therapy should be indicated in the nutritional care plan.

Effects of Drugs on Nutrition

Alteration in Taste, Appetite, and Food Intake
Drugs may affect *taste* in several ways. Many drugs produce a general alteration in taste acuity, or *dysgeusia*. For example, clofibrate (a hypocholesterolemic agent), levodopa (an anti-Parkinson agent), penicillamine (a chelating agent), and sulfasalazine (an antiinflammatory agent) all decrease taste acuity.[1] Each of these belongs to a different class of drugs. The alteration in taste acuity is not necessarily characteristic of other drugs within the same class, however. Some drugs exert a more specific effect by altering sensitivity to one or more of the four basic tastes; amphetamines decrease sensitivity to sweets, while fluorouracil (antineoplastic agent) increases it, and prolonged use of insulin is associated with decreased sensitivity to both salt and sweet tastes.[2] Still other drugs such as allopurinol (an anti-gout drug), penicillin, and quinidine (an anti-arrhythmic agent) leave an unpleasant aftertaste.[1]

Appetite and Food Intake. Side effects of a few drugs include appetite stimulation. Tranquilizers, such as chlorpromazine and diazepam, the antidepressant amitriptyline, corticosteroids, methyldopa (a diuretic), and the sulfonylureas (oral hypoglycemic agents) all tend to increase appetite, resulting in weight gain.[3]

Amphetamines are sometimes used on a temporary basis for their appetite suppressant effects in the treatment of obesity. These drugs stimulate the satiety center of the hypothalamus. Other effects include mood elevation, an increase in motor activity, and slight euphoria. Tolerance to all drugs in this class limits their effectiveness for long-term use in appetite control. The drugs are also sometimes used in hyperkinetic

403

Table 27-1. Some Drugs That Frequently Produce Anorexia, Nausea, and Vomiting

Amphetamines
Anticonvulsants
Antineoplastics
    Asparaginase
    Cisplatin
    Cyclophosphamide
    Methotrexate
    Cytosine arabinoside
    Dactinomycin
Digitalis
Nitrofurantoin
Tetracycline

children in whom they exert a calming effect. Growth retardation occurring in these children has been attributed to diminished food intake and is reversed when the drugs are discontinued.[3]

Many drugs depress appetite indirectly by causing *anorexia* (a decreased desire for food), or nausea. Classes of drugs that are well known for these effects are antineoplastic agents used in cancer therapy and antiinfective agents.[4] (See Table 27-1.) Some dietary suggestions to relieve the unpleasant side effects of these drugs have been offered.[5] Levodopa inhibits gastric emptying, thereby prolonging satiety and depressing appetite.

Alteration in Nutrient Absorption Drugs influence nutrient absorption through several mechanisms, including alterations in gastrointestinal transit time, pH, bile acid activity, enzyme systems, mucosal cells, or by binding to nutrients. Malabsorption may be generalized or specific for particular nutrients.

Transit Time. Gastrointestinal transit time is altered by ganglionic blocking agents, anticholinergics, or cathartics.[6] The ganglionic blocking agents used in treatment of hypertension block the transmission of nerve impulses at the ganglia of the autonomic nervous system. Constipation and paralytic ileus are examples of severe reactions to these drugs. Anticholinergics, sometimes used in management of peptic ulcer and gastrointestinal spasm, may also cause constipation. Cathartics, on the other hand, stimulate the smooth muscles of the bowel, resulting in shortened transit time and possible loss of nutrients.

pH. Reduction of ferric iron to the more easily absorbed ferrous form occurs in the acidic medium of the stomach. Antacids may hinder iron absorption by raising the pH of the gastric contents.

Bile Acid Activity. Prolonged use of drugs that bind bile acids may inhibit absorption of fat-soluble nutrients. Examples of drugs exerting this effect are cholestyramine and clofibrate used in treatment of hypercholesterolemia, and neomycin, an antibiotic.

Enzyme Systems. Decreased activity of intestinal disaccharidases brought about by antiinfectives or clofibrate is another way in which drug therapy may interfere with nutrient absorption. In this case, carbohydrate absorption is decreased. The potential for impaired folate absorption occurs when sulfasalazine is used in treatment of ulcerative colitis.[7] Sulfasalazine inhibits conjugase, an enzyme in the proximal intestine that hydrolyzes the polyglutamate form of folacin to the monoglutamate form for absorption.

Intestinal Mucosal Cells. Drug-induced damage to intestinal mucosal cells is primary or secondary. Primary malabsorption is due to a direct effect of the drug on the mucosal cell, and is exemplified by neomycin and colchicine, which is used in treatment of gout. These drugs produce a generalized malabsorption effect as shown by decreased absorption of vitamin B-12, carotene, cholesterol, lactose, D-xylose, iron, sodium, potassium, calcium, nitrogen, and fat.[8] (See Table 27-2.) Colchicine causes a loss of lactase activity due to altered mucosal structure. Examples of secondary malabsorption are provided by methotrexate and diphenylhydantoin. The antineoplastic drug, methotrexate, interferes with absorption or utilization of folate which, in turn, induces malabsorption of calcium. Phenytoin, an anticonvulsant, hinders absorption of vitamin D with subsequent calcium malabsorption.

Binding with Nutrients. Finally, drugs can interfere with nutrient absorption by binding to nutrients within the lumen. Neomycin binds ionized fatty acids and bile salts, thereby producing fat malabsorption. Tetracyclines form complexes with calcium, magnesium, iron, and zinc, thereby decreasing their absorption.

Alteration in Nutrient Metabolism Classic examples of drug-induced interference with nutrient metabolism are provided by cancer chemotherapeutic agents, antibiotics, anticonvulsants, and oral contraceptive agents.

One class of cancer chemotherapeutic agents acts as antimetabolites. These include analogs of folic acid, pyrimidines, or purines. The folic acid analog, methotrexate, binds to the enzyme dihydrofolate re-

Table 27-2. Some Drugs That Impair Utilization of Vitamins and Minerals*

	Vitamins											Minerals							
	Thiamin	Riboflavin	Pyridoxine	B-12	Folacin	Niacin	Ascorbic Acid	A	D	K	E	Calcium	Magnesium	Iron	Copper	Zinc	Sodium	Potassium	Phosphorus
Alcohol	X		X	X	X								X			X			
Antacids (aluminum hydroxide)								X	X										X
Anticonvulsants			X	X	X		X		X	X		X	X						
Cathartics									X			X						X	
Cholestyramine			X		X			X	X	X	X	X		X					
Clofibrate			X											X					
Colchicine			X		X												X	X	
Corticosteroids		X			X		X		X			X				X		X	X
Coumarin anticoagulants										X									
Digitalis	X											X	X					X	
Estrogens	X	X	X	X	X		X					X				X			
Ethacrynic acid												X	X					X	
Furosemide	X		X									X	X			X	X	X	
Isoniazid			X	X		X								X					
Levodopa			X				X										X	X	
Methotrexate			X		X														
Mineral oil								X	X	X	X	X							X
Neomycin			X	X				X	X	X	X	X		X			X	X	
Penicillamine			X											X	X	X			
Prednisone					X		X		X			X							
Probenecid												X	X				X	X	X
Salicylates	X													X				X	
Sulfasalazine					X									X					
Tetracycline		X			X	X	X		X			X	X			X			
Thyroxine		X																	
Thiazides		X										X	X			X		X	X
Triamterene			X		X							X					X		

* Adapted from the following sources:

Roe, D. A.: "Nutrient and Drug Interactions," *Nutr. Rev.*, **42**:141–53, 1984.

Loebl, S., and Spratto, G.: *The Nurse's Drug Handbook*, 3rd ed. John Wiley & Sons, New York, 1983.

Smith, C. H., and Bidlack, W. R.: "Dietary Concerns Associated with the Use of Medications," *J. Am. Diet. Assoc.*, **84**:901–14, 1984.

Powers, D. E., and Moore, A. O.: *Food–Medication Interactions*, 3rd ed. F-MI Publishing, Tempe, Arizona, 1981.

March, D. C.: *Handbook: Interactions of Selected Drugs with Nutritional Status in Man*, 2nd ed. The American Dietetic Association, 1978.

ductase and prevents the reduction of dihydrofolate to tetrahydrofolate, the active form of the vitamin. Methylene tetrahydrofolate is a methyl donor in the conversion of deoxyuridylate to thymidylate by the enzyme thymidylate synthetase, the rate-limiting step in DNA synthesis. Thus, methotrexate inhibits DNA synthesis.[9] The pyrimidine analog, fluorouracil, binds to thymidylate synthetase and inhibits DNA synthesis. Mercaptopurine, a purine analog, decreases nucleic acid synthesis.

The antibiotic chloramphenicol alters nutrient metabolism by inhibiting mitochondrial protein synthesis. Oral contraceptive agents have several effects on metabolism. Both carbohydrate and tryptophan metabolism are altered, resulting in hyperglycemia, impaired glucose tolerance, decreased serum pyridoxine levels, and increased excretion of tryptophan metabolites. Serum and erythrocyte levels of folate and riboflavin are also decreased. Plasma lipids are often increased when estrogen-containing oral contraceptives are used.

Nutrient metabolism is also altered by drug-induced enzyme induction. In this case, the enzymes that catabolize the drug increase requirements for specific nutrients or affect their metabolism in some other way. For example, prolonged use of phenobarbital is associated with induction of hepatic enzymes which increase the turnover of vitamin D and lead to osteomalacia or rickets. Vitamin D supplements are sometimes needed in persons receiving anticonvulsants.

Alterations in Nutrient Excretion Besides those discussed in the section on alterations in nutrient absorption, several other classes of drugs increase nutrient excretion. Aspirin may uncouple the energy source needed for renal tubular reabsorption of amino acids.[10] Diuretics such as the thiazides and furosemide interfere with renal tubular reabsorption of sodium, potassium, calcium, and magnesium. Penicillamine chelates copper and zinc, and increases their urinary excretion as well as that of pyridoxine. Isoniazid also increases urinary pyridoxine excretion by forming a complex with the vitamin rendering it unavailable to the body. Sodium and water retention may be a side effect of therapy with adrenal corticosteroids, antiinflammatory agents such as phenylbutazone, or the antihypertensives guanethidine and hydralazine.

Effects of Food on Drug Utilization

Alterations in Drug Absorption The absorption of orally administered drugs is influenced by the presence of food in the gastrointestinal tract. Food delays gastric emptying; consequently, drugs are often absorbed more slowly when taken with food. The therapeutic effectiveness of the drug may be compromised or enhanced when taken with food; for example, drug action may be prolonged or the drug may not reach therapeutic levels in the blood. Examples of drugs that are absorbed better in the absence of food are aspirin, antibiotics, and theophylline, an agent used to relieve bronchospasms. (See also Table 27-3.) The

Table 27-3. Influence of Food on Drug Absorption*

Class	Drug	Food
Decreased Drug Absorption When Administered with Food		
Anticoagulant	Warfarin sodium	
Antibiotic	Clindamycin	Pectin
	Erythromycin	
	Lincomycin	Pectin
	Penicillin	
	Sulfadiazene	
	Tetracycline	Dairy products
Analgesic	Acetaminophen	Pectin
Anti-Parkinson	Levodopa	High-protein meal
Antihypertensive	Methyldopa	High-protein meal
Antiarrhythmic	Digoxin	Bran
CNS stimulant	Theophylline	High-protein meals
Increased Drug Absorption When Administered with Food		
Antifungal	Griseofulvin	High-fat meal
Antihypertensive	Hydralazine	
Antiarrhythmic	Propranolol	High-protein meal
Antipsychotic	Lithium	
Diuretic	Spironolactone	
	Chlorothiazide	
Anticonvulsant	Carbamazepine	
Tranquilizer	Diazepam	

* Adapted from the following sources:
Roe, D. A.: "Nutrient and Drug Interactions," *Nutr. Rev.*, **42**:141–53, 1984.
Loebl, S., and Spratto, G.: *The Nurse's Drug Handbook*, 3rd ed. John Wiley & Sons, New York, 1983.
Smith, C. H., and Bidlack, W. R.: "Dietary Concerns Associated with the Use of Medications," *J. Am. Diet. Assoc.*, **84**:901–14, 1984.
Lamy, P. R.: "Effects of Diet and Nutrition in Drug Therapy," *J. Am. Geriatr. Soc.*, **30**:S99–112, 1982.

amebicide metronidazole, digoxin, cimetidine, and alcohol are absorbed more rapidly in the absence of food.[3] Some drugs are absorbed better on an empty stomach, but should be taken with food because of their irritating effect on the gastric mucosa. Included are aspirin, phenytoin, isoniazid, and several diuretics. Some drugs that should be taken with food to enhance absorption are listed in Table 27-3.

Alterations in Drug Metabolism In the intestine drugs are metabolized by mucosal enzymes and by microflora. Diseases of the intestine characterized by mucosal damage can modify intestinal drug metabolism. For example, reduction of brush border enzymes due to mucosal atrophy in gluten enteropathy can decrease the amount of drug that is hydrolyzed and subsequently absorbed.[3]

Diet can also influence the intestinal metabolism of drugs by altering the composition of the microflora or the intestinal transit time. For drugs that are metabolized by the microflora slow intestinal transit time is desired. Diets high in animal protein can influence the composition of the microflora; those high in dietary fiber influence transit time and may modify the therapeutic efficacy of some drugs.

Liver. The components of the hepatic microsomal drug metabolizing system function in electron transport and require specific vitamins and minerals for their activities. (See Chapter 6.) Thus, diet influences drug metabolism in the liver.

In animals, the hepatic degradation of drugs is decreased by high-carbohydrate diets and by deficiencies of calories, protein, ascorbic acid, riboflavin, vitamin E, vitamin A, magnesium, calcium, copper, and zinc. On the other hand, iron deficiency and increased unsaturated dietary fat intake enhance the hepatic degradation of drugs in animals.[8,11] Considerable species variation occurs, however, and the severity of the deficiency, the effect on other nutrient relationships of altering one nutrient, and the response of the target organ must be considered in evaluating these effects for potential clinical significance in humans.

In some individuals high-protein diets increase the rate of hepatic metabolism of drugs such as theophylline. Among other dietary factors that increase hepatic drug metabolism are charcoal broiling of beef, indoles present in cruciferous vegetables, and flavenoids in citrus fruits.[3]

Other. Caffeine enhances the excretion of theophylline by competing with it for metabolic enzymes, and enhances the stimulant effects of theophylline on the cardiovascular, gastrointestinal, and central nervous systems. Caffeine intake should be eliminated in patients taking theophylline.[12] Some common sources of caffeine are shown in Table 27-4.

Citrus juices alkalinize the urine, thereby enhancing reabsorption of the antiarrhythmic quinidine by the kidney and increasing the concentration of the drug in the blood. Patients taking quinidine should be cautioned regarding the potential effects of excess intake of citrus juices. Licorice contains a substance, glycyrrhizic acid, that may cause hypokalemia, sodium retention, and edema in persons taking antihypertensive agents.[5]

Foods with a high content of pressor amines, especially tyramine, may stimulate the release of norepinephrine from storage sites within neurons. Under normal circumstances, circulating monoamine oxidase inactivates dietary tyramine, preventing excessive norepinephrine release. Persons receiving monoamine oxidase (MAO) inhibitors may experience

Table 27-4. Sources of Caffeine in the Diet*

Item	Amount	Caffeine (mg)
Soft drinks		
Coca Cola	12 oz	45
Dr. Pepper	12 oz	40
Dr. Pepper, sugar free	12 oz	40
Mellow Yellow	12 oz	53
Mountain Dew	12 oz	54
Mr. Pibb	12 oz	41
Pepsi Cola	12 oz	38
Pepsi Cola, diet	12 oz	36
Tab	12 oz	47
Coffee		
Brewed	8 oz	88
Instant	8 oz	71
Tea		
Brewed	6 oz	41
Instant	6 oz	29
Milk		
Chocolate	8 oz	8
Other		
Brownie, nut fudge	1¼ oz	8
Cake, chocolate	1/18th of 9 inch	14
Candy, chocolate	1 oz	8
Candy, chocolate covered	1 oz	3
Ice cream, chocolate	⅔ cup	5
Pudding, chocolate	½ cup	6

* Adapted from Council on Scientific Affairs: "Caffeine Labeling," *JAMA*, **252**:803–806, 1984.

severe headaches, and acute hypertension attacks if they consume foods with a high tyramine content. (See Chapter 17, page 247.) Table 27-5 lists foods that should be eliminated from the diet by persons taking MAO inhibitors.

Avoidance of vitamin supplements is indicated with some drug therapies. Pyridoxine inhibits the therapeutic effectiveness of levodopa by catabolizing the drug to dopamine in the blood. Less levodopa is then available for conversion to dopamine in the brain. Patients should be instructed to avoid vitamin supplements containing pyridoxine. Vitamin K supplements are contraindicated in patients receiving coumarin anticoagulants. Supplements containing vitamin A are not advised for patients treated with isotretinoin for cystic acne.[5] Para-aminobenzoic acid is contraindicated in patients receiving methotrexate therapy as the vitamin displaces the drug from plasma protein-binding, possibly increasing the free concentration of the drug in plasma.[5] (See Figure 27-1.)

Alteration in Drug Excretion Diet-induced alkalinization or acidification of the urine may increase excretion of certain drugs. For example, use of a low-

Table 27-5. **Tyramine- and Dopamine-Restricted Diet***

THESE FOODS MUST BE AVOIDED:

Alcoholic beverages, wines, ale, beer

Homemade yeast breads with substantial amounts of yeast; breads or crackers containing cheese

Sour cream

Bananas, red plums, avocado, figs, raisins (allowed on diets not restricted in dopamine); only 1 small orange daily

Aged game, liver, canned meats; yeast extracts; commercial meat extracts; salami, sausage; aged cheese: blue, Boursault, brick, brie, camembert, cheddar, colby, emmentaler, gouda, mozzarella, parmesan, provolone, romano, roquefort, stilton; salted dried fish: cod, herring, camlin; pickled herring

Italian broad beans, green bean pods, eggplant; limit tomato to ½ cup

Yeast concentrates, marmite, soup cubes; products made with concentrated yeast, commercial gravy or meat extracts; soy sauce

* Adapted from American Dietetic Association: *Handbook of Clinical Dietetics.* Yale University Press, New Haven, 1981.

protein diet is associated with a more alkaline urine and may cause increased excretion of the antibiotic nitrofurantoin.[6] On the other hand, increased excretion of the tricyclic antidepressants containing amitriptyline hydrochloride occurs when the urine is more acidic as is the case with a high protein intake. Quinidine toxicity may occur due to altered drug excretion when the diet is excessively alkaline. Lithium toxicity can result if the diet is restricted in sodium while taking the drug as the kidneys reabsorb more of the drug.

Alcohol

Unlike the drugs discussed earlier in this chapter, alcohol is not a prescription drug used in the management of disease. Nevertheless, it is a widely used agent that has many of the characteristics of other drugs. It is the most commonly abused substance in the United States.[13] Alcohol produces alterations in the absorption, metabolism, and excretion of a number of nutrients.

Alcohol and Metabolism   Alcohol is considered to be a food in that it yields 7 kcal per g; however, it does not provide any nutrients to speak of. Alcohol is rapidly and almost completely absorbed. The presence of food in the stomach, as is well known, delays gastric absorption. However, from the small intestine absorption is rapid regardless of whether food is present or not.

Upon absorption alcohol is dispersed rapidly

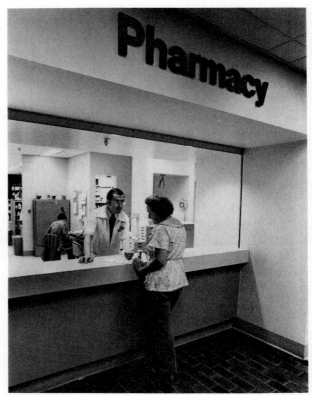

Figure 27-1.   Because food and drug interactions are common, the pharmacist advises a patient regarding not only dosages, but also the time for taking the medication with reference to food intake. (Courtesy, Metropolitan Medical Center, Minneapolis.)

throughout the body water. Less than 10 percent of the alcohol absorbed is eliminated by way of the kidneys and lungs; the rest is oxidized chiefly in the liver. When present, alcohol becomes the preferred fuel for the liver, displacing up to 90 percent of other substrates normally utilized by the liver. The products of oxidation in the liver are hydrogen and acetaldehyde. (See Chapter 6 for a description of the pathways of alcohol oxidation.) Chronic alcohol intake produces a functional disturbance of the mitochondria so that further oxidation of acetaldehyde is reduced. The increases in NADH/NAD ratio and acetaldehyde account for a number of alterations in carbohydrate, lipid, and protein metabolism: elevated levels of lactic acid which lead to acidosis and decreased renal excretion of uric acid, hypoglycemia resulting from impaired gluconeogenesis, triglyceride accumulation, fatty liver, impaired protein secretion, and in some instances, depressed protein synthesis.

Effects of Alcohol on Nutrition   Alcohol has numerous adverse effects on nutrition. It depresses appetite, so that the heavy drinker eats poorly. Chronic use is associated with increased incidence of cancers of the oral cavity and esophagus.[14] It has a direct toxic effect on the esophagus, and may also decrease pressure of the lower esophageal sphincter. In the stomach, alcohol disrupts the mucosal barrier, increases acid secretion, and delays emptying. Alcohol-induced chronic pancreatitis interferes with secretion of bicarbonate and enzymes, resulting in impaired digestion of protein and fats. Alcohol has a direct toxic effect on the liver.

Altered bile salt metabolism further interferes with fat digestion and may result in steatorrhea. Effects of alcohol on the small intestine include inhibition of mucosal enzyme activities, interference with absorption of actively transported substances, increased motility, impaired vitamin B-12 absorption, and interference with folate metabolism. Urinary losses of amino acids, magnesium, potassium, and zinc are increased during periods of drinking. Symptoms of *delerium tremens* have been associated with severe hypomagnesemia.

Alcohol also exerts indirect effects on nutritional status through altered intakes of calories, vitamins, and minerals. Excessive or deficient intake of these substances is manifested as obesity or wasting; hypervitaminosis A and niacin "intoxication" or deficiencies of folacin and thiamin; iron overload or chronic deficiencies of magnesium, zinc, and potassium.[15]

Only about 20 percent of alcoholics develop liver damage. Fatty infiltration is the most common change. With subsequent damage to the liver cells, alcoholic hepatitis occurs. About half of these patients develop alcoholic cirrhosis.

Wernicke's and Korsakoff's Syndromes Wernicke's syndrome and Korsakoff's psychoses are associated with alcoholism and appear to be different phases of the same disease. Wernicke's syndrome is characterized by ophthalmoplegia (paralysis of the eye muscles), ataxia (uncoordinated gait), and mental confusion. Nystagmus (rapid movement of the eyeballs) is a prominent feature. The patient is often unable to stand or walk without support. The eye changes are dramatically corrected, often within hours, by the administration of thiamin.

Korsakoff's syndrome may not be apparent until several weeks after the changes in the eye and gait have become evident. The chief defect is the disturbance in memory and the inability to learn new things so that only the most routine tasks can be performed. Moreover, there is failure to associate past events in their proper sequence. Patients may be confused, anxious, fearful, and even delirious. Vitamin therapy has produced marked effects in restoring the patient to being responsive, alert, and attentive. However, when memory defects are present, they appear to persist despite therapy, suggesting that structural changes in the brain may be irreversible.

References

1. Maslakowski, C. J.: "Drug–Nutrient Interactions/Interrelationships," *Nutr. Suppr. Serv.*, 1:14, 17, November, 1981.
2. Carson, J. A. S., and Gormican, A.: "Disease–Medication Relationships in Altered Taste Sensitivity," *J. Am. Diet. Assoc.*, 68:550–53, 1976.
3. Roe, D. A.: "Nutrient and Drug Interactions," *Nutr. Rev.*, 42:141–53, 1984.
4. Loebl, S., and Spratto, G.: *The Nurse's Drug Handbook*, 3rd ed. John Wiley & Sons, New York, 1983.
5. Smith, C. H., and Bidlack, W. R.: "Dietary Concerns Associated with the Use of Medications," *J. Am. Diet. Assoc.*, 84:901–14, 1984.
6. Lamy, P. R.: "Effects of Diet and Nutrition in Drug Therapy," *J. Am. Geriatr. Soc.*, 30:S99–112, 1982.
7. Halsted, C. H., et al.: "Sulfasalazine Inhibits the Absorption of Folates in Ulcerative Colitis," *N. Engl. J. Med.*, 305:1513–17, 1981.
8. Mueller, J.: "Drug–Nutrient Interrelationships," in Alfin-Slater, R. B., and Kritchevsky, D., (eds.), *Human Nutrition. A Comprehensive Treatise. 3B. Nutrition and the Adult: Micronutrients*, Plenum Press, New York, 1980, pp. 351–65.
9. Kiely, J. M.: "Antineoplastic Agents," *Mayo Clin. Proc.*, 56:384–92, 1981.
10. March, D. C.: *Handbook: Interactions of Selected Drugs with Nutritional Status in Man*, 2nd ed., The American Dietetic Association, 1978.
11. Bidlack, W. R., and Smith, C. H.: "The Effect of Nutritional Factors on Hepatic Drug and Toxicant Metabolism," *J. Am. Diet. Assoc.*, 84:892–98, 1984.
12. Gilman, A. G., et al. eds. *Goodman and Gilman's The Pharmacological Basis of Therapeutics*, 6th ed. Macmillan Publishing Co., Inc., New York, 1980.
13. Halstead, C. H.: "Alcoholism and Malnutrition," *Am. J. Clin. Nutr.*, 33:2705–2708, 1980.
14. Breedon, J. H.: "Alcohol, Alcoholism, and Cancer," *Med. Clin. North Am.*, 68: 163–77, 1984.
15. Roe, D. A.: "Nutritional Concerns in the Alcoholic," *J. Am. Diet. Assoc.*, 78:17–21, 1982.

28

Enteral and Parenteral Nutrition

Normal, Fiber-Restricted (Soft), and Fluid Diets; Formula Diets, Central and Peripheral Parenteral Nutrition

Adaptations of the Normal Diet for Texture

Therapeutic Nutrition Begins with the Normal Diet Normal and therapeutic diets are planned to maintain, or restore, good nutrition in the patient. In diet manuals the normal diet may be designated as *regular, house, normal,* or *full diet.* It consists of any and all foods eaten by the person in health. Fried foods, pastries, strongly flavored vegetables, spices, and relishes are not taboo, but good menu planning means that these foods are used judiciously. The normal diet satisfies the nutritional needs for most patients and also serves as the basis for planning modified diets.

The nutritive contributions of a basic diet composed of recommended levels from the Daily Food Guide were discussed in Chapter 14 and are summarized in Table 4-1. Such a foundation diet may be amplified to provide meal patterns that are typical in many hospitals. For example, an additional cup of milk could be included because it provides important amounts of several nutrients that are likely to be needed in increased amounts by many patients. Contrary to the opinion held by some, milk is one of the best-accepted foods in the hospital dietary.

To use the normal diet as the basis for therapeutic diets is sound in that it emphasizes the similarity of psychologic and social needs of those who are ill with those who are well, even though there may be differences in quantitative or qualitative requirements. Insofar as possible the patient is provided a food allowance that avoids the connotation of a "special" diet that sets him or her apart from family and friends. Moreover, in the home, food preparation is simplified when the modified diet is based upon the family pattern, and the number of items requiring special preparation is reduced to a minimum.

Although it is desirable that the normal diet provide the basis for planning modified diets, it must be remembered that the nutritional requirements of patients are likely to vary widely. The recommended dietary allowances are designed to meet the nutritional needs for almost all healthy persons in the United States, and they should not be interpreted as being appropriate allowances during illness. For any given patient the nutritional requirements depend upon nutritional status, modifications in activity, increased or decreased metabolic demands made by the illness, and the efficiency of digestive, absorptive, and excretory mechanisms.

Many adaptations to the plan presented in Table 4-1 could be devised for varying cultural and socioeconomic circumstances. The calculated values for the basic plan are useful in determining the effects of the omission or addition of foods to such a plan. For example, if a patient is allergic to milk, adjustment would need to be made especially for calcium, riboflavin, and protein. Or, if vegetables and fruits were omitted supplements of vitamin A and ascorbic acid should be prescribed.

Therapeutic Modifications of the Normal Diet The normal diet may be modified (1) to provide change in consistency, as in fluid and soft diets to be described later; (2) to increase or decrease the energy values; (3) to include greater or lesser amounts of one or more nutrients, for example, high-protein and sodium-restricted diets; (4) to increase or decrease bulk—high- and low-fiber diets; (5) to include or exclude specific foods, as in allergic conditions; and (6) to modify the intervals of feeding.

Rationale for Modified Diets The principles for diet therapy in many pathologic conditions are well established, and dietary plans are based on a sound rationale. In such plans the food allowances may vary according to ethnic and socioeconomic factors. It is to be expected that differences in interpretation will be found in the detailed descriptions of diet that are presented in the diet manuals of hospitals. Some of these

---

Regular or Normal Diet

Include These Foods, or Their Nutritive Equivalents, Daily:
2 - 3 cups milk
4 ounces (cooked weight) meat, fish, or poultry; cheese, additional egg or milk, or legumes may substitute in part
1 egg (3 to 4 per week)
4 servings vegetables and fruits including:
   1 serving of citrus fruit, or other good source of vitamin C
   1 serving dark green leafy or deep yellow vegetable
   2 or more servings of other vegetables and fruits, including potatoes
4 or more servings whole-grain cereals or bread
Additional foods such as butter or margarine, soups, desserts, sweets, salad dressings, or increased amounts of foods listed above will provide adequate calories. See calculation in Table 4-1.

Meal Pattern	Sample Menu
BREAKFAST	
Fruit	Sliced banana in orange juice
Cereal, enriched or whole-grain	Oatmeal
Milk and sugar for cereal	Milk and sugar
Egg	Soft-cooked egg
Whole-grain or enriched roll or toast	Whole-wheat toast with margarine
Butter or margarine	
Hot beverage with cream and sugar	Coffee with cream and sugar
LUNCHEON OR SUPPER	
Soup, if desired	
Cheese, meat, fish, or legumes	Cheese soufflé
Potato, rice, noodles, macaroni, spaghetti, or vege-table	Peas with margarine
Salad	Lettuce and tomato salad
Enriched or whole-grain bread	Russian dressing
Butter or margarine	Hard roll with margarine
Fruit	Royal Anne cherries
Milk	Milk
DINNER	
Meat, fish, or poultry	Meat loaf with gravy
Potato	Mashed potato
Vegetable	Carrots with margarine
Enriched or whole-grain bread	Enriched white, rye, or whole-wheat bread with margarine
Butter or margarine	
Dessert	Apple Betty
Milk	Milk
Coffee or tea, if desired	

differences are caused by the fact that some modified diets have only an empirical basis. Research to establish the merits of a particular plan as opposed to another is difficult to control because of the numerous physiologic and psychological variables in human beings. Fortunately, a number of widely varying dietary programs may be equally effective because of the remarkable response of the human body.

Probably no diets are more subject to criticism than those modified for fiber and flavor. In order to reduce the fiber content of a diet, meats may be ground and vegetables and fruits strained. Yet, experience has shown that few patients consume such foods in satisfactory amounts, and the harm to nutritional status is likely to be greater than the possible insult to the mucosa of the gastrointestinal tract.

Some patients experience heartburn, abdominal distention, and flatulence following the ingestion of strongly flavored vegetables, dry beans or peas, and melons. Other patients refuse to eat these foods simply because they have been told that they are poorly digested. There is no evidence that justifies the omission of these foods for all patients. Although dietitians and nurses have a responsibility to correct food misinformation whenever it is encountered, little is gained by coercing someone who is ill into eating a food that he or she dislikes intensely or has a prejudice against.

Diet Manuals and Dietary Patterns The American Dietetic Association has prepared a *Handbook of Clinical Dietetics*, which documents the scientific basis for dietary modification in treatment of specific disorders and includes food lists and sample menus for the various modified diets.[1] Numerous local or regional manuals are available as guides in the standardization of dietary procedures for a given hospital. The best of these manuals have been prepared by committees including representatives of the various medical specialties, nursing, and dietary departments. The manual generally includes statements concerning principles of diet, food allowances with detailed lists of foods to use and to avoid, typical meal patterns, and nutritive evaluations. They serve as a guide for the physician in prescribing a diet, a reference for the nurse, a procedural manual for the dietary department, and a teaching tool for professional personnel.

Although a manual achieves standardization in procedures, it does *not* mean that every patient on a given diet must have exactly the same food allowances as every other patient. In fact, within the guide ample opportunity is provided for individualization of a given patient's plan. The diet manual is *not* an instructional guide for the patient for whom individualized and more detailed aids are necessary. It may, however, serve as the basis for the development of such teaching aids.

Throughout this text dietary plans which are representative of those used in many hospitals are presented. Each description includes a statement of characteristics, lists of foods to include, detailed lists of food permitted and contraindicated, a typical meal pattern, and a sample menu. The student will learn much by comparing one with another and will begin to understand the rationale for diet therapy and how the goals may be achieved in a number of ways.

Nomenclature of Diets Insofar as possible, the nomenclature used in this text will describe the modification in consistency, in nutrients, or in energy; thus *fat-restricted, 1,200-kcal* diet, and so on. When the quantity of one or more nutrients is important to the success of the diet, it is essential that these quantities be specified in the diet prescription. Thus, the term *diabetic diet* has little meaning, but a prescription for 250 g carbohydrate, 85 g protein, and 60 g fat can be accurately interpreted. Likewise, a *sodium-restricted* diet gives no indication of the exact level of restriction required, but the designation *500-mg sodium diet* leaves no room for misinterpretation.

Several undesirable practices have been, and still are, common in the naming of diets. The literature is replete with illustrations of diets named for their originators. The Sippy diet is a classic example, but there have been others from time to time. Unfortunately, such nomenclature tells nothing about the diet, and the practice should be discouraged.

Others have used the name of a disease condition to specify a given diet, such as ulcer, ambulatory ulcer, ulcer discharge, cardiac, and gallbladder diets. Psychologically, this is not good practice, for patients should not need to be reminded of their condition every time they look at a diet on a tray card. Moreover, the diets used for many of these conditions have multiple uses, and the uninitiated may overlook the full usefulness of a given plan with such disease-oriented terminology.

Frequency of Feeding Research on experimental animals and on humans has shown that more than three meals daily may be desirable for some patients. When the patient eats five, six, or more meals a day which are approximately balanced for protein, fat, and carbohydrate, the metabolic load at a given time is less, and the nutrients can be more effectively utilized. It is well known that protein is inefficiently

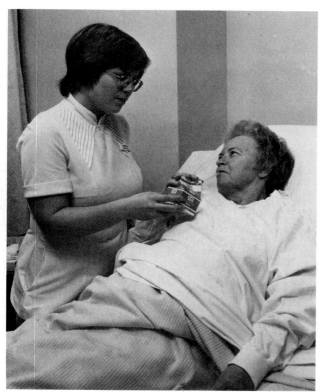

Figure 28-1. Milk is well accepted by most patients and provides important nutrients for liquid diets or between-meal feedings. (Courtesy, University of Minnesota Health Sciences Center, Minneapolis.)

used if the day's allowance is more or less concentrated in one meal. Large amounts of carbohydrate at a given meal require the use of alternate metabolic pathways which favor the deposition of fat.

Sometimes it is desirable to adapt home diets of patients to a six- or seven-meal program. Some protein, fat, and carbohydrate should be given at each meal. Thus, milk or a protein sandwich may be useful for interval feedings, but juices or sweets alone do not satisfy the requirements. The interval between meals should be 1½ to 3 hours, with meals spread throughout the waking hours. Any of the modified diets might be presented in more than three meals. A judicious choice of bedtime snacks apparently does not modify sleep. (See Figure 28-1.)

Mechanical Soft Diet Many persons require a soft diet simply because they have no teeth. It is neither desirable nor essential to restrict the patient to the selection allowed on the customary soft diet (page 414) employed for a postoperative patient or for a patient with a gastrointestinal disturbance. For example,

stewed onions, baked beans, and apple pie are foods considered quite unsuitable for the latter patients but which may be enjoyed by those who simply require foods that are soft in texture. The terms *mechanical soft* and *dental soft* are used in some diet manuals to describe such a dietary modification. The following changes in the normal diet will usually suffice for individuals without teeth:

Meat should be finely minced or ground.,
Soft breads are substituted for crusty breads.
Cooked vegetables are used without restriction, but dicing or chopping may be desirable for some; for example, diced beets, chopped spinach, corn cut from cob.
Most raw vegetables are omitted; raw tomatoes, cut finely, may usually be used. Sometimes finely chopped lettuce in a sandwich may be accepted.
Many raw fruits may be used: banana, orange, grapefruit, soft berries, soft pear, apricots, peaches, grapes with tender skins.
Hard raw fruits such as pineapple and apple are usually avoided; but finely diced apple in fruit cup may be used.
Tough skins should be removed from fruits: raw, soft pear, or baked apple, etc.
Nuts and dried fruits, when used in desserts or other foods, are acceptable if finely chopped.

Fiber-Restricted (Soft) Diet This diet represents the usual dietary step between the full fluid and normal diet. It may be used in acute infections, some gastrointestinal disturbances, and following surgery. The diet is soft in consistency, easy to chew, made up of simple, easily digestible food, and contains no harsh fiber, no rich or highly flavored food. It is nutritionally adequate when planned on the basis of the normal diet.

Liquid Diets Fluid diets are used in febrile states, postoperatively, or whenever the patient is unable to tolerate solid foods. The degree to which these diets are adequate will depend on the type of liquids permitted.

Clear-Fluid Diet. Whenever an acute illness or surgery produces a marked intolerance for food as may be evident by nausea, vomiting, anorexia, distention, and diarrhea, it is advisable to restrict the intake of nutrients. A clear-fluid diet is usually used for 1 to 2 days, at the end of which time the patient is usually able to utilize a more liberal liquid diet.

Tea with lemon and sugar, coffee, fat-free broth, and carbonated beverages are the usual liquids permitted. In addition, strained fruit juices, fruit ices, and plain gelatin are often included. No milk products are used.

Fiber-Restricted (Soft) Diet

Include These Foods, or Their Nutritive Equivalents, Daily:

2-3 cups milk
4 ounces (cooked weight) very tender or ground meat, fish, or poultry; soft cheese, legumes, or additional milk may substitute in part
1 egg (3 to 4 per week)
4 servings vegetables and fruits including:
    2 servings of citrus fruit or juice
    1 serving dark green leafy or deep yellow vegetable—tender chopped or strained
    1 medium potato
    1 or more servings of other tender chopped or strained vegetables, or cooked fruits without skin or seeds, or strained cooked fruit
4 or more servings strained whole-grain cereals or fine whole-grain bread
Additional foods such as butter or margarine, soups, desserts, sweets, or increased amounts of the above wil provide adequate calories.

Nutritive value. See calculation for the normal diet in Table 4-1.

Foods Allowed

All beverages
Bread—white, fine whole-wheat, rye without seeds; white crackers
Cereal foods—dry, such as cornflakes, Puffed Rice, rice flakes; fine cooked, such as cornmeal, farina, hominy grits, macaroni, noodles, rice, spaghetti; strained coarse, such as oatmeal, Pettijohn's, whole wheat
Cheese—mild, soft, such as cottage and cream; cheddar; Swiss
Desserts—plain cake, cookies; custards; plain gelatin or with allowed fruit; Junket; plain ice cream, ices, sherbets; plain puddings, such as bread, cornstarch, rice, tapioca
Eggs—all except fried
Fats—butter, cream, margarine, vegetable oils and fats in cooking
Fruits—raw: ripe avocado, banana, grapefruit or orange sections without membrane; canned or cooked: apples, apricots, fruit cocktail, peaches, pears, plums—all without skins; Royal Anne cherries; strained prunes and other fruits with skins; all juices
Meat—very tender, minced, or ground; baked, broiled, creamed, roast, or stewed: beef, lamb, veal, poultry, fish, bacon, liver, sweetbreads
Milk—in any form
Soups—broth, strained cream or vegetable
Sweets—all sugars, syrup, jelly, honey, plain sugar candy without fruit or nuts, molasses. Use in moderation.
Vegetables—white or sweet potato without skin, any way except fried; young and tender asparagus, beets, carrots, peas, pumpkin, squash without seeds; tender chopped greens; strained cooked vegetables if not tender; tomato juice
Miscellaneous—salt, seasonings and spices in moderation, gravy, cream sauces

Foods to Avoid

Bread—coarse dark; whole-grain crackers; hot breads; pancakes, waffles
Cereals—bran; coarse unless strained

Cheese—sharp, such as roquefort, camembert, limburger
Desserts—any made with dried fruit or nuts; pastries; rich puddings or cake

Eggs—fried
Fats—fried foods

Fruits—raw except as listed; stewed or canned berries; with tough skins

Meat—tough with gristle or fat; salted and smoked meat or fish, such as corned beef, smoked herring; cold cuts; frankfurter; pork

Soups—fatty or highly seasoned
Sweets—jam, marmalade, rich candies with chocolate

Vegetables—raw; strongly flavored, such as broccoli, brussels sprouts, cabbage, cauliflower, cucumber, onion, radish, sauerkraut, turnip; corn; dried beans and peas; potato chips

Miscellaneous—pepper and other hot spices; fried foods; nuts; olives; pickles; relishes

Meal Pattern	**Sample Menu**
BREAKFAST	
Fruit or fruit juice	Orange sections and banana slices
Cereal—strained, if coarse	Oatmeal
Milk and sugar for cereal	Milk and sugar for cereal
Egg	Soft-cooked egg
Soft roll or toast	Toast with margarine
Butter or margarine	
Hot beverage with cream and sugar	Coffee
LUNCHEON OR SUPPER	
Strained soup, if desired	Cream of tomato soup
Mild cheese, tender or ground meat, fish, or poultry	Cheese soufflé
Potato without skin, rice, noodles, macaroni, or spaghetti; or	
Cooked vegetable	Tender peas
Enriched bread	Soft roll
Butter or margarine	Butter or margarine
Fruit	Royal Anne cherries
Milk	Milk
Coffee or tea, if desired	Coffee or tea, if desired
DINNER	
Orange, grapefruit, or tomato juice	Grapefruit juice
Tender or ground meat, fish, or poultry	Meat loaf (no onion or pepper) with gravy
Potato any way except fried	Mashed potato
Cooked vegetable	Carrots with margarine
Enriched bread	Rye bread without seeds
Butter or margarine	Butter or margarine
Dessert	Baked apple without skin; cream
Milk	Milk
Hot beverage with cream and sugar, if desired	Tea with sugar and lemon

The amount of fluid in a given feeding on the clear-fluid diet is usually restricted to 30 to 60 ml per hour at first, with gradually increasing amounts being given as the patient's tolerance improves. Obviously such a diet can accomplish little beyond the replacement of fluids.

Full-Fluid Diet. This diet is indicated whenever a patient is acutely ill or is unable to chew or swallow solid food. It includes all foods liquid at room temperature and at body temperature. It is free from cellulose and irritating condiments. When properly planned, this diet can be used for relatively long periods of time. However, iron is provided at inadequate levels.

Formula Diets

Enteral nutrition by tube is used for patients with a functioning gastrointestinal tract who cannot or should not ingest solid foods. The formula, or tube feeding, can be prepared in the home or hospital or purchased commercially. A wide selection of formulas is available. Selection of the appropriate formula is made on the basis of the patient's digestive and absorptive capacity and on the physical characteristics of the formula.

Some formulas provide balanced amounts of the major nutrients and meet the Recommended Dietary Allowances for all essential nutrients. Examples are meal replacement formulas. Others meet special needs, for example, in gastrointestinal, liver, or renal disease; still others provide selected nutrients and are used as supplements, for example, a protein supplement that can be added to other formulas. Feeding by tube may be required for a short period of time or indefinitely in a variety of circumstances: surgery of the head and neck; esophageal obstruction; gastrointestinal surgery; in severe burns; in anorexia nervosa; and in the comatose patient. For short-term use the feedings are ordinarily given by nasogastric tube, but for long-term use, the feeding is administered through a tube inserted into a new opening ("*-ostomy*") made in the esophagus (esophagostomy), stomach (gastrostomy), or intestine (enterostomy).

Full-Fluid Diet

General Rules
Give six or more feedings daily.

The protein content of the diet can be increased by incorporating nonfat dry milk in beverages and soups. Strained canned meats (used for infant feeding) may be added to broths.

The caloric value of the diet may be increased by: (1) substituting cream for part of the usual milk allowance; (2) adding butter or margarine to cereal gruels and soups; (3) including glucose in beverages; (4) using ice cream as dessert or in beverages.

If a decreased volume of fluid is desired, nonfat dry milk may be substituted for part of the fluid milk.

Include These Foods, or Their Nutritive Equivalents Daily:
6 cups milk

2 eggs (in custards or pasteurized eggnog)

1-2 ounces strained meat

½ cup fine or strained whole-grain cooked cereal for gruel

¼ cup vegetable purée for cream soup

1 cup citrus fruit juice; plus other strained juices

½ cup tomato or vegetable juice

1 tablespoon cocoa

3 tablespoons sugar

1 tablespoon butter or margarine

2 servings plain gelatin dessert, soft or baked custard, ices, sherbets, plain ice cream, or plain cornstarch pudding

Broth, bouillon, or clear soups

Tea, coffee, carbonated beverages as desired

Flavoring extracts, salt

Nutritive values of foods listed in specified amounts kcal, 1,950; protein, 85 g; calcium, 2.1 g; iron, 7.7 mg; vitamin A, 7,150 I.U.; thiamin, 1.1 mg; riboflavin, 3.2 mg; niacin equivalents, 19.1 mg; ascorbic acid, 160 mg.

Meal Pattern	Sample Menu
BREAKFAST	
Citrus juice	Orange juice
Cereal gruel with butter, sugar	Cream of wheat with milk, butter, and sugar
Milk	
Beverage with cream, sugar	Coffee with cream and sugar
MID-MORNING	
Milk, plain, malted, chocolate, or eggnog (pasteurized)	Eggnog, pasteurized
LUNCHEON OR SUPPER	
Strained soup	Beef broth with strained meat
Tomato juice	Tomato juice
Custard, Junket, ice cream, sherbet, ice, gelatin dessert, or plain pudding	Maple Junket
Eggnog, milk, or cocoa	Milk
Tea with sugar, if desired	Tea with sugar and cream
MIDAFTERNOON	
Milk, ice cream, custard, or gelatin dessert	Vanilla milkshake

Meal Pattern	Sample Menu
DINNER	
Strained cream soup	Strained cream of mushroom soup
Citrus juice	Grapefruit juice
Custard, Junket, ice cream, ice, sherbet, or gelatin dessert	Gelatin dessert
Milk or cocoa	Cocoa
Tea, if desired	Tea with sugar and lemon
EVENING NOURISHMENT	
Milk, custard, or juice	Custard

Characteristics of Formula Feedings A satisfactory formula feeding must be (1) nutritionally adequate; (2) well tolerated by the patient so that vomiting is not induced; (3) easily digested with no unfavorable reactions such as distention, diarrhea, or constipation; (4) easily prepared; and (5) inexpensive.

The concentration of the feeding is usually about 1kcal per ml. Lesser concentrations increase the volume which must be given to meet nutrient and energy needs, and greater concentrations are more likely to produce diarrhea. However, formulas supplying 1.5 or 2.0 kcal per ml are sometimes used for severely malnourished patients or for those in whom fluid restriction is necessary. Two to 3 liters per 24 hours is a customary volume.

Nutritional Composition of Formulas The proportion of protein, fat, and carbohydrate should approximate that of the normal diet.

Protein. The most important component of the formula is protein because of its essential role in bodily and cellular functions. Protein sources in enteral formulas are provided as intact protein, protein hydrolysates, or crystalline amino acids. The student is encouraged to review Chapter 5 for a discussion of protein digestion and absorption. *Intact proteins* such as puréed beef or egg white solids require complete digestion to peptides and amino acids before they can be absorbed. Sometimes protein isolates are used. These intact proteins have been separated from the original protein source, for example, lactalbumin, which is derived from whey. Intact proteins are used in patients in whom pancreatic enzyme levels and absorptive capacity of the small intestine are normal. *Protein hydrolysates* are proteins that have been partially hydrolyzed to smaller peptides and amino acids. They are useful in disorders in which there is reduced absorptive area, in certain disorders of amino acid transport and in pancreatic insufficiency. *Crystalline*

amino acids do not require further hydrolysis, and are used in maldigestion or malabsorption, liver and renal diseases.

Fat. The principal sources of fat in formulas are various vegetable oils, medium-chain triglycerides, lecithin, and mono- and diglycerides. In addition to providing a source of essential fatty acids, fat supplies the most concentrated source of calories in the formula. Medium-chain triglycerides (MCT) are composed of 6 to 12 carbons. They are more water soluble than long-chain fats, are hydrolyzed more rapidly, and do not require pancreatic lipase or bile salts to be absorbed. They are useful in disorders of fat absorption occurring in some gastrointestinal diseases and are discussed in more detail on page 444.

Carbohydrate. Several forms of carbohydrate are used in formula diets. *Polysaccharides* (starch) may be in the form of hydrolyzed cereal solids, puréed vegetables or modified food starch, and are used in blenderized formulas. (See page 418 for description of blenderized formulas.)

Hydrolysis of starch yields *glucose polymers* including glucose polysaccharides with 10 or more glucose units, and oligosaccharides, containing up to 10 glucose units, dextrins, and maltose. Glucose polymers are often used in formulas because they are rapidly hydrolyzed and absorbed. A third source of carbohydrate is *disaccharide*, for example, lactose or sucrose. Many commercially available formulas are lactose-free owing to secondary lactose deficiencies occurring in some disorders involving the small bowel mucosa. (See Chapter 31 for more details.)

Vitamins and Minerals. Proprietary formulas that are designed to be nutritionally complete meet the Recommended Dietary Allowances when the recommended volume of full-strength feeding is given. However, when the feeding is diluted, or if the volume given is less than the recommended amount, multivitamin and mineral supplements are needed.

Water. The water content of the formula is important because it is usually the major source of fluid for the tube-fed patient. In very debilitated or unconscious patients the potential for dehydration or hyperosmolality (discussed in the next section) exists if water requirements are not met. Most adults require about 35 ml water per kg body weight daily. Requirements are less in children and in the elderly.[2] Close attention to individual water needs is essential. Commercial formulas supplying 1.5 kcal per ml or less are about 80 percent water by volume; in those over 1.5 kcal per ml about 60 percent of the volume is free water.[2]

Physical Characteristics The physical characteristics of the formula may affect tolerance.

Osmolality. This refers to the number and size of particles present per kilogram of water. The greater the number of particles and the smaller their size, the more osmotic pressure they exert in solution. Amino acids, carbohydrates, minerals, and electrolytes have a significant influence on osmolality—amino acids and glucose because of their small size relative to intact proteins, and glucose polymers and electrolytes because of their small size and tendency to dissociate into ions. The more predigested formulas containing amino acids and glucose are higher in osmolality than those containing intact protein and glucose polymers. Fat does not have a major influence on osmolality.

The normal osmolality of the extracellular fluid is 280 to 300 mOsm; concentrations above this level, or *hyperosmolality*, are associated with a number of clinical manifestations. These may be brought about by feeding formulas of high osmolality. Such formulas cause delayed gastric emptying with associated nausea and vomiting; diarrhea and electrolyte depletion; and an increase in the renal solute load leading to dehydration. The latter is especially likely with use of formulas containing liberal amounts of protein and electrolytes. The kidney requires additional water to excrete the higher solute load imposed by these formulas; thus, the ratio of protein to water in the formula must be lowered in order to correct the hyperosmolality.

Caloric Density. Formulas supplying much more than 1 kcal per ml frequently are not well tolerated by patients. Such feedings delay gastric emptying.

Nutrient Content. Formulas differing markedly from the usual proportions of protein, fat, or carbohydrate may affect tolerance. For example, a formula high in fat may cause a delay in gastric emptying; one high in protein can cause dehydration and hyperosmolality as discussed in the preceding section; those high in carbohydrate can provoke diarrhea.

Fiber. Many formulas contain little or no dietary fiber and are constipating to patients. However, some of the new products include a source of dietary fiber and appear to be well tolerated.*

Types of Formula Feedings Several types of tube feedings are in common use: blenderized, milk-based, lactose-free, and semisynthetic. (See Table 28-1.) In addition, special formulas suitable for use in trauma, liver, or renal diseases are available. Modular components can be adapted for various situations when conventional formulas are unsuitable. A number of commercial products are available for each type of formula feeding. Many of these are also suitable for use as oral supplements. Likewise blenderized and milk-based feedings can be prepared within the hospital or home. Most of these recipes use whole or skim milk, eggs, and vitamin supplements together with some form of carbohydrate such as strained cooked cereals, sugar, or molasses. Vegetable oil or cream and nonfat dry milk are also incorporated to increase the calorie and protein levels, respectively.

Blenderized formulas are made from the ordinary foods of a normal diet by using a high-speed blender. Strained baby meats, fruits, and vegetables are used in addition to the foods listed previously. Blenderized tube feedings are generally well tolerated and are only infrequently associated with diarrhea. Normal functioning of the gastrointestinal tract and normal pancreatic enzyme levels are required with use of these formulas.

Lactose-free preparations contain various carbohydrate sources, for example, maltodextrins, sucrose, glucose oligosaccharides, hydrolyzed cornstarch or corn sirup. Protein sources in these formulas are usually calcium and sodium caseinates, soy protein isolates, lactalbumin or egg albumin. Vegetable oil, and sometimes MCT oil, supply fat. The formulas are low in residue. Lactose-free formulas are used in cases of lactase deficiency or intestinal mucosal damage as in protein-calorie malnutrition, radiation enteritis, in-

---

* Products include Enrich (Ross Laboratories, Columbus, Ohio) and Susta II (Mead Johnson and Company, Evansville, Ind.).

Table 28-1. **Composition of Some Products Suitable for Tube Feeding (per 1,000 ml)***

	Brand A Blenderized	Brand B Milk-Based	Brand C Lactose-Free	Brand D Semisynthetic Fiber-Free
kcal per ml	1	1	1	1
Protein, g/liter	43	58	37	21
Fat, g/liter	37	32	37	2
Carbohydrate, g/liter	141	110	145	231
Nonprotein Calories : Nitrogen	131 : 1	79 : 1	153 : 1	286 : 1
Nutrient source				
Protein	Beef, calcium caseinate	Skim milk, sodium caseinate	Sodium and calcium caseinates, soy protein isolate	L-amino acids
Fat	Corn oil	Corn oil	Corn oil	Safflower oil
Carbohydrate	Hydrolyzed cereal solids, vegetable purée	Lactose, corn syrup, sucrose	Hydrolyzed corn starch, sucrose	Glucose oligosaccharides
mOsm/kg water	300	505 (vanilla flavor)	450 (unflavored)	550 (unflavored)
Volume needed to meet 100 percent of RDAs	1,500	1,250	2,000	1,800

* Brand A: Compleat Modified (Sandoz Nutritionals, Inc., Minneapolis, Minn.).
Brand B: Meritene Liquid (Sandoz Nutritionals, Inc., Minneapolis, Minn.).
Brand C: Ensure (Ross Laboratories, Columbus, Ohio.).
Brand D: Vivonex Standard (Norwich Eaton, Norwich, N.Y.).

flammatory bowel disease, sprue, or drug-induced injury.

Semisynthetic fiber-free preparations are composed principally of carbohydrates from glucose oligosaccharides, maltodextrins, or sucrose. Crystalline amino acids or partially hydrolyzed whey, soy, or meat proteins provide nitrogen. Vegetable oil and MCT supply fat. These formulas are useful in persons with maldigestion or malabsorption. The formula leaves a minimum of residue in the intestinal tract. Patient acceptance of the formulas is limited when taken orally.

Administration of Formula Feedings Most formulas are administered by *intermittent gravity drip* or by *bolus* feeding. These are suitable in patients with a gastrostomy or pharyngostomy in whom gastrointestinal function is normal. Ordinarily rates of about 50 ml per minute and a volume of 350 ml per meal are used. The number of feedings will depend on nutritional need. *Continuous infusion* by means of a pump over periods ranging from 8 to 20 hours is used for jejunostomy formulas. Semisynthetic fiber-free preparations are commonly used. These are begun at a rate of 50 ml per hour, increasing by 25 ml per hour daily until a rate of 125 ml per hour is attained. They are initially diluted to quarter strength or half-strength, and increased to full strength over several days. Each day the rate or the concentration, but not both, will be adjusted until the desirable rate of full-strength feeding is achieved. The concentration is increased first, and then the rate, in gastric feedings; the reverse is true for jejunal feedings.[3] Feedings are generally administered cold from the refrigerator or at room temperature. Heating the formula is not recommended because of the potential for bacterial growth when feedings are heated to room temperature or above, and because overheating may alter protein and vitamins.[2]

A common problem in formula-fed patients is that the amount delivered is less than that prescribed to meet the patient's nutritional needs. Calorie intake should be monitored daily with appropriate adjustments in feeding frequency, rate, or volume.

Complications Associated with Formula Feedings

Gastrointestinal. The most common complications of formula feeding are nausea, vomiting, diarrhea, and constipation. These may relate to a hyperosmolar feeding, rapid infusion, lactose intolerance, fat malabsorption, or protein malnutrition. Dilution, slowing the rate of infusion, elimination of lactose, or reduction of the fat content of the formula are means used to alleviate symptoms.

Metabolic. These include overhydration, dehydration, hyperglycemia, or electrolyte imbalance. Overhydration or dehydration occur with some frequency in formula-fed patients. Overhydration occurs in some malnourished patients upon refeeding, or in those with severe heart, liver, or renal disease. It is corrected by slowing the rate of infusion, then gradually increasing it again. Dehydration is corrected by lowering the osmolality of the feeding. Hyperglycemia requires use of a slower infusion rate. Insulin or an oral hypoglycemic agent is administered to lower the blood glucose level and then the infusion is slowly increased. Intolerance of electrolytes or deficiencies of trace minerals have also been reported.

Infections. Aspiration of the formula feeding is a potential complication in virtually all tube-fed patients and may lead to respiratory distress or failure. Those fed by way of a nasogastric tube are more likely to aspirate the feeding than those fed by gastrostomy or jejunostomy. Measures to prevent aspiration include elevation of the head of the bed to 30°, use of dilute formula initially, with gradual increase in concentration over several days, and checking gastric residuals before each feeding. (See Figure 28-2.) The feeding is stopped if residuals are more than 150 ml in bolus-fed patients, or 10 to 20 percent greater than the infusion rate in those receiving continuous feedings. Resumption of feedings is begun after residuals are cleared.

Infectious complications may also be due to contamination of the feeding solution or tubing. The potential for contamination of the feeding is less in commercially prepared formulas than in those prepared within the hospital or home as the latter are not sterilized.

Mechanical Complications. Those resulting from nasogastric tubes are usually related to the size and positioning of feeding tubes. Examples include nasopharyngeal discomfort, nasal erosions, hoarseness, excessive gagging, esophagitis, and duodenal and intestinal perforation. Complications of gastrostomy include hemorrhage, peritonitis, and premature or delayed closing of the stoma. Jejunostomy complications include dislodgement of the tube, intestinal obstruction, and skin irritation among others.

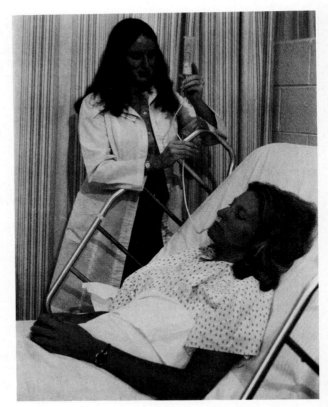

Figure 28-2. The nurse closely monitors the administration of the tube feeding, including position of the patient, the rate of flow and the total intake. (Courtesy, University of Pennsylvania School of Nursing, and Gates Rhodes, photographer.)

Parenteral Nutrition

For patients in whom enteral feedings are contraindicated or are inadequate, parenteral nutrition is used to replete nutritional status. This involves delivery of nutrients such as water, glucose, amino acids, lipids, vitamins, trace minerals, and electrolytes directly into a vein rather than using the gastrointestinal tract. Parenteral nutrition may be used for relatively brief periods, for extended periods, or even for life. Depending on circumstances, it may be used as the only method of feeding or in combination with enteral feeding methods. Supplemental parenteral nutrition solutions are infused into a peripheral vein; total parenteral nutrition solutions are infused into a large diameter central vein, or into a peripheral vein, depending on caloric requirements.

Supplemental Peripheral Nutrition Several types of solutions are used for relatively brief periods to provide fluids and electrolytes. *D5W*, a solution of 5 percent dextrose in water, is often used following surgery to supply calories and water until oral feedings can be resumed. Intravenous dextrose provides only 3.4 kcal per g; thus, 2 or 3 liters supplies 350 to 500 kcal and is insufficient to meet the patient's energy needs.

Isotonic saline contains 0.9 percent sodium chloride and is used to replace electrolytes or in metabolic alkalosis. Sometimes a *hypotonic* saline, 0.45 percent sodium chloride, is used to supply water and electrolytes. *Hypertonic* saline, 3 to 5 percent sodium chloride, is used if there is severe sodium depletion.

Dextrose in saline solutions supply both dextrose and sodium chloride. Usually 5 percent dextrose in normal saline, 0.9 percent is used. In some situations the concentration of dextrose or of sodium chloride is adjusted.

Electrolyte solutions are used to replace losses of sodium, potassium, calcium, chloride and fluid. An example is Ringer's solution. Dextrose and bicarbonate or its equivalent in lactate may also be added to Ringer's solution.

Amino Acid Solutions. Mixtures of amino acids in solutions containing no carbohydrate are used by some as *protein-sparing therapy.* Glucose stimulates insulin secretion and the uptake of amino acids and glucose by skeletal muscle and inhibits fatty acid mobilization. Protein-sparing therapy is based on the theory that infusion of amino acids stimulates less insulin secretion than glucose does, thereby permitting mobilization of endogenous fats and production of ketones for energy while sparing amino acids for visceral protein synthesis.[4] Amino acid solutions are much more expensive than glucose solutions and their use may not be justified unless a clear advantage can be demonstrated. Moreover, the long-term effects of sustained ketosis are not known. Thus, protein-sparing therapy remains controversial.

Total Parenteral Nutrition TPN is used in selected patients when enteral feedings cannot be used and prolonged nutritional support is necessary. Severely debilitated or hypermetabolic patients and those with severe disease of the gastrointestinal tract are likely to benefit from this method of feeding. Nutrients in the form of glucose and lipids for energy, and amino acids are infused by means of an indwelling catheter placed into the internal jugular vein or the subclavian vein and passed into the superior vena cava. (See Figure 28-3.) A large diameter vein with a rapid flow is es-

Figure 28-3. Administration of total parenteral nutrition through a central vein. The catheter is inserted into the subclavian vein and is passed into the superior vena cava, where the rapid blood flow rapidly dilutes the hypertonic solution.

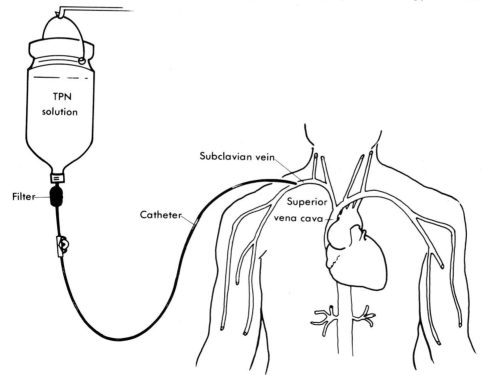

TPN solution

Filter

Catheter

Subclavian vein

Superior vena cava

sential because the nutrient solution is hypertonic. In a hospital setting the nutrient solutions are mixed in the pharmacy using sterile technique. However, pre-mixed solutions are available for patients on home TPN.

Before total parenteral nutrition is initiated, a complete nutritional and metabolic profile is done.[5] This involves determination of resting metabolic expenditure; evaluation of calorie and protein intakes and nitrogen balance; anthropometric measurements including the weight-height index, triceps skinfold and arm muscle circumference; visceral protein status (including albumin, transferrin, prealbumin, and retinol-binding protein) and immune response (delayed hypersensitivity skin testing); and baseline biochemical studies of serum urea nitrogen, glucose, electrolytes, iron, total iron-binding capacity, ferritin, vitamins A, D, and E, magnesium, zinc, triglycerides, cholesterol, white blood cell count, lymphocytes, creatinine excretion, and urinary urea nitrogen.

Once TPN has begun, daily measurements of blood and urinary glucose levels, serum electrolytes, intake and output, body weight, and vital signs are done until the patient is stabilized. Thereafter, routine measurements of electrolytes, liver enzymes, serum urea nitrogen, albumin, creatinine, calcium, magnesium, phosphate, complete blood count, and prothrombin time are done. If fat emulsions are used, serum triglyceride and cholesterol levels are monitored weekly.

Composition of Parenteral Nutrition Solutions

Protein. Crystalline amino acids in solution are available from several pharmaceutical suppliers.* The concentration of amino acids in these products ranges from 2 to 10 percent. A typical solution contains 4.25 percent amino acids and includes all the essential amino acids and several nonessential amino acids such as alanine, arginine, glycine, histidine, and tyrosine. Pediatric solutions contain 2 percent amino acids. Special formulations available for use in renal disease† contain only the essential amino acids plus histidine. Solutions with a high proportion of branched-chain amino acids (isoleucine, leucine, and lysine) and low in methionine are useful in hepatic encephalopathy‡ which is discussed in Chapter 32. High

nitrogen, high branched-chain amino acid solutions are available for use in trauma or sepsis.‡

Carbohydrate. Dextrose is the most commonly used carbohydrate in intravenous solutions and supplies 3.4 kcal per g. Dextrose concentrations range from 5 to 25 percent. The dextrose solution is mixed together with the amino acid solution. A typical solution might contain 1,000 ml of 4.25 percent amino acids with 25 percent dextrose, providing 1,000 kcal per liter.

Excessive amounts of glucose can increase respiratory demands due to increased carbon dioxide production in hypermetabolic and depleted persons. Those with compromised pulmonary function are at increased risk for ventilatory failure when high-carbohydrate solutions are used. Fat emulsions are used in order to lower the amount of glucose used and to lower carbon dioxide production.[6]

Lipids. Intravenous lipid emulsions of soy or safflower oil can be used primarily as a source of essential fatty acids or as a major energy source. For the purpose of preventing essential fatty acid deficiency, 500-ml units are infused every 3 days in adult patients receiving total parenteral nutrition for more than 2 to 4 weeks. Several solutions are available as 10 or 20 per cent fat emulsions, providing 1 or 2 kcal per ml, respectively.¶

If used as a major source of energy fat emulsions can replace from 30 to 60 percent of the total daily calories, depending on the condition being treated. The amount of lipid emulsion administered should not exceed 2.5 g per kg of body weight daily in adults and 4 g/kg in children. The initial infusion rate is 1 ml per minute for 15 to 30 minutes. If tolerated, the rate is increased to provide 500 ml over 4 to 6 hours.

If the fat emulsion is administered into a central vein serum triglyceride and cholesterol determinations should be done before and 4 hours after infusion of the last bottle. Thereafter, serum lipids are measured weekly with blood samples being obtained within 12 hours after infusion of the fat emulsion. In most patients lipids are cleared from the blood within 12 hours. Some patients experience fever, pain in the chest and back, nausea and vomiting, headache, flushing, and dizziness when lipid emulsions are infused.

---

* Aminosyn (Abbott Laboratories, North Chicago, Ill.) Freamine II (American McGaw, Santa Ana, Calif.) and Travasol (Travenol Laboratories, Inc., Deerfield, Ill.).
 †Nephramine (American McGaw, Santa Ana, Calif.).
 ‡ Hepatamine (American McGaw.).

§Freamine HBC (American McGaw.).
 ¶Intralipid (Cutter Medical, Miles Laboratories, Inc., Berkeley, Calif.) Liposyn (Abbott Laboratories, North Chicago, Ill.) and Soyacal (Alpha Therapeutic Corp., Los Angeles, Calif.).

Table 28-2. Protein and Energy Requirements in TPN*

	Calorie Requirements (kcal/kg/day)	Protein Requirements (g/kg/day)
Resting state (adult medical patient)	20–30	0.8–1.0
Uncomplicated postoperative patients	25–35	1.0–1.3
Depleted patients	30–40	1.3–1.7
Hypermetabolic patients (trauma, sepsis, burn)	35–45	1.5–2.0

* Adapted from the following sources:

Long, C. L.: "Energy and Protein Requirements in the Hospitalized Patient," *J.P.E.N.*, **3**:69–72, 1979.

Elwyn, D. H.: "Nutritional Requirements of Adult Surgical Patients," *Crit. Care Med.*, **8**:9–20, 1980.

Most lipid solutions are not mixed with the amino acid–dextrose solution because the resultant mixture is not stable. A separate container and tubing are used to infuse the lipid solution. The tubing from the amino acid–dextrose solution and that from the lipid solution are joined, using a Y connector, just before it enters the vein so that the two solutions mix for only a short time. A newer technique permits the intravenous fat emulsion to be admixed with the other TPN components, under prescribed conditions.*

Energy. Calorie and protein requirements for patients receiving total parenteral nutrition[7,8] are summarized in Table 28–2. The ratio of nonprotein calories to nitrogen in commonly used formulas ranges from 120:1 to 180:1.

Vitamins and Minerals. The precise amounts of vitamins and minerals needed in parenteral nutrition are not known. Several multivitamin preparations are available.* None is complete, however. Vitamin K is administered separately once weekly. Vitamin B-12 may be given in the TPN solution weekly or injected intramuscularly once monthly. Folic acid is often administered separately although it can be put into the parenteral nutrition solution. The fat-soluble vitamins are given in greater than physiologic doses and some cases of toxicity have been reported. Various

* Intralipid (Cutter Medical, Miles Laboratories, Inc., Berkeley, Calif.).

* MVI and MVI Pediatric (Armour Pharmaceutical Co., Kankakee, Ill.); LyphoMed (LyphoMed Inc., Melrose Park, Ill.); and Berocca Parenteral Nutrition and Berocca WS (Roche Laboratories, Nutley, N.J.).

trace mineral deficiencies have occurred in patients receiving TPN for prolonged periods when supplements were not given. The American Medical Association has published guidelines for use of some vitamins and trace minerals in parenteral solutions.[9,10]

Administration of Total Parenteral Nutrition It is essential that the nutrient solution be administered slowly at first because the body must adapt to the high glucose load and hyperosmolar solution. If a 25 percent dextrose solution is used, 1 liter is administered in the first 24 hours, and the rate is gradually increased over the next few days. An infusion pump is used to control the rate of delivery. With these precautions most patients do not require exogenous insulin. A typical daily infusion provides 2,000 to 3,000 kcal, although much higher amounts are possible in unusual situations.

TPN is administered continuously or in a cyclic pattern. In the latter, glucose is not given for a specified portion of the day, often 8 to 10 hours. This permits the blood glucose and insulin levels to fall, thereby promoting mobilization of glycogen and fat.

When the patient is weaned from TPN, the infusion rate should be tapered gradually as enteral intake increases. Clear liquids or formula feedings are often used during the transition period until the patient can tolerate the prescribed diet.

Complications Associated With Total Parenteral Nutrition Complications associated with use of total parenteral nutrition are infectious, metabolic or technical in nature. *Infectious* complications may be bacterial or fungal. These often occur at the catheter insertion site and may enter the bloodstream causing sepsis. The high glucose concentration of the solution provides an excellent medium for growth of bacteria and fungi; thus, it is kept refrigerated until used. The solution should not be hung at room temperature for more than 12 hours. *Metabolic* complications include hyperglycemia resulting from infusion of the solution too rapidly; hypoglycemia occurring when the infusion rate is abruptly decreased; hyperosmolar hyperglycemic nonketotic coma due to excessive glucose load; hypocalcemia, hypokalemia, hypomagnesemia, hyper- or hypophosphatemia, hyperammonemia, acid–base imbalance, elevated liver enzymes, and so on. *Technical* problems include accumulation of air, fluid, or blood in the chest cavity, air leaks into the catheter (embolism), thrombosis (blood clots), and improper placement of the catheter tip sometimes resulting in puncture of the wall of the blood vessel.

Peripheral Parenteral Nutrition This method of feeding avoids some of the risks associated with total parenteral nutrition by way of a central vein. Patients who have moderate protein and calorie deficits, those requiring less than 3,000 kcal per day, or those who require total parenteral nutrition for less than 2 weeks may benefit.

The osmolality of the solution used in peripheral veins is lower than that delivered by way of a central vein. Solutions greater than 600 to 700 mOsm per liter will irritate and damage a peripheral vein. By contrast, osmolality of central vein infusions is two to three times higher. To achieve an osmolality less than 700 mOsm/liter the hypertonic dextrose–amino acid mixture is infused simultaneously with an isotonic lipid emulsion. Vitamins and minerals are added to the solution as previously described.

Case Study 11

Elderly Woman with Gastrostomy

Mrs. D, age 82, is a small woman who emigrated from Czechoslovakia to the United States with her husband and three children 21 years ago. She has since lived in a largely Czechoslovakian speaking community, and, as a result, she has a limited comprehension of English. Mrs. D lives alone in her own home in the same town as her three daughters and their families.

For the past 6 months Mrs. D has had increasing difficulty swallowing. While eating she has frequent bouts of coughing and often regurgitates undigested food particles. For a time she was able to swallow small amounts of soft foods, but now she can handle only small amounts of liquids. She refuses to eat with others because of her dysphagia. Mrs. D has slowly lost weight during the past year and appears emaciated. She now weighs 40 kg (88 lb); height 155 cm (61 in.). Mrs. D finally went to a doctor, who conducted a thorough investigation into the cause of her dysphagia and her recent weight loss.

A barium swallow revealed an irregular lesion in the lower third of Mrs. D's esophagus. Esophagoscopy, biopsy, and cytologic examination resulted in the diagnosis of carcinoma of the esophagus. Since the tumor was inoperable and there was evidence of metastases to the lymph nodes and liver, palliative surgery was done and a gastrostomy was established.

Postoperatively, Mrs. D received amino acid–dextrose solution in combination with a lipid emulsion by peripheral vein. Once bowel sounds were audible, tube feedings were initiated per the gastrostomy. The concentration and rate of administration were gradually increased as tolerated. Peripheral parenteral nutrition was tapered simultaneously with the increasing infusion of enteral feedings and then discontinued when Mrs. D was tolerating full-strength tube feedings in adequate amounts.

In preparation for discharge, a family conference was held. The conference provided the family an opportunity to review treatment plans and ask questions of the oncology team. Plans for radiation therapy on an outpatient basis were discussed.

Mrs. D is weak and unsteady on her feet, and her daughters are concerned about her living alone. However, Mrs. D wants to remain independent and has adamantly refused to move to a nursing home. A compromise was reached when Mrs. D's daughters offered to take turns visiting their mother on a daily basis, and arrangements were made for regular visits by a home care nurse.

Mrs. D and her daughters were instructed in the preparation and administration of the tube feedings. Easy-to-handle equipment was selected, and a commercial tube feeding formula was recommended.

Pathophysiologic Correlations
1. What is a gastrostomy?
2. What physiologic adaptations are made when a tube feeding has a high osmolality?
3. What metabolic alterations may occur when the protein intake and solute load are excessive?

Nutritional Assessment
4. What factors in Mrs. D's history place her at nutritional risk?
5. Using the formula for Resting Metabolic Expenditure (see inside back cover) estimate Mrs. D's calorie needs.
6. Mrs. D's usual weight is 45 kg. How much protein should she have?
7. What should receive first priority in Mrs. D's feeding: protein or calories? Explain.
8. The peripheral parenteral nutrition solution was made up of 4.25 percent amino acid–10 percent dextrose, 1,000 ml; 10 percent fat emulsion, 1,000 ml. Calculate the grams of protein, fat and carbohydrate and the calories provided in the solution. What is the ra-

tio of nonprotein calories to nitrogen in the solution?

9. What components of tube feedings increase osmolality?
10. What are the nutritional effects of radiation therapy of the gastrointestinal tract?

Planning the Diet

11. What is the desirable caloric concentration of tube feedings? What are the consequences of concentrations greater or less than this?
12. What types of foods are appropriate for use in blenderized feedings?
13. What considerations should be kept in mind in planning the content of the tube feeding for protein; carbohydrate; fat; and water?
14. Of the several types of tube feedings, which is the most appropriate for Mrs. D? List several suitable preparations for Mrs. D.
15. Set up a table showing the comparison of three commercial products that you listed for question 14. In this table indicate the values per 1,000 ml for energy; protein; fat; carbo-

hydrate; vitamins; minerals; osmolality; volume required to meet the RDA; and ratio of nonprotein calories per gram nitrogen. Put a circle around all of the items that differ significantly in the three formulas.

16. What is the usual volume of tube feeding given daily?
17. What volume of tube feeding should be given at each feeding?
18. List the methods used to administer tube feedings and the considerations to be kept in mind for each.

Dietary Counseling

19. What feelings should you anticipate that Mrs. D has?
20. How would you attempt to help Mrs. D to accept the gastrostomy feeding?
21. A nurse from the community nursing service visits Mrs. D once a week for 6 weeks and then once a month. What should she observe?

References for the Case Study

Bayer, L. M.: "Psychosocial Aspects of Nutritional Support," *Nurs. Clin. North Am.*, 18:119–28, March 1983.

Hutchinson, M. M.: "Administration of Fat Emulsions," *Am. J. Nurs.*, 82:275–77, 1982.

Kagawa-Busby, K S., et al.: "Effects of Diet Temperature on Tolerance of Enteral Feedings," *Nurs. Res.*, 29:276–80, 1980.

Lichtenstein, V.: "Care of the Acutely Ill Older Adult—Nutritional Management," *Geriatr. Nurs.*, 3:386–91, 1982.

Yasko, J. M.: "Care of the Patient Receiving Radiation Therapy," *Nurs. Clin. North Am.*, 17:631–48, December 1982.

References

1. American Dietetic Association: *Handbook of Clinical Dietetics*. Yale University Press, New Haven, Conn. 1981.
2. Rombeau, J. L., and Caldwell, M. D.: *Enteral and Tube Feeding*. W. B. Saunders Company, Philadelphia, 1984.
3. Freeman, J. B., and Fairfull-Smith, R. J.: "Current Concepts of Enteral Feeding," *Adv. Surg.*, 16:75–112, 1983.
4. "Panel Report on Nutrient-Hormone Interaction," *Am. J. Clin. Nutr.*, 34:1246–59, 1981.
5. Blackburn, G. L., and Harvey, K. B.: "Nutritional Assessment as a Routine in Clinical Medicine," *Postgrad. Med.*, 71:46–59 ff, May 1982.
6. Askanazi, J., et al.: "Nutrition for the Patient with Respiratory Failure," *Anesthesiology*, 54:373–77, 1981.
7. Long, C. L.: "Energy and Protein Requirements in the Hospitalized Patient," *J.P.E.N.*, 3:69–72, 1979.
8. Elwyn, D. H.: "Nutritional Requirements of Adult Surgical Patients," *Crit. Care Med.*, 8:9–20, 1980.
9. American Medical Association, Department of Foods and Nutrition: "Multivitamin Preparations for Parenteral Use. A Statement by the Nutrition Advisory Group," *J.P.E.N.*, 3:258–62, 1979.
10. American Medical Association, Department of Foods and Nutrition: "Guidelines for Essential Trace Element Preparations for Parenteral Use," *JAMA*, 241:2050–54, 1979.

29

Diet in Diseases of the Esophagus, Stomach, and Duodenum

Approximately 10 percent of the United States population, or some 18 million persons, have chronic digestive disease. These diseases account for a significant proportion of all absences from work in the 17- to 64-year-old age group, thus representing an important economic loss to both employers and employees.

Modified diets are commonly prescribed for many digestive diseases, including hiatal hernia, peptic ulcer, gastritis, diarrhea, constipation, malabsorption syndrome, cirrhosis of the liver, cholecystitis, and pancreatitis, among others. Much controversy exists over the role of diet in the treatment of gastrointestinal disturbances. In certain conditions there is a physiologic basis for dietary modification; in others, a sound rationale is lacking and diets traditionally used are of unproven value. For the latter more objective evidence is needed before sound conclusions can be reached in regard to beneficial effects of dietary modification.

Diagnostic Tests in Gastrointestinal Disease

Disorders of the gastrointestinal tract are classified as *functional* or *organic* in nature. Functional disturbances involve no alterations in structure. In organic diseases, on the other hand, pathologic lesions are seen in tissue, as in ulcers or carcinoma. Both types of disorders are characterized by changes in secretory activity and motility. A number of factors including diet are believed to influence these changes. (See Table 29-1.)

Studies of motility and secretion, together with radiologic evidence and, in some instances, biopsy specimens of the affected mucosa, are used in the diagnosis of gastrointestinal disease.

Measurement of Motility Fluoroscopic and x-ray examinations are widely used to determine the emptying time and motility of the intestinal tract, and to locate the site of the disturbance. Following an overnight fast the patient is given a "barium swallow" consisting of a pint of buttermilk or malted milk in which barium sulfate has been mixed. The progress of this opaque "meal" along the intestinal tract can then be visualized by means of fluoroscopy. Roentgenograms taken before and after the meal are studied for filling defects and other abnormalities.

In GASTRIC ATONY, due to lack of normal muscle tone of the stomach, contractions are not of sufficient strength to move the food mass out of the stomach at a normal rate. Larger pieces or fragments of food are not adequately disintegrated and mixed with the stomach juices.

Increased action of the musculature of the stomach and intestine is known as HYPERPERISTALSIS. It may be brought on by excessive amounts of fibrous foods, psychological factors such as worry or fear, or nervous stimulation.

Measurement of Gastric Acidity Tests of gastric secretory function per se are of limited diagnostic value and are most useful in patients in whom a lesion has been demonstrated by radiography or gastroscopy.

Various test meals were formerly used to stimulate gastric secretion. Drugs such as caffeine, histamine, or histalog, which are vigorous stimulants to gastric secretion, are used to determine the amount of acid produced.

Basal acid secretion is measured by collecting gastric juice for a timed period after an overnight fast. Pharmacologic agents such as histamine are then administered to stimulate maximal acid secretion, and

Table 29-1.   Factors That Modify Acid Secretion and Gastrointestinal Motility and Tone

Increased Flow of Acid and Enzyme Production	Decreased Flow of Acid and Enzyme Production
1. Chemical stimulation—meat extractives, seasonings, certain spices, alcohol, acid foods 2. Attractive, appetizing, well-liked foods 3. State of happiness and contentment 4. Pleasant surroundings for meals	1. Large amounts of fat, especially as fried foods, pastries, nuts, etc. 2. Large meals 3. Poor mastication of food 4. Foods of poor appearance, flavor, or texture 5. Foods acutely disliked 6. Worry, anger, fear, pain*

Increased Tone and Motility	Decreased Tone and Motility
1. Warm foods 2. Liquid and soft foods 3. Fibrous foods, as in certain fruits and vegetables 4. High-carbohydrate low-fat intake 5. Seasonings; concentrated sweets 6. Fear, anger, worry, nervous tension	1. Cold foods 2. Dry, solid foods 3. Low-fiber foods 4. High-fat intake, especially as fried foods, pastries, etc. 5. Vitamin B complex deficiency, especially thiamin 6. Sedentary habits 7. Fatigue 8. Worry, anger, fear, pain

* In certain individuals these emotional disturbances may stimulate the flow of gastric juice.

collections of gastric juice are again made for a specified period. Results are reported in terms of maximal acid output or peak acid output. Excess acid secretion is known as HYPERCHLORHYDRIA and is often accompanied by gastric distress. It may be associated with emotional or nervous upsets, or it may accompany organic disease such as peptic ulcer or cholecystitis.

HYPOCHLORHYDRIA denotes a diminished amount of free acid and may be present indefinitely in otherwise healthy persons. The cause should be determined, if possible, since hypochlorhydria also accompanies diseases such as pernicious anemia and is a common finding in sprue, chronic gastritis, and pellagra. It occurs occasionally in cancer, nephritis, cholecystitis, and diabetes. In ACHLORHYDRIA no free acid is present although there is some peptic activity; this finding suggests pernicious anemia and malignant gastric ulcer. ACHYLIA GASTRICA refers to the absence of both acid and enzyme activity.

General Dietary Considerations in Diseases of the Gastrointestinal Tract

Factors in Dietary Management   Many dietary recommendations have been made for the management of gastrointestinal diseases; yet actual knowledge of the specific effects of various foods on the digestive tract is rather limited. Any proposed dietary modifications should take into consideration the possible effects of ingested food upon (1) the secretory activity of the stomach, small intestine, pancreas, liver, and gallbladder; (2) motility of the tract; (3) the bacterial flora; (4) the comfort and ease of digestion; and (5) the maintenance and repair of the mucosal structures. In addition, some disorders interfere with the completeness of digestion or the absorption of one or more nutrients so that the nutrient intake must be modified in order to meet the net requirements of the body.

Influence of Foods on Gastric Acidity   Most foods have a pH between 5 and 7, thus are considerably less acid than gastric juice. No food is sufficiently acid to have an adverse effect on a gastric lesion, although citrus juices and fruits might cause some discomfort to a lesion of the mouth, esophagus, or the achlorhydric stomach.

Gastric secretion is initiated by the sight, smell, and taste of food. As food enters the stomach, the secretion continues and reaches its height sometime later. Protein foods stimulate more acid secretion than carbohydrates and fats.

Protein foods initially have a temporary buffering effect; hence there is less free acid immediately available to erode tissue when protein is fed. Milk has some buffering effect, although this may be outweighed by its ability to stimulate acid secretion. Nevertheless, most patients with active peptic ulcer have progressed well on diets in which frequent milk feedings were used for their neutralizing effect. Regardless of buffering activity, the amount of free acid again is high within ½ to 2 hours following a meal. No diet alone will maintain a 24-hour neutralization of gastric contents.

Fats inhibit gastric secretion. The entrance of fats into the duodenum stimulates the production of enterogastrone, a hormone, which retards gastric secretion and delays gastric emptying.

Meat extractives, tannins, caffeine, and alcohol are well known for their effect in stimulating the flow of acid. Chili powder, cloves, mustard seeds, nutmeg, and black pepper have been shown to be irritating to the gastric mucosa; thus, these spices should be used with discretion by persons with ulcer disease. Black pepper is usually excluded from diets used in the treatment of ulcers. Most other commonly used spices exert no harmful effects and need not be contraindicated.

Influence of Foods on Motility The rate of gastric emptying is related to the caloric density of the food given and is independent of the volume given; that is, isocaloric amounts of carbohydrate and triglyceride are equally effective in slowing gastric emptying. Foods high in fiber increase peristaltic action, and low-fiber foods reduce such motility.

Influence of Foods on Bacterial Flora Experimental studies indicate that increased dietary fiber does not significantly alter the concentration or composition of major groups of fecal bacteria. However, the total output of fecal bacteria is increased as dietary fiber increases.[1]

Foods and Their Effect on Lesions Fibrous foods have often been omitted from diets for diseases of the gastrointestinal tract in the belief that they might mechanically injure or retard the healing of a lesion such as an ulcer. However, it is unlikely that fibrous foods, when sufficiently chewed, would be injurious to a peptic ulcer. Patients should be instructed to chew foods properly. Puréeing of foods is not necessary unless the teeth are poor or absent. The individual can best determine tolerance for specific foods by trial and error.

Influence of Foods on Digestive Comfort Ingestion of certain foods has long been associated with symptoms of belching, distention, epigastric distress, flatulence, constipation, or diarrhea in some persons with digestive disorders. Among these foods are baked beans, cabbage, fried foods, onions, and spicy foods. Tolerance to these and other foods is a highly individual matter. Not all patients react to foods in the same way, nor does the same patient always react to a specific food in the same way.

Disorders of the Esophagus and Stomach

Esophagitis This is an acute or chronic inflammation of the esophageal wall. *Acute* esophagitis is usually characterized by substernal pain brought on by swallowing. It may be a consequence of upper respiratory infections, extensive burns, prolonged gastric intubation, excessive vomiting, ingestion of poisonous substances such as lye, or diseases such as scarlet fever or diphtheria.

Most cases of *chronic* esophagitis are attributed to a sliding hernia that permits the reflux of gastric juice into the esophagus. Mucosal erosions and narrowing of the lumen occur. The disorder occurs most frequently in persons with high gastric acidity, many of whom have a history of duodenal ulcer.

Symptoms. Heartburn, intermittent at first, but becoming progressively worse, is often the chief complaint in esophagitis. Pain following ingestion of very hot or cold foods and spicy or acid foods and eventual dysphagia occur as the disease progresses.

Treatment. The objectives of therapy are to protect the esophagus, to reduce gastric acidity, and to reduce reflux of gastric contents into the esophagus. Antacid preparations are usually prescribed.

Dietary management consists of weight reduction (see Chapter 25) for obese individuals since excess abdominal fat is believed to increase gastric herniation and reflux. Large meals should be avoided in favor of more frequent small meals.

Hiatus Hernia A common disorder affecting the esophagus is the herniation of a portion of the stomach through the esophageal hiatus of the diaphragm. This disorder, known as HIATAL HERNIA, occurs most frequently in persons over 45 years of age. The incidence is greater in persons of stocky build and in overweight persons. Loss of muscle tone weakens muscles around the diaphragm and increased abdominal pressure helps push the stomach through the diaphragm. Symptoms occur when the herniated portion is irritated or injured or is large enough to affect other organs. Tight garments or belts appear to provoke symptoms and should be avoided. Substernal pain, belching, or hiccoughing occurs after meals or while lying down. Eating small amounts at any one time and omitting food for several hours before bedtime are usually recommended. Weight reduction is essential for obese individuals. (See Chapter 25.)

Esophageal Reflux   The lower esophageal sphincter normally maintains a pressure greater than that in the stomach thereby preventing reflux of gastric contents into the esophagus. Incompetence of the sphincter permits postural reflux and may cause esophagitis. Heartburn and dysphagia also occur. The disorder is multifactorial in etiology. Esophageal reflux is not synonymous with a hiatal hernia although both may occur together.

Diagnostic tests for esophageal reflux include an x-ray series following a barium swallow, an acid perfusion test, esophagoscopy, esophageal biopsy, and measurement of lower esophageal sphincter pressure. In the acid perfusion test, a weak solution of acid is given, alternating with saline, to provoke symptoms of gastroesophageal reflux. A combination of two or more of these tests is often used in the diagnosis.

Factors that decrease lower esophageal sphincter pressure include alcohol, caffeine, chocolate, fatty meals, peppermint, and smoking. Proteins and antacids increase sphincter pressure. Carbohydrates appear to have little effect on sphincter pressure.

Treatment.   Several means are used to relieve symptoms. Mechanical measures include elevation of the head of the bed and avoidance of lying down after meals; reduction of abdominal pressure by weight loss, if indicated, and avoidance of tight clothing; and decreasing size of meals. Pharmacologic measures include cholinergics and antacids to increase lower esophageal pressure, and metclopramide, to enhance gastric emptying.

Dietary recommendations include a high-protein diet, restriction of fat, avoidance of substances that lower esophageal sphincter pressure and those that might be irritating to an inflamed mucosa, for example, citrus or tomato juice, and small meals.[2]

Nutritional Effects of Drug Therapy.   Antacids containing aluminum hydroxide or magnesium hydroxide impair absorption of phosphorus and vitamin A, and destroy thiamin.[3]

Achalasia   This disorder of esophageal motility is characterized by absence of peristalsis in the body of the esophagus and failure of the lower esophageal sphincter to relax normally upon swallowing so that food can enter the stomach. Loss or absence of ganglion cells is believed to be involved. The resting lower

esophageal pressure is twice the normal level. Long-continued intraesophageal pressure may lead to dilatation above the point of stricture. The primary symptom is dysphagia with possible vomiting and eventual weight loss.

Treatment consists of dilatation of the stricture. Drug therapy is used to lower esophageal sphincter pressure. Some cases that do not respond to dilatation are treated surgically. The muscle at the lower esophageal sphincter is cut so that the sphincter remains open for passage of food. Gastroesophageal reflux is a common consequence of the surgery. Dietary considerations include avoidance of excessively hot or iced beverages and any foods that may be irritating to the esophagus. If weight loss has been considerable, increased calories and protein are needed. (See Chapter 25.) Some individuals tolerate several small feedings better than larger ones.

Esophageal Obstruction   This may result from a number of causes including pressure from adjacent organs, hiatal hernia, scar tissue formation, foreign bodies, diverticula, and neoplasms. Swallowed foods do not progress beyond the point of stricture owing to narrowing of the lumen. Measures to restore the normal passageway include dilatation, irradiation, or surgical intervention, depending on the nature of the obstruction.

Dietary management is the same for obstruction from any cause. Efforts are directed toward providing foods in suitable form and sufficient amounts to meet the patient's needs. In partial obstruction, liquids should be offered with progression to low-fiber foods (see page 414) as tolerated. Small amounts of food at frequent intervals are preferable. When it is not possible or desirable for food to pass through the esophagus, the patient is fed by means of a gastrostomy. Food is administered through a tube inserted directly into the stomach. (See Chapter 28 for characteristics of tube feedings.)

Indigestion   Indigestion, or dyspepsia, is a functional or organic disease manifested by symptoms of heartburn, acid regurgitation, epigastric pain, "fullness" or bloating especially after meals, flatulence, nausea, or vomiting.

Most cases of indigestion are of functional origin and are usually due to faulty dietary habits or emotional factors. The organic type is associated with diseases affecting the digestive organs; it may also be a symptom of generalized disease as in uremia. Treatment in organic types consists of treating the underlying disease.

Persons with functional dyspepsia need individualized dietary counseling in the essentials of a nutritionally adequate diet. Specific instructions should be given with emphasis on selection of foods from each group in the Daily Food Guide and the importance of regular mealtimes, sufficient time to eat in a relaxed atmosphere, rest after meals, and avoidance of emotional tension.

Gastritis This condition is an inflammation of the mucosa of the stomach, occurring as an acute or chronic lesion with atrophy or hypertrophy in some persons. Causes are toxins of bacterial or metabolic origin (*Salmonella*, *Staphylococcus*, uremia, syphilis); irritation of the gastric mucosa by ingestion of ethyl alcohol, certain drugs (digitalis, glucogenic steroids, salicylates, and others), gastric irradiation, heavy metals, strong alkali or acid; or faulty dietary habits, such as excessive intake of highly seasoned foods. The diagnosis of gastritis is based on biopsies of the gastric mucosa.

ACUTE gastritis is characterized by a general inflammatory reaction of the mucosa with hyperemia, edema, and exudation; in more severe cases, erosion of localized areas and hemorrhages occur. Symptoms vary from anorexia, vague epigastric discomfort, or heartburn, to severe vomiting.

Since acute gastritis usually heals within 3 or 4 days, nutritional management is not the primary concern. Treatment is directed toward removal or neutralization of the offending agent by gastric lavage, antibiotics, withholding of food for 24 to 48 hours to allow the stomach to rest, and replacement of water and electrolyte losses due to severe vomiting. After 1 or 2 days small amounts of clear fluids (100 ml per hour) are administered with gradual progression to soft, easily digested foods. (See page 414.)

CHRONIC gastritis is characterized by altered resistance of the gastric mucosal barrier to hydrogen ions. The resulting tissue damage may be induced by bile reflux or salicylates. Recurrent inflammation leads to glandular atrophy and changes in enzyme activities of the gastric mucosal cells. Complete atrophy results in the inability to absorb vitamin B-12 and in pernicious anemia. Symptoms include epigastric distress, nausea, and vomiting. Chronic gastritis is often directly attributed to dietary indiscretion or indirectly to toxic substances; nevertheless, it may also occur in the absence of any known cause. Gastritis may be the cause of persistent symptoms in patients in whom peptic ulcer has seemingly healed.

Dietary treatment of chronic gastritis consists in correcting faulty dietary habits, providing a relaxed atmosphere at mealtime, and emphasizing adequate caloric intake of soft foods. (See page 414.) Arrangement of meals in four or six small feedings is some times preferred. Iron supplements may be desirable. Once symptoms have abated, progression to a normal diet may be made.

Peptic Ulcer

The term *peptic ulcer* is used to describe any localized erosion of the mucosal lining of those portions of the alimentary tract that come in contact with gastric juice. Most ulcers are found in the duodenum, although they also occur in the esophagus, stomach, or jejunum. Similar symptoms are produced by the ulcer regardless of its location, and response to treatment is essentially the same. The same principles of dietary treatment apply to all regardless of etiology.

Some 3 million persons in the United States suffer from peptic ulcer. Of these, 80 percent have duodenal ulcer, and the remainder have gastric ulcers. Within the past two decades both hospital admissions and death rates for peptic ulcer have declined markedly in the United States. Males were formerly more likely than females to develop peptic ulcer, but females now have a slightly higher prevalence than males.[4]

Etiology In spite of extensive literature on the subject, the exact cause of peptic ulcer has not been determined. In duodenal ulcer, hypersecretion of acid is found, although tissue resistance is normal. Acid hypersecretion is attributed to an increased number of parietal cells, impaired inhibition of gastrin release, and possibly more rapid gastric emptying with loss of buffering effect.[5] In gastric ulcer, both a back diffusion of hydrogen ions into the mucosa and reflux of bile are believed to be involved. An abnormality in the mucosa permits penetration of hydrogen ions. Drugs such as aspirin and indomethacin (used in rheumatoid arthritis) can alter the gastric mucosal barrier by increasing backdiffusion of hydrogen. Bile acids can destroy the gastric mucosal barrier. Reflux of bile acids from the duodenum due to an incompetent pyloric sphincter leads to chronic gastritis and subsequent ulceration. In both gastric and duodenal ulcers, then, the net effect is an excess of acid and pepsin for the amount of local tissue resistance.

Personality type plays a role—highly nervous and emotional individuals seem to be more susceptible to the disease. Anxiety, worry, and strain may cause hypersecretion of acid and hypermotility. A positive family history of recurrent pain is not uncommon.

Symptoms and Clinical Findings Epigastric pain occurring as deep hunger contractions 1 to 3 hours after meals is often the chief complaint. The pain may be described as dull, piercing, burning, or gnawing and is usually relieved by the taking of food or alkalies. The basis for the pain may be the action of unneutralized hydrochloric acid on exposed nerve fibers at the site of the ulcer. Pain is also associated with hypermotility of the stomach or gastric distention following ingestion of large amounts of food or liquids.

Low plasma protein levels are often present and delay rapid and complete healing of the ulcer. Weight loss and iron-deficiency anemia are common. The intake of iron, ascorbic acid, and the B-complex vitamins, particularly thiamin, may be less than desirable because of self-imposed limitation of leafy green vegetables and other food sources of these nutrients. (See Chapters 9, 12, and 13.)

In some instances, hemorrhage is the first indication of an ulcer and requires surgical intervention. Other complications such as intractability, obstruction, perforation, and carcinoma of gastric ulcer are treated surgically.

Rationale for Treatment Individualized attention to the whole person rather than to the ulcer per se is extremely important in the management of persons with ulcer disease. The patient must be taught to accept responsibility for progress since medical and dietary therapies produce only symptomatic improvement. In general, treatment consists of drugs, rest, and diet.

Drugs. A histamine hydrogen receptor antagonist, cimetidine, inhibits basal and stimulated acid secretion and increases the rate of ulcer healing.[6] It is taken with meals and at bedtime. *Antacids* are prescribed to neutralize excess acid, but usual dosages do not influence the rate of healing. These are taken between meals and at bedtime but should not be taken simultaneously with cimetidine.[7] *Anticholinergic* drugs inhibit acid secretion, and *antispasmodics* delay gastric emptying. Nutritional side effects of these drugs are listed in Appendix Table B.

Rest. Good physical and mental hygiene is basic if the person is to learn to cope with his or her problems constructively. Mental and physical rest is important; modification of living and work habits is needed when overwork and physical stress cause exacerbations of the disease. Control of emotional stress is equally important.

Diet. The development of potent drugs, such as cimetidine, has largely replaced the role of diet in treatment of peptic ulcer. Most clinicians agree that diet does not influence the rate of healing of an ulcer, that regularity of mealtimes is essential, and that individualization of the diet is important. Patients are generally advised to avoid caffeine-containing beverages and alcohol from the diet. Pepper and highly seasoned foods are omitted due to their irritating effect on the gastric mucosa.

For most patients hospitalized for an active peptic ulcer, some type of fiber-restricted "bland" or soft diet is commonly used, although there is much variation in composition of these diets. The diet must be nutritionally adequate in order to correct any preexisting deficiencies and to promote healing. In some instances, intakes of nutrients in excess of the recommended dietary allowances are desirable, with emphasis on high quality protein, ascorbic acid and iron.

Nutritional Effects of Drug Therapy. Prolonged use of cimetidine may interfere with absorption of vitamin B-12; thus, supplements may be indicated. Most antacids contain substantial amounts of sodium, which may be excessive for persons on sodium-restricted diets. Antacids containing large amounts of calcium may cause hypercalcemia. Those containing magnesium hydroxide or aluminum hydroxide cause malabsorption of phosphorus and vitamin A, and destruction of thiamin. Anticholinergics cause generalized malabsorption.

DIETARY COUNSELING

The patient needs to know which foods are needed for a nutritionally adequate diet and the importance of including these daily. He or she should be taught to select an essentially normal diet from a wide variety of foods, omitting those foods known to be distressing to the patient. Moderate use of seasonings is permitted and may greatly enhance the flavor of foods. The patient should be instructed to establish regularity of mealtimes and to use moderation in amounts eaten. If the diet to be used at home is planned with the patient, giving consideration to his or her cultural pattern, the patient is more likely to follow recommendations made. Meals eaten in restaurants should pose no particular problems if the individual uses good judgment in food selection.

Dietitians or nurses should stress the importance of eating meals in a relaxed atmosphere with a happy frame of mind and advise the patient to try to forget personal or family problems while eating. A short rest before and after meals may be conductive to greater enjoyment of meals.

Ulcers frequently recur even after complete healing is believed to have taken place. To prevent recurrence of symptoms prompt treatment is advisable following great stress. In periods of great emotional strain careful compliance with medical therapy is especially important.

Modification of Diet in Bleeding Ulcer The degree of dietary modification in bleeding ulcer depends on the peculiarities of the individual case. In severe hemorrhage, it is customary to give no food until the bleeding has been controlled and the patient's condition is stabilized. If hemorrhage is not severe, and if nausea and vomiting are not a problem, the patient may desire food and tolerate it well. In many hospitals initial dietary treatment consists of frequent small feedings of easily digested foods, such as egg, custards or simple puddings, toast, crackers, and tender cooked fruits and vegetables. Gradual progression in amounts and types of foods is made as the patient improves.

CASE STUDY 12

Career Woman with Duodenal Ulcer

Ms. F, age 35, was divorced a year ago and has custody of her three children: two sons, ages 3 and 7, and a 9-year-old daughter. She is committed to becoming financially independent so that she can provide for the future of her children. She is a high-strung individual and a perfectionist at whatever she does.

Ms. F has been under a lot of pressure with her new job. Three months ago she was promoted to the position of a correspondent for a nationally circulated magazine. Her work entails traveling away from home about 6 days a month, usually for 2 or 3 days at a time. She feels guilty about being away from home so much. Arrangements for a live-in babysitter have not worked out very well. She has had three babysitters within the past 3 months. Ms. F has had difficulty finding a dependable person whose discipline style is similar to her own. Since she started traveling, Ms. F has not had time for hobbies and outside interests. She used to enjoy an occasional game of tennis or taking the children on excursions to the park or zoo.

While away from home Ms. F's meals are business-related engagements. Breakfast consists of midmorning coffee and a sweet roll. Most of her meetings occur around coffee and sometimes cocktails; many of the people in the meetings smoke. At noon she has a cocktail and a large meal. She frequently has indigestion after eating fried foods and when she must rush from lunch to another appointment. Because she does not like to eat by herself, she often skips dinner when she gets back to her hotel.

When in town Ms. F keeps busy, irregular office hours. She has little time for food preparation at home and eats hurried meals. She is a heavy coffee drinker and smokes excessively when she is nervous. She also has a history of frequent tension-related headaches for which she takes salicylates.

Periodically during the past 6 months Ms. F experienced a persistent gnawing sensation in the right epigastric area about an hour after eating. The pain subsides after she has something to eat or after taking an antacid. When the pain became so severe that she was waking up in the early hours of the morning, she consulted her physician.

Diagnostic studies revealed a duodenal ulcer. Ms. F was placed on Tagamet (cimetidine). She was advised to avoid gastrointestinal irritants in her diet as well as alcoholic beverages, coffee, nicotine, and salicylates.

Pathophysiologic Correlations
1. What are the stressful situations in Ms. F's history that may have contributed to ulceration?
2. What are some possible alterations to mechanisms in gastric physiology that may contribute to duodenal ulcer?
3. What are the effects of smoking, alcohol, and caffeine on the gastrointestinal mucosa?
4. Why does Ms. F get relief when she eats something or takes an antacid?
5. What adverse effects, if any, does aluminum hydroxide gel have on nutrition?

Nutritional Assessment
6. What nutrients, if any, is Ms. F likely to be consuming in less than desirable amounts?
7. Ms. F has lost 2.2 kg (5 lb) during the past year. She now weighs 50.5 kg (111 lb) and her height is 167 cm (66 in.); she has a small body frame. What is an appropriate weight for her?
8. Estimate Ms. F's caloric needs.
9. What are the nutritional effects of cimetidine? salicylates? antacids?

Planning the Diet

10. Does Ms. F's diet need to be modified from the normal diet? Explain.
11. List several suggestions for more nutritious, easy to prepare meals for Ms. F.
12. Should Ms. F's daily meal plan include frequent small meals? Explain.

Dietary Counseling

13. Outline the points that you would emphasize in counseling Ms. F about her diet.
14. Ms. F is afraid that she will gain weight if she stops smoking. How would you advise her?

15. List several behavior modification strategies that might be appropriate to recommend to Ms. F.
16. Ms. F asks whether she can have decaffeinated coffee and tea. What would you tell her?
17. Ms. F's father had an ulcer 12 years ago for which a milk-based bland diet was described. Ms. F was somewhat surprised that she was not given the same diet. Explain.
18. Ms. F's recovery rests in part on the solution of problems relating to child care and to her new job. What referrals for assistance in these matters might be helpful?

References for the Case Study

BURNSTEIN, A. V.: "Peptic Ulcer Disease: Medical and Surgical Considerations," *Crit. Care Q.*, 5:1–7, September 1982.

GROSSMAN, M. I., et al.: "Peptic Ulcer. New Therapies, New Diseases," *Ann. Intern. Med.*, 95:609–27, 1981.

KRATZER, J. B., et al.: "What to Teach Your Patient about His Duodenal Ulcer," *Nursing '78*, 8:54–56, January 1978.

References

1. Bornside, G. H.: "Stability of Human Fecal Flora," *Am. J. Clin. Nutr.*, 31:S141–S144, 1978.

2. Richter, J. E., and Castell, D. O.: "Gastroesophageal Reflux," *Ann. Intern. Med.*, 97:93–103, 1982.
3. Moore, A. O., and Powers, D. E.: *Food-Medication Interactions*, 3rd ed. FMI Publishing, Tempe, Arizona, 1981.
4. "Mortality from Peptic Ulcers in the United States," *Stat. Bull. Met. Life Found.*, 63:7–9, April–June 1982.
5. Isenberg, J. I.: "Peptic Ulcer," *DM*:28:1–58, December 1981.
6. Isenberg, J. I., et al.: "Healing of Benign Gastric Ulcer with Low Dose Antacid or Cimetidine," *N. Engl. J. Med.*, 308:1319–24, 1983.
7. Steinberg, W. M., et al.: "Antacids Inhibit Absorption of Cimetidine," *N. Engl. J. Med.*, 307:400–404, 1982.

30

Diet in Disturbances of the Small Intestine and Colon

High-Fiber Diet

The functions of the small intestine may be unfavorably influenced by diseases affecting the tract itself or those organs closely related to the digestive process—the liver, gallbladder, and pancreas. In addition, many seemingly unrelated pathologic conditions, to be discussed in chapters that follow, have profound effects on the functioning of the gastrointestinal tract, for example, renal diseases. Depending on the nature of the disease, there may be disturbances in motility, adequacy of enzyme production or release, hydrolytic activity, integrity of the mucosal surfaces, transport mechanisms, and so on. Any of these abnormalities interferes with the efficiency and completeness of absorption and hence the nutritional status of the individual. This chapter includes a discussion of alterations in bowel motility and inflammatory diseases of the mucosa. The malabsorption syndrome will be discussed in Chapter 31 and diseases of the liver, gallbladder, and pancreas in Chapter 32.

Alterations in Bowel Motility

Diarrhea   This is the passage of stools with increased frequency, fluidity, or volume compared to the usual for a given individual. A reduction in segmental activity of the sigmoid colon lowers intraluminal pressure and peripheral resistance, permitting more rapid passage of intestinal contents.[1] The number of stools varies from several per day to one every few minutes. Diarrhea is a symptom of underlying functional or organic disease and is acute or chronic in nature. Some causes of diarrhea are shown in Table 30-1.

Acute diarrhea is characterized by the sudden onset of frequent stools of watery consistency, abdominal pain, cramping, weakness, and sometimes fever and vomiting. Since the duration is usually 24 to 48 hours, nutritional losses are not a prime concern. Acute diarrhea may be the presenting symptom of systemic infection or chronic gastrointestinal disease such as regional enteritis or ulcerative colitis.

Diarrhea is chronic when it persists for 2 weeks or longer. Nutritional deficiencies eventually develop because the rapid passage of the intestinal contents does not allow sufficient time for absorption. Mechanisms that increase fluid loss are (1) osmotic, as when poorly absorbed water-soluble molecules remain in the intestinal lumen and retain water, for example, lactase deficiency or laxative abuse; (2) secretory, in which the mucosa of the large intestine is stimulated to secrete, rather than absorb fluids, as in cholera; and (3) exudative, which is caused by the outpouring of serum proteins, blood, or mucus from sites of inflammation, as in inflammatory bowel disease.

Nutritional Considerations in Diarrheas   Fluid, electrolyte, and tissue protein losses are usually severe if diarrhea is prolonged.

Fluids.   Losses of fluids should be replaced by a liberal intake to prevent dehydration, especially in susceptible age groups such as the very young or elderly persons. Parenteral fluids are often administered to these individuals.

Electrolytes.   Losses of sodium, potassium, and other electrolytes account for the profound weakness associated with severe diarrhea. Potassium loss, in particular, is detrimental as potassium is necessary for normal muscle tone of the gastrointestinal tract. Anorexia, vomiting, listlessness, and muscle weakness

Table 30-1. Some Causes of Diarrhea

Acute Types	Chronic Types
1. Chemical toxins, such as arsenic, lead, mercury, or cadmium	1. Malabsorptive lesions of anatomic, mucosal, or enzymatic origin
2. Bacterial toxins, such as *Salmonella* or staphylococcal food poisoning	2. Metabolic diseases, such as diabetic neuropathy, uremia, or Addison's disease
3. Bacterial infections, such as *Streptococcus, E. coli,* or *Shigella*	3. Alcoholism
4. Drugs, such as quinidine, colchicine, or neomycin	4. Carcinoma of small bowel or colon
5. Psychogenic factors, such as emotional instability	5. Postirradiation to small bowel or colon
6. Dietary factors, such as food sensitivity or allergy	6. Cirrhosis
	7. Laxative abuse

may occur unless losses are replaced by a liberal intake of fluids such as fruit juices that are high in potassium. (See Chapter 40.)

Nutrient Malabsorption. Long-continued diarrhea may result in depletion of tissue proteins and decreased serum protein levels. Fat losses are considerable in certain disorders with consequent loss of calories and fat-soluble vitamins. Intake of calories must be great enough to replace losses and may need to be as high as 3,000, with 100 to 150 g protein, 100 to 120 g fat, and the remainder as carbohydrate. (See Chapter 33.)

Vitamin deficiencies frequently seen in chronic diarrheas are related to the decreased intake of vitamins and the increased requirements because of losses in the stools. A temporary reduction of synthesis of some B-complex vitamins also occurs when antibiotic therapy is used. Vitamin B-12, folic acid, and niacin deficiencies have been observed in various diarrheas.

Iron deficiency is a prominent finding in patients with chronic diarrhea owing to the increased losses of iron in the feces, the occasional blood losses, and the reduced intake of iron-rich foods because of fear that some foods might aggravate an existing lesion. Patients often show remarkable improvement when given supplemental iron therapy.

Dietary Considerations. Any dietary modification in diarrheal states depends on the nature of the underlying defect. In acute diarrhea, current recommendations include ad libitum oral intake of glucose-electrolyte solutions for those able to drink, with progression to foods as tolerated in small frequent feedings, as appetite improves.[2]

Many patients with chronic diarrhea of a functional or organic nature do not tolerate milk or foods high in fat or fiber content. Generally speaking, however, the need is for a diet high in protein and calories, with adequate amounts of vitamins and minerals, and liberal amounts of fluids. (See Chapter 33.)

Constipation In this condition, hypermotility of the sigmoid colon increases resistance to movement of intestinal contents; consequently, there is distention and infrequent or difficult evacuation of feces from the intestine. An accurate definition is related to personal habits since the frequency of bowel movements varies greatly among individuals. For some, daily elimination is normal; in other equally healthy persons, regular evacuation occurs every second or third day.

Infrequent or insufficient emptying of the bowel may lead to malaise, headache, coated tongue, foul breath, and lack of appetite. These symptoms usually disappear after satisfactory evacuation has taken place.

Temporary or chronic constipation can be due to any one of a number of factors such as: (1) failure to establish regular times for eating, adequate rest, and elimination; (2) faulty dietary habits, such as inadequate fluid intake or use of highly refined and concentrated foods that leave little residue in the colon; (3) interference with the urge to defecate brought on by poor personal hygiene or injury to the nervous mechanism; (4) changes in one's usual routine brought on by illness, nervous tension, or a trip away from home; (5) chronic use of laxatives and cathartics; (6) difficult or painful defecation due to hemorrhoids or fissures; (7) poor muscle tone of the intestine and stasis due to lack of exercise occurring especially in bedridden patients, invalids such as arthritics, the aged, and others; (8) organic disorders, such as diverticulosis or obstruction from adhesions or neoplasms; (9) ingestion of drugs, large amounts of sedatives, ganglionic blocking agents, or opiates; and (10) spasm of the intestine due to presence of irritating material, psychogenic influences, or others.

Determination of the cause is important so that proper treatment can be given. Correction of constipation depends in large measure on establishing regularity in habits—eating, rest, exercise, and elimination.

Dietary Considerations. Attention to diet may be beneficial in *atonic* and *spastic* constipation. (See Irritable Colon Syndrome, following.) In the atonic type the diet should contain sufficient fiber to induce peristalsis and to contribute bulk to the intestine. A regular diet with an abundance of both raw and cooked fruits and vegetables is suitable for such patients. Whole-grain breads and cereals should be substituted for refined ones. Bran is useful for some patients but excesses are to be avoided since it may act as an irritant to sensitive intestinal tracts. Fat-containing foods such as bacon, butter, cream, and oils are useful for some because of the stimulating effect of the fatty acids on the mucous membranes. Excesses may cause diarrhea and should be avoided. Mineral oil if used should not be taken at mealtime because of its interference with the absorption of fat-soluble vitamins.

A fluid intake of 8 to 10 glasses a day is useful in keeping the intestinal contents in a semisolid state for easier passage along the tract. Some individuals find that 1 or 2 glasses of hot or cold water, plain or with lemon, are helpful in initiating peristalsis when taken before breakfast.

Irritable Colon Syndrome This condition, also known as *spastic colon*, is a functional disorder involving a disturbance in normal motor activity of the colon. This disorder probably accounts for 50 to 70 percent of all gastrointestinal complaints. It is considered by some to be a forerunner of diverticular disease.

Etiology. Many factors contribute to this functional disorder. Included are excessive use of laxatives or cathartics; antibiotic therapy; food allergy; inadequate dietary fiber; poor hygiene in regard to rest, work, fluid intake, and elimination; and emotional upsets. Nervous, tense individuals are especially sensitive to gastrointestinal neurosis.

Symptoms. The most frequent symptom is pain, due to gaseous distention or to vigorous contractions of the colon. Pain is described as dull aching, cramping, or sharp and intermittent and may be accompanied by anorexia, nausea, and vomiting. Headache, palpitation, and heartburn sometimes occur. Constipation, or diarrhea, or both may occur in the same individual. Weight loss is uncommon.

Treatment. The underlying causes should be determined and corrected. Most patients need help in developing good personal and mental hygiene. Through counseling the individual will hopefully gain insight into the relationship between tension and the symptoms. Faulty eating habits must be corrected and the use of laxatives forbidden. Regular vigorous exercise should be encouraged.

Dietary treatment for those patients with irritable colon syndrome who are constipated should consist of foods that increase intestinal residue enough to aid in evacuation. Increased amounts of fruits, vegetables, and whole-grain cereals provide additional bulk. Some persons experience relief of symptoms when unprocessed bran is added to the diet.

In recurrent diarrhea, a diet restricted in fiber and residue allows the colon the most rest. (See page 414.)

Intestinal Obstruction The movement of the intestinal contents is impaired or prevented by many causes such as tumors, impaction of material in the intestine, or paralytic ileus following surgery. As a rule, the obstruction must be removed by surgical intervention before an adequate diet can be administered. The postoperative diet should be fiber free for a period of time, after which a soft diet is usually ordered.

Inflammatory Disease of the Mucosa

Regional Enteritis *(Crohn's Disease)* This chronic, nonspecific inflammatory disease involves chiefly the terminal ileum, but affects any part of the intestine. The cause is unknown, although genetic and environmental factors have been implicated. The incidence and prevalence of the disease appear to be increasing throughout the world.[3] In the United States incidence peaks at ages 20 to 29, 50 to 59, and 70 to 79[4]. The onset may be acute or insidious; the latter is typical in children.

The inflammatory reaction extends through the entire intestinal wall causing edema and fibrosis. It may be confined to one segment or involve multiple segments with normal areas in between. Patients with long-standing Crohn's disease of more than 7 years' duration are at increased risk for large bowel cancer.[5]

Symptoms and Clinical Findings. Characteristic symptoms include abdominal pain, cramping, diarrhea, steatorrhea, weight loss, fever, and weakness. Systemic complications, malnutrition, and fistula formation are common. Intestinal protein loss, negative nitrogen balance, and anemia occur in a high proportion of patients. Deficiencies of a number of vitamins and minerals are frequent as a consequence of inadequate intake, increased losses, interference with absorption by drugs, or increased requirements. Growth failure in children is usually secondary to insufficient calorie intake.

Conservative management is used unless obstruction or other complications make surgical intervention (ileal resection) necessary. (See Chapter 34.)

Dietary Considerations. The maintenance of good nutrition is an essential component of therapy in this disease. During acute attacks semisynthetic fiber-free diets (see Chapter 28) are used in order to rest the bowel and to prevent danger of obstruction. Alternatively, parenteral nutrition is sometimes used. Progression to a regular diet is made, eliminating only those foods known by the patient to aggravate symptoms. Elimination or restriction of lactose is needed if there is lactose intolerance; likewise, fiber is restricted if strictures are present.

The diet should provide 1.0 to 1.5 g of protein and 40 to 50 kcal per kg of ideal body weight in order to overcome losses due to exudation and malabsorption. (See Chapter 33.) Medium-chain triglyceride therapy (see Chapter 31) is effective in reducing steatorrhea and electrolyte losses in some patients. Foods high in potassium should be given in cases of prolonged diarrhea. (See Chapter 40.) Supplementary B vitamins and minerals such as calcium and iron are often advised. For selected patients with extensive disease and malnutrition, home enteral or parenteral nutrition provides additional nutritional support.[6]

Nutritional Consequences of Drug Therapy. Prednisone, often used in the treatment of regional enteritis, interferes with the utilization of calcium[7] and increases requirements for ascorbic acid, folate, pyridoxine, and vitamin D.[8] Sulfasalazine interferes with folate absorption. Besides supplements of B vitamins, iron supplementation is indicated if anemia is present.

Diverticulosis In this condition, many small mucosal sacs, called DIVERTICULA, protrude through the intestinal wall. Most diverticula are found in the sigmoid colon, although they have been demonstrated throughout the length of the gastrointestinal tract. Diverticulosis is fairly common and the incidence increases with age.

The underlying defect is attributed to abnormal thickening of the muscle layers of the sigmoid colon resulting in narrowing of the lumen and increased intraluminal pressure. Contraction of the colon further increases pressure within the lumen and leads to herniation of the mucosa through the intestinal wall at

points where it is weakened by penetration of blood vessels. Intraluminal pressure is greater when the diet is low in residue. On the other hand, foods that leave a high residue increase the volume and weight of materials reaching the sigmoid colon, and, by distending the colon, may prevent development of high-pressure segments. For this reason, foods high in fiber (see following) have been recommended for use in diverticulosis. Low-residue diets formerly used in this disorder are now considered to be contraindicated.

DIVERTICULITIS occurs when one or more diverticula become inflamed and perforate. Inflammation usually results from accumulation of food particles or residues in the sacs and subsequent bacterial action. Symptoms include steady pain in the lower left abdomen, abdominal distention, changes in bowel habits—usually as constipation, colonic spasm, and occasionally fever. Steatorrhea and megaloblastic anemia, often associated with small bowel diverticula, are due to stasis.

DIETARY COUNSELING

Persons with diverticular disease who are placed on high-fiber diets need careful counseling in regard to the purpose of the diet. Those accustomed to restricting fiber intake may be especially apprehensive about such a drastic change in their diets and need frequent reassurance from the dietitian and the nurse. For most patients, increasing the fiber content of the diet should be made gradually. Whole-grain cereals should be used, and breads and other baked goods made with 100 percent whole-wheat or whole-rye flour substituted for those made with white flour. Generous amounts of fruits and vegetables such as raw carrots, apples, oranges, and lettuce, stewed fruits, potatoes cooked in skins, and so on should be encouraged. Some physicians may recommend the use of bran, the amount depending on the fiber content of the rest of the diet. It is usually best to start with 1 tablespoon of bran per day in a liquid such as milk or juice, gradually increasing the amount of bran until one soft stool is produced daily or until symptoms are relieved. Some patients experience flatulence and distention at first, but the diet should not be discontinued because of these temporary problems. Coarsely ground bran is preferable to finely ground wheat bran.[5] Bran can be mixed with foods such as cereals, soup, or puddings or added to homemade breads, muffins, and cakes.

Bran inhibits iron absorption; thus, the iron status of individuals regularly consuming large amounts should be monitored.

The management of acute attacks of diverticulitis includes bedrest, antibiotics, and clear liquids with progression to a fiber-restricted diet. In recurrent or persistent attacks, surgical resection of the involved portion of colon may be necessary. Complications, such as obstruction, perforation, or fistula formation, also necessitate surgical intervention.

Ulcerative Colitis This diffuse inflammatory and ulcerative disease of unknown etiology involves the mucosa and submucosa of the large intestine. No single etiologic factor has been identified, although genetic and autoimmune factors are thought to be involved.

High-Fiber Diet

Characteristics
This diet is essentially a regular diet with fiber content increased as follows:
1. Substitute at least four servings whole-grain bread and cereals for refined breads and cereals.
2. Emphasize raw fruits and vegetables that are high in fiber.
3. Add 1 to 2 tablespoons bran each day.

The substitution of fibrous foods should be made gradually; for example, whole-grain breads and cereals are added first, then fibrous cooked fruits and vegetables followed by raw fruits and vegetables.

Foods Allowed
Beverages—all
Breads—breads, muffins, or rolls made from 100 per cent whole-wheat or whole-rye flour; graham, wheat, or rye crackers; Ry-Krisp
Cereals—whole-grain such as oatmeal, rolled oats; bran flakes, granola; grapenuts; Shredded Wheat, wheat flakes; brown rice; bran, in moderation
Cheese—all
Desserts—all, with fruit and nuts, if tolerated
Eggs—all
Fats—all
Fruits—all, including dried; preferably raw
Meats—all
Soups—all, preferably vegetable
Sweets—jam, marmalade, preserves
Vegetables—all, especially raw; potatoes in skin
Miscellaneous—condiments and seasoning in moderation

Sample Menu

BREAKFAST
Orange sections
Oatmeal with milk and brown sugar
Poached egg
Bran muffins
Butter or margarine
Marmalade
Coffee

LUNCHEON OR SUPPER
Vegetable soup
Club sandwich:
  Sliced turkey
  Bacon
  Whole-wheat bread
  Lettuce and tomato
  Mayonnaise
Baked apple with raisin stuffing
Milk

DINNER
Brown beef stew
  Onions
  Carrots
Oven-browned potato
Coleslaw with pineapple
Rye bread
Butter or margarine
Apricot fruit crisp
Tea with lemon and sugar

BEDTIME SNACK
Milk
Fresh pear
Graham crackers

Symptoms and Clinical Findings.   Ulcerative colitis may occur at any age but predominates in young adults. The onset is insidious in most cases, with mild abdominal discomfort, an urgent need to defecate several times a day, and diarrhea accompanied by rectal bleeding. Loss of water, electrolytes, blood, and protein from the colon produces systemic symptoms such as weight loss, dehydration, fever, anemia, and general debility. In early stages the mucosa is edematous and hyperemic. In more severe disease, necrosis and frank ulceration of the mucosa occur. The severity of the symptoms does not necessarily correlate with the extent of the disease. Patients with localized disease can be very seriously ill; on the other hand, persons with very troublesome symptoms may have mild disease. Approximately 20 to 25 percent of patients require proctocolectomy (removal of the colon and rectum) and ileostomy for complications.[9] The risk of cancer of the colon and rectum is increased in cases lasting more than 7 years.[9]

Dietary Considerations.   One of the most important factors in the dietary management of this disorder is the individual attention given to the patient. Frequent visits by the dietitian and the nurse can do much toward convincing the patient of a sincere interest in his or her welfare. Many individuals with this disease are extremely apprehensive about what they can eat and seem to need constant reassurance. Mealtime visits provide an excellent opportunity to give encouragement and support.

Much patience and understanding are needed in helping ulcerative colitis patients with dietary problems. The diet must be highly individualized and yet be nutritionally adequate. Genuine efforts to meet the patient's requests must be made; the patient must never be made to feel that numerous questions and frequent demands are troublesome. On the other hand, gentle, but firm guidance must be given in helping the patient select a nutritionally adequate diet. It must be understood that he or she is expected to eat the entire meal. Many patients have poor appetites, and it may be preferable to provide six or eight small feedings; for others, however, having less frequent meal intervals is a more satisfactory approach.

Liberal amounts of high-quality protein (1 to 1.5 g per kg of desirable body weight) are needed, since nitrogen losses from the bowel may be considerable. (See Chapter 33.) Emphasis should be on tender meats, fish, poultry, and eggs for those patients who are allergic or intolerant to milk. Intakes of 40 to 50 kcal per kg desirable body weight are necessary to replace losses due to steatorrhea, and to promote weight gain. A semisynthetic fiber-free diet may be used at first. In intractable cases, total parenteral nutrition is used to bring about remission. When oral feedings are gradually resumed, some degree of fiber restriction is usually needed as many ulcerative colitis patients do not tolerate raw fruits or vegetables, and further damage to an already inflamed mucosa must be prevented. Supplementary vitamins and minerals are usually indicated to compensate for gastointestinal losses and inadequate dietary intake. Especially important are iron salts when anemia is present, and calcium salts if milk is not tolerated.

Nutritional Effects of Drug Therapy.   Sulfasalazine, frequently used in treatment of ulcerative colitis, inhibits a number of steps in the metabolism of folates. Thus, the drug should be taken between meals rather than with meals. Folate supplements are recommended.[10]

CASE STUDY 13

Man with Diverticulosis

Mr. C is a 55-year-old black man who lives with his family in Detroit. He has been laid off for the past 3 months from his job on an automobile assembly line. His wife works rotating shifts as a nursing assistant in a nearby nursing home.

For several months, Mr. C has been troubled by intermittent cramping pain in his left lower abdomen that worsens after eating. He has also noted a change in his bowel habits with a tendency toward constipation. When the pain became intolerable, Mr. C went to his doctor. In addition to left lower quadrant abdominal pain, Mr. C's presenting symptoms included a low-grade fever, chills, leukocytosis, nausea, and flatulence. His doctor recommended rest, antibiotic therapy, and a liquid diet as treatment measures for acute diverticulitis. As his symptoms subsided Mr. C gradually increased his diet to one low in fiber.

After Mr. C recovered from the acute attack, further diagnostic studies were conducted that confirmed the presence of diverticula in the large bowel. His doctor then prescribed a prophylactic regimen of a high-fiber diet and a bulk laxative, psyllium hydrophilic mucilloid (Metamucil). A program of vigorous exercise several times weekly was recommended.

Pathophysiologic Considerations

1. What are diverticula? Where are they found?
2. Describe the mechanisms that are believed to be involved in diverticula formation.
3. A barium enema was ordered for Mr. C. What was the purpose of this test?
4. Does diet play a role in the etiology of diverticulosis? Explain.
5. What effects does fiber have in the colon?

Nutritional Assessment

6. What was the purpose of the fiber-restricted diet ordered for Mr. C?
7. Explain the rationale for the high-fiber diet once the acute attack subsided.
8. List some nutritional consequences of therapy with Metamucil.

Planning the Diet

9. Is a low-residue diet synonymous with a low-fiber diet? Explain.

10. What is meant by dietary fiber? List the constituents.
11. Do all constituents of dietary fiber have the same effect on gastrointestinal physiology? Explain fully.
12. List six foods that are high in fiber.

Dietary Counseling

13. The physician recommended that Mr. C use 2 tablespoons of bran daily, but Mr. C believes the bran will be "too scratchy." How would you explain the importance of bran to him?
14. Mr. C experienced distention after a few days using bran and refused to take it further. What would you advise?
15. Suggest some ways that Mr. C can incorporate bran into his diet.
16. The C family cannot afford to purchase either the bran, Metamucil, or fresh fruits and vegetables. What suggestions can you offer that will bring about the desired changes in the large bowel?

References for the Case Study

BURAKOFF, R.: "An Updated Look at Diverticular Disease," *Geriatrics*, 36:83–91, March 1981.

DAVIS, W. D.: "Lower Bowel Disorders. 2. Diverticular Disease," *Postgrad. Med.*, 68:60–62, October 1980.

CASE STUDY 14

College Student with Ulcerative Colitis and an Ileostomy—Short-Term Use of Total Parenteral Nutrition

Jim, age 20, is a college student majoring in political science and mathematics. He lives in a fraternity house on the university campus where he eats all his meals. He has a steady girl friend, and they plan to announce their engagement next spring. Jim is the only child in the family and he does not get along well with his parents.

At the age of 15 Jim was diagnosed as having chronic ulcerative colitis. Primary medical treatment has included rest, a high-protein low-residue diet, and sulfonamide and steroid drugs. A combination of prednisone and sulfasalazine (Azulfidine) had effectively controlled the disease for some time.

In spite of prolonged intensive medical management, Jim has suffered frequent exacerbations and has required repeated hospitalizations in the past year. He has missed many classes because of his illness, and the cost of medical care has severely drained the family's financial resources. After a recent relapse Jim elected surgical treatment consisting of a total colectomy and ileostomy. A member of the ostomy club visited him and discussed several of Jim's concerns and questions.

The major preoperative goals were to improve Jim's nutritional status and to correct fluid and electrolyte imbalances. Jim was weak, cachectic, and dehydrated on admission. The presenting symptoms included lower abdominal cramps and tenderness, frequent bloody diarrhea, and weight loss of 9 kg (20 lb) during the past year. Jim is 178 cm (70 in) tall and weighs 66 kg (145 lb). The total serum protein was 5.2 g per dl; serum albumin, 3.0 g per dl; serum potassium 2.7 mEq per liter; and hemoglobin, 8.0 g per dl. Stool specimens contained blood, pus, and mucus, but no pathogens.

In preparation for the surgery, Jim was given

blood transfusions and then placed on total parenteral nutrition (TPN). His weight, urine and blood glucose levels, fluid balance, and nutritional needs were closely monitored. Two weeks later he had gained 1 kg (2.2 lb) and his symptoms had subsided, so surgery was performed.

Once peristalsis returned postoperatively, Jim was placed on a progressive diet beginning with clear liquids and advancing as tolerated to one low in fiber and high in protein and calories. A multivitamin was prescribed. Intravenous hyperalimentation was discontinued 1 week after surgery.

Jim's postoperative course was uncomplicated. In preparation for discharge he was instructed in the care of his ileostomy, diet, and medications. The importance of follow-up care and the need for vitamin B-12 injections were explained. He was cautioned about potential sodium and water imbalances that might occur secondary to flu or through excessive perspiration in extremely hot weather or with strenuous exercise. He was advised to avoid alcoholic beverages and foods that provoke diarrhea or flatus.

Pathophysiologic Correlations

1. In addition to weight loss and hypochromic anemia, list six other systemic manifestations of ulcerative colitis.
2. On admission Jim's serum potassium level was 2.7 mEq per liter. How do you explain this deficit?
3. By closely monitoring some physical and biochemical measurements, the risks of TPN are reduced. What are some possible risks associated with TPN?

Nutritional Assessment

4. What are the factors in Jim's history that indicate he may have moderately severe protein-calorie malnutrition?
5. Calculate Jim's deviation from his "ideal" body weight and also from his usual body weight.

$$\frac{\text{"Ideal" weight} - \text{actual weight}}{\text{"Ideal" weight}} \times 100 = \begin{array}{l}\text{percent}\\ \text{deviation}\\ \text{from "ideal"}\\ \text{weight}\end{array}$$

$$\frac{\text{Usual weight} - \text{present weight}}{\text{Usual weight}} \times 100 = \begin{array}{l}\text{percent}\\ \text{deviation}\\ \text{from usual}\\ \text{weight}\end{array}$$

6. What additional measurements might be used to confirm the presence of protein-calorie malnutrition?
7. What factors in Jim's history contribute to fluid and electrolyte imbalance?
8. Why is TPN indicated for Jim?
9. List the nutritional considerations following ileostomy.
10. Explain why Jim will require periodic injections of vitamin B-12.

Planning the Diet

11. What are the usual components of a solution for total parenteral nutrition?
12. Calculate Jim's calorie and protein needs. (NOTE: Use the formula for Resting Metabolic Expenditure inside back cover to predict energy needs; use Table 28-2, page 423, for protein requirements.)
13. The solution given to Jim supplied 1,000 kcal per liter and 6.0 g nitrogen per liter. Was Jim's energy and protein requirement met by the end of the third day if he received 3 liters per day?
14. What was the ratio of nonprotein calories to nitrogen in the TPN solution?
15. Why was the solution of TPN introduced gradually over 3 days?
16. Why is it important to maintain the prescribed rate of solution flow?
17. When full fluids were allowed, the dietitian first provided a low-lactose formula. Why?
18. As tissue repletion occurs, what mineral elements are needed in increased amounts?
19. What nursing care before meal service might improve Jim's ability to consume his food?

Dietary Counseling

20. Outline the dietary recommendations you would make to Jim in preparation for discharge.
21. When Jim first went home his diet was fairly restricted until adjustment could be made to the ileostomy.
    a. Would it be advisable to prescribe vitamin–mineral supplements? If so, explain.
    b. What suggestions can you give Jim for liberalizing his diet?
22. Suggest some measures that might reduce Jim's discomfort after eating.
23. The dietitian has recommended that Jim eat foods that are high in potassium. List several foods that are good sources of potassium yet low in fiber.

References for the Case Study

MITCHELL, C., and SCOTT, S.: "Total Parenteral Nutrition: A Nursing Perspective," *Heart Lung*, 11:426–29, 1982.

MONRO-BLACK, J.: "The ABC's of Total Parenteral Nutrition," *Nursing '84*, 14:50–56, February 1984.

PERKEL, M. S.: "Acute Inflammatory Bowel Disease," *Crit. Care Q.*, 5:21–27, September 1982.

SIMMONS, M. A.: "Using the Nursing Process in Treating Inflammatory Bowel Disease," *Nurs. Clin. North Am.*, 19:11–25, March 1984.

STOTTS, N. A., et al.: "Care of the Patient Critically Ill with Inflammatory Bowel Disease," *Nurs. Clin. North Am.*, 19:61–70, March 1984.

References

1. Parks, T. G.: "Colonic Motility in Man," *Postgrad. Med. J.*, 49:90–99, 1973.
2. Hirschhorn, N.: "The Treatment of Acute Diarrhea in Children. An Historical and Physiological Perspective," *Am. J. Clin. Nutr.*, 33:637–63, 1980.
3. Janowitz, H. D.: "Crohn's Disease—50 Years Later," *N. Engl. J. Med.*, 304:1600–1602, 1981.
4. Garland, C. F., et al.: "Incidence Rates of Ulcerative Colitis and Crohn's Disease in 15 Areas of the United States," *Gastroenterology*, 81:1115–24, 1981.
5. Shorter, R. G.: "Risks of Intestinal Cancer in Crohn's Disease," *Dis. Colon Rectum*, 26:686–89, 1983.
6. Heymsfield, S. B., et al.: "Home Nasoenteric Feeding for Malabsorption and Weight Loss Refractory to Conventional Therapy," *Ann. Intern. Med.*, 98:168–70, 1983.
7. Sitrin, M. D., et al.: "Nutritional and Metabolic Complications in a Patient with Crohn's Disease and Ileal Resection," *Gastroenterology*, 78:1069–79, 1980.
8. Moore, A. O., and Powers, D. E.: *Food–Medication Interactions*, 3rd ed., F-MI Publishing, Tempe, Arizona, 1981.
9. Kirsner, J. B., and Shorter, R. G.: "Recent Developments in Nonspecific Inflammatory Bowel Disease," *N. Engl. J. Med.*, 306:775–81, 1982.
10. Halstead, C. H., et al.: "Sulfasalazine Inhibits the Absorption of Folates in Ulcerative Colitis," *N. Engl. J. Med.*, 305:1513–17, 1981.

31

Malabsorption Syndrome

Medium-Chain Triglyceride Diet; Lactose-Restricted Diet; Sucrose-Restricted Diet; Gluten-Restricted Diet

General Characteristics and Treatment

The term *malabsorption syndrome* is used to describe a number of disorders that are characterized by steatorrhea and multiple abnormalities in absorption of nutrients. Malabsorption in these disorders may be due to defects in (1) the intestinal lumen, resulting in inadequate fat hydrolysis or altered bile salt metabolism; (2) the mucosal epithelial cells, affecting absorbing surfaces and interfering with transport functions; or (3) intestinal lymphatics (See Table 31-1). Malabsorption is also often associated with infectious disease, as in tropical sprue, or with certain metabolic and endocrine disorders.

Symptoms and Laboratory Findings Symptoms present to a variable degree in most persons with this

Table 31-1. Some Malabsorptive Disorders Responsive to Dietary Modification

Abnormalities in the Intestinal Lumen	Abnormalities in the Mucosa
Inadequate lipid hydrolysis*	Specific defects
Pancreatic insufficiency	Lactase insufficiency
Gastric resection	Sucrase-isomaltase deficiency
	Glucose-galactase deficiency
	A-beta-lipoproteinemia
Alteration of bile salt	Nonspecific defects*
metabolism*	Short-bowel syndrome
Hepatobiliary disease	Gluten enteropathy
Intestinal resection	Radiation enteritis
Bacterial overgrowth	Intestinal lymphatic
Drug therapy	obstruction*
	Lymphangiectasia

* MCT therapy effective in disorders in this group.

syndrome include (1) pale, bulky, frothy, and offensive stools due to abnormally high fat content; (2) muscle wasting and progressive weight loss due to steatorrhea, diarrhea, and anorexia; (3) abdominal distention in children, less marked in adults; (4) evidence of vitamin and mineral deficiencies, such as macrocytic anemia due to inadequate absorption of folic acid and vitamin B-12, iron-deficiency anemia, hypocalcemic tetany, glossitis, and so on.

Laboratory findings include decreases in serum concentrations of electrolytes, albumin, and carotene; impaired absorption of D-xylose, glucose, folic acid, and vitamin B-12; and increased fecal fat and nitrogen.

Diagnostic Tests The diagnosis of malabsorption syndrome is based on findings from absorption tests, intestinal mucosal biopsy, and radiologic studies.

Direct tests of absorption involve measurement of *fecal fat*. The balance study method is widely used and involves the chemical analysis of a 72-hour stool collection. The patient is fed a diet containing a known amount of fat, usually 50 to 100 g, for several days before and during the collection period. Stools are then analyzed for fat. Normal excretion is less than 7 g per 24 hours. Alternatively, a fatty meal absorption test followed by measurement of serum triglycerides and chylomicrons is performed.[1] Stool collections are also used to measure fecal radioactivity following administration of a test dose of ^{131}I-labeled triolein. The triolein is mixed with a marker and stools are collected until the marker is no longer visible. Normal fecal radioactivity is less than 7 percent of the test dose.

The *serum carotene* level is a useful screening test,

443

and malabsorption is suspected if levels of less than 60 μg per dl are found.

Oral tolerance tests provide indirect evidence of malabsorption. Most commonly used are D-*xylose* and *lactose*. Urinary excretion of D-*xylose* following ingestion of a 25 g load is used as an indication of carbohydrate absorption. Excretion of less than 4.5 g in 5 hours in patients with normal renal function indicates decreased absorptive capacity. The *lactose tolerance test* is used in suspected lactase deficiency. Administration of lactose, 2 g per kg body weight, or a maximum of 50 g, is followed by determination of blood glucose levels for 2 hours.[2] *Lactose malabsorption* is indicated if the blood glucose rises less than 26 mg. per dl. Symptoms of abdominal distention, cramping, and diarrhea may occur following ingestion of the lactose in persons with *lactose intolerance*.[2]

Measurement of breath hydrogen following a lactose load is a more sensitive test for lactose malabsorption. Unabsorbed lactose undergoes bacterial fermentation in the colon with production of hydrogen gas, part of which is excreted through the lungs. An increase in breath hydrogen in expired air samples collected at specified intervals indicates lactose malabsorption.[3] In another breath test, excretion of carbon dioxide following administration of certain fats labeled with stable isotopes is used as a screening test for fat malabsorption.[4,5]

The *Schilling test* is frequently used as an index of vitamin B-12 absorption; an oral dose of radioactive vitamin B-12 is administered followed at 2 hours by an intramuscular injection of nonradioactive B-12. Urinary excretion of less than 5 to 8 percent of the radioactive dose indicates malabsorption.

The *folic acid test* consists of assaying urine for 24 hours following injection of the vitamin and again after it is given orally 48 hours later. In malabsorption, excretion of folic acid is less after an oral dose than after injection.

Biopsy specimens of the jejunal mucosa showing villous atrophy provide nonspecific evidence of disturbances in absorptive function. Radiologic evidence of intestinal dilatation, altered motility, and bone demineralization may also be seen in malabsorption.

Treatment Therapy is directed toward alleviation of symptoms by correction of the basic defect insofar as possible, dietary modification in accordance with the nature of the defect, vitamin and mineral supplements, and prevention or correction of complications by administration of appropriate agents.

Dietary Modification Generally speaking, the diet in malabsorption syndrome should be high in protein and calories. (See Chapter 33.) In a few of the disorders elimination of specific carbohydrates or proteins is necessary and the dietary management is outlined in the sections that follow. Modification of fat intake is often indicated. Vitamin and mineral supplementation is usually needed. A soft diet or fiber-restricted diet is useful for patients with persistent diarrhea. (See Chapter 28.)

Fat absorption can be improved in some malabsorptive disorders by changing the type of fat ingested. Food fats are composed principally of fatty acids containing 12 to 18 carbon atoms (long-chain triglycerides). By contrast, fats composed almost entirely of fatty acids containing 8 and 10 carbon atoms (medium-chain triglycerides) have been synthesized. Substitution of medium-chain triglycerides (MCT) for longer-chain fats (LCT) is associated with reduced steatorrhea and decreased losses of calcium, sodium, and potassium in many of the disorders comprising the malabsorption syndrome. (See Table 31-1.)

The effectiveness of MCT over long-chain fats appears to be due to differences in the rate of hydrolysis, absorption, and route of transport.[6] Medium-chain fats are hydrolyzed much more rapidly than long chain fats by intestinal and pancreatic lipases. A mucosal enzyme system, specific for medium-chain triglyceride hydrolysis, has been described. Medium-chain triglycerides are transported by way of the portal vein as free fatty acids bound to albumin, whereas long-chain fats must undergo esterification and chylomicron formation and are transported by way of the lymph.

Side effects of nausea, abdominal distention or cramps, and diarrhea have been noted in about 10 percent of patients receiving MCT supplements. Symptoms are attributed to the hyperosmolar load produced by rapid hydrolysis of MCT and possible irritating effects of high levels of free fatty acids in the stomach and intestine. These symptoms can be overcome by slow ingestion of small amounts of the supplement.

Medium-chain triglycerides are available commercially as an oil preparation* or as a powdered formula.† A number of recipes have been developed for incorporating these products into the diet.‡ The oil provides a concentrated source of calories, and can be

---

* MCT from fractionated coconut oil (Mead Johnson & Co., Evansville, Ind.): Provides 8.3 kcal per gram, or approximately 225 kcal per 30 ml.

† Portagen (Mead Johnson & Co., Evansville, Ind.): An 8-ounce glass of the product reconstituted to 20 kcal per ounce provides 5.6 g protein from sodium caseinate, 18.4 g carbohydrate from corn syrup solids and sucrose, and 7.75 g fat from MCT and corn oil.

‡ These recipes are available from Mead Johnson & Co., Evansville, Ind.

used in frying and in recipes such as salad dressings, hot breads, and desserts. It is a clear, odorless oil with a bland taste. The powder, on the other hand, is useful as a calorie-protein supplement to an otherwise very low fat diet. A proprietary formula containing MCT is available for infants.§

Dietary Management From 50 to 70 percent of the fat is supplied as MCT and the remainder as foods

§ Pregestimil (Mead Johnson & Co., Evansville, Ind.).

containing long-chain triglycerides. To maintain this ratio, foods containing LCT are limited to the following:

> 4 ounces of meat, fish, or poultry
> 1 egg
> 3 teaspoons butter

This provides about 25 g LCT per day.

The following diet is adapted from the plan described by Schizas et al.[7]

Medium-Chain-Triglyceride (MCT) Diet

Characteristics and General Rules
This diet provides for a reduction in long-chain triglycerides by substituting an oil containing medium-chain triglycerides as a source of fat. The diet is adjusted to provide 50 to 70 percent of the fat calories as MCT.

The protein intake may be increased by adding nonfat dry milk to fluid skim milk, skim cottage cheese, egg whites, and cereal products.

The caloric level may be increased by adding high-carbohydrate foods such as fruits, sugar, jelly, and fat-free desserts.

Modifications in fiber and consistency may be made by applying restrictions concerning the soft diet (see Chapter 28) to the following listed foods.

Initially, small amounts of MCT should be taken with meals and gradually increased according to individual tolerance. Between-meal feedings may be desirable if large amounts of food are not tolerated.

Include These Foods Daily:
2 or more cups skim milk
4 ounces (cooked weight) lean meat, poultry, or fish
1 egg
3 or more fruits including:
    1-2 servings citrus fruit or other good source of ascorbic acid
    1-2 other fruits
3-4 servings vegetables including:
    1 dark green or deep yellow
    1 potato
    1-2 other vegetables, raw or cooked, as tolerated
5 servings bread and cereals
3 teaspoons butter
MCT oil in amounts prescribed (usually 2 ounces)

Nutritive Value On the basis of these specified amounts of foods: protein, 75 g (13 percent of calories); fat, 35 g (13 percent of calories); carbohydrate, 315 g (53 percent of calories); MCT, 60 g (21 percent of calories); 2,400 kcal.

Foods Allowed
Beverages—cereal beverages, coffee, tea, soft drinks
Breads and substitutes—hamburger rolls, hard rolls, white enriched, whole-wheat, pumpernickel, or rye bread. Bread products contain some LCT but are permitted to add palatability and variety to the diet. Cooked or dry cereals, macaroni, noodles, rice, spaghetti

Foods to Avoid

Commercial biscuits, coffeecake, corn bread, crackers, doughnuts, muffins, sweet rolls

Foods Allowed

Cheese—skim cottage cheese
Desserts—angel cake, gelatin, meringues, any made from MCT special recipes

Egg—egg whites as desired; whole eggs and egg yolks only in prescribed amounts
Fats—butter in prescribed amounts, gravies made from clear soups and MCT oil
Fruits—all except avocado
Meats—lean meat, fish, and poultry only in prescribed amounts
Milk—skim milk

Soups—fat-free broth, bouillon, consommé
Sweets—jelly, syrups, sugars
Vegetables—all to which no fat is added except MCT
Miscellaneous—any special recipe in which MCT is substituted for long-chain fats

Foods to Avoid

Cheese made from whole milk.
Commercial cakes, pies, cookies, pastries, puddings and custards; mixes allowed only if they contain no LCT
Whole eggs and egg yolks except as prescribed

Oils and shortenings of all types, sauces and gravies except those made with MCT oil
Avocado
Fatty meats, fish, frankfurters, cold cuts, sausages

Buttermilk, partially skim milk, whole milk, light, heavy, or sour cream
Cream soups, others
Butter, chocolate, coconut, or cream candies
Creamed vegetables, or those with fats other than MCT added
Creamed dishes; commercial popcorn; frozen dinners; homemade products containing eggs, whole milk, and fats; mixes for biscuits, muffins, and cakes; olives

Sample Menu

BREAKFAST
Fresh grapefruit—1 half
MCT waffle—1
Butter—1 teaspoon
Maple syrup—2 tablespoons
Sugar—1 teaspoon
Coffee or tea

LUNCHEON OR SUPPER
Chicken sandwich
  Chicken—2 ounces
  MCT mayonnaise—1 tablespoon
  Whole-wheat bread—2 slices
  Lettuce and tomato
Fresh fruit cup—½ cup
MCT brownie—1
Skim milk—1 cup

DINNER
Veal chop—2 ounces
MCT scalloped potatoes—½ cup
Carrots—½ cup
  With lemon butter—2 teaspoons
Mixed green salad—1 serving
MCT Italian dressing—2 teaspoons
Angel cake—¹/₁₆ of 8 inch diameter
Fresh strawberries—1 cup
Coffee or tea

EVENING SNACK
Skim milk—1 cup
MCT sugar cookies—2

DIETARY COUNSELING

The patient must understand the importance of using the recommended amounts of MCT in the diet. He or she should be cautioned to take the oil slowly in small amounts; no more than 1 tablespoon of MCT should be taken at any given feeding. The diet to be used at home should be planned with consideration given to the individual's cultural background and usual meal pattern. The patient must be taught to use cuts of meat that are low in fat and to select only lean meats. Suggestions for incorporating the MCT oil into meals should be offered and suitable recipes supplied. Some persons prefer to take the oil mixed in fruit juice or as a "milkshake" composed of skim milk, fruit ice, and the oil. Others prefer to add the oil to solid foods such as cooked cereals, mashed potatoes, or sauces. The oil imparts a golden color to foods when used in frying; care should be taken to see that all the oil is removed from the frying pan, however, and actually consumed. Meals eaten away from home need not be a problem if the individual orders clear soups, lean meats trimmed of all visible fat, vegetables without cream sauces or other added fat, and so on. Desserts such as fruits, angel cake, and gelatin are suitable and usually available.

Abnormalities in the Intestinal Lumen

Inadequate Digestion Any condition that interferes with normal secretion or activity of pancreatic lipase causes inadequate hydrolysis of lipids in the intestinal lumen and results in malabsorption.

Pancreatic Insufficiency. Inadequate production of lipase occurs in pancreatic insufficiency. This disorder may result form chronic pancreatitis, cystic fibrosis, carcinoma, pancreatectomy, or destruction of exocrine function by ligation of the duct. Steatorrhea and symptoms of generalized malabsorption occur due to poor utilization of fats and protein. Weight loss may be significant in spite of a good appetite. Deficiencies of fat-soluble vitamins are seen.

The diet is designed to prevent further weight loss and to control gastrointestinal symptoms. From 2,500 to 4,000 kcal is required. The protein intake should be 100 to 150 g. Carbohydrate (400 g or more) is the chief source of calories, since fat is poorly tolerated. Generally, long-chain fatty acids should be restricted to 30 to 60 g per day. Pancreatic enzymes are given with meals to aid in fat absorption. MCT can be used to increase the calorie intake. (See page 445.)

Gastric Resection. Steatorrhea sometimes follows gastric resection because of inadequate mixing of food with pancreatic juice and bile or bacterial overgrowth in an afferent loop of intestine. In addition, anemia is frequently seen because of limited intake or impaired absorption of iron, vitamin B-12, and folic acid. Weight loss is common and persistent. Improved absorption of fats may be achieved by supplementing the diet with MCT. Other dietary considerations are described on page 485.

Altered Bile Salt Metabolism Steatorrhea occurs if adequate amounts of conjugated bile salts are not available for micelle formation and is frequently associated with the following conditions.

Hepatobiliary Disease. Decreased amounts of bile salts in the lumen in hepatobiliary disease are due to impaired synthesis of bile acids or biliary stasis.

Ileal Resection. Removal of the ileum reduces the bile salt pool thereby lowering the concentration of conjugated bile salts in the jejunum available for hydrolysis of fats. Unabsorbed fatty acids and bile salts may provoke diarrhea. Parenteral administration of vitamin B-12 is indicated if the distal ileum is not functional.

Bacterial Overgrowth (Blind Loop Syndrome). Intestinal stasis is associated with changes in the bacterial flora. Deconjugation of bile salts by bacteria prevents adequate micelle formation. In some instances steatorrhea can be corrected by feeding conjugated bile salts. Bacteria also bind vitamin B-12 so that it is unavailable for absorption, and replacement therapy is needed.

Effects of Drug Therapy. Certain drugs bind ionized fatty acids and bile salts in the proximal intestine with subsequent fat malabsorption. Other mechanisms involved in drug-induced malabsorption are decreased disaccharidase activity, interference with absorption of nutrients and increased fecal losses of nutrients.[8,9] Drugs exerting this multifactorial influence on absorption include neomycin, cholestyramine, colchicine, and para-aminosalicylic acid, among others.[9]

Abnormalities in Mucosal Cell Transport—Specific Disorders

Absence or deficiency of specific enzymes or failure of proper regulation of enzyme activity in the cell interferes with the absorption of certain nutrients and produces symptoms of malabsorption.

Lactose Intolerance Inability to utilize lactose may be due to lactase deficiency or may be secondary to conditions that produce alteration in absorptive surfaces. In the absence of lactase lactose is not hydrolyzed to glucose and galactose. The accumulation of lactose in the intestine causes fermentation, abdominal pain, cramping, and diarrhea. Failure to gain weight is an important symptom in infants.

Congenital lactose intolerance is a rare disorder characterized by absent brush border lactase activity. Symptoms occur following ingestion of milk by the infant. A strict lactose-free formula is used, several commercial products being available.* All products containing lactose in any form whatsoever are rigidly excluded.

Intestinal lactase activity is normally high during infancy but declines after weaning to low levels in adults. The decline in lactase activity is determined by an autosomal recessive mechanism and is not influenced by dietary lactose intake.[10] Throughout most of

---

* Isomil (Ross Laboratories, Columbus, Ohio); MBF (meat-base formula) (Gerber Products Company, Fremont, Mich.); Nutramigen and ProSobee (Mead Johnson & Company, Evansville, Ind.)

the world the majority of adults are unable to digest lactose, and they develop symptoms of distention, cramping, and diarrhea following its ingestion. These individuals, who have no history of gastrointestinal disease or childhood intolerance to milk, are described as having *primary* lactose intolerance. In the United States, from 60 to 95 percent of adult blacks, American Indians, Jews, Mexican Americans, and Orientals are lactose malabsorbers compared to 5 to 15 percent for whites.

Several hypotheses have been proposed to explain the differences in ability to utilize lactose among various ethnic groups. One theory holds that a genetic mutation occurring as a result of some selective advantage may permit high levels of lactase to persist into the adult years in certain populations, primarily those from northern and western Europe.[10]

Adults with primary lactose intolerance can usually tolerate the amounts of milk in many prepared foods such as breads, lunch meats, and even cream soups and cream sauces provided that the lactose source is spaced through the day. Those who experience classical symptoms following excessive milk or lactose ingestion, can be kept asymptomatic by limiting their intake of milk products. A controlled lactose diet that restricts only obvious sources of lactose is used. The quantity of lactose allowed is a matter of individual tolerance.

Several studies with lactose malabsorbers indicate that subjects experience significantly fewer symptoms following ingestion of lactose-hydrolyzed milk than regular milk.[11,12] A commercially available enzyme,* when added to milk, hydrolyzes about 75 percent of the lactose, thus permitting intake of a larger quantity of milk without provoking symptoms.

Secondary lactose intolerance is often observed following gastrectomy or extensive small bowel resection, and in celiac disease, sprue, colitis, enteritis,

* Lact-Aid (SugarLo Company, Atlantic City, N.J.)

cystic fibrosis, kwashiorkor, and malnutrition. In these conditions it may be necessary to omit obvious sources of lactose initially, but a strict lactose-free diet is usually not required.

DIETARY COUNSELING

Adults who become symptomatic after excess lactose ingestion should be advised to limit intake of milk, cream soups, puddings, custards, ice cream, and so on. Some find that milk is better tolerated if taken in small amounts several times daily, especially with meals, and at room temperature rather than cold. Many persons remain symptom free by limiting their intake of milk to one glass per day. Chocolate milk is sometimes tolerated better than plain milk; this may be related to a slower rate of emptying from the stomach.[13] Individuals failing to respond to a lactose-controlled diet may need to further restrict lactose intake. When improvement is noted small amounts of lactose-containing foods are tested, one at a time (for example, one fourth cup of milk at a meal) to determine levels that may be tolerated. Fermented dairy products such as yogurt, buttermilk, and many cheeses may be included if tolerated.

Persons on lactose-restricted diets should be advised to carefully check labels on all commercial products. Foods containing milk in any form, butter, and margarine are to be avoided. Typical sources of lactose include breads, candies, cold cuts, mixes of all types, powdered soft drinks, preserves, soups, and so on. Fruit juices or water can be substituted for milk in many recipes. Meals eaten away from home should include foods prepared without breading, cream sauces, gravies, and so on. Broiled or roasted meats, baked potato, vegetables without added fat, salads, and desserts such as plain angel cake, fresh fruit, and gelatin are good choices. Kosher-style foods are suitable.

Lactose-Restricted Diet

Characteristics and General Rules

This diet is designed to eliminate all sources of lactose.

All milk and milk products must be eliminated.

Lactose is used in the manufacture of many foods and medicines. It is essential to read labels of commercial products before use.

The diet is inadequate in calcium and riboflavin. Supplements of these nutrients should be prescribed.

The protein intake may be increased by adding meat, fish, poultry, or eggs, lactose-free milk substitutes, or breads and cereals from those allowed.

The caloric level may be increased by adding high-carbohydrate foods such as fruits, sugar, jelly, and desserts free of lactose.

Modifications in fiber and consistency may be made by applying restrictions concerning the soft diet (see Chapter 28) to the foods listed here.

Include the Following Foods Daily:
7 ounces meat, fish, or poultry
1 egg
3 or more fruits including:
    1-2 servings citrus fruit or other good source of ascorbic acid
    1-2 other fruits
3-4 servings vegetables including:
    1 dark green or deep yellow
    1 potato
    1-2 other vegetables, raw or cooked, as tolerated
6 servings enriched bread or cereals
6 teaspoons fortified milk-free margarine
Other foods as needed to provide calories

Foods Allowed

Beverages—carbonated drinks, fruit drinks, coffee, tea

Breads and cereals—breads and rolls made without milk, cooked cereals, some prepared cereals (check labels), macaroni, spaghetti, soda crackers

Cheese—none

Desserts—angel cake, cakes made with vegetable oils, gelatin, puddings made with fruit juices, water, or allowed milk substitutes, water ices

Eggs—prepared any way except with milk or cheese

Fats—lard, peanut butter, pure mayonnaise, vegetable oils, margarines without milk or butter added, some cream substitutes (check labels)

Fruits—all except canned and frozen to which lactose is added

Milk—none

Meat, fish, or poultry—all kinds, cold cuts (check labels for added nonfat dry milk), kosher frankfurters

Vegetables—fresh, canned, or frozen—plain or with milk-free margarine (check labels of canned or frozen)

Soups—meat and vegetable only (check labels)

Miscellaneous—corn syrup, honey, nuts, nut butters, olives, pickles, pure seasonings and spices, pure jams and jellies, pure sugar candies, some cream substitutes, sugar

Foods to Avoid

Cereal beverages, cocoa, instant coffee (check label)

Bread with milk added, crackers made with butter or margarine, French toast, mixes of all types, pancakes, some dry cereals (read labels), waffles, zwieback

All types

Cakes, cookies, pies, puddings or other desserts made with milk and butter or margarine, commercial fruit fillings, commercial sweet rolls, custards, custard and cream pies, ice cream, pie crust made with butter or margarine, sherbets

Any prepared with milk or cheese

Butter, cream substitutes, cream, sweet and sour, margarine with butter or milk added, salad dressings

Canned or frozen prepared with lactose

All types, infant food formulas, simulated mother's milk, yogurt

Breaded or creamed dishes, cold cuts and frankfurters containing nonfat dry milk, liver sausage

Canned or frozen vegetables prepared with lactose, commercial french-fried potatoes, corn curls, creamed vegetables, instant or mashed potatoes, any seasoned with butter or margarine

All others

Ascorbic acid and citric acid mixtures, butterscotch, caramels, chewing gum, chocolate candy, cream sauces, cream soups, diabetic and dietetic preparations, dried soups, frozen cultures, frozen desserts, gravy, health and geriatric foods, monosodium glutamate extender, party dips, peppermints, powdered soft drinks, spice blends, starter cultures, sweetness reducers in candies, fruit pie fillings, icings, and preserves, toffee

Sample Menu

BREAKFAST
Orange Juice
Cornflakes with cream substitute and sugar
Soft-cooked egg
French bread, toasted enriched
Margarine—milk free
Coffee with cream substitute and sugar

LUNCH
Baked chicken breast
Parslied potato
Asparagus tips
Sliced tomato and lettuce
French or Italian bread, enriched
Margarine—milk free
Grape jelly
Canned peach halves
Tea with lemon and sugar

DINNER
Roast beef sirloin
Baked potato
Diced carrots
French or Italian bread, enriched
Margarine—milk free
Apple jelly
Fresh fruit cup
Tea with lemon and sugar

Sucrase-Isomaltase Deficiency Deficiencies of these enzymes lead to symptoms similar to those seen in lactase insufficiency following ingestion of significant amounts of sucrose and isomaltose. A sucrose tolerance test is used to confirm the diagnosis. The sucrose breath hydrogen test has also been reported to be a reliable indicator of sucrose malabsorption in this disorder.[14]

Sucrose is added to many foods during processing and preparation. In addition, naturally occurring sucrose is present in a number of foods, making a strict sucrose-free diet impractical. Nevertheless, elimination of foods containing relatively large amounts of sucrose should be made. (See Table 31-2.) Glucose is substituted as a sweetening agent. Products containing wheat and potato starches should be avoided, as these yield more isomaltose upon hydrolysis than do other starches such as rice and corn.

Table 31-2. Foods Containing More Than 5 g Sucrose per 100 g Edible Portion*

Apricots	Jams and jellies	Puddings
Bananas	Macadamia nuts	Syrups
Candy	Mangoes	Sorghum
Cane sugar	Milk chocolate	Soybeans
Cake	Molasses	Soybean flour or meal
Chestnuts, Va.	Oranges	Sugar beets
Chocolate, sweet	Pastries	Sweet breads and rolls
Condensed milk	Peaches	Sweet pickles
Cookies	Peanuts	Sweet potatoes
Dates	Peas	Tangerine
Honeydew melon	Pineapple	Watermelon
Ice cream	Prune plums, Italian	Wheat germ

* Adapted from Hardinge, M. G., et al.: "Carbohydrates in Foods," *J. Am. Diet. Assoc.*, **46**:197–204, 1965.

Increased sucrase activity following fructose feeding has been reported in this disorder, thus permitting ingestion of small amounts of sucrose without provoking symptoms. Infants with the disorder have responded to a strict sucrose-free diet within 24 hours, and after about 1 week are permitted gradual additions of foods low in sucrose.[15]

Glucose-Galactase Deficiency This rare disease is characterized by inability to absorb any carbohydrate that yields glucose or galactose upon hydrolysis. Substitution of fructose as the sole source of carbohydrate in the diet leads to improvement in symptoms. A special formula containing 4 to 8 percent fructose has been devised for infants.[16] This formula is used almost exclusively for the first few months, after which it is gradually decreased and addition of foods low in starch is begun. By the age of three, a regular diet for age is usually tolerated with limited amounts of milk and starch-containing foods. Some degree of dietary restriction is necessary throughout life in order to prevent recurrence of symptoms of diarrhea. If a galactose-free diet is ordered, the lactose-free diet (see page 448) is used; sugar beets, peas, and Lima beans must also be avoided. Liver, brains, and sweetbreads store galactose and are usually avoided.

A-Beta Lipoproteinemia This rare congenital disorder is believed to involve a defect in the release or synthesis of beta-lipoprotein. As a result fat is not transported from the intestinal cells into the lacteals. Total beta-lipoprotein deficiency is manifested by steatorrhea and failure to thrive among other symptoms in infants. The malabsorption of fats is associated with extremely low serum concentrations of beta-lipoprotein, cholesterol, vitamin A, and phospholipids.

Substitution of medium-chain triglycerides for long-chain fats in the diet results in improved fat absorption, since the shorter chain fats are absorbed by way of the portal vein rather than by lymph.

Abnormalities in Mucosal Cell Transport—Nonspecific Disorders

Reduction in the absorptive surface area by massive intestinal resection or by damage to the villi produced by disease may have profound effects on nutrient uptake and absorption.

Short-Bowel Syndrome This term is used to describe those patients who are in metabolic imbalance as a consequence of massive resection of the small intestine. Removal of large portions of the bowel shortens the transit time of the contents through the intestine, thereby reducing the time for absorption. Attempts to increase absorption by delaying transit time include dietary modification and drug therapy. In this syndrome, the length of the remaining bowel is generally less than 8 feet. The amount of bowel left intact and the site of resection have an important bearing on the patient's nutritional status.

Nutrients normally absorbed in the proximal intestine are shown in Figure 31-1. Following removal of the jejunum, some absorption of these nutrients may take place in the ileum by virtue of its ability to act as a functional intestinal reserve. On the other hand, the jejunum has a limited capacity to absorb water and electrolytes and cannot compensate for the massive losses that occur when the ileum is removed. Following ileal resection of more than 100 cm, steatorrhea occurs because of bile salt deficiency.

Typically, the patient goes through three stages after massive resection of the bowel. In the immediate postoperative period, diarrhea and fluid and electrolyte imbalance may be so severe as to be life threatening. Total parenteral nutrition is used as the sole source of nutrients for 1 or 2 months. Oral food intake is contraindicated due to massive diarrhea, exceeding two liters of fluid loss per day. The patient surviving this period enters the second stage when nutritional concerns are of prime importance. Steady weight loss occurs as a result of anorexia, diarrhea, and steatorrhea. Osteomalacia and anemia may develop. Parenteral nutrition is continued for a time. Elemental or semi-synthetic fiber-free diets are used in the transi-

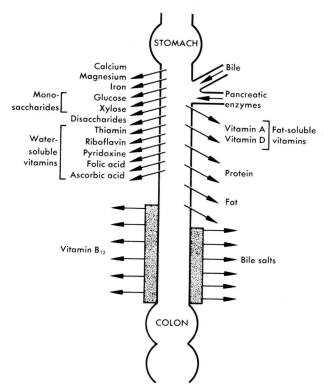

Figure 31-1. Sites of absorption in the small bowel. Most nutrients are absorbed from the proximal portion of the small intestine. (Adapted from Booth, C. C.: "Effect of Location Along Small Intestine on Absorption of Nutrients," in *Handbook of Physiology. Alimentary Canal.* Vol. 1. American Physiological Society, Washington, D.C., 1967.)

tion from parenteral to oral feedings. Alternatively, tube feedings are used. When the oral intake exceeds 2,000 kcal without exacerbating diarrhea, parenteral nutrition is tapered.

Carbohydrates and proteins are used first when oral feedings are begun. The diet is low in lactose, sucrose, and fiber as these are poorly tolerated. From 50 to 100 g carbohydrate per day is used initially. After the patient tolerates carbohydrate and proteins, small amounts of fat are gradually introduced. For many patients a maximum of 40 g fat is tolerated. Amounts greater than this increase steatorrhea. Supplements of pancreatic lipase are given when fats are incorporated into the diet. Finally, after several months to 1 year, the patient's condition stabilizes usually at a substantially lower weight. The fat intake can usually be increased to 50 to 60 g per day.

The extreme losses of all nutrients in this syndrome require greatly increased intakes of calories, protein, vitamins, and minerals. Especially important are calcium, magnesium, iron, and zinc. Up to 5,000 kcal and 175 g of protein may be needed to prevent further weight loss. Substitution of medium-chain triglycerides for long-chain fats has led to decreased diarrhea and electrolyte losses and improvement in nutritional status. Frequent small meals are tolerated best. Dietary oxalate is restricted together with fat to compensate for enhanced oxalate absorption by colonic mucosa.[17,18] Calcium supplements can minimize oxalate absorption by binding to oxalate and preventing its absorption.

Gluten Enteropathy This is a disease of genetic origin characterized by intolerance to the gliadin fraction of gluten with consequent malabsorption. The disorder is known as *celiac disease* in childhood and as *adult celiac disease* or *nontropical sprue* in later life. The mechanism of the sensitivity to gluten is not understood. Current hypotheses hold that a primary mucosal defect permits gluten to exert a toxic effect in genetically predisposed individuals[19] or that immune factors are involved. According to the latter theory, gluten binds to cell-surface receptors and interacts with lymphocytes to produce antibodies and other immune products which damage the cell.[19] The diagnosis is made by intestinal biopsies initially, after 3 months of a gluten-free diet and after a gluten challenge.[20]

The onset of this disease is insidious and is manifested by diarrhea, steatorrhea, weight loss, and other symptoms of the malabsorption syndrome. Stools are characteristically loose, pale, and frothy (due to fermentation of undigested carbohydrate) and contain excessive amounts of fat. Biopsy specimens of the mucosal surface have a flattened appearance; the villi become shorter and club shaped and appear to be fused. A marked decrease in the number of microvilli in the brush border drastically reduces the absorptive surface. Laboratory findings are consistent with those of the malabsorption syndrome. (See page 443.)

Exacerbations and remissions are common in this disorder. Symptoms are provoked by ingestion of gluten from wheat, rye, barley, buckwheat, and, in some instances, oats.

Elimination of gluten from the diet (see Gluten-Restricted Diet) should be given a trial of at least 6 weeks. Regeneration of villi and return of enzyme activity occur in most cases following strict adherence to a gluten-restricted diet. Lack of response to the diet in some cases may be due to failure to follow the diet or to secondary lactose intolerance resulting from mucosal damage. In this case, a gluten-restricted, lactose-free diet leads to improved fat and carbohydrate absorption.

The diet should provide 100 g or more protein to replace wasted tissue. Some moderation in fiber content and fat intake may be needed initially as these are usually poorly tolerated. Improved fat absorption can be achieved through the üse of MCT. Supplementary vitamins and minerals are needed to overcome nutritional deficiencies resulting from excessive losses in the stools.

Gluten-Restricted Diet

Characteristics and General Rules
This diet excludes all products containing wheat, rye, oats, and barley. Read all labels carefully.
Aqueous multivitamins are usually prescribed in addition to the diet.
The diet may be progressed gradually; that is, small amounts of unsaturated fats may be used at first, adding harder fats later. Fiber may be reduced initially by using only cooked fruits and vegetables. Strongly flavored vegetables may be poorly tolerated at first.

Include These Foods, or Their Nutritive Equivalents, Daily:
4 cups milk
6-8 ounces (cooked weight) lean meat, fish, or poultry
1 egg
4 vegetables including:
    1 dark green or deep yellow
    1 potato
    2 other vegetables
    Other to be served raw, if tolerated
3 fruits including:
    1-2 servings citrus fruit or other good source ascorbic acid
    1-2 other fruits

4 servings bread and cereals: corn, rice, soybean
No wheat, rye, oats, barley
2 tablespoons fat
Additional calories are provided by using more of the foods listed, dessert, soups, sweets

Nutritive Value of Listed Foods protein, 105 g; fat, 110 g; carbohydrate, 200 g; 2,200 kcal. Minerals and vitamins in excess of recommended allowances.

Foods Allowed

Beverages—carbonated, cocoa, coffee, fruit juices, milk, tea

Breads—corn bread, muffins, and pone with no wheat flour; breads made with cornmeal, cornstarch, potato, rice, soybean, wheat-starch flour

Cereals—cooked cornmeal, Cream of Rice, hominy or grits, rice; ready to eat: corn or rice cereals such as cornflakes, rice flakes, Puffed Rice.

Cheese—cottage; later, cream cheese

Desserts—custard, fruit ice, fruit whips, plain or fruit ice cream (homemade), plain or fruit gelatin, meringues; homemade puddings—cornstarch, rice, tapioca; rennet desserts; sherbet; cakes and cookies made with allowed flours

Eggs—as desired

Fats—oil: corn, cottonseed, olive, sesame, soybean; French dressing, pure mayonnaise, salad dressing with cornstarch thickening. Later additions: butter, cream, margarine, peanut oil, vegetable shortening

Flour—cornmeal, potato, rice, soybean

Fruits—all cooked, canned, and juices; fresh and frozen as tolerated, avoiding skin and seeds initially

Meat—all lean meats, poultry, fish: baked, broiled, roasted, stewed

Milk—all kinds

Soups—broth, bouillon, cream if thickened with cornstarch, vegetable

Sweets—candy, honey, jam, jelly, marmalade, marshmallows, molasses, syrup, sugar

Vegetables—cooked or canned: buttered; fresh as tolerated

Miscellaneous—gravy and sauces thickened with cornstarch; olives, peanut butter, pickles, popcorn, potato chips

Foods to Avoid

Beverages—ale, beer, instant coffee containing cereal, malted milk, Postum, products containing cereal

Breads—all containing any wheat, rye, oats, or barley; bread crumbs, muffins, pancakes, rolls, rusks, waffles, zwieback; all commercial yeast and quick bread mixes; all crackers, pretzels, Ry-Krisp

Cereals—cooked or ready-to-eat breakfast cereals containing wheat, oats, barley; macaroni, noodles, pasta, spaghetti, wheat germ

Desserts—cake, cookies, doughnuts, pastries, pie; bisques, commercial ice cream, ice cream cones; prepared mixes containing wheat, rye, oats, or barley; puddings thickened with wheat flour

Fats—bacon, lard, suet, salad dressing with flour thickening

Flour—barley, oat, rye, wheat—bread, cake, entire wheat, graham, self-rising, whole-wheat, wheat germ

Fruits—prunes, plums, and their juices; those with skins and seeds at first

Meat—breaded, creamed, croquettes, luncheon meats unless pure meat, meat loaf, stuffings with bread, scrapple, thickened stew
Fat meats such as corned beef, duck, frankfurters, goose, ham, luncheon meats, pork, sausage
Fatty fish such as herring, mackerel, sardines, swordfish, or canned in heavy oil

Soups—thickened with flour; containing barley, noodles, etc.

Sweets—candies with high fat content, nuts; candies containing wheat products

Vegetables—creamed if thickened with wheat, oat, rye, or barley products. Strongly flavored if they produce discomfort: baked beans, broccoli, brussels sprouts, cabbage, cauliflower, corn, cucumber, lentils, onions, peppers, radishes, turnips

Miscellaneous—gravies and sauces thickened with flours not permitted

Sample Menu

BREAKFAST
Tomato juice
Rice Krispies
Milk, sugar
Southern corn muffins
Butter or margarine
Currant jelly
Scrambled eggs
Coffee, with cream, sugar

LUNCH
Beef stew (not thickened)
  Beef cubes
  Potato
  Carrots
  Onions

Tossed green salad
French dressing
Rice-flour bread
Butter or margarine
Milk
Vanilla cornstarch pudding with sliced frozen peaches

DINNER
Broiled lamb patties (all meat)
Mint jelly
Rice with saffron seasoning
Buttered asparagus
Celery and olives
Milk
Lemon meringue pudding (thickened with cornstarch)
Coffee with cream, sugar

DIETARY COUNSELING

Proteins from lean meats, poultry, fish, cottage cheese, egg white, and skim milk are well utilized and should be encouraged. Individual tolerance for fibrous foods and strongly flavored vegetables should determine whether or not these foods are included. The patient should be advised to read labels on all commercial food products in order to avoid any foods containing wheat, rye, oats, or barley. Besides cereals and breads as obvious sources, many other foods contain wheat or other flour as a thickener. Canned soups, cheese spreads, cooked salad dressing, cold cuts, breaded meats, mixes of all kinds, catsup, ice cream, and pastries are but a few of the many foods that contain cereal products. Hydrolyzed vegetable protein used as a flavor enhancer in commercially prepared soups may be made from soy, wheat, or other proteins. Some authorities permit it in the diet, as the quantities used are small. Information on prepared and packaged foods known to be gluten free is available for patients.* Many standard cookbooks contain suitable recipes utilizing cornstarch, cornmeal, potato, rice, or tapioca instead of flour. Sources of special recipes utilizing arrowroot starch or wheat starch (from which the gluten is removed) should be supplied to the patient.* However, patients should be cautioned that mere substitution of other flours for wheat will not produce satisfactory

* Available from companies such as General Foods, General Mills, and others.

results; other adjustments in mixing technique, baking time, and temperature are also needed. When meals are eaten away from home, plain foods, without breading, gravies, cream sauces, and so on, should be selected. Persons who are not intolerant to oats should be permitted to add this cereal to the diet.

Radiation Enteritis Radiation to the abdomen damages the intestinal mucosa resulting in flattened villi and depressed enzyme activities, thus interfering with absorption of many nutrients. (See also Chapter 35.)

Abnormality of Intestinal Lymphatics

Intestinal Lymphangiectasia This is a congenital defect in which obstruction of intestinal lymphatics is associated with leakage of chylomicron fat and plasma proteins into the intestinal lumen. In addition to decreased serum protein levels and associated edema and ascites formation, steatorrhea occurs. Protein losses are reduced considerably by use of medium-chain triglycerides or a fat-restricted diet. (See page 465.)

Tropical Sprue This disorder is a form of the malabsorption syndrome that occurs chiefly in the West Indies, Central America, and the Far East. In some respects it is similar to nontropical sprue, but the onset is more acute and it responds to different therapy. Both disorders are characterized by steatorrhea and secondary enzyme deficiencies in the intestinal mucosa. In tropical sprue there is also ileal involvement. Hypocalcemia with tetany and osteomalacia do not occur as commonly as in nontropical sprue; however, nutritional deficiencies of folic acid and vitamin B-12 do occur and are manifested as macrocytic anemia. Dramatic improvement in symptoms is often shown following administration of folic acid and vitamin B-12.

The diet in tropical sprue should be high in protein and calories and restricted in fiber and in fat. The substitution of medium-chain triglycerides for some of the fat has resulted in weight gain and disappearance of steatorrhea. The restriction of gluten for patients with tropical sprue does not usually lead to further improvement.

CASE STUDY 15

Baby with Gluten Enteropathy

Pamela, the newest addition to the W family, was adopted when she was 6 months old. The parents and their two boys, Jason, 5, and Paul, 3, had eagerly awaited Pamela's arrival ever since the adoption papers were approved. The W family lives on a cattle ranch in Montana.

At the time of adoption Pamela appeared to be in good physical condition except for a mild anemia (hemoglobin, 9.8 g). Since Pamela's previous dietary history was not known, the pediatrician recommended an iron-fortified proprietary formula by bottle, then transfer to a cup with gradual introduction of cereals, fruits, vegetables, meats, and strained egg yolks.

During the first month with the W family Pamela was irritable and vomited on occasion. Mrs. W thought perhaps Pamela was having difficulty adjusting to her new home. But as the weeks went on Pamela did not improve. Her appetite was poor and she appeared pale. Mrs. W then took her to a physician for a checkup. Pamela weighed 8.2 kg (18 lb 1 oz); length, 68.5 cm (27 in.). Six weeks earlier, at the time of her adoption, her weight was 7.8 kg (17 lb, 4 oz); length, 67 cm (26-3/8 in.) Pamela's abdomen was distended and Mrs. W reported that Pamela had frequent, foul-smelling, foamy, light-colored stools and that she was irritable and easily fatigued. She noted that Pamela's symptoms began after solids such as oatmeal and teething biscuits were introduced. The pediatrician recommended that the baby be hospitalized for a series of tests.

A diagnostic workup provided the following information: serum carotene, 38 μg per dl; total serum protein, 4.6 g per dl; negative sweat test. Stool specimens were found to contain a high percentage of fat, fatty acids, and calcium soaps. Biopsy of the small intestinal mucosa showed subtotal villous atrophy. A provisional diagnosis of celiac sprue was made.

Pamela was placed on a high-protein, high-calorie, gluten-restricted diet. Water-miscible preparations of Vitamin A and D together with iron supplementation were prescribed. Pamela's appetite and well-being improved rapidly, and she started to gain weight soon after the gluten-restricted diet was begun. Before Pamela's discharge, Mrs. W reviewed with the nutritionist the detailed list of permitted foods and was given a recipe booklet. She was also informed of resources available through the American Celiac Society.

On a follow-up visit at age 10 months, Pamela's condition was markedly improved. Mrs. W brought along a record of Pamela's intake, which she discussed with the pediatrician and nutritionist. She remarked that she has to watch to be sure that the boys do not offer snacks that contain gluten to Pamela. Pamela has responded well to the gluten-restricted diet as demonstrated by her weight gain, improved appetite, and fewer fatty stools.

Pathophysiologic Correlations
1. List the symptoms of gluten-induced enteropathy that were observed in Pamela.
2. Describe the pathologic changes that occur in the small intestine in this disorder.
3. Describe fully the effects of the change in the mucosal surface on nutrient absorption.
4. What is gluten? What part of gluten is specifically involved in this disease?
5. What theories have been proposed to explain the effect of gliadin?
6. Suggest some probable causes for the diarrhea observed in celiac disease.
7. How was the diagnosis of gluten enteropathy established?

Nutritional Assessment
8. What are the acceptable values for each of the following tests for a child of Pam's age: hemoglobin; serum total protein; plasma carotene; stool fat?
9. List some manifestations that are evidence of

nutritional deficiency for each of these organ systems: hematopoietic; skeletal; muscular; nervous; endocrine; integument. Indicate for each the probable nutrient lacks.

10. Compare the dietary allowances for Pamela at 10 months with those for a healthy 10-month baby.

11. At 6 months what would Pam's weight be if she were at the 50th percentile? At 10 months? What would be her height both at 6 months and at 10 months at the 50th percentile?

12. What is the likelihood that Pam will outgrow her sensitivity to gluten?

13. Mrs. W can no longer use enriched breads in Pam's diet. Which nutrients are provided by enriched breads? Suggest some alternate sources of these nutrients.

Planning the Diet

14. Outline the objectives you would set in planning Pam's diet.

15. List some considerations that are important in the nutritional management of the child with gluten enteropathy.

16. Circle which of the following foods must be omitted from Pamela's diet: ice cream; oatmeal; vanilla wafers; zwieback; instant mashed potato; junior chopped vegetables and chicken dinner; spaghetti with meat sauce; chocolate custard pudding; creamed carrots. For each food that you have circled indicate an appropriate substitution.

Dietary Counseling

17. The W family likes spaghetti with meat sauce, macaroni and cheese, and other pasta dishes. Suggest some appropriate alternatives that could also be used for Pam.

18. Mrs. W enjoys baking sweet breads and desserts. Suggest some baked items that would be suitable for Pamela as well as the rest of the family.

19. Mrs. W found some recipes in which wheat starch was needed. Can wheat starch be included in Pam's diet? Explain.

20. Mrs. W asks whether she should continue the supplements of vitamins A and D when Pam goes home. What would you tell her?

References for the Case Study

DODGE, J. A.: "Gluten Intolerance, Gluten Enteropathy, and Clinical Disease," *Arch. Dis. Child.*, **55**:143–45, 1980.

HARTWIG, M. S.: "Sticking to a Gluten-Free Diet," *Am. J. Nurs.*, **83**:1308–9, 1983.

McCREERY, M.: "Diet: First–Line Defense Against Celiac Disease," *R.N.*, **39**:50–52, February 1976.

References

1. Goldstein, R., et al.: "The Fatty Meal Test: An Alternative to Stool Fat Analysis," *Am. J. Clin. Nutr.*, **38**:763–68, 1983.

2. Committee on Nutrition: "The Practical Significance of Lactose Intolerance in Children," *Pediatrics*, **62**:240–45, 1978.

3. Solomons, N. W., et al.: "Hydrogen Breath Test of Lactose Absorption in Adults: The Application of Physiological Doses and Whole Cow's Milk Sources," *Am. J. Clin. Nutr.*, **33**:545–54, 1980.

4. Newcomer, A. D., et al.: "Triolein Breath Test. A Sensitive and Specific Test for Fat Malabsorption," *Gastroenterology*, **76**:6–13, 1980.

5. Goff, J. S.: "Two-Stage Triolein Breath Test Differentiates Pancreatic Insufficiency from Other Causes of Malabsorption," *Gastroenterology*, **83**:44–46, 1982.

6. Bach, A. C., and Babayan, V. K.: "Medium-Chain Triglycerides: An Update," *Am. J. Clin. Nutr.*, **36**:950–62, 1982.

7. Schizas, A. A., et al.: "Medium-Chain Triglycerides—Use in Food Preparation," *J. Am. Diet. Assoc.*, **51**:228–32, 1967.

8. Mueller, J. F.: "Drug–Nutrient Interrelationships," in Alfin-Slater, R.B., and Kritchevsky, D., eds. *Human Nutrition. A Comprehensive Treatise. 3B. Nutrition and the Adult: Micronutrients.* Plenum Press, New York, 1980.

9. Green, P. H. R., and Tall, A. R.: "Drugs, Alcohol and Malabsorption," *Am. J. Med.*, **67**:1066–76, 1979.

10. Newcomer, A. D., and McGill, A. B.: "Clinical Importance of Lactase Deficiency," *N. Engl. J. Med.*, **310**:42–43, 1984.

11. Nielsen, O. H., et al.: "Calcium Absorption and Acceptance of Low Lactose Milk Among Children with Primary Lactase Deficiency," *J. Pediatr. Gastroenterol. Nutr.*, **3**:219–23, 1984.

12. Pedersen, E. R., et al.: "Lactose Malabsorption and Tolerance of Lactose-Hydrolyzed Milk," *Scand. J. Gastroenterol.*, **17**:861–64, 1982.

13. Welsh, J. D.: "Diet Therapy in Adult Lactose Malabsorption: Present Practices," *Am. J. Clin. Nutr.*, **31**:592–96, 1978.

14. Ford, R. P. K., and Barnes, G. L.: "Breath Hydrogen Test and Sucrase-Isomaltase Deficiency," *Arch. Dis. Child.*, **58**:595–97, 1983.

15. Ament, M. E., et al.: "Sucrase-Isomaltase Deficiency—A Frequently Misdiagnosed Disease," *J. Pediatr.*, **83**:721–27, 1973.

16. Lindquist, B., and Meeuwisse, G.: "Diets in Disaccharidase Deficiency and Defective Monosaccharide Absorption," *J. Am. Diet. Assoc.*, 48:307–10, 1966.

17. Greenberger, N. J.: "State of the Art: The Management of the Patient with Short Bowel Syndrome," *Am. J. Gastroenterol.*, 70:528–40, 1978.

18. Tilson, M. D.: "Pathophysiology and Treatment of Short Bowel Syndrome," *Surg. Clin. North Am.*, 60:1273–84, 1980.

19. Falchuk, Z. M.: "Update on Gluten-Sensitive Enteropathy," *Am. J. Med.*, 67:1085–96, 1979.

20. Lebenthal, E., and Branski, D.: "Childhood Celiac Disease—A Reappraisal," *J. Pediatr.*, 98:681–90, 1981.

32

Diet in Disturbances of the Liver, Gallbladder, and Pancreas

High-Protein, High-Carbohydrate, Moderate-Fat Diet; Fat-Restricted Diet

Diseases of the Liver— General Considerations

The liver is the largest and most complex organ in the body. It performs many functions that have an important bearing on one's nutritional state. Diseases of this organ may therefore markedly affect health.

Functions The role of the liver in intermediary metabolism with reference to proteins, fats, and carbohydrates has been described in Chapters 5, 6 and 7 and is briefly summarized as follows:

1. Protein metabolism (Chapter 5)—synthesis of plasma proteins; deaminization of amino acids; formation of urea.
2. Carbohydrate metabolism (Chapter 6)—synthesis, storage, and release of glycogen; synthesis of heparin.
3. Lipid metabolism (Chapter 7)—synthesis of lipoproteins, phospholipids, cholesterol; formation of bile; conjugation of bile salts; oxidation of fatty acids.
4. Mineral metabolism (Chapter 9)—storage of iron, copper and other minerals.
5. Vitamin metabolism (Chapter 11)—storage of vitamins A and D; some conversion of carotene to vitamin A, and of vitamin K to prothrombin.
6. Detoxification of bacterial decomposition products, mineral poisons, and certain drugs and dyes.

Etiology Liver diseases may have a number of causes: infectious agents, toxins, metabolic or nutritional factors, biliary obstruction, and carcinoma. The pathologic changes in the liver parenchymal cells are similar regardless of the etiology for the disease. Basic changes include atrophy, fatty infiltration, fibrosis, and necrosis.

Symptoms and Clinical Findings *Jaundice* is a symptom common to many diseases of the liver and biliary tract and consists of a yellow pigmentation of the skin and body tissues because of the accumulation of bile pigments in the blood. *Obstructive jaundice* results from the interference of the flow of bile by stones, tumors, or inflammation of the mucosa of the ducts. *Hemolytic jaundice* results from an abnormally large destruction of blood cells such as occurs in yellow fever, pernicious anemia, and so forth. *Toxic jaundice* originates from poisons, drugs, or virus infections.

Other symptoms commonly seen in liver diseases include lassitude, weakness, fatigue, fever, anorexia, and weight loss; abdominal pain, flatulence, nausea, and vomiting; hepatomegaly; ascites and edema; and portal hypertension.

Nutritional Considerations in Liver Disease Protection of the parenchymal cells is the foremost consideration in all types of liver injury. Since the liver is so intimately involved in the metabolism of foodstuffs, a nutritious diet is an important part of therapy and should be designed to protect the liver from stress and to enable it to function as efficiently as possible. With the exception of hepatic coma, generous amounts of high-quality protein should be provided for tissue repair and for prevention of fatty infiltration and degeneration of liver cells. A high-carbohydrate intake ensures an adequate reserve of glycogen, which, together with adequate protein stores, has a protective effect. Moderate amounts of fat are indicated for many persons. Signs of nutritional deficiency such as glossitis, nutritional anemia, or peripheral neuropathy are not uncommon in patients with liver disease. Generous amounts of vitamins, especially of the B-complex, must be provided to compensate for deficiencies. If edema and ascites are present, sodium restriction may be necessary.

Hepatitis

Etiology and Symptoms   This is an infectious disease characterized by inflammatory and degenerative changes of the liver. Two classes are recognized, *viral* and *drug induced*. The viral type is more common and occurs as *type A* (formerly called *infectious*), *type B (serum)*, or *type C* (posttransfusion). Specific viruses have been identified for types A and B. Type A is transmitted either by fecal contamination of water or food or parenterally. Epidemics occur from time to time in young people and are usually traced to a breakdown in sanitation. Type B is transmitted chiefly by the parenteral route through improperly sterilized needles but also by saliva, blood, and semen. Type C accounts for a high percentage of cases of posttransfusion hepatitis in hospitalized patients; it, too, is frequently seen in male homosexuals. Type A viral hepatitis is usually mild and rarely progresses to chronic hepatitis whereas Type B is often more severe and more likely to progress to a potentially serious liver disorder, chronic active hepatitis, which is associated with a number of pathologic lesions.

Drug-induced hepatitis may be due to alcohol, heroin, marijuana, or hashish, or to hypersensitivity to sulfa compounds or penicillin, or to a direct toxic effect on the liver by agents such as carbon tetrachloride.

Aside from mode of transmission and period of incubation, the two classes of hepatitis are similar. Nonspecific symptoms such as anorexia, fatigue, nausea and vomiting, diarrhea, fever, weight loss, and abdominal discomfort usually precede the development of jaundice, which ordinarily subsides after 1 to 2 weeks. Complete recovery may take several months. Treatment consists of adequate rest, nutritious diet, and avoidance of further damage to the liver.

Dietary Modification   The objectives of dietary treatment are to aid in the regeneration of liver tissue and to prevent further liver damage. This can be accomplished by providing a nutritious diet and enticing the patient to eat it. The patient must be convinced of the importance of the diet in promoting recovery and preventing relapses. Anorexia is frequently a problem; hence every effort must be made to encourage the patient to eat. Foods must be well prepared and attractively served with consideration given to the individual's food preferences.

Initially, foods of liquid-to-soft consistency (see Chapter 28) may be preferable if there is anorexia in the acute stages of the illness, progressing to a wider selection of foods with convalescence. Sufficient calories should be provided to maintain weight, or to bring about weight gain, if needed. A liberal intake of carbohydrate and fat as tolerated is required to reduce protein catabolism. At least 1 g protein or more per kilogram of body weight daily is needed to overcome negative nitrogen balance, to promote regeneration of parenchymal cells, and to prevent fatty infiltration of the liver. Judicious use of spices and condiments may help stimulate the appetite. Small to moderate portions at mealtime with between-meal supplements of high-protein beverages are frequently more acceptable than larger meals. Some individuals need assistance in feeding themselves and should be allowed adequate time to eat at a leisurely pace. The following high-protein, moderate-fat, high-carbohydrate diet is appropriate to meet the nutritional goals for patients whose appetite has returned.

High-Protein, Moderate-Fat, High-Carbohydrate Diet

Characteristics and General Rules
The caloric level may be increased by adding high-carbohydrate foods. Small amounts of cream and ice cream may be used when tolerated.
The protein intake may be increased by adding nonfat dry milk to liquid milk.

Modifications in fiber and consistency may be made by applying restrictions concerning the soft diet (Chapter 28) to the foods listed here.

Six or more small feedings may be preferred when there is lack of appetite.

When sodium restriction is ordered, all food must be prepared without salt. Low-sodium milk should replace part or all of the prescribed milk. See Sodium-Restricted Diets, Chapter 39.

Include These Foods Daily:

1 quart milk
8 ounces lean meat, poultry, or fish
1 egg
4 servings vegetables including:
    2 servings potato or substitute
    1 serving green leafy or yellow vegetable
    1 - 2 servings other vegetable
    One vegetable to be raw each day
3 servings fruit including
    1 serving citrus fruit or other good source of ascorbic acid
    2 servings other fruit
1 serving enriched or whole-grain cereal
6 slices enriched or whole-grain bread
2 tablespoons butter or margarine
4 tablespoons sugar, jelly, marmalade, or jam
Additional foods to further increase the carbohydrate as the patient is able to take them

Nutritive Value of Above Food List: protein, 135 g; fat 106 g; carbohydrate, 236 g; kcal, 2,590; calcium, 2.53 g; iron, 18.3 mg; vitamin A, 18,770 IU; thiamin, 2.11 mg; riboflavin, 3.39 mg; niacin, 27.6 mg; ascorbic acid, 159 mg.

Typical Food Selection

Beverages—carbonated beverages, milk and milk drinks, coffee, tea, fruit juices, cocoa flavoring
Breads and cereals—all kinds
Cheese—cottage, cream, mild cheddar
Desserts—angel cake, plain cake and cookies, custard, plain or fruit gelatin, fruit whip, fruit pudding, Junket, milk and cereal desserts, sherbets, ices, plain ice cream
Eggs—any way
Fat—butter, margarine, cream, cooking fat, vegetable oils
Fruits—all
Meat—lean beef, chicken, fish, lamb, liver, pork, turkey
Potato or substitute—hominy, macaroni, noodles, rice, spaghetti, sweet potato
Seasonings—salt, spices, vinegar (in moderation)
Soups—clear and cream
Sweets—honey, jam, jelly, sugar, sugar candy, syrups
Vegetables—all

Foods to Avoid

No foods are specifically contraindicated. Many patients complain of intolerance to the following groups of foods: strongly flavored vegetables; rich desserts; fried and fatty foods; chocolate; nuts; and highly seasoned foods. Although such complaints cannot always be explained on a physiologic basis, nothing is gained by giving the offending foods to the patient.

Meal Pattern	**Sample Menu**
BREAKFAST	
Fruit	Half grapefruit
Cereal with milk and sugar	Wheatena with milk and sugar
Egg	Scrambled egg
Whole-grain or enriched toast—2 slices	Whole-wheat toast
Butter or margarine—2 teaspoons	Margarine
Marmalade—1 tablespoon	Orange marmalade
Beverage with cream and sugar	Coffee with cream and sugar

Meal Pattern	Sample Menu
LUNCHEON OR SUPPER	
Lean meat, fish, or poultry—4 ounces	Broiled whitefish
Potato or substitute	Escalloped potatoes
Cooked vegetable	Asparagus with margarine
Salad	Celery and carrot strips
Whole-grain or enriched bread—2 slices	Whole-wheat bread
Butter or margarine—2 teaspoons	Margarine
Jelly—1 tablespoon	Grape jelly
Fruit	Sliced banana
Milk	Milk
MIDAFTERNOON	
Milk with nonfat dry milk	High-protein milk with strawberry flavor
DINNER	
Lean meat, fish, or fowl—4 ounces	Roast beef
Potato	Mashed potato
Vegetable	Baked acorn squash
Whole-grain or enriched bread—2 slices	Dinner rolls
Butter or margarine—2 teaspoons	Margarine
Jelly—1 tablespoon	Apple jelly
Fruit, or dessert	Raspberry sherbet
Milk—1 glass	Milk
Tea, if desired	
EVENING NOURISHMENT	
Milk beverage	High-protein milk flavored with caramel
	Bread-and-jelly sandwich

Cirrhosis

Etiology   This chronic disease of the liver is characterized by diffuse degenerative changes, fibrosis, and nodular regeneration of the remaining cells. The causes include infectious hepatitis in a small percentage of patients, chronic alcoholism in association with malnutrition, underlying metabolic disturbances such as hemochromatosis or Wilson's disease, hepatotoxins derived from certain plants and fungi, and prolonged biliary stasis.

Laennec's Cirrhosis.   The most common type of cirrhosis in the United States is Laennec's (*alcoholic, portal*) cirrhosis. The exact etiology has not been established although alcohol and relative or absolute malnutrition are implicated in the majority of patients. Alcohol has a direct toxic effect on the liver, but the extent to which malnutrition promotes this effect is not clear.[1] Only about 10 percent of alcoholics develop cirrhosis, and it occurs after years of excessive alcohol intake in individuals whose diets are less than optimal in a number of nutrients. Pathologic changes include fatty infiltration, necrosis, and proliferation of fibrous tissue.

Symptoms and Clinical Findings   The onset of cirrhosis may be gradual, with gastrointestinal disturbances such as anorexia, nausea, vomiting, pain, and distention. As the disease progresses, jaundice and other serious changes occur.

Ascites.   Ascites is the accumulation of abnormal amounts of fluid in the abdomen. It may develop as a consequence of portal vein hypertension, obstruction of the hepatic vein, a fall in plasma colloid osmotic pressure due to impaired albumin synthesis, increased sodium retention, or impaired water excretion.

Esophageal Varices (varicose veins).   Varices in the esophagus and upper part of the stomach may develop as a complication of portal hypertension. Hemorrhage is then an ever-present danger and may be provoked by roughage of any kind. The hemorrhage itself may be fatal, or the blood may provide for the accumulation of ammonia and subsequent hepatic coma.

Modification of the Diet   Regeneration of parenchymal cells occurs if appropriate diet therapy is initiated before the disease is well advanced. The high-protein, high-carbohydrate diet outlined for infectious hepatitis is satisfactory. In advanced cirrhosis, however, further dietary modification is needed.

Protein. Individual requirements for protein must be considered, and intake must be adjusted as the disease progresses or improves. Most clinicians recommend an initial protein intake high enough to maintain nitrogen equilibrium, but low enough to prevent hepatic coma (approximately 35 to 50 g per day). Protein intake is restricted to less than 35 g per day if signs of impending coma develop.

Fats. Malabsorption of fats occurs in many cirrhotics. For some patients the substitution of medium-chain triglycerides for part of the dietary fat is effective in reducing steatorrhea. (See Chapter 31.)

Carbohydrate. The carbohydrate content of the diet will be high, 300 to 400 g per day, in order to provide sufficient calories so that protein is not used for energy.

Calories. From 35 to 50 kcal per kg, or 2,500 to 3,500 kcal per day for a 70-kg man, is needed. Most patients find it difficult to consume adequate calories because of anorexia and nausea. Individual food preferences should be taken into consideration and a sincere attempt made to provide the patient with food that is appealing. For some, several small meals are preferable to three large meals daily.

Vitamins and Minerals. Malabsorption of fat-soluble and B-complex vitamins occurs in alcoholic and biliary cirrhosis. Serum calcium, magnesium, and zinc are decreased. Potassium supplements are sometimes needed to correct deficiency resulting from nausea, vomiting, diarrhea, antibiotic therapy, or a reduced protein intake. Vitamin supplements may be advisable to replenish liver stores and repair tissue damage, especially if the patient has anorexia.

Sodium. Sodium restriction is prescribed if edema and ascites are present. Severe restriction of sodium for many months is often necessary for effective removal of excess fluid accumulation. Diets restricted to less than 500 mg sodium per day are not uncommon in this disorder. On such strict low-sodium diets, all food used must be naturally low in sodium and prepared without sodium-containing compounds. Milk is limited to 1 pint per day. Close attention to food selection is needed in order to provide an adequate protein intake without exceeding the sodium allowance. (See Chapter 39.)

Fluid. Some clinicians restrict fluid intake to an amount equivalent to the previous day's urinary output; however, fluids may not need to be severely limited if sodium restriction is effective in correcting edema and ascites.

Consistency. Reduction in fiber content of the diet is necessary in advanced cirrhosis when there is danger of hemorrhage from esophageal varices. A liquid or soft diet with small meals is used. (See Chapter 28.)

Hepatic Coma

Etiology This complex syndrome is characterized by neurologic disturbances that may develop as a complication of severe liver disease. Although the precise cause of hepatic coma is not clear, it is characterized by (1) elevated blood ammonia levels, as the failing liver loses the ability to utilize ammonia for synthesis of urea; (2) entrance of nitrogen-containing compounds, including ammonia, into the cerebral circulation without having been metabolized first by the liver, attributed to shunting of portal blood around the damaged liver; (3) high blood concentrations of aromatic amino acids, especially phenylalanine, tyrosine, and tryptophan, perhaps resulting from failure of the diseased liver to deaminate them; and (4) low levels of branched-chain amino acids in plasma. Aromatic amino acids compete with branched-chain amino acids for transport across the blood-brain barrier, where they then promote the synthesis of false neurotransmitters. The altered balance of neurotransmitters in the brain may be responsible for development of encephalopathy.[2] One hypothesis holds that excess ammonia, which is toxic to the brain, reacts with glutamic acid to form glutamine. The latter, in turn, is exchanged for aromatic amino acids, increasing their concentration in the brain and, ultimately, altering the balance of neurotransmitters.[3]

Symptoms Signs of impending coma include confusion, restlessness, irritability, inappropriate behavior, delirium, and drowsiness. There may also be incoordination and a flapping tremor of the arms and legs when extended. Electrolyte imbalance occurs. The patient may go into coma and may have convulsions. The breath has a fecal odor (*fetor hepaticus*). Prompt treatment is imperative or death occurs.

Treatment Conventional treatment consists of dietary protein restriction, cleansing of the bowel with enemas or laxatives to reduce the nitrogenous load, or antibiotics to suppress bacterial growth. Lactulose is sometimes used to increase motility. This is a synthetic disaccharide containing galactose and fructose, which is metabolized by colonic bacteria to acetic and lactic acids and which lowers the pH of the colon, thereby favoring diffusion of ammonia from blood to the colon. Oral, enteral, or intravenous administration of branched-chain amino acids* have reportedly improved both the plasma amino acid pattern and the encephalopathy.[4-6] Branched-chain amino acids are believed to decrease the transport of aromatic amino acids into the brain and also serve as an energy source in muscle, thereby lessening efflux of amino acids into the circulation.[4]

Dietary Modification The fundamental principle in the dietary management of hepatic coma is to reduce the protein intake to a minimum, thus decreasing the amount of ammonia produced. Catabolism of tissue proteins must also be avoided.

Calories. About 1,500 to 2,000 kcal is needed to prevent breakdown of tissue proteins for energy and is provided chiefly in the form of carbohydrates and fats. Although anorexia may occur, attempts should be made to keep the caloric intake as high as is practical to minimize tissue breakdown.

Protein. Some clinicians omit protein completely for 2 or 3 days, and others permit 20 to 30 g per day. As the patient improves, the protein intake is gradually increased by 10 to 15 g at a time until a maximum of 1 g per kg of body weight is reached. The patient must be carefully watched following each increment lest signs of coma recur.

Levels of 40 to 50 g protein per day may be used for long periods of time without detriment to nutritional status provided the diet supplies sufficient calories to maintain weight. Nitrogen balance can be achieved on protein intakes as low as 35 g per day if high-quality protein is used and caloric intake is adequate. Some advocate use of diets composed of vegetable protein, 40 g, because these are lower in certain amino acids and other compounds implicated in the etiology of encephalopathy.[7]

Dietary Management These patients pose problems in feeding because of anorexia and behavioral patterns ranging from apathy, drowsiness, and confusion to irritability and hyperexcitability. Restrictions of protein, sodium, and fluid may make the diet unacceptable to the patient. The challenge to entice the patient to consume sufficient calories sometimes cannot be met by conventional foods. A number of flavored liquid formulas, high in branched-chain amino acids and low in sodium and providing 1.0 to 1.5 kcal per ml are available. Alternatively, oral or enteral modular feedings are useful in this disorder and can be planned to include 40 g or more of protein and 2,000 kcal or more.[8] As tolerance to conventional foods improves, diets providing 20, 40, or 60 g protein (see page 567) may be gradually introduced.

Diseases of the Gallbladder

Incidence Gallbladder disease affects some 15 to 20 million adults in the United States. The exact prevalence is not known because many persons have asymptomatic gallbladder disease and never seek medical care. However, gallbladder disease is the fifth leading cause of hospitalization in the United States, and cholecystectomy is one of the most frequently performed surgical procedures. Gallstones are frequently found at autopsy in persons who were not known to have gallbladder disease. The incidence of gallbladder disease is higher in northern Europe and North and South America than in the Orient and other parts of the world. The American Indian, in particular, is at increased risk for the disease, and a genetic predisposition has been postulated.[9] Studies among the Pima Indians in the Southwest indicate that 70 percent of the women eventually develop gallstones; about half have gallstones by age 25.[10]

In most populations the incidence of gallbladder disease is higher in females than in males. Obesity correlates strongly with the disease, and the prevalence increases with age. Gastrointestinal disorders involving malabsorption of bile acids, such as ileal disease, resection, or bypass, and prolonged use of total parenteral nutrition[11] are frequently associated with gallstone development. Certain drugs, such as clofibrate and estrogens, increase the risk for gallstone formation.

Function of the Gallbladder The gallbladder concentrates bile formed in the liver and stores it until needed for digestion of fats. The entrance of fat into the duodenum stimulates secretion of the hormone *cholecystokinin* by the intestinal mucosa. The hormone is carried by way of the bloodstream to the gallbladder and forces it to contract, thus releasing bile into the common duct, and then into the small intes-

---

*Hepatic-aid (McGaw Laboratories, Irvine, Calif.); Stresstein (Sandoz Nutrition, Minneapolis, Minn.); Traum-Aid HBC (McGaw Laboratories, Irvine, Calif.); Travasorb Hepatic (Travenol Laboratories, Deerfield, Ill.); Vivonex T.E.N. (Norwich Eaton, Norwich, N.Y.).

tine, where it is needed for the emulsification of fats. Interference with the flow of bile occurring in gallbladder disease may cause impaired fat digestion.

Inflammation of the gallbladder is known as CHOLECYSTITIS. Gallstone formation, or CHOLELITHIASIS, occurs when cholesterol, bile pigments, bile salts, calcium, and other substances precipitate out of the bile. CHOLEDOCHOLITHIASIS refers to stones lodged in the common duct.

Diagnostic Tests The most widely used test for the diagnosis of gallbladder disease is oral cholecystography. This involves administration of an iodine contrast dye which is taken up and concentrated by the gallbladder. Presence of stones can then be visualized by roentgenogram. When a diseased gallbladder is not visualized, intravenous cholangiography is sometimes used. Injection of an iodine contrast medium permits visualization of the biliary ducts. Ultrasonography or computed tomography (CT scan) are also used to visualize the biliary tree and gallbladder.

Pathophysiology In the United States and Canada, the principal component of the vast majority of gallstones is cholesterol. Growth of the stones involves several stages, each of which is a prerequisite for the next: (1) a genetic and metabolic stage in a susceptible individual; (2) a chemical stage, in which bile becomes supersaturated with cholesterol; (3) a physical stage, in which the supersaturated bile is nucleated and growth of cholesterol crystals begins; (4) aggregation of microscopic crystals into stones; and (5) a symptomatic stage occurring when stones initiate cholescystitis or block the cystic or common bile duct.[10]

Limited data suggest that enhanced activity of HMA-CoA reductase, the rate-limiting enzyme in hepatic cholesterol synthesis, occurs in individuals with cholesterol gallstones.[12] In obese persons there is increased hepatic cholesterol secretion. Conversion of cholesterol to bile acids is increased in these individuals but apparently not in sufficient amounts to solubilize the excess cholesterol. Persons of normal weight with cholesterol gallstones have a decreased bile acid pool size. It is not clear whether the decrease in bile acid pool size is a cause or consequence of cholelithiasis.[13]

In western countries, about 10 percent of gallstones are pigment stones. This type occurs more frequently in countries where malnutrition and parasitic infection are common. The chief pigment in these stones is bilirubin. Biliary tract infections and hemolytic disorders predispose to increased formation of free bilirubin, which complexes with calcium in bile to form insoluble stones.

Symptoms and Clinical Findings Acute cholecystitis is usually associated with a gallstone lodged in the cystic duct and is accompanied by mild to severe pain, abdominal distention, nausea and vomiting, and fever. The pain occurs whenever the gallbladder contracts. Ingestion of fatty foods may thus cause discomfort, and fat digestion may be impaired because of the diminished flow of bile. Intolerance to certain strongly flavored vegetables, legumes, melons, and berries occurs in many persons with gallbladder disease, but the reason for this is not known.

Treatment of Gallbladder Disease Dietary, medical, or surgical intervention is used, depending on the individual case. Conservative treatment includes dietary management, although the importance of dietary factors in the etiology of gallbladder disease is

Table 32-1. Food Allowances for Two Levels of Fat Restriction
(Approximately 1,500 kcal)

	20 g Fat	50 g Fat
Milk, skim	2 cups	2 cups
Meat, fish, poultry (lean)	6 ounces*	6 ounces*
Eggs (3 per week)	½	½
Vegetables		
Dark green leafy or deep yellow	1 serving	1 serving
Potato	1 serving	1 serving
Other	1 or more servings	1 or more servings
Fruits		
Citrus	1 serving	1 serving
Other	3 servings	3 servings
Bread and cereals		
Cereals	1 serving	1 serving
Breads	6 slices	3 slices
Fats, vegetable	None	6 teaspoons
Sweets	3 tablespoons	2 tablespoons
Total fat, g	20	50
Cholesterol, mg	270†	270†
Protein, g	85	80
kcal (approximate)	1,500	1,500

* Only lean cuts of meat, fish, poultry made be used. Each ounce is equivalent to 8 g protein and 3 g fat.

† Cholesterol level would be reduced to about half this level if eggs were not used. If butter is used instead of vegetable fat, the cholesterol level would be increased.

not known. The principal aim is to reduce discomfort by providing a diet restricted in fat.

Energy. Excess caloric intake appears to be a risk factor for development of gallbladder disease. The disease is much more common among the obese than in persons of normal weight. Persons at increased risk for gallbladder disease should be encouraged to achieve and maintain normal weight through controlled dietary intake and a regular exercise program. For many, strict dieting is not needed if smaller portion sizes are used, and energy-dense snacks and desserts are replaced by low-calorie vegetables and fruits or other foods high in fiber. (See Chapter 25.)

Fat. The patient receives no food initially during acute attacks of cholecystitis. Progression to a 20- to 30-g fat diet is then made. If this is tolerated the fat can then be increased to 50 to 60 g per day, thus im-

proving palatability of the diet. In chronic cholecystitis some degree of fat restriction is usually necessary. With restriction of fats, carbohydrates are used more liberally.

Cholesterol. Several studies have found no relationship between serum cholesterol levels and gallstone formation. High-cholesterol diets increase biliary cholesterol; however, much more cholesterol is synthesized in the body from fragments of carbohydrates, amino acids, and fat metabolism. Dietary restriction of cholesterol, therefore, is probably not very effective in prevention of gallstones. If a reduction in cholesterol content of the diet is ordered, egg yolks, liver, and other organ meats are omitted, and skim milk and margarine are substituted for whole milk and butter. See Table A-5 for cholesterol content of foods. Food allowances for two levels of fat restriction are shown in Table 32–1.

Fat-Restricted Diet

Foods Allowed

Beverages—skim milk as desired; coffee, coffee substitute, tea; fruit juices

Breads—all kinds except those with added fat

Cereals—all cooked or dry breakfast cereals, except possibly bran; macaroni, noodles, rice, spaghetti

Cheese—cottage only

Desserts—angel cake; fruit whip; fruit pudding; gelatin; ices and sherbets; milk and cereal puddings using part of milk allowance

Eggs—3 per week

Fats—vegetable oil or margarine

Fruits—all kinds when tolerated

Meats—broiled, baked, roasted, or stewed without fat: lean beef, chicken, lamb, pork, veal, fish

Seasonings—in moderation: salt, pepper, spices, herbs, flavoring extracts

Soups—clear

Sweets—all kinds: hard candy, jam, jelly, marmalade, sugars

Vegetables—all kinds when well tolerated; cooked without added butter, or cream

Foods to Avoid

Beverages—with cream; soda-fountain beverages with milk, cream, or ice cream; whole milk

Breads—griddle cakes; sweet rolls with fat; French toast

Cheese—all whole-milk cheeses, both hard and soft

Desserts—any containing chocolate, cream, nuts, or fats: cookies, cake, doughnuts, ice cream, pastries, pies, rich puddings

Eggs—fried

Fats—cooking fats, cream, salad dressings

Fruits—avocado, raw apple, berries, melons may not be tolerated

Meats—fatty meats, poultry, or fish: bacon, corned beef, duck, goose, ham, fish canned in oil, mackerel, pork, sausage; organ meats. Smoked and spiced meats if they are poorly tolerated

Seasonings—sometimes not tolerated: pepper; curries; meat sauces; excessive spices; vinegar

Soups—cream, unless made with milk and fat allowance

Sweets—candy with chocolate and nuts

Vegetables—strongly flavored may be poorly tolerated: broccoli, brussels sprouts, cabbage, cauliflower, cucumber, onion, peppers, radish, turnips; dried cooked peas and beans

Miscellaneous—fried foods; gravies; nuts; olives; peanut butter; pickles; popcorn; relishes

Meal Pattern (20 g fat)

BREAKFAST

Fruit
Cereal with skim milk and sugar
Egg—1 only (3 per week)
Enriched or whole-grain toast
Jelly
Beverage with skim milk and sugar

LUNCHEON OR SUPPER

Lean meat, fish, poultry, or cottage cheese
Potato or substitute
Vegetable
Salad; no oil dressing

Enriched or whole-grain bread
Dessert or fruit
Milk, skim— ½ cup

DINNER

Lean meat, poultry, or fish
Potato or substitute
Vegetable
Enriched or whole-grain bread
Jelly
Dessert or fruit
Milk, skim—1 glass

Sample Menu

BREAKFAST

Stewed apricots
Cornflakes with skim milk and sugar
Poached egg
Whole-wheat toast with jelly

Coffee with skim milk and sugar

LUNCHEON OR SUPPER

Tomato bouillon
Fruit salad plate:
    Cottage cheese
    Sliced orange
    Tokay grapes
    Pear
    Romaine
Whole-wheat roll
Vanilla pudding (using milk allowance)
Tea with milk, sugar

DINNER

Roast lamb, trimmed of fat
Boiled new potatoes; no added fat
Zucchini squash
Parkerhouse roll
Jelly
Angel cake with sliced peaches
Milk, skim—1 glass

Fiber.   The association of gallbladder disease in populations consuming low-fiber diets and the relative lack of the disease in those populations that habitually consume diets high in fiber has led to speculation that fiber plays a role in prevention of the disease. Some evidence suggests that interactions among certain components of fiber, bile salts, and intestinal flora, alter the composition of the bile acid pool, leading to increased chenodeoxycholic acid, which enhances solubility of biliary cholesterol.[14] More research is needed to determine whether dietary fiber has a sustained influence on biliary saturation.

Diet Following Cholecystectomy   Some fat restriction is indicated for several weeks following removal of the gallbladder. Thereafter, most individuals can tolerate a regular diet.

Dissolution of Gallstones   For selected patients oral administration of chenodeoxycholic acid induces dissolution of gallstones. In the National Cooperative Gallstone Study, a small percentage of patients experienced complete dissolution of gallstones after receiving 750 mg of chenodeoxycholic acid daily for 2 years; another 27 percent experienced partial dissolution of stones.[15]

DIETARY COUNSELING

Restriction of dietary fat influences the methods of food preparation permitted. The patient should be advised to prepare meats by baking, broiling, roasting, or stewing and to use only lean meats trimmed of all visible fats. Meat drippings, cream sauces, and so on are not allowed, but spices and herbs in moderation can be used to enhance flavor of foods. Use of fortified skim milk and inclusion of green leafy or yellow vegetables is needed to help ensure adequate intake of vitamin A. The small amounts of fat permitted should be taken as butter or margarine. Any foods known to cause distention should be omitted. Most individuals need guidance in selecting suitable substitutes for desserts that are high in fat.

Pancreatic Disorders

Pancreatic disease may be due to congenital or inflammatory diseases, trauma, or tumors. Disorders of the pancreas usually involve inadequate production of enzymes needed for normal digestive processes. Interference with this process leads to impaired digestion and is manifested by the presence of excess fat and undigested protein in the stools. Some starch may also be present. Dietary treatment of pancreatic disorders depends on the nature and extent of digestive impairment rather than on the disease itself.

Acute Pancreatitis Acute inflammatory disease of the pancreas results from interference with the blood supply to the organ or from obstruction to the outflow of pancreatic juice. The usual causes are alcoholism and biliary tract disease; however, acute pancreatitis may also be due to trauma, virus infections, tumors, nutritional deficiency, certain vascular diseases, and a number of metabolic diseases. Alcohol is implicated in about half the cases of acute pancreatitis in the United States.[16] Acute pancreatitis and severe fat intolerance are also seen in Types 1 and 5 hyperlipoproteinemias. (See Chapter 38.)

Acute pancreatitis may range from a mild inflammatory reaction to severe illness. The most predominant symptom is severe upper-abdominal pain radiating to the back and is aggravated by eating. Epigastric tenderness, distention, constipation, nausea, and vomiting occur.

Increased pressure in the ducts causes the activated pancreatic enzymes to escape into the interstitial tissues, leading to elevations in serum amylase and lipase. Other clinical findings include hyperlipemia and hypocalcemia. Alteration of structure or function of the pancreas or adjacent organs may be demonstrated radiographically. The islets of Langerhans are not necessarily involved.

Treatment. Conservative management is used. Aims are to alleviate pain, to keep pancreatic secretory activity at a minimum, and to replace fluids and electrolytes. Dietary management usually consists of giving the patient nothing by mouth for several days during acute attacks. Progression from clear liquids or a semisynthetic fiber-free to a regular diet is made as tolerated.

Chronic Pancreatitis This disease may be described as relapsing, recurrent, or continuous in nature. As in acute pancreatitis, alcoholism is the most common cause of attacks but the basic defect is not known. Alcohol indirectly stimulates pancreatic secretions, and may also obstruct pancreatic outflow. Obstruction of the ducts leads to chronic changes, including destruction of the islets of Langerhans in some patients, fibrosis, pseudocyst, and pancreatic calcification. When enzyme secretion is only 10 percent of normal, impaired digestion leads to steatorrhea, creatorrhea, and deficiency of the B-complex and fat-soluble vitamins.

The chronic form is characterized by recurrent attacks of burning epigastric pain, especially after meals containing alcohol and fat. Other symptoms include flatulence, anorexia, weight loss, nausea, and vomiting.

Treatment. Conservative management is used unless the patient has unremitting pain or complications necessitating partial or complete pancreatectomy. Medications to alleviate pain and to inhibit pancreatic secretion are used.

The aim of dietary treatment is to minimize gastric secretion because of its stimulating effect on secretin output. Diet during attacks is the same as that in acute pancreatitis. Thereafter a diet high in protein and calories, and low in fat, should be used. Six small meals are better tolerated than large meals. Pancreatic extract is used to aid in fat absorption. Medium-chain triglycerides (MCT) and semisynthetic fiber-free diets have been useful in the disease. Alcohol is forbidden.

Case Study 16

Alcoholic with Laennec's Cirrhosis

Mr. Y, age 50, has been drinking excessively for the past 10 years. His family and friends have tried without success to get him into a chemical dependency treatment program. Within the past 6 months, he has lost his job and has been divorced.

Mr. Y now rents a hotel room downtown that has a small refrigerator and a hot plate; however, he has little incentive to cook for himself. Occasionally he eats a meal in a diner or fast-food place. There are days when his only intake is alcohol. He works now and then as a day laborer with a temporary labor pool.

Ten days ago Mr. Y was arrested for driving under the influence of alcohol and was taken to a detoxification unit. There he received meals and lodging, a physical examination, and counseling. The physical findings included hepatomegaly, ataxia, jaundice, ascites, pedal edema, palmar erythema, spider angiomas, and evidence of muscle wasting. Mr. Y weighed 71 kg (156 lb); height, 180 cm (71 in.). He was hospitalized for further evaluation and treatment.

Mr. Y recalled no exposure to hepatotoxic drugs

or chemicals other than alcohol. He is a heavy smoker and has trouble getting to sleep at night. Over a period of weeks he has experienced abdominal pain, fatigue, chronic dyspepsia, and anorexia, and he has noticed deepening jaundice. He admits to being lonely and is upset about the loss of his job and family.

Evidence of liver dysfunction, fluid retention, and portal hypertension led to the diagnosis of Laennec's cirrhosis. Folic acid, thiamin, and zinc deficiencies were also identified.

Rest, withdrawal of alcohol, diet, and diuretic therapy were important elements of treatment. A 1,000-mg sodium, 60-g protein, 3,000-kcal soft diet was prescribed with a fluid restriction of 1,000 ml per day. Since Mr. Y was anorectic, frequent small feedings were offered. His food preferences were considered in planning his diet. He was also given a multivitamin preparation, folacin, and zinc sulfate. To promote diuresis Mr. Y was given spironolactone (Aldactone) in combination with furosemide (Lasix). Fluid and electrolyte levels were carefully monitored. Daily measurements of weight, abdominal girth, and intake and output were made.

Four days after admission Mr. Y was lethargic, confused, and forgetful. Other manifestations of impending hepatic coma included flapping tremor (asterixis), characteristic EEG changes, and elevated blood levels of ammonia. Mr. Y's serum potassium was 3.0 mEq per liter.

Treatment for hepatic encephalopathy included restriction of dietary protein to 20 g, and administration of magnesium citrate, oral neomycin, lactulose, and enemas. Diuretics were discontinued for several days. Potassium chloride was given to correct the hypokalemia. When the symptoms had subsided protein was added to his diet in increments of 5 g every few days until a level of 50 g was reached. No untoward symptoms appeared.

The steps taken to lower the serum ammonia levels were effective. Eventually the sodium restriction and diuretics reduced Mr. Y's ascites and edema. Plans for discharge are to transfer Mr. Y to an alcoholic treatment center.

Pathophysiologic Correlations

1. Describe the functions of the liver with respect to the utilization of each of the following: carbohydrate; fat; protein; minerals; vitamins.
2. What are the pathologic characteristics of Laennec's cirrhosis?
3. What is the basis for the fatty liver seen in cirrhosis?
4. What possible etiologic factors might explain the jaundice?
5. Explain the basis for the ascites.
6. Why are the daily measurements of weight important?
7. List the basis for other clinical symptoms commonly seen in cirrhosis.
8. Identify the abnormality in liver function that is measured with each of these tests: serum proteins; prothrombin time; ammonia; blood urea nitrogen; SGOT.
9. What signs might alert the dietitian or the nurse that the patient is approaching hepatic coma?
10. Explain the etiology of hepatic encephalopathy.
11. What are some precipitating factors that lead to hepatic coma?
12. What means are used to reduce the accumulation of ammonia? Explain the action of each.

Nutritional Assessment

13. List the findings in Mr. Y's history that suggest faulty nutrition.
14. Identify other characteristic symptoms presented by patients with cirrhosis of the liver that suggest nutritional deficiency.
15. In what ways does chronic alcoholism interfere with nutritional status?
16. When Mr. Y is drinking he consumes 750 ml whiskey (86 proof) daily. About how many calories are provided?
17. Assume that Mr. Y has a total plasma volume of 3,500 ml. Since the total serum protein deficit is 2.2 g per dl, what is the total deficit in his circulation?
    Assuming that each gram of serum protein deficit represents a body tissue deficit of 30 g, what is the total body protein deficit?
    If Mr. Y's diet enables him to synthesize 5 g protein per day, how long will it take him to replace his tissues?
18. List some problems generally associated with protein deficiency.
19. What symptoms might suggest that the patient may have a zinc deficiency?
20. What are some nutritional side effects of neomycin therapy?
21. What hazards must be kept in mind with severe sodium restriction?
22. Before his hospitalization Mr. Y occasionally ate in fast-food restaurants. Suggest a typical meal that he might have ordered, and indicate the nutritional contribution it made to his diet.

Planning The Diet

23. State two aims of diet therapy for Mr. Y.
24. List the characteristics of a successful diet for Mr. Y. Explain the rationale for each.

25. What problems should be anticipated in providing a satisfactory diet for Mr. Y?
26. What dietary steps must be taken immediately when hepatic coma is present?
27. Why is the multivitamin supplement ordered for Mr. Y essential?

Dietary Counseling

28. List the aspects of assistance and dietary counseling that should be provided for Mr. Y when he returns home.
29. Enumerate the points you would emphasize during the counseling session with Mr. Y insofar as his diet is concerned. Explain the reason for each of these points.
30. With limited storage facilities, and little inclination to cook, give some suggestions for snacks that Mr. Y could have on hand to increase his caloric intake.
31. List examples of sodium compounds found in foods that Mr. Y should avoid in his diet.
32. What are some hidden sources of sodium that Mr. Y should avoid?
33. Can Mr. Y use salt substitutes? Explain.
34. The 1,000-mg sodium diet cannot be provided at the treatment center nor is this level realistic for Mr. Y when he goes home. What is a realistic level to recommend?

References for the Case Study

Brodsley, L.: "The Hospitalized Alcoholic. Avoiding a Crisis: The Assessment," *Am. J. Nurs.*, 82:1865–71, 1982.

Fredette, S. L.: "When the Liver Fails," *Am. J. Nurs.*, 84:64–7, 1984.

Gannon, R. B., and Pickett, V.: "Jaundice," *Am. J. Nurs.*, 83:404–7, 1983.

Guenter, P., and Slocum, B.: "Hepatic Disease: Nutritional Implications," *Nurs. Clin. North Am.*, 18:71–80, March 1983.

Thompson, M. A.: "Managing the Patient with Liver Dysfunction," *Nursing '81*, 11:101–7, November 1981.

References

1. Lieber, C. S.: "Alcohol, Protein Metabolism, and Liver Injury," *Gastroenterology*, 79:373–90, 1980.
2. Review: "Muscle Protein Catabolism in Cirrhotic Patients Reduced by Branched Chain Amino Acids," *Nutr. Rev.*, 41:146–49, 1983.
3. Review: "Hepatic Encephalopathy: A Unifying Hypothesis," *Nutr. Rev.*, 38:371–73, 1980.
4. Freund, H., et al.: "Chronic Hepatic Encephalopathy. Long-Term Therapy with a Branched-Chain Amino-Acid-Enriched Elemental Diet," *JAMA*, 242:347–49, 1979.
5. Keohane, P. P., et al: "Enteral Nutrition in Malnourished Patients with Hepatic Cirrhosis and Acute Encephalopathy," *J.P.E.N.*, 7:346–50, 1983.
6. Cerra, F. B., et al.: "Cirrhosis, Encephalopathy, and Improved Results with Metabolic Support," *Surgery*, 94:612–19, 1983.
7. Weber, F. L.: "Therapy of Portal-Systemic Encephalopathy: The Practical and the Promising," *Gastroenterology*, 81:174–77, 1981.
8. Smith, J., et al.: "Enteral Hyperalimentation in Undernourished Patients with Cirrhosis and Ascites," *Am. J. Clin. Nutr.*, 35:56–72, 1982.
9. Morris, D. L., et al.: "Gallbladder Disease and Gallbladder Cancer Among American Indians in Tricultural New Mexico," *Cancer*, 42:474–77, 1978.
10. Small, D. M., et al.: "Diseases of the Gallbladder and Biliary Passages," *Gastroenterology*, 69:1121–30, 1975.
11. Roslyn, J. J., et al.: "Gallbladder Disease in Patients on Long-Term Parenteral Nutrition," *Gastroenterology*, 84:148–54, 1983.
12. Redinger, R. N.: "Cholelithiasis," *Postgrad. Med.*, 65:56–62 ff, June 1979.
13. Roslyn, J. J., et al.: "Chronic Cholelithiasis and Decreased Bile Salt Pool Size," *Am. J. Surg.*, 139:119–24, 1980.
14. Story, J. A., and Kritchevsky, D.: "Bile Acid Metabolism and Fiber," *Am. J. Clin. Nutr.*, 31:S199–S202, 1978.
15. Palmer, R. H., and Carey, M. C.: "An Optimistic View of the National Cooperative Gallstone Study," *N. Engl. J. Med.*, 306:1171–74, 1982.
16. Toskes, P. P., and Greenberger, N. J.: "Acute and Chronic Pancreatitis," *DM*, 29:1–81, 1983.

33

Immunity, Stress, and Infections

High-Protein Diet; High-Protein Fluid Diet

Poor nutritional status has an adverse effect on immune function and on the ability to cope with the stress of infections and fevers. Protein depletion, in particular, compromises recovery from the stress of illness. Included in this chapter are a discussion of some aspects of immune function, the influence of stress on nutrient utilization, and nutritional needs during stress.

Immunity

The Immune System The body protects itself against disease by (1) physical barriers, such as the skin and mucous membranes, which form a first line of defense against entry of microorganisms or foreign substances; and (2) systemic immunity by which specialized cells respond to invasion of foreign materials such as bacteria, viruses, or fungi, or to unwanted substances arising from within the body, such as neoplastic cells. Cells involved in the immune system are located throughout the body. Some are in fixed tissues, such as the thymus, lymph nodes, bone marrow, spleen, lymphoid tissues of the respiratory, gastrointestinal, and genitourinary tract, Kupffer cells of the liver, and Peyer's patches of the small intestine. Others, such as leukocytes and lymphocytes, are mobile, and are released into the blood and carried to the site where they are needed when microorganisms have invaded the tissue.

Types of Immune Responses The immune response involves interactions of multiple cell types. Systemic immune responses are classified as nonspecific or specific. A *nonspecific* immune response involves a generalized defensive response to any foreign substance, or *antigen*, entering the tissue. Two types

of leukocytes are involved in nonspecific immune responses: polymorphonuclear leukocytes and monocytes. Polymorphonuclear leukocytes are mature cells that circulate freely in the blood with the ability to function as phagocytes—that is, they engulf microorganisms and cellular debris and release digestive enzymes known as lysosomes to destroy the invading microorganism. Monocytes also circulate freely in the blood, but upon entering tissues they enlarge and form macrophages which also function as phagocytes.

Unlike the phagocytic response, which is innate, the *specific* immune response is acquired. A highly selective response is mediated by lymphocytes for each type of antigen that invades the tissues. Upon initial exposure to the antigen, the response is weak. However, subsequent exposures trigger specialized "memory" cells that recognize the antigen and produce a stronger immune response. There are two types of specific immunity: cell mediated and humoral. Some antigens evoke a cell-mediated immune response, while others elicit a humoral immune response; reasons for this are unknown.

Cell-Mediated Immunity. This type of immunity is mediated by thymus-dependent lymphocytes, or T cells, which are derived from the thymus after maturation from stem cells produced by the bone marrow. T cells are the predominant type of lymphocyte found in the blood and lymph. The cell-mediated immune response is initiated when T cells become sensitized by contact with an antigen. The sensitized T cell reacts directly with the antigen. (See Figure 33-1.) T cells produce mediators known as *lymphokines*, which aid in the destruction of the antigen. Several subgroups of T cells have specific functions in the immune response. These cells include memory, cytotoxic, helper, and suppressor cells.

470

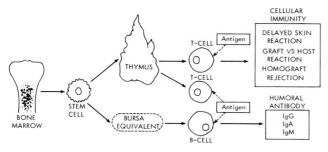

Figure 33-1. Origins of T cells and B cells and their role in immunity. (From O'Loughlin, J. M.: "Infections in the Immunosuppressed Patient," *Med. Clin. North Am.*, **59**:495–501, used with permission.)

Cellular immunity is measured clinically by *delayed hypersensitivity* skin testing. A small amount of antigen to which the patient has been previously exposed, is injected under the skin, and the injection site is observed for redness (erythema) and hardening (induration) at 24 and 48 hours. A normal positive response is manifested by presence of both erythema and induration, indicating that T lymphocytes and phagocytes have migrated to the area as part of the body's immune response. Usually three or more antigens are injected. Failure to respond to any of these is termed *anergy*. (See page 392.) Anergy occurs in protein-calorie malnutrition but is also seen in burns, cancer, various bacterial and viral infections, liver disease, uremia, chemotherapy, and so on.[1]

Humoral Immunity. This type of immune response is mediated by B- lymphocytes, or B cells. The site in which B cells are formed after maturation from stem cells is not known. (See Figure 33-1.) The humoral immune response does not involve a direct interaction between the lymphocyte and the antigen. Upon stimulation by an antigen, a B cell specific to the antigen differentiates into plasma cells. These produce *antibodies* or immunoglobulins (Ig) that react directly with the antigen. Five major classes of immunoglobulins are known: IgG, IgM, IgA, IgD, and IgE. Each is involved in a different kind of immune reaction. Antibodies are carried in the body fluids to the site of the invading antigen where they bind to it. The antigen–antibody complex is then phagocytized by polymorphonuclear leukocytes, monocytes, and macrophages. Antibodies also activate the blood complement system, consisting of a series of nine proteins that react sequentially in a cascade type of system, to bring about destruction of the antigen. Several mediators also participate in the humoral response. Examples are histamine, serotonin, and bradykinin.

Nutrition and Immune Function Malnutrition is the most common cause of secondary immunodeficiency.[2] Deficiencies of protein, vitamin A, B-complex, ascorbic acid, and zinc lead to characteristic skin lesions that serve as entry points for bacteria and subsequent infections. Protein and vitamin A deficiencies lead to damage to the intestinal mucosa with alterations in the number and type of flora. A review of the effect of specific nutrient deficiencies on immune function is included in the references at the end of this chapter.[3] Adequate protein synthesis is especially critical for immune function. Decreased immunocompetence is often seen in nutritionally depleted individuals or in those in whom protein catabolism exceeds protein synthesis. Among the changes that might occur with undernutrition are the following:

Cell-mediated immunity—lymphocyte T cells: depressed

Specific antibody production: often impaired. Skin tests to many antigens are frequently negative. Immunization of children who are severely malnourished may not be effective.

Humoral immunity—B cells: immunoglobulins IgG, IgM, and IgA are usually normal in malnutrition alone; in the presence of infection these immunoglobulins are usually elevated. Secretory IgA (S-IgA) secreted in the tears, nasal secretions, and saliva: depressed with malnutrition

Polymorphonuclear leukocytes and macrophages: normal levels in malnutrition, but bacterial killing may be impaired because of enzyme deficiency.

Complement system, except for C4, concentrations are depressed.

Physiologic Stress

Physiologic stress occurs in many hospitalized patients as a consequence of infections, fever, surgery, burns, or other trauma. Many patients are unable to ingest sufficient energy and protein to meet the increased needs imposed by stress. Compromised nutritional status has been shown to increase susceptibility to infection, to prolong the hospital stay, and to increase mortality rates.[4] The metabolic response during stress differs from that in fasting or starvation.

The Metabolic Response in Starvation The normal healthy person adapts to total fasting or starvation by utilizing bodily reserves to meet energy needs. Although the greatest reserves occur in the form of adipose tissue, the body preferentially utilizes glycogen as a potential source of glucose. Glycogen reserves are normally exhausted in less than 24 hours, however, after which protein from skeletal muscle is the primary source of energy. Amino acids are deaminated in the liver and the carbon skeleton is used for the synthesis of glucose. Nitrogen is excreted in the urine, resulting in a substantial negative nitrogen balance, approximating 12 g nitrogen per day, which represents a loss of about 75 g protein per day. After several days, the body attempts to conserve nitrogen and begins utilizing fatty acids for energy. Serum insulin levels fall, thereby permitting mobilization of fatty acids. The liver also converts fatty acids to ketones. Nitrogen losses decrease to about 4 g per day. As starvation continues, all tissues including the brain adapt to using ketones for energy. Urinary nitrogen losses show a further slight decrease. The metabolic rate and energy expenditures are lowered. Ultimately, in prolonged starvation fat reserves are depleted, visceral and plasma proteins are used for energy, and death results.

The Metabolic Stress Response The tendency of the body to conserve protein in the healthy individual undergoing starvation is reversed when physiologic stress is superimposed on starvation. An increase in the metabolic rate and accelerated tissue catabolism, mediated by hormonal changes, characterize the metabolic response to stress, as illustrated by the many changes that occur in infection (see the section on the metabolic consequences of infection following).

Infections

Nutrition and Infection The interaction between nutrition and infection is synergistic—that is, nutritional deficiency lowers resistance to infection, and infection aggravates existing malnutrition. Persons who are chronically undernourished not only succumb to infections more readily but have a longer period of recovery than do the well nourished. In the United States the vulnerable groups are the elderly who are poor or who lack incentive to eat properly, the chronically ill who have poor appetites, the young child living in a low-income area, and the teenager who follows a poor pattern of food intake. In the developing countries infants and preschool children are the most vulnerable.

Infection may have significant effects on nutritional status. The extent of the changes depends upon the nature and severity of the infectious disease, its duration, the presence of fever, and the previous nutritional status of the individual. Nutrient needs are generally increased during infection by the following mechanisms: (1) the stress reaction induces a catabolic response with increased losses of nitrogen, magnesium, potassium, phosphate, and zinc; (2) in severe infections or if fever is present, the increased metabolic rate raises energy needs; (3) anorexia decreases food intake; (4) nutrient losses may be increased due to increased perspiration, vomiting, or diarrhea; and (5) malabsorption, in enteric infections, may interfere with nutrient utilization.

Metabolic Consequences of Infection A number of metabolic, biochemical, and hormonal responses favor protein catabolism and altered fluid and electrolyte balance during infections. Several factors contribute to negative nitrogen balance: losses of urinary nitrogen are increased during catabolism; the resting metabolic expenditure is increased, especially if there is fever; and anorexia limits food intake. Although energy needs are increased, the utilization of glucose and fat in peripheral tissues is reduced; consequently, skeletal muscle is catabolized and amino acids are used for gluconeogenesis in the liver.

Responses of several hormones are altered in an attempt to meet the increased energy needs in infection. Increased levels of glucocorticoids, growth hormone, catecholamines, and glucagon work synergistically to increase glycogenolysis and gluconeogenesis. Normally ketogenesis is also enhanced by these hormones. During infection, however, ketogenesis is suppressed, probably due to high levels of circulating insulin, which inhibits lipolysis and ketone formation.[5,6] In spite of increased insulin levels glycogenolysis and gluconeogenesis persist, and hyperglycemia results. Impaired glucose utilization or insulin resistance by muscle results in catabolism of skeletal muscle protein for energy.

Branched-chain amino acids (leucine, isoleucine, valine) are oxidized in muscle to their ketoderivatives to provide energy for muscle function. The amino group is transaminated with pyruvate in muscle to form alanine and is transported to the liver. There alanine is deaminated and the nitrogen is converted to urea and is excreted; the remaining carbon skeleton undergoes gluconeogenesis and glucose is returned to muscle. Non-branched-chain amino acids from muscle are transported to the liver and used for gluconeogenesis. Available nitrogen is used for the synthesis of constituents needed for the immune response: lymphocytes, phagocytes, antibodies, components of the complement system, and lymphokines. Synthesis of a group of proteins called *acute-phase reactants* occurs also. These proteins increase in serum at the onset of the inflammatory response and are believed to modulate the immune response.[7] The increased synthesis of acute phase proteins is accompanied by decreased synthesis of albumin, leading to hypoalbuminemia.[5]

Losses of potassium, magnesium, and phosphorus during acute infections accompany nitrogen losses. Retention of salt and water occur due to the influence of mineralocorticoid and antidiuretic hormones. Shifts in plasma levels of certain minerals occur. For example, plasma zinc and iron levels fall while copper increases.[5] These appear to be protective mechanisms. Both zinc and iron are believed to be involved in the immune process, altering phagocytosis and bactericidal activity. Zinc is also needed for globulin synthesis and repair of tissue damage. Microorganisms require iron for growth; during infection leukocytes secrete lactoferrin, an iron-binding protein, thus making iron less available for promotion of bacterial growth.[8] During the acute phase of an infection provision of large amounts of iron may be detrimental.

Nutritional Considerations Perhaps the most important nutritional consequence of infection is the catabolic effect on protein metabolism. Even in mild infections some protein depletion occurs whether or not fever is present. Because of the body's decreased ability to utilize fat during an infection nitrogen losses may be substantial. Restoration of body cell mass is thus the primary goal of nutritional therapy.

The nitrogen losses that accompany stress are inevitable. Increasing the protein intake will not prevent negative nitrogen balance from occurring during the peak catabolic period following severe stress (5 to 10 days postinjury); however, it can improve nitrogen balance. Depending on the nature and severity of the infection, nitrogen losses may be as high as 16 to 18 g per day during the peak catabolic period.[9] Protein requirements during this period are based on measured urinary losses, with correction for integumental and fecal losses. When urinary nitrogen losses are not measured, the protein requirement can be estimated by determining the energy requirement, and providing a calorie to nitrogen ratio of 150:1 during stress.[9] This provides approximately 16 percent of calories as protein. For the moderately stressed patient, 1.5 to 2.0 g protein per kg will be needed.[9] In severe stress the ratio may range from 100:1 to 150:1.

In mild infections energy needs are estimated to be 20 percent over the resting metabolic expenditure, whereas energy expenditure in sepsis has been shown to increase as much as 70 percent.[9] Various formulas can be used to predict the approximate daily energy expenditure in patients with infections and other types of physiologic stress.[9,10] The formulas are based on the Harris–Benedict equation for predicting basal metabolic rate[11] and include factors for activity and injury or stress. One such formula is shown inside the back cover of this text.[9] Just as the activity factor increases with convalescence, the injury factor gradually subsides and energy expenditure decreases, necessitating a reduction in calorie and protein intake. Daily monitoring of weight can be used as a guide in determining appropriateness of the calorie intake. Some recommend that the calorie to nitrogen level should be maintained at 150:1 during the period of convalescence.[9]

Energy and protein needs for recovery from mild infections in previously well-nourished persons can usually be met by supplements to the regular diet. A variety of proprietary products is available, most providing about 1 kcal per ml. The carbohydrate sources in these products should be considered because those high in mono- and disaccharides present a high osmolar load to the intestine, and those high in lactose may not be well tolerated. (See Chapter 31.)

Individuals with marginal nutritional status with regard to vitamins are at increased risk for deficiencies of these vitamins during infectious disease. For these individuals, liberal intakes, two to three times the recommended dietary allowances, are needed.[12] No advantage of increased vitamin intake during simple infection has been demonstrated for those whose previous intake has been satisfactory.[13] Vitamin requirements are increased if infection is accompanied by inflammation and necrosis of tissue.

Nutritional Effects of Drug Therapy. Many antibiotics and antiinfectives cause mild gastrointestinal disturbances including nausea, vomiting, and diarrhea. Some specific side effects of the various drugs on nutrient utilization are outlined in Appendix B.

Fevers

Classification of Fevers FEVER is an elevation in body temperature above the normal which may occur in response to infection, inflammation, or unknown causes. It may be due to exogenous agents, such as bacteria or fungi, or to endogenous factors, such as antigen–antibody reactions, malignancy, or graft rejection. Exogenous factors produce fever through activation of phagocytes in bone marrow to release a fever-inducing hormone, endogenous pyrogen.[14] This hormone, in turn, is believed to induce synthesis of prostaglandins, which act as mediators in the initiation of fever by somehow influencing the thermoregulatory center in the anterior hypothalamus to increase its normal "setpoint" for body temperature. Drugs such as aspirin are effective in reducing fever because they inhibit prostaglandin synthesis.[14]

The duration of fever may be (1) short as in acute fevers of colds, tonsillitis, influenza, and so on or (2) chronic as in long-standing tuberculosis, or it may be intermittent as in malaria.

Metabolism in Fevers The metabolic effects of fevers, proportional to the elevation of body temperature and the duration, include the following:

1. An increase in the metabolic rate amounting to 13 percent for every degree Celsius rise in body temperature (7 percent for each degree Fahrenheit); an increase also in the restlessness and hence a greatly increased calorie need
2. Decreased glycogen stores and decreased stores of adipose tissue
3. Increased catabolism of proteins, especially in typhoid fever, malaria, typhus fever, poliomyelitis, and others; the increased nitrogen wastes place an additional burden on the kidneys
4. Accelerated loss of body water owing to increased perspiration and the excretion of body wastes
5. Increased excretion of sodium and potassium.

General Dietary Considerations The diet in fevers depends on the nature and severity of the pathologic conditions and upon the length of the convalescence. In general it should meet the following requirements:

Energy. The caloric requirement may be increased as much as 50 percent if the temperature is high and the tissue destruction is great. Restlessness also increases the caloric requirement. Initially, the patient may be able to ingest only 600 to 1,200 kcal per day, but this should be increased as rapidly as possible.

Protein. About 100 g protein or more is prescribed for the adult when a fever is prolonged. This will be most efficiently utilized when the calorie intake is liberal. High-protein beverages may be used as supplements to the regular meals.

Carbohydrates. Glycogen stores are replenished by a liberal intake of carbohydrates. Any sugars such as glucose, corn syrup, and cane sugar may be used. However, glucose is less sweet than some other sugars and consequently more of it can be used. Furthermore, it is a simple sugar which is absorbed into the bloodstream without the necessity for enzyme action.

Lactose, in some individuals, may increase fermentation in the small intestine resulting in diarrhea.

Fats. The energy intake may be rapidly increased through the judicious use of fats, but fried foods and rich pastries may retard digestion unduly.

Minerals. A sufficient intake of sodium chloride is accompanied by the use of salty broth and soups and by liberal sprinkling of salt on food. Generally speaking, foods are a good source of potassium, but a limited food intake might result in potassium depletion whenever fever is high and prolonged. Fruit juices and milk are relatively good sources of this element.

Vitamins. Fevers apparently increase the requirements for vitamin A and ascorbic acid, just as the B-complex vitamins are needed at increased levels proportionate to the increase in calories; that is, 0.5 mg thiamin, 0.6 mg riboflavin, and 6.6 mg niacin equivalents per 1,000 additional kcal. Oral therapy with antibiotics and drugs interferes with synthesis of some B-complex vitamins by intestinal bacteria, thus necessitating a prescription for vitamin supplements for a short time.

Fluid. The fluid intake must be liberal to compensate for the losses from the skin and to permit adequate volume of urine for excreting the wastes. From 2,500 to 5,000 ml per day is necessary, including beverages, soups, fruit juices, and water.

Ease of Digestion. Bland, readily digested foods should be used to facilitate digestion and rapid absorption. The food may be soft or of regular consistency. Although fluid diets may be used initially, there are some disadvantages: (1) most fluid diets occupy bulk out of all proportion to their caloric and nutrient values, so that reinforcement of liquids is essential; (2) a liquid diet sometimes increases abdominal distention to the point of acute discomfort, whereas solid foods may be better tolerated; (3) many patients experience less anorexia, nausea, and vomiting when they are taking solid foods.

Intervals of Feeding. Small quantities of food at intervals of 2 to 3 hours will permit adequate nutrition without overtaxing the digestive system at any one time. With improvement, many patients consume more food if given three meals and a bedtime feeding.

Diet in Fevers of Short Duration The duration of many fevers has been shortened by antibiotic and drug therapy, and nutritional needs are usually met without difficulty. During an acute fever the patient's appetite is often very poor, and small feedings of soft or liquid foods as desired should be offered at frequent intervals. (See Chapter 28.) Sufficient intake of fluids and salt is essential. If the illness persists for more than a few days, high-protein, high-calorie foods will need to be emphasized. (See High-Protein Diet, page 478.)

Diet in Tuberculosis Tuberculosis is an infectious disease caused by the bacillus *Mycobacterium tuberculosis*. It affects the lungs most often but may also be localized in other organs, such as the lymph nodes or kidneys, or it may be generalized. The initial infection is believed to be a rather benign process in which the tubercle bacilli enter the body but are kept in check by the body's cell-mediated immune system, and the disease heals spontaneously. The presence of the organisms constitutes a potential risk of active disease that often occurs years after the initial attack in susceptible persons.

Tuberculosis is a major cause of illness and death worldwide, with at least 3 million people dying each year.[15] The incidence in the United States has declined sharply since the turn of the century, with a case rate of 11.0 per 100,000 reported in 1982.[16]

The reduced incidence has been attributed to more effective chemotherapeutic agents, better housing, and improved nutrition, yet there is still concern among the elderly and those with increased susceptibility to disease, and in areas where inadequate housing, poverty, and poor sanitation prevail.

Pulmonary tuberculosis is accompanied by wasting of tissues, exhaustion, cough, expectoration, and fever. The acute phase resembles pneumonia, with high fever, and increased circulation and respiration. The chronic phase is accompanied by low-grade fever, and the metabolic rate is lower than in acute fevers. Because of the protracted illness, wasting may be considerable.

The individual with chronic tuberculosis often has increased energy needs in order to achieve desirable weight. From 2,500 to 3,000 kcal per day is usually satisfactory. A protein intake of 75 to 100 g helps regenerate the serum albumin levels, which are often low. Calcium is needed to promote healing of the tuberculous lesions. At least a quart of milk, or its equivalent, should be taken daily. Iron supplementation may be necessary if there has been hemorrhage. Carotene appears to be poorly converted to vitamin A so that the diet should provide as much preformed vitamin A as possible. In addition, a vitamin A supplement may be necessary. Ascorbic acid deficiency is frequently present, and additional amounts of citrus fruits or ascorbic acid supplementation are essential.

Nutritional Effects of Drug Therapy. Prolonged administration of chemotherapeutic agents used in the treatment of tuberculosis may have an adverse effect on certain of the B-complex vitamins. Isoniazid is an antagonist of vitamin B-6 and may inhibit the folate-dependent interconversion of glycine and serine. Low serum folate and megaloblastic anemia have been noted in patients receiving this therapy. Supplements of vitamin B-6 are indicated to prevent the peripheral neuritis characteristic of B-6 deficiency. See Appendix B for side effects of other chemotherapeutic agents.

Selection of Foods. During the acute state of the illness, a high-protein high-calorie fluid diet may be given as in other acute fevers, progressing to the soft and regular diets when improvement occurs. Most of these patients have very poor appetites. For some, a six-meal routine is best, whereas others eat better if they receive three meals and a bedtime feeding. Those responsible for planning meals should respect the patient's food idiosyncrasies. To this end, a selective menu from which the patient chooses foods each day is helpful. Other patients may eat better when they are not consulted in advance about their diets, thus introducing an element of surprise. Needless to say, every attention must be given to make meals as appetizing in appearance and taste as possible.

DIETARY COUNSELING

Failure of the patient to follow the prescribed drug regimen leads to great increases in recurrence and repeated hospitalization. Good nutrition is likewise important in preventing recurrence. The characteristics of a normal diet, with special emphasis on a liberal milk intake, protein-rich foods, fruits, and vegetables, must be pointed out. To increase the calcium and protein intake, 3 to 5 tablespoons of nonfat dry milk may be added to each 8 ounces of whole milk. If desired, fruit flavors or chocolate syrup may be added. This beverage supplementation is conveniently prepared, provides substantial nutritive value at minimum bulk, and is low in cost.

Because many of the patients with tuberculosis have low incomes, some assistance is necessary in providing practical measures to purchase the necessary foods. This entails not only additional welfare allowances in some instances but guidance in budgeting the food money. In families with low incomes it may not be practical to improve the diet of the patient alone, for additional allowances of money may be spent for the children's diet rather than for the patient. In such situations the best prophylaxis may well be the improvement of the diet for all members of the family.

Emphysema This lung disorder is characterized by enlargement of the air spaces beyond the terminal bronchioles and pathologic changes in the walls of the alveoli. Emphysema ranks second to coronary artery disease as a cause of disability compensation in the United States and accounts for 20,000 deaths each year in this country.[17] It occurs primarily in men over 40 years of age who have a long history of cigarette smoking and bronchitis. Other possible causes are air pollution and respiratory infections. Exertional dyspnea is often the first symptom and may be accompanied by chronic cough, wheezing, and fatigue. The course of the disease may be slow over many years or it may progress rapidly to the terminal stage in a few years. In early stages some patients may be obese, and the distress in breathing is further accentuated. Some improvement is noted when weight is brought within desirable levels.

Shortness of breath places a severe limitation on the ability to ingest an adequate diet, with the result that weight loss and tissue wasting are common. Chewing and swallowing require further effort, and the patient often stops short of satisfactory intake. Not infrequently the purchase and preparation of food, or seeking a place to eat a meal, require more effort than the patient can expend. Because the patient is unable to work, there may be insufficient income to purchase adequate food.

A soft high-calorie diet is usually indicated. Patients are especially short of breath after a night's sleep and experience difficulty in eating breakfast. Small, frequent feedings of concentrated foods should be used. High-protein commercial supplements are useful because they are concentrated, palatable, easy to prepare, and easy to ingest. Too many fibrous fruits and vegetables or meats requiring much chewing may necessitate an energy expenditure beyond that justified by the nutrient values obtained. The patient will eat very slowly, and should refrain from talking while eating, since the swallowing of air is responsible for much of the discomfort.

Protein Deficiency

Incidence and Etiology Findings from both the Ten-State Nutrition Survey and the Health and Nutrition Examination Survey (HANES) indicate that the vast majority of Americans receive sufficient protein, and severe protein deficiency is rare. The intake of protein may be inadequate under certain conditions. Strict weight-reduction diets, especially those that require fasting, can lead to depletion of tissue proteins. Chronic alcoholism and drug addiction also interfere with a satisfactory food intake, in part because the cost of the habit often leaves insufficient money for the purchase of an adequate diet. Ignorance of the essentials of an adequate diet and child neglect are contributing factors to malnutrition in children. Protein-calorie malnutrition as a principal world health problem in children has been discussed in Chapter 24.

Many pathologic conditions are aggravated by nutritional deficiency; conversely, an existing deficiency is likely to become more severe during illness.

1. Disturbances of the gastrointestinal tract frequently initiate nutritional deficiency because of interference with intake, digestion, or absorption of foods. Anorexia, nausea, vomiting, the discomfort of ulcers, the abdominal distention present in many illnesses, and the cramping associated with diarrhea preclude a satisfactory food intake. Many patients are afraid to eat and restrict their choice to a few foods that do not meet nutritional requirements. Even though the food intake may be adequate under normal circumstances, the increased motility that accompanies some disturbances does not permit sufficient time for digestion and absorption so that excessive amounts of nutrients are lost. In the malabsorption syndrome—sprue, for example—a reduction in the digestive enzymes and in the absorptive surfaces leads to great losses of all nutrients from the bowel.

2. Excessive protein losses result from proteinuria in certain renal diseases, from hemorrhage, from increased nitrogen losses in the urine during the catabolic phase accompanying injury and immobilization, and from exudates of burned surfaces or draining wounds. The increased catabolism that follows immobilization is not fully understood, but is related, at least in part, to an increased production of adrenocortical hormones. After an injury healthy individuals show greater nitrogen losses than do persons who have more limited reserves. During the acute stage of catabolism high-

protein high-calorie diets seem to have little effect on reducing the losses. Eventually, of course, such losses must be replaced.

3. An increased metabolic rate in fevers and in thyrotoxicosis is accompanied by increased destruction of tissue proteins.
4. In diseases of the liver the synthesis of plasma proteins may be reduced even though the supply of amino acids is satisfactory.

Clinical and Biochemical Signs of Protein Undernutrition Fatigue, loss of weight, and lower resistance to infection are among the symptoms presented by patients with protein deficiency. Because these are common to many pathologic conditions they are of little diagnostic value.

Underweight together with a history of recent weight loss is of particular concern in many disease conditions. Weight loss entails loss of tissue proteins as well as adipose tissue. Recovery from illness is often slow, and wound healing is prolonged because the essential amino acids for tissue repair are lacking. Anemia is sometimes observed because of a reduced synthesis of the protein globin. The immune response is impaired as patients become protein depleted.

After prolonged protein deficiency the concentration of the plasma proteins and the circulating blood volume are decreased. Low albumin levels indicate visceral protein deficit. Moreover, since plasma albumin is particularly important for the maintenance of oncotic pressure, severe hypoalbuminemia may result in nutritional edema. When edema occurs it is necessary to rule out impaired circulation and excretion that occur in cardiac or renal failure. Edema is a rather inconstant finding that is not directly related to the plasma protein level. Thus, an individual may be severely depleted of proteins and show no signs of edema. The serum transferrin level is a more sensitive indicator of visceral protein deficit than is albumin. Because of the shorter half-life of transferrin, 5 to 7 days, compared to a half-life of approximately 20 days for albumin, a decrease in transferrin levels can occur before a significant fall in albumin. Low levels of serum albumin and transferrin are associated with an increased incidence of anergy. Anergic patients are more susceptible to increased morbidity and mortality from infectious diseases.

Although the liver has an amazing ability to carry out its functions even under adverse conditions, a prolonged nutritional deficiency gradually reduces the regeneration of liver cells as well as the synthesis of many regulatory compounds. A deficit in the lipotropic factors and of the lipoproteins leads to a decreased mobilization of fats from the liver, and thus fatty infiltration reduces the efficiency of the organ. The liver is less able to neutralize the effects of toxic substances, and its cells may be damaged—sometimes beyond repair.

Nutritional Considerations Protein and energy requirements are increased in stress, infection, and trauma. Protein repletion cannot be accomplished by giving a patient a high protein diet for a few days. A diet adequate in calories and somewhat liberalized in protein is essential for several weeks to several months. The levels of protein and calories are equally important in achieving satisfactory tissue synthesis. If the calorie intake is insufficient, protein will be utilized to meet energy needs. On the other hand, protein intake beyond the body's need for essential amino acids will be wasted since the body has no capacity to store protein in the sense that it stores carbohydrate as glycogen or fat as adipose tissue.

Protein. A nitrogen-to-calorie ratio of 1 : 300 is satisfactory for maintenance; for anabolism the ratio is adjusted to 1 : 150. In stress, protein utilization is less efficient than during convalescence, thus, provision of 16 percent of the calculated energy needs as protein is customary. Most pre- and postoperative patients probably experience mild stress, whereas those with severe burns or multiple trauma would be described as severely stressed. During infection optimal protein intake is 1.5 to 2.0 g protein per kg per day.[9]

Energy. Several approaches are used to estimate energy needs, depending somewhat on personnel available. Some estimate the basal energy expenditure (BEE) on the basis of the patient's height, weight, age, and sex. Others calculate the basal energy total daily expenditure using the formula shown inside the back cover of this text.[9] The calorie requirement for anabolism is expressed as a multiple of the basal energy expenditure. Feedings given by way of the enteral route are used more efficiently than those administered parenterally; thus, the energy requirement is greater when intravenous feeding is used. Oral intakes of 35 kcal per kg per day result in positive nitrogen balance whereas 40 kcal per kg daily is needed if parenteral feeding is used.[18]

Management of the Diet A high-protein diet furnishes 100 to 125 g protein and includes at least 2,500 kcal. To consume these amounts is not difficult for an individual with a good appetite. Most patients who require these liberal diets have had an impaired appetite for some time, and only the continuous and determined effort on the part of the nurse and others working with the patient can help the patient toward the goal of adequate intake. Some patients prefer small meals with between-meal feedings, whereas for others three meals and an evening snack are more suitable. High-protein beverages aid in achieving maximum protein intake with a minimum increase in volume. A number of palatable, inexpensive, and convenient proprietary compounds using nonfat dry milk and casein as the principal sources of protein are also available.

For emaciated patients the amount of food and the concentration of protein are increased gradually until the gastrointestinal tract again becomes accustomed to handling more food, and until the heart and circulatory system can cope with the additional demands made on it. When the food intake by these patients is rapidly increased, circulatory failure and even death can occur.

DIETARY COUNSELING

Dietary counseling is initiated by an evaluation of the patient's present meal pattern and food intake. The patient needs to know why adequate calorie and protein intakes are essential. Practical suggestions are given for increasing the calorie intake (see page 379) and the protein intake. With a list of protein equivalents from which to choose, the patient is guided toward developing a meal pattern that more nearly meets his or her needs.

Protein Equivalents (6-8 g protein per unit)
1 cup milk or buttermilk
⅓ cup nonfat dry milk
1 ounce American-type cheese
¼ cup cottage cheese
1 egg
1 ounce meat, fish, or poultry
2 tablespoons peanut butter
8 ounces ice cream
⅔ cup milk pudding

From such a list patients select a combination that will be acceptable to them. Some will prefer additional amounts of milk, whereas others find larger portions of meat to be more acceptable. A high-protein diet need not strain the food budget since nonfat dry milk can be used in substantial amounts. Most patients, and those who cook for them, need practical suggestions, including recipes, for incorporating dry milk into eggnogs, milk shakes, custards, puddings, cream soups, and other prepared foods.

The individual who requires a high-protein high-calorie diet is likely to be one who finds it difficult to consume a large volume of food. One who has a daily intake of 55 g protein and 1,600 kcal does not readily consume 120 g protein and 2,500 kcal. The physician, nurse, and dietitian can help the patient recognize his or her needs, but only the patient can set goals that are realistic. Perhaps a regular meal pattern requires emphasis; skipping breakfast, for example, makes it difficult to consume enough food for the rest of the day. Possibly a high-protein high-calorie beverage can be substituted for a low-calorie beverage, or an additional portion of dessert can be eaten at bedtime.

Patients need to know whether their efforts are successful. Probably one of the better guides for the patient is gradual weight gain—1 to 2 pounds per week being a reasonable expectation. With improvement in the state of protein nutrition the patient will experience a greater sense of well-being.

High-Protein Diet

Characteristics and General Rules
Select ½ to ⅔ of the day's protein allowance from complete protein foods. Include some complete protein at each meal.
Divide the protein allowance as evenly as practical among the meals of the day.
To increase the protein content of liquid milk add 2 to 4 tablespoons nonfat dry milk to each cup of milk.

Include These Foods, or Their Nutritive Equivalents, Daily:
4 cups (1 quart) milk
7-8 ounces (cooked weight) meat, fish, poultry, or beans
2 eggs
6 servings vegetables and fruits including:
　1 serving green or yellow vegetable
　1 to 2 servings potato

1 to 2 servings other vegetable
One vegetable to be eaten raw daily
    1 serving citrus fruit—or other good source of ascorbic acid
    1 serving other fruit
6 servings bread and cereals including:
    1 serving whole-grain or enriched cereal
    5 slices whole-grain or enriched bread
Additional foods from the Fats-Sweets group including butter or margarine, sugars, desserts, or more of the
    listed foods to meet caloric needs.

Nutritive Value On the basis of specified amounts of foods above: protein, 125 g; kcal, 2,500. All vitamins
and minerals in excess of normal diet—see page 411.

Sample Menu

Breakfast
Fruit	Half grapefruit
Cereal	Oatmeal
Egg—1	Fried egg
Bread, whole-grain or enriched	Whole-wheat toast
Butter or margarine	Butter
Milk to drink and for cereal	Milk
Beverage	Coffee

Luncheon or Supper
Meat or substitute of egg, cheese, fish or poultry—large serving	Chicken soufflé / Mushroom sauce
Potato, macaroni, spaghetti, noodles or vegetable	Buttered green beans
Salad with dressing	Shredded carrot and raisin salad
Bread with butter or margarine	Whole-wheat roll and butter
Fruit	Fresh peaches
Milk—1 glass	Milk

Dinner
Meat, fish, or poultry—large serving	Broiled trout with parsley garnish
Potato	Creamed potato
Vegetable	Buttered spinach
Bread with butter or margarine	Rye bread with butter
Dessert	Lemon-flake ice cream
Milk	Brownies
Beverage	Milk
	Tea with lemon

Evening Nourishment
Eggnog—1 glass	Chocolate eggnog
Sandwich with cheese or equivalent	American cheese and tomato sandwich

High-Protein Fluid Diet

Characteristics and General Rules

From 2 to 4 tablespoons nonfat dry milk may be added to each cup of milk or it may be used in custards or
    cream soups.
Eggs are sometimes contaminated with *Salmonella*. Pasteurized eggnogs may be purchased and are prefer-
    able to those made with raw eggs.
The calorie intake is increased by adding butter to gruels and cream soups; adding sugar to beverages; and
    substituting light cream for part of the milk allowance.

Include These Foods, or Their Nutritive Equivalents, Daily:

6 cups milk
⅔ cup nonfat dry milk
4 eggs
1 - 2 ounces strained meat
½ cup strained cereal for gruel
1 cup citrus juice
½ cup tomato juice
¼ cup vegetable purée for cream soup
2 servings plain dessert—gelatin, Junket, custard, cornstarch pudding, ice cream, sherbet
2 - 3 tablespoons sugar
1 - 2 tablespoons butter or margarine
Cream for coffee, for gruel, and in milk
Tea, coffee, decaffeinated coffee, cocoa powder, carbonated beverages
Flavoring extracts

Nutritive Value protein, 110 g; kcal, 2,100.

Sample Menu

BREAKFAST
Citrus fruit juice
Cereal gruel with milk and sugar
Poached or soft-cooked egg
Hot beverage with cream, sugar

MIDMORNING
High-protein beverage

LUNCHEON OR SUPPER
Cream soup with butter
Tomato juice
High-protein milk, plain or flavored
Fruit-juice gelatin, cornstarch pudding, ice cream, or custard

MIDAFTERNOON
Malted milk or eggnog

DINNER
Broth with strained meat
Strained fruit juice
Milk, high-protein milk, or eggnog
Ice cream, Junket, custard, gelatin or plain pudding

EVENING
Eggnog, milk, shake, or plain milk
Ice cream, gelatin, or custard

References

1. Shizgal, H. M.: "Nutrition and Immune Function," *Surg. Annu.*, 13:15–29, 1981.
2. Chandra, R. K.: "Nutrition and Immune Responses," *Can. J. Physiol. Pharmacol.*, 61:290–94, 1983.
3. Beisel, W. R., et al.: "Single-Nutrient Effects on Immunologic Functions," *JAMA*, 245:53–58, 1981.
4. Weinsier, R. L., et al.: "A Prospective Evaluation of General Medical Patients During the Course of Hospitalization," *Am. J. Clin. Nutr.*, 32:418–26, 1979.
5. Keusch, G. T.: "Nutrition and Infections," *Compar. Ther.*, 8(5):7–15, 1982.
6. Bistrian, B. R.: "Interaction of Nutrition and Infection in the Hospital Setting," *Am. J. Clin. Nutr.*, 30:1228–30, 1977.
7. Beisel, W. R.: "Effects of Infection on Nutritional Status and Immunity," *Fed. Proc.*, 39:3105–08, 1980.
8. Weinberg, E. D.: "Infection and Iron Metabolism," *Am. J. Clin. Nutr.*, 30:1485–90, 1977.
9. Long, C. L.: "The Energy and Protein Requirements of the Critically Ill Patient," in Wright, R. A., and Heymsfield, S., eds. *Nutritional Assessment.* Blackwell Scientific Publications, Inc., Boston, 1984, pp. 157–81.
10. Apelgren, K. N., and Wilmore, D. W.: "Nutritional Care of the Critically Ill Patient," *Surg. Clin. North Am.*, 63:497–507, 1983.
11. Harris, J. A., and Benedict, F. G.: *A Biometric Study of Basal Metabolism in Man.*, Carnegie Institution of Washington. Pub. No. (279) 189–90, Washington, D.C., 1919.
12. Dionigi, R., et al.: "Nutrition and Infection," *J.P.E.N.*, 3:62–68, 1979.
13. Vitale, J. J.: "The Impact of Infection on Vitamin Metabolism: An Unexplored Area," *Am. J. Clin. Nutr.*, 30:1473–77, 1977.
14. Baracos, V., et al.: "Stimulation of Muscle Protein Degradation and Prostaglandin E_2 Release by Leukocytic Pyrogen (Interleukin-1). A Mechanism for the In-

creased Degradation of Muscle Protein During Fever," *N. Engl. J. Med.*, **308**:553–58, 1983.

15. Grzybowski, S.: "Tuberculosis: A Look at the World Situation," *Chest*, **84**:756–61, 1983.

16. Anonymous: "Tuberculosis—United States, 1982," *MMWR*, **32**:478–80, 1982.

17. Hoidal, J. R., and Niewoehner, D. E.: "Pathogenesis of Emphysema," *Chest*, **83**:679–85, 1983.

18. Blackburn, G. L., et al.: "Nutritional and Metabolic Assessment of the Hospitalized Patient," *J.P.E.N.*, **1**:11–22, 1977.

34

Nutrition in Surgical Conditions

High-Protein, High-Fat, Low-Carbohydrate Diet

Significant advances have been made in the area of surgical nutrition within the past two decades. A better understanding of the effects of stress on metabolism in infections, surgery, and trauma has had a major impact on nutritional management of surgical patients. This chapter will discuss nutritional considerations in selected surgical conditions and in the management of the trauma patient. Numerous preparations suitable for oral, enteral, or parenteral administration are now available for nutritional support of surgical patients. These were described in Chapter 28. The student is encouraged to review the material and to study supplementary material that describes specific characteristics of various proprietary products.

The Surgical Patient— General Considerations

Effects of Surgery on the Nutritive Requirements Good nutrition before and after surgery ensures fewer postoperative complications, better wound healing, shorter convalescence, and lower mortality. The patient whose preoperative nutritional state is poor is at increased risk when undergoing major surgery. Persons with chronic diseases are especially likely to have less than optimal nutriture. Serious malabsorption of nutrients may occur especially in liver diseases and those involving the gastrointestinal tract. Extensive losses of nutrients and fluids may have occurred through hemorrhage, vomiting, or diarrhea.

The extent of the deficiency is manifested by weight loss, poor wound healing, decreased intestinal motility, anemia, edema, or dehydration, and the presence of decubitus ulcers. The circulating blood volume and the concentration of the serum proteins, hemoglobin, and electrolytes may be reduced.

After surgery or injury the need for nutrients is increased as a result of loss of blood, plasma, or pus from the wound surface; hemorrhage from the gastrointestinal or pulmonary tract; vomiting; and fever. During immobilization, the loss of some nutrients such as protein is accelerated.

A fairly simple operation often involves moderate deficiency in food intake for a few days after the operation. Some nutrients may be supplied by parenteral fluids, but the full needs of the body usually are not met by that means alone. Provided that adequate oral intake is rapidly resumed, the metabolic losses are not of serious consequence. On the other hand, adequate oral intake is often delayed for a considerable period after cardiac or gastrointestinal surgery. Metabolic losses are great and alternative methods of nutritional support are needed.

Preoperative Nutritional Assessment Evaluation of nutritional status should be a routine part of preoperative assessment. A brief dietary history and clinical observations, together with anthropometric and biochemical measurements identify those likely to be at increased risk for complications. (See Chapters 23 and 26.) One group has developed a formula based on serum albumin and transferrin levels, triceps skinfold, and delayed hypersensitivity skin testing measurements to predict risk of complications in patients undergoing gastrointestinal surgery.[1] Actual morbidity and mortality increase significantly as predicted risk increases.

Nutritional Considerations The objectives in the dietary management of surgical conditions are (1) to improve the preoperative nutrition whenever the operation is not of an emergency nature, (2) to maintain correct nutrition after operation or injury insofar as possible, and (3) to avoid harm from injudicious choice of foods.

Protein. A satisfactory state of protein nutrition ensures rapid wound healing by providing the correct assortment and quantity of essential amino acids, increases the resistance to infection, exerts a protective action on the liver against the toxic effects of anesthesia, and reduces the possibility of edema at the site of the wound. The presence of edema is a hindrance to wound healing and, in operations on the gastrointestinal tract, may reduce motility, thus leading to distention.

The protein status of surgical patients is of special concern because the postoperative complication rate is increased in patients who are protein depleted.[2] It is not always realistic to fully replace protein losses before surgery because the disease process itself may be such as to preclude a satisfactory intake of food. For selected patients, parenteral administration of amino acids and adequate calories is useful. The extent to which surgery should be delayed in order to improve the nutritional state is obviously a highly individual matter.

Protein catabolism is increased for several days immediately after surgery or injury; patients are characteristically in negative nitrogen balance even though the protein intake may be appreciable. Well-nourished persons lose more nitrogen than poorly nourished persons whose labile protein stores are already depleted. The degree of negative balance can be reduced at higher intakes of protein and calories.

The level of protein to be used in preoperative and postoperative diets depends on the previous state of nutrition, the nature of the operation, and the extent of the postoperative losses. Intakes of 1.0 to 1.5 g per kg, or about 100 g protein, are satisfactory for elective general surgery patients.[3]

Energy. The weight status is an important pre- and postoperative consideration, for it serves as a guide to the caloric level to be recommended. Without sufficient caloric intake, tissue proteins cannot be synthesized. Excessive metabolism of body fat may lead to acidosis, whereas depletion of the liver glycogen may increase the likelihood of damage to the liver. Some recommend 35 to 45 kcal per kg per day for maximal utilization of amino acids for protein synthesis.[4]

Obesity constitutes a hazard in surgery. Whenever possible, it should be corrected, at least in part, by using one of the calorie-restricted diets. (See page 372.) Rapid weight loss results in loss of lean body mass and should be avoided.

Vitamins. Ascorbic acid is especially important for wound healing and should be provided in increased amounts before and after surgery. Vitamin K is of concern to the surgeon, since the failure to synthesize vitamin K in the small intestine, the inability to absorb it, or the defect in conversion to prothrombin is likely to result in bleeding. Hemorrhage is especially likely to occur in patients who have diseases of the liver.

Minerals. Phosphorus and potassium are lost in proportion to the breakdown of body tissue. In addition, derangements of sodium and chloride metabolism may occur subsequent to vomiting, diarrhea, perspiration, drainage, anorexia, and diuresis or renal failure. The detection of electrolyte imbalance and appropriate parenteral fluid therapy requires careful study of clinical signs and biochemical evaluation.

Iron-deficiency anemia occurs in association with malabsorption or excessive blood loss. Diet alone is ineffective in correction of anemia, but a liberal intake of protein and ascorbic acid, together with administration of iron salts, is of value in convalescence. Transfusions are usually required to overcome severe reduction in hemoglobin level. Zinc losses are increased by stress. Deficiency may impair cell-mediated immunity and may interfere with wound healing.

Fluids. The sources of water and the large amounts of fluids lost daily by the normal individual are outlined on page 139. The fluid balance may be upset before and after surgery owing to failure to ingest normal quantities of fluids and to increased losses from vomiting, exudates, hemorrhage, diuresis, and fever. A patient should not go to operation in a state of dehydration, since the subsequent dangers of acidosis are great. When dehydration exists prior to operation, parenteral fluids are administered if the patient is unable to ingest sufficient liquid by mouth. After major surgery the fluid balance is maintained by parenteral fluids until satisfactory oral intake can be established.

Planning the Preoperative Diet Patients who have lost much weight prior to surgery benefit considerably by ingesting a high-protein, high-calorie diet (see page 379) for even a week or two before surgery. The diet may be of liquid, soft, or regular consistency depending on the nature of the pathologic condition. Parenteral nutrition or semisynthetic fiber-free diets are sometimes used. In addition, the maintenance of metabolic equilibrium as in diabetes or other diseases must not be overlooked.

When surgery is delayed in order to improve the nutritional status, each day's intake should represent such improvement in nutrition that the delay is justified. This necessitates constant encouragement by the nurse and dietitian; it likewise requires imagination in varying the foods offered to the patient and ingenuity in getting the patient to eat. Foods that provide a maximum amount of nutrients in a minimum volume are essential. Small feedings at frequent intervals are likely to be better accepted than large meals that cannot be fully consumed.

For additional protein, milk beverages may be fortified with nonfat dry milk or commercial protein supplements. Strained meat in broth may be used when patients are unable to eat other meats. Fruit juices fortified with glucose polymers and butter incorporated into foods are also useful for increasing the calorie intake.

Food and fluids are generally allowed until midnight just preceding the day of operation, although a light breakfast may be given when the operation is scheduled for afternoon and local anesthesia is to be used. It is essential that the stomach be empty prior to administering the anesthesia so as to reduce the incidence of vomiting and the subsequent danger of aspiration of vomitus. When an operation is to be performed on the gastrointestinal tract, a diet low in residue (page 414) may be ordered 2 to 3 days before operation. In acute abdominal conditions such as appendicitis and cholecystitis, no food is allowed by mouth until nausea, vomiting, pain, and distention have passed in order to prevent the danger of peritonitis.

Planning the Postoperative Diet Resumption of oral intake depends on the nature of the surgery and the individual's progress. After minor surgery, liquids are often tolerated within a few hours and rapid progression to a normal diet is made. After major surgery, however, oral intake may be delayed for days. Alternative methods for partial or complete nutritional support are provided by conventional intravenous feedings, semisynthetic fiber-free diets, tube feedings, or total parenteral nutrition. (See Chapter 28.)

Progression of Oral Feeding. Motility of the gastrointestinal tract is diminished after abdominal surgery. Small intestine motility recovers rapidly but return of

gastric motility may take 24 hours or longer, and colonic motility 3 to 5 days. Patients are given nothing by mouth for the first 24 hours after surgery. Oral feeding is begun after gastrointestinal secretions are being produced and peristalsis resumes. Feeding should not be delayed once such function has returned. The accumulation of gastrointestinal secretions may result in a feeling of fullness. Moreover, the wound strength is sufficient to permit digestion of food.

Progression from ice chips to sips of water, then clear liquids and full liquids is made in accordance with the patient's tolerance. Patients usually respond better once they are given solid foods. Initially, the feedings are small and may be restricted to a low-residue diet. (See also Chapter 30.) Foods high in protein and fat are believed to be less distending than those which are high in carbohydrate. Perhaps of greater importance is the emphasis on eating slowly and in small amounts to reduce the amount of air which is swallowed. As the patient improves, the selection of foods is that of a soft or regular diet, depending on the nature of the surgery.

Diet in Specified Surgical Conditions

Upper Alimentary Tract The period between full extraction of teeth and satisfactory adjustment to new dentures may take several weeks. For 1 or 2 days after the surgery, it may be necessary to restrict the diet to liquids taken through a drinking tube. Thereafter, any soft foods that require little if any chewing may be used for 3 weeks or longer.

Radical surgery of the mouth necessitates the use of full fluids or puréed foods, but immediately after surgery one of the regimens for formula feeding described in Chapter 28 may be used. After an operation on the esophagus, a gastrostomy formula feeding is used.

After tonsillectomy the patient is given cold fluids including milk, bland fruit juices, ginger ale, plain ice cream, and sherbets. Tart fruit juices and fibrous foods must be avoided. On the second day, soft foods such as custard, plain puddings, soft eggs, warm but not hot cereals, strained cream soups, mashed potatoes, and fruit and vegetable purées may be tolerated. As a rule, the regular diet is swallowed without difficulty within the week.

Gastric Restrictive Surgery Surgical treatment is used for selected patients who meet certain criteria and in whom conventional management of obesity has failed. Some groups consider patients eligible if their weight is 100 pounds or more over the "ideal";

others use 100 percent over the "ideal" weight as a criterion. Gastric surgery has largely replaced the jejunoileal bypass procedure for obesity because of serious long-term consequences associated with the latter. Both gastric bypass and gastric partitioning, or gastroplasty, are used. These procedures exclude 90 percent of the gastric reservoir.

Gastric Bypass.   In this procedure, the stomach is divided by means of several rows of staples into a small proximal pouch of 50- to 60-ml capacity, and a nonfunctioning distal compartment. The small proximal pouch is then anastomosed to the jejunum. (See Figure 34-1.) *Gastroplasty* retains normal anatomical structure by incomplete staple division of the stomach. A small opening, approximately 12 mm or ½ inch in diameter, permits passage of food between the small upper pouch and the distal stomach. A modification of this procedure is the vertical banded gastroplasty. These procedures result in rapid filling and slow emptying of the stomach, giving a feeling of satiety and forcing the individual to eat small meals. Weight loss is attributed to the reduction in food intake. Nausea and vomiting follow overindulgence. Ingestion of hypertonic sweets can provoke symptoms of the dumping syndrome and diarrhea. A number of complications, including malnutrition, have been associated with these procedures.[5] Negative nitrogen balance for periods up to 3 months and reduced intake of all nutrients are contributing factors. Gastric bypass is associated with more frequent operative risk and postoperative complications, but weight loss is more predictable than with gastroplasty.[6,7]

Dietary Management.   After gastric surgery, the usual progression is nothing by mouth until bowel sounds are heard, followed by hourly sips of water, then clear liquids for 24 to 48 hours, after which blenderized foods thin enough to go through a straw are permitted. Liquid and blenderized foods are used for 8 weeks. Gradual introduction of very soft foods are then made with progression to solids. The volume of the feeding is small so as not to cause distention. Frequent feedings are needed in order to meet energy and protein needs. Dietary considerations are similar to those in the dumping syndrome. (See page 486.) Close monitoring of intake is needed. Multivitamins, especially of the B-complex, iron, and other mineral supplements, are used.

Gastrectomy   A number of problems arise after gastrectomy, and their treatment should be anticipated. Weight loss is common, and most patients fail to regain weight to desirable levels. The loss of a reservoir for food means that small feedings given at frequent intervals must be used if sufficient nutrients are to be ingested. Moreover, the absence of pepsin and hydrochloric acid entails the entire digestion of protein by the enzymes of the small intestine. Fat utilization is often impaired because of inadequate biliary and pancreatic secretions or defective mixing of food with the digestive juices. Intestinal motility is frequently increased. After total gastrectomy the lack of gastric acidity may permit bacterial overgrowth that disrupts the vitamin B-12–intrinsic factor complex and deconjugates bile salts, resulting in malabsorption. This was discussed in Chapter 31.

Iron is less readily absorbed and hypochromic microcytic anemia is common. After total gastrectomy the absence of intrinsic factor eventually leads to macrocytic anemia unless injections of vitamin B-12 are given. Disturbed bone mineral metabolism due to vitamin D deficiency and calcium malabsorption have been reported following gastrectomy.[8]

Proximal gastric vagotomy inhibits gastric secretion but leaves the pylorus intact so that gastric emptying is nearly normal. Nutritional consequences are thus minimized.

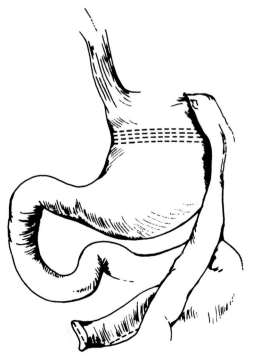

Figure 34-1.   Gastric bypass. The stomach is divided into a small proximal pouch and a nonfunctioning distal pouch. The proximal pouch is then anastomosed to the jejunum. (From Bothe, A., et al.: "Energy Regulation in Morbid Obesity by Multidisciplinary Therapy," *Surg. Clin. North Am.*, **59**:1017-31, 1979, used with permission.)

Dietary Progression. Oral feedings vary widely from one patient to another. The usual sequence consists of hourly feedings of 60 to 90 ml fluids for several days with progression from water to full liquids by the third day. Thereafter, the diet increases from day to day according to the individual's tolerance for food. By the fourth or fifth day, soft low-fiber foods are used. Eggs, custards, thickened soups, cereals, crackers, milk, and fruit purées are suitable. Tender meats, cottage cheese, and puréed vegetables are the next foods added. Meals are divided into five or six small feedings daily with emphasis on foods high in protein and fat; carbohydrate is kept relatively low. The selection of foods allowed for the Fiber-Restricted Diet (Chapter 28) may be used initially. In some cases, milk, fruit, and vegetables are temporarily omitted from the diet. Many patients progress more satisfactorily if no liquids are taken with meals, and if the diet continues to be low in carbohydrate, especially the simple sugars. Patients who have had proximal gastric vagotomy usually need not restrict their diet.

Dumping Syndrome After convalescence from gastric surgery a relatively high proportion of patients experience distressing symptoms about 10 to 15 minutes after eating. There is a sense of fullness in the epigastrium with weakness, nausea, pallor, sweating, and dizziness. The pulse rate increases and the patient seeks to obtain relief by lying down for a few minutes. Vomiting and diarrhea are infrequently present. Weight loss is common because of insufficient intake and malabsorption. A small percentage of patients who develop this syndrome continue to have severe symptoms as long as 10 years after the surgery. The late postprandial dumping syndrome, occuring 1½ to 3 hours after eating, is less common and is characterized by symptoms of reactive hypoglycemia.

The exact etiology of the dumping has not been established but may be partly explained as follows: Ingestion of large amounts of easily hydrolyzed carbohydrates following loss of the pylorus rapidly introduces a hyperosmolar mixture into the proximal intestine. Fluid withdrawn from the extracellular space to dilute this mixture leads to distention and the cardiovascular symptoms. Both the gastrointestinal and the vasomotor symptoms have been attributed to release of vasoactive hormones from the small intestine. Newer operative procedures such as proximal gastric vagotomy are usually not accompanied by symptoms of dumping.

Modification of the Diet. Dietary regimens developed to alleviate the symptoms of the dumping syndrome emphasize the following: (1) avoidance of sugar and concentrated forms of carbohydrate, (2) liberal protein, (3) small frequent feedings, and (4) dry meals with fluids taken only between meals.

To control early postprandial symptoms, carbohydrate is limited to 100 to 120 g per day. With carbohydrate restriction dietary fat is increased to provide needed calories and to retard gastric emptying. Six small meals are given daily; meals must be eaten regularly without omission. Liquids low in carbohydrate are taken 30 to 60 minutes after meals. Foods and beverages should be of moderate temperature. The diet is individualized in accordance with the patient's food tolerances; many do not tolerate milk. Meals should be eaten slowly and followed by a short rest.

In the late dumping syndrome, carbohydrate is initially limited to 50 g per day and gradually increased to 60 to 80 g per day for the first year after surgery. Thereafter, up to 100 g carbohydrate daily is permitted. Frequent small feedings are needed to prevent symptoms of hypoglycemia. Fluids at meals need not be restricted.

High-Protein, High-Fat, Low-Carbohydrate Diet

Characteristics and General Rules
1. Initially, the amount of carbohydrate permitted is severely restricted; it is gradually increased as the patient's condition warrants. Carbohydrates must be measured accurately.
2. Liberal portions of proteins and fats are used.
3. Six small meals are given daily.
4. Liquids are taken 30 to 60 minutes after meals.
5. Multiple vitamin and mineral supplements are prescribed.
6. Rest before and after meals, eating slowly, and chewing well are essential.
7. Foods to avoid include milk, ice cream and other frozen desserts; sugars, sweets, candy, syrup, chocolate; gravies and rich sauces.
8. The composition of the two routines is approximately:

	Routine I	Routine II
Carbohydrate, g	95	125
Protein, g	95	125
Fat, g	83	110
kcal	1,500	2,000

Foods Allowed

Meat, fish, poultry—all kinds: broiled, baked, poached, stewed, grilled; luncheon meats without cereal filler
Eggs—2 to 3; poached, scrambled, coddled, shirred, hard cooked
Bread—enriched toast, zwieback, melba toast; only one slice with each feeding.
Bread substitutes—lima beans, sweet corn, cooked dried beans and peas; saltines, soda crackers; grits, noodles, macaroni, rice, spaghetti; parsnips, boiled potato, mashed potato, sweet potato. See Table A-4, Bread List, for equivalents.
Cereals—thick, cooked, only one serving
Vegetables—all kinds, not more than one serving per meal
Fruits—fresh, canned, or frozen without sugar. Drained of all liquid. Fruit juices may be taken 30 to 60 minutes after meals.
Fats—butter or margarine, crisp bacon, cream cheese, whipping cream
Nuts—when tolerated, plain or salted. Chew thoroughly.
Miscellaneous—olives, pimiento, salt, lemon or lime juice on fish, and so on.

Sample Menu Plans for Patients with Dumping Syndrome

Routine I

MORNING
2 eggs, poached
1 slice toast with
1 teaspoon butter or margarine

MIDMORNING
2 tablespoons smooth peanut butter
3 saltines

NOON
3 ounces ground round
¼ cup noodles with
1 teaspoon butter or margarine
2 halves unsweetened peaches

MIDAFTERNOON
¼ cup tuna with
1 teaspoon mayonnaise on
1 slice bread

EVENING
3 ounces roast leg of lamb
½ cup mashed potato with
1 teaspoon butter or margarine
½ cup carrots with
1 teaspoon butter or margarine
1 half unsweetened pear

BEDTIME
2 ounces cold chicken on
    1 slice bread

Routine II

Same
Same
Same

Same
6 saltines

4 ounces ground round
½ cup noodles
Same
Same
½ cup asparagus with
1 teaspoon butter or margarine

½ cup tuna with
2 teaspoons mayonnaise
Same

4 ounces roast leg of lamb
Same
Same
Same
Same
½ cup unsweetened applesauce

2 ounces cold chicken on
    1 slice bread with
    1 teaspoon mayonnaise
    1 half unsweetened pear

Intestinal Surgery Obstruction, persistent ileitis or diverticulitis, perforation, and malignancy are among the reasons for removal of a section of the ileum (ILEECTOMY) or colon (COLECTOMY). A permanent opening is made in the abdominal wall for elimination of wastes. Following removal of part of the ileum and colon, the proximal end of the ileum is attached to the opening (ILEOSTOMY). Because the absorptive function of the colon has been eliminated by the surgery, the waste material is fluid and continuous. Fluid, sodium, and potassium losses may be considerable, fat absorption is often poor, and vitamin B-12 absorption is reduced or absent.

A COLOSTOMY consists in attaching the proximal end of the resected colon to the opening in the abdominal wall. Some ability to absorb water is retained so that feces are more or less formed, and bowel regularity can be reestablished.

After any operation on the small intestine or colon, the initial oral intake is restricted to clear fluids and followed with a low-residue diet as a rule. Patients with an ileostomy are usually young and require a good deal of guidance and support from the nurse and dietitian. Gradually, they may add foods moderately low in fiber, but each food should be tested for tolerance before introducing a second. Many patients find that they cannot tolerate the following foods: nuts, seeds and skins of fruits, onion, lettuce, cabbage, peas, cucumber, sweet corn, mushrooms, and raisins.[9] Weight loss may be considerable, and a high-protein, high-calorie diet is generally required. Vitamin B-12 injections are required to prevent the occurrence of macrocytic anemia in later years. Good food sources of sodium and potassium should be recommended to the patient with an ileostomy to compensate for increased losses.

After extensive small bowel resection, as in Crohn's disease, absorption of dietary oxalates is increased, hyperoxaluria occurs, and may be accompanied by fat malabsorption, increasing the possibility of renal stones.[10] A diet low in fat and restricted in oxalates is used.

Removal of the ileum reduces the bile salt pool, thereby lowering the concentration of conjugated bile salts in the jejunum for hydrolysis of fats. Unabsorbed fatty acids and bile salts may provoke diarrhea. Parenteral administration of vitamin B-12 is indicated.

Colostomy is performed more frequently on elderly persons. In time they may resume an essentially normal diet, but usually they require some counseling concerning the foods required for nutritive adequacy. They too require emotional support as well as assurance that foods will not be harmful.

Other Abdominal Operations The principles outlined on page 484 pertain to the planning of diet following appendectomy, cholecystectomy, and other abdominal operations. Adynamic ileus is present longer following cholecystectomy and hysterectomy than after removal of the appendix. Patients who have had the gallbladder removed may require a fat-restricted diet for several weeks after which a regular diet is used.

Following peritonitis and intestinal obstruction, nothing whatever is given by mouth until gastrointestinal function has been resumed. Drainage of the stomach and upper intestine is essential until there is reduction of distention and passage of gas. This may require several days, during which time nutrition is maintained by intravenous therapy. When the patient shows tolerance for water, broth, and weak tea, a low-residue diet is introduced cautiously.

See Chapters 38 and 40 for nutritional considerations following coronary bypass surgery for advanced coronary artery disease and renal transplantation, respectively.

Fractures Following fractures there is a tremendous catabolism of protein, which may not be reversed for several weeks. Nitrogen loss is accompanied by loss of phosphorus, potassium, and sulfur. Fever and infection may further accentuate such losses.

Calcium loss is also great but calcium therapy may lead to the formation of renal calculi and should not be attempted until the cast is removed and some mobilization is possible.

A liberal intake of protein is essential to permit restoration of the protein matrix of the bone, so that calcium can be deposited. Sufficient calories to permit maximum use of the protein for synthesis should be provided.

The Trauma Patient

Trauma is the fourth leading cause of death in the United States and the leading cause of death for persons aged 1 to 38 years. About 12 percent of hospital beds are occupied by trauma patients. The economic cost in terms of death, disability, and loss of productivity due to trauma amounts to more than $83 billion annually.[11]

In many areas availability of excellent emergency care, regional trauma centers, and specialty intensive care units has made possible the survival of patients with major injuries from automobile accidents, gunshot wounds, industrial accidents, fires, and so on. Of great concern after these patients are stabilized is prevention of late mortality due to sepsis or multiple organ failure. Early administration of aggressive nutritional support can improve the likelihood of survival by providing energy, protein to ameliorate the catabolic response and for synthesis of acute-phase proteins, and other nutrients essential for the immune response.

The Hormonal Response   The initial period following trauma, referred to as shock, is accompanied by decreases in the metabolic rate and energy expenditure as well as reductions in blood volume and blood pressure. This phase is somewhat transitory and is followed by a period of days or weeks during which protein and fat catabolism persist, sodium and water are retained, and potassium is excreted. The metabolic consequences of hormonal action in response to stress were discussed in Chapter 33. This section will focus on a brief description of the specific actions initiated by each of the four major hormones involved in the stress response.

Antidiuretic Hormone.   A reduction in blood volume activates the hormonal response following trauma. Release of antidiuretic hormone (ADH) from the pituitary results in decreased water clearance in the kidneys and subsequent water retention and may be manifested clinically by oliguria. Return of ADH levels to normal occurs when blood volume is restored.

Adrenocorticotropic Hormone.   ACTH causes the release of aldosterone and cortisol from the adrenals. Aldosterone is of primary importance in regulation of interstitial fluid volume and control of blood pressure. Through its action, the kidney retains sodium and excretes potassium. (See page 521.) After injury or trauma, one of the earliest changes is an increase in the plasma cortisol level. Cortisol stimulates gluconeogenesis by increasing liver enzymes. At the same time, it enhances muscle protein catabolism and lipolysis so that amino acids and fatty acids are available as energy substrates. The net effect is that glucose production has priority over muscle protein conservation.

Catecholamines.   The catecholamines, epinephrine and norepinephrine, are released from the adrenal medulla in response to trauma and stress. These hormones, sometimes called the hormones of stress, act in two ways. They stimulate release of free fatty acids from adipose tissue for use as an energy substrate in the liver, kidney, lung, heart, and skeletal muscle. The liver can also form ketone bodies from the fatty acids,

thereby providing another energy source. (See page 92.) In spite of increased plasma levels of fatty acids, peripheral tissue uptake is reduced, however. In addition to their role in gluconeogenesis, catecholamines contribute to the hyperglycemia often seen in trauma patients. Through catecholamine release, glycogenolysis occurs, insulin release from the pancreas is suppressed while that of glucagon is increased, and impaired glucose utilization or insulin resistance by muscle occurs.

Glucagon.   Increased levels of glucagon in trauma patients are brought about by the action of ACTH and catecholamines. The increased amount of glucagon relative to insulin has a catabolic effect. Glucagon acts to increase the blood glucose level by hepatic gluconeogenesis and by enhancing glycogenolysis and oxidation of fats.

Through the synergistic action of these four hormones the metabolic response to trauma and stress results in loss of ability to conserve protein, lipid catabolism, retention of sodium and water to increase the blood volume, and enhanced potassium excretion. Prolonged catabolism of muscle protein and of fat due to the hormonal response may lead to muscle wasting, respiratory failure, and death. The hormonal response subsides when appropriate action is initiated, such as correction of fluid and electrolyte imbalance, drainage of sepsis, and surgical intervention.

Levels of Stress   The magnitude of the metabolic changes associated with stress vary with the nature, severity, and duration of stress, and the individual patient. Characteristic changes include increases in urinary nitrogen excretion, blood levels of glucose and lactate, the glucagon-to-insulin ratio, and oxygen consumption. On the basis of these metabolic changes, several levels or stages of stress have been described.[3] (See Table 34-1.)

Energy and Protein Requirements.   The energy requirements for the various levels of stress are not precisely known. However, the hypermetabolic patient is now thought to require fewer calories than was formerly believed. Even in major burns, the most severe form of stress, the resting metabolic expenditure rarely increases more than twofold.[12] Protein needs, on the other hand, may be greater than previously thought. Twenty percent or more of calories as protein has been recommended in the treatment of stress.[3] This corresponds to a nonprotein calorie-to-nitrogen ratio of 100:1. The nutritional needs of the trauma patient and the critically ill are often pro-

Table 34-1. **Classification of Stress***

	Level of Stress			
Factor	0 Uncomplicated Starvation	1 Elective General Surgery	2 Multiple Trauma	3 Sepsis
Urinary nitrogen, g per day	5	5–10	10–15	>15
Plasma lactate, μM/liter	100 ± 5	1,200 ± 200	1,200 ± 200	2,500 ± 500
Plasma glucose, mg/dl	100 ± 20	150 ± 25	150 ± 25	250 ± 50
Oxygen-consumption index, ml/m^2	90 ± 10	130 ± 6	140 ± 6	160 ± 10
Glucagon : insulin	2 ± 0.5	2.5 ± 0.8	3.0 ± 0.7	8 ± 1.5
Respiratory quotient	0.7	0.85	0.85	0.85 early 1.00 late

* Adapted from Cerra, F. B.: *Pocket Manual of Surgical Nutrition.* The C. V. Mosby Company, St. Louis, 1984.

vided by means of total parenteral nutrition. Guidelines for energy and protein requirements of these patients are presented in Table 34-2.

Most conventional solutions infused by way of a central vein are extremely high in carbohydrate. (See Chapter 28.) In recent years greater appreciation of the consequences of overfeeding the critically ill patient with high glucose loads has led to new theories regarding the appropriate proportions of carbohydrate, protein, and lipid in these solutions.[13,14] The optimal amounts of these nutrients are currently believed to vary in specific states of organ failure. Some examples follow.

Burns Tremendous losses of protein, salts, and fluid take place when large areas of the body have been burned. Energy expenditure following major burns is increased up to 200 percent above basal needs, and the greatly increased nutritive requirements continue for weeks or months. Several formulas for estimating daily energy needs of burn patients are available.[16] One such formula is shown inside the back cover of this text.[12] Another commonly used formula[17] for burns covering more than 20 percent of the body surface is as follows:

Adults: 25 kcal (preburn weight in kilograms) + 40 kcal (percent burn)
Children: 40 to 60 kcal (preburn weight in kilograms) + 40 kcal (percent burn)

Thus, a patient weighing 70 kg who has sustained a

Table 34-2. **Energy and Protein Needs in Stress***

	Level of Stress				
	0	1	2	3 (early)	3 (late)
Estimated energy needs					
Basal energy expenditure	BEE	BEE × 1.3	BEE × 1.3	BEE × 1.5	BEE × 2.0
Total calories, kcal per kg	28	28–32	32	40	50
Nonprotein kcal, per kg	25	25	25	30	35
Nonprotein kcal : N	150 : 1	100 : 1–150 : 1	100 : 1	80 : 1	80 : 1
Amino acid needs, g/kg	1.0	1.0–1.5	1.5	2.0	2.0–2.5
Distribution of calories, percent					
Amino acids	15	15–20	20	25	30
Glucose	60	50–60	50	40	70
Lipid	25	25–30	30	35	—

* Adapted from Cerra, F. B.: *Pocket Manual of Surgical Nutrition.* The C. V. Mosby Company, St. Louis, 1984.

40 percent burn would require $25(70) + 40(40) = 3,350$ kcal.

The extent to which full-thickness burns influence energy requirements is not known. Severe hypoproteinemia, edema at the site of injury, failure to obtain satisfactory skin growth, gastric atony, and weight loss are among the nutritional problems encountered. In patients with serious weight loss and inadequate oral intake, total parenteral nutrition or formula feeding, or both, may be needed to establish caloric equilibrium.[17] From 2.0 to 4.0 g protein per kg body weight is needed in major burns during the peak catabolic phase.[12]

The optimal ratio of calories-to-nitrogen is unknown. Research has shown that a nonprotein calorie-to-nitrogen ratio of 150:1 is sufficient to achieve positive nitrogen balance in patients with burns covering less than 10 percent of the body surface area. A lower ratio, 100:1, is needed in burns covering a larger area.[18]

When oral feedings are tolerated, high-protein meals supplemented with high-protein beverages are used. (See Chapter 33.) The need for as much as 1.0 g ascorbic acid has been definitely established, and additional B-complex viatmins are also considered essential. Pharmacologic doses of vitamin A are sometimes used to prevent occurrence of stress ulcers.

Acute Respiratory Failure

Conventional 5 percent dextrose solutions administered to mildly stressed patients are insufficient to meet energy needs; consequently, endogenous fat, which is oxidized with a respiratory quotient (RQ) of 0.7 is utilized to meet energy needs. Glucose supplied in excess of energy needs is converted to fat. Lipogenesis requires a large increase in carbon dioxide production, resulting in an RQ above 1.0.[19] The severely stressed or hypermetabolic patient receiving total parenteral nutrition utilizes glucose (RQ 1.0) as an energy source. In patients with compromised pulmonary function, high glucose loads are associated with marked increases in carbon dioxide production and can precipitate respiratory failure.[20,21] The increase in carbon dioxide production may be a factor in those patients who are difficult to wean from respirators.[19] Substitution of calories from fat for part of the carbohydrate lowers carbon dioxide production and the respiratory quotient; thus, the lung has less carbon dioxide to excrete.[22] Some recommend that carbohydrate be limited to 60 percent of calories in patients with compromised pulmonary function.[23] Others, citing the high cost of intravenous lipids, suggest that glucose be used to provide all the nonprotein calories for critically ill patients, with care to avoid calories in excess of requirements so that lipogenesis does not occur.[24]

Acute Renal Failure

This may be a consequence of direct trauma, shock or nephrotoxic drugs in the critically ill patient. Aggressive fluid resuscitation has diminished the incidence of acute failure following trauma; however, when it does occur, the mortality rate approaches 50 percent. Before dialysis, concentrated calorie sources low in protein are used. Substantial losses of amino acids in hemodialysis and of protein in peritoneal dialysis, together with the increased protein requirements brought about by trauma, necessitate provision of at least 1 g protein per kg per day, and preferably 1.5 g per kg.[13] (See Chapter 40.) Both enteral and parenteral solutions containing only essential amino acids are designed for use in renal failure.* It is not yet known, however, whether use of these products is any more cost effective than conventional mixtures of non-essential and essential amino acids.

Hepatic Insufficiency

Injury, surgery, shock, sepsis, or anesthesia can result in hepatic insufficiency in the trauma patient. Hepatic encephalopathy may result in altered ratios of branched-chain and aromatic amino acids in serum. Some evidence suggests that, in selected patients, use of formulas with a high content of branched-chain amino acids* is associated with improvement of amino acid profiles, protein synthesis, and decreased skeletal muscle catabolism.[13] Improvement in nitrogen retention and immune competence has been reported with use of these formulas in patients with moderate- to high-level surgical stress.[25] The formulas are not recommended for patients in the absence of significant stress or for those who do not have liver failure; standard formulas that supply a balanced mixture of amino acids are used in these situations. Further research is needed to determine whether the clinical results achieved with these specialized formulas are cost effective.

---

* Amin-aid (McGaw Laboratories, Santa Ana, Calif.); Travasorb Renal (Travenol Laboratories, Inc., Deerfield, Ill.); Nephramine (American McGaw).

* Hepatic-aid (McGaw Laboratories, Irvine, Calif.); Stresstein (Sandoz Nutrition, Minneapolis, Minn.); Traum-Aid HBC (McGaw Laboratories, Irvine, Calif.); Travasorb Hepatic (Travenol Laboratories, Deerfield, Ill.); Vivonex T.E.N. (Norwich Eaton, Norwich, N.Y.).

CASE STUDY 17

Salesman with Gastrectomy and Dumping Syndrome (Greek American)

For the past 40 years Mr. E, age 60, has been employed as an insurance salesman. Both Mr. and Mrs. E are Greek Americans. Mrs. E is a very good cook and prepares many Greek pastries of which Mr. E is very fond. Mr. E drinks six to seven cups of black coffee every day with lots of sugar. He does not drink milk, but each day he has some yogurt that Mrs. E prepares. Mr. E has always liked fruits and vegetables but now finds that onions and cabbage do not agree with him.

Recently Mr. E has been increasingly bothered by symptoms of periodic pain in his upper left quadrant after meals as well as nausea and vomiting associated with a chronic gastric ulcer. In the past 6 months he has lost 6 kg (13 lb). He now weighs 62 kg (136 lb); height is 167 cm (66 in.). Since the ulcer was no longer responsive to medical management, surgical intervention was recommended.

A subtotal gastrectomy with a Billroth II reconstruction was performed. Mr. E returned from the operating room with a nasogastric tube in place, which was attached to low, intermittent suction. While food and fluids were withheld, Mr. E was maintained on intravenous fluids. Once peristalsis returned to normal, the nasogastric tube was removed. Mr. E's diet was gradually increased from hourly feedings of clear liquids to small feedings of full liquids and eventually to six small meals of a fiber-restricted diet.

Ten days after surgery, Mr. E became weak and dizzy shortly after dinner. He perspired profusely, appeared pale, and experienced nausea and epigastric fullness. He felt better after lying down. Mr. E called his physician, who suggested measures to lessen the possibility of recurrent symptoms related to early dumping syndrome.

Pathophysiologic Correlations

1. List some factors that increase acid secretion and enzyme production and some that decrease production.
2. Which digestive enzymes may be reduced after gastrectomy? List the enzyme substrates and the products formed.
3. List the hormones that affect the digestive processes. Indicate the stimuli needed for their production, and the action exerted. Which of these hormones may be affected by gastrectomy? Explain.
4. Give examples of drugs that may induce gastric ulceration.
5. What is accomplished by vagotomy?
6. What is the Billroth II procedure? How does it differ from the Billroth I procedure? Draw a diagram of each.
7. What is meant by the dumping syndrome?
8. List five characteristic symptoms of the dumping syndrome.
9. Discuss the physiologic changes and the possible mechanisms that explain the symptoms seen in the dumping syndrome. What mechanisms may explain the changes in the late dumping syndrome?

Nutritional Assessment

10. What factors in Mr. E's history place him at nutritional risk?
11. Compare Mr. E's usual weight with that given in life insurance tables, and with the average for his age, height, and build. Assume that he has a medium frame.
12. Estimate Mr. E's energy and protein needs.
13. At 24 hours before surgery Mr. E was placed on a liquid diet. What was the rationale for this?
14. Describe fully the effect of the surgery on nitrogen balance.
15. How long will the negative nitrogen balance last?
16. What are the criteria that indicate when oral feeding can be resumed?
17. What effects would partial removal of the stomach have on Mr E's ability to eat and digest foods? Explain fully the functions of the stomach that might be affected.
18. In view of the above functions of the stomach, list the changes that Mr. E will probably need to make in his postoperative diet.
19. What are some long-range problems in nutritional status that should be anticipated?
20. What are some potential nursing diagnoses that might apply in this case?
21. Identify some appropriate nursing interventions for each of the diagnoses you listed in the previous question.

Planning the Diet

22. List the important goals of preoperative nutritional care for Mr. E.
23. The following diet has been planned for Mr. E. Using the Exchange Lists (Table A-4) calculate the protein, fat, and carbohydrate value of the diet. Exchanges: meat, 15; fat, 8;

fruit, 2; vegetables, 2; bread, 6. How many calories does this diet provide? Is the diet sufficient to meet Mr. E's energy needs? If not, how could it be adjusted?

24. What is the rationale for the above proportions for protein, fat, and carbohydrate?
25. Evaluate the nutritional adequacy of the diet outlined in question 23.
26. Show how the number of exchanges could be distributed throughout the day to provide six meals.
27. Write a menu for one day based on the diet prescription Mr. E will use. Show how *shashlik* and *pilavi* could be included in this menu.

Dietary Counseling

28. Outline the points you would emphasize in counseling Mr. E about his diet.

29. State some prophylactic measures that might be taken to prevent symptoms of dumping from occurring.
30. List five foods that Mr. E should avoid if there is any indication of the dumping syndrome.
31. The following are among Mr. E's favorite foods. Describe the nature of each, and indicate whether it is likely that he may have them at home: *bourglour*, *baklava*, lentil soup, *moussaka*, apricot candy, pistachio nuts, yogurt. (See Chapter 16).
32. What suggestions would you offer for adding new foods to Mr. E's diet?
33. Mr. E wonders whether he may have a small glass of wine or coffee with meals. What would you tell him?

References for the Case Study

HILL, G. L.: "Surgically Created Nutritional Problems," *Surg. Clin. North Am.*, 61:721–28, 1981

HOPPE, M. C., et al.: "Gastrointestinal Disease. Nutritional Implications," *Nurs. Clin. North Am.*, 18:47–56, 1983.

PASSARO, E., and STABILE, B. E.: "Late Complications of Vagotomy in Relation to Alterations in Physiology," *Postgrad. Med.*, 63:135–37ff, April 1978.

RODMAN, M. J.: "Current and Coming Treatment for Peptic Ulcers," *R.N.*, 40:74–79, February 1979.

CASE STUDY 18

Car Accident Victim with Severe Burns (Vietnamese)

Three weeks ago Mr. K, age 32, was severely burned after a head-on car collision with a truck. His car burst into flames and the back of his body caught fire as he ran from the car. He rolled on the ground to extinguish the flames, but still he suffered extensive burns. After emergency first-aid treatment, Mr. K was transferred by air ambulance to a regional burn center.

On admission to the burn unit Mr. K's systolic blood pressure was 90 and his pulse 110, weak, and thready. He complained of thirst and was restless but alert. His unburned skin was pale and cool. Mr. K sustained partial- and full-thickness burns on his back, hands, and both arms and legs (42 percent) of his body surface. There was no evidence of respiratory distress. He weighed 55 kg (121 lb); height 163 cm (64 in.). Before the accident he weighed 59 kg (130 lb).

Initially Mr. K was treated for burn shock. Small doses of morphine were given intravenously for relief of pain. A central venous line was inserted and fluid replacement therapy was begun.

Mr. K's fluid and electrolyte status was closely monitored. The amount of fluids given during the first 48 hours was designed to ensure a urine output of 30 to 50 ml per hour. A Foley catheter was inserted and the volume of urine was measured hourly. With fluid replacement therapy, Mr. K's blood pressure improved and he was less restless. Cimetidine (Tagamet) and antacids were given during the period of fluid resuscitation.

Once the shock was under control, Mr. K's wounds were cleansed and debrided. They were then dressed with silver sulfadiazene-impregnated gauze. The burn team closely monitored Mr. K's nutritional status. After active bowel function returned, a soft silastic feeding tube was placed in Mr. K's upper jejunum. Formula feedings were initiated in small volumes and at a dilute strength. When Mr. K tolerated the full-strength formula, the volume was increased in increments until the desired flow rate was achieved. As Mr. K's condition improved, formula feedings were supplemented with a diet high in calories and protein. As his oral intake increased, formula feeding rates were slowly decreased. Once Mr. K was able to meet his nutritional needs orally, the feeding tube was removed.

Mr. K faces a long hospitalization with the need for grafting procedures and rehabilitation. Mr.

and Mrs. K and their three children immigrated from South Viet Nam to the United States five years ago with his parents. They live together on a limited income. Mrs. K has stayed with her husband much of the time at the hospital. The other family members have not seen him since the accident because their home is 100 miles from the burn center.

Pathophysiologic Correlations

1. Explain the immediate effects of thermal injury on each of the following: extracellular fluid; intracellular fluid; hematocrit; cardiac output; blood pressure; renal function; blood urea nitrogen; gastrointestinal function.
2. Describe the alterations that occur in the metabolism of carbohydrate, protein, and fat following severe injury.
3. Explain the sequence of events leading to shock following a major burn.
4. Why is it important to estimate the size and the extent of the burned surfaces promptly?
5. What are the usual components of fluid therapy within the first 24 hours?
6. What observations would help determine whether fluid and electrolyte therapy are adequate?
7. At what point does water loss return to normal levels?
8. What is the rationale for withholding oral fluids during the first 24 to 48 hours following a major burn?
9. List the findings that indicate dehydration.
10. What symptoms would suggest that the patient might have hypokalemia?
11. List the factors involved in the catabolic processes of nitrogen following thermal injury.
12. What are some causes of renal failure in burn patients?
13. After the acute period has passed, what are the general principles of therapy for burn patients?
14. State three hazards of long-term immobilization.
15. List the problems associated with prolonged negative nitrogen balance.

Nutritional Assessment

16. Enumerate the problems that the dietitian and nurse are likely to encounter in meeting Mr. K's nutritional needs.
17. Outline the steps you would use to monitor whether the burn patient's needs are being met.
18. Mr. K excreted 25 g nitrogen in the urine. How much protein was catabolized? Does this account for the total amount of protein lost? Explain.
19. Calculate Mr. K's energy requirements using the formula inside the back cover of this text.
20. Why does the caloric requirement for a burned patient increase so greatly?
21. How much protein should be provided in Mr. K's feedings?
22. Explain the rationale for a high caloric intake in reducing the likelihood of hypoproteinemia.
23. Estimate the vitamin requirements during the period of recovery. State the reasons for your estimates.
24. List the long-range problems that must be faced for Mr. K's rehabilitation.
25. List the nutritional effects of the medications that Mr. K received.

Planning the Diet

26. What are the goals of early nutritional management of the burn patient?
27. List some precautions to prevent gastrointestinal complications in patients receiving tube feedings.
28. What techniques might help achieve an adequate food intake?
29. After the feeding tube was removed, Mr. K was given a 2,500-kcal 125 g protein diet. Using the exchange lists (Table A-4), calculate a food allowance that will meet these levels.
30. The diet was to be advanced as tolerated until Mr. K's daily caloric intake fully met his calculated needs (see Nutritional Assessment, question 19) and his protein intake was 2.5 g per kg. What additions could you make to the diet calculated above?
31. List five nutritionally complete proprietary products that will enhance Mr. K's caloric and protein intakes. List the calories and protein per 250 ml of each.
32. List the nutrients provided by each of the following Vietnamese foods: *chao gio*; *banh cuon*; *thit kho*; *canh cai*; *ca kho*; *cha tom*.
33. Which groups in the Daily Food Guide are represented by the above foods?
34. Cranberry juice or prune juice was included daily in Mr. K's diet. What was the purpose?

Dietary Counseling

35. Summarize the principles of nutritional care during the rehabilitative phase following thermal injury.
36. Mr. K's hands are bandaged and he cannot

feed himself, yet he resents being fed. How would you handle this situation?

37. After several weeks Mr. K is tired of hospital food. What solutions can you offer?

38. Suggest some snacks that Mr. K might enjoy and that would be tasty and nutritious.

39. Suggest some ways Mr. K could be actively involved in his own nutritional care.

40. How can the social worker, nurse, and dietitian help solve some of the psychologic problems Mr. K faces?

References for the Case Study

CRANE, N. T., and GREEN, N. R.: "Food Habits and Food Preferences of Vietnamese Refugees Living in Northern Florida," *J. Am. Diet. Assoc.*, 76:591–93, 1980.

DECROSTA, T.: "What Burn Centers Want You To Know," *Nurs. Life*, 4:44–49, January–February, 1984.

FORLAW, L.: "The Critically Ill Patient: Nutritional Implications," *Nurs. Clin. North Am.*, 18:111–17, March 1983.

HOPPE, M. C., "Nutritional Management of the Trauma Patient," *Crit. Care. Q.*, 6:1–6, June 1983.

KONSTANTINIDES, N. M., et al.: "Tube Feeding: Managing the Basics," *Am. J. Nurs.*, 83:1312–20, 1983.

KRAVITZ, M., et al.: "The Use of the Dobhoff Tube to Provide Additional Nutritional Support in Thermally Injured Patients," *J. Burn Care Rehab.*, 3:226–28, 1982.

VANOSS, S.: "Emergency Burn Care: Those Crucial First Minutes," *R.N.*, 45:45–49, October 1982.

References

1. Buzby, G. P., et al.: "Prognostic Nutritional Index in Gastrointestinal Surgery," *Am. J. Surg.*, 139:160–7, 1980.
2. Mullen, J. L., et al.: "Implications of Malnutrition in the Surgical Patient," *Arch. Surg.*, 114:121–5, 1979.
3. Cerra, F. B.: *Pocket Manual of Surgical Nutrition.* The C. V. Mosby Company, St. Louis, 1984.
4. Wolfe, B. M., et al.: "Evaluation and Management of Nutritional Status Before Surgery," *Med. Clin. North Am.*, 63:1257–69, 1979.
5. Martin, E. W., et al.: "Complications of Gastric Restrictive Operations in Morbidly Obese Patients," *Surg. Clin. North Am.*, 64:1181–90, 1983.
6. Anonymous: "Gastric Restrictive Surgery for Morbid Obesity," *JAMA*, 251:3011, 1984.
7. Lenner, J. H.: "Comparative Effectiveness of Gastric Bypass and Gastroplasty," *Arch. Surg.*, 117:695–700, 1982.
8. Hoikka, V., et al.: "The Effect of Partial Gastrectomy on Bone Mineral Metabolism," *Scand. J. Gastroenterol.*, 17:257–61, 1982.
9. Bingham, S., et al.: "Diet and Health of People with an Ileostomy. I. Dietary Assessment," *Br. J. Nutr.*, 47:399–406, 1982.
10. Kirsner, J. B., and Shorter, R. G.: "Recent Developments in 'Nonspecific' Inflammatory Bowel Disease," *N. Engl. J. Med.*, 306:775–81, 1982.
11. Frey, C. F.: "Accidents and Trauma Care—1983," *Surg. Annu.*, 16:59–69, 1984.
12. Long, C. L.: "The Energy and Protein Requirements of the Critically Ill Patient," in Wright, R. A., and Heymsfield, S., eds. *Nutritional Assessment*, Blackwell Scientific Publications, Boston, 1984, pp. 157–81.
13. Abbott, W. C., et al.: "Nutritional Care of the Trauma Patient," *Surg. Gynecol. Obstet.*, 157:585–97, 1983.
14. Teasley, K. M., et al.: "Nutrition and Metabolic Support of the Surgical Patient," *Urol. Clin. North Am.*, 10:119–29, 1983.
15. Fischer, J. E.: "Nutritional Support in the Seriously Ill Patient," *Current Prob. Surg.*, 17:469–531, 1980.
16. Morath, M. A., et al.: "Interpretation of Nutritional Parameters in Burn Patients," *J. Burn Care Rehab.*, 4:361–6, 1983.
17. Curreri, P. W., and Luterman, A.: "Nutritional Support of the Burned Patient," *Surg. Clin. North Am.*, 58:1151–6, 1978.
18. Matsuda, T., et al.: "The Importance of Burn Wound Size in Determining The Optimal Calorie: Nitrogen Ratio," *Surgery*, 94:962–8, 1983.
19. Hunker, E. D., et al.: "Metabolic and Nutritional Evaluation in Patients Supported with Mechanical Ventilation," *Crit. Care Med.*, 8:628–32, 1980.
20. Askanazi, J., et al.: "Nutrition for the Patient with Respiratory Failure," *Anesthesiology*, 54:373–7, 1981.
21. Covelli, H. D., et al.: "Respiratory Failure Precipitated by High Carbohydrate Loads," *Ann. Intern. Med.*, 95:579–81, 1981.
22. Baker, J. P., et al.: "Randomized Trial of Total Parenteral Nutrition in Critically Ill Patients: Metabolic Effects of Varying Glucose–Lipid Ratios as the Energy Source," *Gastroenterology*, 87:53–9, 1984.
23. Apelgren, K. N., and Wilmore, D. W.: "Nutritional Care of the Critically Ill Patient," *Surg. Clin. North Am.*, 63:497–507, 1983.
24. Clouse, R. E., and Alpers, D. H.: "Energy Sources in Total Parenteral Nutrition Patients: Would Sugar Suffice?" *Gastroenterology*, 87:226–7, 1984.
25. Nuwer, N., et al.: "Does Modified Amino Acid Parenteral Nutrition Alter Immune Response in High Level Surgical Stress?," *J.P.E.N.*, 7:521–4, 1983.

35

Nutrition for the Cancer Patient

Cancer is the second leading cause of death in the United States, exceeded only by ischemic heart disease, and accounting for 20 percent of all deaths.[1] Some 80 to 90 percent of the cancer cases in the United States are believed to be due to environmental factors; one such factor is diet. The role of diet in the etiology of malignant disease is not clear. Epidemiologic evidence suggests a possible indirect role for dietary factors in certain types of cancer.

Nutritional status is adversely affected by cancer. A high proportion of patients exhibit protein-calorie malnutrition, characterized by depletion of visceral protein stores. Loss of visceral protein is associated with increased morbidity and mortality in cancer patients. The malnutrition affects tissue function and repair, immune status, and metabolism of drugs.

The discussion in this chapter is limited to dietary factors associated with increased risk for cancer in humans, some metabolic effects of cancer, the influence of cancer therapy on nutritional status, and dietary management for patients with cancer.

Role of Dietary Factors in Cancer Incidence

A number of dietary factors have been implicated in the etiology of cancer, based on experimental research in animals and on epidemiologic studies. Animal studies often involve drastic dietary manipulations; furthermore, experimentally induced tumors in animals may not be comparable to spontaneous tumors in humans. Extrapolation of data from animal studies to humans should be made with great caution. Epidemiologic studies suggest possible relationships between diet and cancer but do not prove a cause and effect relationship. Additional limitations of epidemiologic studies that relate diet to cancer have recently been reviewed.[2,3]

Epidemiologic Studies Compared with the incidence in the United States, the incidence of colon and breast cancer in Japan is low whereas that of stomach cancer is high. Studies of Japanese who have migrated to the United States show that within two or three generations the cancer incidence patterns in Japanese Americans resemble those prevalent in the United States. This shift has been correlated with adoption of a westernized diet high in calories and fat.[4] Homogeneous population groups, such as Seventh Day Adventists in California, have a lower incidence of colon cancer than the general population. This has been attributed to a difference in lifestyle—the Adventists are a nonsmoking vegetarian population whose diet is lower in meat and fat and higher in dietary fiber, vitamins A and C, than that of most Americans.[5] However, lower mortality from colon cancer in Adventists is reportedly unrelated to decreased meat intake.[5]

Lower cancer incidence has also been reported in Mormons in Utah[6] but cannot be attributed solely to diet because dietary habits of this group do not differ markedly from those of the rest of the population. Worldwide correlations have shown higher mortality from breast and colon cancer in countries with a high habitual dietary fat intake. The studies are based on food disappearance data, and may not be indicative of actual consumption. Nevertheless, the United States is among the highest in the world for fat intake and mortality from these cancer types. Among population groups the correlations appear to be stronger for total fat than for type of fat intake but data on the latter are limited.[7]

Dietary Factors A number of laboratory and epidemiologic studies have implicated various dietary factors in the etiology of specific cancers.

Calories. Animal studies have shown that severe calorie restriction inhibits growth of most types of tumors, possibly because insufficient energy is available for tumor formation or for replication of malignant cells. However, the intake of all nutrients is decreased in calorie-restricted diets, and the reduction in tumor incidence could be due to the reduction of a specific nutrient. Calorie restriction is not a means of preventing tumor formation in humans.

Limited epidemiologic evidence relating total calorie intake to cancer incidence is available. However, an excess of calories in humans is associated with increased risk for endometrial and possibly for gallbladder cancer.[8]

Protein. In laboratory experiments tumor growth is suppressed at protein intakes at or below the minimum required for optimal growth. Protein intakes two to three times the minimum are associated with enhanced tumor growth in chemically induced cancers; however, results from various studies are not consistent.

Epidemiologic studies suggest that risk for cancer increases with high protein intakes. Cancer of the breast and colon occur with greater frequency in the industrialized nations and some have suggested a possible association between high intakes of total protein or animal protein and the risk of these specific cancers.[7] In the United States lower rates of colon cancer have been reported in vegetarian Seventh Day Adventists.[5] It is not known which of several dietary factors might be most important in this regard: lower intakes of meat and fat or increased dietary fiber. Insufficient evidence is available at present to conclude that a high meat intake per se increases risk for these cancers or that a vegetarian diet lowers risk.

Fat. Both the type and amount of fat are believed to influence tumor formation in animals. A high percapita fat intake in humans has been epidemiologically linked to increased risk for breast and colon cancer. One theory relates a high fat intake to increases in intestinal anaerobic bacteria and biliary steroid secretion.[9] Anaerobic bacteria are capable of synthesizing estrogens, which are believed to be potential carcinogens in mammary tissue, from biliary steroids. In addition, bile acids are degraded by intestinal bacteria to the secondary bile acids, deoxycholate and lithocholate; these may act as carcinogens in the colon. Another theory holds that *trans* fatty acids are more carcinogenic than *cis* conformations.[10]

Fiber. Dietary fiber is postulated to exert a protective effect against colon cancer by several mechanisims: shortening intestinal transit time, thereby re-

ducing the exposure time of epithelial surfaces to potential carcinogens; influencing bile acid metabolism, resulting in decreased formation or enhanced excretion of potential carcinogens; influencing intestinal flora with decreased degradation of bile acids and neutral sterols; and diluting potential carcinogens in the bowel.[8,9] Underdeveloped countries have a low incidence of cancer of the colon, and the diet in these countries is generally high in dietary fiber compared with that in the United States. Differences in other aspects of the diet or lifestyle must also be considered before concluding that dietary fiber accounts for the differences in cancer incidence between underdeveloped countries and Western nations. The effects of dietary fiber on colonic function vary with the nature and quantity of fiber, and other components of the diet, especially fat. Knowledge of the effects of specific components of fiber is too limited to conclude that any exert a protective effect against cancer.

Vitamin A. Laboratory experiments have shown that increased susceptibility to chemically induced cancer occurs in vitamin A deficiency and that increased intake of vitamin A exerts a protective effect in most cases. Synthetic analogs of vitamin A, *retinoids*, also inhibit chemically induced tumors. Data on the anticarcinogenic effect of carotenes are limited.

Epidemiologic evidence suggests that intake of foods rich in preformed vitamin A or its carotenoid precursors is associated with reduced risk for cancers at certain sites. Several studies have related low serum vitamin A levels to increased cancer incidence.[11]

Vitamin C. In laboratory studies vitamin C has been shown to inhibit formation of carcinogenic nitroso compounds, to prevent malignant transformation of cells grown in culture, and to lead to regression of transformed cells. In humans, several studies have shown that consumption of foods containing appreciable amounts of vitamin C is associated with a lower risk of esophageal and gastric cancer. However, data are inconclusive regarding an important role for vitamin C in prevention of cancer.

Selenium. High levels of selenium intake have been found to be antitumorigenic in animals, but the applicability of the data to humans is not clear.[12] Limited epidemiologic evidence suggests that cancer risk is inversely related to blood selenium levels, per capita intake, or levels in drinking water. However, further research using controlled clinical trials is needed before conclusions can be drawn.

Alcohol. The incidence of cancers of the mouth, pharynx, larynx, and esophagus is significantly increased in heavy smokers who consume large amounts of alcohol. In nonsmokers use of alcohol is not associated with increased risk for these cancers. Excessive beer drinking has been associated with an increased risk of colorectal cancer in the United States.[13]

Other Nutritional Factors. Other factors associated with increased risk for various cancers in humans include intake of salt-cured, pickled, and smoked foods; nonnutritive compounds in cruciferous vegetables, coffee, artificial sweeteners, and low serum cholesterol levels.

Cured and smoked foods contain nitrites that may be converted to carcinogenic nitrosamines during cooking or in vivo. Likewise polycyclic aromatic hydrocarbons in smoked foods, in charcoal-broiled meats, and in fish are carcinogenic in animals and are mutagenic. In humans frequent consumption of cured, smoked, or pickled foods is associated with increased incidence of cancers of the esophagus and stomach.[7,14]

Nonnutritive compounds, such as indoles, flavenoids, phenols, and aromatic isothiocyanates in cruciferous vegetables (broccoli, brussels sprouts, cabbage, carrots, cauliflower), inhibit chemically induced cancers in laboratory animals. Some epidemiologic evidence indicates that frequent consumption of these vegetables is inversely associated with cancers of the stomach and colon.[7,11]

Coffee has been associated with increased risk for bladder cancer in several case-control studies, although the data are inconclusive.[7] Increased risk for pancreatic cancer has also been associated with coffee consumption.[15] Among Seventh Day Adventists, mortality from cancer of the colon is significantly greater in those who drink two or more cups of coffee daily than in non-coffee drinkers.[5] Data are too limited to permit conclusions to be drawn regarding a cause-and-effect relationship between coffee drinking and cancer.

Artificial sweeteners have been the subject of much controversy. Experimental studies relating large doses of saccharin to bladder cancer in animals have prompted a great deal of publicity over the safety of artificial sweeteners. No studies in humans have demonstrated an increased risk of bladder cancer with use of saccharin. The most recently approved sweetener, aspartame, has not been reported to be carcinogenic in animals. No long-term studies of its use in humans have been reported.

Serum cholesterol levels have also been related to cancer risk. Naturally occurring low levels of serum cholesterol have been reported in some studies to be associated with increased risk for colon cancer.[16] However, it has been postulated that this association is due to metabolic changes accompanying undetected cancer at the time of the serum cholesterol determination rather than the cause of cancer.[17]

Interim Dietary Guidelines In 1982 the Committee on Diet, Nutrition, and Cancer of the National Academy of Sciences issued interim dietary guidelines based on review of experimental and epidemiologic evidence relating diet to the etiology and prevention of cancer. (See Table 3-4.) The American Institute for Cancer Research has published a food guide for health care professionals to aid in implementing the dietary guidelines.[18]

Metabolic Effects of Cancer

Cancer Cachexia In advanced disease, this complex metabolic syndrome is a major cause of morbidity and mortality. Anorexia, early satiety, weight loss, wasting, and weakness characterize the syndrome. The etiology is uncertain but according to one theory may be due to the systemic effects of peptides and other small metabolites produced by the cancer.[19] Alterations in energy, carbohydrate, protein, and fat metabolism, acid-base balance, enzyme activities, endocrine homeostasis, and immunologic status are seen. The metabolic rate is usually increased, as in Hodgkin's disease and leukemia. There are impaired glucose tolerance, decreased insulin production, and insulin resistance. Marked loss of body fat due to mobilization of free fatty acids from adipose tissue is seen. Skeletal muscle mass is reduced and hypoalbuminemia is common. Negative nitrogen balance occurs in spite of sufficient intake. Fluid retention may mask true weight loss; urinary excretion of sodium and potassium is increased. Enzyme changes in liver and muscle occur. The marked wasting in the syndrome is due to inadequate energy intake, which may be secondary to altered metabolism, anorexia, impaired digestion and absorption, tumor–host competition for nutrients, and increased energy expenditure by the host.[19]

Anorexia A frequent but poorly understood finding in advanced cancer is anorexia. It may be related to the disease process, to adverse effects of cancer therapy, or to emotional and psychologic reactions to cancer. The weight loss experienced by many patients with cancer is often due to reduction in food intake associated with anorexia.

Alterations in taste and smell are common in advanced cancer. Some patients have an increased threshold for sweet or sour tastes. Addition of sugar or other sweeteners, or lemon can make food more acceptable to these patients. Some patients experience a reduction in threshold for bitter tastes. Most meats, but especially red meats, are associated with a bitter taste. Substitution of other protein sources (eggs, fish, milk, legumes) should be made so that protein intake is not compromised.

Insulin stimulates appetite. The reduction in insulin secretion in cancer patients may thus have an adverse effect on appetite. Lactic acid and products of anaerobic metabolism of glucose cause anorexia and nausea. Amino acid imbalance can suppress appetite. Anorexia is often due to radiation therapy or to various chemotherapuetic agents. It is likely that the anorexia of most cancer patients is multifactorial.

Nutritional Effects of Cancer Therapy

Obstruction by a tumor may interfere with nutritional intake or digestive or absorptive functions. Nutritional status may be further compromised by surgery, radiation therapy, chemotherapy, or immunotherapy.

Surgery The site and extent of surgery determine the nutritional consequence. For example, interference with chewing and swallowing mechanisms follow surgery of the head and neck regions; impaired absorption of nutrients, especially of fat, follows gastrointestinal surgery; and diabetes mellitus may occur secondary to pancreatectomy.[20]

Radiation Therapy The nutritional problems associated with radiation therapy depend on the site and dose of irradiation. Adverse effects of irradiation to the upper alimentary tract include xerostomia (dry mouth) due to impaired salivary secretion, dental caries, loss of teeth, altered taste sensations, loss of appetite, dysphagia, sore mouth and throat, and esophageal irritation. Patients receiving radiation to the abdominal and pelvic areas commonly experience nausea, and diarrhea.[21] Gastric ulcer, enteritis, malabsorption, and weight loss are other consequences of radiation.

Chemotherapy Virtually all chemotherapeutic agents cause nausea and vomiting. Reduced food intake, generalized weakness, fluid and electrolyte imbalance, and weight loss ensue. Mucosal damage may be manifested as mucositis, stomatitis, glossitis, cheilosis, and esophagitis. Constipation or diarrhea are associated with some agents. Weight loss may be severe in prolonged therapy. Appetite suppression, malabsorption syndromes, and vitamin deficiencies occur with some drugs. Hormonal therapy may lead to fluid and electrolyte disturbances.[22] (See Appendix B.)

Immunotherapy Immunotherapy is used to stimulate the immune system and may induce a flulike syndrome, with chills, fever, malaise, nausea, and body aches.

Nutritional Considerations

The various modes of cancer therapy—surgery, radiation, and chemotherapy—all have nutritional consequences. Assessment of nutritional status of cancer patients is, therefore, essential in order to determine those patients who are likely to be at increased risk for nutritional problems during treatment, and to provide a basis for planning appropriate nutritional support. Periodic monitoring of nutritional status should continue during therapy.

Appropriate nutritional support can help reduce weight loss, provide an improved sense of well-being, and improve immunocompetence. Weight loss is associated with a significantly shortened survival time in patients with non-Hodgkins lymphoma, sarcoma, cancer of the breast, lung, stomach, prostate, and colon.[23] Well-nourished patients tolerate cancer therapy better than the malnourished.[24] Improved nutrition of the host causes an increased rate of tumor growth; thus, nutritional support should be accompanied by appropriate antitumor therapy.[21] The goals of nutritional therapy are to minimize weight loss and to correct nutrient imbalances and deficiencies. When oral feedings are contraindicated, formula feedings or parenteral feeding are used. These were discussed in Chapter 28.

Little is known of nutrient requirements in cancer. One group estimates the requirement for protein to be 1.2 to 1.5 g per kg body weight, whereas that for energy is 30 to 35 kcal per kg per day when enteral feeding is used, and 35 to 45 kcal per kg using parenteral feeding.[25] Others suggest that energy and protein requirements are increased by approximately 20 percent in cancer patients and can be estimated as follows[26]:

Protein: desirable weight in pounds × 0.77
Calories: desirable weight in pounds × 20 (males) or 18 (females)

Vitamin deficiencies are not uncommon in cancer patients; however, the therapeutic use of vitamins in treatment has been controversial. Deficiency of minerals, especially trace minerals, is likely in any patient whose dietary intake is inadequate in other respects.

Alternative Nutritional Therapies For various reasons, some cancer patients resort to alternative therapies such as greatly increased intakes of specific vitamins, minerals, or other substances purported to have nutritional benefits, such as Laetrile. Amygdalin (Laetrile) is promoted as vitamin B-17 but, in fact, is not a vitamin. It is a compound found in the seeds of certain fruits and nuts: apricots, peaches, plums, almonds, and macadamias. In the popular press, Laetrile is credited with improvement in cancer patients, often after conventional treatment has failed. Controlled clinical trials have not borne out this claim.[27] Others embrace the macrobiotic diet and way of life advocated by Kushi, which condemns conventional treatment of cancer as artificial and toxic.[28] The American Cancer Society has stated that there is no scientific evidence that macrobiotic diets are effective in treating cancer, and cautions that such diets, if improperly planned, are nutritionally inadequate.[28]

Hospice Care

A movement that has grown immensely in the United States over the past decade is that of hospice care. The hospice concept promotes whole-person medical care for terminally ill persons and their families.[29] While many of the patients have cancer, hospice care is not limited to this group. Hospices may be hospital based, home health agency based, or free standing. Characteristics of most programs include (1) health care and services provided to the terminally ill, that is, those with a stated life expectancy of 6 months or less; (2) a unit of care comprising the patient and family, or others responsible for the patient's care; (3) care available 24 hours a day, 7 days a week; (4) an interdisciplinary approach toward provision of care, with medical supervision of the team required; (5) care directed toward providing physical, emotional, and spiritual support of terminal illness; and (6) trained volunteers providing support as needed.[30]

In 1982 Congress approved Medicare reimbursement for hospice care based on the premise that costs are less than for conventional care of terminally ill patients. Under the provisions of the law, up to $6,500 per patient is reimbursable; no more than 20 percent of care can cover an inpatient setting.

Many patients who qualify for hospice care are likely to have serious nutritional problems such as those described on pages 498–99, arising as a consequence of the disease or the therapy. Dietary counseling is covered under the Medicare hospice benefit and should include the points discussed in the following section.

DIETARY COUNSELING

Most cancer patients need a good deal of guidance and encouragement in order to cope with the nutritional problems that arise during and following cancer therapy. Initially, the diagnosis of cancer may so overwhelm the patient and family that the importance of maintaining good nutritional status is not appreciated. Most have no understanding of the devastating effects that cancer therapy has on

Table 35-1. Some Side Effects of Cancer Therapy and Suggested Dietary Management

Nausea and vomiting	Clear, cold, and carbonated beverages with added Polycose*
	Sipping beverages slowly through a straw
	Small, frequent meals low in fat
	Dry crackers or toast before arising
	Tart or salty foods
	Cold foods—meat plates, fruit plates, cottage cheese, popsicles, gelatin desserts
	Liquids 30 to 60 minutes before eating
Dry mouth	Drinking at least 2 quarts of liquid daily
	High-calorie beverages are preferable to water
	Sauces, gravies, broth to moisten foods, and to make them easier to swallow
	Chewing sugar-free gum or sugar-free candy to stimulate salivation
	Artificial saliva
Taste alterations	Experimenting with different flavors and seasonings
	Substitution of other proteins for red meats
	Marinating meats in wine, fruit juices, etc.
Loss of appetite	Small, frequent feedings
	High-calorie, high-protein snacks and beverages
Sore mouth and throat	Soft, nonacid foods
	Blended or liquefied foods
	Foods and beverages at room temperature
	Using straw with liquids
	Avoiding highly seasoned foods
Swallowing problems	Liquid feedings or puréed foods
	Frequent feedings
	Formula feedings may be needed in some cases
	Adding butter and sauces to foods
	Finely chopped foods or foods cut into small pieces
Early satiety	Small frequent meals
	Chewing foods well and eating slowly
	Avoiding foods excessively high in fat, rich sauces
	Liquids 30 to 60 minutes before meals, not at meals

*Polycose (Ross Laboratories, Columbus, Ohio).

one's ability and willingness to eat. The dietitian and nurse can provide invaluable assistance to patients and their families by offering suggestions to make dietary management easier.

Before cancer therapy is started, guidance in the essentials of a nutritionally adequate diet should be given. The patient also needs to know what to expect from the various forms of cancer therapy, and should be informed of typical dietary problems experienced by others undergoing similar therapy. Some nutritional side effects of cancer therapy and suggested means for coping with them are shown in Table 35-1. Omitting food for several hours before radiation or chemotherapy treatments may prevent some of the nausea and food aversions that develop in many patients.

The importance of weight maintenance should be stressed. Patients should be encouraged to take advantage of times when they are feeling well to prepare food that can be frozen for later use. Convenience foods, mixes, casseroles, and snack items prepared in advance are useful for those times when nausea and fatigue limit ability and desire to prepare meals.

The atmosphere at mealtimes should be conducive to enjoyment of food. An attractively set table, relaxing music, pleasant conversation, and perhaps a glass of wine before dinner can help turn the patient's thoughts away from how he or she is feeling. Families should encourage, but not pressure, the patient to eat. Appropriate use of antiemetics and pain medication before meals permits eating to be more pleasant. Zinc supplements may improve taste acuity.

The diet is modified in texture and composition as needed. For example, for a patient who has had a laryngectomy, custards, and puréed fruits and vegetables are tolerated better than more coarse foods. One who is undergoing radiation to the abdomen may need foods low in lactose, fiber, and fat. Constipation is sometimes a problem and may be due to emotional stress, pain medications, or

chemotherapeutic drugs. Dietary fiber can easily be increased by use of bran cereals, whole-grain breads, fruits and vegetables, and use of snack foods such as granola bars, date bars, oatmeal cookies, and so on. (See Chapter 30.) For some patients, diarrhea may necessitate reduction in fibrous foods and provision of those high in potassium.

Most patients fare better with small, frequent meals. Nutritious snacks, should be readily available. A compromise must be reached between the need for high-protein, high-calorie foods and avoidance of excessive amounts of sugars and fats. A number of proprietary balanced formulas are suitable. Some patients find certain of these to be too sweet; thus, it is important to try a variety of formulas to find those acceptable to the patient. Taste preferences often change during therapy, and it may be preferable to keep on hand a supply of bland-tasting formulas which can be easily flavored with coffee, brandy, lemon, chocolate, and so on as the patient desires. Beverages kept on ice in a place readily accessible to the patient are more likely to be consumed. Ingenuity in varying the form and texture of supplements (e.g., beverages, puddings, soups) will enhance their appeal to the patient.

The protein content of the diet can be increased by adding skim milk powder to soups, gravies, and sauces; using milk in place of water for canned cream soups, and instant cocoa; adding diced meat to soups and casseroles; adding grated cheese to sauces, vegetables, soups, and so on. Calories can be increased by adding butter or margarine to soups, vegetables, or cooked cereals; adding honey to tea or cooked cereal; adding brown sugar and raisins to cooked cereals, and so on. (See also Chapter 25.) The National Cancer Institute has compiled a booklet of recipes and tips for better nutrition for cancer patients.[31] Similar booklets are available from local and regional cancer referral centers, and others.[32]

Woman with Adenocarcinoma of the Stomach

Mrs. L, age 71, is a second-generation Swede who has lived in Minneapolis all her life. After her husband's death a year ago Mrs. L sold the house where they had lived for many years and moved into a high-rise apartment building for senior citizens. She has a one-bedroom apartment with a narrow galley kitchen.

Mrs. L has been lonely and despondent since her husband's death and has had a difficult time adjusting to the apartment building. She does not join in any of the group activities sponsored for the residents of the building and finds living with elderly people to be very depressing. Her only hobby is reading.

Independence is very important to Mrs. L, and she is concerned about becoming a burden to others. For this reason she has turned down an offer from her only son and his family to live with them in their home in Oregon. Social Security checks and a small monthly income from savings are her sources of income. Prior to marriage Mrs. L had been an elementary school teacher, but she never returned to teaching.

On a visit to her doctor 6 weeks ago Mrs. L complained of mid-epigastric pain after meals, early satiety, and a distaste for meat. She stated that she had lost her interest in eating. Her weight was 50 kg (110 lb); height, 163 cm (64 in.). She has lost 9 kg (20 lb) during the past year.

During the physical examination, a palpable mass was found in the epigastrium. Significant laboratory data included elevated liver enzymes, hypoalbuminemia, a hemoglobin level of 9.0 g per dl, and hematocrit, 35 percent. The doctor recommended hospitalization for further evaluation.

Roentgenograms, fluoroscopy, and gastroscopy revealed a tumor in the antrum of the stomach. Occult blood was found in several stool specimens. Exploratory surgery showed adenocarcinoma of the stomach, regional lymph node involvement, and metastasis to the liver so a palliative resection was done. The omentum, spleen, and regional lymph nodes were removed. After surgery, the oncologist recommended a course of combination chemotherapy consisting of fluorouracil (5-FU), doxorubicin (Adriamycin), and mitomycin (Mutamycin).

Two weeks after the initial chemotherapy treatment, Mrs. L complained of a sore mouth and a burning sensation of the lips and tongue. Her lips were dry and cracked. Mild erythema and edema of the oral mucosa were observed. Mrs. L was given a prescription for viscous lidocaine (Xylocaine), a topical anesthetic, to be used before meals. The importance of frequent oral hygiene was stressed.

Mrs. L has experienced anorexia and some nausea and vomiting following chemotherapy. Prochlorperazine (Compazine) has helped relieve the nausea, and she has been able to tolerate small, frequent meals. A nutritional supplement, Ensure, was prescribed in conjunction with a high-calorie, high-protein diet.

Pathophysiologic Correlations

1. In what ways are the metabolism of carbohydrate, protein, and lipid altered in the presence of cancer?
2. What other metabolic abnormalities are commonly seen in cancer?

3. Compare Mrs. L's hematologic findings with the normal.
4. In what ways might the gastric resection influence Mrs. L's nutritional status?
5. List some of the nutritional consequences of chemotherapy.
6. Besides those experienced by Mrs. L, what other side effects are common with the chemotherapeutic agents prescribed in this case?

Nutritional Assessment

7. Compare Mrs. L's usual weight and her weight just prior to admission with the average. (NOTE: Use NHANES percentiles; see Table A-18.)
8. Calculate the percentage of weight loss for Mrs. L. How would you categorize the extent of depletion in this case? (Use table inside back cover of this text.)
9. Mrs. L's daily intake is approximately 1,100 kcal and 40 g protein. How does this compare with her requirements?
10. What are some potential nursing diagnoses that might apply in Mrs. L's case?
11. Identify some appropriate nursing interventions for each of the nursing diagnoses you listed in question 10.

Planning the Diet

12. Based on the protein deficit calculated in question 9, plan several combinations of foods that Mrs. L might add to her diet to bring her protein intake to the desired level.
13. Suggest several ways in which Mrs. L could bring her calorie intake to the desired level, assuming she has already made the changes recommended in question 12.

Dietary Counseling

14. Based on the information you have, what positive findings might provide a good starting point for counseling Mrs. L?
15. What suggestions would you offer Mrs. L for ways to maintain good nutrition even though she experiences anorexia?
16. Suggest some dietary guidelines to alleviate Mrs. L's nausea and vomiting.
17. How would you counsel Mrs. L regarding ways to manage the change in taste acuity she has experienced?

References for the Case Study

BERSANI, G, and CARL, W.: "Oral Care for Cancer Patients," *Am. J. Nurs.*, 83:533–6, 1983.
FREDETTE, S. L., and GLORIANT, F. S.: "Nursing Diagnoses in Cancer Chemotherapy. In Theory," *Am. J. Nurs.*, 81:2013–20, 1981.
KNOX, L. S.: "Nutrition and Cancer," *Nurs. Clin. North Am.*, 18:97–109, March 1983.

OBERFELL, M. S.: "The Challenge: Nutritional Support of the Patient with Gastrointestinal Cancer," *Am. J. I.V. Ther. Clin. Nutr.*, 10:6–10, June 1983.

OSTCHEGA, Y.: "Preventing and Treating Cancer Chemotherapy's Oral Complications," *Nursing '80*, 10:47–52, August 1980.

PETTON, S.: "Easing the Complications of Chemotherapy," *Nursing '84*, 14:58–63, February 1984.

SCOGNA, D. M., and SMALLEY, R.: "Chemotherapy-Induced Nausea and Vomiting," *Am. J. Nurs.*, 79:1562–4, 1979.

References

1. "Mortality for Leading Causes of Death, U.S.—1979," *Ca—A Cancer Journal for Clinicians*, 34:8, January–February 1984.
2. Lyon, J. L., et al.: "Methodological Issues in Epidemiological Studies of Diet and Cancer," *Cancer Res. (Suppl.)*, 43: 2392s–2396s, 1983.
3. Block, G., and Hartman, A. M.: "Understanding the Results of Epidemiologic Studies," *Semin. Oncol.*, 10: 257–63, 1983.
4. Gori, G. B.: "Dietary and Nutritional Implications in the Multifactorial Etiology of Certain Prevalent Human Cancers," *Cancer*, 43:2151–61, 1979.
5. Phillips, R. L., and Snowdon, D. A.: "Association of Meat and Coffee Use with Cancers of the Large Bowel, Breast, and Prostate Among Seventh-Day Adventists: Preliminary Results," *Cancer Res. (Suppl.)* 43:2403s–2408s, 1981.
6. Lyon, J. L., and Sorenson, A. W.: "Colon Cancer in a Low-Risk Population," *Am. J. Clin. Nutr.*, 31:S227–S230, 1978.
7. Palmer, S., and Bakshi, K.: "Diet, Nutrition, and Cancer," *J. Natl. Cancer Inst.*, 70:1151–70, 1983.
8. Willett, W. C., and MacMahon, B.: "Diet and Cancer—An Overview," *N. Engl. J. Med.*, 310:697–703, 1984.
9. Wynder, E. L., and Reddy, B. S.: "Dietary Fat and Fiber and Colon Cancer," *Semin. Oncol.*, 10:264–72, 1983.
10. Enig, M. G., et al.: "Dietary Fat and Cancer Trends—A Critique," *Fed. Proc.*, 37:2215–20, 1978.
11. Kummet, J., and Meyskens, F. L.: "Vitamin A: A Potential Inhibitor of Human Cancer," *Semin. Oncol.*, 10:281–9, 1983.
12. Committee on Diet, Nutrition, and Cancer: "Executive Summary. Diet, Nutrition, and Cancer," *Nutr. Today*, 17:20–5. July–August 1982.
13. Broitman, S. A., et al.: "Ethanolic Beverage Consumption, Cigarette Smoking, Nutritional Status, and Digestive Tract Cancers," *Semin. Oncol.*, 10:322–29, 1983.
14. Weisburger, J. H., et al.: "Possible Genotoxic Carcinogens in Foods in Relation to Cancer Causation," *Semin. Oncol.*, 10:330–41, 1983.
15. Review: "Coffee Consumption and Cancer of the Pancreas," *Nutr. Rev.*, 40:262–63, 1982.
16. Sidney, S., and Farquhar, J. W.: "Cholesterol, Cancer, and Public Policy," *Am. J. Med.*, 75:494–508, 1983.
17. Stamler, R., and Dyer, A.: "Circulating Cholesterol Level and Risk of Death From Cancer in Men Aged 40–69 Years," *JAMA*, 248:2853–59, 1982.
18. American Institute for Cancer Research: *Planning Meals That Lower Cancer Risk: A Reference Guide*, Washington, D.C., 1984.
19. Theologides, A.: "Cancer Cachexia," *Cancer*, 43: 2004–12, 1979.
20. Rivlin, R. S., et al.: "Nutrition and Cancer," *Am. J. Med.*, 75:843–54, 1983.
21. Shils, M. E.: "How to Nourish the Cancer Patient," *Nutr. Today*, 16:4–15, May–June, 1981.
22. Ohnuma, T., and Holland, J. F.: "Nutritional Consequences of Cancer Chemotherapy and Immunotherapy," *Cancer Res.*, 37:2395–2406, 1977.
23. Kisner, D. L.: "The Nutrition of the Cancer Patient," *Cancer Treatm. Rep.*, (Suppl. 5), 65:1–2, 1981.
24. Donaldson, S. S.: "Effect of Nutritional Status on Response to Therapy," *Cancer Res. (Suppl.)*, 42:754s–55s, 1982.
25. Harvey, K. B., et al.: "Nutritional Assessment and Patient Outcome During Oncological Therapy," *Cancer*, 43:2065–69, 1979.
26. Rosenbaum, E. H., and Rosenbaum, I. R.: "Principles of Home Care for the Patient with Advanced Cancer," *JAMA*, 244:1484–87, 1980.
27. Moertel, C. G., et al.: "A Clinical Trial of Amygdalin (Laetrile) in the Treatment of Human Cancer," *N. Engl. J. Med.*, 306:201–6, 1982.
28. Anonymous: "Unproven Methods of Cancer Management, Macrobiotic Diets," *Ca—A Cancer Journal for Clinicians*, 34:60–2, January–February, 1984.
29. Mount, B. M., and Scott, J. F.: "Whither Hospice Evaluation," *J. Chron. Dis.*, 36:731–6, 1983.
30. Keller, C. D., and Bell, H. K.: "The New Hospice Medicare Benefit," *Postgrad. Med.*, 75:71–3ff, February 1984.
31. *Eating Hints, Recipes and Tips for Better Nutrition During Treatment.* NIH Pub. No. 80-2079, U.S. Department of Health, Education and Welfare, PHS 1980.
32. Margie, J. D., and Bloch, A. S.: *Nutrition and the Cancer Patient*, Chilton Book Company, Radnor, Pa., 1983.

36

Diabetes Mellitus

Diabetes mellitus is a chronic disease that has affected humankind throughout the world. The records of the ancient civilizations of Egypt, India, Japan, Greece, and Rome describe the symptoms of the disease and usually include recommendations for treatment. The wasting away of flesh, copious urination, and the sweet taste of the urine were frequently noted by the ancient medical writers. Aretaeus of Cappadocia, who lived between A.D. 30 and 90, not only named the disease *diabetes*, which means "to run through or to siphon," but also recommended milk, cereals, starch, autumn fruits, and sweet wines.[1] The term *mellitus*, which means honeylike, was added by a London physician, Willis, in 1675.

The Nature of Diabetes

Insulin and Metabolic Defects Diabetes has been defined as a genetically and clinically heterogeneous group of disorders all of which show glucose intolerance.[2] It is characterized by a partial or total lack of functioning insulin and alterations in carbohydrate, protein, and fat metabolism.

The insulin defect may be a failure in its formation, liberation, or action. Since insulin is produced by the beta cells of the islets of Langerhans, any reduction in the number of functioning cells will decrease the amount of insulin that can be synthesized. Many diabetics can produce sufficient insulin, but some stimulus to the islet tissue is needed in order that secretion can take place. Especially in the early stages of the disease the insulinlike activity (ILA) of the blood is often increased, but most of this insulin appears to be bound to protein and is not available for transport across the cell membrane and action within the cell.

The hormones of the anterior pituitary, adrenal cortex, thyroid, and alpha cells of the islets of Langerhans are glucogenic; that is, they increase the supply of glucose. Just how these hormones are involved in the etiology of diabetes is not fully understood. Possibly they could increase the demand, decrease the secretion, or antagonize and inhibit the action of insulin.

Scope of the Problem Diabetes mellitus is an important public health problem in the United States. Although the exact prevalence is not known, various surveys indicate that about 2 percent of the population, or some 4 million persons, have the disease. About 400,000 cases are diagnosed annually, most of whom are over 40 years of age and are also affected by one or more chronic conditions of the vascular system, including heart disease, high blood pressure, neuropathy, nephropathy, and retinopathy.

The life span of diabetics is shorter than that of nondiabetics at nearly all ages. Diabetes is listed as the principal cause of death in about 2 percent of all deaths in the United States annually. Diabetes is a major socioeconomic ill costing some $6 billion annually in loss of earnings and costs of hospitalization, physicians' fees, medication, and rehabilitation. The disease is much more prevalent in lower economic groups.

Classes of Diabetes Three distinct classes, each of which has subtypes, have been identified.

1. DIABETES MELLITUS. This class of diabetes is characterized by fasting hyperglycemia or elevated plasma glucose levels during an oral glucose tolerance test. Three subtypes are known:
   a. *Type I, insulin-dependent diabetes mellitus:* Various genetic and environmental or acquired factors have been implicated in the etiology: altered frequency of certain human lymphocyte antigens (HLA) on chromosome 6, abnormal immune responses, autoimmunity, and islet cell antibodies. In some cases viral infectious diseases such as measles or mumps may trigger the autoimmune response.
   b. *Type II, noninsulin-dependent diabetes mellitus:* Genetic factors include familial aggregation of cases and autosomal dominant inheri-

504

tance in some cases. Environmental factors, such as obesity, superimposed on a genetic susceptibility, may precipitate the disease.

   c. *Diabetes secondary to other conditions:* Includes pancreatic disease; endocrine disorders, such as acromegaly, Cushing's syndrome, primary aldosteronism, and others; drug therapy including diuretics, oral contraceptives, thyroid hormones, antidepressants, or catecholamines. This subtype may also be associated with abnormalities in insulin receptors or certain genetic syndromes.

2. IMPAIRED GLUCOSE TOLERANCE. In this class of diabetes hyperglycemia occurs but the fasting plasma glucose level is less than that seen in classic diabetes (140 mg per dl) and the plasma glucose level during an oral glucose tolerance test is intermediate between normal and diabetic. This type may be a stage in the development of type I or type II diabetes, although many do not go on to develop clinical diabetes. Many elderly persons fall into this group.

3. GESTATIONAL DIABETES. This class includes women who develop glucose intolerance during pregnancy. Known diabetics who become pregnant are excluded from this class. Complex hormonal and metabolic changes are probably involved in the etiology, and insulin resistance may play a part.

Factors Influencing the Risk of Diabetes Two additional classes identify those who are known to be at increased risk for diabetes.

1. *Previous abnormality of glucose tolerance:* Individuals who now have normal glucose tolerance but who have a history of impaired glucose tolerance are included. Such persons were formerly described as being prediabetic or latent diabetics. Women who have had gestational diabetes and formerly obese diabetics whose weight has returned to normal are included in this group.

2. *Potential abnormality of glucose tolerance:* Persons in this group have never had abnormal glucose tolerance but are at greatly increased risk for development of diabetes. They include persons who are identical twins, siblings, or children of diabetics; mothers of infants weighing more than 9 pounds at birth; obese individuals; or certain racial or ethnic groups with a high prevalence of diabetes, such as American Indians. The Pima tribe has an especially high incidence.

Clinical Characteristics INSULIN-DEPENDENT DIABETES (TYPE I) is characterized by an absolute defi-

ciency of endogenous insulin and susceptibility to ketosis. Thus, type I diabetics depend on exogenous insulin to sustain life. The onset is usually abrupt and is seen most frequently in juveniles, but may occur at any age. Most patients are of normal weight or underweight. They manifest the classic symptoms of diabetes.

    POLYURIA, or frequent urination and an abnormally large volume of urine

    POLYDIPSIA, or excessive thirst

    POLYPHAGIA, or increased appetite

    Loss of weight

    KETOSIS is sometimes the abnormality that brings the patient to the physician. It is a condition in which the accumulation of lower fatty acids in the blood leads to the excretion of ketones in the urine. The ketonuria is accompanied by loss of base, acidosis, dehydration, and eventually coma.

Exogenous administration of insulin is necessary to control symptoms. In the early stages after metabolic control has been restored, endogenous insulin secretion appears to be restored and symptoms abate. This period, often called the "honeymoon" phase, is only temporary and is followed by a period of exacerbation in which symptoms are difficult to control, and finally by lifelong dependence on exogenous insulin. The extent to which residual insulin secretory ability is maintained is important in stability of diabetes control. Individuals with a severe insulin secretory defect are often termed "brittle" diabetics because their blood sugar levels are difficult to control and they fluctuate between diabetic coma and hypoglycemia.

The insulin secretory defect is less severe in TYPE II DIABETES MELLITUS. Basal insulin levels are usually normal or increased while glucose-stimulated insulin is diminished. Individuals with this type often do not present with the classic symptoms, usually are not dependent on exogenous insulin, and are not ketosis prone. Hyperglycemia is controlled with diet, oral hypoglycemic agents, or insulin. Onset is generally after the age of 40.

Type II diabetes has been subdivided into type IIa and type IIb.[3] Type IIa individuals are thin, while type IIb diabetics are usually obese. The latter type accounts for about 80 percent of all diabetics. Persons in either group may or may not require insulin to control hyperglycemia, but they are not insulin dependent in the sense that the type I diabetic is.

Insulin resistance is characteristic of most type IIb patients and is related to (1) abnormalities in the cell membrane resulting in a decreased number of insulin receptors, decreased binding of insulin to receptors, abnormal receptors, or antibodies to the receptor; or

(2) defects within the cell, such as the second messengers or the receptors on the second messenger. Many obese diabetics have type IV hyperlipidemia. (See Chapter 38.)

Laboratory Studies Several tests are used in the diagnosis of diabetes.

Glycosuria, or the presence of an abnormal amount of sugar in the urine, should be regarded as evidence of diabetes until proved otherwise. Sugar is present in the urine in many other conditions including pentosuria as a result of the body's failure to use the 5-carbon sugars; lactosuria in nursing mothers; alimentary glycosuria from excessive dietary loads of carbohydrate; fructosuria and galactosuria, resulting from enzyme deficiencies; and renal glycosuria because of a reduced ability of the tubules to reabsorb glucose.

Hyperglycemia, a high blood sugar, may be detected after a fast of 12 hours. A fasting plasma glucose of more than 140 mg per deciliter is suggestive of diabetes. Many older persons have slightly elevated blood sugar levels without having diabetes.

The ORAL GLUCOSE TOLERANCE TEST measures the body's ability to utilize a known amount of glucose. The test is done in the morning after 3 days of a diet containing at least 150 g of carbohydrate daily. The subject must have nothing to eat or drink, except water, for 10 to 16 hours preceding the test. A fasting blood sample is drawn, after which a solution containing a weighed amount of glucose is given. The glucose dose for nonpregnant adults is 75 g. For children, 1.75 g per kg of ideal body weight, up to a maximum of 75 g is used. A flavored commercial preparation is given* or the glucose is dissolved in flavored water, 25 g glucose per dl. Blood samples are taken at ½, 1, 1½, and 2 hours after the ingestion of glucose. Under the conditions of the test, according to the National Diabetes Data Group criteria,[2] diabetes is present if both the 2-hour glucose concentration and an intermediate value exceed the values shown in Table 36-1 on more than one occasion. In children the fasting level must also be greater than those indicated. Typical glucose tolerance curves are shown in Figure 36-1.

Ketonuria, or excretion of ketones, occurs when fatty acids are incompletely oxidized in the body.

Glycosylated Hemoglobin. Glycosylated hemoglobin, sometimes called hemoglobin A_{1c}, is formed in red blood cells by a reaction of hemoglobin A with

* Trutol (Sherwood Medical Industries, St. Louis, Mo.).

Table 36-1. Whole Blood and Plasma Glucose Concentrations During Oral Glucose Tolerance Test for Nonpregnant Adults*

	Normal	Impaired Glucose Tolerance	Diabetes
		mg per dl	
Fasting			
Whole blood	<100	<120	≥120
Plasma	<115	<140	≥140
½, 1, or 1½ hours			
Whole blood	<180	≥180	≥180
Plasma	<200	≥200	≥200
2 hours			
Whole blood	<120	120–180	≥180
Plasma	<140	140–200	≥200

* Adapted from National Diabetes Data Group: "Classification and Diagnosis of Diabetes Mellitus and Other Categories of Glucose Intolerance," *Diabetes*, **28**:1039–57, 1979.

glucose. The rate of formation increases when the blood glucose level is elevated as in uncontrolled diabetes mellitus. The reaction is irreversible; thus, the hemoglobin A_{1c} (HbA_{1c}) level falls only as red blood cells are replaced by new red blood cells. Since the average life span of the red blood cell is 3 to 4 months, measurement of the HbA_{1c} level can be used as an index of blood glucose control over time. In the nondiabetic, HbA_{1c} represents about 5 percent of the total hemoglobin. In poorly controlled diabetes, the HbA_{1c} level may be over 10 percent.[4]

Figure 36-1. Glucose tolerance curve in various metabolic disorders.

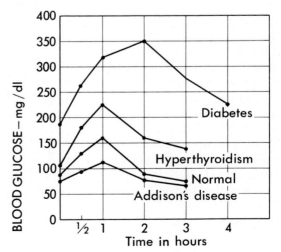

Diagnostic Criteria The oral glucose tolerance test is not always needed to establish the diagnosis. In adults, the diagnosis of diabetes is based on the presence of any one of the following: classic symptoms of diabetes and unequivocal elevation of plasma glucose; elevated fasting plasma glucose levels (140 mg per dl) on more than one occasion; sustained plasma glucose elevation during an oral glucose tolerance test on more than one occasion. Values at 2 hours after the ingestion of glucose and at some other time between 0 and 2 hours must be 200 mg per dl or greater.[2] In children, presence of the classic symptoms and a random plasma glucose greater than 200 mg per dl is diagnostic. In asymptomatic children there must be fasting plasma glucose of 140 mg per dl and sustained plasma glucose elevation during an oral glucose tolerance test on more than one occasion using the same criteria described above for adults.[2] The criteria for impaired glucose tolerance are indicated in Table 36-1.

Metabolism in Diabetes To understand the changes in metabolism that occur in diabetes, the student should first review the normal metabolism of proteins, carbohydrates, and fats. (See Chapters 5, 6, and 7.) A deficient supply of functioning insulin affects the metabolism of carbohydrates, fats, proteins, electrolytes, and water, and the consequences of the impairments are complex. (See Table 36-2.)

When insulin is not being produced or is ineffective, the formation of glycogen is decreased, and the utilization of glucose in the peripheral tissues is reduced. As a consequence the glucose that enters the circulation from various sources is removed more slowly and hyperglycemia follows. This is further accentuated by gluconeogenesis through which about 58 percent of the protein molecule and 10 percent of the fat molecule can yield glucose. When the blood glucose level exceeds the renal threshold (about 160 to 180 mg per dl), glycosuria occurs. The loss of glucose in the urine represents a wastage of energy and entails an increased elimination of water and sodium. Ordinarily thirst and the increased ingestion of liquids compensate for the water loss, but interference with the intake such as occurs in nausea or through vomiting could lead to rapid dehydration.

With a deficiency of insulin lipogenesis decreases and lipolysis is greatly increased, these effects being of both immediate and long-range consequence. The fatty acids released from adipose tissue or available by absorption from the intestinal tract are oxidized by the liver to form "ketone bodies" including acetoacetic acid, beta-hydroxybutyric acid, and acetone. The liver utilizes only limited quantities of the ketones and releases them to the circulation. Normally the peripheral tissues metabolize the ketones at a rate equal to their production by the liver so that the blood level at any given time is minimal. In diabetes mellitus the ketones are produced at a rate that far exceeds the ability of the tissues to utilize them and the concentration in the blood is greatly increased (KETONEMIA). Acetone is excreted by the lungs and gives the characteristic fruity odor to the breath. Acetoacetic acid and beta-hydroxybutyric acid are excreted in the urine (KETONURIA). Being fairly strong organic acids, these ketones combine with base so that the alkaline reserve is depleted, and acidosis results. The accompanying dehydration leads to circulatory failure, renal failure, and coma if not corrected. (See page 515.)

The rapid release of fatty acids into the blood circulation often results in a hyperlipemia and the blood serum may have a milky opalescent appearance. The blood levels of cholesterol are usually increased either because of increased synthesis or because of decreased destruction by the liver. The development of atherosclerosis in diabetic individuals occurs at an earlier age than in the nondiabetic and is more pronounced. (See page 529.)

Muscle protein catabolism is accelerated in uncontrolled diabetes; thus, amino acids, especially alanine, are released to the liver for gluconeogenesis. Protein catabolism also increases the amount of nitrogen that must be excreted as a result of deaminization. The catabolism of protein tissues is accompanied by the release of cellular potassium and its excretion in the urine.

Table 36-2. Some Metabolic Effects of Insulin Deficiency

Clinical Effect	Mechanism
Hyperglycemia	↓uptake of glucose by liver, muscle, adipose tissue
	↑glucose production by liver due to glycogenolysis and gluconeogenesis
	↑release of substrate by muscle: ↑glycogenolysis, ↑ amino acid release
Hypertriglyceridemia	↓triglyceride uptake by adipose tissue
Ketonemia	↑fatty acid mobilization by adipose tissue
	↑conversion of fatty acids to ketones by the liver
	↓uptake by muscle of ketones produced in liver
Hyperaminoacidemia	↓hepatic uptake of branched-chain amino acids

Treatment for Diabetes Mellitus

Dietary control is central to success in treatment of diabetes. It is accompanied, when necessary, by insulin or oral hypoglycemic drugs. A regulated program of exercise and attention to personal hygiene are important to the total program. The many aspects of therapy require a continuing program of education for the patient together with periodic evaluation by the physician, nutritionist, and other specialists in health care.

Insulin When the islets of Langerhans are unable to produce insulin it must be supplied by injection. It cannot be taken orally because the insulin molecule, being protein in nature, would be hydrolyzed in the digestive tract and thus inactivated.

Specific circumstances vary the insulin requirement considerably. Exercise reduces the need and infections increase the need. Emotional upsets may also modify the utilization of insulin. The types of insulin and their action are listed in Table 36-3.

Several approaches to insulin therapy are used. For most patients a *conventional* approach is used. This involves injection of a single morning dose or twice daily injections. In selected patients intensive conventional therapy, sometimes called *multiple daily injections* (MDI), is used along with home self-monitoring of blood glucose levels. The individual administers an intermediate or long-acting insulin to maintain a steady basal insulin level throughout the day and night and injects regular insulin before each meal and at bedtime. Although this approach requires several insulin injections daily, it permits the individual to maintain the blood glucose level near the normal level. Persons using this method must measure their blood glucose before meals and at bedtime using one of several commercial kits. Blood is obtained by finger stick. The insulin dose is then based on the blood glucose level.

The availability of portable programmable insulin pumps that provide a *continuous subcutaneous insulin infusion* (CSII) permits even closer control of the blood glucose level. A small device worn on the belt or under clothing delivers insulin through a small tube and a tiny needle inserted subcutaneously into the abdomen or thigh. A continuous infusion of regular insulin is delivered by the pump in order to maintain a steady low level of basal insulin. About half the total insulin dose is administered in this manner. Larger bolus doses are delivered by activation of the pump before mealtimes. The amount delivered is based on the results of blood glucose monitoring done before meals. Usually the bolus dose is planned to provide 35 percent before breakfast, 25 percent before lunch and dinner and 15 percent before bedtime.[5] To prevent the "dawn phenomenon" of hypoglycemia, monitoring of blood glucose at 3:00 A.M. is recommended.[5]

In addition to closer control of blood glucose levels, use of the insulin pump is reported to lower elevated levels of serum cholesterol and triglycerides and to permit greater flexibility in timing of meals.[6]

Oral Hypoglycemic Drugs Sulfonylurea compounds increase the release of insulin from the beta cells of the pancreas. These agents are sometimes used in the management of noninsulin-dependent diabetes that cannot be controlled by diet alone. Since function of the beta cells is required for these compounds to be effective, they are not used in type I insulin-dependent diabetes. Several preparations are available,* which differ from one another chiefly in potency and duration of action. These drugs may produce hypoglycemia if food intake is delayed; thus regularity of meals is important. The second generation sulfonylureas are much more potent drugs that potentiate insulin action through an effect on insulin receptor binding and enhancing tissue responsiveness to insulin.[7] These drugs are not yet approved for use in the United States.

Table 36-3. Types of Insulin and Their Action*

Type	Onset	Peak Action	Duration
		hours	
Rapid action, short duration			
Regular crystalline	½–1	2–5	6–8
Semilente	½–1½	5–10	12–16
Intermediate action and duration			
Lente	1–1½	8–12	24
NPH	1–1½	8–12	24
Delayed action, prolonged duration			
Protamine zinc	4–8	14–20	24–36
Ultralente	4–8	10–30	36+

* Adapted from Cannon, M.L.: "Insulin Products Commercially Available in 1984: A Summary," *Parenterals*, **2**:3, January/February 1984.

* Tolbutamide (Orinase) (The Upjohn Company, Kalamazoo, Mich.; Chlorpropamide (Diabinese) (Charles Pfizer & Co., Inc., New York, N.Y.); Acetohexamide (Dymelor) (Eli Lilly Company, Indianapolis, Ind.; Tolazamide (Tolinase) (The Upjohn Company, Kalamazoo, Mich.).

Rationale for Dietary Management The American Diabetes Association lists several goals for the dietary management of diabetes: (1) to improve the overall health of the patient by attaining and maintaining optimum nutrition; (2) to attain and maintain an ideal body weight; (3) to provide for normal physical growth in the child, and for adequate nutrition during pregnancy and lactation; (4) to maintain plasma glucose as near the normal physiologic range as possible; (5) to prevent or delay the development of chronic complications of diabetes: cardiovascular, renal, retinal, and neurologic; (6) to modify the diet as needed for complications of diabetes and for associated diseases; (7) to make the diet prescription as attractive and realistic as possible.[8] There are three points of view concerning the degree of dietary control needed.

Chemical Control. A measured diet and insulin dosage are carefully regulated so that the blood sugar is kept within normal limits and the urine is free or nearly free of sugar at all times. Such control is believed to reduce the incidence and severity of degenerative complications. One criticism sometimes leveled against it is that the treatment may tend to be directed to the diabetes and not to the person as a whole.

Clinical Control. Hyperglycemia and glycosuria are disregarded, and insulin is used to control ketosis. The diet differs little if any from that of normal persons and is controlled only to the point of maintenance of normal weight. Some physicians use these so-called free diets in the most liberal sense, but others restrict concentrated carbohydrate foods, especially those from sources contributing no other nutrients. Those who favor clinical control believe that the patient has an increased sense of well-being and that the degenerative complications are not more frequent.

Intermediate Control. The majority of physicians adopt a regimen that falls between the preceding two. The objectives are: (1) to treat the patient as an individual and not on the basis of the diabetes alone; (2) to provide adequate nutrition for the maintenance of normal weight, a sense of well-being, and a life of usefulness; (3) to keep the blood sugar almost at normal levels for a large part of the day by using insulin as needed and by avoiding hypoglycemia; (4) to keep the urine sugar free or with only traces of sugar for most of the day.

Nutritional Needs Dietary control is an integral part of management for the diabetic. The diet should always provide the essentials for good nutrition, and adjustments must be made from time to time for changing metabolic needs, for example, during growth, pregnancy, or modified activity.

Energy. Control of calorie intake to achieve normal weight is a primary objective for all diabetics. The calorie allowance is essentially the same as that for normal individuals of the same activity, size, and sex. Obese individuals should be placed on a calorie-restricted diet until the desirable weight for height and age is attained. Such weight loss in middle-aged obese patients very often leads to return of normal glucose tolerance. From 30 to 40 percent of diabetics do not need insulin if their diets are controlled.

One approach to planning the calorie level is to determine the patient's present food intake and to use it as a guide for the calculated diet. The patient's continuing weight status determines whether the diet, in fact, is satisfactory in its calorie level—assuming, of course, that the patient is adhering to it. A convenient guide for planning the energy level is as follows:

	kcal per kg	kcal per pound (Desirable Weight)
For weight loss	20	9
For a bed patient	25	11
For light work	30	14
For medium work	35	16
For heavy work	40	18

Protein. The recommended dietary allowance for protein for each age and sex category is satisfactory for the diabetic individual. The American Diabetes Association recommends that 12 to 20 percent of calories should be from protein.[8] Up to 25 percent is permitted using the Canadian recommendations.[9]

Carbohydrate. A level of 100 g carbohydrate will prevent ketosis. Several studies have shown that raising the carbohydrate intake does not adversely affect fasting blood glucose levels, glucose tolerance, or insulin requirements, provided that total calories are not increased. Insulin needs are more closely correlated with total calorie intake than with the carbohydrate level in the diet. Consequently, liberalization of the carbohydrate intake to more closely approximate that of typical diets in the United States and Canada has been recommended. For most diabetics in the United States, 50 to 60 percent of calories as carbohydrate, mostly of the complex type, is recommended.[8] For the 20 percent or so of adult diabetics with hypertriglyceridemia, carbohydrate should be limited to 35 percent of calories.[9]

Some research has shown that the increases in plasma insulin and glucose levels produced by carbohydrate-containing foods vary considerably from one food to another.[10] For example, isocaloric amounts of glucose from dextrose and potato yield similar postprandial blood glucose responses that are higher than those produced by bread or rice.[11] In other research, test meals, each containing a different type of carbohydrate but providing similar amounts of carbohydrate, protein, and fat, were used. The increase in plasma glucose level was not significantly higher when sucrose was used in preference to other carbohydrates. The smallest increase in plasma glucose was produced by a fructose-containing meal.[12] Although research in this area is of interest to health professionals who work with diabetics, other factors that influence glycemic response must be considered before these data can be applied in the day-to-day dietary management of persons with diabetes.[13]

Fat.   After protein and carbohydrate levels have been established, the fat allowance makes up the remaining calories. For most diets, 30 to 35 percent of the calories as fat is satisfactory. Foods high in saturated fat and cholesterol should be limited.[8,9] The level of saturated fat recommended is less than 10 percent of total calories, with polyunsaturated fat providing up to 10 percent of total calories. This entails use of skim milk, low-fat meats, and polyunsaturated fats in calculating the diet and planning the daily meals. (See Table A-4.) Fat intake should be appropriately reduced when alcohol is ingested so that the energy intake will not be excessive. Carbohydrate intake should also be reduced to compensate for any carbohydrate in the alcoholic beverage.

Fiber.   Short term studies with high fiber diets have been associated with reductions in postprandial glucose, serum cholesterol, and triglycerides, and insulin requirements in persons with type II diabetes.[14] The American and Canadian Diabetes Associations recommend substitution of foods containing unrefined carbohydrate with fiber for highly refined carbohydrate foods that are low in fiber.

Regularity of Meals Day-to-day consistency in amounts and distribution of carbohydrate, protein, and fat is needed especially for persons taking insulin

or oral hypoglycemic agents. Meals should be spaced to coincide with the availability of insulin. A delay in eating may produce hypoglycemia. On the other hand, hyperglycemia, brought on by eating an excess of rapidly hydrolyzed carbohydrate, is to be avoided. Physical activity influences insulin requirements and adjustments in the diet may be needed as well.

Determination of the Diabetic Diet Prescription A number of procedures may be used to arrive at the diet prescription. This is the responsibility of the physician, but the nurse and dietitian should have an understanding of the basis for the calculation. Following is described one of the methods often used.

Let us assume that a diet is to be planned for a secretary who is 25 years old and 170 cm (67 in.) tall. According to the table of heights and weights (Table A-16), her desirable weight is 63 kg (139 pounds) (medium frame).

1. Calories:30 kcal per kg (14 per pound) of desirable body weight
$$63 \times 30 = 1,890 \text{ kcal per day}$$
2. Protein: 12 to 20 percent of total calories
$$1,890 \times 18 \text{ percent} = 340 \text{ kcal}$$
$$340 \text{ kcal} \div 4 = 85 \text{ g protein daily}$$
3. Carbohydrate: 50 to 60 percent of total calories
$$1,890 \times 53 \text{ percent} = 1,002 \text{ kcal}$$
$$1,002 \div 4 = 250 \text{ g carbohydrate per day}$$
4. Fat calories: Total calories minus calories from protein and carbohydrate
$$1,890 - (340 + 1,002) = 548 \text{ kcal}$$
5. Fat: fat calories divided by 9
$$548 \div 9 = 61 \text{ g fat per day}$$

By rounding off the numbers, the prescription is: protein 85 g; carbohydrate, 250 g; fat 60 g.

Procedure for Calculating the Diet Once the diet prescription is determined, the number of servings from each of the exchange lists is calculated. The procedure was described in Chapter 4. Table 36-4 illustrates one way in which the diet prescription described above could be met.

Distribution of Calories Calories, especially those from carbohydrate, are distributed so as to coincide with the type of insulin being used and modified according to each patient's needs in order to achieve the best possible regulation of carbohydrate utilization. When intermediate or long-acting insulins are used, a portion of the carbohydrate—usually 20 to 40 g—is

Table 36-4. Sample Calculation of Diet Using Food Exchange Lists*

List	Food	Measure	Carbohydrate (g)	Protein (g)	Fat (g)
1	Starch/Bread	9 exchanges	135	27	—
2	Meat, lean	2 exchanges		14	6
	medium fat	3 exchanges		21	15
3	Vegetables	3 exchanges	15	6	
4	Fruit	5 exchanges	75	—	—
5	Milk, skim	2 cups	24	16	—
6	Fat	8 exchanges		—	40
			249	84	61

* Carbohydrate, 250 g; protein, 85 g; fat, 60 g. See prescription, page 510.

reserved for a midafternoon or bedtime feeding or both. This carbohydrate must be in slowly available form and should be accompanied by a portion of the day's protein. For example, a patient receiving an intermediate-acting insulin such as NPH, might receive 1/7, 2/7, 1/7, 2/7, 1/7 of the total carbohydrate and calories for breakfast, lunch, afternoon snack, dinner, and evening snack, respectively. (See Table 36-5.) Some prefer to have a distribution in tenths, thus 2/10, 3/10, 1/10, 3/10, 1/10 for the previous example.

Planning the Meal Pattern The dietitian and the nurse must translate the prescription into terms of common foods, keeping the following points especially in mind.

1. The diet should be planned with the patient so that it can be adjusted to his or her pattern of living. This requires consideration of the patient's economic status, the availability and cost of food, national, religious, and social customs, personal idiosyncrasies, occupation, facilities for preparing or obtaining meals, and so on. The diabetic diet need not be an expensive one, and ideally, it should be so planned that it fits in with the menus of the rest of the family. However, if the family diet is a

poor one, the entire family will benefit when the basic food groups become the center about which meals are planned. The diet for the diabetic person does not require many special foods; thus, the rest of the family should not be deprived.

2. The adequacy of the diet for minerals and vitamins is most easily ensured if one includes basic amounts of foods from the Daily Food Guide.

3. Including some of the protein and fat in each meal helps to provide satiety and balance of food selection.

4. The food exchange lists (Table A-4) permit reasonable dietary constancy from day to day and considerable flexibility in meal planning.

5. The meal distribution of the carbohydrate can be adjusted to within 7 or 8 g without using fractions of exchanges. The protein and fat should be adjusted within meals so that maximum flexibility is possible in meal planning. For example, the inclusion of milk at breakfast permits either cereal or bread to be selected from the bread exchanges; meat exchanges are wisely divided among the three meals with somewhat larger amounts being allocated to dinner. An example of the distribution of food exchanges into meal patterns is shown in Table 36-6 for the diet calculation illustrated on page 510.

Table 36-5. Typical Meal Distribution of Calories and Carbohydrate

Type of Insulin	Breakfast	Noon	Midafternoon	Evening	Bedtime
None	1/3	1/3		1/3	Usually none
	1/5	2/5		2/5	
Short-acting (before breakfast and dinner)	2/5	1/5		2/5	Usually none
Intermediate-acting NPH	1/7	2/7	1/7	2/7	1/7
Long-acting	1/5	2/5		2/5	20–40 g carbohydrate
With regular insulin at breakfast	1/3	1/3		1/3	20–40 g carbohydrate

Table 36-6. Meal Pattern and Sample Menu*

Meal Pattern	Exchange	C (g)	P (g)	F (g)	Sample Menu
Breakfast					
Milk, list 5	½	6	4	—	Skim milk—½ cup
Fruit, list 4	1	15	—	—	Orange—1
Meat, med. fat, list 2	1	—	7	5	Soft cooked egg—1
Bread, list 1	1	15	3	—	Whole wheat toast—1 slice
Fat, list 6	1	—	—	5	Margarine—1 teaspoon
Coffee or tea					
		36	14	10	290 kcal = 15 percent
Luncheon					
Bread, list 1	3	45	9	—	Broth with saltines—6
					Whole wheat bread—2 slices
Meat, low fat, list 2	2	—	14	6	Sliced chicken—2 ounces
Vegetables, list 3	2	10	4	—	Sliced tomato/lettuce
(see also free list)					Carrot and celery sticks
Fat, list 6	2	—	—	10	Mayonnaise—2 teaspoons
Fruit, list 4	1	15	—	—	Banana—½ (9 in. long)
Coffee or tea					
		70	27	16	532 kcal = 29 percent
Midafternoon					
Bread, list 1	1	15	3	—	Graham crackers—3 squares
Fat, list 6	1	—	—	5	Margarine—1 teaspoon
Fruit, list 5	1	15	—	—	Grapes, small—15
Milk, skim, list 5	½	6	4	—	Skim milk—½ cup
		36	7	5	217 kcal = 12 percent
Dinner					
Meat, med. fat, list 2	2	—	14	10	Chopped beef—2 ounces
Bread/starch, list 1	3	45	9	—	Rice—2/3 cup
					Dinner roll—1
Vegetables, list 3	1	5	2	—	Wax beans—½ cup
(free list)					Sliced cucumbers
Fruit, list 4	1	15	—	—	Strawberries—1¼ cups
Milk, list 5	½	6	4	—	Skim milk—½ cup
Fat, list 6	2	—	—	10	Margarine—2 teaspoons
Coffee or tea					
		71	29	20	580 kcal = 31 percent
Evening Snack					
Bread/starch, list 1	1	15	3	—	Popcorn—3 cups
Fat, list 6	2	—	—	10	Margarine—2 teaspoons
Fruit, list 4	1	15	—	—	Apple—1 (2 inch)
Milk, list 5	½	6	4	—	Skim milk—½ cup
		36	7	10	262 kcal = 14 percent
Totals, g		249	84	61	1,881 kcal = 100 percent
Percentage of kcal		53	18	29	

* Calorie and carbohydrate division: breakfast, $1/7$; luncheon, $1/7$; midafternoon, $1/7$; dinner, $2/7$; evening snack, $1/7$.

DIETARY COUNSELING

Essential Knowledge The diabetic patient needs to know about (1) the nature of diabetes and the reasons for the measures that will be recommended, (2) the importance of weight control, (3) the details of the dietary program, (4) the amounts, time intervals, and method of adminis-tration of insulin or oral drugs, if needed, (5) skin care and personal hygiene, (6) procedures for testing the urine, (7) signs of hypoglycemia or acidosis and what steps to take in the event they occur, (8) emergency measures to take during infection and illness until medical help is available, and (9) the importance of periodic visits to the physician. (See Figure 36-2.)

Insofar as diet is concerned, the diabetic patient

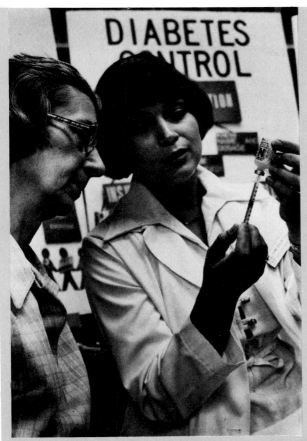

Figure 36-2. The nurse teaches the diabetic patient the importance of carefully measuring the prescribed insulin dose, the technique to use in administering insulin, the importance of rotating injection sites, and proper timing of the insulin injection. (Courtesy, Metropolitan Medical Center, Minneapolis, and Jeffry Grosscup, Photojournalist.)

needs to be taught the importance of the timing of meals, the calorie content of food, the amount of food to use at each meal, how to interpret labels when purchasing food, how to prepare food for meals, and sources for information on foods.

The individual with type I diabetes should be encouraged to be reasonably consistent in timing of meals and amounts of food eaten at each meal. The mealtimes should correlate with the peak action time of the insulin. The use of foods high in complex carbohydrate and low in fats should be encouraged. Patients should be instructed in regard to effects of foods and exercise on the blood glucose level so that they can make adjustments when needed.

Emphasis on weight control is the highest priority in the dietary management of most type II diabetics. Many need instruction in controlling food portions. Various means can be used to teach portion control. The exchange lists are not necessarily appropriate for all patients. Some do better by not changing their dietary pattern, but simply reducing portion sizes.

For elderly persons newly diagnosed with diabetes, the diet should be changed as little as possible. Reduction of simple sugars is sufficient to lower blood glucose levels in some. An increase in dietary fiber may be beneficial, especially if the patient is troubled with constipation or diverticulosis.

Responsibility for Education The physician, nurse, and dietitian share the responsibility for counseling the patient. The physician explains the nature of diabetes and the factors of importance in maintaining control. He or she also makes referrals to the dietitian and nurse for detailed aspects of education. In the hospital or outpatient clinic the dietitian usually initiates dietary instruction and arranges for a continuing program of education. The nurse instructs the patient regarding insulin administration, urine testing, and hygiene. The nurse is a valuable assistant for dietary counseling and may be fully responsible for dietary instruction in some situations where no dietitian is available.

Experience has shown that the majority of diabetics fail to understand their diets. Satisfactory counseling of the patient includes individualized instruction which may be supplemented by group instruction. The patient must be involved throughout in order to fully understand and adopt the program necessary. Frequent follow-up visits with the dietitian or public health nurse are essential to reinforce motivation, to answer questions, and to give added information.

Not only the patient but members of the family must be included in the counseling sessions. Each member of the family needs to understand that the diet for the diabetic patient is essentially a normal one, but that a regulated routine of meals and of the quantities of food is a vital aspect of the program. Members of the family also need to be aware of the complications that could arise and should know what to do in emergencies.

Teaching Aids The booklet, *Exchange Lists for Meal Planning*, published by the American Diabetes Association and the American Dietetic Association, is an excellent guide for the client. It includes food selection from each of the six lists, a list of "free" foods, seasoning suggestions, a list of combination foods, foods for occasional use, and guides for dietary planning. The booklet should always be used in conjunction with personal counseling.

The patient's tray at each meal constitutes one of the best visual aids. If the patient has been introduced to the food exchange lists, the foods on the tray can be located in these lists and the amounts served identified in number of exchanges. Needless to say, careful checking of the tray before it is brought to the patient is important to emphasize dietary control. Measuring cups, measuring spoons, and various sizes of glasses and cups used for table service should be demonstrated during the instruction of the patient. Paper and plastic food models are useful in demonstrating menu planning and may be used by the patient for practice sessions in planning his or her own diet. In a relatively short time most patients can learn to estimate the portion sizes allowed on their diets.

Programmed instruction, when available, can be an important teaching aid. Slides, filmstrips, and movies pertaining to the many aspects of diabetic care are especially useful for group instruction. Each patient should be encouraged to participate in some group events not only for their instructional value, but to afford the opportunity to share experiences with others.

Some Problems in Education of the Diabetic Patient Lack of education, inability to read English, and failing vision are among the problems encountered in the use of printed materials. Sometimes a member of the family can assist in using printed materials. Poster, tapes, films, and food models may be used. The nurse and dietitian must expect to spend more time with patients who present these problems, but repeated verbal instruction can be successful.

About half the diabetic patients are from families with very limited incomes. Although the diabetic diet need not be more expensive than a normal diet, the daily meal pattern must be carefully planned to make the best use of inexpensive foods. Most patients and their families can profit by advice in the wise purchase of foods.

Patients often ask about the use of dietetic foods. Water-packed fruits sweetened with artificial sweetener or those packed in natural juice without sugar are available in most supermarkets at costs only slightly above that of regular packs and are useful when fresh fruits are out of season. Many water-packed fruits are sweetened with artificial sweeteners.

Dietetic foods such as cookies, candies, ice cream, and gluten breads are not needed since most diabetic diets are sufficiently liberal to include a wide choice of foods. Some of the specialty products are expensive. Although low in carbohydrate, most of them contain protein and fat, thus contributing available glucose and calories. Some prefer to teach the patient to figure in the regular item (e.g., ice cream) and to adjust the insulin accordingly.[15] Short-term studies suggest that fructose or sorbitol is absorbed from the gastrointestinal tract more slowly than glucose and therefore does not elevate fasting plasma glucose, but long-term studies are needed.[16] Products containing fructose or sorbitol should not be used freely as the calorie value of these sugars is equivalent to that of glucose. The patient who wishes to use such products should be advised about the specific changes which need to be made in his or her meal pattern. Other sweeteners, such as saccharin and aspartame provide negligible calories and are used in many foods, beverages, chewing gum, and snack foods. These should be used with discretion because the long-term effects are not known. (See Chapter 6.)

Some patients ask about the use of alcoholic beverages. If the physician permits their use, the caloric equivalent of the beverage, as fat, is first subtracted from the day's allowance, and the balance of the diet is calculated accordingly. Diabetics using alcohol should limit their intake to two equivalents, equal to two fat exchanges, daily. Examples of an equivalent are 1.5 ounces whisky, gin, or vodka; 3 ounces of dry sherry; 4 ounces of dry wine; or 12 ounces of light beer.[17]

Initially the patient should become thoroughly familiar with the kinds and amounts of foods allowed from the exchange lists. Once confidence has been developed in the use of these lists, the patient needs to be given some assistance in the use of food mixtures. A number of cookbooks have been prepared specifically for diabetic patients and include calculations of nutritive values. Some food processors have developed tables showing how their products can fit into the food exchanges. Patients usually need some assistance in the interpretation of these printed materials.

Persons using the insulin pump or multiple daily injections of insulin often believe that they can eliminate the need for diet control with these therapies. In most respects, however, the dietary management is the same for these patients as it is for those on conventional therapy. Weight control, consistency in meal size from day to day, regularity of meal times, and avoidance of concentrated sweets are basic to dietary management in diabetes, regardless of the type of therapy used. The insulin pump permits more flexibility in timing of meals and eliminates the need for snacks, since it is not necessary to eat at specific times to cover the insulin peak of intermediate-acting insulin. Most investigators recommend that a bedtime snack be included, however.

Acute Complications of Diabetes

Hypoglycemia Insulin shock or hypoglycemia is caused by an overdose of insulin, a decrease in the available glucose because of delay in eating, omission of food, or loss of food by vomiting and diarrhea, or an increase in exercise without accompanying modification of the insulin dosage.

The patient going into insulin shock becomes uneasy, nervous, weak, and hungry. He or she is pale, the skin is moist, and perspiration is excessive. There may be trembling, dizziness, faintness, headache, and double vision. Movements may be uncoordinated. Emotional instability may be indicated by crying, by hilarious behavior, or by belligerency. Occasionally nausea and vomiting or convulsions may occur. Without treatment coma follows and death is impending. Laboratory studies show a blood sugar below 50 mg per dl.

Orange juice or other fruit juices, sugar, candy, syrup, honey, a carbonated beverage, or any readily available carbohydrate may be given. If absorption is normal, recovery follows in a few minutes. If there is stupor, intravenous glucose is necessary. Some patients are now using one or another of the slowly acting insulins, in which case reactions may recur after a few hours. To avoid such subsequent reactions, it is necessary to follow the initial carbohydrate therapy in 1 or 2 hours and at later intervals with foods containing carbohydrate which is slowly absorbed—such as in milk and bread.

The patient must be impressed with the importance of balance between diet and insulin dosage and the importance of close adherence to the physician's orders. The patient should always carry some sugar or hard candy to avert symptoms when they are still mild.

Diabetic Acidosis and Coma Diabetic ketoacidosis is a state of severe insulin deficiency which is characterized by hyperglycemia, elevated glucagon levels, acidosis, and elevated blood ketones, and which may progress to coma. Coma often originates because the patient consumed additional foods for which the insulin did not provide, or because he failed to take the correct amount of insulin or omitted it entirely. The presence of diabetes is first detected in some persons who were not aware of the disease until coma occurred. Infection is an especially sinister influence since even a mild infection reduces the carbohydrate tolerance and severe acidosis may sometimes occur before the insulin dosage has been appropriately increased. Trauma of any kind, whether an injury or surgery, aggravates the diabetes so that acidosis is more likely.

Some of the signs of diabetic acidosis and coma are similar to those of insulin shock, and a differentiation cannot be made without information concerning the patient prior to the onset of the symptoms, together with blood and urine studies. The patient complains of feeling ill and weak; he or she may have a headache, anorexia, nausea and vomiting, abdominal pain, and aches and pains elsewhere. The skin is hot, flushed, and dry; the mouth is dry and the patient is thirsty. An acetone odor on the breath, painful, rapid breathing, and drowsiness are typical signs. Symptoms of shock, unconsciousness, and death follow unless prompt measures are taken. Sugar, acetone, and acetoacetic acid are present in the urine, blood lipids and blood glucose are elevated, and the blood carbon dioxide content is decreased.

When early signs of ketosis are present, small repeated doses of insulin are given together with small carbohydrate feedings. Diabetic coma, however, is a medical emergency best treated in a hospital, where close nursing care can be given. The physician directs the therapy, which includes large doses of regular insulin with smaller doses repeated as needed every hour or so until the urine sugar is reduced and the blood sugar is lowered to less than 200 mg per dl; saline infusions for the correction of dehydration; gastric lavage if the patient has been vomiting; and alkali therapy for the correction of the severe acidosis.

When the urine sugar decreases and the blood sugar begins to fall, glucose is given by infusion in order to avoid subsequent hypoglycemic reactions. As soon as fluids can be taken orally, the patient is given fruit juices, ginger ale, tea, and broth. All are useful for their fluid content; fruit juice and ginger ale provide carbohydrate; broth contains sodium chloride; and fruit juices and broth contribute potassium. These fluids may be given in amounts of 100 ml, more or less, every hour or so during the first day. By the second day, the patient is usually able to take a soft diet, which is calculated to contain 100 to 200 g carbohydrate, and by the third day the patient may take the diet that meets his or her particular requirements.

Chronic Complications of Diabetes

Large Vessel Disease Atherosclerosis of the coronary, cerebral, and lower extremity arteries is accelerated in all age groups. The likelihood of cardiovascular disease is two to three times greater, with higher morbidity and mortality than in nondiabetics. Obese women with diabetes are at especially high risk for cardiovascular disease.

Small Vessel Disease Generalized thickening of the capillary basement membranes occurs in long-standing diabetes and precedes the development of retinopathy and nephropathy.

Changes in vessels of the retina may lead to cataracts, retinopathy, or blindness. Diabetes is the leading cause of new cases of blindness in the United States. Retinopathy is seen in about 20 percent of those who have had the disease for 10 years and in nearly half of those with diabetes for 25 years or more.

Renal disease accounts for about half the deaths in persons with insulin-dependent diabetes of many years' duration. Glomerulosclerosis, vascular changes, hypertension, albuminuria, and edema are characteristically seen in Kimmelstiel-Wilson's disease, a syndrome occurring in diabetes.

Neuropathy Peripheral nerve dysfunction is a common finding in diabetes. Several hypotheses have been proposed to explain the etiology: (1) ischemic vascular disease; (2) biochemical changes in nerves and structural changes in Schwann cells, leading to demyelination (loss of myelin could slow the rate of nerve conduction); or (3) damage to the neurons followed by degeneration of axons and eventual nerve demyelination.[18] Because of the sensory impairment good foot care is essential. Even minor trauma can lead to infection and gangrene.

It is not known how important the control of blood glucose levels is in preventing or delaying development of chronic complications of diabetes. Some investigators believe that large vessel changes are related primarily to obesity and abnormal lipid metabolism, whereas small vessel disease and neuropathy are more closely related to hyperglycemia. Control of blood glucose levels may have a favorable effect in decreasing the latter type of complications, although this is still controversial.[19-22]

The National Institutes of Health are conducting a multicenter trial (The Diabetes Control and Complications Trial) designed to study the relationship between metabolic controls and chronic complications of diabetes.[23]

Special Situations

Exercise Exercise is an important component of diabetes management because of the improvement in glucose metabolism that follows. For the obese diabetic, a regular exercise program combined with caloric restriction may be sufficient to promote weight loss and improve blood glucose control. Insulin-dependent type I diabetics or insulin-requiring type II diabetics should take snacks containing simple carbohydrates before short-duration exercise and protein and complex carbohydrates before prolonged exercise

in order to prevent hypoglycemia. Reduction of the usual insulin dose may also be needed. Carbohydrate such as candy, juice, or soft drinks should be available to treat hypoglycemic symptoms if needed.

Minor Illness The stress of acute illnesses such as flu requires adjustments in insulin and diet. Patients sometimes mistakenly believe they can omit their insulin if nausea and vomiting prevent them from eating as usual. They should be instructed to continue the usual dose of insulin and to test the urine for sugar and acetone at least four times per day.[24] Regular insulin should be used if additional insulin is needed. Liquids should be taken frequently throughout the day. If the regular diet is not tolerated, soft or liquid foods can provide the appropriate amount of carbohydrate. The physician should be notified if the illness persists more than 3 days, if the regular diet is not tolerated, and if glycosuria and ketonuria persist.

Surgery Ideally, the diabetic patient who is having surgery should have a normal blood sugar, no glycosuria, and no ketosis. A glycogen reserve is essential and can be ensured only if sufficient carbohydrate is included up to 12 hours before the operation and if insulin is supplied in great enough amounts for the utilization of the carbohydrate. Fluids in abundance are indicated. When emergency surgery is needed, parenteral glucose is usually ordered.

Carbohydrate feedings should begin within 3 hours after operation, as a rule. Initially glucose may be given parenterally. When liquids can be taken by mouth, tea with sugar, orange juice, and ginger ale may be used. When a full fluid or soft diet can be tolerated, the diet can be calculated to provide the protein and fat as well as the carbohydrate allowances.

Infection The guidance of a physician is important when a diabetic patient has an infection. An infection lowers the carbohydrate tolerance and increases the insulin requirement. A mild diabetic may become a severe case, and infections may precipitate coma. The physician sometimes orders insulin for patients who are not ordinarily required to use insulin.

Pregnancy Diabetes increases the hazards of pregnancy because of the dangers of glycogen depletion, hypoglycemia, acidosis, and infection. Despite the increased hazards the diabetic woman can have an uneventful pregnancy and a healthy baby. She should have medical guidance throughout her pregnancy with emphasis on control of the rate of weight gain and the prevention of edema. The nutritional requirements are similar to those of the nonpregnant diabetic woman. An optimum weight gain of 22 to 30 lb (10 to 13 kg) is recommended with a 2 to 4-lb increase in the first trimester and a gain of 0.5 to 1.0 lb each week thereafter.[25] Addition of 50 g carbohydrate and 30 g protein to the prepregnancy meal plan will provide the additional calories needed. The protein allowance for young teens and older adolescents is slightly higher than that for biologically mature women.[26] The importance of regularity in mealtimes and snacks should be emphasized. Insulin requirements are usually increased late in pregnancy. A bedtime snack with at least 25 g carbohydrate is needed to lessen the possibility of overnight hypoglycemia.[26]

CASE STUDY 20

Woman with Noninsulin-Dependent Diabetes Mellitus

Mrs. I, age 45, is the mother of three teenagers. She works full time as a counselor in a job placement bureau. Recently Mrs. I noticed that she has difficulty reading street signs and fine print. Thinking that she needed a new pair of glasses, she made an appointment with her ophthalmologist. A significant refractive change and evidence of premature cataracts were found during the eye examination. The ophthalmologist suspected that Mrs. I's eye problems were complications related to diabetes and referred her to an internist.

The internist found no evidence of cardiovascular, neurologic, or renal impairment. Mrs. I's blood pressure was 120/70; height 165 cm (65 in.); and weight 74 kg (163 lb). A 2-hour postprandial blood glucose level was 200 mg per dl. Mrs. I made an appointment for a glucose tolerance test the following week. Her fasting blood sugar was 130 mg per dl. Glucose tolerance test values were 300 mg per dl at 1 hour, 248 mg per dl at 2 hours, and 195 mg per dl at 3 hours.

In terms of significant history, Mrs. I's mother has noninsulin-dependent diabetes, and two of Mrs. I's children weighed over 4.5 kg (9 lb, 14 oz) at birth. The only symptoms Mrs. I recalled were recurrent blurred vision and thirst. She had not experienced any hypoglycemic symptoms.

The history, physical examination, and laboratory studies confirmed the diagnosis of type II diabetes mellitus. Mrs. I was placed on a 1,200-kcal diet. The clinic nurse demonstrated glucose monitoring and record keeping. Mrs. I was encouraged to exercise daily to help her achieve her weight goal and help reduce hyperglycemia.

The clinic dietitian assisted Mrs. I with exchange meal planning. In the course of the diet history the dietitian learned that Mrs. I pays little attention to her food intake. Mrs. I often snacks when she is nervous and is a compulsive eater. She enjoys baking bread and pastries for her family and she does not feel that she should deprive them of their favorite foods, especially sweets. She has a difficult time not tasting what she is preparing. Mr. and Mrs. I often have wine with their dinner. The dietitian gave Mrs. I exchange lists and several sample menus. She suggested helpful recipe books and answered Mrs. I's many questions about her diet.

Mrs. I also participated in group classes one evening a week with other new diabetics, in which topics such as the nature and treatment of diabetes, acute and chronic complications, and what to do in case of illness were covered. Mrs. I was invited to join a group of diabetics trying to lose weight. She was informed of the many resources available to her. She decided to join the local chapter of the American Diabetes Association and will receive *Forecast* magazine through that organization.

Pathophysiologic Correlations

1. What factors in Mrs. I's history suggest that she might eventually become diabetic?
2. Which of the following terms apply to most persons with noninsulin dependent diabetes: hyperglycemia; stable; labile; have lost weight; produce some insulin; usually require some insulin; prone to ketoacidosis; may be hyperinsulinemic.
3. Why are obese persons more susceptible to diabetes?
4. Why would Mrs. I's diabetes be more easily controlled with weight loss?
5. Mrs. I was instructed to maintain her usual activity pattern and to consume a high-carbohydrate diet for the 3 days preceding her glucose tolerance test. What was the purpose of this?
6. List some factors that may result in an abnormal glucose tolerance test.
7. In noninsulin-dependent diabetes there is a lack of effective insulin in the body. What reasons can you suggest for Mrs. I's lack of effective insulin?
8. List some of the chronic complications of diabetes mellitus.

Nutritional Assessment

9. Assuming a large body frame, what should Mrs. I weigh? (NOTE: Use the Metropolitan

Life Insurance Table, Appendix A-16.) Using the HANES I data, how does Mrs. I's weight compare with that of other women of her height and age?

10. What is a reasonable goal for the length of time needed for Mrs. I to achieve her desired weight?

11. What problems do you face in helping Mrs. I to become motivated to follow a diet?

Planning the Diet

12. List the objectives you would set up when planning Mrs. I's diet.

13. A 1,200-kcal diet was prescribed for Mrs. I. The caloric distribution of the diet was as follows: carbohydrate, 55 percent; protein, 15 percent; fat, 30 percent. Calculate the grams of carbohydrate, protein, and fat to be included in the diet.

14. Based on your calculations in the preceding question, calculate the number of exchanges of food that might be included in Mrs. I's diet. See Table A-4 for exchange values.

15. Using the calculations in question 14, plan a menu for one day for Mrs. I. Keep the calorie and carbohydrate distribution between the three meals as even as possible. Indicate measures of foods to be used.

Dietary Counseling

16. List the points you would emphasize in counseling Mrs. I about her diet.

17. Because Mrs. I gets so much pleasure from baking rich desserts, is it realistic to expect her to give up pastries, cakes, and so on? What suggestions can you make?

18. Mrs. I asks about the use of dietetic canned foods. How would you advise her?

19. Would you recommend that she use dietetic cookies, ice cream, and candies? Explain.

20. What advice can you give concerning the use of fructose instead of sucrose in the diet?

21. Mrs. I asked her physician if she could have wine. The physician suggested that she might try it occasionally. If Mrs. I substitutes 3 ounces wine for fat exchanges, how many fat exchanges would she need to omit?

22. Mrs. I asks whether there is anything that she can do to prevent the occurrence of diabetes in her children. What would you tell her?

23. One of Mrs. I's co-workers is on a high-protein, low-carbohydrate, "quick weight loss" diet. Would this type of diet be suitable for Mrs. I? Explain.

References for the Case Study

HEINS, J. M.: "Dietary Management in Diabetes Mellitus," *Nurs. Clin. North Am.*, 18:631–43, December 1983.

McDONALD, J.: "Alcohol and Diabetes," *Diabetes Care*, 3:629–37, 1980.

NEMCHIK, R.: "A Very Different Diet; A New Generation of Oral Drugs," *R.N.*, 45:41–45ff, 1982.

NUTTAL, F. Q.: "Diet and the Diabetic Patient," *Diabetes Care*, 6:197–207, 1983.

POPKESS-VAWTER, S.: "The Adult Living with Diabetes Mellitus," *Nurs. Clin. North Am.*, 18:777–89, December 1983.

References

1. Stowers, J. M.: "Nutrition in Diabetes," *Nutr. Abstr. Rev.*, 33:1–15, 1963.

2. National Diabetes Data Group: "Classification and Diagnosis of Diabetes Mellitus and Other Categories of Glucose Intolerance," *Diabetes*, 28:1039–57, 1979.

3. Lipson, L. G., and Lipson, M.: "The Therapeutic Approach to the Obese Maturity-Onset Diabetic Patient," *Arch. Intern. Med.*, 144:135–8, 1984.

4. Guthrie, D. W., and Guthrie, R. A.: "The Disease Process of Diabetes Mellitus. Definition, Characteristics, Trends, and Developments," *Nurs. Clin. North Am.*, 18:617–30, December 1983.

5. Bergman, M., and Felig, P.: "Newer Approaches to the Control of the Insulin-Dependent Diabetic Patient," *DM*, 29:8–65, April 1983.

6. Loewenstein, J. E.: "Insulin Pumps and Other Recent Advances in the Outpatient Treatment of Diabetes," *Arch. Intern. Med.*, 144:755–8, 1984.

7. Shuman, C. R.: "Glipizide: An Overview," *Am. J. Med.*, 75 (5B):55–9, 1983.

8. American Diabetes Association: "Principles of Nutrition and Dietary Recommendations for Individuals with Diabetes Mellitus: 1979," *Diabetes*, 28:1027–30, 1979.

9. Arky, R., Wylie-Rosett, J., and El-Beheri, B.: "Examination of Current Dietary Recommendations for Individuals with Diabetes Mellitus," *Diabetes Care*, 5:59–63, January–February 1982.

10. Jenkins, D. J. A.: "Dietary Carbohydrates and their Glycemic Responses," *J. Am. Diet. Assoc.*, 251: 2829–31, 1984.

11. Crapo, P. A., et al.: "Comparison of Serum Glucose, Insulin, and Glucagon Responses to Different Types of Complex Carbohydrates in Noninsulin-Dependent Diabetic Patients," *Am. J. Clin. Nutr.*, 34:184–90. 1981.

12. Bantle, J. T., et al.: "Postprandial Glucose and Insulin Response to Meals Containing Different Carbohydrates in Normal and Diabetic Subjects," *N. Engl. J. Med.*, 309:7–12, 1983.

13. Crapo, P. A.: "Theory vs. Fact. The Glycemic Re-

sponse to Foods," *Nutr. Today*, **19**:6–11, March–April 1984.

14. Munoz, J.: "Fiber and Diabetes," *Diabetes Care*, **7**:297–300, May–June 1984.

15. Nathan, D. M., et al.: "Ice Cream in the Diet of Insulin-Dependent Diabetic Patients," *JAMA*, **251**: 2825–7, 1984.

16. Brunzell, J. D.: "Use of Fructose, Sorbitol, or Xylitol as a Sweetener in Diabetes Mellitus," *J. Am. Diet Assoc.*, **73**:499–506, 1978.

17. Franz, M. J.: "Diabetes Mellitus. Considerations in the Development of Guidelines for the Occasional Use of Alcohol," *J. Am. Diet. Assoc.*, **83**:147–52, 1983.

18. Clements, R. S.: "Diabetes Neuropathy—New Concepts of Its Etiology," *Diabetes*, **28**:604–11, 1979.

19. Raskin, P., et al.: "The Effect of Diabetes Control on the Width of Skeletal-Muscle Capillary Basement Membrane in Patients with Type I Diabetes Mellitus," *N. Engl. J. Med.*, **309**:1546–50, 1983.

20. Siperstein, M. D.: "Diabetic Microangiopathy and the Control of Blood Glucose," *N. Engl. J. Med.*, **309**: 1577–9, 1983.

21. Gerich, J. E.: "Role of Growth Hormone in Diabetes Mellitus," *N. Engl. J. Med.*, **310**:848–9, 1984.

22. Holman, R. R., et al.: "Prevention of Deterioration of Renal and Sensory Nerve Function by More Intensive Management of Insulin-Dependent Diabetic Patients," *Lancet*, **1**:204–8, 1983.

23. Salans, L. B.: "NIH Plans Study of Diabetes Control and Complications," *N. Engl. J. Med.*, **307**:1527–8, 1982.

24. Bovington, N. M., et al.: "Management of the Patient with Diabetes Mellitus During Surgery or Illness," *Nurs. Clin. North Am.*, **18**:661–71, December 1983.

25. Ney, D., and Hollingsworth, D. R.: "Nutritional Management of Pregnancy Complicated by Diabetes. Historical Perspective," *Diabetes Care*, **4**:647–55, 1981.

26. Franz, M.: "Nutritional Management in Diabetes and Pregnancy," *Diabetes Care*, **1**:264–70, 1978.

37

Various Metabolic Disorders
Purine-Restricted Diet

Many diseases for which dietary modification is an effective part of treatment are deviations of normal metabolic pathways in the body. They occur because of abnormal production of one or more hormones, a deficiency of an enzyme, or a modification of excretion. Those which are discussed in this chapter fall into one or another of these categories but otherwise bear little, if any, relation to each other.

Hypoglycemia

Etiology   HYPOGLYCEMIA refers to an abnormally low blood glucose level and may be of organic or functional origin. Organic causes include the following: (1) hyperinsulinism due to tumors or hyperplasia of islet cells; surgery rather than dietary management is essential; (2) hepatic diseases involving enzyme defects (see Chapter 42), alcoholism, or cirrhosis; and (3) endocrine disorders such as hypothyroidism and adrenocortical or pituitary insufficiency. Functional hypoglycemias are more common and may produce symptoms in the fasting state (spontaneous type) or, more frequently, in response to food intake (reactive type). An example of the latter is functional hyperinsulinism, in which there is oversecretion of insulin following carbohydrate ingestion, with the following effects on the blood glucose level: (1) a normal fasting blood sugar; (2) hypoglycemia 2 to 4 hours after meals, especially in the forenoon and late afternoon; (3) no hypoglycemia following fasting or the omission of meals; and (4) a glucose tolerance curve (see Figure 36-1), which shows a normal fasting sugar, initially elevated glucose level after taking the glucose, and a sharp fall to very low sugar levels generally less than 50 mg per dl.

Functional hypoglycemia may occur following gastrectomy or gastroenterostomy when nutrients are absorbed at an extremely rapid rate. In such situations the food reaches the small intestine much more rap-

idly than is normal, is very quickly absorbed, and the sudden elevation of the blood sugar serves as an extra stimulus to the islet cells and a subsequent hypoglycemia. (See Chapter 34 for description of the dumping syndrome.) Functional hypoglycemia may also be a manifestation of early noninsulin-dependent diabetes, may be induced by drug therapy such as salicylates or sulfonylureas, or may be idiopathic in nature.

Symptoms   Rapid fall of the blood glucose level causes release of epinephrine and produces symptoms of weakness, nervousness, trembling, perspiring freely, rapid heartbeat, hunger, or nausea and vomiting. As a result of inadequate delivery of glucose to the brain, the person with chronic, severe hypoglycemia may experience headache, incoordination, irritability, confusion, emotional instability, and even coma.

Contrary to popular belief, occurrence of these symptoms does not necessarily indicate functional (reactive) hypoglycemia. Criteria for the diagnosis include occurrence of symptoms when the blood glucose is at its lowest point (nadir) and relief of symptoms by glucose ingestion.[1]

Modification of the Diet   A diet prescription to meet each patient's needs is planned.

Carbohydrate.   In hypoglycemias associated with some hepatic enzyme deficiencies or liver diseases, carbohydrate supplements are needed. In postprandial hypoglycemias the carbohydrate serves as a stimulus to further insulin secretion and is provocative of the hypoglycemic attack; thus, it is usually restricted to 100 g or less. A diet low in refined carbohydrates is used; and complex carbohydrates are substituted.[2]

Protein.   A high-protein diet is essential, since there is no appreciable increase in the blood sugar level following high-protein meals even though protein furnishes approximately 50 percent of its weight in available glucose. This available glucose is released to the bloodstream so gradually that there is little stimulation to the islets of Langerhans.

Fat. When the levels of carbohydrate and protein have been established, the remaining calories are obtained from fat. Because the carbohydrate is so severely restricted, the fat level is, of necessity, high.

DIETARY COUNSELING FOR POSTPRANDIAL HYPOGLYCEMIA

The exchange lists (see Table A-4) may be used for calculation of the diet prescription. Since carbohydrates are drastically restricted, the bread exchanges will usually be omitted. In order to include adequate amounts of fruits and vegetables, milk is limited to 2 or 3 cups; children should receive calcium supplements.

In order that absorption from the intestine will be gradual, the daily allowances of protein and fat, as well as carbohydrate, are divided into three approximately equal parts. Midmorning, midafternoon, and bedtime feedings are often desirable, in which case part of the food planned for the preceding meal can be used for the interval feeding. Carbohydrate-containing foods must be carefully measured. Alcohol is not recommended because of its glucose-lowering effect.

Adrenocortical Insufficiency

Addison's disease is a comparatively rare condition resulting from an impairment of the functioning of the adrenal cortex.

Sometimes adrenalectomy is necessary in which event the resultant metabolic effects are those of Addison's disease. Since the pituitary governs the activity of the adrenal cortex, hypophysectomy will also lead to characteristic symptoms of adrenal insufficiency.

Metabolic Effects and Related Symptoms Clinical manifestations usually do not occur until 90 percent of the adrenal cortex has been destroyed. The symptoms of insufficiency are directly related to the absence of hormones produced by the adrenal cortex.

Glucocorticoids. The principal action of these hormones, chiefly cortisol, is on the regulation of the metabolism of carbohydrate, protein, and fat. Upon stimulation of cortisol, the liver forms glycogen from the amino acids supplied by the tissues. The hormone increases the rate of protein catabolism and decreases the permeability of the muscle cells to amino acids. On the other hand, the permeability of the liver cells is increased and the amino acids released as a result of protein catabolism are transported to the liver and may be used for synthesis of new protein. The glucocorticoids also influence the deposition of fatty tissue or the mobilization of fats.

In the absence of glucocorticoids rapid glycogen depletion occurs, followed by hypoglycemia a few hours after meals. Such hypoglycemia may be severe in a patient who has had no food for 10 or 12 hours. A glucose tolerance test shows a lower maximum blood sugar and a more rapid return to normal fasting levels than is obtained in normal individuals. (See Figure 36-1.)

The production of glucocorticoids by the adrenal gland is governed by the adrenocorticotropic hormone (ACTH) of the pituitary. In the event hypophysectomy is performed, the adrenal cortex atrophies and glucocorticoids are not produced, just as they are not elaborated in Addison's disease.

Mineralocorticoids. Mineralocorticoids, of which aldosterone is of primary importance, are concerned with maintaining electrolyte homeostasis, especially for sodium and potassium. This production is regulated by the levels of sodium and potassium in the circulation. Aldosterone production leads to increased retention of sodium and greater excretion of potassium. Unlike the glucocorticoids, aldosterone production is not influenced by the pituitary. A deficiency of aldosterone, as seen in Addison's disease, leads to excessive excretion of sodium and increased retention of potassium. With the large salt loss much water is also excreted, thus leading to dehydration, hemoconcentration, reduced blood volume, and hypotension. In severe deficiency the patient experiences profound weakness and may have a craving for salt.

Androgenic Hormones. Androgenic hormones stimulate protein synthesis. In their absence, tissue wasting, weight loss, reduction of muscle strength, and fatigue are present.

Patients with adrenal insufficiency frequently experience anorexia, nausea, vomiting, abdominal discomfort, and diarrhea. Most of the patients have an increased pigmentation of the skin, often that of a deep tan or bronze. This results from the excessive production of *melanophore-stimulating hormone* by the pituitary when the adrenal steroids are lacking to exert an inhibitory effect.

Diagnostic Tests Adrenal insufficiency is detected by determination of plasma cortisol levels and by an ACTH stimulation test.

Treatment Replacement of glucocorticoids and mineralocorticoids is necessary. Cortisone (or hydrocortisone) is the primary drug; however, supplementary mineralocorticoid as fludrocortisone is sometimes needed. A liberal salt intake is needed especially during periods of excessive physical exercise, very hot weather, or gastrointestinal upsets.

DIETARY COUNSELING

A diet high in protein and relatively low in carbohydrate reduces the stimulation of insulin and helps avoid the episodes of hypoglycemia. Meals should be given at frequent intervals—allowing between-meal feedings and a late bedtime feeding. Each of the feedings should include protein in order to reduce the rate of carbohydrate absorption. Simple carbohydrates—candy, sugar, and other sweets—are best avoided because of their rapid digestion and absorption and their stimulation of excessive insulin production. Patients should be advised to take cortisone with meals or with milk to prevent irritation of the gastric mucosa by the drug.[4]

Metabolic Effects of Adrenocortical Therapy

The adrenocorticotropic hormone of the anterior pituitary gland (ACTH) and the steroids of the adrenal cortex are used for the treatment of a wide variety of diseases such as arthritis, allergies, skin disturbances, adrenal insufficiency, many gastrointestinal diseases, and others. Although the various products used may vary somewhat in the degree of their effects on metabolism, it is important to be aware of possible nutritional implications of long-continued use of these hormones.

Water and Electrolyte Metabolism Adrenocortical steroids in excess lead to retention of sodium and water and loss of potassium, as seen in Cushing's syndrome. Some sodium restriction is necessary for many patients. Usually, it is sufficient to avoid salty foods and to use no salt at the table, but a 1,000-mg-sodium diet may occasionally be required. (See Chapter 39.) When the patient is eating well, the amounts of potassium in the diet are liberal. Foods especially high in potassium include broth, fruit juices, vegetables, whole-grain cereals, and meats.

Protein Metabolism A negative nitrogen balance may result when large doses of cortisone are used. This can be prevented when the diet is sufficiently liberal in carbohydrate to exert a maximum protein-sparing effect and when high-protein intakes are emphasized.

Carbohydrate Metabolism Cortisone therapy increases the storage of glycogen by increasing the amount of glycogen formation from protein. There also appears to be an insensitivity to insulin, as indicated by hyperglycemia and glycosuria. In diabetic patients, who are also receiving cortisone, additional insulin may be required.

Gastrointestinal System Hydrochloric acid secretion is increased following adrenocortical steroid therapy, and peptic ulceration may develop. In such a situation, the dietary modification described for peptic ulcer should be used. (See Chapter 29.)

Several tests can be used to diagnose Cushing's disease. These include measurement of basal A.M. and P.M. plasma cortisol, urinary free cortisol, urinary 17-hydroxysteroids, and a dexamethasone suppression test.[3]

Hyperthyroidism

Symptoms and Clinical Findings Hyperthyroidism is a disturbance in which there is an excessive secretion of the thyroid gland with a consequent increase in the metabolic rate. It is believed to be an autoimmune disease occurring in genetically predisposed persons. The disease is also known as exophthalmic goiter, thyrotoxicosis, Graves' disease, or Basedow's disease. The chief symptoms are weight loss sometimes to the point of emaciation, excessive nervousness, prominence of the eyes, and a generally enlarged thyroid gland. The appetite is often increased, weakness may be marked, and signs of cardiac failure may be present.

Metabolism All the metabolic processes in the body are accelerated in hyperthyroidism. Serum protein-bound iodine values are elevated. The basal metabolic rate may be increased 50 percent or more in severe cases. Moreover, the patient tends to be restless so that the total energy metabolism is further increased. When the level of calories is insufficient, the liver store of glycogen is rapidly depleted. This is especially serious just prior to surgery, since postoperative shock is more likely.

The increased level of nitrogen metabolism leads to destruction of tissue proteins. Unless both protein and calorie levels are adequate, loss of weight may be rapid.

The excretion of calcium and phosphorus is greatly increased in hyperthyroidism. Osteoporosis and bone fractures are associated with severe losses. The increased level of energy metabolism increases the requirement for B-complex vitamins. For reasons not fully understood, the utilization of vitamin A and ascorbic acid is also speeded up.

Treatment   Hyperthyroidism is treated by radioactive iodine, antithyroid drugs, or surgery. Antithyroid drugs reduce the basal metabolic rate to normal, but a liberal diet is still indicated because patients have usually experienced severe malnutrition before therapy.

DIETARY COUNSELING

Until normal nutrition is restored, approximately 4,000 to 5,000 kcal and 100 to 125 g protein should be allowed. (See High-Calorie Diet, Chapter 25.) Frequent feedings will help satisfy hunger. A liberal calcium intake is desirable and may be provided as calcium salts in addition to the liberal use of milk. The diet itself will include generous allowances of vitamin A, the B complex, and ascorbic acid, but supplements are often prescribed.

Hypothyroidism

Decreased production or activity of the thyroid hormone, or hypothyroidism, is a relatively common problem. It occurs most often in adult women. It is known as myxedema when severe in the adult, or cretinism when its symptoms become apparent shortly after birth. (See Chapter 9.) Myxedema is characterized by a lowered rate of energy metabolism—often 30 to 40 percent below normal, muscular flabbiness, puffy face, eyelids, and hands, sensitivity to cold, marked fatigue with slight exertion, and a personality change including apathy and dullness. Decreased gastrointestinal motility often results in constipation. Blood lipids are often elevated.

Treatment.   Replacement of thyroid hormone by medication is the customary therapy. Obesity is a problem for some patients with hypothyroidism, since they may continue in their earlier patterns of eating even though the energy metabolism has been significantly reduced. In other patients, the appetite may be so poor that undernutrition results. For overweight persons, reduction of calories is necessary. (See Chapter 25.) Reduction of dietary cholesterol may be indi-

cated. Adequate fluids and foods high in dietary fiber are needed to overcome constipation.

Joint Diseases

Incidence   Arthritis is the principal crippler in the United States. It affects more than 30 million Americans, of whom some 3 million persons are limited in their usual activity.[5] The incidence is higher in women, in people with low incomes, in the later years of life, and among residents of rural areas. Most cases of arthritis occur in persons over 45 years of age.

Symptoms and Clinical Findings   The terms *arthritis* and *rheumatism* are applied to many joint diseases. Rheumatic fever is a special threat to the child or young adult because inadequate treatment may permanently damage the heart. Gout, another of the joint diseases, is an error of uric acid metabolism and is discussed on page 524.

The most common form of arthritis is *osteoarthritis* or *degenerative* arthritis. Theories regarding etiology hold that it is (1) primarily a degenerative disease of cartilage, which leads to subsequent changes in bone; or (2) due to pathologic changes in bone, which increase stress on cartilage and lead to its breakdown. The earliest pathologic changes occur in joint cartilage and subsequent new bone spurs develop at the edges. Joint stiffness is characteristic. Pain is confined to joints and is associated with motion or weight bearing and is relieved by rest. Joints of the fingers, knees, hip, and spine are frequently involved. Degenerative joint disease may also occur secondary to obesity, trauma, and metabolic and endocrine diseases, among others.

Rheumatoid arthritis is a highly inflammatory and very painful condition having its onset in young adults, especially women. Autoimmunity and an infectious process have been proposed as etiologic factors. Rheumatoid arthritis is characterized by fatigue, pain, stiffness, deformity which may be severe, and limited function. The disease is progressive, but the symptoms may spontaneously disappear only to reappear again at a later time. With early diagnosis the disabling effect can be delayed but there is no known cure.

Treatment   Probably few diseases have had more theories offered concerning therapy. Arthritics spend over $950 million annually on phony diets and devices.[5] None of the claims made by promoters has been supported by research. Over the years numerous diets have been tried by clinicians, but none has been effective in modifying the course of the disease. These trials have included diets high or low in protein, fat, and carbohydrate; modified for acid or alkaline ash; or supplemented with vitamins, especially ascorbic acid and vitamin D.

A number of drugs beginning with aspirin bring relief to the arthritic patient. Nonsteroidal antiinflammatory drugs and gold salts have been effective for many. Corticosteroids are used in severe cases. Since these may bring about undesirable side effects, their use for each patient must be carefully evaluated.

Patients whose deformities limit their activities can be helped by physical and occupational therapy. The occupational therapist, home economist, dietitian, and nurse can help patients to greater independence by teaching them how to use many self-help devices. (See Figure 37-1.) Homemakers need counseling on ways to accomplish their housekeeping activities with less effort. Sometimes a rearrangement of kitchen equipment is sufficient; in other instances some modi-

fication of the design of the kitchen itself is needed. (See also pages 397 to 399.)

Nutritional Effects of Drug Therapy. Some individuals experience gastric irritation or even ulceration from aspirin or steroid therapy. These effects can be prevented by taking these medications with meals and with a bedtime snack containing protein foods for their buffering capacity. Steroid therapy also leads to sodium retention in some in which case mild sodium restriction is indicated. Usually it is sufficient to omit salty foods and the use of salt at the table; sometimes, a 1,000-mg-sodium diet may be required. Continued steroid therapy adversely affects the calcium balance, leading to gradual bone demineralization. A liberal intake of milk, contrary to popular opinion, is desirable.

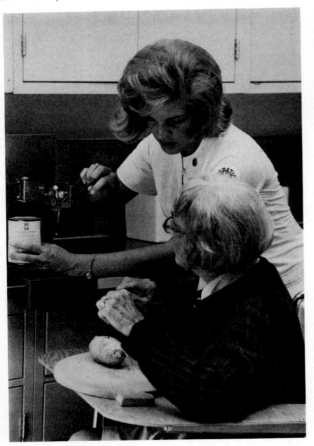

Figure 37-1. An occupational therapist shows a handicapped homemaker how to modify food preparation procedures for her physical limitations. (Courtesy, The Arthritis Foundation.)

DIETARY COUNSELING

Arthritic patients require the same foods for health that other persons need. When patients are of normal weight and in good nutritional status, the normal diet is suitable.

Obesity is a common problem in osteoarthritis, and weight loss should be brought about in order to reduce the added stress on weight-bearing joints. (See Chapter 25 for low-calorie diets.)

Many patients with rheumatoid arthritis have lost weight and are in poor nutritional status. For them a high-calorie high-protein diet is indicated until good nutritional status has been achieved. (See pages 379 and 478.)

Gout

This is a disorder of purine metabolism occurring principally in middle-aged and older men. Women are more susceptible after the menopause. It is characterized by hyperuricemia, recurrent attacks of acute inflammatory arthritis, and deposits of sodium urate (tophi) in joints, cartilage, and kidneys. Uric acid nephrolithiasis occurs in many patients. Hyperuricemia is due to impaired ability of the kidney to excrete the normal urate load presented to it, with a consequent rise in serum uric acid. A smaller percentage of cases are attributed to overproduction of uric acid precursors.[6]

Nature and Occurrence of Uric Acid Cellular material of both plant and animal origin contains *nucleoproteins*. Glandular organs such as liver, pancreas, and kidneys are among the richest sources;

meats and the embryo or germ of grains and legumes, together with the growing parts of young plants, also furnish appreciable amounts. During digestion nucleoproteins are first split into proteins and nucleic acid. Further cleavage of nucleic acid leads to several products, one group of which are the purines. The latter in turn are oxidized to uric acid.

In addition to the uric acid available from the metabolism of nucleic acid, the body can synthesize purines from the simplest carbon and nitrogen compounds such as carbon dioxide, acetic acid, and glycine. Thus any substances from which these materials originate, namely carbohydrate, fat, and protein, give rise to a considerable production of uric acid. Even in the fasting state there is a constant production of uric acid from cellular breakdown.

The liver and tissues store uric acid and its precursors for variable lengths of time and release them later. As a normal constituent of urine, uric acid represents a part of the daily nitrogenous excretion. Some uric acid is also excreted via the bile into the intestinal tract.

Symptoms and Clinical Findings The range of serum uric acid in normal individuals is 2 to 7 mg per dl, whereas in those with susceptibility to gout the concentration is above 7 mg per dl and may reach as high as 20 mg per dl. A large percentage of individuals with hyperuricemia sooner or later will have acute attacks of gout characterized by sudden inflammation and swelling accompanied by severe pain of the joints, especially the metatarsal, knee, and toe joints. The acute attack usually responds dramatically in 24 to 48 hours to treatment with colchicine.

Acute attacks may be precipitated by rapid weight loss, overindulgence in food or alcohol, high-fat diets, ketoacidosis, and drugs, such as thiazide diuretics. Both lactic acid, resulting from heavy alcohol use, and keto acids favor urate retention by the kidney and hyperuricemia.

Treatment A number of drugs are effective in the treatment of gout, and diet is considered an adjunct to drug therapy. Colchicine and a number of other drugs provide effective relief from the pain that accompanies the acute attack. In addition, these drugs reduce the frequency of attacks when they are also used as interval therapy.

Uricosuric drugs (probenecid and others) increase the excretion of uric acid, thereby bringing plasma levels within a normal range. With the lowering of the plasma uric acid levels, sodium urate deposits in the joints are gradually dissolved out. These drugs are not effective in reducing the pain of the acute attack and may exacerbate the symptoms during an attack. Therefore, they are used during the quiescent periods of the disease.

Allopurinol is a drug that inhibits the action of the enzyme *xanthine oxidase*, which is responsible for the formation of uric acid from xanthine and hypoxanthine. Therefore, the excretion of uric acid is diminished and that of xanthine is increased. Inasmuch as xanthine can precipitate out to form kidney stones, it is essential that the patient have a liberal fluid intake and excrete a urine that is neutral or slightly alkaline.

Nutritional Effects of Drug Therapy. Drugs such as colchicine, allopurinol, and probenecid, used in the treatment of gout, should be taken with water close to mealtimes to prevent irritation of the gastrointestinal tract. Damage to the intestinal mucosa induced by these drugs can lead to reduced absorption of sodium, potassium, fat, carotene, riboflavin, vitamin B-12, and lactose.[7]

Modification of the Diet During the acute attacks a low-purine diet is sometimes ordered in addition to drug therapy. Some physicians also recommend moderate restriction of purines as interval therapy for patients receiving uricosuric drugs.

DIETARY COUNSELING

Data on the purine content of foods are limited. Foods have been grouped into three categories in Table 37-1. As may be seen from this classification, all flesh foods and extractives from them

Table 37-1. **Purine Content of Foods per 100 g**

Group I (0–15 mg)	Group II (50–150 mg)	Group III (150 mg and over)
Breads and cereals	Beans, dry	Anchovies
Butter and other fats*	Fish	Asparagus*
Caviar*	Lentils	Brains*
Cheese	Meats	Gravies*
Eggs	Oatmeal*	Kidney
Fish roe*	Peas, dry	Liver
Fruits	Poultry*	Meat extracts
Gelatin*	Seafood	Mincemeat*
Milk	Spinach	Mushrooms*
Nuts*		Sardines
Sugar, sweets*		Sweetbreads
Vegetables		

* Adapted from Turner, D.: *Handbook of Diet Therapy*, 5th ed. University of Chicago Press, Chicago, 1970, p. 117. Starred items are additions to Turner's list.

such as gravies and soups must be eliminated for the low-purine diet. If purine restriction is also prescribed for interval therapy, the allowance of meat, poultry, and fish is limited to 2 to 3 ounces on each of 3 to 5 days.

Energy   The overweight individual should gradually lose weight but should not be placed on a low-calorie diet during acute attacks of gout, since the catabolism of adipose tissue reduces the excretion of uric acid. Rapid weight loss effected by starvation or by extremely low-calorie diets can precipitate an attack of gout. Usually, men can lose weight satisfactorily when their diets are restricted to 1,200 to 1,600 kcal. (See Chapter 25.)

Protein, Fat, and Carbohydrate   Because the nitrogen of the purine nucleus is supplied by protein, the intake is restricted to about 1 g per kg.

Fat is often restricted to about 60 g per day. When the food intake is poor because of illness, it is essential that high-carbohydrate fluids be given so that adipose tissue is not excessively catabolized.

Fluid   The daily intake of fluids should be at least 3 liters. Coffee and tea may be used in moderate amounts. These beverages contain methylated purines which are oxidized to methyl uric acid. The latter is excreted in the urine and is not deposited in the tissues. Hence, the customary omission of coffee and tea may impose an unnecessary hardship.[8] Some clinicians forbid use of alcohol, whereas others permit small amounts occasionally.

To effect an alkaline urine when antigout drugs are prescribed, the diet should be liberal in its content of fruits and vegetables.

Purine-Restricted Diet

General Rules
For a diet essentially free of exogenous purines, use foods only from group 1, Table 37-1.
For a low-purine level, allow 3 to 5 small servings of lean meat, poultry, and fish from group II each week.
If a low-fat regimen is ordered, the butter is omitted, and skim milk is substituted for the whole milk.

Include These Foods Daily:
3-4 cups milk; 1-2 ounces cheese
2 eggs; allow 2 to 3 ounces lean beef, veal, lamb, poultry, or fish 3 to 5 times a week during interval therapy
3-4 servings vegetables including:
   1 medium potato
   1-2 servings green leafy or yellow vegetable
   1 serving other vegetable
2-3 servings fruit including:
   1 serving citrus fruit
   1-2 servings other fruits
   1 serving enriched cereal
4-6 slices enriched bread
   2 tablespoons margarine or butter
Additional calories are provided as needed by increasing the amount of potato, potato substitutes such as
   macaroni, rice, noodles, bread, sugars, sweets, fruits, and vegetables.

Nutritive Value of Basic Foods Above: calories, 1,850; protein, 68 g; fat, 80 g; carbohydrate, 220 g; calcium, 1,400 mg; iron, 11.3 mg; vitamin A, 11,350 IU; thiamin, 1.3 mg; riboflavin, 2.3 mg; niacin, 10 mg; ascorbic acid, 145 mg.

Foods to Avoid
All foods high in purines (see group III, Table 37-1)
Alcohol
For low-fat diets:
   Pastries and rich desserts
   Cream and ice cream
   Fried foods
Eggs not to exceed 2 daily; hard cheese not to exceed 1 ounce. Severe purine restriction may require the
   omission of eggs, whole milk, cheese, and butter. Skim milk and cottage cheese must then be used in ample amounts to provide the necessary protein.

CASE STUDY 21

Young Adult with Suspected Hypoglycemia

Susan is a thin, anxious, 28-year-old graduate student enrolled part time in a MBA program at the University. Besides her classes, Susan enjoys painting and is active in the Jaycees wives. Her husband, Tom, is branch manager of a bank near their home. Susan felt faint one evening after dinner, and Tom convinced her to see a doctor because this happened for the third time in recent weeks.

Susan usually omits breakfast. Because she does not like to cook, she frequently has lunch, consisting of a salad and diet soda, in the student union before her 1:00 P.M. class. Sometimes she has a candy bar instead of lunch if she needs time to read her class assignment. For dinner she has meat, salad, and milk. She usually has a can of soda pop and a snack later in the evening.

Susan's presenting symptoms included occasional sudden onset of headache and dizziness. She remarked that symptoms ceased after she drank soda pop or had something to eat. Upon questioning by the physician, Susan attributed her symptoms to hypoglycemia. Approximately 6 months earlier she had seen a TV talk show on which hypoglycemia was discussed. One of the guests on the show stated that millions of people have undiagnosed hypoglycemia and that a low-carbohydrate diet would relieve symptoms.

The physical examination was unremarkable. There was no history of alimentary, hormonal, or metabolic abnormalities that would cause hypoglycemia. The physician scheduled a 5 hour oral glucose tolerance test for the following week. Susan's fasting blood sugar was 83 mg per dl. Blood glucose values at ½, 1, 2, 3, and 5 hours were 145, 100, 65, 73, and 80 mg per dl, respectively. Between the second and third hour of the test, Susan complained of a headache and dizziness. No significant elevation of plasma cortisol or growth hormone secretion in response to stress was noted following the glucose nadir.

The physician informed Susan that the results of her tests did not substantiate a diagnosis of hypoglycemia. He referred her to a nutritionist for dietary counseling.

Pathophysiologic Correlations

1. What criteria are used for the diagnosis of hypoglycemia?
2. Compare spontaneous hypoglycemia and reactive hypoglycemia.
3. How does the glucose tolerance curve differ in diabetes mellitus and functional hypoglycemia?
4. What factors might contribute to Susan's fatigue?
5. What symptoms are associated with a rapid fall in blood sugar level in hypoglycemia? What is the basis for these symptoms?
6. What symptoms are associated with a slow fall in blood sugar level in hypoglycemia? What is the basis for these symptoms?

Nutritional Assessment

7. Using the Daily Food Guide evaluate Susan's diet for nutritional adequacy.
8. Which nutrients are likely to be provided in less than desirable amounts if carbohydrate intake is limited to 100 g?
9. What additional information is needed in order to recommend an appropriate calorie level for Susan?
10. Are supplementary vitamins and minerals indicated for Susan? Explain.

Planning the Diet

11. Plan a meal pattern for Susan.
12. Outline the points you need to consider in planning Susan's nutritional care.
13. List some problems you foresee in planning Susan's diet.

Dietary Counseling

14. What dietary adjustments are usually indicated for functional hypoglycemia?
15. What is the purpose of keeping protein intake constant at each meal?
16. List the points you would emphasize in counseling Susan about her diet.
17. Identify some nutritious, easy-to-prepare snacks that Susan can carry with her.

References for the Case Study

AMERICAN DIABETES ASSOCIATION: "Statement on Hypoglycemia," *Diabetes Care*, **5**:72–73, January—February 1982.

LEV-RAN, A., and ANDERSON, R. W.: "The Diagnosis of Postprandial Hypoglycemia," *Diabetes*, **30**:996–99, 1981.

SANTIAGO, J. V., et al.: "Fasting Hypoglycemia in Adults," *Arch. Intern. Med.*, **142**:465–68, 1982.

Problems and Review

1. You are assigned to care for Mr. J, a 58-year-old patient with Addison's disease.
   a. What modifications of mineral and water metabolism are present in Addison's disease? In what way is this corrected by hormone therapy?
   b. Why is a sodium-restricted diet occasionally ordered for a patient receiving hormone therapy in Addison's disease? Under what circumstances would an increase in sodium intake be used?
   c. On the basis of your understanding of the metabolism in Addison's disease, what are some of the functions of the adrenal gland in the normal individual? What is the effect of the activity of the pituitary?

2. A patient with hyperthyroidism was seen in the metabolism clinic and was asked to return in 1 month for surgery. The nutritionist instructed the patient on a diet to provide 5,000 kcal and 125 g protein.
   a. What are some of the characteristic symptoms of hyperthyroidism? of hypothyroidism?
   b. Compare the diet that might be used in a hyperthyroid patient who is well controlled with antithyroid drugs and one who has an elevated metabolic rate.
   c. Suggest five ways in which the calories for a patient with hyperthyroidism might be increased.
   d. Why does a surgeon so frequently insist that a patient gain weight before an operation on the thyroid?
   e. What is myxedema? What is its chief cause? How can you explain the frequent occurrence of overweight?

3. Your grandmother shows you an ad in a booklet with a diet "guaranteed" to cure arthritis and aid in weight reduction.
   a. What would you tell her about the role of diet in arthritis?
   b. Outline briefly the dietary considerations in arthritis.
   c. What are the dietary implications of long-term use of cortisone in this disease or in other conditions?

4. You are asked to teach Mr. O about his diet for gout. Consider the following questions in planning your remarks:
   a. What are sources of uric acid in the body? In what ways is uric acid metabolism disturbed in gout?
   b. How can you explain the fact that a person who has gout may have an acute attack following surgery or during an acute infection?
   c. What is the basis for restricting the protein intake to 1 g per kg in dietary planning for a patient with gout?
   d. What problems are entailed when a purine-free diet is ordered for a patient, insofar as nutritional adequacy is concerned?
   e. Plan a menu for 1 day for a low-purine diet.

5. What is the role of each of these hormones in protein and mineral metabolism: thyroxine; parathormone; androgen; cortisone?

References

1. Gastineau, C. F.: "Is Reactive Hypoglycemia a Clinical Entity?" *Mayo Clin. Proc.*, **58**:545–49, 1983.
2. Lev-Ran, A., and Anderson, R. W.: "The Diagnosis of Postprandial Hypoglycemia," *Diabetes*, **30**:996–99, 1981.
3. Burke, M. D.: "Adrenal Dysfunction. Test Strategies for Diagnosis," *Postgrad. Med.*, **69**:155–59ff, January 1981.
4. Smith, C. M., and Bidlack, W. R.: "Dietary Concerns Associated with the Use of Medications," *J. Am. Diet. Assoc.*, **84**:901–14, 1984.
5. Price, J. H.: "The Public's Perceptions and Misperceptions of Arthritis," *Arthritis Rheum.*, **26**:1023–28, 1983.
6. Boss, G. R., and Seegmiller, J. E.: "Hyperuricemia and Gout. Classification, Complications, and Management," *N. Engl. J. Med.*, **300**:459–68, 1979.
7. Moore, A. O. and Powers, D. E., *Food-Medication Interactions*, 3rd ed. F-MI Publishing, Tempe, Arizona, 1981.
8. American Dietetic Association, *Handbook of Clinical Dietetics*. Yale University Press, New Haven, Conn., 1981.

38

Hyperlipidemia and Atherosclerosis

Fat-Modified Diet in Three Phases;
Diets for Hyperlipoproteinemias

Cardiovascular Disease, A Major Public Health Problem

Cardiovascular diseases represent an enormous medical, social, and economic burden to the American public. Some statistics illustrate this point.

Some 42 million Americans have some form of heart or blood vessel disease. Many have more than one cardiovascular disease.

    37   million have high blood pressure
    4.5 million have coronary heart disease
    1.9 million have rheumatic heart disease
    1.8 million have stroke

Cardiovascular diseases accounted for half of all deaths in the United States in 1980.

Some 1.5 million Americans experience a heart attack each year. Another 0.5 million suffer stroke.

Approximately 1.5 million Americans undergo cardiovascular operations and procedures each year.

The estimated economic cost of cardiovascular diseases in this country is $60 billion for medical expenses, lost wages, and lost productivity.[1]

Cardiovascular diseases are the leading cause of Social Security disability. They account for more hospital bed days than any other cause except cancer.

The mortality rates from cardiovascular diseases in the United States are among the highest in the world. Heart attack is the leading cause of deaths due to cardiovascular diseases, and accounts for over a half million deaths each year. Some 170,000 more are attributed to stroke.

Since the mid-1960s the mortality rate from major cardiovascular diseases has been decreasing in the United States and Canada, while that in most of the world is unchanged or increasing. From 1969 to 1979 the age-adjusted death rates for cardiovascular diseases, coronary heart disease, and stroke fell 31 percent, 29.4 percent, and 41.6 percent, respectively.[2] Several changes in lifestyle and risk factors among the population as a whole have no doubt contributed to the decline in mortality: (1) a change in eating habits whereby the intake of saturated fat and cholesterol is lower now than it was during the 1950s; (2) over the last two to three decades mean serum cholesterol levels in middle-aged men have fallen from about 240 mg per dl 25 years ago to about 215 mg per dl; (3) millions of Americans have given up smoking; (4) regular exercise has become a way of life for many; (5) hypertension detection and treatment has improved substantially during the last decade; (6) most hospitals have coronary care units; and (7) emergency medical services are now available in many areas.

Ischemic heart disease may occur at any age, but it is not common until middle age at which time it assumes practically epidemic proportions. Males over 45 years of age are highly susceptible. Except for those who have hypertension or diabetes mellitus, ischemic heart disease is not common in women until after the menopause.

Multiple Risk Factors in Coronary Disease   No single factor is an absolute cause either of atherosclerosis or of coronary disease. Many factors are interrelated and to the extent that they are present they increase the risk of disease. Major risk factors are elevated serum cholesterol, hypertension, cigarette smoking, diabetes mellitus, and marked obesity. Other risk factors include a family history of early heart disease, other lipid abnormalities, certain personality–behavior patterns, lack of physical activity, and stress.

Coronary Disease and the Role of Diet

The discussion in this chapter is concerned with (1) the rationale for dietary modification to reduce the incidence of atherosclerosis and coronary disease, (2) the fat modified diet, and (3) diets for five types of hyperlipoproteinemia. The dietary management of acute episodes of illness is discussed in the chapter that follows. The student should review normal fat and carbohydrate metabolism in order to understand the effects of altered physiology and biochemistry in coronary disease. (See Chapters 6 and 7.)

Ischemic Heart Disease MYOCARDIAL ISCHEMIA is a cardiac disability resulting from an inadequacy of the coronary arterial system to meet the needs of the heart muscle for oxygen and nutrients. It may be manifested as sudden death, myocardial infarction, or angina pectoris.

An *infarct* is a localized area of necrosis that results when the supply of blood to that area is inadequate for cellular survival. An infarct of the heart is known as a MYOCARDIAL INFARCTION (heart attack), and one in the brain as a CEREBROVASCULAR ACCIDENT (stroke). If the infarct is small, the remainder of the organ can

Figure 38-1. Gradual development of atherosclerosis in a coronary artery, leading to a heart attack. (Courtesy, American Heart Association.)

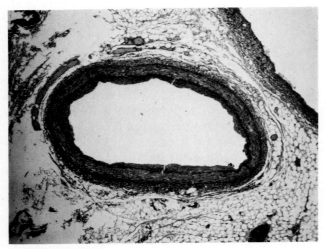

A. Normal artery

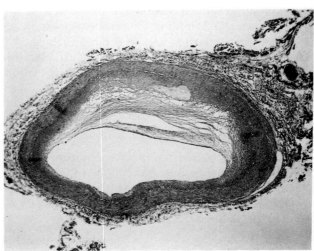

B. Deposits formed in inner lining of artery

function and healing takes place with the formation of scar tissue. The functional capacity of the organ is curtailed to the extent that tissue has been lost. Thus, repeated myocardial infarctions continue to reduce the functional capacity of the heart.

ANGINA PECTORIS refers to the tight, pressing, burning, and sometimes severe pain across the chest that follows exertion and that is a result of inadequate oxygen to the myocardium. As the coronary arteries become increasingly occluded, the pain develops with less and less exertion.

ATHEROSCLEROSIS is a disease of the blood vessels resulting from the interaction of multiple factors such as heredity and the individual's environment (e.g., diet, activity, smoking, lifestyle). Atheromatous plaques

begin as soft, mushy accumulations of lipid material in the intima of the blood vessels. These plaques consist of a proliferation of the blood vessel wall of connective tissue into which lipids are deposited. The lipids include free cholesterol, cholesterol esters, and triglycerides in proportions that approximate those of the circulating blood lipids.

Atherosclerosis begins in the first decades of life and is almost universally present in people who live in affluent, highly developed countries. It develops gradually with increasing thickening of the arterial wall, loss of elasticity, and narrowing of the lumen. Finally, some event brings about occlusion of the vessel and ischemia of the affected part. (See Figure 38-1.)

Most myocardial infarctions are due to atheroscle-

(Figure 38-1. continued.)

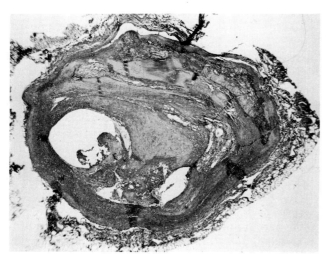

C. Deposits harden

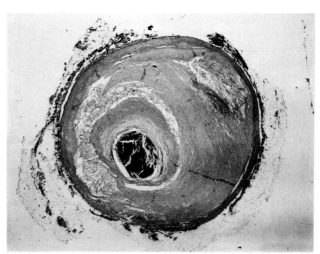

D. Channel is blocked by a blood clot

rosis of the major coronary arteries, but many people with atherosclerosis do not develop clinical disease. The conditions that bring about occlusion are not well understood. In some instances ulceration of the atheroma and hemorrhage into the lumen with clot formation occur. The anatomic location of the atheroma, the extent to which the lumen has been narrowed, the changes in the clearing of the blood lipids, and decrease in fibrinolytic activity are probably involved in the process.

Blood Studies Related to Coronary Disease Measurements of various blood constituents can be used not only to determine the presence of abnormal concentrations but also to evaluate the effects of changes in diet and other therapy on the levels of these components. HYPERLIPIDEMIA is a general term that denotes an elevation of plasma lipids. HYPERCHOLESTEROLEMIA refers to an elevation of serum cholesterol and HYPERTRIGLYCERIDEMIA to increased triglycerides. Although the specific levels separating normal from abnormal cannot be known precisely for all members of the population, epidemiologic studies indicate that the risk for coronary heart disease increases sharply when plasma cholesterol levels exceed 220 mg per dl.[3] Plasma triglyceride levels about 250 mg per dl indicate clinical hypertriglyceridemia.[4] HYPERLIPOPROTEINEMIA refers to elevation of any one of the classes of lipoproteins. (See Chapter 7.) Five types of hyperlipoproteinemia have been described.[5] The differentiation is based on the appearance of the serum, the concentrations of cholesterol and triglyceride, and the classes of lipoproteins that serve as the vehicle for the lipids. HYPERTENSION, or elevated blood pressure, is generally considered to be present when the systolic pressure is 160 mm Hg or greater and the diastolic pressure is 95 mm Hg. The risk of coronary heart disease is increased two- to threefold at these levels. Readings of 140/90 represent borderline hypertension; coronary heart disease rates are increased by 50 percent at these levels, and there is a threefold increase in stroke.[6]

Determination of serum cholesterol is considered by some to be the best single measurement for estimating risk of atherosclerosis. Data from the Framingham Study indicate that total cholesterol is not a useful predictor of risk in individual cases because values in persons free of coronary disease overlap those of persons who develop coronary heart disease. However, the ratio of total cholesterol to high-density lipoprotein cholesterol was found to be a good predictor of risk for coronary heart disease. The desirable ratio is less than 4.5.[6]

Long-Term Studies on Modified Diets Numerous studies have established that serum cholesterol can be lowered by dietary modification. Many investigators have sought to determine whether dietary modification could also lessen morbidity and mortality from coronary disease.[7-10] Most of the studies have been criticized for experimental design, small sample size, lack of randomization, or relatively short duration. Nevertheless, sustained reduction of serum cholesterol by long-term dietary modification was associated with a decline in morbidity and mortality from coronary disease although the results were not statistically significant in all the studies.

Two long-term studies by the National Heart, Lung, and Blood Institute have recently been reported. The Multiple Risk Factor Intervention Trial (MRFIT) was a randomized primary prevention study involving 12,000 men aged 35 to 57 years who were followed for an average of 7 years. The men were at risk for coronary heart disease because of elevated serum cholesterol, high blood pressure, and cigarette smoking. Half were assigned to a special intervention group and received counseling for reduction of risk factors throughout the study. The other half received their health care from their usual sources. Reduction of all three risk factors occurred in both groups, but to a greater extent in the special intervention group. The decline in coronary heart disease mortality was less than expected and was not significantly different between the two groups.[11] Some possible reasons for this outcome have been proposed.[12] In both groups, mortality rates due to coronary heart disease were substantially higher when either smoking or hypertension or both were present in addition to hypercholesterolemia. Persons with elevated cholesterol levels and who smoked but who did not have hypertension appeared to benefit most from the special intervention. The mortality rate from coronary heart disease in this group was nearly 50 percent less than in the usual care group.[11]

The Lipid Research Clinics Coronary Primary Prevention Trial was designed to determine whether drug-induced reduction of elevated serum cholesterol levels in otherwise healthy men would prevent development of coronary heart disease. Some 3,800 men, aged 35 to 59 years, were followed for an average of 7 years and were randomly assigned to a treatment group that received cholestyramine (a drug that binds bile acid and enhances its excretion) or to a control (placebo) group. Both groups were on a low-cholesterol diet providing less than 300 mg per day. Among the findings were the following: (1) the reduction in plasma total cholesterol levels was less than 5 percent in the control group and nearly 14 percent in the drug–diet treated group, and (2) the drug–diet group experienced a 19 percent decrease in the incidence of nonfatal myocardial infarction and a 24 percent reduction in coronary heart disease mortality. The decline in coronary heart disease incidence was related to the fall in total cholesterol and LDL-cholesterol levels. A 10.4 percent decrease (22.3 mg per dl) in LDL-cholesterol levels was associated with a 16 to 19 percent reduction in risk for coronary heart disease.[13,14]

Dietary Adjustments for Hyperlipidemias Health professionals are not in unanimous agreement concerning dietary recommendations for prevention of coronary heart disease. Most believe that persons *at increased risk* should make specific dietary changes as outlined below to lower fat and cholesterol intake. The American Heart Association has stated that such dietary modifications are appropriate for the general population.[15,16] Others are of the opinion that drastic changes in the diet are not necessary for the general public.[17,18] See page 32 for discussion of the Dietary Guidelines for Americans. The rationale for dietary adjustments in hyperlipidemias follows.

Calorie Balance. Obesity has long been recognized as one of the risk factors in cardiovascular disease. In the Framingham Study weight was a powerful predictor of cardiovascular disease.[6] When overweight is associated with diabetes mellitus, the serum cholesterol and triglyceride levels are customarily high, thereby increasing risk. Reduction in body weight and blood lipids is accomplished by lowering calorie intake and substituting polyunsaturated fats for part of the saturated fats in the diet.

Increased body weight probably has its greatest effect by increasing the work load of the heart. A mild stenosis associated with obesity can be critical in a situation of added stress.

Normal weight is maintained only when energy intake and output are equal. Therefore, early in life it is important to develop a program of regular exercise that can be continued throughout the years. (See Chapter 25.) A regular program of modest exercise is also effective in raising serum HDL-cholesterol levels.

Fats. Dietary fat is the single most important factor requiring adjustment in programs of prevention and control. (See also Figure 1-2.) The typical American diet furnishes about 40 percent of the calories from fat. The saturated fat in the diet is about twice as high as the polyunsaturated fat.

For the prevention of hyperlipidemia the total fat content should be reduced to about 30 to 35 percent of calories. The content of saturated fat should be limited to 10 percent of calories and polyunsaturated fat should not exceed 10 percent of calories. Large increases in polyunsaturated fat intake are not recommended because of an association with increased formation of gallstones following prolonged use of such diets.[19]

Cholesterol. The cholesterol content of American diets ranges from 500 to 1,000 mg per day, depending largely on the number of eggs that are consumed. (See Table A–5.) Most dietary plans now restrict the cholesterol intake to 300 mg or less when hypercholesterolemia is present.

Carbohydrate. A sudden increase of carbohydrate in the diet produces a temporary elevation of plasma triglycerides in both normal and hyperlipidemic persons; however, there is no evidence that the amount of carbohydrate has a sustained effect on blood lipid levels.[20] Sucrose may have a hyperlipidemic effect in persons with hypertriglyceridemia; thus, complex carbohydrates are recommended in place of sucrose. For the general population, 45 to 55 percent of calories as carbohydrate, with emphasis on complex carbohydrates, has been recommended.[16]

Dietary Fiber. Pectins, gums, and soluble fibers have a serum cholesterol lowering effect. Wheat bran and cellulose have little influence on serum cholesterol levels. Mechanisms proposed to explain the hypocholesterolemic effect of these fibers include (1) altered intestinal absorption, metabolism, and release of cholesterol, through an influence on bile acids; (2) altered hepatic metabolism and release of cholesterol, with increased excretion of bile acids reducing the size of the bile acid pool, and less cholesterol available for incorporation into lipoproteins and subsequent release into the circulation; and (3) altered peripheral metabolism of lipoproteins. Fiber may alter the proportion of cholesterol incorporated into chylomicrons and lipoproteins.[21]

Alcohol. The effect of alcohol on blood lipid levels appears to vary with the individual. In some persons, plasma triglycerides increase after alcohol intake. On the other hand, alcohol has been reported to increase HDL-cholesterol levels and to protect against coronary heart disease when taken in modest amounts.[22,23]

Other Dietary Factors. Soy protein has a hypocholesterolemic effect compared with animal protein in both normal and hypercholesterolemic subjects.[24,25] Habitual high salt intake increases risk for hypertension in susceptible persons. Lowering salt intake has been proposed to reduce risk. The American Medical Association has stated that moderation in salt intake is desirable for the entire population.[26] The role of minerals in cardiovascular disease is uncertain. The mortality rate from cardiovascular diseases is significantly lower in areas where the drinking water is hard than in those areas where the water is soft. Sufficient evidence is lacking to incriminate specific minerals; however, some data suggest that higher concentrations of calcium and magnesium in hard water may have a protective effect.[27,28] Patients dying suddenly from ischemic heart disease have been found to have lower concentrations of magnesium and potassium in myocardial tissue than patients dying of causes unrelated to heart disease.[29] Interactions of copper and zinc have been proposed.[30] Alterations of copper balance are also associated with irregularities in electrocardiograms and respond to administration of copper salts.[31,32]

Fat-Modified Diets

Three-Phase Diet The American Heart Association has recommended dietary changes for the general public based on the concept that modification of risk factors will lower risk for coronary heart disease.[16] A three-phase diet, suitable for the general public and for persons with hyperlipidemias is proposed.[33]

Phase 1, for the general public, permits 30 to 32 percent of calories as fat. Saturated fat is limited to about 10 percent of calories; polyunsaturated fat intake should not exceed 10 percent of calories. Cholesterol intake is less than 300 mg per day. Carbohydrate comprises about 45 to 50 percent of calories; complex carbohydrates are emphasized. Egg yolks are limited to two per week. Butterfat, lard, and most organ meats are omitted. Soft margarine, vegetable oils, shortening, skim milk, and egg white are substituted for butter, lard, whole milk, and eggs.

Phase 2 permits 30 percent of calories as fat, with equal amounts of the three types of fatty acids. Carbohydrate supplies 50 percent of calories. Cholesterol is restricted to less than 200 mg per day. Meat, poultry, and seafoods are limited to 5 to 6 ounces daily. Only very lean meats and skim milk cheeses are permitted. Increased amounts of legumes, grains, fruits, and vegetables are used.

Phase 3 restricts fat intake to 20 to 25 percent of calories with equal amounts of each class of fatty acids, and cholesterol to 100 mg per day. From 55 to 60 per-

Table 38-1. Food Allowances for Three Fat-Modified Diets for 1,800 kcal (Number of servings per day).

Food Groups	Phase 1	Phase 2	Phase 3
Meat, poultry, seafood	6	4	3
Meatless alternatives	0	1	3
Eggs (per week)	2	0	0
Milk and cheese	3	3	3
Fats and oils	7	8	5
Breads, cereals, starchy	6	7	8
Vegetables	4	4	4
Fruits	4	4	4
Sweets	1	1	1

cent of calories are from carbohydrate. Meat, shellfish, and poultry are limited to 3 ounces daily.

For all phases, adjustment of calorie intake is made to achieve and maintain desirable body weight. Reduction of salt intake is encouraged for persons with high blood pressure. The diet is adequate in all essential nutrients. However, large amounts of dietary fiber may interfere with absorption of some minerals. (See Chapter 6.)

The dietary changes are phased in gradually in order to improve compliance, and because response to a given level of dietary fat and cholesterol varies from one individual to another. In some persons reduction in serum lipids is achieved with moderate restriction of fat and cholesterol; in others, more drastic dietary changes are needed to reduce the risk for atherosclerosis. Plans for fat-modified meals at 1,200, 1,500, 2,000, and 2,300 calories for each of the three phases

Table 38-2. Composition of Three 1,800-Calorie Fat-Modified Diets

	Phase 1	Phase 2	Phase 3
Calories	1793	1808	1808
Fat, percentage of kcal	30.6	29.9	21.9
Saturated	8.3	7.6	6.3
Monounsaturated	10.7	10.2	7.9
Polyunsaturated	9.4	10.8	7.7
P/S	1.1	1.4	1.2
Cholesterol, mg	230*	148	91
Carbohydrate, percentage of kcal	48.9	50.2	58.8
Starch	23.6	28.5	31.6
Fructose, lactose, etc.	18.7	18.6	22.1
Sucrose	6.7	3.1	4.9
Protein, percentage of kcal	20.5	19.9	19.2
Animal, percent	82.6	68.0	64.0
Vegetable, percent	17.4	32.0	36.0

*Weighted average, assuming 2/7 of one egg per day.

Table 38-3.   Sample Menus for Three 1,800-kcal Fat-Modified Diets

	Phase 1	Phase 2	Phase 3
Breakfast			
Orange slices, ½ cup	1	1	1
Wheat flakes, ¾ cup	1	1	1
Muffin with 1 tsp. oil	1	0	0
Toast, slice	0	2	2
Soft-cooked egg	1	0	0
Egg substitute, ¼ cup	0	1	0
Margarine, tsp.	1	2	2
Skim milk, cup	1	1	1
Sugar, tsp.	2	1	1
Jelly, Tbsp.	0	0	1
Lunch			
Split pea soup, cup	0	1	1
Saltines, 6 per serving	0	1	0
Roast chicken, ounces	3	1	0
Sliced cheese, ounces	0	0	2
Mashed potato, ½ cup	1	0	0
Rye bread, slice	1	0	1
Summer squash, ½ cup	1	1	1
Tossed salad, cup	1	1	1
French dressing, tsp.	1	1	1
Mayonnaise, tsp.	0	2	0
Margarine, tsp.	1	0	0
Skim milk, cup	1	1	1
Baked apple	1	1	1
With 1 Tbsp. sugar	1	0	0
Dinner			
Veal baked in tomato sauce, ounces	3	3	2
With oil, tsp.	1	1	1
Rice, ½cup	1	1	1
Dinner roll	1	1	2
Asparagus, ½ cup	1	1	1
Sliced cucumbers, ½ cup	1	1	1
Skim milk, cup	1	1	1
Margarine, tsp.	2	2	1
Fresh peach	1	1	1
Grapes, 12 per serving	1	1	1

of the diet have been published by the American Heart Association.[34] Details of the diet and food lists have been published for the layman.[33] The food listings are summarized on pages 535 to 538. Table 38-1 illustrates the number of servings from each food group for an 1,800-kcal diet. Nutrient composition and sample 1,800-kcal menus for each of the three phases of the diet are shown in Tables 38-2 and 38-3.

Alternative Diets   A diet plan similar in principle to the one described above but slightly lower in fat has been described.[20] A progressive reduction in dietary fat intake is made—35, 25, and 20 percent of calories as fat in phases 1, 2, and 3, respectively. Emphasis is placed on increased use of vegetable proteins in place of animal sources of protein. Meat is used only once a day in phase 2; beans, grains, and low-fat fish and cheeses are used in place of meat. Meat is used mainly as a condiment in phase 3; intake is limited to 3 to 4 ounces daily. Sucrose intake is lowered to about 10 percent of calories. Dietary fiber is increased from 10 to 12 g in the usual American diet to 48 to 60 g per day.[20]

Pritikin Diet.   Another dietary approach to prevention of cardiovascular disease is the Pritikin diet.[35] Stringent reductions in fat and cholesterol intake are made. Less than 10 percent of calories are from fat. In the regression diet, which is used until the individual's plasma cholesterol falls below 160 mg per dl, the diet provides about 25 mg cholesterol. The maintenance diet supplies 100 mg cholesterol. Carbohydrate comprises about 75 to 80 percent of calories and is chiefly in the form of complex carbohydrates. Emphasis is on use of whole grains, legumes, and fruit. Alcohol and caffeine are eliminated from the diet, and calories are sharply limited.

Food Lists for Fat-Modified Diets*

Foods Allowed	**Foods to Avoid**

Milk and Cheese
Milk
Skim milk or 1 percent low-fat milk; buttermilk made from skim or 1 percent low-fat milk; nonfat or 1 percent low-fat dry milk; evaporated skim milk

Buttermilk made from whole milk; chocolate milk; condensed milk; dried whole milk; evaporated milk; low-fat milk with 1 ½ percent or more butterfat; whole milk; half-and-half; nondairy sour cream; sour cream

Creamers
Nondairy creamers made from polyunsaturated fat

Nondairy coffee creamers (liquid, powder, frozen)

* Adapted from Food Lists in *Eating for a Healthy Heart*, American Heart Association, Dallas, Texas, 1983.

Foods Allowed	**Foods to Avoid**
Cheese All containing 2 g fat or less per ounce: dry curd or low-fat cottage cheese; natural or processed cheeses with up to 8 percent butter fat	Cheese, all varieties made with whole or cream (containing more than 8 percent butterfat); cottage cheese, creamed; cream cheese
Yogurt Skim or low fat: plain yogurt	Frozen or fresh yogurt made from whole milk
Desserts All made with low-fat or skim milk (1 percent butterfat or less): puddings, custards, (made with egg white or egg substitute); ice milk, soft or hard; sherbet; frozen or fruited yogurt	Ice cream; Mellorine; nondairy whipped toppings (tub, powdered, aerosol, or frozen); whipping cream
Beverages Cocoa, homemade or commercial made with skim milk (1 percent butterfat or less); low-calorie hot cocoa mix; low-calorie flavored milk drink mix; fortified milk drink powders mixed with skim or low-fat milk (1 percent butterfat or less); powdered milk flavorings	
Meat, Poultry, and Seafood All lean, well trimmed: beef, veal, pork, lamb; chicken and turkey without skin; fish, shellfish; wild game—duck, rabbit, pheasant, venison; organ meats; liver (limit to 3 ounces per month)	*Beef*—all prime grade or heavily marbled meats or untrimmed cuts; beef sausage; brisket; chili; corned beef; regular ground beef; pastrami; plate ribs—short or spare; rib eye steak, standing rib roast *Veal*—breast riblets *Pork, fresh*—Boston (roast or steak); ground; loin back ribs; shoulder arm or blade; spareribs; *Pork, cured*—canned deviled ham; ham-country, dry cure; neckbones; pigs' feet, pickled; salt pork; sausage—all kinds; smoked pork jowl, shoulder, picnic or roll *Lamb*—ground; mutton *Fish and shellfish*—caviar; commercially fried fish or shellfish *Poultry*—poultry skin *Game and other meats*—duck, domestic; goose; oppossum; raccoon; venison sausage *Luncheon meat*—bologna; canned and packaged luncheon meats; frankfurters; head cheese; salami *Organ meats*—brains, chitterlings, gizzard, heart, kidney, pork maws *Miscellaneous*—commercially fried meat, poultry, seafood; meats canned or frozen in gravy or sauce; pork and beans
Meatless Alternatives *Beans*—aduki, black, cranberry, fava, garbanzo, great northern, kidney, lima, pinto, marrow, mung, navy, pea, soy (tofu) *Peas*—black-eyed, chick, cow, field, split, lentils *Whole grains*—barley, corn (cornbread, grits), oats, rice, rye, wheat	

Foods Allowed	**Foods to Avoid**
Nuts and seeds—almonds, beechnuts, Brazil, filberts, pecans, pine, walnuts, pumpkin, sunflower *Peanut butter, cheeses,* up to 8 percent fat *Egg substitute* *Tofu* (soybean curd)	

Fruit
See List 2, Table A-4

Vegetables
See List 3, Table A-4   All prepared with butter or cream sauce

Breads, Cereals, and Starchy Foods
Bread, Cereal, Pasta and Starchy Vegetables

Bread—all varieties; English muffin, bagel, hamburger bun, tortilla *reals*—cooked or dry; macaroni, noodles, rice, spaghetti; potato; lima beans; peas; winter squash; corn; sweet potatoes, yams	Bagels made with eggs or cheese; butter rolls; cheese breads; commercial doughnuts, muffins, sweet rolls, biscuits, waffles, and pancakes; croissants, egg breads; granola type cereals containing coconut or coconut oil; chow-mein noodles, fried vegetables; vegetables prepared with cream sauce

Crackers and Snacks Bread sticks; crackers: animal, graham, rye, saltines, oyster; melba toast; flatbread, matzo, pretzels, popcorn, rusk, zwieback	Other commercial crackers such as butter or cheese crackers; those made with coconut or palm oil

Soup Made with water: broth or bouillon; chicken noodle; clam chowder, Manhattan style; minestrone; onion; split pea; vegetable; vegetarian vegetable	Cream of celery, cheese, chicken, mushroom, potato, tomato; chunky type; vichyssoise

Modified Fat Desserts All modified to contain low fat (1 percent) or skim milk, margarine, vegetable oil, egg substitutes: cake, cupcakes, cookies, pie	Commercial cake, cookies, pie, frozen pie crust; cheesecake; sweet rolls

Quick Breads All modified to contain 1 percent low-fat or skim milk, margarine, egg substitute: banana bread, biscuits, cornbread, French toast, muffins, pancakes, soft rolls, waffles	All except those made with allowed ingredients

Fats and Oils

Margarines—stick, tub, or squeeze margarine listing liquid corn, safflower, or sunflower oil as the first ingredient	All other stick or tub margarines; those made with animal fat; butter
Oils—Corn, cottonseed, safflower, sunflower, or soybean	Bacon drippings, coconut, palm or palm kernel oil
Salad dressings and mayonnaise made with allowed oils; low-calorie salad dressings	Blue cheese: green goddess, roquefort, those made with sour cream or cheese
Miscellaneous—pumpkin, sesame, or sunflower seeds; avocado; olives; peanut butter	Chocolate; gravy made from meat drippings; ham hocks; lard; meat drippings; meat fat; salt pork; shortening; suet; cashew, macadamia, or pistachio nuts

Foods Allowed	Foods to Avoid
Sweets Candies, hard; carbonated beverages; fudgesickles; gelatin, flavored; honey; ices, fruit; jams, jellies, marmalade, molasses, preserves, syrups; popsicles; punch-fruit flavored; lemonade; sugar	All not listed on allowed lists

Hyperlipoproteinemias

Types I to V Some hyperlipoproteinemias are induced by an excess of endogenous or exogenous fat, others by an intolerance to carbohydrates, especially sugars, and still others are influenced by dietary cholesterol. These disorders of lipid metabolism may be hereditary or they may be caused by an intake of an abnormal diet. They are frequently associated with diabetes mellitus. Some types predispose to early atherosclerosis. Xanthomas are frequent, and in types I and V abdominal pain and acute pancreatitis may occur. In all types diet is the primary therapy. When diet alone is ineffective, drug therapy is used, except in type I.

Type I. An extremely high triglyceride concentration in the serum is characteristic of this type, with the serum cholesterol being normal to high. There is an inability to clear chylomicrons (dietary fat) from the blood, probably as a result of a genetic deficiency of lipoprotein lipase. The condition is rare, usually familial, and seen early in life. It may be associated with diabetes mellitus.

The diet must be very low in fat—25 to 35 g per day for adults and about 15 g for children. Cholesterol is not restricted. The carbohydrate is necessarily high in order to supply the needed calories. Alcohol is contraindicated because it increases the serum triglyceride levels when it is metabolized. The elimination of table spreads, cooking fats, and oils results in a dry diet. Medium-chain triglycerides are sometimes prescribed by the physician since they increase the calorie intake and may be used in food preparation (See page 444.)

Types IIa and IIb. In both types IIa and IIb decreased clearance of low-density lipoprotein (LDL) causes increased serum cholesterol levels. In type IIa, very-low-density lipoprotein (VLDL) and triglycerides are normal, but in type IIb both are elevated.

Primary type IIa, sometimes called familial hypercholesterolemia, is a common hereditary disorder that involves a genetic defect in the catabolism of LDL

possibly due to inability to synthesize adequate numbers of LDL receptors. It is inherited as an autosomal dominant trait. One of every 500 persons is a heterozygote for the disorder. In these individuals total plasma cholesterol is moderately elevated from birth and usually ranges from 300 to 600 mg per dl. Clinical symptoms usually do not develop until adulthood when tendon xanthomas and premature coronary disease develop. Type IIa may occur secondary to excessive cholesterol intake, nephrosis, myxedema, or liver disease.

Primary type IIb, also known as familial combined hyperlipidemia, does not involve a defect in LDL receptors. However, both LDL and VLDL levels are elevated. Individuals with this type tend to be overweight.

Calories are not restricted in type IIa, but weight reduction is often indicated in type IIb. The cholesterol content of the diet is restricted to less than 300 mg per day. Egg yolks are not permitted. The only source of cholesterol is the meat. Protein is not restricted. Saturated fats are decreased and polyunsaturated fats increased, so that a high P/S ratio is achieved. Carbohydrates and fats are limited to 40 percent of calories in type IIb, and concentrated sweets are restricted. Alcohol may be used with discretion in both types.

Type III. This relatively uncommon disorder is also known as broad beta disease or dysbetalipoproteinemia. It is believed to be due to a defect in the catabolism of lipoprotein remnants.[36] It is characterized by increases in LDL and VLDL. The latter are also abnormal in structure. Xanthoma formation of the elbows, knees, and buttocks are common. The incidence of premature cardiovascular disease is increased. Overweight is frequent, and a calorie-restricted diet is indicated until the desirable weight is attained. The fat and carbohydrate are each limited to not more than 40 percent of the calories. Concentrated sweets are eliminated, and polyunsaturated fats are substituted for saturated fats. Cholesterol is restricted to 300 mg per day. Alcohol may be substituted for up to two servings bread or cereal.

Type IV. This very common pattern, also known as exogenous hypertriglyceridemia, is characterized by an increase in VLDL. The abnormality is attributed to overproduction and impaired clearance of VLDL. Triglycerides are elevated but the serum cholesterol is often normal. Many patients in this group have an abnormal glucose tolerance and some have hyperuricemia. This disorder may be hereditary or associated with diabetes mellitus or another metabolic disorder. Obesity and the complications of atherosclerosis are frequent.

Initially the calories are restricted until desirable weight is achieved. Weight loss alone usually lowers the serum lipids, sometimes to normal. The maintenance diet provides not more than 45 percent of the calories from carbohydrates and eliminates concentrated sweets. A P/S ratio of about 1 is maintained by substituting polyunsaturated fats for saturated fats. Cholesterol is restricted to 300 to 500 mg per day. Alcohol may be used at the physician's discretion.

Type V. Chylomicrons and VLDL are elevated in this type, indicating intolerance to both endogenous and exogenous sources of fat. As with type IV, glucose tolerance and blood uric acid levels are often abnormal. This disorder is commonly associated with diabetic acidosis, nephrosis, alcoholism, and obesity. The liver and spleen may be enlarged, and abdominal pain is relatively common.

Calorie restriction is emphasized until the desired weight is achieved. The fat in the maintenance diet is kept as low as practical, but not more than 25 to 30 percent of the calories. The P/S ratio, although not important, is somewhat higher than in typical diets because polyunsaturated fats are substituted for saturated fats. Cholesterol is restricted to 300 to 500 mg per day. The carbohydrate intake is not more than 50 percent of the calories, thus necessitating a protein intake of 20 to 25 percent of calories. Concentrated sweets and alcohol are contraindicated.

Nutritional Effects of Drug Therapy. The primary treatment for the hyperlipoproteinemias is diet. However, drug therapy is used in some cases that do not show a satisfactory response to diet. Cholestyramine, colestipol, clofibrate, and nicotinic acid should be taken with food. Cholestyramine may cause constipation unless additional fluids and sufficient dietary fiber are taken. Most of the drugs cause nausea and vomiting. Vitamin and mineral status should be monitored in patients receiving these drugs, as decreased absorption of carotene, fat-soluble vitamins, B-12, folacin, calcium, and iron are possible side effects.[37,38]

Dietary Plans A committee of the Heart, Lung, and Blood Institute, National Institutes of Health, has developed detailed dietary plans for the five types of hyperlipoproteinemia described here.[39] These are available in separate booklets for the patient, including individualized dietary plans for the patient, food lists, guidelines for the purchase and preparation of foods, and suggestions for eating out. The daily food allowances for the five diets are summarized in Table 38-4. The sample menus for diets for type I, type IIa,

Table 38-4.   Food Allowances for Types I to V Hyperlipoproteinemia*

Food	Type I	Type IIa	Type IIb, III	Type IV	Type V
Skim milk, cups	4	2	2	2	4
Meat, poultry, fish, ounces	5	6–9	6	6	6
Egg yolks as substitute for 1 ounce meat	3/week	None	None	3/week	3/week
Bread, cereals, servings	6+	7+	7	3	10
Potato or other starchy vegetable, servings	1+	1+	1	2	1
Vegetables, servings			2	2	Ad lib.
Dark green or yellow, daily	5	5			
Fruit, servings			3	3	3
Citrus, daily					
Fat, teaspoons	None	6–9	12	10	9
Sugar, sweets	Ad lib.	Ad lib.	None	None	None
Low-fat dessert	Ad lib.	Ad lib.	None	None	None
Alcohol	None	With discretion	Subst.†	Subst.†	None

* Adapted from Fredrickson, D. S., et al.: *Dietary Management of Hyperlipoproteinemia.* Pub. No. (NIH) 76–110. U.S. Department of Health, Education and Welfare, Washington, D.C., 1975.
† In these diets up to two servings of alcoholic beverages may be substituted for 2 slices bread. One slice of bread is equal to 1 ounce gin, rum, vodka, or whiskey; 1½ ounces sweet or dessert wine; 2½ ounces dry wine; or 5 ounces beer.

Table 38-5. Sample Menus for Three 1,800-kcal Diets in Hyperlipoproteinemias*

Type IIa	Type I	Type IV
Breakfast		
Orange slices—½ cup	Same	Same
Whole-wheat cooked cereal—½ cup	Same	Same
Brown sugar—1 teaspoon	Same	None
Skim milk—1 cup	Same	Same
Homemade muffin—2	Toast—2 slices	Toast—2 slices
Soft margarine—2 teaspoons	None; use jelly—2 teaspoons	Margarine—2 teaspoons
Coffee	Same	Same
Sugar for coffee—2 teaspoons	Same	None
Luncheon or Supper		
Roast chicken—3 ounces	Roast chicken—2 ounces; no fat	Broiled chicken—3 ounces; brushed with 1 teaspoon oil
Mashed potato with 1 teaspoon margarine	Mashed potato; no fat	Mashed potato—with 1 teaspoon margarine
Ripe tomato wedges	Tomato wedges; no fat	Tomato wedges
Tossed green salad	Same	Same
French dressing—1 tablespoon	None	French dressing—1 tablespoon
Rye bread—1 slice	Same	Bread—2 slices
Soft margarine—1 teaspoon	None; add jelly—1 teaspoon	Margarine—1 teaspoon
Skim milk—1 cup	Same	Same
Baked apple with 1 tablespoon sugar	Same	Fresh apple
Dinner		
Veal—3 ounces, baked in tomato sauce with oil—1 teaspoon	Same	Veal—3 ounces baked in sauce with oil—2 teaspoons
Rice—½ cup	Same	Same
Asparagus with pimiento	Same	Same; add 1 teaspoon oil
Dinner roll	Hard roll	Dinner roll
Soft margarine—1 teaspoon	None; use jelly—1 teaspoon	Margarine—2 teaspoons
Skim milk—1 cup	Same	Same
Fresh peach	Gelatin, ⅔ cup	Fresh peach
Angel cake—small slice	Same	None
Tea or coffee	Same	Same
Snack		
None	Skim milk—1 cup	None
	Fresh peach	
	Bread; jelly—1 teaspoon	

* See Table 38-4 for food allowances.

and type IV hyperlipoproteinemia are shown in Table 38-5 to illustrate the variations that are applicable for a given menu.

DIETARY COUNSELING

Dietary modification for the correction of hyperlipidemia requires substantial changes in food selection and preparation for many individuals. Nevertheless, the diet is a palatable one that fits into family menus, the foods are readily available in any food market, and numerous recipes are available for meal planning. The diet need not cost more than conventional diets.

Food Lists   The food lists must be meticulously followed with respect to the kinds and amounts of food that may be used and also those that must be avoided. Once the patient is familiar with the lists a great deal of flexibility is both possible and desirable. The food habits must be permanently changed if the diet is to be effective.

Motivation   Because the serum lipids generally respond within a few weeks following dietary modification, the lowering of lipid levels usually encourages dietary adherence. On the other hand, the patient needs to know that the full benefits of diet on the incidence of clinical disease may not become apparent for up to 2 or even 3 years. Usually the patient who has had a heart attack is more highly motivated to adhere to a modified diet than is the coronary-prone individual. Periodic visits to the physician and the dietitian or nurse are helpful in giving support to the patient as well as in giving greater depth to the level of instruction.

Some Special Problems Some patients find it difficult to restrict meat, shellfish, and poultry to 3 to 4 ounces per day. The market supply of fish and veal in some locations is limited, and some people dislike fish and poultry.

Food preparation: More food preparation "from scratch" is a key rule for these modified diets. Frozen dinners, casseroles, baked foods, and cake, bread, and pudding mixes usually contain more saturated fat than is permitted. Although home preparation implies that more time must be spent in the kitchen, the results can be rewarding by creating numerous dishes that are delicious and lower in cost than the convenience foods of comparable quality. The person responsible for food preparation often needs some guidance in adapting recipes to the needs of the diet. Home economists for processors of fats and oils have developed many excellent recipes, and the dietitian or nurse should give the homemaker guidance in using those that are appropriate for the diet prescription.

The following guidelines may be helpful:

1. Select only lean cuts of meat. Trim any visible fat. Remove skin before cooking poultry.
2. Prepare meat using low-fat preparation methods. Broil or bake instead of frying.
3. Use meatless alternatives for one major meal each day.
4. Use smaller portions of shrimp and sardines, as they are higher in cholesterol than other seafoods.
5. Avoid organ meats. Liver may be used occasionally because it is a good source of iron.
6. When including soups or stews prepare them a day before use. Chill them thoroughly, and remove the fat when it is hardened.
7. Egg yolks including those used in baked foods are limited or omitted depending on the phase of fat-modified diet (see Table 38-1) or the type of hyperlipoproteinemia (see Table 38-4).
8. Use only skim milk or 1 percent low fat milk for drinking and food preparation.

Eating away from home: Adhering to a fat-modified diet is more difficult in a restaurant, partly because the composition of foods is unknown and partly because the varied menu may be too tempting for the dieter. Nevertheless, an occasional meal away from home should be enjoyed. Those who must eat all their meals in a restaurant will need to determine which ones can best meet their dietary requirements. Some restaurants may be able to give a regular customer some special consideration if his or her needs are made known. The dieter can safely choose from these foods: fruit, fruit juice, or clear soup; roasted or broiled meat, fish or poultry without gravy; plain vegetables (many restaurants do not add much seasoning); tossed or fruit salad with or without dressing (no cheese dressing); hard rolls; fruit, plain gelatin, or fruit ice. Sauces, cream soups, butter, cream, ice cream, pastries, and puddings should be avoided.

Many ethnic foods are low in cholesterol and fat: Oriental, Mexican, Italian, and Middle Eastern dishes use little meat in dishes.

Surgery for Coronary Artery Disease Surgical intervention is sometimes undertaken when severe atherosclerosis of the coronary arteries produces myocardial ischemia and disabling angina. The occluded vessels are bypassed by constructing new sources of blood supply to the heart by using portions of a vein or artery grafted from elsewhere in the body. In the immediate postoperative period fluids and sodium are restricted to prevent development of pulmonary edema or congestive heart failure. (See Chapter 39.) Thereafter, restriction of calories and a diet low in saturated fat and cholesterol are usually recommended to prevent recurrence or progression of the coronary artery disease.[40] Many patients become anemic after surgery; oral iron salts are recommended for 4 to 6 weeks after surgery and should be taken with meals to minimize gastrointestinal side effects.

CASE STUDY 22

Business Executive at High Risk with Type IIa Hyperlipoproteinemia

Mr. R is an aspiring business executive who, at age 35, is proud of his many achievements. He claims that he thrives on the pressures of work. He is president of the Chamber of Commerce and is active in the Rotary Club. When his schedule permits, Mr. R enjoys playing baseball and basketball with his two children. Other favorite activities include hunting and camping.

Mr. R recently applied for additional life insurance and was required to have a health examination. He has been in good health and had not seen a physician in several years. Mr. R is a heavy smoker and drinks about 10 cups of coffee a day. During the examination it was noted that Mr. R's blood pressure was 140/90; pulse, regular at 72 per minute; height, 178 cm (70 in.); weight 82 kg (180 lb, and wrist circumference, 6⅜ inches. His electrocardiogram was normal. Laboratory findings included hemoglobin, 15 g per dl; blood urea nitrogen, 10 mg per dl; creatinine, 1.2 mg per dl; total cholesterol, 300 mg per dl; HDL-cholesterol, 35 mg per dl; and triglycerides, 120 mg per dl. A xanthoma was noted on his Achilles' tendon.

Subsequent blood pressure readings and laboratory studies confirmed the diagnoses of borderline hypertension and Type IIa hyperlipoproteinemia. Mr. R was advised to quit smoking, to reduce his intake of caffeine, and to increase his participation in sports and outdoor activities.

Mr. R's wife and two children were screened for hyperlipoproteinemia. The 9-year-old son had a serum cholesterol level of 260 mg per dl, indicative of type IIa hyperlipoproteinemia. His triglyceride level was within normal limits. Mr. R stated that his father died of a myocardial infarction at the age of 47.

The family physician recommended that Mr. R and his son sharply reduce their dietary intake of cholesterol and saturated fat. Mrs. R has decided to plan the entire family's menu around a type IIa diet.

Mr. R was referred to a coronary prevention group staffed by a multidisciplinary team. The team monitors each member's cardiovascular status and provides instruction aimed at reducing the individual's risk of heart disease. For example, the dietitian helped Mrs. R. develop menus consistent with the prescribed type IIa diet and the family's food preferences.

Pathophysiologic Correlations

1. Mr. R is at increased risk of a heart attack or a cerebrovascular accident. List the risk factors that are presented in his history.
2. The physician explained atherosclerosis to Mr. R. What are atheroma?
3. What are the principal constituents of atheroma?
4. What are the principal abnormal findings in type IIa hyperlipoproteinemia?
5. Why did Mr. R's physician recommend screening for the rest of the family?
6. What is the relationship between HDL-cholesterol and risk of coronary heart disease? What steps can be taken to improve the HDL-cholesterol level?
7. What is the likelihood that Mr. R's serum cholesterol level will return to normal levels through diet modification alone?
8. Would you expect dietary modification alone to be effective in lowering his son's serum cholesterol level? Explain.

9. List the mechanisms of action and the side effects of therapy for the following hypolipidemic agents: beta-sitosterol; clofibrate; nicotinic acid; cholestyramine; colestipol.
10. Compare the laboratory findings on Mr. R with normal values for individuals of his age.

Nutritional Assessment

Mr. R indicated his typical daily intake to be as follows:

Breakfast—Fruit juice, usually orange juice; 2 eggs with bacon and sausage, 2 slices toast with butter, jelly; coffee with whole milk and sugar. On weekends he has pancakes, or waffles, or sweet rolls.

Lunch—Eaten in a restaurant: soup such as split pea with crackers, corned beef on rye bread, marbled mocha spice cake or ice cream, coffee with whole milk and sugar.

Dinner—Generous portion of meat such as beef, ham, occasionally chicken; seldom eats fish but enjoys lobster, shrimp, oysters; mashed or baked potato with butter or sour cream, peas, corn, or green beans with butter; gelatin salad about three times a week; pudding, pie, or ice cream.

Snacks—evening only—apple and cheese, pretzels, corn chips, soft drink.

Alcohol—3 to 4 cocktails a week.

11. Based on the pattern of food intake, how would you evaluate Mr. R's diet for calories; protein; iron; ascorbic acid; riboflavin; ratio of polyunsaturated fats to saturated fats.
12. Which foods in Mr. R's diet contribute important amounts of saturated fat?
13. Which foods in Mr. R's diet contribute important amounts of cholesterol?
14. Which foods in Mr. R's diet contribute important amounts of polyunsaturated fat?
15. What should Mr. R weigh?

Planning the Diet

16. List the important characteristics of the diet for type IIa hyperlipoproteinemia.
17. List the changes that are essential to meet the requirements of Mr. R's diet with respect to milk; meat, poultry, fish; eggs; fruits; vegetables; breads and cereals; fats; desserts.
18. Write a menu that incorporates the suggested changes but that retains as much as possible of the plan Mr. R is now using.
19. Indicate several ways by which Mr. R's typical intake can be adjusted to lower the energy intake by 500 kcal per day. About how long will it take him to reach his weight goal if he lowers his energy intake by 500 kcal/day?

Dietary Counseling

20. Check the fats that are appropriate for Mrs. R to use in cooking: olive oil; peanut oil; veg-

etable shortening; safflower oil; corn oil; butter; soybean oil; cottonseed oil. What reason can you give for your choices?

21. Suggest what Mrs. R. should look for when she purchases margarine.

22. Mr. R's physician recommended moderate sodium restriction (1,000 to 1,500 mg per day). What points would you emphasize in counseling Mr. R about sodium in foods?

23. Mrs. R states that her family would really miss pie for Sunday dinner. What could you suggest to her?

24. Mrs. R asks whether the diet will prevent Mr. R from having a heart attack. How would you respond?

25. As president of the Chamber of Commerce and an active Rotary member, Mr. R eats many meals away from home. Is it realistic for him to try to adhere to any diet? What suggestions can you offer for meals away from home?

26. Mr. R has read that he should have more vitamin E in his diet. He wonders whether he should take vitamin E supplements. Explain what his action should be.

27. A popular paperback describes the role of fiber in the diet. Among the claims made in this book is that low-fiber diets are related to a higher incidence of heart attacks. What possible role might fiber have in the body's use of fat and cholesterol?

28. Suggest some exercise Mr. R can participate in on a regular basis.

29. Is there any contraindication to use of the type IIa diet by the entire R family?

References for the Case Study

BROWN, M. S., and GOLDSTEIN, J. L.: "Lowering Plasma Cholesterol by Raising LDL-Receptors," *N. Engl. J. Med.*, **305**:515–17, 1981.

HUNNINGHAKE, D. B.: "Pharmacologic Therapy for the Hyperlipidemic Patient," *Am. J. Med. (Suppl. 5A)*, **74**:19–22, 1983.

KUO, P. T.: "Hyperlipoproteinemia and Atherosclerosis: Dietary Intervention," *Am. J. Med. (Suppl. 5A)*, **74**:15–18, 1983.

SLOAN, R. W.: "Hyperlipidemia," *Am. Fam. Physician*, **28**: 171–82, September 1983.

References

1. *Heart Facts, 1983*. American Heart Association, Dallas, Texas 1983.
2. Stamler, J., and Stamler, R.: "Intervention for the Prevention and Control of Hypertension and Atherosclerotic Diseases: United States and International Experience," *Am. J. Med (Suppl. 2A)*, **76**:13–36, 1984.
3. American Heart Association Special Report: "Recommendations for Treatment of Hyperlipidemia in Adults," *Circulation*, **69**:1065A–1090A, 1984.
4. National Institutes of Health Consensus Development Panel: "Treatment of Hypertriglyceridemia," *Arteriosclerosis*, **4**:269–301, 1984.
5. Fredrickson, D. S., et al.: "Fat Transport in Lipoproteins—An Integrated Approach to Mechanisms and Disorders," *N. Engl. J. Med.*, **276**:34–44; 94–103; 148–56; 215–26; 273–81; 1967.
6. Castelli, W. P., et al.: "Epidemiology of Coronary Heart Disease. The Framingham Study," *Am. J. Med. (Suppl. 2A)*, **26**:4–12, 1984.
7. Christakis, G., et al.: "The Anti-Coronary Club. A Dietary Approach to the Prevention of Coronary Heart Disease—A Seven-Year Report," *Am. J. Publ. Health*, **56**:299–314, 1966.
8. Review: "Los Angeles Veterans Administration Diet Study," *Nutr. Rev.*, **27**:311–16, 1969.
9. Turpeinen, O., et al.: "Dietary Prevention of Coronary Heart Disease. Long-Term Experiment. I. Observations on Male Subjects," *Am. J. Clin. Nutr.*, **21**:255–76, 1968.
10. Leren, P.: "Effect of Plasma Cholesterol Lowering Diet in Male Survivors of Myocardial Infarction," *Bull. N.Y. Acad. Med.*, **44**:1012–20, 1968.
11. Multiple Risk Factor Intervention Trial Research Group: "Multiple Risk Factor Intervention Trial. Risk Factor Changes and Mortality Results," *JAMA*, **248**:1465–77, 1982.
12. Lundberg, G. D.: "MRFIT and the Goals of the *Journal*," *JAMA* **248**:1501, 1982.
13. Lipid Research Clinics Program: "The Lipid Research Clinics Coronary Primary Prevention Trial Results. I. Reduction in Incidence of Coronary Heart Disease," *JAMA*, **251**:351–64, 1984.
14. Lipid Research Clinics Program: "The Lipid Research Clinics Coronary Primary Prevention Trial Results. II. The Relationship of Reduction in Incidence of Coronary Heart Disease to Cholesterol Lowering," *JAMA*, **251**:365–374, 1984.
15. American Heart Association Committee Report: "Risk Factors and Coronary Heart Disease," *Circulation*, **62**:449A–455A, 1980.
16. AHA Committee Report: "Rationale of the Diet-Heart Statement of the American Heart Association," *Circulation*, **65**:839A–854A, 1982.
17. Reiser, R.: "Oversimplification of Diet: Coronary Heart Disease Relationships and Exaggerated Diet Recommendations," *Am. J. Clin. Nutr.*, **31**:865–75, 1978.
18. Reiser, R.: "A Commentary on the Rationale of the Diet–Heart Statement of the American Heart Association," *Am. J. Clin. Nutr.*, **40**:654–8, 1984.
19. Sturdevant, R. A. L., et al: "Increased Prevalence of Cholelithiasis in Men Ingesting a Serum Cholesterol-Lowering Diet," *N. Engl. J. Med.*, **288**:24–7, 1973.

20. Connor, W. E., and Connor, S. L.: "The Dietary Treatment of Hyperlipidemia. Rationale, Technique, and Efficacy," *Med. Clin. North Am.*, 66:485–518, 1982.
21. Anderson, J. W., and Chen, W.-J. L.: "Plant Fiber, Carbohydrate and Lipid Metabolism," *Am. J. Clin. Nutr.*, 32:346–63, 1979.
22. St. Leger, A. S., et al.: "Factors Associated with Cardiac Mortality in Developed Countries with Particular Reference to the Consumption of Wine," *Lancet*, 1:1017–19, 1979.
23. Castelli, W. P., et al.: "Alcohol and Blood Lipids," *Lancet*, 2:153–5, 1977.
24. Carroll, K. K., et al.: "Hypocholesterolemic Effect of Substituting Soybean Protein for Animal Protein in the Diet of Healthy Young Women," *Am J. Clin. Nutr.*, 31:1312–21, 1978.
25. Descovich, G. C., et al.: "Multicentre Study of Soybean Protein Diet for Outpatient Hypercholesterolaemic Patients," *Lancet*, 2:709–12, 1980.
26. Council on Scientific Affairs: "American Medical Association Concepts of Nutrition and Health," *JAMA*, 242:2335–8, 1979.
27. Dawson, E. B., et al.: "Relationship of Metal Metabolism to Vascular Disease Mortality Rates in Texas," *Am. J. Clin. Nutr.*, 31:1188–97, 1978.
28. Punsar, S., et al.: "Coronary Heart Disease and Drinking Water," *J. Chron. Dis.*, 28:259–87, 1975.
29. Johnson, C. J., et al.: "Myocardial Tissue Concentrations of Magnesium and Potassium in Men Dying Suddenly from Ischemic Heart Disease," *Am. J. Clin. Nutr.*, 32:967–70, 1979.
30. Klevay, L. M.: "Interactions of Copper and Zinc in Cardiovascular Disease," *Am. J. Nutr.*, 32:967–70, 1979.
31. Klevay, L. M., et al.: "Effects of a Diet Low in Copper on a Healthy Man," *Clin. Res.*, 28:758A, 1980.
32. Spencer, J. C.: "Direct Relationship Between the Body's Copper/Zinc Ratio, Ventricular Premature Beats, and Sudden Coronary Death," *Am. J. Clin. Nutr.*, 32:1184–5, 1979.
33. *Eating for a Healthy Heart.* American Heart Association, Dallas, Texas 1983.
34. *Counseling the Patient with Hyperlipidemia.* American Heart Association, Dallas, Texas, 1984.
35. Pritikin, N.: "The Pritikin Diet," *JAMA*, 251:1160–1, 1984.
36. Gregg, R. E., et al.: "Type III Hyperlipoproteinemia: Defective Metabolism of an Abnormal Apolipoprotein E," *Science*, 211:584–86, 1981.
37. Moore, A. O., and Powers, D. E.: *Food–Medication Interactions.* F-MI Publishing, 3rd ed. Tempe, Arizona, 1981.
38. Smith, C. H., and Bidlack, W. R.: "Dietary Concerns Associated with the Use of Medications," *J. Am. Diet. Assoc.*, 84:901–14, 1984.
39. *Dietary Management of Hyperlipoproteinemia.* A Handbook for Physicians and Dietitians. National Heart and Lung Institute, Bethesda, Md., 1973.
40. Paterson, C. R.: "Dietary Counseling for Patients Admitted for Coronary Artery Bypass Graft," *J. Am. Diet. Assoc.*, 68:158–9, 1976.

39

Dietary Management of Acute and Chronic Diseases of the Heart

Sodium-Restricted Diet

Diseases of the Heart

Clinical Findings Related to Dietary Management
Heart disease affects people of all ages, but it is most frequent in those of middle age and is most often caused by atherosclerosis. (See Chapter 38.) Diseases of the heart may affect (1) the pericardium or outer covering of the organ, (2) the endocardium or membranes lining the heart, or (3) the myocardium or the heart muscle. In addition, the blood vessels within the heart or those leaving the heart or the heart valves may be diseased. Heart disease may be acute with no prior warning, as in a coronary occlusion, or chronic with progressively decreasing ability to maintain the circulation.

The heart may be only slightly damaged so that nearly normal circulation is maintained to all parts of the body; this is a period of *compensation*. The patient is able to continue normal activities with perhaps some restriction of vigorous activity. On the other hand, in severe damage, or *decompensation*, the heart is no longer able to maintain the normal circulation to supply nutrients and oxygen to the tissues, or to dispose of carbon dioxide and other wastes. Prompt measures including bed rest, oxygen, and drug therapy are essential to relieve the strain.

Impairment of the heart is manifested by dyspnea on exertion, weakness, and pain in the chest. In severe failure there is a marked dilation of the heart with enlargement of the liver. The circulation to the tissues and through the kidney is so impaired that sodium and water are held in the tissue spaces. Edema fluid collects first in the extremities and, with increasing failure, in the abdominal and chest cavities. This is referred to as CONGESTIVE HEART FAILURE.

Infections, obesity, hypertension, and constipation complicate and make the treatment of diseases of the heart more difficult. Moreover, the heart is located close to several other organs, especially the stomach and intestines, and distention taking place in either of these organs is likely to press against and interfere with the functioning of the heart. Loss of appetite, nausea, vomiting, and other digestive disorders are common symptoms of heart disease.

Modification of the Diet   Objectives in the dietary management of cardiac patients include (1) maximum rest for the heart, (2) prevention or elimination of edema, (3) maintenance of good nutrition, and (4) acceptability of the program by the patient. The following modifications of the diet are necessary to achieve these goals.

Energy.   Loss of weight by the obese leads to considerable reduction in the work of the heart because the imbalance between body mass and strength of the heart muscle is corrected. There are a slowing of the heart rate, a drop in blood pressure, and thereby improved cardiac efficiency. Some physicians recommend a mild degree of weight loss even for the cardiac patient of normal weight. Usually a 1,000- to 1,200-kcal diet is suitable for an obese patient in bed; rarely is it necessary to reduce calories to a level below this.

Those patients whose weight is at a desirable level are permitted a maintenance level of calories during convalescence and their return to activity. Usually

1,600 to 2,000 kcal will suffice, with slight increases as the activity becomes greater.

Nutritive Adequacy.   Normal allowances of protein, minerals and vitamins are recommended. The proportions and kinds of fat and carbohydrate may be modified so that polyunsaturated fatty acids and/or complex carbohydrates are increased. (See Chapter 38.) When sodium is restricted, other sources of iodine should be prescribed especially for pregnant women and children. A severe restriction of sodium also reduces the intake of vitamin A because carrots and some of the deep green leafy vegetables that are high in sodium must be omitted.

Sodium.   A sodium-restricted diet is indicated when there is retention of fluid and sodium. Usually a restriction of sodium to 1,600 to 2,300 mg (70 to 100 mEq) is satisfactory in patients with congestive heart failure who are receiving diuretics, but occasionally sodium needs to be reduced further.[1] Some patients who have associated renal disease are unable to reabsorb sodium in a normal fashion; these "salt wasters" become depleted of sodium on a severely restricted diet.

Fluid.   The restriction of fluid is not required as long as the sodium is restricted. Less work is required by the kidney when ample fluid is available for the excretion of wastes. Because of the homeostatic mechanisms afforded by adrenal and pituitary hormones, water is retained only when there is sufficient sodium to maintain physiologic concentrations. (See also page 148.) An intake of 2 liters of fluid daily is usually permitted.

In advanced congestive failure, especially with excessive use of diuretics, water may be retained even though the sodium intake is low. The hormonal controls are no longer balanced, and the sodium concentration of extracellular fluid is low even though the total body content of sodium is high. Such a circumstance necessitates the restriction of fluid as well as sodium.

Amount of Food.   Small amounts of food given in five or six meals are preferable to bulky, large meals that place an excessive burden on the heart during digestion. Part of the food normally allowed at mealtime may be saved for between-meal feedings.

Consistency.   When decompensation occurs, liquid or soft, easily digested foods that require little chewing should be used. During the early stages of illness, the patient may need to be fed. When the patient's condition improves, he or she should be given foods that are easy to chew and to digest.

Choice of Food.   Abdominal distention must be avoided. Until the patient's food tolerances are known, it is best to omit vegetables of the cabbage family, onions, turnips, legumes, and melons. Occasionally a patient may complain that milk is distending. Because of its relaxing effect, the physician may prescribe small amounts of alcohol.

Constipation must be avoided by the judicious use of fruits and vegetables, prune juice, and a sufficient fluid intake.

Progression of the Diet   During severe decompensation, as in coronary occlusion, rest is the primary consideration, and all attempts to feed the patient are avoided for the first few days. Liquids are then used for 2 or 3 days. All liquids are served at room temperature. Extremes of temperature such as very hot or iced beverages are contraindicated because they may induce dysrhythmias. Beverages containing caffeine are usually omitted because of their stimulating effect on the heart rate. A number of nutritionally complete proprietary formulas that are low in sodium and fluid content are suitable.* When the acute phase has passed, more solid foods are permitted and small feedings of easily digested foods are given as tolerated. The foods may be selected from those permitted for the Fiber-Restricted Diet, page 414, giving only small amounts at each of five to six feedings. Mild sodium restriction (2 g) is usually prescribed. During this phase calories are usually limited to 1,000 to 1,200 daily. Cholesterol and saturated fat are restricted. (See Chapter 38 for adjustments made in hyperlipoproteinemias.) In the rehabilitative stage, calories are adjusted as necessary to bring about weight change if needed. The fat-modified diet (see Chapter 38) is used with sodium restriction if needed. If decompensation is severe, sodium may be restricted to 500 mg or less per day.

Nutrition Following Cardiac Transplantation   During the immediate postoperative period energy and protein needs are increased substantially. Three meals with liquid supplements between meals are used.

The primary goal in long-term management is to achieve and maintain ideal body weight. Excess

---

* Magnacal (Biosearch Medical Products, Inc., Somerville, N.J.); Ensure Plus (Ross Laboratories, Inc., Columbus, Ohio); Travasorb MCT (Travenol Laboratories, Inc., Deerfield, Ill.).

weight is not only a burden for the new heart, but is frequently associated with hypertension and elevated serum lipids. Dietary adjustments include reduction of calories, sodium (2 g per day), cholesterol (less than 300 mg per day), total fat (35 percent of calories), and concentrated sweets. The ratio of polyunsaturated to saturated fats is increased to 1.0 and dietary potassium is increased if needed.[2]

Nutritional Effects of Drug Therapy. Cyclosporin, an immunosuppressive agent, should be taken mixed with milk, juice, or water. Steroid-induced diabetes or peptic ulcer may occur secondary to prednisone therapy. Nutritional considerations in management of type II diabetes mellitus were discussed in Chapter 36, and peptic ulcer was discussed in Chapter 29.

Hypertension

Hypertension, or elevation of the blood pressure above normal, is a symptom that accompanies many cardiovascular and renal diseases. It is a major risk factor that increases morbidity and mortality from cardiovascular diseases. Some 37 million Americans are known to have hypertension.[3] The prevalence in blacks is considerably higher than that in whites. Hypertension occurs at any age but is found most frequently in those over 40 years of age. About 85 to 90 percent have ESSENTIAL HYPERTENSION, for which the cause is unknown. Both genetic and environmental factors have been implicated. Emotional disturbances, excessive smoking, certain kidney diseases, and adrenal tumors account for a small proportion of cases. Hypertension is diagnosed when the diastolic pressure is consistently 90 mm Hg or more or the systolic pressure exceeds 140 mm Hg on several occasions. Diastolic pressure of 90 to 104 mm Hg is classified as *mild* hypertension; readings of 105 to 114 mm Hg indicate *moderate* hypertension; and those of 115 mm Hg or more, *severe* hypertension.[4]

Prevention Some 10 to 30 percent of the U.S. population is genetically predisposed to hypertension.[5] Some clinicians recommend lifelong modest sodium restriction as a means of delaying onset of the disorder and preventing its complication in persons who are genetically susceptible.[4,5]

The Food and Nutrition Board recommends that those with a family history of hypertension or who have borderline hypertension should limit sodium intake to *less* than 1,600 to 2,300 mg (70 to 100 mEq) per day.[1] The Dietary Guidelines for Americans propose a reduction in daily salt intake as a preventive measure.[6] The Food and Drug Administration is encouraging food manufacturers to lower the amounts of sodium added to foods where this is safe and feasible, and to provide information to consumers about the sodium content of foods.[7]

Role of Dietary Factors The role of dietary factors in the etiology of hypertension is not settled. Obesity is often associated with hypertension, although it is not necessarily causative. A strong correlation has been shown between weight and blood pressure and between increases in weight and increases in blood pressure. Even a modest sustained weight loss of 10 pounds or more is sufficient to produce a substantial fall in blood pressure.[4]

Epidemiologic evidence indicates that in populations with low habitual salt intake, the prevalence of hypertension is low. However, other factors in these groups could also have an influence, such as physical activity patterns, homogeneity, and differences in lifestyle, and other dietary factors such as potassium and fiber intake. On the other hand, countries in which the population has a markedly high salt intake, such as Japan, have a high incidence of hypertension. Prolonged very high salt intake can cause elevated blood pressure even in normal subjects.

Sodium restriction is effective in lowering blood pressure in some persons; when used alone, however, except in patients with mild hypertension, the level of sodium permitted is so low as to be impractical for most persons. The combination of modest weight reduction and sodium restriction brings about a greater fall in blood pressure than either one alone.

Some evidence in this country has indicated that persons with hypertension have lower intakes of potassium or calcium than non-hypertensive individuals.[8-10] Potassium supplementation has been reported to reduce blood pressure in hypertensive persons.[11]

In other short-term studies a reduction in blood pressure has been reported in hypertensive patients when a low-sodium high-potassium diet was used.[8] The long-term effectiveness of this approach has not been tested. One hypothesis holds that the dietary sodium to potassium ratio may be a major controlling factor in blood pressure.[12]

Results of one study suggested that persons with mild hypertension who were placed on a diet of very low total fat intake (less than 25 percent of calories), with a polyunsaturated to saturated fat ratio of 1.0 experienced a reduction in blood pressure.[13] So far there is no evidence that persons in the general population who consume diets with increased amounts of polyunsaturated fats achieve similar reductions in blood pressure. It should be noted, however, that the total fat intake in this study was considerably lower than that of the general population in the United States and Canada. Elimination of alcohol intake from hypertensive heavy drinkers also reportedly lowers blood pressure.[11]

Much more information is needed before it can be concluded that alteration of specific dietary factors is important in the prevention and control of hypertension. It is more likely that dietary changes for those at risk need to be multifactorial—for example, adjustments to lower intake of calories, fat, sodium, and alcohol, and possibly to increase potassium, calcium, and dietary fiber.

Dietary Modification The primary means of treating hypertension is through use of diuretics. Some evidence suggests that excessive intake of sodium may block the antihypertensive effects of these drugs. For this reason the committee on Sodium-Restricted Diets of the Food and Nutrition Board recommends use of sodium-restricted diets in combination with diuretics in the treatment of hypertension. The suggested intake is 1,600 to 2,300 mg (70 to 100 mEq).[1] Sodium restriction also enhances the effects of diuretic therapy and permits smaller doses of such drugs. The Joint National Committee on Detection, Evaluation, and Treatment of High Blood Pressure has recommended mild sodium restriction, 2 g (70 to 90 mEq), for patients with essential hypertension.[4]

Nutritional Effects of Drug Therapy. Most diuretics and antihypertensive drugs cause nausea, vomiting, and abdominal cramps. These drugs should be taken with food to minimize gastric irritation. Good food sources of potassium should be recommended to patients receiving diuretics such as thiazides, furosemide, and ethacrynic acid. A few examples of potassium-rich foods that are also low in sodium are apricots, bananas, prunes, raisins, broccoli, brussels sprouts, baked squash, and baked potato. Dried fruits and legumes are especially good sources for those who are not on calorie-restricted diets. The amount of potassium needed has not been determined but a reasonable goal is 100 mEq (3,900 mg) daily.[1] Potassium supplements such as potassium chloride may be necessary to achieve this level of intake. Most salt substitutes contain approximately 60 mEq (2,350 mg) of potassium per teaspoon.[14] Some physicians may approve use of these for patients without renal disease.

Diuretics have been shown to produce increases in triglycerides and plasma cholesterol.[15] Use of the beta-blocker propranolol together with diuretics raises triglyceride levels even more[15] and lowers HDL-cholesterol. Patients receiving these drugs should be counselled regarding dietary changes to prevent further elevation of blood lipids. (See Chapter 38.) Reduction of saturated fat and cholesterol intake may be needed.

Triamterene and spironolactone are potassium-sparing diuretics. Excessive intake of potassium-containing foods should be avoided when these drugs are used. Triamterene is known to be a weak folacin antagonist; low levels of serum folate and vitamin B-12 have been reported following use of the drug; thus levels of these vitamins should be monitored.[16]

DIETARY COUNSELING

Failure to comply with therapy is a major problem in management of hypertension. In addition to the considerations described on pages 549 to 553 the importance of weight control should be stressed at regular follow-up visits. Review of food records at periodic visits will give an indication of compliance with sodium restriction. Recommendations for changes in types or amounts of food eaten, or in methods of preparation should be phased in gradually. Some require months to adapt to the reduction in salt intake, and time is needed to find acceptable substitutes for favorite foods or new flavoring agents. (See page 552.) The client must be helped to understand the importance of the dietary changes and should actively participate in planning for each step required and evaluating the outcome.

Sodium-Restricted Diets

Levels of Sodium Restriction Sodium-restricted diets are used for the prevention, control, and elimination of edema in many pathologic conditions, and occasionally for the alleviation of hypertension. Since sodium is the ion of importance, it is incorrect to designate a diet as "salt free," "salt poor," or "low salt." Moreover, to call a diet "low sodium" or "sodium-restricted" is misleading, since any amount of sodium below the normal sodium intake would satisfy such a description, but would not necessarily be at therapeutic levels. Sodium-restricted diets should be prescribed in terms of milligrams of sodium, for example, 500 to 700 mg-sodium diet.

Because of the wide range of sodium in single foods, precision in determining actual sodium intake is not possible in the usual clinical situation. For most patients sodium restriction entails major changes in lifestyle because of the extra care required in shopping and in preparing meals that are appealing yet sufficiently low in sodium to meet the therapeutic goal. The Food and Nutrition Board has stated that the level of sodium used should involve the least amount of restriction necessary to achieve the desired clinical response.[1] Four levels of sodium restriction are used.

The normal diet contains about 3 to 6 g of sodium daily, although a liberal intake of salty food results in considerably higher sodium levels. The normal diet is modified for its sodium content as described in the following paragraphs.

200 to 300 mg (9 to 13 mEq*); extreme sodium restriction: No salt used in cooking; careful selection of foods low in sodium; low-sodium milk substituted for regular milk. This diet is used in conditions such as cirrhosis of the liver with ascites to induce a diuresis, and in congestive heart failure if severe sodium restriction is ineffective.[1]

500 to 700 mg (22 to 30 mEq); severe sodium restriction: No salt used in cooking; careful selection of foods in measured amounts; regular milk. This level is used for severe congestive heart failure; occasionally in severe renal disease with edema if patients are not being dialyzed, or in cirrhosis with ascites.[1]

1,000 to 1,500 mg (43 to 65 mEq); moderate sodium restriction: No salt in cooking; careful selection of foods low in sodium, but may include measured amounts of salt, or salted bread and butter. this level is suggested for those with a strong family history of hypertension or patients with borderline hypertension.[1]

2,000 to 3,000 mg (87 to 130 mEq); mild sodium restriction: Some salt may be used in cooking, but no salty foods are permitted; no salt is used at the table. This level is used as a maintenance diet in cardiac and renal diseases.

Sources of Sodium The sodium-restricted diet must be planned with respect to the amount of naturally occurring sodium in foods and the sodium added in food preparation and processing. Sodium values for common foods are given in Table A-2. Most prepared foods show wide variations in sodium content, depending on conditions of growth and processing of the food, sodium content of water used in preparation, and others. The values listed in any table should not be considered absolute, but they do give reasonable

* One milliequivalent of sodium is 23 mg; thus 200 mg ÷ 23 = 9 mEq.

approximations of foods which may be used and which should be avoided.

Naturally Occurring Sodium in Foods. The natural sodium content of animal foods is relatively high and reasonably constant. Thus, meat, poultry, fish, eggs, milk, and cheese are the foods which, although nutritionally essential, must be used in measured amounts. Organ meats contain somewhat more sodium than muscle meats. Shellfish of all kinds are especially high in sodium, but other saltwater fish contain no more sodium than freshwater fish. A few plant foods, especially greens like spinach, chard, and kale, contain significant amounts of sodium and are omitted in the more severely restricted diets.

Fruits, cereals, and most vegetables are insignificant sources of sodium. Likewise, sugars, oils, shortenings, and unsalted butter and margarine are negligible sources of sodium.

The drinking water in many localities contains appreciable quantities of sodium, either naturally or through the use of water softeners. When the sodium content is in excess of 20 mg per liter, the daily intake from water alone may be appreciable.[1]

Sodium Added to Foods. Table salt is by far the most important source of sodium in the diet. Each gram of salt contains about 400 mg sodium; thus, a teaspoon of salt would furnish 2,000 mg sodium. Salt is not only used in cooking and at the table but it also finds its way into many products through manufacturing processes: as in the preservation of ham, bacon, frozen and dried fish; in the brining of pickles, corned beef, and sauerkraut; in koshering of meat; as a rinse to prevent discoloration of fruits in canning; as a means of separating peas and lima beans for quality before freezing or canning. Canned foods (except fruits), frozen casseroles, dinners, and baked foods, biscuit, bread, cookie, dessert, and sauce mixes contain high levels of salt.

Baking powder and baking soda are widely used in food preparation. Potassium bicarbonate may be used in place of sodium bicarbonate, and sodium-free baking powder may be substituted for regular baking powder.

Numerous sodium compounds other than sodium chloride, baking soda, and baking powder are used in food manufacture: sodium benzoate as a preservative in relishes, sauces, margarine; disodium phosphate to shorten the cooking time of cereals; sodium citrate to enhance the flavor of gelatin desserts and beverages; monosodium glutamate (MSG) as a widely used seasoning in restaurants and in food processing; sodium

Table 39-1. **Nutritive Values of Food Lists for Planning Sodium-Restricted Diets***

List	Amount	Energy (kcal)	Protein (g)	Fat (g)	Carbohydrate (g)	Sodium (mg)
1. Milk, whole	1 cup, regular	170	8	10	12	120
	1 cup, low sodium	170	8	10	12	7
Milk, nonfat	1 cup, regular	85	8	—	12	120
	1 cup, low sodium	85	8	—	12	7
2. Vegetables						
List 2	½ cup	25	2	—	5	9
Starchy vegetables	Varies with choice	70	2	—	15	5
3. Fruits	Varies with choice	40	—	—	10	2
4. Low-sodium breads, cereals	Varies with choice	70	2	—	15	5
5. Meat, poultry, fish, eggs, or cheese	1 ounce meat or equivalent	75	7	5	—	25
6. Fats	1 teaspoon butter or equivalent	45	—	5	—	tr

* Arranged from *Your 500 Milligram Sodium Diet*, American Heart Association, New York, 1977.

propionate in cheeses, breads, and cakes to retard mold growth; sodium alginate for smooth texture in chocolate milk and ice cream; and sodium sulfite as a bleach in the preparation of maraschino cherries and to prevent discoloration of dried fruits. (See Figure 39-1.)

Label Information. Standards of identity have been established for many food products by the Food and Drug Administration. Such products do not need to carry a listing of ingredients. Thus, the fact that salt is not listed is no guarantee that it is a low-sodium product. Mayonnaise, catsup, and canned vegetables are examples of foods ordinarily prepared with salt but that belong in the category of foods for which a standard of identity has been set up.

Foods specially produced for sodium-restricted diets must be labeled according to regulations set up by the Food and Drug Administration. The label must indicate the sodium content in an average serving and also in 100 g of the food. Although foods may have been processed without added sodium compounds, some of them may exceed the limits allowed for a given category. For example, a vegetable that contains 50 mg sodium per serving is much higher than the average sodium content of vegetables. (See Table 39-1 also page 551.)

Sodium in Drugs. Many laxatives, antibiotics, alkalizers, cough medicines, and sedatives contain sodium, and the physician needs to determine whether the amount of a given drug will nullify the effects of a prescribed diet. Patients need to be especially warned against self-medication with sodium bicarbonate or antacids.

Unit Lists for Sodium-Restricted Diets A joint committee of the American Dietetic Association, the American Heart Association, and the U.S. Public Health Service has grouped foods for sodium-restricted diets in *Unit Lists*. Each list corresponds closely to the meal exchange lists (Table A-4, Appendix), but foods that are not to be used are also listed. The group C vegetables of the unit lists are those included in the bread exchange lists. (See Table 39-1.)

Meal Planning with Unit Lists A 500 mg sodium diet at three caloric levels is shown in Table 39-2.

Table 39-2. **Food Allowances for 500-mg Sodium Diet***

Food List	1,200-kcal units	1,800-kcal units	Unrestricted Calories
Milk	2 (skim)	2 (2% fat)	2 (whole)
Vegetables, List 2	2	2	2 or more
Starchy vegetables	1	1	1 or more
Fruit	4	6	2 or more
Bread	4	8	4 or more
Meat	5	5	5 only
Fat	4	7	as desired
Distribution of kcal:			
Protein, percent	21	16	
Fat, percent	30	33	
Carbohydrate, percent	49	51	

* Adapted from *Your 500 Milligram Sodium Diet*, American Heart Association, New York, 1977. Allowances calculated to provide less than 500 mg sodium in order to allow for sodium in water used for cooking and drinking. Sodium content of water assumed to be 5 mg per dl.

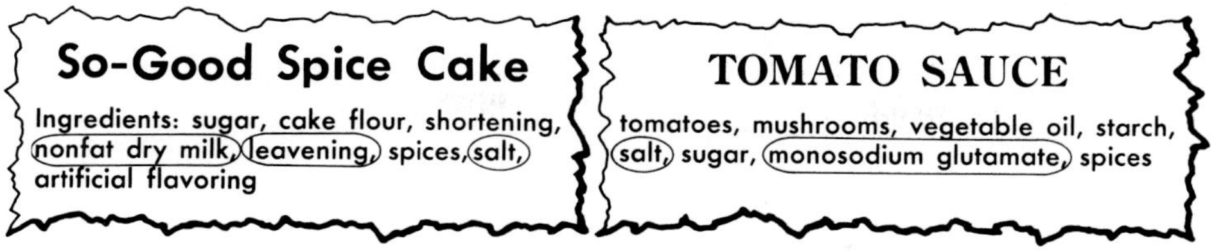

Figure 39-1. Watch for the words *salt* and *sodium* on labels when selecting foods for sodium-restricted diets. Leavenings and nonfat dry milk also contribute significant amounts of sodium.

Food Lists for Sodium-Restricted Diets *

See Table A-4, pages 662-666 for food groupings and portion sizes. For each list, note the following items that must be avoided.

Foods Allowed	Foods to Avoid
LIST 1. MILK Skim, whole, evaporated, low sodium	Commercial foods made with milk—chocolate milk, condensed milk, ice cream, malted milk, milk mixes, milk shakes, sherbet
LIST 2. VEGETABLES Fresh, frozen, or dietetic canned with no salt or other sodium compounds (See list 2, page 663)	Canned vegetables or juices except low-sodium dietetic Artichoke, beet greens, celery, chard (Swiss), dandelion greens, kale, mustard greens, sauerkraut, spinach Beets, carrots, frozen peas if processed with salt, white turnips
Starchy vegetables (see Bread list, pages 664)	Frozen lima beans if processed with salt, hominy, potato chips
LIST 3. FRUITS Fresh, frozen, canned, or dried (See list 3, page 663)	Crystallized or glazed fruit, maraschino cherries, dried fruit with sodium sulfite added
LIST 4. BREAD Low-sodium breads, cereals, and cereal products Breads and rolls (yeast) made without salt; quick breads made with sodium-free baking powder or potassium bicarbonate and without salt, or made from low-sodium dietetic mix	Yeast bread, rolls, or Melba toast made with salt or from commercial mixes; quick breads made with baking powder, baking soda, salt or MSG or made from commercial mixes
Cereals, cooked unsalted; dry cereals: Puffed Rice, Puffed Wheat, Shredded Wheat	Quick-cooking and enriched cereals which contain a sodium compound. Read the label. Dry cereals except as listed
Barley; cornmeal; cornstarch; crackers, low sodium; matzo, plain, unsalted; waffle, yeast	Graham crackers or any other except low-sodium dietetic; salted popcorn; self-rising flour; pretzels; waffles containing salt, baking powder, baking soda, or egg white
LIST 5. MEAT Meat, poultry, fish, eggs, and low-sodium cheese and peanut butter	
Meat or poultry: fresh, frozen, or canned low sodium	Brains or kidneys

* Adapted from *Your 500 Milligram Sodium Diet*, American Heart Association, New York, 1977.

Foods Allowed

Liver (only once in 2 weeks)
Tongue, fresh

Fish or fish fillets, fresh only
Bass, bluefish, catfish, cod, eels, flounder, halibut, rockfish, salmon, sole, trout, tuna
Salmon, canned low-sodium dietetic
Tuna, canned low-sodium dietetic

Cheese, cottage, unsalted
Cheese, processed, low-sodium dietetic
Egg (limit 1 per day)
Peanut butter, low-sodium dietetic

LIST 6. FAT
Spreads, oils, cooking fats unsalted

MISCELLANEOUS FOODS
Beverages
Alcoholic with doctor's permission
Cocoa made with milk from diet
Coffee, instant, freeze dried, or regular; coffee substitutes
Lemonade; Postum; tea
Candy, homemade, salt free, or special low sodium
Gelatin, plain unflavored

Leavening agents
Cream of tartar; sodium-free baking powder; potassium bicarbonate; yeast
Rennet dessert powder (not tablets)

Foods to Avoid

Canned, salted, or smoked meat: bacon, bologna, chipped or corned beef, frankfurters, ham, kosher meats, luncheon meat, salt pork, sausage, smoked tongue, etc.
Frozen fish fillets
Canned, salted, or smoked fish: anchovies, caviar, salted and dried cod, herring, canned salmon (except low-sodium dietetic), sardines, canned tuna (except low-sodium dietetic)
Shellfish: clams, crabs, lobsters, oysters, scallops, shrimp, etc.
Cheese, except low-sodium dietetic

Egg substitutes, frozen or powdered
Peanut butter unless low-sodium dietetic

Salted butter or margarine, bacon and bacon fat; salt pork; olives; commercial French or other dressing except low sodium; commercial mayonnaise, except low sodium; salted nuts

Fountain beverages; instant cocoa mixes; prepared beverage mixes, including fruit-flavored powders

Commercial candies, cakes, cookies
Commercial sweetened gelatin desserts
Mixes of all types
Pastries

Regular baking powder; baking soda (sodium bicarbonate)
Rennet tablets; pudding mixes; molasses

Flavoring Aids Allowed

Allspice
Almond extract
Anise seed
Basil
Bay leaf
Bouillon cube (low sodium)
Caraway seed
Cardamom
Chives
Cinnamon
Cloves
Cocoa (1 - 2 teaspoons)
Cumin
Curry
Dill
Fennel
Garlic
Ginger
Horseradish (prepared without salt)
Juniper
Lemon juice or extract
Mace
Maple extract
Marjoram
Mint
Mustard, dry
Nutmeg
Onion, fresh, juice or sliced
Orange extract
Oregano
Paprika
Parsley
Pepper

Flavoring Aids to Avoid

Barbecue sauce
Bouillon cube, regular
Catsup
Celery salt, seed, leaves
Chili sauce
Cyclamates
Garlic salt
Horseradish prepared with salt
Meat extracts, sauces, tenderizers
Monosodium glutamate
Mustard, prepared
Olives
Onion salt
Pickles
Relishes
Salt

Flavoring Aids Allowed

Peppermint extract	Sesame seeds
Poppy seed	Sorrel
Poultry seasoning	Sugar
Purslane	Tarragon
Rosemary	Thyme
Saccharin	Turmeric
Saffron	Vanilla extract
Sage	Vinegar
Salt substitutes (with physician's approval)	Wine, if allowed by physician
Savory	Walnut extract

Flavoring Aids to Avoid

Soy sauce
Sugar substitutes containing sodium
Worcestershire sauce

Sample Menu for 500-mg Sodium Diet

1,200 kcal	**1,800 kcal**
BREAKFAST	
Honeydew melon, ⅛ medium	Same
Shredded Wheat, 1 biscuit	Same
Low-sodium corn muffin, 1	2
Unsalted margarine, 1 teaspoon	2
Milk, 1 cup skim	1 cup 2 percent
Coffee or tea, no sugar	Same
LUNCHEON OR SUPPER	
Toasted sandwich:	
Low-sodium bread, 2 slices	Same
Low-sodium tuna fish, 2 ounces	Same
Low-sodium mayonnaise, none; use lemon juice	Same
Lettuce	Same
Tomato	Same
Mixed green salad	Same
Low-sodium, low-calorie dressing, 1 tablespoon	Same
Fresh apple, medium	Baked apple with stuffing:
	Raisins, 2 tablespoons
	Brown sugar, 2 teaspoons
Milk, skim, 1 cup	1 cup 2 percent
DINNER	
Broiled pork chop, 3 ounces	Same
Baked potato, small	Same
Baked acorn squash, ½ cup	Same
Low-sodium dinner roll, none	2
Low-sodium margarine, 2 teaspoons	3 teaspoons
Fruit cup:	
Fresh pineapple, ¼ cup	½ cup
Fresh strawberries, ½ cup	1 cup
Coffee or tea, no sugar	Same

Adjustments for Sodium Level   The 500-mg sodium diet in Table 39-2 may be adjusted for lower or higher levels of sodium as follows:

200 to 300 mg (9 to 13 mEq): substitute low-sodium milk for regular milk.

1,000 to 1500 mg (43 to 65 mEq): substitute limited amounts of ordinary salted bread (contains 100 to 125 mg sodium per slice) and salted butter or margarine (contains 50 mg sodium per teaspoon); or a carefully measured amount of salt placed in a shaker and used for cooking or at table (¼ teaspoon salt contains approximately 500 mg sodium).

2,000 to 3,000 mg (87 to 130 mEq): At 1,200 kcal use lightly salted food and allow ordinary salted bread and regular milk. When 1,800 kcal or more are allowed, it is possible to keep the sodium level around 2,000 to 3,000 mg only by omitting salt in food preparation. Omit salting of food at the table. Omit salty foods such as potato chips, salted popcorn, and nuts, olives, pickles, relishes, meat sauces, smoked and salted meats.

Dangers of Sodium Restriction Diets that are very low in sodium must be used with caution since there is occasional danger of depletion of body sodium. Hot weather may bring about great losses of sodium through the skin, and vomiting, diarrhea, surgery, renal damage, or the use of mercurial diuretics also increases the amounts of sodium lost from the body. Sodium depletion is characterized by weakness, abdominal cramps, lethargy, oliguria, azotemia, and disturbances in the acid-base balance. Patients must be instructed to recognize the symptoms of danger and to consult a physician immediately when they occur.

DIETARY COUNSELING

Perhaps no diet provides greater obstacles with respect to acceptance for taste appeal and understanding of the permissible food choices than does the sodium-restricted diet. Skilled counseling of the patient by dietitian, nurse, and physician is essential from the time the diet is first prescribed. Far too many patients have assumed that the omission of salt merely represented poor cookery and have eaten forbidden foods brought in by well-meaning but uninformed relatives and friends.

When a sodium-restricted diet is to be continued in the home, the patient should be given some understanding of the purposes of the diet and some indication regarding the length of time it needs to be used. The patient needs information on the foods that are permitted on the diet, what foods are contraindicated, where foods may be purchased, and how to prepare palatable foods with flavoring aids. He or she should not expect foods to taste the same as those that are salted, but in time most patients learn to adjust to the change in flavors.

The individual responsible for meal preparation must be included in all phases of dietary counseling so that he or she understands the importance of the diet and learns what modifications in planning, purchasing, and preparation are required.

The American Heart Association has published detailed booklets concerning three levels of sodium restriction and low-calorie and maintenance energy allowances. For patients who find the details confusing, concise leaflets have also been prepared. Neither of these teaching aids should take the place of individualized instruction, nor should the patient be expected to comprehend all the information in one or two counseling sessions.

Cultural patterns must be considered, inasmuch as favorite dishes are often high in sodium. Usually, these dishes may be adapted within the sodium restriction rather than omitting them entirely.

The patient and the homemaker must be taught to read labels of food products, looking especially for the words *salt* and *sodium*. (See Figure 39-1.)

Preparation of Food Ingenuity is required in the preparation of foods for sodium-restricted diets so that they will be accepted by the patient. A number of salt substitutes are available, but they should be used only upon the recommendation of the physician since many of them contain substantial amounts of potassium, which may be contraindicated when there is renal damage.

Numerous flavoring aids are available (see page 552 for list) to provide taste appeal. Herbs and spices are especially useful, but they should be used with a light touch.

Delicious yeast breads, muffins, waffles, and doughnuts may be prepared using part of the milk and egg allowance of the diet. Low-sodium baking powder must be substituted for regular baking powder. When low-sodium milk is required in the diet, recipes may be successfully prepared by substituting low-sodium milk for regular milk. The calcium and thiamin levels of low-sodium milk are lower, and the potassium level much higher than those of regular milk. In other nutrients low-sodium milk compares favorably with whole milk.

The sodium content of kosher meats is too high for sodium-restricted diets. Orthodox Jewish patients should salt their meats lightly and allow them to stand for a minimum length of time to draw out the blood. Thoroughly washing with water will remove much of the salt. Then meats are simmered in a large volume of water, and the cooking liquid is discarded. The leaching is more effective if the meat is cut into pieces before cookery. Thorough rinsing of some foods can reduce the sodium content substantially, and may be suitable for mild or moderate sodium restriction.[17]

Restaurant Meals Meals eaten in restaurants and fast-food chains contribute substantially to the sodium intake. For persons on mild sodium-restricted diets, occasional meals in fast-food chains are permissible if discretion is used in choice of foods. Items such as beef or chicken on a bun (without ketchup or barbeque sauce), cole-slaw or lettuce and tomato, milk, juice, coffee, or tea could be ordered. French fries, onion rings, milkshakes, and pastries should be avoided. Foods that might be ordered in more traditional restaurants could include broiled meat or fish except shellfish, baked potato, plain vegetables, salads without dressing, juice, fruit, or sherbet. Broth-based soups, cheeses, crackers with salted tops, and most bakery products should be omitted.

CASE STUDY 23

Woman with Congestive Heart Failure (Italian)

Mr. and Mrs. N, both second-generation Italians, owned and operated a restaurant specializing in Italian food in the heart of the city for 35 years. The N's did well in their business, as the restaurant was well known for its good food and friendly atmosphere. After Mr. N's death 15 years ago, Mrs. N sold the restaurant since she did not feel that she could handle the business herself and wanted to retire.

Mrs. N has been living with her youngest daughter and her family for the past 3 years.

In spite of the fact that she is hard-of-hearing and blind in the right eye, Mrs. N is very active for her 84 years. She particularly enjoys her involvement in church and community activities, and she maintains her interests in cooking, painting, and gardening.

Recently Mrs. N noticed that she tired more easily and was frequently short of breath after walking short distances. Mrs. N has a history of arterial hypertension that has been fairly well controlled with hydrochlorothiazide (Hydro-diuril), but she has not adhered to the 2,000-mg sodium-restricted diet recommended by her physician. At the age of 60 Mrs. N had an inferior myocardial infarction. During the past 5 years she has been hospitalized twice for the treatment of congestive heart failure.

About 3:00 one morning Mrs. N awakened, gasping for air. Hearing a disturbance, her daughter checked on her mother and immediately noticed her labored and gurgly breathing. She became frightened when her mother started to cough up blood-tinged sputum, and she called an ambulance.

Mrs. N was admitted to the coronary care unit with the diagnosis of acute pulmonary edema. She appeared cyanotic, diaphoretic, dyspneic, and extremely anxious. Hepatomegaly, ascites, distended neck veins, and pitting edema in the lower extremities were noted during the physical examination. Mrs. N, a petite, small-boned woman of 160 cm (63 in.), weighed 57 kg (125 lb).

Initially Mrs. N was placed on a liquid 500 to 700-mg sodium diet. Because of massive edema, fluids were restricted to 1,000 ml per day. Treatment included rotating tourniquets, oxygen therapy, digitalization, and the administration of furosemide and morphine sulfate. These measures effectively relieved the pulmonary edema.

On her second hospitalization day the fluid restriction was removed and Mrs. N was placed on a 500 to 700-mg sodium 1,000-kcal soft diet. She was less dyspneic, but she complained of pain in the upper right side of her abdomen and a poor appetite.

During the remainder of her hospitalization, Mrs. N's activity was gradually increased. Treatment of the edema resulted in a weight loss of 4.6 kg. (10 lb).

In the process of discharge planning the nurse learned that Mrs. N is home alone during the day and prepares her own lunch. Mrs. N's daughter usually prepares the evening meals for the household. The R family enjoys highly spiced foods, pasta, sausages, and cheeses. They use many vegetables and fruits. Upon discharge Mrs. N is to be on a 2,000-mg sodium diet with emphasis on foods that are rich in potassium. Take-home medications include furosemide (Lasix), potassium chloride (K-Lyte), and digoxin (Lanoxin).

Pathophysiologic Correlations
1. In regard to congestive heart failure, which of these alterations in the mechanisms for fluid and electrolyte equilibrium have proba-

bly taken place? Put a circle around each correct answer.

Decreased	Increased
a. Cardiac output	i. Venous hydrostatic pressure
b. Colloidal osmotic pressure	j. Blood volume
c. Volume of interstitial fluid	k. Secretion of aldosterone and antidiuretic hormone
d. Venous hydrostatic pressure	l. Reabsorption of sodium and water
e. Blood volume	m. Glomerular filtration rate
f. Reabsorption of sodium and water	n. Excretion of sodium and water
g. Excretion of sodium and water	
h. Glomerular filtration rate	

2. Compare the concentrations, in mEq per liter and mg per dl, for sodium and potassium in extracellular and intracellular body fluids. (NOTE: 1 mEq sodium = 23 mg sodium; 1 mEq potassium = 39 mg potassium.)
3. List three important functions of sodium.
4. List three important functions of potassium.
5. What is the effect of edema on the nutrition of tissues?
6. What is the effect of the medications prescribed for Mrs. N on fluid and electrolyte balance: furosemide (Lasix); digoxin (Lanoxin); potassium chloride (K-Lyte)?

Nutritional Assessment

7. Within each group of the Daily Food Guide, list foods that are typical of the Italian cuisine.
8. List several seasonings widely used in the Italian diet.
9. What are the psychosocial factors that must be considered in planning Mrs. N's diet when she goes home?
10. What problems in the use of a sodium-restricted diet should be anticipated when Mrs. N goes home?

Planning the Diet

11. For the first day Mrs. N was given a 500 to 700-mg sodium fluid diet not to exceed 1,000 ml. What beverages would be contraindicated? Why?
    Write a menu for the initial diet prescribed.
12. List the objectives implied in the order for the 500 to 700-mg sodium 1,000-kcal soft diet in six meals ordered for Mrs. N.
13. Write a day's menu for the 500 to 700-mg sodium 1,000-kcal soft diet.
14. How does a 500 to 700-mg sodium diet compare with a typical day's intake of sodium?
15. List 10 foods to which considerable amounts of sodium are added in processing or preparation.
16. List five foods that are naturally high in sodium.
17. Mrs. N was told to emphasize foods high in potassium. List 10 such foods.

Dietary Counseling

18. While still in the hospital Mrs. N's daughter brought some homemade minestrone soup because she noticed her mother had not been eating well and didn't like the hospital food. How would you respond to this situation?
19. Mrs. N drinks little milk but is fond of cheese. What cheeses might be included in her home diet?
20. Mrs. R asks about selection and preparation of foods for Mrs. N. Suggest some guidelines under each of the following heads: milk group; meat group; vegetable–fruit group; bread–cereal group; fats; seasonings. Assume that she has a 2,000-mg sodium allowance.
21. Mrs. R asks whether her mother could use MSG (monosodium glutamate) or "light salt" in place of regular salt. How would you reply?
22. Why is it important for Mrs. N's weight to be checked at least once a week?

References for the Case Study

COHEN, S.: "New Concepts in Understanding Congestive Heart Failure, Part 2: How the Therapeutic Approaches Work," *Am. J. Nurs.*, 81:357–80, 1981.

ENGSTROM, A. M., and TOBELMANN, R. C.: "Nutritional Consequences of Reducing Sodium Intake," *Ann. Intern. Med.*, 98:870–72, 1983.

FELDMAN, E.: "Does Nutrition Play a Role in Cardiovascular Disease?" *Geriatrics*, 35:65–66, 71–75, July 1980.

MCCAULEY, K.: "Probing the Ins and Outs of Congestive Heart Failure," *Nursing '82*, 12:60–5, November 1982.

MCCAULEY, K., and WEAVER, T. E.: "Cardiac and Pulmonary Disease: Nutritional Implications," *Nurs. Clin. North Am.*, 18:81–96, March 1983.

TODD, B.: "When The Patient Has a Potassium Deficiency," *Geriatr. Nurs.*, 2:373, 376, 1981.

Man with Hypertension and Type IV Hyperlipoproteinemia (Jewish)

Mr. G, age 45, is editor-in-chief of a city newspaper, and typically works 10 to 12 hours a day, 6 days a week. His position is a demanding one, but he enjoys his work. He commutes to work from his home in a Boston suburb.

Mr. G is married and the father of three sons: ages 13, 15, and 17. The G's are a close-knit family who enjoy eating out and attending sports events.

While shoveling snow one evening Mr. G was troubled by a heavy, dull, aching substernal chest pain. After resting a few minutes, the chest pain disappeared. He first attributed the discomfort to indigestion, as he had just eaten a large meal. Earlier in the week he had experienced the same sensations after climbing two flights of stairs. Mr. G has become very anxious about the cause of his chest pains. Two close associates have had heart attacks within the past year, and Mr. G has stated, "I think I'm next in line." His concern prompted him to see a cardiologist.

Mr. G's blood pressure was 180/110. The electrocardiogram indicated a normal sinus rhythm. Laboratory findings included the following: serum cholesterol, 250 mg per dl; triglycerides, 400 mg per dl; blood urea nitrogen, 12 mg per dl; and an abnormal glucose tolerance test. Mr. G had no complaint of pain or discomfort. There was no evidence of edema or respiratory distress. The diagnoses were angina pectoris, essential hypertension, and type IV hyperlipoproteinemia.

Mr G had not had a physical examination since his herniorrhaphy 5 years ago. At that time there was no evidence of hypertension or angina. Yearly physicals were recommended then as the family history indicated that Mr. G's father died of a myocardial infarction at the age of 53. His mother has noninsulin-dependent (type II) diabetes and hypertension. Except for an occasional attack of gout, Mr. G has been in good health. Probenecid (Benemid) has kept the gout under control.

An 1,800-kcal 2,000-mg sodium diet with cholesterol moderately restricted (300 to 500 mg) and carbohydrate limited to 45 percent of calories was prescribed. Mr. G was encouraged to begin a program of daily exercise and was advised to quit smoking. He was given prescriptions for chloro-thiazide (Diuril) and nitroglycerin. Counseling regarding diet and the use of medications was provided. Mr. G was invited to join the Heart Health Club sponsored by a local hospital for members of the community.

Both Mr. and Mrs. G are overweight. Mr. G is is 183 cm (72 in.) tall and has never been concerned about his weight of 113.6 kg (250 lb). He is not looking forward to the diet his cardiologist has recommended. Mr. G eats many of his meals in restaurants and tends to snack at work when trying to meet deadlines. He does not feel that he will be able to limit himself to 1,800 kcal per day.

Mrs. G enjoys cooking for her family. She is very concerned about her husband's health and thinks that this would be a good time for both of them to lose weight. In the past few years she has tried several "crash" reducing diets without success. Mrs. G plans to prepare separate meals for the boys.

The G family strictly observes the Orthodox Jewish dietary laws in their home. Koshered meat and poultry are purchased from a local meat market. When eating in restaurants or other homes they accept foods that are not strictly within the limits of the dietary laws.

Pathophysiologic Correlations

1. Which factors in Mr. G's history place him at risk for angina? for hypertension?
2. What is the etiology of type IV hyperlipoproteinemia?
3. What are the characteristic findings in type IV hyperlipoproteinemia?
4. What is the rationale for the use of probenecid even though Mr. G has no symptoms of gout?

Nutritional Assessment

5. How does Mr. G's weight compare with the average weight for a man of his age and height? (Use the NHANES I tables.)
6. Assuming a medium body frame, what is an appropriate weight for Mr. G?
7. If Mr. G maintains his weight with a 2,600-kcal intake, how long would it take him to reach his goal weight on an 1,800-kcal intake?
8. Why is rapid weight loss contraindicated for Mr. G?
9. Summarize the dietary changes Mr. G will need to make and the rationale for each.
10. What is the effect of high intakes of each of the following on uric acid excretion: carbohydrate; fat; fluid?

11. Identify the characteristics of the Orthodox Jewish dietary pattern in terms of the following groups: milk; meat; vegetables–fruits; breads–cereals; fats; desserts.

12. Suggest some means by which Mr. G might increase his exercise two or three times weekly.

Planning the Diet

13. Outline the general goals of treatment for hypertension.

14. State the principles of dietary management of type IV hyperlipoproteinemia.

15. What dietary modifications are needed for a 2-g sodium diet?

16. Which features of the kosher diet make it difficult to adapt to a sodium-restricted diet?

17. Plan a menu for one day for Mr. G, using a work day when he eats in a restaurant.

Dietary Counseling

18. What basic knowledge do hypertensive patients need in order to manage their diets successfully?

19. List some specific guidelines you would keep in mind as you prepare to teach Mr. G about his 2-g sodium diet.

20. Suggest some dessert items that could be substituted for a bread exchange in the type IV diet.

21. Suggest some snack foods that Mr. G could enjoy without going off his diet.

22. Does Mrs. G need to prepare separate meals for the boys? Explain.

23. Mrs. G recalls that her grandfather had gout and was on a restricted diet. She asks what foods her husband should omit. How would you advise her?

24. Mrs. G asks whether Mr. G's diet would be suitable for her in order that she could lose weight. How would you respond?

25. What advice should be given to Mrs. G concerning kosher meats?

26. Among the favorite foods used by the G family are the following. Briefly describe each, and indicate whether Mr. G may continue to include them in his diet: gefilte fish; knishes; blintzes; bagels; borscht; lox; matsoh; bubke; schmalts.

References for the Case Study

BRAITHWAITE, J. D., and MORTON, B. G.: "Patient Education for Blood Pressure Control," *Nurs. Clin. North Am.*, 16:321–39, June 1981.

BURDEN, L. L., and ATWELL, K.: "The Treacherous Waters of Unstable Angina Pectoris," *Nursing '83*, 13:50–55, December 1983.

HILL, M.: "Helping the Hypertensive Patient Control Sodium Intake," *Am. J. Nurs.*, 79:906–9, 1979.

KERN, L. S., and GAWLINSKI, A.: "Stage-Managing Coronary Artery Disease," *Nursing '83*, 13:34–40, April 1983.

TANNENBAUM, R. P., et al.: "Angina Pectoris: How to Recognize It; How to Manage It," *Nursing '81*, 11:44–51, September 1981.

References

1. Committee on Sodium-Restricted Diets, Food and Nutrition Board, National Research Council: *Sodium-Restricted Diets and the Use of Diuretics. Rationale, Complications, and Practical Aspects of their Use.* National Academy of Sciences, Washington, D.C., 1979.

2. Kumar, M., and Coulston, A. M.: "Nutritional Management of the Cardiac Transplant Patient," *J. Am. Diet. Assoc.*, 83:463–5, 1983.

3. American Heart Association: *Heart Facts, 1983.* Dallas, Texas, 1983.

4. The Joint Committee on Detection, Evaluation, and Treatment of High Blood Pressure: "The 1984 Report of the Joint National Committee on Detection, Evaluation, and Treatment of High Blood Pressure," *Arch. Intern. Med.*, 144:1045–57, 1984.

5. Freis, E. D.: "Salt, Volume, and the Prevention of Hypertension," *Circulation*, 53: 589–95, 1976.

6. "Nutrition and Your Health. Dietary Guidelines for Americans," *Nutr. Today*, 15:14–18, March/April 1980.

7. Hayes, A. H., Jr.: "FDA's Dietary Sodium Initiative in the War Against Hypertension. A New Weapon," *Pub. Health Rep.*, 98:207–10, May/June 1983.

8. Heyden, S., et al.: "The Role of Potassium Manipulation in Blood Pressure Control," *Arteriosclerosis*, 3:302–6, 1983.

9. Grim, C. E., et al.: "Racial Differences in Blood Pressure in Evans County, Georgia. Relationship to Sodium and Potassium Intake and Plasma Renin Activity," *J. Chron. Dis.*, 33:87–94, 1980.

10. McCarron, D. A., et al.: "Assessment of Nutrition Correlates of Blood Pressure," *Ann. Intern. Med.*, 98(P2): 715–19, 1983.

11. Stamler, J., and Stamler, R.: "Intervention for the Prevention and Control of Hypertension and Atherosclerotic Diseases: United States and International Experience," *Am. J. Med.*, 76(P2A):13–36, 1984.

12. Langford, H. G.: "Dietary Potassium and Hypertension: Epidemiologic Data," *Ann. Intern. Med.*, 98(P2):770–2, 1983.

13. Puska, P., et al.: "Controlled Randomized Trial of the Effect of Dietary Fat on Blood Pressure," *Lancet*, 1:1–5, 1983.

14. Sopko, J. A., and Freeman, R. M.: "Salt Substitutes as a Source of Potassium," *JAMA*, 238:608–10, 1977.

15. Lasser, N. L., et al.: "Effects of Antihypertensive Therapy on Plasma Lipids and Lipoproteins in the Multiple Risk Factor Intervention Trial," *Am. J. Med.*, 76(2A): 52–65, 1984.

16. Smith, C. H., and Bidlack, W. R.: "Dietary Concerns Associated with the Use of Medications," *J. Am. Diet. Assoc*, 84:901–14, 1984.

17. Vermeulen, R. T., et al.: "Effect of Water Rinsing on Sodium Content of Selected Foods," *J. Am. Diet. Assoc.*, 82:394–6, 1983.

40

Diseases of the Kidney

Controlled Protein, Sodium, Potassium, and Phosphorus Diet; Calcium-Restricted Diet

Renal Function and Disease The important function of the kidneys is to maintain the normal composition and volume of the blood. They accomplish this by the excretion of nitrogenous and other metabolic wastes, by regulation of electrolyte and fluid excretion so that water balance is maintained, by making the final adjustment of acid-base balance, and by the synthesis of enzymes and other substances that influence metabolic activities. In view of the central role of the kidneys in maintaining the constant internal environment it is not surprising that renal disease and eventually renal failure affect every system and tissue in the body. A review of the functions of the normal kidney (see pages 145 to 147) is recommended before the student begins the study of dietary management in renal diseases.

Disease may affect the glomeruli, the tubules, or both. NEPHRITIS means literally an inflammation of the nephrons. Although GLOMERULONEPHRITIS indicates that the glomeruli are particularly affected, the functioning of the tubules will also be disturbed. Renal disease may be acute, subacute or latent, or chronic. The majority of patients with acute glomerulonephritis recover completely but a small group progress to chronic nephritis. In some patients disease may be in a latent stage for months or even years during which the individual is asymptomatic. Obviously, for each patient a careful evaluation must be made of the etiology, the presenting symptoms, and the level of renal function before any treatment including dietary control can be initiated.

Acute Glomerulonephritis

Symptoms and Clinical Findings Acute glomerulonephritis, also known as *hemorrhagic nephritis*, is primarily confined to the glomeruli. It occurs mostly in children and young adults as a frequent sequel to streptococcic infections such as scarlet fever, tonsillitis, pneumonia, and respiratory infections. In some patients the renal infection is so mild that the disease is not apparent until symptoms resulting from permanent damage appear much later. Others notice some swelling of the ankles and puffiness around the eyes and complain of headache, anorexia, nausea, and vomiting. Varying degrees of hypertension, dimness of vision, and even convulsions may occur. Usually there is diminished urinary volume, hematuria, some albuminuria, and some nitrogen retention.

The acute phase of the illness lasts from several days to a week, but renal function returns to normal much more slowly. Full recovery is the rule, provided that treatment is prompt and appropriate. The recovery time varies from 2 to 3 weeks to several months, as determined by renal function tests.

Modification of the Diet During the acute phase of illness when nausea and vomiting are present it is unrealistic to provide a diet that fully meets nutritional requirements. An effort should be made to maintain fluid balance and to provide non-protein calories, either orally or parenterally, to minimize the catabolism of tissue proteins. High-carbohydrate, low-electrolyte supplements,* fruit juices sweetened with glucose, sweetened tea, ginger ale, fruit ices, and hard candy contribute to the carbohydrate intake. Excessive amounts of sweet foods, however, may contribute to the nausea.

As the patient improves and the appetite returns, the following dietary modifications are appropriate.

* Controlyte (Sandoz Nutritionals, Minneapolis, Minn.); Moducal (Mead Johnson and Company, Evansville, Ind.; Polycose (Ross Laboratories, Columbus, Ohio); Pro-Mix Carbohydrate Supplement (Navaco Laboratories, Phoenix, Arizona); Sumacal (Chesebrough-Pond's, Inc., N.Y.).

Energy. The recommended dietary allowances (page 26) provide a general guide to the caloric requirement for persons of various ages and body size. In the absence of fever and at bedrest, these allowances can be reduced somewhat if the patient is not malnourished.

Protein. Unless oliguria or renal failure develops, protein is not restricted. If it is determined that protein restriction is necessary, a diet not exceeding 40 g protein daily is used initially. Gradual increases are made over the next 2 weeks in accordance with individual tolerance. When there is marked albuminuria, the protein intake should be increased by the amount of protein lost in the urine.

Sodium. If there is edema or hypertension, sodium restriction to 500 or 1,000 mg may be prescribed. Sodium restriction is also used if there is danger of congestive failure and pulmonary edema.

Fluid. In the presence of oliguria, fluids are restricted to prevent further edema. The volume permitted depends on the previous day's output. Usually 500 to 1,000 ml more fluid than the previous day's output is allowed. Larger amounts of fluid are given to replace losses by vomiting, diarrhea, or excessive perspiration.

Selection of foods The food allowances for 20 g-, 40 g- and 60 g-protein diets listed in Table 40-2 (page 567) are used as the basis for meal planning. The emphasis is on protein foods of high biologic value, especially eggs and milk; however, the amounts of each must be carefully controlled. Peas, lima beans, dried beans and peas, nuts, peanut butter, and gelatin are high in protein of poor biologic value and should be omitted.

Achieving a satisfactory caloric intake is doubly difficult; the limitations placed upon protein intake necessitate restriction of breads, cereals, potatoes, and similar foods that are good sources of calories, and poor appetite often interferes with food intake. The caloric intake can be increased by using appropriate supplements, low-protein desserts, sugars, jellies, hard candy, butter or margarine, vegetable oils, and carbonated beverages. Cream may be substituted for part of the milk allowance.

When sodium restriction is ordered, the food lists on pages 551 to 553 should be consulted. Regular milk can be used in the amounts listed, but all foods must be prepared without salt or other sodium-containing compounds for any restriction of 1,000 mg or less.

Chronic Glomerulonephritis

Clinical Findings Most cases of chronic glomerulonephritis have an immunologic basis of unknown etiology. Patients may be asymptomatic for months or even years. The nephritis may be detected only by laboratory studies. As the disease progresses there is gradually increasing involvement: proteinuria, hematuria, hypertension, and vascular changes in the retina. The kidneys are unable to concentrate urine and there are both frequent urination and nocturia. Although the specific gravity of the urine is low, the large volume of urine makes possible the excretion of the metabolic wastes. In some patients the nephrotic syndrome (see following) characterized by massive edema and severe proteinuria develops. Hypoproteinemia and anemia are sometimes encountered. Eventually the symptoms of renal failure occur (see page 562).

Modification of the Diet The objectives of dietary management are (1) to maintain a state of good nutrition; (2) to control or correct protein deficiency; (3) to prevent edema; and (4) to provide palatable, easily digested meals adjusted to the individual patient's needs.

During the period when the kidneys are able to excrete wastes adequately the normal daily allowance of protein plus the amount of protein lost in the urine is allowed. With progression of the disease, elevated blood urea nitrogen levels may necessitate restriction of protein to 40 g or less daily.

Sufficient carbohydrate and fat should be provided so that the energy needs of the body can be met without the breakdown of body protein. The daily caloric needs for the adult will usually range from 2,000 to 3,000 kcal.

Sodium restriction to 500 or 1,000 mg is indicated only when edema is present. Some clinicians recommend a mild level of sodium restriction (see page 549) even when there is no edema. During the diuretic phase of nephritis increased amounts of sodium may be excreted because of the kidney's inability to reabsorb the ion. Thus, a markedly restricted sodium diet could lead to body depletion with its attendant weakness, nausea, and symptoms of shock.

Nephrotic Syndrome

Glomerular injury from a number of causes may lead to massive proteinuria, hypoalbuminemia, and edema. Hypercholesterolemia is often marked but the mechanism involved is not clear. Large urinary losses of albumin and other plasma proteins lead to tissue wastage, malnutrition, fatty liver, edema, and increased suspectibility to infection. Besides a fall in plasma oncotic pressure that accompanies loss of albumin, other factors contribute to the edema, including reductions in plasma volume and renal blood flow. Consequently, enhanced renal renin production leads to increased aldosterone secretion. Aldosterone favors sodium reabsorption and further contributes to the edema.

Sodium. Diuretics and sometimes sodium restriction are used to prevent further accumulation of edema fluid. The level of sodium permitted is usually less than 2 g per day, and even as low as 500 mg per day. The sodium intake is liberalized when edema is corrected. Modest restriction may be used to prevent recurrence of edema.

Protein and Energy. Studies in patients with prolonged proteinuria have shown that positive nitrogen balance is associated with use of high protein intake, which suggests that a general body protein deficit is involved. The reduced serum protein level is one manifestation of this deficit.

Protein, 120 g per day, and a high calorie intake (50 to 60 kcal per kg) are needed for tissue repletion. High-protein supplements are useful for some patients provided the sodium content does not exceed the permitted intake.* In some areas palatable low-sodium milk is available and can be used to increase the protein intake.

Fat. Types IIa, IIb, and V hyperlipoproteinemia have been observed in nephrotic syndrome. Dietary measures to reduce plasma lipids in these disorders are appropriate and were discussed in Chapter 38.

Nephrosclerosis

Nephrosclerosis, or hardening of the renal arteries, occurs in adults after 35 years of age, as a rule, and is associated with arteriosclerosis. The disease may run a benign course for many years. During late stages some albuminuria, nitrogen retention, and retinal changes develop. Death usually results from circulatory failure. In a small number of younger persons nephrosclerosis runs a stormy, rapid course leading to

uremia and death. This is called *malignant hypertension.*

Modification of the Diet Weight reduction of the obese is desirable. A 200-mg-sodium diet has been used successfully in some instances. The protein intake is kept at a normal level until marked nitrogen retention indicates that the kidney is no longer able to eliminate wastes satisfactorily. The diet presented in Table 40-2 may be used with or without sodium restriction when a lower level of protein becomes necessary.

Renal Failure

Symptoms and Biochemical Findings Chronic glomerulonephritis, nephrosclerosis, and chronic pyelonephritis are the principal diseases of the kidney leading to renal failure. This is a condition in which the kidneys are no longer able to maintain the normal composition of the blood. UREMIA, a general term applied to the syndrome arising from the failing function of the kidney, refers to the retention of urea and other urinary constituents in the blood. It is accompanied by nausea and vomiting, hyperkalemia, azotemia, oliguria, and bone disease. AZOTEMIA is a more specific term for the accumulation of nitrogenous constituents in the blood. OLIGURIA denotes a scanty output of urine (less than 500 ml), and ANURIA is the minimal production or absence of urine (less than 100 ml per day).

Acute Renal Failure This is characterized by a rapid fall in glomerular filtration rate and a progressive rise in serum creatinine and urea concentrations. Oliguria or even anuria occur. Acute renal failure occurs in extensive burns, severe acute glomerulonephritis, following inhalation or ingestion of poisons such as carbon tetrachloride or mercury, crushing injuries, or shock from surgery. The mortality rate is nearly 50 percent. Dialysis is often employed until the kidney again resumes its function.

Dietary treatment is directed toward correction of fluid and electrolyte imbalances and maintenance of adequate nutritional status in order to minimize endogenous protein catabolism and subsequent uremia.

Energy. In the initial period when vomiting and diarrhea preclude oral intake, intravenous glucose, 100 g per 24 hours, is administered to reduce protein catabolism. In some cases, total parenteral nutrition, using hypertonic glucose and amino acids is appropri-

---

* Casec (Mead Johnson and Company, Evansville, Ind.); Pro-Mix (Navaco Laboratories, Phoenix, Arizona); Propac (Chesebrough-Pond's, Inc., N.Y.).

ate. When oral intake is permitted a high calorie intake is needed to prevent catabolism of proteins to meet energy needs.

Protein. Traditionally, severe protein restriction has been used in acute renal failure, but in recent years use of dialysis to remove accumulated nitrogen wastes has permitted a more liberal protein intake. Initially a protein-free diet is used in the non-dialyzed patient. Intravenous glucose with the essential amino acids added has also been used successfully. In the diuretic phase, 20 to 40 g protein is permitted, with gradual increases to a normal intake as renal function improves. Losses into the dialysate must be replaced for those on peritoneal or hemodialysis.

Fluid. The fluid allowance is regulated in accordance with the urinary output, any additional losses from vomiting or diarrhea, and an allowance for insensible water losses. During the oliguric phase, the fluid permitted is less than 400 ml daily for non-dialyzed patients. In the diuretic phase that follows accurate measurement of urinary output is essential so that appropriate fluid replacement can be made.

Potassium. The potassium allowance is individualized in accordance with serum levels and whether the patient is being dialyzed.

Sodium. The dietary sodium allowance is based on frequent measurements of the ion in serum and urine. For the nondialyzed patient in the oliguric phase, restriction of sodium to 500 to 1,000 mg per day is usually necessary. Patients on dialysis are permitted a more liberal sodium intake, 1,500 to 2,000 mg per day.

Chronic Renal Failure In chronic renal failure symptoms appear when the glomerular filtration rate (GFR) is inadequate to excrete nitrogenous wastes. When the GFR is less than 10 ml per minute (normal 120 ml per minute) and the serum urea nitrogen (SUN) is more than 90 mg per dl (normal 8 to 18 mg per dl), dietary modification usually brings about improvement in symptoms. Some restrict protein intake when the SUN reaches 60 mg per dl because patients reportedly feel better if the SUN is maintained below this level.[1] When the GFR is more than 25 ml per minute and the SUN is only mildly elevated, patients usually do not experience symptoms, and therefore, dietary restrictions may not be needed.

Daily protein intake is restricted progressively as the GFR fails, thus:

GRF (ml per min)	Protein (g)
20–25	60–90
15–20	50–70
10–15	40–55

About 60 percent of the protein should be of high biologic value. When the GFR falls below 4 to 5 ml per minute, dietary control alone is inadequate and dialysis is necessary.[1] Protein intake is increased gram for gram when there are urinary protein losses.

Symptoms involving the gastrointestinal tract are often present in chronic renal failure and are especially trying because of the discomfort associated with them and the constant interference with food intake. The sight or smell of food may bring about nausea or vomiting. The breath has an ammoniacal odor that interferes with the taste of food. Ulcerations of the mouth and hiccups also interfere with food intake.

The nervous system is usually affected. Patients are irritable or drowsy and eventually sink into coma. Headache, dizziness, muscular twitchings, neuritis, and even failing vision occur, especially if there is also hypertension.

The functioning of the heart is seriously disturbed. Congestive failure occurs when the heart failure is associated with retention of sodium and water. Death results when HYPERKALEMIA (elevated serum potassium) blocks the contraction of the heart.

Many alterations in metabolic and endocrine function occur in end-stage renal disease. Patients with terminal uremia have a progressively worsening anemia. There is interference with the clotting mechanism, the capillaries are fragile, ulcerations in the gastrointestinal tract may lead to bleeding, the life span of the red cells is reduced, hemolysis occurs readily, and hematopoiesis is reduced. Because the anemia reduces the effective exchange of oxygen and carbon dioxide at the tissues and in the lungs, fatigue and weakness are ever present.

When the GFR falls to 25 ml per minute, the serum phosphorus level is elevated and hypocalcemia occurs. Parathyroid hormone secretion is increased to compensate for the elevated phosphorus. This hormone decreases the reabsorption of phosphorus by the kidney and increases calcium resorption from bone. In spite of elevated parathyroid hormone production phosphorus accumulates and hypocalcemia results. Besides the secondary hyperparathyroidism induced by the disturbed calcium and phosphorus metabolism, RENAL OSTEODYSTROPHY occurs. This term is used to encompass osteomalacia, other bone deformities, and deposition of calcium in soft tissues. The kidney is unable to convert 25-hydroxy vitamin D_3 to its active form, 1,25-dihydroxy vitamin D_3, so that calcium absorption from the intestine is decreased. (See Chapter 11 and Figure 11-5). Excess fluoride may also play a role in the bone demineralization seen in uremia. Hyperglycemia and impaired glucose tolerance occur possibly due to peripheral insulin insensitivity and an increase in hormones antagonistic to insulin. Elevation of serum triglycerides (type IV hyperlipoproteinemia) is frequent and may increase the risk of premature cardiovascular disease. About half of all deaths in patients on long-term hemodialysis are due to atherosclerotic vascular disease. Excessive hepatic synthesis of triglycerides may be a consequence of insulin resistance. Deficient lipolysis may also be a factor in the hypertriglyceridemia. As the function of the kidneys further deteriorates, hyperkalemia and acidosis become increasingly severe, and edema is marked. Progressive weakness, itching, and jaundice occur. Mental disorientation, severe gastrointestinal symptoms, bleeding, and coma are characteristic of the final stages.

Nutritional Assessment Ongoing assessment of nutritional status is essential in patients with chronic renal failure because of the wasting and malnutrition seen in many patients. In addition to the usual anthropometric and biochemical parameters discussed in Chapters 23 and 26, determinations of the serum urea nitrogen to serum creatinine ratio and the amount of urea nitrogen excreted are useful in determining optimal protein intake.

Dialysis

In the management of end-stage renal disease, whether acute or chronic, dialysis is often used on a temporary or permanent basis. In *hemodialysis* the patient's blood circulates outside the body through coils or sheets of semipermeable membranes that are constantly bathed by a hypotonic dialyzing fluid so that the nitrogenous wastes are removed into the dialysate. The membranes do not permit bacteria to enter the blood nor can proteins escape from the blood. However, some amino acids are lost into the dialysate.

Although hemodialysis is a lifesaving measure, the patient does not return to a full normal life. He or she must be attached to a dialyzer for perhaps 18 hours each week. With dialysis for 4 to 6 hours three times weekly, blood urea levels that range from 100 to 170

mg per dl fall to 20 to 40 mg per dl. Dialysis does not eliminate the need for dietary control, however. Between dialyses nitrogenous end products, potassium, and sodium accumulate. If the diet is uncontrolled, dialysis will need to be more frequent. Since the artificial kidney does not correct the endocrine failure of the kidneys, most of the patients have severe anemia and hypertensive disease.

Dialysis and the associated diet require a great deal of the patient in terms of emotional stability, motivation, and intelligence. Those who are under 21 years of age especially resent the program, and those between 21 and 41 years seem to adapt best to the program. If home dialysis is used, the husband or wife, father or mother, or other relative or friend is trained to operate the dialyzer, and must also be able to provide moral support to the patient. Other considerations such as the scarcity of the equipment and the great cost limit the program to only a small number of those who could benefit.

Peritoneal Dialysis. This consists of introducing 1 to 2 liters of dialysis fluid into the peritoneal cavity and 30 to 90 minutes later withdrawing the fluid. The process is repeated until the blood urea level drops to tolerable levels.

Some blood proteins (10 to 44 g per dialysis period) as well as amino acids are lost through peritoneal dialysis and compensation must be made for this loss in order to avoid severe hypoproteinemia.

In *continuous ambulatory peritoneal dialysis* (CAPD), the dialysate is introduced into the abdominal cavity three to five times each day through a permanent indwelling catheter. The dialysate remains in the abdominal cavity from 4 to 8 hours after which it is drained and fresh dialysate is instilled. Protein losses occur, but are easily replaced by dietary protein.

General Dietary Considerations in Chronic Renal Failure

The objectives of nutritional management are (1) to maintain optimal nutritional status, (2) to minimize uremic toxicity, (3) to prevent net protein catabolism; (4) to improve the patient's well being, (5) to delay the progression of renal failure, and (6) to delay the need for dialysis.[2] Present-day management of the diet in chronic renal disease is based on the principles outlined by Giordano[3] and Giovannetti[4] during the early 1960s. These investigators found that essential amino acid requirements could be met by providing diets containing limited amounts of high biologic value protein such as egg and milk. Other protein-containing foods were sharply restricted. Such a diet provides a minimum of nonessential amino acids theoretically enabling the patient to utilize accumulated urea nitrogen for protein synthesis. Subsequent studies by others have shown that recycling of urea is only a minor source of nitrogen for protein synthesis. Nevertheless, such diets are accompanied by lowering of the blood urea nitrogen level and symptomatic improvement. Simultaneous provision of adequate nonprotein calories is essential to enhance protein utilization and to prevent endogenous protein catabolism. Restriction of fluids, sodium, potassium, and phosphorus are also employed.

A number of suitable diets have been developed utilizing the principles just described. In general, all of these aim for provision of adequate calories, regulation of protein, sodium, potassium, and fluid intake, restriction of phosphate, and supplements of calcium, iron, trace minerals, ascorbic acid, and the B vitamins.

Energy. The importance of adequate calories cannot be overemphasized, for without an adequate calorie intake body tissues will be rapidly catabolized, thus increasing the blood urea and potassium levels beyond the capacity of the kidney to excrete them. For adults, caloric needs range from 35 to 45 kcal per kg of ideal body weight, or about 2,000 to 3,000 kcal per day for chronically uremic patients and for those undergoing maintenance hemodialysis or peritoneal dialysis.[2] Patients receiving chronic ambulatory peritoneal dialysis absorb significant amounts of glucose from the dialysate and excess weight gain is a potential problem.[5] Lower energy intakes are required for these patients, for the obese, and for those with hypertriglyceridemia.

Carbohydrates are the main source of calories and should be ingested simultaneously with the protein so that the protein will not be utilized for energy. High-carbohydrate supplements that are protein free and low in electrolytes can greatly increase caloric intake if accepted by the patient.* In addition, high-calorie supplements containing the essential amino acids plus histidine are available.†

---

* Controlyte (Sandox Nutritionals, Minneapolis, Minn.); Moducal (Mead Johnson and Company, Evansville, Ind.); Polycose (Ross Laboratories, Columbus, Ohio); Pro-Mix Carbohydrate Supplement (Navaco Laboratories, Phoenix, Arizona); Sumacal (Chesebrough-Pond's, Inc., N.Y.).
† Amin-aid (McGaw Laboratories, Santa Ana, Calif.); Travasorb Renal (Travenol Laboratories, Inc., Deerfield, Ill.).

Protein. The optimal level of protein intake in advanced renal failure is not known. Some recommend 0.6 g protein per kg of body weight on the basis that this level is associated with improved nitrogen balance and a greater sense of well-being in nondialyzed uremic patients. More restricted intakes may induce wasting.[1] Use of a low-protein diet (less than 25 g) plus essential amino acids and ketoacids is associated with improved nitrogen utilization in renal failure.[6] Hemodialysis patients need 1.0 g protein per kg body weight daily to compensate for losses of amino acids in the dialysate. Some recommend 1.2 g protein per kg with additional supplements during complications such as bleeding or infection; or 1.0 g protein per kg plus 0.2 g per kg of high biologic value protein or essential amino acids per dialysis.[1,7] In intermittent or chronic ambulatory peritoneal dialysis greater protein losses into the dialysate increase the protein requirement to 1.2 to 1.5 g per kg.[8,9] Children on dialysis need 1.5 to 2.0 g high biologic value protein per kg per day.[10] Generally, the aim is to provide about half of the protein allowance as high biologic value protein.

Semisynthetic diets low in protein (19 to 23 g per liter) and electrolytes are available for use in renal disease.* These supply protein in the form of essential amino acids, carbohydrate as glucose oligosaccharides or sucrose, and fat as soybean, MCT, or sunflower oil. Modular feedings can also be used to meet individual requirements for patients in whom oral intake from conventional foods is unsatisfactory.

Carbohydrate and Fat. Type IV hyperlipoproteinemia is common in patients with chronic renal disease. Elevated serum triglycerides can be lowered by controlling carbohydrate intake, restriction of dietary cholesterol, and increasing the intake of polyunsaturated fat. (See Chapter 38).

Potassium. Excess or deficiency of potassium is detrimental to the patient, but in chronic renal failure hyperkalemia is the rule. The potassium allowance is individualized in accordance with the patient's blood chemistries, urinary output, and the amount of potassium in the dialysate. For nondialyzed patients, potassium intake is generally limited to 1,500 to 2,000 mg, depending somewhat on the protein allowance. The upper limit permitted for hemodialysis patients is 2,700 mg, or 70 mEq. In peritoneal dialysis, 75 to 90 mEq or 3.0 to 3.5 g is used.[1] Foods high in animal pro-

---

* Amin-aid (McGaw Laboratories, Santa Ana, Calif.); Travasorb Renal (Travenol Laboratories, Inc., Deerfield, Ill.).

tein are usually high in potassium and many fruits and vegetables must be sharply limited or excluded from the diet because of their high potassium content. Kayexalate,† a potassium-binding agent, is often prescribed in addition to dietary potassium restriction. Potassium restriction is not needed for patients on chronic ambulatory peritoneal dialysis.

Sodium. Dietary sodium intake depends on amounts in serum and urine. Restriction is often needed because of edema, hypertension, and threat of congestive heart failure. Nondialyzed patients who are hypertensive may be permitted less than 1 gm sodium, 40 mEq, daily; those who are depleted of sodium need to increase their intake to about 2 gm daily (90 mEq). Patients on hemodialysis are usually permitted intakes of 1.0 to 1.5 g (43 to 65 mEq), whereas those on peritoneal dialysis receive 2 to 3 g (85 to 130 mEq).[1] The sodium allowance in children is 50 mg per kilogram per day.[10] Patients on chronic ambulatory peritoneal dialysis generally do not need to restrict sodium as sodium balance and blood pressure control are improved. On the contrary, the sodium intake may need to be increased if there is hypotension.

Phosphorus. Serum levels of phosphorus gradually increase in the uremic patient, thus contributing to the acidosis as well as to metastatic calcification. Restriction of dietary phosphorus to 600 to 1,200 mg per day is made in order to control serum levels. Dairy products are restricted because of their high phosphorus content, thereby lowering the calcium content of the diet. Aluminum hydroxide gel is often prescribed to bind some of the phosphate in the intestinal tract, thereby reducing the absorption. Concern over use of this drug has arisen because aluminum is absorbed and is believed to contribute to dialysis dementia, a lethal degeneration of the central nervous system. Control of serum phosphorus levels is greatly improved in chronic ambulatory peritoneal dialysis; thus, phosphorus restriction is not used, although foods excessively high in phosphorus are limited in order to keep phosphorus intake below 1,200 mg per day.[5]

Calcium. The hypocalcemia seen in renal failure is often made worse by the use of diets restricted in protein and phosphorus, as such diets tend to be low in calcium as well. The serum calcium level should be monitored closely, and supplements should be given once the serum phosphorus levels return to normal.

† Kayexalate (Winthrop Laboratories, New York, N.Y.).

Patients with chronic uremia require about 1.2 to 1.6 g per day, those on maintenance dialysis, 1.0 g per day. Although the specific level required by patients on CAPD has not been determined, supplementation is needed.[5]

Trace Minerals. Diet alone cannot meet the iron and trace mineral requirements; supplements should be prescribed. Decreased taste acuity (hypogeusia) is common in chronic renal failure. Zinc supplements have been reported to improve the sense of taste in some patients but not in others. Plasma zinc levels do not seem to correlate with the taste deficit.[11] More research is needed before conclusions regarding the therapeutic effectiveness of zinc supplements can be made.

Vitamins. Losses of ascorbic acid and many of the B vitamins occur during dialysis. In addition, intake of these vitamins is likely to be low because raw fruits and vegetables are restricted and because foods may be cooked in large volumes of water to reduce the potassium content. Folic acid and pyridoxine requirements may be increased because of antagonistic effects of drug therapy. Impaired vitamin D metabolism occurs because the nonfunctioning kidney cannot convert the vitamin into its active form. Supplements of all these vitamins are needed.

Fluids. Intake of fluids needs to be monitored closely in chronic renal failure. If there is not hypertension or edema, the daily allowance is usually 500 ml over the urinary output. From 1.5 to 3 liters is permitted. If anuria or oliguria is present, fluid is restricted to less than 1.5 liters.[1] Weight gain of about 1 pound per day for patients on dialysis is permitted. Patients on CAPD do not need to restrict fluid intake because they can control the amount of fluid removed by adjusting the quantity of hypertonic glucose solution used in the dialysate.[5]

Controlled Protein, Sodium, Potassium, and Phosphorus Diet

Food Lists A number of dietary plans have been described for the control of protein, potassium, and sodium. Each of these plans is based on food groupings in which the foods within a given list are of approximately the same protein, potassium, and sodium value. Food choices for daily menus can therefore be made from a given group in the amounts specified. Generally speaking, the broad food groupings used in the various plans are similar, but they differ in the

Table 40-1. Protein, Sodium, Potassium, and Phosphorus Values for Food Lists

Food List	Household Measure	Weight (g)	Protein (g)	Sodium* (mg)	Potassium (mg)	Phosphorus (mg)
Milk	1 cup	240	8	120	350	245
Meat or substitute	1 ounce	30	7	25	100	65
Vegetables						
Group I	½ cup	100	1	5–10	110–190	15–20
Group II	½ cup	100	2	2–10	120–185	30–35
Group III	½ cup	100	3	15	175	50
Fruits						
Group I	½ cup	100	trace	1–3	100–185	10–15
Group II	½ cup	100	1	2	115–210	15–20
Bread or substitute	Varies	Varies	2		30	30
Fats	Varies	Varies	—	—	—	—

* Except for milk, the values listed for sodium are those that apply when no salt is used in processing or preparation of the food. Also, certain high-sodium items in the meat and vegetable lists would be omitted for diets restricted in sodium.

specific foods included and the portion sizes, depending on the criteria used in setting them up. For example, oranges are relatively high in potassium and are omitted from some lists; they are included in other lists in controlled amounts because of their popular appeal, their relatively low cost, and their content of ascorbic acid. Potatoes are excluded in some lists but included in others, provided that they are prepared by methods to minimize their potassium content. When the directions for the use of any of these plans are explicitly followed any one of them will lead to satisfactory results.

Dietitians, nurses, and physicians must be aware of the many factors that modify the sodium and potassium content of foods. Actual diet contents may be higher or lower than published values. The methods of food preparation significantly modify the electrolyte levels. Those factors that enter into the sodium content of foods have been discussed in Chapter 39.

With respect to potassium, considerable leaching out occurs when foods are cooked in large volumes of water. The amount lost to the water is greater if food is cut into small pieces.

One dietary plan for these controlled diets is described in detail in the pages that follow. Table 40-1 lists the composition of the food groups that follow. Table 40-2 indicates the food allowances for four levels of protein. Each of these plans must be individualized according to the patient's caloric requirement, the nutritional status, and the level of biochemical control.

The 20- and 40-g-protein diets are used only for patients whose renal function has deteriorated so much that they are no longer able to avoid the gastrointestinal and other symptoms of renal failure, and who are not being dialyzed. These diets should be supplemented with B-complex vitamins, calcium, iron, vitamin D, and trace minerals.

Table 40-2. Food Selection for Controlled Protein, Sodium, Potassium, and Phosphorus Diets

Food List	Measure	Protein			
		20 g	40 g	60 g	70 g
Milk, whole or skim	1 cup	¾	1	1	1
Meat or substitute	1 ounce	1	3	5	6
Vegetable, Group I	½ cup	2	2	2	3
Fruit, Group I	½ cup	3	3	3	3
Group II	½ cup	—	—	—	1
Bread or substitute	Exchange	1	3	5	6
Low-protein bread	Slice	5	—	—	—
Low-protein beverage	1 cup	1	1	1	1
Low-protein cookies	Each	2	2	2	2
Fat	Exchange	Ad lib	Ad lib	Ad lib	Ad lib
Jelly, sweets	Varies	Ad lib	Ad lib	Ad lib	Ad lib

Food Lists for Controlled Protein, Sodium, Potassium, and Phosphorus Diets*

Foods Allowed

LIST 1. MILK

1 cup equals 8 g protein, 350 mg potassium, 245 mg phosphorus

Evaporated milk, reconstituted
Nonfat dry milk, reconstituted
Skim milk
Whole milk
Yogurt

LIST 2. MEAT OR SUBSTITUTE

1 ounce cooked equals 7 g protein, 100 mg potassium, 65 mg phosphorus

Beef, chicken, duck, lamb, liver, pork, tongue (unsalted), turkey, veal

Cod, flatfish (flounder and sole), kingfish (whiting), haddock, perch; canned salmon and tuna (omit on sodium-restricted diet)

Clams, crab, lobster, oysters, scallops, shrimp (all omitted on sodium-restricted diet)

Egg (1 egg equals 7 g protein, 60 mg potassium, 90 mg phosphorus)

Cheese (1 ounce equals 7 g protein, 25 mg potassium, 280 mg phosphorus), cheddar, cottage, American, Swiss (Omit on sodium-restricted diets.)

LIST 3. VEGETABLES

Group I

1 g protein, 110 mg potassium, 15 mg phosphorus per serving

½ cup servings of raw cabbage, cucumber, lettuce, onion, tomato

Group IA

1 g protein, 125 mg potassium, 25 mg phosphorus per serving

½ cup servings of canned green or wax beans, carrots (+), spinach (+), fresh cooked cabbage, eggplant, mustard greens, onion, summer squash

Group IB
The following may be used for diets with liberal potassium allowance:

1 g protein, 190 mg potassium, 20 mg phosphorus per serving

½ cup servings of canned beets (+), turnips (+), frozen summer squash, winter squash

Foods to Avoid

Commercial foods made of milk:
    Chocolate milk
    Condensed milk
    Ice cream
    Malted milk
    Milkshake
    Milk mixes
    Sherbet

Brains, kidneys
Canned, salted, or smoked meats as: bacon, bologna, chipped beef, corned beef, frankfurters, ham, kosher meats, luncheon meats, salt pork, sausage, smoked tongue
Frozen fish fillets
Canned, salted, or smoked fish: anchovies, caviar, cod (dried and salted), herring, halibut, sardines, salmon, tuna

All items marked (+) if diet is sodium restricted
Artichokes
Beans, baked
Beans, dried
Beans, lima
Beet greens
Broccoli, fresh
Brussels sprouts
Carrot, raw
Celery, raw
Chard
Endive, raw
Parsnips
Peas
Potato in skin, or frozen
Sauerkraut
Spinach, fresh or frozen
Squash, baked winter

Foods Allowed

Group II

2 g protein, 120 mg potassium, 30 mg phosphorus per serving

½ cup servings of canned asparagus, fresh or frozen green or wax beans, okra

Group IIA

The following may be used for diets with liberal potassium allowance:

2 g protein, 185 mg potassium, 35 mg phosphorus per serving

½ cup servings of fresh or frozen cauliflower; cooked dandelion greens (+); potato, boiled (pared before cooking) or mashed

Group III

3 g protein, 175 mg potassium, 50 mg phosphorus per serving

½ cup servings of kale (+), frozen asparagus, broccoli, collards (+), mixed vegetables (+), whole kernel corn

List 4. Fruits

Group I

Less than 0.5 g protein, 100 mg potassium, 10 mg phosphorus per serving

Apple, raw, 1 small

Grapes, European, 12

½ cup servings of canned applesauce, pears, pineapple, watermelon (diced)

½ cup of these juices: apple, grape, peach nectar, pear nectar, orange-apricot, pineapple-grapefruit, pineapple-orange

Group IA

The following may be used for diets with liberal potassium allowance:

Less than 0.5 g protein, 185 mg potassium, 15 mg phosphorus per serving

½ cup servings of apricot nectar, pineapple juice, canned fruit cocktail, peaches, purple plums

Group II

1 g protein, 115 mg potassium, 15 mg phosphorus per serving

Pear, raw, 1 small

Tangerine, 1 small

½ cup servings of fresh or frozen blackberries, blueberries, boysenberries, canned cherries, figs, canned or fresh grapefruit, frozen red raspberries

Group II A

The following may be used for diets with liberal potassium allowance:

1 g protein, 210 mg potassium, 20 mg phosphorus per serving

Orange, 1 small

Peach, raw, 1 small

Plums, fresh, 2 medium

Strawberries, fresh, ⅔ cup

½ cup servings of cantaloupe, honeydew, frozen melon balls, fresh or frozen rhubarb

Foods to Avoid

All dried and frozen fruits with sodium sulfite added

Apricots, fresh

Avocado

Bananas

Glazed fruits

Maraschino cherries

Nectarines

Prunes

Raisins

Foods Allowed

½ cup of these juices: grapefruit, grapefruit-orange, orange, tomato

LIST 5. BREADS AND SUBSTITUTES

2 g protein, 30 mg potassium, 30 mg phosphorus per serving

Bread, 1 slice
Cereals, dry, 1 cup
  Cornflakes, Puffed Rice, Puffed Wheat, Shredded Wheat
Cereals, cooked, ½ cup
  cornmeal, farina, oatmeal, rice, rolled wheat
Crackers, soda, 3 squares
Flour, 2 tablespoons
Grits, 1 cup
Macaroni, noodles, or spaghetti, ¼ cup
Rice, ½ cup

LIST 6. FATS

Negligible protein, potassium, and phosphorus content

Butter
Cream, light or heavy (1 ounce contains 35 mg potassium, 20 mg phosphorus)
Fat or cooking oil
Margarine
Salad dressings: French or mayonnaise

Miscellaneous Foods

Cornstarch
Flavoring extracts (see list, page 552)
Ginger ale
Hard candies
Herbs (see list, page 552)
Honey
Jam or jelly
Jellybeans
Rice starch
Spices (see list, page 552)
Sugar, white, confectioners'
Syrup
Tapioca, granulated
Vinegar
Wheat starch

Foods to Avoid

Avoid tomato juice if diet is sodium restricted

Yeast breads or rolls or melba toast made with salt or from commercial mixes
Quick breads made with baking powder, baking soda, or salt, or made from commercial mixes
Commercial baked products
Dry cereals except as listed
Self-rising cornmeal
Graham or other crackers except low-sodium dietetic
Self-rising flour
Salted popcorn
Potato chips
Pretzels
Waffles containing salt, baking powder, baking soda, or egg white

Salted fats on sodium-restricted diets
Avocado
Bacon, bacon fat
Olives
Nuts
Salt pork

Antacids, laxatives
Bouillon, broth
Canned, dried, frozen soups
Chocolate
Cocoa, instant cocoa mixes
Coconut
Consommé
Fruit-flavored powders and prepared beverage mixes
Fountain beverages
Commercial candies except as listed
Commercial gelatin desserts
Regular baking powder and soda
Rennet tablets
Molasses
Pudding mixes
Peanut butter
Most carbonated beverages

Flavoring Aids to Avoid

Catsup, celery leves, celery salt, chili sauce, garlic salt, prepared horseradish, meat extracts, meat sauces, meat tenderizers, monosodium glutamate, prepared mustard, onion salt, pickles, relishes, salt, and salt substitutes, soy sauce, Worcestershire sauce

---

* Adapted from American Dietetic Association, *Handbook of Clinical Dietetics.* Yale University Press, New Haven, Conn., 1981.

DIETARY COUNSELING

Importance of Adequate Guidance Dietary treatment in renal failure, with or without dialysis, is an integral part of therapy. Although the dietary modification cannot lead to improvement in kidney function, it can do much toward alleviation of uncomfortable symptoms that interfere with adequate food intake. The rigid controls required make this diet as complex as any that can be prescribed. Particularly at 20- and 40-g-protein levels, the diet lacks much in palatability, especially if sodium restriction is also severe, and the level of motivation of the patient and those who care for him or her must be high.

Many hours of dietary instruction are required for the patient and for those who will prepare the food at home. The counseling started in the hospital must be continued either in the outpatient clinic or by home visitation.

What the Patient Needs to Know Each patient needs to know why the diet is important, and what risks will be encountered if he or she fails to follow the diet. The patient must understand that it is important to include the exact amounts of high-quality protein foods that have been prescribed. Likewise he or she needs to know the importance of eating sufficient quantities of low-protein low-electrolyte foods so that body weight is maintained and tissue catabolism does not take place.

High-calorie foods such as sugars, jams, honey, hard candies, butter, or margarine should be used. Patients must be reminded frequently to make liberal use of these items. Growth failure is a common problem in children on dialysis whose calorie intake in inadequate.

The patient (or person preparing food for the patient) must be thoroughly familiar with the food lists and the amounts of foods that may be used from each. Some practice in planning the daily meals from these lists is essential. If special products such as wheat starch are needed, the patient must be told where they can be purchased and how much they will cost. Recipes for the use of these special products are needed together with precautions to take in food preparation.

Food Preparation The extraction of gluten from wheat flour yields a low-protein wheat starch that is also practically electrolyte free. With sodium and potassium restriction yeast must be used as a leavening agent; regular leavening agents are too high in sodium, and low-sodium leavening agents are too high in potassium. Breads and other products made from wheat starch do not have the same texture as those made from wheat flour because of the absence of the elastic gluten. Some patients find the bread more acceptable when toasted, served with butter and jelly or jam, or prepared as cinnamon toast or French toast.

If potatoes are allowed in the diet, they should be cut into small pieces and boiled in a large volume of water. Following this they may be pan fried with some of the fat or mashed with part of the milk and fat allowance. Meats that are simmered in a large volume of water also lose some of their potassium to the cooking liquid, but these cooking procedures also result in greater losses of the water-soluble vitamins and of some other mineral elements.

Canned fruits are used, for the most part, instead of fresh raw fruits. Since part of the potassium has leached out into the syrup, only the solid fruit should be used.

Salt substitutes containing potassium are prohibited, since they contain as much as 60 mEq, or about 2,350 mg, per teaspoon.[12]

Diet Following Renal Transplantation Following successful renal transplantation most of the previous dietary restrictions are no longer needed. Mild sodium restriction (see Chapter 39) is usually necessary because prolonged administration of steroids favors fluid retention. Potassium supplements are recommended in order to overcome steroid-induced potassium excretion. Other side effects of long-term immunosuppressive therapy such as obesity, diabetes mellitus, and atherosclerosis may make further dietary modifications necessary.

Hypokalemia

Occurrence Although the emphasis in the preceding discussion has been upon the problems of elevated levels of blood potassium, there are renal and extrarenal circumstances in which the plasma or serum level of potassium is below 3.3 mEq per liter. One situation in which this occurs is by dilution of the extracellular fluid volume. This results when the fluid intake exceeds the ability of the kidney to excrete it as in olioguria and anuria. The total amount of the ion in the extracellular fluid remains the same, but the concentration is lowered because of the expanded volume.

In the diuretic stage of nephritis, the kidneys do not conserve potassium as effectively as normal, and potassium depletion occurs, especially if the intake is low because of a poor appetite. Adrenocortical steroids and many diuretics are likely to accentuate the renal losses of potassium.

Hypokalemia also occurs when there is rapid uptake of potassium by the cells. Growth, cellular repair, cellular dehydration, glycogen formation, and administration of glucose and insulin in diabetic acidosis promote entrance of potassium into the cell. In dehydration and in the correction of diabetic acidosis emergency measures are required to replace the extracellular potassium.

Excessive losses of potassium occur with vomiting, diarrhea, and gastrointestinal drainage. Unless these losses are replaced the plasma levels are often lowered to dangerous levels.

Treatment If hypokalemia is severe, the correction will require the parenteral administration of potassium-containing fluids. This is followed by therapy with potassium-containing syrups and emphasis on foods that are rich in potassium. When the appetite is good, any varied diet will supply a considerable amount of potassium. A few foods that are especially good sources of potassium include orange juice, tomato juice, milk, baked potato, and banana. Most salt substitutes contain substantial amounts of potassium (10 to 12 mEq per g) and can increase the potassium intake considerably.[12]

Urinary Calculi

Nature of Calculi Urinary CALCULI (kidney stones) may be found in the kidney, ureter, bladder, or urethra. They consist of an organic matrix with interspersed crystals and vary in size from fine gravel to large stones.

About 90 percent of all stones contain calcium as the chief cation. More than half the stones are mixtures of calcium oxalate and magnesium ammonium phosphate. Uric acid stones account for about 10 percent of renal stones in the United States. Xanthine stones are extremely rare. Cystine stones are unique in that they are often pure and are a hereditary defect.

Incidence and Etiology The incidence of renal calculi in the United States is unknown. In Thailand, India, and Turkey (known as stone belts) bladder stones are a common occurrence in children, especially small boys. Most of these are urate and oxalate stones and their cause is unknown. The incidence of bladder stones in adults is high in Syria, Bulgaria, India, China, Madagascar, and Turkey, but low in Africa. The reasons for these geographic variations are not known.

Renal calculi are more prevalent in sedentary people than in those who are active. No dietary relationship has been established, but kidney dehydration may be a factor and more fluid intake and exercise are urged as prophylaxis.

The formation of stones is more probable in the presence of urinary tract infections, during periods of high urinary excretion of calcium, in certain gastrointestinal disorders, following intestinal bypass, surgery, and in disorders of cystine, oxalate, or uric acid metabolism. High urinary excretion of calcium occurs in hyperparathyroidism, following overdosage with vitamin D, in long periods of immobilization, in osteoporosis, or following excessive ingestion of calcium and of absorbable alkalies. Excessive intakes of ascorbic acid may induce formation of calcium oxalate stones in susceptible individuals. In disorders involving fat malabsorption and especially after intestinal bypass surgery, an excess of fatty acids in the intestinal lumen binds available calcium, thereby decreasing the calcium available to bind oxalate. Increased absorption of oxalate from the bowel and subsequent hyperoxaluria may contribute to stone formation.

Rationale of Treatment When the cause of urinary calculi is known, the physician can effectively direct treatment toward the correction of the disorder. However, in a large percentage of urinary calculi, the cause is not known or the disorder is not easily corrected.

A liberal fluid intake and drug therapy are the primary means of treatment. A liberal fluid intake is essential—3,000 ml or more daily—to prevent the production of a urine at a concentration where the salts precipitate out. The patient should be impressed with the importance of taking fluids throughout the day, so that the urine dilution is maintained.

Calcium Oxalate Stones. These may be due to (1) idiopathic hypercalciuria related to increased intestinal absorption of calcium or to defective reabsorption of calcium in the renal tubule; (2) hyperuricosuria; or (3) intestinal hyperoxaluria. In the absorptive type of hypercalciuria, excessive intestinal calcium absorption results in high normal serum calcium levels, in turn suppressing parathyroid hormone and increasing the filtered load of calcium presented to the kidney. With suppression of parathyroid hormone, renal tubular reabsorption of calcium is lowered; as the filtered load increases, urinary calcium excretion is enhanced. In the renal type, defective tubular calcium reabsorption produces a mild hypocalcemia and stimulates parathyroid hormone secretion. An increase in 1,25-dihydroxycholecalciferol production by the kidney then leads to increased intestinal calcium absorption and subsequent hypercalciuria. The aims of therapy are to decrease calcium absorption from the intestine and to promote the reabsorption of calcium from the renal tubule.[13] In the renal type of hypercalciuria, thiazide diuretics are used to stimulate urinary calcium reabsorption. In the absorptive type, a low-calcium diet is used along with an ion-exchange resin that binds calcium in the intestine and prevents its absorption.[14]

In some persons calcium oxalate stone formation occurs as a result of increased uric acid excretion (HYPERURICOSURIA). This is usually attributed to excessive dietary purine intake. Mechanisms proposed to explain stone formation in these persons are that uric acid or monosodium urate crystals provide a nidus for growth of calcium oxalate crystals or that uric acid interferes with an inhibitor of crystal growth.[13] Allopurinol is used to decrease the formation of uric acid from precursors.

Intestinal hyperoxaluria occurring after small bowel resection or bypass can also result in calcium oxalate stone formation. Such patients are treated with cholestyramine, which adsorbs oxalate; the diet is modified as well, as discussed in the next section.[14]

Uric Acid Stones. The aim of treatment in uric acid stones is to raise the urinary pH. Sodium bicarbonate is used, and a high fluid intake is encouraged in order to maintain a dilute urine.

Cystine Stones. These are usually due to congenital cystinuria. Sodium bicarbonate is used to maintain an alkaline urine since the stones form in acid urine. Alternatively, penicillamine, which forms a complex with cystine and reduces its excretion in the urine, is used. A liberal fluid intake is essential.

Modification of the Diet No diet of itself is effective in bringing about solution of stones already formed. However, for the predisposed individual it is thought that diet may be of some value in retarding the growth of stones or preventing their recurrence, although the effectiveness of such prophylaxis has not been fully established.

Calcium Restriction. In idiopathic hypercalciuria some investigators recommend a liberal fluid intake and reduction of calcium intake to 600 mg or less per day in order to reduce hypercalciuria and to prevent calcium oxalate stone formation.[15] (See Table 40-3.) Others prefer to lower the intake of dairy products, limit the intake of meats to 8 ounces or less per day and to encourage the use of foods high in fiber to bind excess intestinal calcium.[13]

Oxalate Restriction. For calcium stones induced by intestinal hyperoxaluria, a low oxalate diet is used in combination with calcium supplements (1 g daily) and a fat-restricted diet (less than 50 g).[14] Oxalate rich foods include green and wax beans, beets and

Table 40-3. Calcium-Restricted Diet

Include These Foods Daily*		Protein (g)	Fat (g)	Carbohydrate (g)	Calcium (mg)
Milk	1 cup	8	10	12	290
Egg	1 whole	7	5	—	25
Meat, fish, poultry	6 ounces	42	30	—	20
Vegetables					
Potato	1 small	2	—	15	15
Leafy or yellow	½ cup	2	—	5	25
Other	½ cup	2	—	5	25
Fruits					
Citrus	½ cup	—	—	10	30
Other	2 servings	—	—	20	25
Cereal, refined, without added calcium	2 servings	4	—	30	5
Bread, refined, without added calcium	6 slices	12	—	90	20
Fats	2 tablespoons	—	30	—	—
Sugars, sweets	2 tablespoons	—	—	30	—
		79	75	217	480

* Protein, fat, and carbohydrate values on the basis of meal exchange lists, Table A-4. Calcium values have been rounded off to the nearest 5 mg. Values for vegetables, fruits, cereals, and breads are averages of those permitted. Individual selections vary somewhat from these averages.

beet greens, chard, endive, okra, spinach, sweet potatoes; currants, figs, gooseberries, Concord grapes, plums, rhubarb, raspberries; almonds, cashew nuts; chocolate, cocoa, tea.

Fiber. Rao and co-workers consider a reduction in the nutrient density of the diet to be important in the management of patients with idiopathic stone formation.[16] Some 340 patients, of whom 40 percent had increased excretion of calcium, oxalate, or uric acid,

were studied. Significant reduction in the excretion of these occurred when the diet was high in fiber and low in sugar and other refined carbohydrates, and protein.

Nutritional Effects of Drug Therapy. All the drugs used in the management of renal stones have potential adverse effects on nutritional status. Allopurinol was discussed in Chapter 37, cholestyramine in Chapter 38, and thiazides in Chapter 39.

Calcium-Restricted Diet

Characteristics and General Rules
The diet provides a maintenance level of calcium. Milk constitutes the main source of calcium in the diet. (See Table 40-3.)
When further restriction of calcium is desired, the milk and egg may be eliminated. The calcium level is then reduced to 165 mg and the protein level to 64 g.

Foods Allowed
Beverages—Milk in allowed amounts; coffee, tea

Breads—French or Italian without added milk; pretzels; saltines, matzoh; water rolls

Cereals—cornflakes, corn grits, farina, rice, rice flakes, Puffed Rice; macaroni, noodles, spaghetti; cornmeal, cornstarch, tapioca, white flour

Cheese—½ ounce cheddar or Swiss cheese may be used instead of ½ cup milk
Desserts—angel cake, white sugar cookies, gelatin, fruit pies, fruit tapioca, fruit whip, pudding with allowed milk and egg, shortbread, water ices

Eggs—1 whole; whites as desired
Fats—butter, cooking oils and fats, lard, margarine, French dressing
Fruits—all, but restricting dried fruits to dates (3), prunes (2), raisins (1 tbsp.)
Meats—beef, ham, lamb, pork, veal; chicken, duck, turkey; bluefish, cod, haddock, halibut, scallops, shad, swordfish, tuna
Milk—1 cup daily
Soups—broth of allowed meats; consommé; cream soups using allowed milk
Sweets—sugar, syrup, jam, jelly, preserves, hard candy, marshmallows, mints without chocolate
Vegetables—artichokes, asparagus, beans—green or wax, brussels sprouts, cabbage, carrots, cauliflower, corn, cucumber, eggplant, escarole, lettuce, onions, peppers, potatoes—white and sweet, pumpkin, radishes, romaine, squash, tomatoes, turnips
Miscellaneous—pickles, mustard, salt, spices

Foods to Avoid
Beverages—chocolate; cocoa; fountain beverages; proprietary beverages containing milk powder
Breads—biscuits; breads: brown, corn, cracked wheat, raisin, rye, white with nonfat dry milk, whole wheat; rye wafers; muffins; pancakes; waffles
Cereals—bran, bran flakes, corn and soy grits, oatmeal, wheat flakes, wheat germ, Puffed Wheat, Shredded Wheat; rye flour, soybean flour, self-rising flour, whole wheat flour

Desserts—cakes and cake mixes, custard, doughnuts, ice cream, Junket, pies with cream filling or milk and eggs, milk puddings—except when daily allowance is used

Fats—mayonnaise, sweet and sour cream

Meats—clams, crab, herring, lobster, mackerel, oyster, fish roe, salmon, sardines, shrimp; brains, heart, kidney, liver, sweetbreads

Soups—cream in excess of milk allowance; bean, lentil, split pea
Sweets—caramels, fudge, milk chocolate, molasses, dark brown sugar
Vegetables—dry beans; kidney, lima, navy, pea, soybean; beet greens, broccoli, chard, collards, chickpeas, dandelion greens, kale, okra, parsnips, peas—fresh and dried, rutabagas, soybeans, soybean sprouts, spinach, turnip greens, watercress
Miscellaneous—chocolate, cocoa, nuts, olives, brewer's yeast

Sample Menu

BREAKFAST
Fresh raspberries
Cornflakes
Milk— ½ cup
Soft-cooked egg
Toasted Italian bread
Butter or margarine
Apple jelly
Coffee

LUNCHEON OR SUPPER
Cold sliced turkey
Potato salad (potato, diced cucumber, minced green pepper and onion, French dressing) on lettuce; tomato wedges
Italian bread
Butter or margarine
Angel cake with fresh strawberries
Milk— ½ cup only

DINNER
Roast pork
Buttered noodles
Zucchini squash
Hard rolls, made without milk
Butter or margarine
Fruit gelatin
Tea with lemon

CASE STUDY 25

Woman with Chronic Renal Failure (Chinese)

Mrs. M, age 40, is a thin Chinese woman who lives with her family in a small four-room apartment in a low-income area of San Francisco. The family group consists of Mr. and Mrs. M, their teenage son and daughter, and Mr. M's mother. Mr. M has a meager income as a cook in a hotel. Mrs. M completed high school, but she has not been able to work because of ill health.

Mrs. M has a history of recurrent glomerulonephritis and secondary hypertension. She has been hospitalized on two occasions for chronic renal failure. A diet controlled in protein, sodium, and potassium was prescribed. The order specified 25 g protein, 1.5 g sodium, and 1.5 g potassium. Mrs. M finds the diet hard to accept, especially the sodium restriction.

Because of economic difficulties Mrs. M did not seek further medical help in spite of continued symptoms. She had waited several months to see if her symptoms of severe headache, dyspnea, pitting edema in her hands and legs, failing vision, poor appetite, nausea and vomiting, abdominal pain, and fatigue would let up on their own. At home she often used home remedies to alleviate her symptoms, such as sodium bicarbonate for indigestion. Recently, her husband had noticed that she was confused and insisted that she see a physician.

Mrs. M was admitted to the University Hospital because of her need for kidney dialysis. Admitting diagnoses included azotemia, congestive heart failure, metabolic acidosis, normocytic normochromic anemia, and hypertension. Evidence of peripheral neuropathy and osteomalacia was also found. On admission Mrs. M weighed 44 kg (97 lb); height, 160 cm (63 in.).

She complained of insomnia, muscle cramping and twitching, pruritus, and numbness and tingling in her hands and feet. Laboratory findings included total protein, 5.2 g per dl; serum albumin, 3.0 g per dl; serum transferrin, 155 mg per dl; serum urea nitrogen, 130 mg per dl; serum creatinine, 14 mg per dl; serum potassium, 5.5 mEq per liter; calcium, 6 mg per dl; hematocrit, 18 percent; and total iron-binding capacity, 200 μg per dl. Triceps skinfold was 8 mm; arm muscle circumference, 18 cm.

A team consisting of a physician, nurse, dietitian, and social worker planned Mrs. M's medical management. Peritoneal dialysis, diet, and medications were used to treat the renal failure. The medications included oral supplements of folacin, vitamin D, and calcium; methyldopa (Aldomet); and furosemide (Lasix). She was placed on docusate sodium (Colace) to prevent constipation.

Initially Mrs. M was placed on a controlled diet consisting of 45 g protein, 1.5 g sodium, and 1.5 g potassium. Fluids were restricted to 600 ml per day. Several factors, including nausea and vomiting, bleeding gums, a metallic taste, and ammonia odor to her breath, affected her appetite. Even the smell of food provoked nausea at times.

She was thirsty and had a difficult time allocating her fluids throughout the day. After she had been on dialysis for several weeks, Mrs. M's protein allowance was increased to 60 g per day, and fluids were increased to 1 liter per day.

Dialysis alleviated many of Mrs. M's symptoms. It was determined that she would need to be maintained on dialysis, and plans were made to teach Mr. and Mrs. M how to do home chronic ambulatory peritoneal dialysis. Instruction regarding the principles of CAPD and the dialysis procedure itself was begun. Mr. and Mrs. M were counseled regarding diet and medications. The social worker advised Mr. and Mrs. M that federal funds are available to help defray the costs of chronic renal disease; she will follow through to see that this assistance is provided to them. Mr. M is very nervous and overwhelmed by his wife's illness, but he has consented to learn how to do the dialysis procedure.

Pathophysiologic Correlations

1. List some etiologic factors in the development of chronic renal failure. Which of these were probably involved in Mrs. M's case?
2. In addition to the symptoms Mrs. M showed, what others are characteristic of chronic renal failure?
3. Compare Mrs. M's blood values with normal ranges: SUN: creatinine; hematocrit; potassium; calcium.
4. List two findings in Mrs. M's history that might account for her edema.
5. What alterations in metabolism probably explain Mrs. M's indigestion?
6. Explain the basis for Mrs. M's fatigue and weakness; anemia; bone demineralization.
7. Why is hyperkalemia a dangerous finding in the renal patient?
8. What is the role of the kidneys in hormonal control?
9. What are the nutritional implications related to the hormonal control exercised by the kidney?

Nutritional Assessment

10. For each of the following compare Mrs. M's values with acceptable standards: total protein; serum albumin; serum transferrin; total iron-binding capacity; hematocrit; triceps skinfold; midarm muscle circumference; weight. How would you assess Mrs. M's overall nutritional status?
11. List the goals for nutritional care for Mrs. M.
12. What are the recommended allowances for each of the following for a person of Mrs. M's body build and age: energy; protein; calcium; iron; ascorbic acid; folacin? What changes in these allowances are probably indicated for Mrs. M? Explain your reasons for any suggested changes.
13. Compare Mrs. M's dietary allowances before and after chronic ambulatory peritoneal dialysis: energy; protein; sodium; potassium; fluids. What are the bases for change?
14. How is Mrs. M's phosphorus intake controlled?
15. List the vitamin and mineral supplements that might be ordered for Mrs. M. Explain why each was ordered.
16. List the possible side effects on nutrition of these medications prescribed for Mrs. M: docusate sodium; methyldopa; furosemide.
17. Use the Daily Food Guide to list foods that are typical of the Chinese dietary pattern.

Planning the Diet

18. List the principles of dietary management for Mrs. M.
19. Indicate some of the psychosocial factors to be considered in planning Mrs. M's diet.
20. What concerns do you need to consider in planning an appropriate calorie intake for Mrs. M?
21. What other factors should be considered for patients on CAPD?

Dietary Counseling

22. Mrs. M is to return to the outpatient clinic once a month for a checkup and for further counseling. Summarize the information that is important for you to obtain at these visits.
23. Which aspects of the diet are likely to be the most difficult for Mrs. M?
24. List several recommendations you would make to overcome these difficulties.

References for the Case Study

BODNAR, D. M.: "Rationale for Nutritional Requirements for Patients on Continuous Ambulatory Peritoneal Dialysis," *J. Am. Diet. Assoc.*, 80:247–9, 1982.

CHAMBERS, J. K.: "Bowel Management in Dialysis Patients," *Am. J. Nurs.*, 83:1051–2, 1983.

MURPHY, L. M., AND COLE, M. J.: "Renal Disease: Nutritional Implications," *Nurs. Clin. North Am.*, 18:57–70, March 1983.

REED, S. B.: "Giving More Than Dialysis," *Nursing '82*, 8:58–63, April 1982.

RODRIGUEZ, D. J., AND HUNTER, V. M.: "Nutrition Intervention in the Treatment of Chronic Renal Failure," *Nurs. Clin. North Am.*, 16:573–85, Sept. 1981.

References

1. Kopple, J. D.: "Nutritional Therapy in Kidney Failure," *Nutr. Rev.*, 39:193–205, 1981.
2. Burton, B. T., and Hirschman, G. H.: "Current Concepts of Nutritional Therapy in Chronic Renal Failure: An Update," *J. Am. Diet. Assoc.*, 82:359–63, 1983.
3. Giordano, C.: "Use of Exogenous and Endogenous Urea for Protein Synthesis in Normal and Uremic Subjects," *J. Lab. Clin. Med.*, 62:231–46, 1963.
4. Giovannetti, S., and Maggiore, Q.: "A Low Nitrogen Diet with Proteins of High Biological Value for Severe Chronic Uremia," *Lancet*, 1:1000–3, 1964.
5. Bodnar, D. M.: "Rationale for Nutritional Requirements for Patients on Continuous Ambulatory Peritoneal Dialysis," *J. Am. Diet. Assoc.*, 80:247–9, 1982.
6. Mitch, W. E., et al.: "Long-Term Effects of a New Ketoacid-Amino Acid Supplement in Patients with Chronic Renal Failure," *Kidney Int.*, 22:48–53, 1982.
7. Kluthe, P., et al.: "Protein Requirements in Maintenance Hemodialysis," *Am. J. Clin. Nutr.*, 31:1812-20, 1978.
8. Blumenkrantz, M. J., et al.: "Nutritional Management of the Adult Patient Undergoing Peritoneal Dialysis," *J. Am. Diet. Assoc.*, 73:251–6, 1978.
9. Blumenkrantz, M. J., et al.: "Metabolic Balance Studies and Dietary Protein Requirements in Patients Undergoing Continuous Ambulatory Peritoneal Dialysis," *Kidney Int.*, 31:849–61, 1982.
10. Holliday, M. A., et al.: "Nutritional Management of Chronic Renal Disease," *Med. Clin. North Am.*, 63: 945–62, 1979.
11. Review: "Decreased Taste Acuity in Chronic Renal Patients," *Nutr. Rev.*, 39:207–9, 1981.
12. Sopko, J.A., and Freeman, R. M.: "Salt Substitutes as a Source of Potassium," *JAMA*, 238:608–10, 1977.
13. Menon, M., and Krishnan, C. S.: "Evaluation and Management of the Patient with Calcium Stone Disease," *Urol. Clin. North Am.*, 10:595–615, 1983.
14. Coe, F. L., and Favus, M. J.: "Treatment of Renal Calculi," *Adv. Intern. Med.*, 26:373–92, 1981.
15. Smith, L. H., et al.: "Nutrition and Urolithiasis," *N. Engl. J. Med.*, 298:87–9, 1978.
16. Rao, P. N., et al.: "Dietary Management of Urinary Risk Factors in Renal Stone Formers," *Br. J. Urol.*, 54:578–83, 1982.

41

Diet in Allergic and Skin Disturbances

Elimination Diets

Food Allergies

More than one in six persons in the United States or some 35 million persons, suffer from some form of allergy. This high incidence of allergic diseases is an important health and economic problem in terms of days lost from work and school. Food allergies account for a relatively small proportion of all allergies, but allergies to major food groups present serious problems in meal planning and in adequate nutrition. Moreover, many people who suffer from nonfood allergies find it difficult to ingest an adequate diet—the individual with severe asthma, for example.

Definition Terms commonly used to describe an adverse reaction to foods include food allergy, hypersensitivity, sensitivity, and intolerance. Strictly speaking, these terms are not synonymous. Food ALLERGY or HYPERSENSITIVITY denotes an adverse immunologic response to a specific substance with characteristic symptoms whenever the food is ingested. Food SENSITIVITY is a slightly broader term applied to conditions in which an abnormal reaction occurs following ingestion of specific foods and in which an immunologic etiology is likely, but not proven. Food INTOLERANCE, on the other hand, does not involve an immunologic mechanism, and may be due to an enzyme deficiency or other factors.[1] In food allergy, symptoms are produced within minutes or a few hours following ingestion of the food and the reaction occurs whenever the food is ingested. In food sensitivity or intolerance symptoms may occur hours or days after ingestion of the food substance, and the condition tends to improve spontaneously or following a period of elimination of the food.

The substance responsible for initiation of the allergic reaction is an ALLERGEN or ANTIGEN. It is usually a protein, but may be a polysaccharide, or a substance that binds to a protein to form a complex which becomes the active allergen. The reaction may be brought about by (1) *ingestion* of food or drugs; (2) *contact* with foods, pesticides, drugs, adhesive, fur, hair, feathers, molds, fungi, and so on; (3) *inhalation* of pollens, dust, molds, fungi, cosmetics, perfumes; and (4) *injection* of vaccines, serums, antibiotics, and hormones.

In most individuals, food antigens are destroyed in the gastrointestinal tract; however, in *atopic* persons, those with a predisposition to allergy, after repeated exposure to the allergen, the antigen is absorbed from the gastrointestinal tract and enters the circulation. In infants and young children food allergy is usually attributed to an immature gastrointestinal tract which permits passage of the antigenically active substance into the circulation.

Immunologic Aspects The body has two mechanisms for coping with the presence of the antigen: (1) HUMORAL IMMUNITY, in which protection is conferred by formation of antibodies specific for certain antigens; and (2) CELL-MEDIATED IMMUNITY, which does not depend on antibody formation. Antibodies are chiefly gamma-globulins, belonging to the group of substances known as immunoglobulins (Ig). Several classes of immunoglobulins are known: IgE, IgA, IgM, IgG, and IgD.

Hypersensitivity Reactions. Four types of hypersensitivity reactions are known. *Type I*, or *immediate*, is IgE mediated; it results from an interaction between antigen and target cells sensitized by IgE, with release of mediators such as histamine from mast cells and basophils. Mediators act on blood vessels, smooth muscle, and mucous glands to produce symptoms that appear within minutes to a few hours following exposure to a small quantity of the allergen, and usually clear up in 24 to 48 hours. IgE-mediated reactions are usually associated with respiratory tract symptoms such as hay fever and asthma due to inhalants. Foods less commonly cause this type of reaction. However, individuals who are highly sensitive to foods, such as eggs or nuts, experience immediate, violent symptoms following ingestion of even small amounts of the food.

Type II, or *cytotoxic*, involves binding of IgG or IgM to an antigen bound to a cell, activation of complement, and cell lysis. This type of reaction is not due to food hypersensitivity. *Type III*, or *immune-complex disease*, involves the deposition of an antigen–antibody complex in tissues, activation of complement, and destruction of the antigen. Strong evidence linking food hypersensitivity with this type of reaction is lacking. *Type IV*, or *delayed cell-mediated*, is cellular in nature and involves a reaction of sensitized lymphocytes with antigens, release of lymphokines and subsequent lysis of the antigen. The reaction occurs 24 to 72 hours following exposure to the allergen and lasts for several days. This type may be involved in some cases of gastrointestinal food sensitivity or intolerance. The reaction to milk is often delayed. The whole food protein is believed to be the allergen in the immediate type of reaction, and a breakdown product formed during digestion of the food in delayed reactions. The reaction time toward a given substance always remains the same in an individual; that is, if the reaction to eggs is immediate, it will always be so, and not delayed. An individual may have an immediate reaction toward one substance and a delayed response to another.

Etiology Heredity is important in the development of allergies. The incidence is increased in children whose parents have allergies, especially if both parents are affected. The child does not inherit a sensitivity to a specific substance or an identical manifestation of the allergy. The parent may be sensitive to wheat, for example, and the child to pollens.

Any kind of physical or emotional stress increases the severity of allergic reactions. However, stress situations do not cause the allergy. Other factors that may influence the allergic reaction include the frequency of eating the food, the amount eaten, the physical state of the food, and the season.

Food Allergens Any food may produce reactions, but the most frequent offenders are milk, eggs, wheat, citrus fruits, chocolate or cola, legumes, corn, fish, shellfish, and some spices.[2] The increasing incidence of food allergies due to use of soy products and food additives is of some concern.[3]

Foods unlike in flavor and structure but belonging to the same botanic group may result in allergic manifestations. For example, buckwheat is not of the cereal family but in a group that includes rhubarb. The sweet potato is not related to the white potato but is a member of the morning glory family. Spinach, a frequent reactor, is in the same family with beets. The following botanic classification of a few common foods illustrates the relationship of foods that at first appear to be dissimilar.

Cereal—wheat, rye, barley, rice, oats, malt, corn, sorghum, cane sugar
Lily—onion, garlic, asparagus, chives, leeks, shallots
Gourd—squash, pumpkin, cucumber, cantaloupe, watermelon
Cabbage and mustard—turnips, cabbage, collards, cauliflower, broccoli, kale, radish, horseradish, watercress, brussels sprouts

Symptoms of Food Allergies Manifestations of allergy may occur in any part of the body. The tissues of these systems are frequently involved: cutaneous, gastrointestinal, respiratory, and neurologic. The symptoms are consequently varied depending on the parts affected.

1. Skin manifestations may include canker sores, dermatitis, edema, fever blisters, pruritus, and urticaria (hives).
2. Common gastrointestinal manifestations include cheilitis, stomatitis, colic in infants, abdominal distention, constipation, diarrhea, dyspepsia, and nausea and vomiting. The symptoms may be suggestive of appendicitis, colitis, gallbladder disease, or ulcers, and there may be confusion in diagnosis.
3. Respiratory symptoms include allergic rhinitis, asthma, bronchitis, and nasal polyps among others.
4. Neurologic symptoms such as migraine, neuralgias, and the tension-fatigue syndrome are sometimes due to food allergy. The latter syndrome is characterized by anxiety, fatigue, irritability, muscle and joint aching, restlessness, stomach pains, and so on.
5. Miscellaneous symptoms such as anaphylactic reactions, arthralgias, arthritis, and edema have been attributed to food allergy.

Diagnosis of Food Allergies   The procedures used include a complete history, skin testing, possibly other tests, and trials with restricted diets.

History.   A complete history is the single most important diagnostic tool. When a severe reaction occurs immediately, the patient is usually aware of the circumstances leading up to it. However, when reactions are delayed or when allergies are multiple in nature, the elucidation of the offending factors is often exceedingly difficult. The history must include a complete evaluation of the physical status and the conditions and events preceding the attack.

The patient is asked to keep a detailed diary of all foods ingested and of the occurrence of any symptoms. Individual likes and dislikes must be taken into consideration. One patient may like a food well enough to risk an allergic reaction by eating it, while another may claim to be allergic to a food he or she dislikes.

Skin Tests.   Skin tests are sometimes used to confirm presence of allergies but their usefulness in the case of food allergy is limited. Skin tests include (1) *scratch* tests, in which a small amount of solution containing the antigen is placed into a series of scratches made on the skin; (2) *prick* or *puncture* tests, in which the antigen is placed on the skin and a superficial break is then made in the epidermis with a sharp needle; and (3) *intradermal* tests, which involve injection of a small amount of dilute antigen extract beneath the skin. Reactions to skin tests are checked immediately and at specified intervals thereafter, usually 24 to 48 hours. Positive reactions are usually characterized by a small area of circumscribed edema surrounded by erythema at the test site. A positive skin test does not necessarily indicate that the individual is clinically sensitive to the material. It may represent past or potential sensitivity. On the other hand, a negative skin reaction does not necessarily eliminate the possibility of food allergy, for symptoms may be manifested in other tissues. Verification of results from skin tests is made by recurrence of symptoms following ingestion of the food in a symptom-free patient.

Other Tests.   In vitro measurements of specific antibodies are another means of diagnosing allergies. For example, elevated serum IgE levels have been reported in individuals allergic to milk.[4] The radioallergosorbent test (RAST) is used to detect specific IgE antibodies to a variety of antigens and is considered by some to be useful in the diagnosis of IgE-mediated food allergy. However, the test results must be correlated with clinical observations. The RAST test is not considered more sensitive than skin tests and is more expensive.[5] It is useful in cases in which direct testing of foods might risk an anaphylactic reaction.[6] Many other tests have been reported, but are not widely available or are not sufficiently reliable for routine use.

Restricted Diets.   Many variants of restricted diets have been proposed as diagnostic aids. For infants and very young children it is relatively simple to determine whether allergic symptoms are due to foods by allowing only milk and crystalline vitamins. If a food other than milk is responsible, symptoms such as eczema will be relieved in a few days; but if milk or nonfood allergy is responsible, no improvement will occur and further testing will be necessary. An approach used for older children and adults is to restrict the patient to a list of foods to which no skin reactions were shown. The restricted diet may be tested for 1 to 3 weeks, after which new foods are added, one at a time, at 3-day intervals. If symptoms develop following addition of a food, it is eliminated for a time and reintroduced later.

A number of *elimination diets* have been developed, based on the principle that only those foods that are seldom responsible for allergy are included in the trial diet. Many elimination diets are modifications of the regimen advocated by Rowe (see following diets), who recommends its use for a minimum of 3 months in the diagnosis of food allergy.[7]

Rowe's patients are first placed on a cereal-free elimination diet. This diet eliminates all cereal grains, milk, egg, beef, pork (except bacon), fish, and a number of fruits and vegetables. Soybean oil is the only oil permitted; milk-free margarine made from soy oil is used. Bakery products are made from soy, lima, or potato starch. Soymilk or meat-based formulas are used for infants. Calcium and vitamin supplements are needed. When the patient is free of allergic symptoms, fruits and vegetables are added, one at a time, every 2 to 5 days. Cereals are added in the following order: rice, oats, corn, rye, and wheat. Beef is added after 1 to 2 months. Tolerance for condiments and spices is determined by challenge testing. Subsequent additions of specified oils and other foods are made on recommendation by the physician.

A fruit-free cereal-free elimination diet is used for patients who are allergic to fruits, spices, or condiments. On this diet careful planning is needed to ensure adequate calories, vitamins, and minerals, especially ascorbic acid, calcium, potassium, magnesium, iron, and iodine. A number of recipes suitable for use on cereal-free or fruit-free elimination diets are available.

Cereal-Free Elimination Diet*

Beverages—fruit juices: apricot, grapefruit, peach, pineapple, prune, or tomato
Breads—lima-potato, soy-potato; muffins made from allowed flours; pancakes or waffles made from soy-potato flours; soy crackers
Desserts—cakes, cookies, cupcakes made from soy or potato flours; gelatin, plain; soy ice cream; puddings made from allowed flours; water ices made with allowed fruits
Flours and starches—lima, potato, soy; pearl tapioca
Fruits—fresh, cooked, or canned apricots, grapefruit, peaches, pears, pineapple, lemon, prunes
Fats—sesame oil, soy oil, milk-free margarine made with soy oil
Gravy—thickened with potato starch
Meats—bacon; Canadian bacon; chicken (no hens); lamb; lamb liver
Soups—broth, chicken or lamb; lima bean; split pea; tomato
Sweets—brown sugar, beet or cane sugar; jams, jellies, preserves made from allowed fruits; maple syrup; maple sugar candy, plain fondant
Vegetables—artichokes, asparagus, carrots, lettuce, lima beans, peas, potatoes, spinach, squash, string beans, sweet potatoes, tomatoes, yams
Miscellaneous—baking powder (no cornstarch or tartaric acid); baking soda, cream of tartar, lemon extract, salt, vanilla extract, white vinegar

Sample Menu for Cereal-Free Elimination Diet

BREAKFAST
Half grapefruit with brown sugar
Canadian bacon
Hash brown potatoes
Muffins, using soy-potato flour
Milk-free soy margarine
Peach preserves
Hot lemonade, pineapple, apricot, or prune juice

LUNCH OR SUPPER
Tomato juice with lemon wedge
Fried chicken, using soy oil, potato flour
New potato, boiled
Peas
Mixed fruit cup with peach, pear, pineapple
Lemon gelatin salad with grated carrot and crushed pineapple
Soy-potato bread

Milk-free soy margarine
Jam or preserves from allowed fruits
Soy ice cream with caramel sauce
Soy cookies
Lemonade or apricot juice

DINNER
Broiled lamb chops
Baked potato
Mashed squash
Lettuce and tomato salad
Salad dressing, using soy oil, lemon juice, salt
Soy-potato bread
Milk-free soy margarine
Jam or preserves from allowed fruits
Pineapple upside-down cake, using soy-potato flour
Lemonade, apricot, or tomato juice

* Adapted from Rowe, A. H.: *Food Allergy. Its Manifestations and Control and the Elimination Diets. A Compendium.* Charles C Thomas, Publisher, Springfield, Ill., 1972.

Fruit-Free Cereal-Free Elimination Diet*

Beverages—tea, if permitted by physician
Breads—lima-potato, soy-potato; muffins made from allowed flours; pancakes or waffles from potato or soy flour
Desserts—cakes, cookies, cupcakes made from soy or potato flours; gelatin, plain; soy ice cream; puddings made from allowed flours.
Fats—sesame oil; soy oil; milk-free soy margarine
Gravy—thickened with potato starch
Meats—bacon; Canadian bacon; chicken (no hens); lamb; lamb liver
Soups—broth, lamb or chicken; lima bean, split pea

Fruit-Free Cereal-Free Elimination Diet*

Flours and starches—lima, potato, soy; pearl tapioca
Sweets—beet or cane sugar; brown sugar; syrup made with cane sugar
Vegetables—artichokes, carrots, lima beans, peas, potatoes, string beans, squash, sweet potatoes, yams
Miscellaneous—corn-free tartaric acid baking powder; salt

Sample Menu for Fruit-Free Cereal-Free Elimination Diet

BREAKFAST
Waffles, using soy-potato flour
Bacon
Pearl tapioca cooked with water and sugar
Milk-free soy margarine
Maple syrup
Tea, if permitted

LUNCHEON OR SUPPER
Split pea soup with bacon crumbs
Soy crackers
Sliced chicken sandwich on soy-potato bread
Milk-free soy margarine
Gelatin salad with shredded carrots
Frosted soy cupcake
Tea, if permitted

DINNER
Chicken broth with carrots, peas, lima beans
Soy crackers
Roast lamb
String beans
Mashed potato, using milk-free soy margarine, salt
Gravy, thickened with potato starch
Soy-potato muffin
Milk-free soy margarine
Carrot marmalade
Soy ice cream
Butterscotch sauce, using milk-free soy margarine
Tea, if permitted.

* Adapted from Rowe, A. H.: *Food Allergy. Its Manifestations and Control and the Elimination Diets. A Compendium.* Charles C Thomas, Publisher, Springfield, Ill., 1972.

Milk Sensitivity　A special problem in infants and young children is milk sensitivity. From 1 to 2 percent of all children are sensitive to cow's milk.[6] In many instances this may be associated with infection and emotional stress; in others genetic factors may be a cause. (See Galactosemia, Chapter 42, and Lactose Intolerance, Chapter 31.)

In infants with true milk allergy the response to the ingestion of milk is immediate and may lead to colic, spitting up of the feeding, irritability, diarrhea, and respiratory disorders. In others, a delayed reaction may occur hours to days following the ingestion of milk, and thus it becomes difficult to determine the exact cause.

The incidence of hypochromic anemia in some infants has been attributed to sensitivity to milk. Following the ingestion of milk by these sensitive infants, some blood is lost from the gastrointestinal tract. This may average several milliliters per day and may go unnoticed until the anemia becomes apparent months later. Some infants may have a sufficiently high intake of other iron-rich foods so that the anemic tendency is counteracted. (This is discussed in more detail in Chapter 43.)

Each of the common proteins in milk has been found to be allergenic, but beta-lactoglobulin is the most common.[8] Several hypoallergenic formulas are available, with a casein hydrolysate, meat, or soybean often used as the protein source.*

Dietary Treatment of Food Allergy　Especially for children, it is always necessary to consider the relative importance of the allergic disturbance in relation to the diet. It is better management, for example, to treat a mild case of eczema locally than to subject the child to the dangers of an inadequate diet with its far more serious consequences.

If a single food such as strawberries or grapefruit is implicated, the food is easily omitted from the diet. If allergy involves more than one food, the initial diet contains only those foods that produce no reactions. Thus, if improvement has occurred on an elimination diet, simple, not mixed, foods are added, one at a time, to the allowed list of foods. Several days to a week must elapse between the addition of each new food. A given food should be tested on at least two, preferably three, occasions before it is permanently added to, or eliminated from, the diet. Because wheat, eggs, and milk are frequent allergens, these foods are added last.

Dietary adequacy becomes a matter of great con-

*Nutramigen (Mead Johnson and Co., Evansville, Ind.); MBF (Meat-base formula) (Gerber Products Company, Fremont, Mich.).

cern when important foods are eliminated for a long period of time. This is especially true in infants and young children and care must be taken to ensure inclusion of acceptable foods similar in nutrient content to the one omitted.

In milk sensitivity changing the form of the milk sometimes improves tolerance—that is, boiled, powdered, acidulated, or evaporated milk may be satisfactory when fresh cow's milk is not. Some children will tolerate no milk whatsoever, and a hypoallergenic formula must be substituted. Many youngsters outgrow their sensitivity to milk but others need to continue a milk-free diet indefinitely.

Hyposensitization consists of decreasing the sensitivity to a given substance by giving minute doses of the allergen in gradually increasing amounts. It is a very tedious procedure and is seldom used in food allergy, and then only when a major food group is involved.

Dietary Management for Asthmatic Patients. Those who have severe asthma often find it difficult to consume an adequate diet. The meals should be small and eaten slowly in an environment free from stress. Interval feedings are necessary to bolster the calorie intake. Fluid intake should be encouraged. Usually breakfast and lunch are the best meals of the day, and particular attention should be paid to their nutritional quality and attractiveness. A rest period after meals is helpful. Ordinarily, late-evening feedings are not advisable. Some clinicians routinely eliminate highly allergenic foods such as chocolate, nuts, shellfish, and so on. Milk products are sometimes omitted because of their tendency to form mucus.

DIETARY COUNSELING

The diet counselor should stress the importance of reading labels on food products every time purchases are made. Formulations change periodically and current ingredients are listed on the label. However, even conscientious checking of labels is not always adequate protection for the individual with food allergy. Foods for which a standard of identity has been established by the Food and Drug Administration need not be labeled with a complete listing of ingredients; only optional ingredients must be listed. For example, mayonnaise contains small amounts of egg, but this is not indicated on the label. A number of breads have been included under standards of identity, and thus the label would not indicate that milk is an ingredient.

Many patients may not be aware of the great number of food mixtures containing milk, eggs, cereal, or soy products. The patient should be provided with detailed lists showing typical uses of these foods and should be encouraged to ask specific questions concerning ingredients used in foods when in doubt. Examples of foods to be omitted for wheat, egg, milk, corn, or soy-free diets follow.

Recipes and helpful hints on substitutions should be offered the patient. For example, water or fruit juices can usually be substituted in recipes using milk. Quick breads can be made from rice, potato, rye, or other flours, but adjustments in baking temperature and time must be made. The proportion of baking powder is increased because of the lack of gluten in these flours. The finished products differ in texture from those prepared from wheat. They should be stored in a freezer rather than in the refrigerator as they tend to dry out quickly.

Patients should be cautioned that improperly washed utensils or use of the same stirring or serving spoon in foods for allergic and non-allergic persons may be sources of prohibited foods for the food-sensitive individual.

Suggestions for ordering foods when eating away from home are useful for patients. Broiled meats, baked potato, plain vegetables without sauces, lettuce salads, and fruits for dessert are usually acceptable.

Diet Without Wheat—Foods to Avoid

Beverages—beer; Cocomalt; coffee substitutes; instant coffee unless 100 percent coffee; gin; malted milk; whiskey

Breads, crackers, and rolls—all breads including pumpernickel, rye, oatmeal, and corn; baking powder biscuits; crackers; gluten bread; griddle cakes; hot breads and muffins; matzoh; pretzels; rusk; waffles; zwieback

Cereals—All-bran, bran flakes, Cheerios, Cream of Wheat, farina, Granola type, Grape-nuts, Grape-nuts flakes, Kix, Maltex, New oats, Pettijohn's, Puffed Wheat, Ralston cereals, Shredded Wheat, Special K, Total, Wheatena, Wheat flakes, wheat germ, Wheaties, Wheat Chex

Diet Without Wheat—Foods to Avoid

Desserts—cake or cookies, homemade, from mixes, or bakery; doughnuts; ice cream, ice cream cones; pies; popovers; puddings
Flour—all purpose; graham, white, whole wheat
Gravies and sauces—thickened with flour
Meat—canned meat dishes such as stews, chili; frankfurters, luncheon meats, or sausage in which wheat has been used as a filler; prepared with bread, cracker crumbs or flour, such as croquettes and meatloaf; stews thickened with flour or made with dumplings; stuffings and commercial stuffing mixes
Pastas—macaroni, noodles, spaghetti, vermicelli, and so on
Salad dressings—thickened with flour
Soups—bouillon cubes; commercially canned

Diet Without Eggs—Foods to Avoid

Eggs—or commercial egg substitutes in any form
Beverages—Cocomalt; eggnog; malted beverages; Ovaltine; root beer; wine
Bread and rolls—containing eggs; crust glazed with egg; French toast; griddle cakes; muffins; pretzels; sweet rolls; waffles; zwieback
Desserts—cake; cookies; cream-filled pies, coconut, cream, custard, lemon, pumpkin; custard; doughnuts; ice cream; meringue; puddings; sherbet
Meat—breaded meats dipped in egg; meat loaf
Noodles
Salad dressings—cooked dressings; mayonnaise
Sauces—hollandaise, tartar
Soups—bouillon; broth, consommé
Sweets—many cake icings: candies; chocolate, cream, fondant, marshmallow, nougat; whips
Miscellaneous—baking mixes; baking powder; cake flour; dessert powders; fondue; fritters; pastries; soufflé

Diet Without Milk—Foods to Avoid

Milk—all forms: buttermilk; evaporated; fresh whole or skim; malted; yogurt
Beverages—chocolate; cocoa; Cocomalt; Ovaltine
Breads and rolls—any made with milk (most breads contain milk); bread mixes; griddle cakes; soda crackers; waffles; zwieback
Cereals—some dry (read labels)
Cheese—all kinds; cheese dips and spreads
Desserts—cakes; cookies; custard; doughnuts; ice cream; mixes of all types; pie crust made with butter or margarine; pies with cream fillings such as chocolate, coconut, cream, custard, lemon, pumpkin; puddings with milk; sherbets
Fats—butter, cream, margarine
Meat—frankfurters, luncheon meats, meat loaf—unless 100 percent meat
Sauces—any made with butter, margarine, milk, or cream
Soups—bisques; chowders; cream
Sweets—caramels; chocolate candy
Vegetables—au gratin; mashed potatoes; seasoned with butter or margarine; scalloped; with cream sauces

Diet Without Corn—Foods to Avoid

Corn sugar (dextrose) and syrup are widely used in commercially prepared foods. Cornstarch is also used as a binder and thickening agent in many commercial products. Labels should be carefully checked.

Beverages—ale; beer; carbonated; coffee lighteners; gin; grape juice; instant tea; milk substitutes; soy milks; whiskey

Breads, crackers, and rolls—corn breads or muffins; enchiladas; English muffins; corn chips; tacos; tortillas; graham crackers

Cereals—cornmeal; hominy; ready-to-eat: cornflakes; Corn Chex, Grape-nuts, Kix

Desserts—cakes; candied fruits; canned or frozen fruit or juices; cream pies; ice cream; pastries; pudding mixes; sherbet

Fats—corn oil; corn oil margarine; gravies, salad dressings thickened with cornstarch; mayonnaise, salad dressings, and shortenings unless source of oil is specified

Flours and thickeners—cornmeal; cornstarch

Meats—bacon; hams (cured, tenderized); luncheon; sausage

Soups—all commercial; homemade thickened with cornstarch

Sweets—candy; cane sugar; corn syrups, corn sugars; imitation maple syrups; imitation vanilla; jams, jellies, preserves

Vegetables—Harvard beets, (thickened with cornstarch); corn; mixed vegetables containing corn; succotash

Miscellaneous—baking powder; batters for frying; catsup; chewing gum; cheese spreads; Chinese foods; commercial mixes of all types: baking, cake, pancake, pie crust, pudding; confectioner's sugar; distilled vinegar; monosodium glutamate; peanut butter; popcorn; sandwich spreads; sauces; toppings; vitamin capsules; yeast

Diet Without Soy—Foods to Avoid

Soy products are widely used in commercial food preparations. Omit all products for which labels state: soy, soybean oil, soy flour, soy milk, soy curd; vegetable protein; protein isolate; lecithin. Look for these terms especially on the following:

Beverages—beer, chocolate or cocoa mixes, coffee whiteners, soy milk, wine

Breads, crackers, or rolls—many commercial breads; frankfurter or hamburger rolls; dinner rolls; English muffins; biscuit/pancake mixes; bread or cereal stuffings

Cereals—natural or Granola type; flavored rice mixes; macaroni, spaghetti, noodle, or pizza mixes (canned or dry)

Desserts—cake and cake mixes; prepared frostings; chocolate pudding mixes

Fats—cooking oils, margarines, mayonnaise, salad oil, salad dressings, shortenings in which the type of oil is not specified

Flour—soy

Meat—meat extenders; frankfurters; luncheon meats; pork sausage; fish canned in oil

Soups—bouillon cubes; canned, dried, instant soups

Sweets—candy; chocolate chips; semisweet chocolate; caramels; some pancake syrups

Vegetables—frozen in sauces; au gratin potato mixes; instant mashed potatoes; prepared fried potatoes; potato chips

Miscellaneous—Baco's; pretzels; seasoned sauces: mushroom, soy, steak, tabasco, Worcestershire; dip mixes; powdered seasonings

Diseases of the Skin

The quality of the diet is a determining factor in skin health. Deficiencies of one or more nutrients are known to produce various cutaneous disorders. For example, there are the dermatitis associated with pellagra and resulting from lack of niacin (see page 186), the eruptions that accompany severe vitamin A deficiency (see page 160), the cheilosis of riboflavin lack (see page 184), and the eczema that occurs in infants with essential fatty acid deficiency (see page 87).

Some individuals may be allergic to certain substances and thus manifest skin disorders such as eczema or urticaria. Whenever allergy is suspected, it is essential to determine the offending agent as described in the preceding part of this chapter. No single food or food group predominates in producing allergic skin disorders.

Acne vulgaris is a particular problem during adolescence, and many boys and girls try bizarre diets in an effort to correct the situation. High-fat and concentrated carbohydrate diets have been considered to be undesirable. Chocolate, milk, nuts, cola, and iodized salt are among foods commonly implicated in exacerbation of symptoms. However, controlled studies show that dietary restriction is less effective than other forms of therapy, such as antibiotics, benzoyl peroxide, or vitamin A acid therapy.[9]

Dietary emphasis in skin disorders should be placed on nutritional adequacy; that is, the diet should contain sufficient milk, meat, eggs, fruits, vegetables, and whole-grain or enriched cereals and breads. Attention should be directed to improving the general hygiene, including skin cleanliness, regular meal hours, sufficient fluid intake, adequate rest, proper elimination, and psychological support. There is no harm in excluding candies and sweets, fried foods, chocolate, and rich desserts, but such exclusion probably is most useful in that these foods are replaced by others that are more nutritionally satisfactory.

Nutritional Effects of Drug Therapy. Some reports indicate that as many as 40 percent of patients treated with cis-retinoic acid for acne experience elevation of serum triglycerides and lowering of HDL-cholesterol, both of which appear to be dose related.[10,11] Reduction of dietary triglycerides has been recommended for the duration of the drug therapy.[11]

CASE STUDY 26

Pregnant Woman with Milk and Egg Allergy

Mr. and Mrs. Q have been eagerly anticipating the arrival of their first child and attending prenatal classes together. During a class on "Nutritional Needs During Pregnancy," Mrs. Q expressed concern about including enough protein in her diet for the baby and herself because of food allergies.

Mrs. Q has had a milk and egg allergy since infancy. She was born with a rash, and the pediatrician cautioned her mother to watch for possible allergic reactions. She reacted to the milk-based formula, so was placed on a meat-based formula instead. Each food added to her diet was given in small amounts, with only one new food introduced in any given week. Her mother kept a record of her intake and noted the type of symptoms and time of onset. At 8 months she reacted violently to the addition of egg yolk. Skin tests at that time were positive for milk and eggs. When eggs were reintroduced a few months later, she again experienced untoward symptoms, so she was placed on a milk-free, egg-free diet.

Through the years, Mrs. Q has been gradually desensitized to milk. She is now able to tolerate up to 1 cup skim milk daily but has adverse reactions to whole milk, ice cream, cream, and cottage cheese. Her reactions to milk products are less severe than those toward eggs. She tends to experience gastrointestinal disturbances about four to eight hours after she has ingested foods or beverages containing milk.

However, Mrs. Q still experiences immediate, severe reactions with any exposure to eggs or egg products. A few minutes after eating even a small amount of egg she experiences nausea. Later symptoms include vomiting, abdominal pain, and diarrhea. The symptoms subside within 4 to 5 hours. If she inhales egg particles while eggs are being prepared her eyes become red and swollen and she also has asthmalike symptoms.

Food selection presents challenges for Mrs. Q. She usually eats her noon meal in the cafeteria of the bank building where she works. She has learned to inquire about ingredients and avoids casseroles, sauces, and gravies. When shopping for food she carefully reads labels. She does not enjoy cooking and tires of preparing the same foods over and over again. Her husband likes to cook and often prepares the dinner meal.

Pathophysiologic Correlations
1. Briefly describe the sequence of events in immediate and delayed hypersensitivity.
2. What is the role of the immune reaction?
3. What is meant by the term anaphylaxis?
4. In what ways are allergic reactions induced?
5. List some ways in which food allergies are manifested in various body systems.
6. What behavioral factors might aggravate or bring on an allergic reaction?
7. Are food intolerance and food allergy synonymous? Explain.
8. List the common food allergens.

9. Why is a history the first step in diagnosing allergy?
10. Describe the principles involved in each of these diagnostic procedures: challenge test; elimination diet; skin tests.

Nutritional Assessment

11. Compare the Recommended Dietary Allowances for the nonpregnant woman, for pregnancy, and for lactation for the following: energy, protein, ascorbic acid, vitamin A, folacin, calcium, iron, zinc.
12. Which nutrients might be provided at inadequate levels in Mrs. Q's diet because of her allergies?
13. If Mrs. Q does not get enough calcium in her diet, will her baby be deficient in calcium?

Planning the Diet

14. List some problems you foresee in planning Mrs. Q's diet.
15. Outline the objectives in planning Mrs. Q's diet.
16. Plan a day's protein intake for Mrs. Q. List sources and amounts to be used at each meal in order to meet her daily needs during pregnancy.
17. a. Could Mrs. Q use commercial egg substitutes as protein sources?
    b. Mrs. Q. uses a liquid cream substitute for her cereal and coffee. How much protein would this provide?
    c. Mrs. Q is accustomed to using French or Vienna bread because of her milk allergy. How does this bread compare with white enriched bread or whole wheat bread in protein content?
    d. List several low-cost protein sources that Mrs. Q might include in her diet.

Diet Counseling

18. List some important dietary sources of calcium other than milk and milk products.
19. Should Mrs. Q depend on these foods to supply all her calcium needs? Explain.
20. Since the tendency to allergy is inherited, Mrs. Q's baby may well have some allergies.
    a. Would the baby inherit the same allergies and the same manifestations?
    b. List the foods to which infants are frequently allergic.
    c. Outline the procedures Mrs. Q should follow when introducing new foods to the baby.
21. What precautions are especially important in the potentially allergic infant if the baby is breast fed?

References for the Case Study

BUCKLEY, R. H., and METCALFE, D.: "Food Allergy," *JAMA*, 248:2627–31, 1982.

HENLEY, E. C., et al.: "Symposium on Maternal and Newborn Nutrition Across the Woman's Life Cycle," *Nurs. Clin. North Am.*, 17:99–110, March 1982.

WHITE, J. E., and OWSLEY, V.: "Helping Families Cope with Milk, Wheat, and Soy Allergies," *MCN*, 8:423–8, 1983.

References

1. McCarthy, E. P., and Frick, O. L.: "Food Sensitivity: Keys to Diagnosis," *J. Pediatr.*, 102:645–52, 1983.
2. Speer, F.: "Food Allergy: The Ten Common Offenders," *Am. Fam. Physician*, 13:106–12, February 1976.
3. Halpin, T. C., et al.: "Colitis, Persistent Diarrhea, and Soy Protein Intolerance," *J. Pediatr.*, 91:404–7, 1977.
4. Bahna, S. L., and Gandhi, M. D..: "Milk Hypersensitivity. II. Practical Aspects of Diagnosis, Treatment and Prevention," *Ann. Allergy*, 50:295–301, 1983.
5. Atkins, F. M.: "The Basis of Immediate Hypersensitivity Reactions to Foods," *Nutr. Rev.*, 41:229–34, 1983.
6. Dannaeus, A.: "Management of Food Allergy in Infancy," *Ann. Allergy*, 51:303–6, 1983.
7. Rowe, A. H.: *Food Allergy. Its Manifestations and Control and the Elimination Diets. A Compendium.* Charles C Thomas, Publisher, Springfield, Ill., 1972.
8. Bahna, S. L., and Gandhi, M. D.: "Milk Hypersensitivity. I. Pathogenesis and Symptomatology," *Ann. Allergy*, 50:218–23, 1983.
9. Hurwitz, S.: "Acne Vulgaris. Current Concepts of Pathogenesis and Treatment," *Am. J. Dis. Child.*, 133:536–44, 1979.
10. Schachner, L.: "The Treatment of Acne: A Contemporary Review," *Pediatr. Clin. North Am.*, 30:501–10, 1983.
11. Spear, K. L., and Muller, S. A.: "Treatment of Cystic Acne with 13-cis-Retinoic Acid," *Mayo Clin. Proc.*, 58:509–14, 1983.

42

Inborn Errors of Metabolism

Many professional and lay groups have united in their efforts to understand the nature of the ever-growing number of inborn errors of metabolism and to seek methods of prevention and treatment. To the physician, the problems are those of diagnosis, of early detection before damage has occurred, and of effective treatment. To the biochemist falls the task of identifying the metabolic defect so that a possible rationale of therapy can be developed. To the nurse and dietitian fall the practical aspects of nursing care and of dietary planning and implementation. The problem of control through genetic counseling belongs to the geneticist. Most of all, to the parent of a child affected the problem is immediate and urgent; in some disorders treatment is effective, but in others no remedy is available.

Nature of Inborn Errors The term INBORN ERROR was coined at the beginning of this century by Sir Archibald E. Garrod who wrote a book in which he described four diseases of a hereditary nature.[1] These were alkaptonuria, a defect of phenylalanine metabolism in which a metabolite excreted into the urine becomes dark upon standing; albinism, also a defect in phenylalanine metabolism characterized by a lack of pigmentation; cystinuria, or an excessive excretion of cystine because of a defect in the renal tubules that prevents the reabsorption of the amino acid cystine; and pentosuria, characterized by the presence of pentose in the urine owing to the lack of an enzyme in metabolism.

Inborn errors of metabolism include well over 100 disorders that originate in one or more mutations of the gene so that normal function is disrupted. These diseases are also referred to as *genetic diseases* or as *hereditary molecular diseases*. The effects of genetic mutation vary widely and may alter the metabolism of specific amino acids, carbohydrates, lipids, vitamins, or minerals. They may affect the synthesis of a body product, interfere with the transport of materials across a cell membrane, or produce toxic effects on tissues because of the accumulation of intermediate products.

Some errors of metabolism result in no serious limitations on the individual; others lead to rapid changes in the central nervous system so that mental retardation is severe; still others may be lethal shortly after birth. Some become evident a few days after birth, whereas other hereditary diseases such as diabetes mellitus and gout may show no signs until adult life. Dietary management is effective in the control of many disorders but no known therapy is yet available for others.

Some of the inborn errors of metabolism are characterized by serious mental retardation if the condition is not treated promptly. During the first years of life the brain is developing so rapidly that any interference with its growth cannot be fully corrected at a later time. Thus, diagnosis at a very early age is important if effective treatment is to take place before serious damage has occurred. Inexpensive screening tests may be applied to some conditions during the first weeks of life.

Several conditions for which dietary treatment has been successful are discussed in this chapter. For some of these disorders the diet is built around specialized formulas that supply most of the energy, protein, and other nutrients needed, but which are designed to be low in specific amino acids in accordance with the metabolic defect. Small amounts of natural foods are also used to provide a controlled intake of protein and certain amino acids in addition to other required nutrients. For some disorders specialized food equivalency lists are available in which all foods within a given group provide approximately the same amount of particular amino acids and protein. The detailed lists are not included in this chapter but are cited in the references. The diet for phenylketonuria serves as an example of the considerations that must be kept in mind when planning highly specialized diets.

Children with inborn errors of metabolism such as phenylketonuria are treated primarily in specialty clinics of major medical centers where a team of highly skilled specialists monitor the child's progress on a regular basis. Since the numbers of patients are small, health team members learn to know the child and parents and their ability to cope with the problems involved in management of the disorder. Dietary management is a special challenge for the dietitian and family alike. The importance of accuracy in calculating amounts of various foods permitted cannot be overemphasized for, in some instances, excessive amounts can lead to neurological damage. On the other hand, insufficient amounts of specific nutrients can impair normal growth and development. The child's progress must be monitored closely and the diet adjusted in accordance with physical and biochemical changes. The diet must be nutritionally adequate for all nutrients except the one(s) which must be limited. The dietitian must be aware of new food products and their nutrient composition as they become available in order to adequately counsel patients and their families regarding their use. The nurse is usually not directly involved in the planning of highly specialized diets, but must be aware of the child's progress on the diet and any problems encountered. The nurse must understand the general principles of the diet and should be cognizant of food sources of the nutrients that are restricted in order to be able to answer questions and evaluate information relayed by the family concerning the diet. Day-to-day dietary management is every bit as challenging for the parents and family as the technical aspects of management are for the health professional. The family must ensure strict adherence to the diet by the child, plan special menus, and encourage the child to eat specialized products.

The information presented in this chapter is not sufficient to enable the dietitian or nurse to competently plan nutritional care for children with inborn errors of metabolism. The material presented is intended to give an overview of some conditions requiring highly complex diets, the importance of careful dietary planning in these disorders, and the need for continuing counseling of parents regarding the child's nutritional management.

Phenylketonuria

PHENYLKETONURIA (often abbreviated PKU) was first diagnosed by Asbjörn Fölling, a Norwegian biochemist, in 1934, and has been successfully treated with a phenylalanine-restricted diet since 1952. When the disorder is discovered early in infancy and is treated with the phenylalanine-restricted diet, mental development is normal.

Incidence About 1 child in each 11,000 Caucasian births has phenylketonuria, although 1 person in 50 is a carrier of the trait.[2] About 1 percent of all patients in mental institutions are estimated to be phenylketonurics.

Phenylketonuria is transmitted by an autosomal recessive gene. Thus, each of the parents would have one defective gene and would be clinically normal. Each birth from the mating of two heterozygotes involves a one in four chance that the child will be phenylketonuric, two chances that he or she will be a heterozygote but clinically normal, and one chance that he or she will be entirely normal.

Biochemical Defect An enzyme, *phenylalanine hydroxylase*, is absent in the individual with classic phenylketonuria. As a consequence the hydroxyl (OH) grouping cannot be incorporated into the phenylalanine molecule to form tyrosine. Tyrosine levels remain normal, but phenylalanine and several metabolites accumulate in the blood circulation and are excreted in the urine. One of these is phenylpyruvic acid, a ketone, for which the condition is named—that is—phenyl–keton–uria. Another intermediate product is phenylacetic acid, which accounts for the characteristic "wild," "gamey," or "mousy" odor from the skin and urine of these patients. (See Figure 42-1.)

Testing for Phenylketonuria Most states require that newborn infants be screened for phenylketonuria. In normal infants the serum phenylalanine level is less than 2 mg per dl. Elevation of phenylalanine levels in serum above 2 mg per dl at 12 to 48 hours of age, and above 4 mg per dl at 3 days or more requires monitoring.[3]

In some children phenylalanine hydroxylase is not missing but is present in reduced amounts and there is consequent elevation of serum phenylalanine levels. Neurologic development in these youngsters is usually normal. Occasionally infants have an initial elevation of serum phenylalanine that later returns to normal. Other infants, especially prematures, show a slight elevation of serum phenylalanine, and sometimes tyrosine, because of delayed maturation of the tyrosine-oxidizing system. Usually this is corrected by the administration of ascorbic acid. It is important to distinguish these conditions from true PKU so that children are not subjected to the phenylalanine-restricted diet unnecessarily.

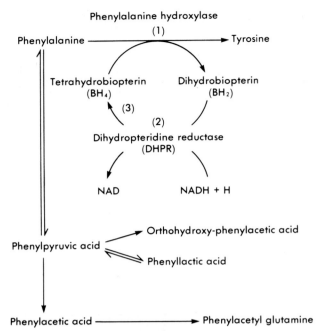

Figure 42-1. In classic phenylketonuria, there is a deficiency of phenylalanine hydroxylase (1). Variant forms are due to deficiency of dihydroxpteridine reductase (2), or deficiency of tetrahydrobiopterin or defective recycling of BH$_4$ due to DHPR deficiency (3).

Hyperphenylalaninemia may also occur due to deficiencies of two other components of the phenylalanine hydroxylase system, dihydropteridine reductase and tetrahydrobiopterin. (See Figure 42-1.) These cofactors are necessary for the synthesis of the neurotransmitters serotonin, dopamine, and norepinephrine. Deficiency of either component leads to elevated serum phenylalanine levels and neurological dysfunction.[4]

Clinical Changes   Mental retardation in untreated subjects is usually severe with most patients having an intelligence quotient below 50. The child appears to be normal at birth but within the first few days or weeks of life the various intermediate products of faulty phenylalanine metabolism accumulate and can be detected in the blood and urine. If treatment is not initiated promptly, progressive irreversible brain damage occurs. Although the faulty phenylalanine metabolism is clearly understood as the cause of the brain damage, it is not yet known just how this change takes place.

Because of the block in tyrosine formation, the production of pigments is reduced. Consequently, these children are usually blond, blue eyed, and have a fair skin, even though their parents may be of a darker skin, eye, and hair coloring. Eczema is a common finding.

The behavior of untreated children is considerably altered. They are hyperactive, wave their arms, rock back and forth, and grind their teeth. They show poor coordination, are irritable, immature, and overdependent. At times they may have seizures. Their behavior can be extremely trying even to the most loving parents.

Treatment   The successful treatment of PKU depends on (1) early diagnosis; (2) restriction of phenylalanine intake to maintain an acceptable range of serum phenylalanine; (3) a nutritionally adequate diet adjusted from time to time to meet the requirements for normal growth and development; (4) continuing clinical and biochemical monitoring; and (5) a comprehensive program of education of the parents. Children for whom such treatment is begun within the first few weeks or months of life show apparently normal mental and physical development. The team approach is essential, including the physician, nurse, clinical chemist, social worker, dietitian, parents, and sometimes others.

Ordinarily use of a low-phenylalanine diet is not necessary if the serum phenylalanine level is below 15 mg per dl; however, it is used when the serum phenylalanine is more than 30 mg per dl. The use of dietary treatment if serum phenylalanine levels are between these levels is controversial.[5] However, such infants may benefit if phenylalanine intake is adjusted to reduce serum levels to less than 15 mg per dl during the period of brain development in the first 1 to 2 years.[6]

A delay in the initiation of the diet reduces the likelihood of satisfactory mental development. Once brain damage has occurred reversal does not take place. After 3 years of age, little improvement in mental development can be expected. However, even for the older child the phenylalanine-restricted diet is believed to be of some benefit in modifying the behavior characteristics.

Hyperphenylalaninemia due to deficiency of dihydropteridine reductase or tetrahydrobiopterin is treated with neurotransmitter therapy—that is, by DOPA and 5-hydroxytryptophan and a low phenylalanine diet.[2]

Modification of the Diet   The allowances for protein and for calories are essentially the same as those for normal children. Phenylalanine needs to be restricted but it cannot be totally eliminated from the diet since it is an essential amino acid. Proteins contain 4 to 6 percent phenylalanine, which is excessive for the child with PKU. Several commercial preparations are available.* *Lofenalac* has 95 percent of the phenylalanine removed and is designed for infants as the chief source of protein. *Phenyl-free* and PKU-AID, for older children, contain no phenylalanine, thus they permit the use of more natural foods containing phenylalanine.

Clinical experience has shown that a balance must be maintained between the amount of low-phenylalanine formula and the amount of natural foods that are fed. The formula supplies most of the energy, protein, and other nutrients, and if inadequate amounts are fed, the amino acid and other nutritional requirements of the child will not be met. On the other hand, if insufficient amounts of natural foods are given, the phenylalanine intake will be too low to meet growth requirements. Catabolism of tissue proteins then leads to a temporary increase in the serum phenylalanine level.

The signs of inadequate phenylalanine intake include anorexia, vomiting, listlessness, inconsistent growth or failure to grow, pallor, and skin rash.

Management of the Diet The diet is so unlike a normal diet that many problems are encountered in its administration. A skillful approach by physician, nurse, and nutritionist is required to achieve acceptance on the part of the parent as well as the child.

Considerations in planning the diet are as follows:

1. Estimate the daily protein, calorie, and phenylalanine requirements in accordance with the child's age and weight.
2. Calculate the amount of special formula required to meet the protein and calorie allowances.
3. Determine amounts of other foods needed to meet the phenylalanine allowance.

Lofenalac provides the basis for the diet in infants. Except for phenylalanine, this preparation is nutritionally complete, containing amino acids, unsaturated fat, carbohydrate, vitamins, and minerals. It is a satisfactory substitute for milk and other protein foods. Measured amounts are used to supply protein and calories for the young infant who is not yet receiving other foods, and to provide 85 percent of the protein needs for the older child. To meet the phenylalanine requirement for the infant, from 1 to 2 ounces of milk are added to the *Lofenalac* formula. Milk contains about 55 mg percent phenylalanine and should always be incorporated into the formula so that the

infant does not develop a taste for milk. The diet should be progressed as for a normal infant and child. Appropriate amounts of fruits, vegetables and cereal foods are introduced as the child grows, and *Lofenalac* may be incorporated into these and other allowed foods. A variety of recipes have been developed for such use. Planning the diet is made easier by the use of special serving lists in which all foods within a given group provide the same amount of phenylalanine, protein, and calories when given in the specified amounts.[7]

The optimal age for discontinuing the diet is not known. For psychologic reasons it is usually discontinued about the time the child enters school. A survey of phenylketonuria centers in the United States revealed that subtle changes in cerebral function may occur when the diet is discontinued. Children participating in the survey were randomly assigned, at age 6, to discontinue the phenylalanine-restricted diet or to continue the diet until age 8. The IQ scores did not change in children after age 6 whether they were on the low-phenylalanine diet or not. However, school performance was better in those children who continued the diet until age 8. Concern that the cumulative effects of lowered school performance may jeopardize the child's future has led some to recommend that the low phenylalanine diet be continued until adolescence or even later.[8]

Phenylalanine restriction is recommended during pregnancy of the phenylketonuric woman; however, some evidence suggests that such restriction may need to be in effect at the time of conception in these women in order to reduce the risk of infants with mental retardation, microcephaly, and congenital heart disease.[9] Guidelines for dietary management have been described.[10]

DIETARY COUNSELING

Eating problems are encountered frequently in the phenylketonuric children. These may be the result of great parental anxiety and feelings of guilt. The parent may overemphasize diet and allow it to dominate the relationships with the child. Initially, the acceptance of Lofenalac may be poor. If it is forced at first, or if the parent or brothers and sisters indicate dislike for the diet, the child may continue to refuse the formula. It is best to offer the formula at the beginning of the feeding when the child is hungry, and to avoid any show of concern if it is not fully accepted. When parents begin to see the improvement in the child, encouragement is provided for the considerable effort needed to maintain careful vigilance in regard to the diet.

---

* Lofenalac (Mead Johnson and Company, Evansville, Ind.); Phenyl-free (Mead Johnson and Company); and PKU-AID (Ross Laboratories, Columbus, Ohio, manufactured in England).

Both parents must receive detailed information concerning the amounts of phenylalanine permitted daily and the amounts of foods that will provide them. They should be asked to demonstrate the measurement and preparation of the formula and to plan a series of daily menus showing the phenylalanine, protein, and calorie content. The diet must be continually monitored. A record of the child's daily intake should be kept and brought along each time the child is seen in the PKU clinic so that the physician and nutritionist can assess the child's progress in relation to the diet. A program of home services is invaluable in assuring that the diet is being used as planned. The public health nurse often supervises the home care and also consults with the dietitian or nutritionist in the planning and in problems of dietary management. Printed recipe materials should be carefully explained to the parent.

Tyrosinemia

Hereditary tyrosinemia is transmitted as an autosomal recessive gene. A deficiency of *parahydroxyphenylpyruvic acid oxidase* places a block on the conversion of tyrosine to homogentisic acid. The plasma tyrosine, phenylalanine, and sometimes methionine levels are elevated, and increased amounts of tyrosine, parahydroxyphenylpyruvic acid, methionine, other amino acids, and phosphates are excreted in the urine.

Patients with this deficiency show extensive liver and renal damage, failure to thrive, cataracts, hypoglycemia, rickets, and mental retardation. Newborn infants sometimes have a transient form of tyrosinemia and tyrosyluria. These abnormalities occur especially in premature infants and are directly correlated with the level of protein intake. This appears to be a benign condition and is not associated with specific symptoms. The increased tyrosine levels in the blood and in the urine return to normal as the infant matures. The blood levels are reduced if adequate ascorbic acid is given early.

Dietary Modification Initially a hydrolysate low in phenylalanine and tyrosine* is used with small amounts of milk added to provide these amino acids. If blood methionine levels are elevated, a synthetic

* Low Phe/Tyr Diet Powder (Product 3200 AB) (Mead Johnson & Company, Evansville, Ind.).

mixture of amino acids without tyrosine, phenylalanine, and methionine is used together with a protein-free supplement† to provide carbohydrate, fat, vitamins, and minerals. A diet low in phenylalanine, tyrosine, and methionine has been described.[11]

Maple Syrup Urine Disease

This inborn error of metabolism derives its name from the maple syrup odor of urine, a valuable clue in the diagnosis. The disease is also known as *branched-chain ketoaciduria*, a term that relates to the biochemical defect. It was first recognized in the United States in 1954 and since then has been described in several other countries. It is transmitted as an autosomal recessive trait. The worldwide frequency is estimated to be about 1 per 225,000 newborns.

Biochemical Defect Three branched-chain amino acids, namely, leucine, isoleucine, and valine, are normally metabolized to ketoacids and then further degraded through decarboxylation to simple acids. In maple syrup urine disease an *oxidative decarboxylase* in the white blood cells is missing. Because the carboxyl group cannot be removed, the amino acids and their keto acids accumulate in the blood and are excreted in excessive amounts in the urine. A metabolite related to isoleucine is believed to be responsible for the odor of the urine and of the sweat.

Clinical Changes In the classic form of the disease, infants begin to show symptoms within the first few days. They are unable to suck and swallow satisfactorily, respiration is irregular, and there are intermittent periods of rigidity and flaccidity. Seizures of the grand mal type may occur. In untreated infants, mental retardation is severe. Hypoglycemia is common. Frequent infections lead to increased tissue catabolism and thus to a further accumulation of the offending metabolites in the circulation.

Dietary Treatment A diet restricted in leucine, isoleucine, and valine is used.[12] A special formula, consisting of one of several commercially available mixtures of amino acids without the branched-chain amino acids,* small amounts of milk, and a protein-

† Protein-Free Diet Powder (Product 80056) (Mead Johnson & Company).
* Gibco Amino Acid Mix minus Branched-Chain Amino Acids (Grand Island Biological Company, Grand Island, N.Y.); MSUD Diet Powder (Mead Johnson & Company, Evansville, Ind.); MSUD-AID (Ross Laboratories, Columbus, Ohio, manufactured in England). This product contains no carbohydrate or fat and should be used with an appropriate source, such as Product 80056.

free supplement,* has been described.[12] Fruits, vegetables, and cereals low in protein are added in controlled amounts as the child grows.[12,13] A variant form of the disorder responds to pharmacologic doses of thiamin.[14] The dietary modifications are needed permanently.

Homocystinuria

Biochemical and Clinical Findings   This is a disorder of methionine metabolism. The enzyme *cystathionine synthetase* is essential for the conversion of homocysteine to cystathionine, both of which are intermediate products formed in the metabolism of methionine. When the enzyme is lacking, increased amounts of methionine and homocysteine are found in the plasma, and large amounts of homocystine are excreted in the urine. Lack of the enzyme is an autosomal recessive trait. Other rarer forms of homocystinuria involve defects in the folate remethylating pathway. These disorders are characterized by elevated plasma homocysteine and normal or low methionine levels. Common features of homocystinuria include mental retardation, dislocated lenses, skeletal deformities, thromboembolism, and early atherosclerosis.

Treatment   Some patients with classic homocystinuria respond to pharmacologic doses of pyridoxine, a coenzyme for cystathionine synthetase. For others, a regimen of pyridoxine, folic acid, and betaine or choline is associated with improved clinical response and decrease in plasma homocysteine levels.[15] Folic acid and betaine have also been used in homocystinuria due to defects in the folate remethylating pathway.

Dietary Modification   For patients who respond to pyridoxine therapy, a normal, but not excessive, protein intake is recommended. For those unresponsive to pyridoxine, a low-methionine diet supplemented with cystine is used. A special formula, low in methionine, is used.† Considerations in planning the diet are similar to those in phenylketonuria—calculating the amount of formula needed to meet protein and calorie requirements, and determining amounts of other foods permitted. Methionine exchange lists and recipes have been described.[13]

* Protein-Free Diet Powder (Product 80056) (Mead Johnson & Company, Evansville, Ind.).

† Low Methionine Diet Powder (Product 3200-K) (Mead Johnson & Company, Evansville, Ind.).

Leucine-Induced Hypoglycemia

A relatively rare inborn error of metabolism, *leucine-induced hypoglycemia* becomes apparent after about the fourth month of life. Convulsions may be the first indication of an abnormality. Infants with this disorder fail to thrive and show some evidence of delayed mental development. Signs typical of Cushing's syndrome—acne, hirsutism, obesity, and osteoporosis—are often present.

When L-leucine is given in a test dose to the infant, a profound lowering of the blood glucose occurs in the leucine-sensitive infant. The precise reason for the increased sensitivity is not known. Among the several theories suggested, the most likely one appears to be that leucine may act as a stimulus to insulin production or to enhance insulin utilization.

Dietary Management   A diet low in leucine is used,[16] but the minimum leucine requirement of 150 to 230 mg per kg must be included. Protein foods are sources of leucine and must be restricted. The diet is planned to furnish the minimum requirements of protein for normal development. Fruits and vegetables are added to the diet according to the infant's normal feeding schedule. To counteract the hypoglycemic effects of the leucine, a carbohydrate feeding (equivalent to 10 g) is given 30 to 40 minutes after each meal. By the age of 5 to 6 years the disease has run its course, and from that time on the child is able to tolerate a normal diet. A proprietary product low in leucine is available.*

Galactosemia

Biochemical Defect   Galactosemia is caused by the absence of an enzyme *galactose-1-phosphate uridyl transferase*, sometimes abbreviated P-Gal-transferase, which is needed in the liver for the conversion of galactose to glucose. Galactose is derived from the hydrolysis of lactose in the intestine. It is absorbed normally in this inborn error, but in the absence of transferase, galactose, galactose 1-phosphate, and galactitol accumulate in the blood and tissues. Analysis of the red blood cells shows little or no transferase in those who have the disease, and only half the normal levels in carriers of the defect. Urine tests show the presence of galactose, albumin, and amino

* MSUD Diet Powder (Mead Johnson & Company, Evansville, Ind.).

acids. A galactose tolerance test helps to establish the diagnosis. Mothers of galactosemic infants have a diminished ability to metabolize galactose. If they drink unlimited amounts of milk during pregnancy, the possibility of damage to the fetus exists since galactose may pass the placenta. The enzyme defect is inherited as an autosomal recessive trait.

Clinical Changes The disease becomes apparent within a few days after birth by such symptoms as anorexia, vomiting, occasional diarrhea, drowsiness, jaundice, puffiness of the face, edema of the lower extremities, and weight loss. The spleen and liver enlarge, and in some there may be evidence of liver failure within a short time leading to ascites, bleeding, and early death. Mental retardation becomes evident very early in the course of the disease, and cataracts develop within the first year.

Dietary Treatment Milk is the important dietary source of lactose, which in turn yields galactose. Human milk is especially high in galactose, and thus the breast-fed infant who lacks the necessary enzyme shows symptoms very early. The substitution of a non-milk formula leads to rapid improvement as a rule. All the symptoms disappear except that mental retardation that has already occurred is not reversible. Damage to the central nervous system is greatest during the first few weeks and months of life, when growth is rapid. Therefore, the prompt initiation of therapy is essential.

A number of nonmilk formula products are available. These include Nutramigen,* ProSobee,* and a meat-base formula.†

The formulas are supplemented with calcium gluconate or chloride, iron, and vitamins. Since milk is the only food that supplies lactose, other foods may be introduced into the infant's diet at the appropriate times. These include breads, crackers, and cereals made without milk, eggs, meat, poultry, fish, fruits, vegetables, and gelatin desserts. All foods that contain milk must be rigidly excluded: most commercial breads, cookies, cakes, puddings, pudding mixes, some ready-to-eat cereals, all cheeses, cream, ice cream, butter, margarine churned with milk, chocolate, cold cuts, and others. See the list of foods to avoid for lactose free diets, page 449. Liver, brains,

---

* Nutramigen and ProSobee (Mead Johnson & Co., Evansville, Ind.).
† Meat-base formula (Gerber Products Company, Fremont, Mich.).

and pancreas store galactose and are usually avoided. The stachyose present in soybeans, beets, lima beans, and peas is not hydrolyzed to free galactose; thus, is not absorbed. Nevertheless, these foods are not included in the first year.

As with phenylketonuria, dietary counseling is of paramount importance. Infants accept the substitute formulas quite well, but older children may refuse them for a time. Parents must avoid showing too much anxiety about refusal of food. They need to become thoroughly familiar with lists of foods that contain milk and must learn to read labels with care. The diet is successful only when repeated opportunities are available for follow-up, whether in the clinic or in the home. Such follow-up visits not only reinforce dietary instruction but provide encouragement to the parents.

Complete elimination of galactose is necessary for the very young child but breads and other prepared foods containing milk are usually permitted when the child enters school. Milk must be permanently excluded from the diet, however.

Hereditary Fructose Intolerance

This is an inborn error in which there is a deficiency of *fructose-1-phosphate aldolase*, which splits fructose-1-phosphate into glyceraldehyde and dihydroxyacetone phosphate. The accumulation of fructose-1-phosphate prevents replenishment of cellular inorganic phosphate needed for regeneration of ATP.[17] The introduction of sucrose or fructose in the infant's diet before 6 months of age results in anorexia, vomiting, failure to thrive, hypoglycemic convulsions, and dysfunction of the liver and kidney. Older children with the defect are often asymptomatic or they may have spontaneous hypoglycemia. When an oral dose of fructose is given, the blood fructose and magnesium levels rise, but the levels of glucose and phosphate fall. The hypoglycemia that occurs is believed to be caused by reduced glycogenolysis and gluconeogenesis. The breath hydrogen test has also been used to diagnose the condition.[18]

Treatment This condition is controlled by a diet that eliminates all sources of fructose from the diet. Most fruits contain some fructose, and the intestinal hydrolysis of sucrose also yields fructose. Sorbitol is oxidized to fructose; thus, foods containing this sugar should be avoided. Glucose should be used in place of sucrose, and starches are utilized normally. For the infant a formula is calculated to meet normal requirements, using glucose as the source of carbohydrate. A formula that is mono- and disaccharide free is used.* Unsweetened cereals, egg yolk, strained meats, and strained vegetables are added at intervals as in normal infant feeding. Sugar beets, sweet potatoes, and peas contain appreciable amounts of sucrose. (See also Table 31-2.) Most patients learn to avoid sweets.

Wilson's Disease

HEPATOLENTICULAR DEGENERATION, or Wilson's disease, is an example of an inborn error of mineral metabolism. It is an hereditary disorder transmitted by an autosomal recessive gene. The characteristic triad includes Kayser-Fleischer rings, a greenish brown discoloration in the eye, neurologic dysfunction, and low levels of ceruloplasmin, the copper-containing protein in blood. Increased deposits of copper in the brain, liver, and kidney are due to decreased biliary excretion. Because of renal intoxication by the copper, there is a marked aminoaciduria and a negative phosphate balance.

Clinical Findings In adults the disorder most often presents as neurologic disease while, in children, hepatic disease is seen. The onset of symptoms is correlated with the time required for sufficient copper to accumulate in the tissues to produce damage. They may appear as early as 4 or 5 years of age, or as late as the thirties. Signs and symptoms include splenomegaly, jaundice, liver enlargement, easy bruisability, and neurologic involvement. The common neurologic signs include indistinct speech, a fixed unblinking stare, hypertonus or rigidity, tremor, seizures, and dementia.

Treatment A chelating agent such as penicillamine is used to increase the urinary excretion of copper. Patients are usually advised to avoid foods that are excessively high in copper such as organ meats, shellfish, mushrooms, legumes, whole-grain cereals, bran, chocolate, and nuts. (See Table A-2.) The normal copper intake is about 2 to 3 mg. To establish negative copper balance, a more restricted intake is necessary, usually 1.5 mg or less. For such diets, distilled water must be used if the water supply contains more than 1 ppm copper. Cooking utensils

* Mono- and Disaccharide-Free Diet Powder (Product 3232A) (Mead Johnson & Company, Evansville, Ind.).

made of copper cannot be used. A paucity of data on the copper content of foods introduces difficulty in planning a diet that is reliably low in copper. Because of the presence of copper in most foods, it is difficult to maintain a sufficiently high caloric intake.

Nutritional Effects of Drug Therapy Penicillamine is the drug of choice in Wilson's disease. It should be taken on an empty stomach. Side effects may include decreased taste sensation for salty and sweet foods, anorexia, nausea, and vomiting. Pyridoxine excretion is increased, and supplements may be needed for patients whose dietary intake of the vitamin is insufficient.[19]

Oral zinc therapy is recommended by some as an alternative to penicillamine. Zinc induces synthesis of metallothionein in the intestine; copper binds to metallothionein and is not absorbed.[20] Zinc also competes with iron for absorption; thus, the iron status of patients receiving zinc should be monitored.[21]

Familial Hypercholesterolemia

This disorder involves a genetic defect in the catabolism of low-density lipoprotein (LDL). It is characterized by elevated plasma LDL-cholesterol levels, and deposits of LDL-cholesterol in tendons and arteries. It is inherited as an autosomal dominant trait. One of every 500 persons is a heterozygote for the disorder; the frequency of homozygotes is 1 per million population. The total plasma cholesterol for heterozygotes usually ranges from 300 to 600 mg per dl. The plasma cholesterol is moderately elevated from birth but the individual does not develop clinical symptoms until adulthood when tendon xanthomas and premature coronary disease develop. In homozygotes plasma cholesterol ranges from 650 to 1,000 mg per dl, and clinical symptoms occur in the very young child. Coronary disease is often fatal before adulthood is reached.

Attempts to delay the atherosclerotic changes by dietary intervention in young children involve use of very low cholesterol intakes. Diets containing less than 150 mg cholesterol daily and a P/S ratio of 1.5 : 1 are effective in lowering serum cholesterol to normal levels in hypercholesterolemic children.[22] See Chapter 38 for diets restricted in cholesterol.

See Chapter 31 for discussion of the following genetic errors characterized by malabsorption: lactose intolerance; invertase–isomaltase deficiency; glucose–galactose malabsorption.

CASE STUDY 27

Preschool Boy with Phenylketonuria

Bryan U is an active, blond, blue-eyed 2½-year-old. He is the only child in the family. At birth Bryan weighted 2.1 kg (4 lb. 10 oz). After several feedings a routine test for phenylketonuria revealed elevated serum phenylalanine levels. At 2 weeks of age Bryan's serum phenylalanine level was 40 mg per dl, and phenylpyruvic acid was identified in the urine.

With the confirmation of the diagnosis of phenylketonuria, Bryan was started on Lofenalac formula at age 2 weeks. During the first year of life he was seen at frequent intervals at the PKU clinic for phenylalanine determinations and formula adjustment.

Bryan's diet is carefully supervised by the pediatrician and nutritionist at the PKU clinic. They closely monitor his nutritional status and adjust his diet to meet growth needs. Dietary management has been individualized on the basis of urine and blood levels of phenylalanine, his level of physical and mental development, and the absence of physical symptoms. Bryan's neurologic development has been normal.

Now at age 2½, Bryan is due for another checkup. He weighs 12.3 kg (27 lb); he is 89 cm (35 in.) tall. His blood phenylalanine is 20 mg per dl. He has been in good health and appears well nourished. However, Mrs. U states that Bryan's appetite is poor, and she describes him as a picky eater. Mealtimes are very unpleasant, as Mr. U becomes upset when Bryan won't eat and Mrs. U continues to coax him to eat.

Mrs. U says that Bryan has not had "forbidden foods" until recently. Problems arise when playmates offer him foods he should not eat. Mrs. U brought a 3 day diet record for evaluation and review with the nutritionist.

The pediatrician recommended that Bryan attend nursery school. Mrs. U has found one in the neighborhood where she can be confident that Bryan's diet will be followed.

Pathophysiologic Correlations

1. The physician discussed with Mr. and Mrs. U the nature of the defect in phenylketonuria (PKU) when she was certain of the diagnosis shortly after Bryan's birth. She also described the necessary diet and the prognosis. Give your understanding of the points that she covered.

2. What is meant by an inborn error of metabolism?

3. What failure in metabolism occurs in PKU?

4. State the name of the enzyme that is deficient.

5. Why is early screening for PKU important?

6. Why did the physician wait a few days before ordering the test for PKU?

7. Why were Bryan's tests repeated at the end of 2 and 4 weeks?

8. What is the normal range for blood phenylalanine?

9. If Bryan had not been treated early with a low-phenylalanine formula, what symptoms might have been expected?

10. Mr. and Mrs. U have brown eyes and dark hair. How do you explain Bryan's light coloration?

11. What abnormal excretion products are found in the urine of children who are not treated?

12. Since PKU is transmitted through an autosomal recessive gene, would you expect either parent to have PKU?

13. What is the likelihood that Mrs U's next baby will have PKU?

14. Why are the first and second years of life especially critical for the treatment of PKU?

Nutritional Assessment

15. The nutritionist evaluated the 3-day food intake record Mrs. U had kept for Bryan and found his intake to average 1,125 kcal, 26 g protein, and 320 mg phenylalanine. His dietary needs had been calculated to be 1,450 kcal, 36 g protein, and 430 to 490 mg phenylalanine (35 to 40 mg per kg). How can you explain the elevated blood phenylalanine level despite the fact that apparently he has not exceeded his diet?

16. Would you expect the phenylalanine level to remain high? Explain.

17. Why is it important to include some phenylalanine in the diet?

18. State the criteria for judging the correctness of the phenylalanine level in the diet.

19. Describe the consequences of an inadequate intake of phenylalanine.

20. List some possible reasons for Bryan's poor appetite.

Planning the Diet

21. The phenylalanine content of proteins in foods averages about 5 percent. Assuming a protein intake of 36 g from the usual animal and plant foods, how much phenylalanine would this furnish?

22. How does this compare with Bryan's prescription?
23. List eight foods that are low in phenylalanine.
24. Describe the composition of Lofenalac. How does Phenyl-free compare with Lofenalac?
25. The following diet plan was calculated for Bryan.

	Servings	Phenylalanine (mg)	Protein (g)	Energy (kcal)
Lofenalac	21 measures	158	31.5	903
Water to make	24 ounces			
Special Food Serving Lists				
Vegetables	4	60	1.2	20
Fruits	4	60	0.8	320
Bread	5	150	2.5	100
Fat	1	5	0.1	45
"Free" foods	Varies			Varies
Totals		433	36.1	1,388

Using this plan, and the special food lists for the diet in phenylketonuria, write a menu for 1 day for Bryan. Allow for three meals and midmorning and midafternoon snacks. Be sure to specify amounts of each food he may have.

26. Why is it important to distribute foods fairly evenly throughout the day?
27. List the foods that are omitted entirely from Bryan's diet.

Dietary Counseling

28. State the reason for counseling both parents about the details of Bryan's disease and care.
29. Determine the cost of a 2½ pound can of Lofenalac in a local pharmacy. Assuming 21 measures (220 g) is used each day for Bryan, calculate the cost for each day's supply of Lofenalac.
30. List some flavorings that might lend variety to the Lofenalac.
31. List some ways that Lofenalac can be used other than as a beverage.
32. Mrs. U is reluctant to give candy and soft drinks to Bryan in the belief that they are not good for him. How can the nutritionist justify their use?
33. Since Bryan receives a morning snack and lunch at the nursery school, what arrangements must Mrs U make with the school personnel?
34. Bryan begs to taste foods that other children have. Would there be any harm if Mrs. U allows "just a taste"?
35. What suggestions can you give Mr. and Mrs. U to correct the feeding problems that Bryan now presents?

References for the Case Study

Acosta, P. B., and Wenz, E.: *Diet Management of PKU for Infants and Preschool Children*, DHEW Pub. No. (HSA) 77-5209, U. S. Department of Health, Education and Welfare, PHS, HSA, Bureau of Community Health Services, Rockville, Md., 1977.

Heffernan, J. F., and Trahms, C. M.: "A Model Preschool for Patients with Phenylketonuria," *J. Am. Diet. Assoc.*, **79**:306–8, 1981.

Management of Newborn Infants with PKU. DHEW Pub. No. (HSA) 78-5211. U. S. Department of Health, Education and Welfare, PHS, Health Services Administration, Bureau of Community Health Services, 1978.

Review: "The Dietary Treatment of Phenylketonuria," *Nutr. Rev.*, **41**:11–14, 1983.

Reyzer, N.: "Diagnosis: PKU," *Am. J. Nurs.*, **78**:1895–8, 1978.

References

1. Garrod, A. E.: *Inborn Errors of Metabolism*. Frowde, Hodder & Stoughton, London, 1909.
2. Scriver, C. R., and Clow, C. L.: "Phenylketonuria: Epitome of Human Biochemical Genetics," *N. Engl. J. Med.*, **303**:1394–1400, 1980.
3. McCabe, E. R. B., et al.: "Newborn Screening for Phenylketonuria. Validity as a Function of Age," *Pediatrics*, **72**:390–8, 1983.
4. Kaufman, S.: "Differential Diagnosis of Variant Forms of Hyperphenylalaninemia," *Pediatrics*, **65**:840–1, 1980.
5. Berry, H. K., et al.: "Diagnosis of Phenylalanine Hydroxylase Deficiency (PKU)," *Am. J. Dis. Child.*, **136**:111–14, 1982.
6. Berry, H. K., et al.: "The Diagnosis of Phenylketonuria," *Am. J. Dis. Child.*, **135**:211–13, 1981.
7. Acosta, P. B., and Wenz, E.: *Diet Management of PKU for Infants and PreSchool Children*, DHEW Pub. No. (HSA) 77-5209, U.S. Department of Health, Education and Welfare, PHS, HSA, Bureau of Community Health Services, Rockville, Md., 1977.
8. Koch, R., et al.: "Preliminary Report on the Effects of Diet Discontinuation in PKU," *J. Pediatr.*, **100**:870-5, 1982.
9. Lenke, R. R., and Levy, H. L.: "Maternal Phenylketonuria—Results of Dietary Therapy," *Am. J. Obstet. Gynecol.*, **142**:548–53, 1982.
10. Acosta, P. B., et al.: "Nutrition in Pregnancy of

Women with Hyperphenylalaninemia," *J. Am. Diet. Assoc.*, **80**:443–50, 1982.

11. Michals, K., et al.: "Dietary Treatment of Tyrosinemia Type I," *J. Am. Diet. Assoc.*, **73**:507–14, 1978.

12. Bell, L., et al: "Dietary Management of Maple-Sirup-Urine Disease: Extension of Equivalency Systems," *J. Am. Diet. Assoc.*, **74**:357–61, 1979.

13. Acosta, P. B., and Elsas, L. J.: "Dietary Treatment of Branched Chain Ketoaciduria (MSUD)," in *Dietary Management of Inherited Metabolic Disease: Phenylketonuria, Galactosemia, Tyrosinemia, Homocystinuria, Maple Sirup Urine Disease.* ACELMU Publishers, Atlanta, 1976.

14. Elsas, L. J., and Danner, D. J.: "The Role of Thiamin in Maple Sirup Urine Disease," *Ann. N.Y. Acad. Sci.*, **378**:404–21, 1982.

15. Wilcken, D. E. L., et al.: "Homocystinuria—The Effects of Betaine in the Treatment of Patients Not Responsive to Pyridoxine," *N. Engl. J. Med.*, **309**:448–53, 1983.

16. Roth, H., and Segal, S.: "The Dietary Management of

Leucine Sensitive Hypoglycemia with Report of a Case," *Pediatrics*, **34**:831–68, 1964.

17. Mock, D. M., et al.: "Chronic Fructose Intoxication after Infancy in Children with Hereditary Fructose Intolerance," *N. Engl. J. Med.*, **309**:764–70, 1983.

18. Barnes, G., et al.: "Detection of Fructose Malabsorption by Breath Hydrogen Test in a Child with Diarrhea," *J. Pediatr.*, **103**:575–7, 1983.

19. Moore, A. O., and Powers, D.E.: *Food–Medication Interactions*, 3rd ed. FMI Publishing, Tempe, Arizona, 1981.

20. Brewer, G. J., et al.: "Oral Zinc Therapy for Wilson's Disease," *Ann. Intern. Med.*, **99**:314–20, 1983.

21. Review: "Oral Zinc Therapy for Wilson's Disease," *Nutr. Rev.*, **42**:184–6, 1984.

22. Stein, E.A., et al.: "Changes in Plasma Lipid and Lipoprotein Fractions After Alteration in Dietary Cholesterol, Polyunsaturated, Saturated, and Total Fat in Free-Living Normal and Hypercholesterolemic Children," *Am. J. Clin. Nutr.*, **35**:1375–90, 1982.

43

Nutrition in Children's Diseases

Nutrition for the Sick Child

Although the principles of normal and therapeutic nutrition that apply to the adult are also applicable to the sick child, additional factors that must be carefully considered for the child are (1) growth needs; (2) stage of physical, emotional, and social development; (3) the presence of physical handicaps in some; and (4) the more rapid nutritional deterioration which occurs.

The essentials of normal nutrition provide the baseline for planning meals for the sick child. (See Chapters 20 and 21.) The factors affecting food acceptance must be considered (see Chapter 15), and the principles of nutritional care and counseling are similar to those for adults. (See Chapter 26.) The principles of dietary modification for many conditions are similar for adults and for children, and the preceding chapters pertaining to therapeutic nutrition should be consulted for specific regimens. The discussion that follows supplements the descriptive material set forth in the earlier chapters.

Feeding Problems of the Sick Child   Like adults, children face many obstacles in illness. Eating a satisfactory diet may be difficult because of fatigue, nausea, lack of appetite occasioned by the illness and by drugs, and pain. Children often regress to an earlier stage of feeding; for example, the child who has learned to accept chopped foods may refuse them, or the child who can feed himself or herself may refuse to eat unless someone feeds him or her. Older children especially may experience a sense of failure and express it by excessive eating or refusal to eat. Illness produces emotional tensions in the child as well as in the adult. The child who must be placed in a hospital is also faced with the separation from home and parents. The principles of feeding the normal child apply in even greater degree to the child who is ill.

Insofar as possible the feeding program should establish a pattern of continuity with that to which the child is accustomed. A record of the child's feeding history is a first requisite, so that the normal or therapeutic diet makes allowances for individual likes and dislikes. The period of a child's illness is no time in which to introduce new foods or to provide equipment that the child does not know how to handle.

Even though careful menu planning takes into consideration the usual likes and dislikes of children and includes variations in both flavor and textures, foods may be refused. The illness itself and the strange environment are sufficient cause for such refusal; sometimes portions are a bit too large, or there may be a slight change in the flavoring or texture of a familiar food. Regardless of the reason for refusal, nothing can be gained by trying to force a child to eat.

Nurses and nutritionists must like children and must enjoy working with them if they expect to achieve good results in nutritional care. They must be observant of the child's behavior, of the acceptance or rejection of food, and of what the child says about the food. They have a special responsibility to communicate with the parents. From the parents they learn about the child's food habits at home, and about his or her attitudes toward food. In turn the parents are kept informed about the child's progress in food acceptance while in the hospital, and about changes that may be required after discharge.

Children often eat better when they are fed in groups. Family-style service in the pediatric ward to children who are well enough to sit up is more successful than individual tray service. Older children enjoy selecting their foods from a cafeteria arrangement whenever that is possible. Every advantage should be taken of birthdays and holidays to provide favorite foods and special treats. Many children are encouraged to eat when the mother can bring a favorite food, provided it does not contradict the dietary

599

regimen that has been ordered. Most hospitals now encourage parents to visit at any time they wish, and a young child fed by a parent may respond better than one who is fed by a stranger.

Parents and children who are old enough to understand are jointly counseled regarding dietary modifications that will be required at home. Much less friction is likely to occur at home when the child is included in the interview. Parents assume the primary responsibility for nutritional care of the young child, but the child needs to know what is expected. As early as possible the child should begin to assume some responsibility for his or her care. Older children under parental guidance gradually assume full responsibility for their own diets. In counseling it is important to direct the interview and the instructions to the child rather than to the parent. (See Figure 43-1.)

One important aspect of counseling is to determine the attitudes of the parent toward the development of food habits, and likewise the child's attitudes not only toward the food but also toward his or her parents. Not infrequently the child uses food to achieve various ends.

If a modified diet will be required indefinitely as for diabetes mellitus, every effort must be made to plan this within the framework of the normal life pattern of the child; the diet must not become the dominating factor that interferes with the child's psychosocial development. Being like one's peers is very important to the child, and for many rea-sons the child may be reluctant to disclose that he or she is in any way different. Insofar as possible the diet should be planned so that it can include foods that are popular with other children. The child must be helped to understand that the condition does not make him or her abnormal in relations with others. Selecting foods from those offered by the school lunch would be better for the diabetic child, for example, than carrying a lunch.

Sometimes the hospital stay is sufficiently long that some nutrition education can be included in a group situation. A number of movies appropriate for young children are available from the National Dairy Council and other sources. Other children often view movies with interest in the hospital playroom that they might consider to be boring in the school situation. The teacher assigned to the hospital schoolroom may also be involved in the dietary instruction. For example, children can learn to keep records, to score their diets, and to learn about their needs for basic foods. The calculation of a diet with meal exchanges may be used as an arithmetic assignment. Eye-catching fliers on patient's trays have been used to introduce new ideas about foods such as a food custom of an ethnic group or a simple recipe.

Gastrointestinal Diseases in Infants and Children

Celiac Disturbances The celiac syndrome includes gluten enteropathy, or celiac disease, and cystic fibrosis. Both are characterized by similar symp-

Figure 43-1. The dietitian consults with a young diabetic child and her parents. The child's meal plan is planned around the family pattern. The importance of snacks and avoidance of concentrated sweets is emphasized. (Courtesy, Metropolitan Medical Center, Minneapolis.)

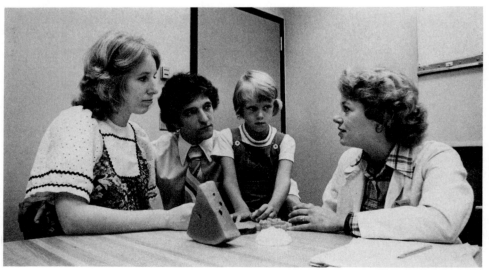

toms, malabsorption, and nutritional deficiencies. The general characteristics, diagnostic tests, and dietary modification for gluten enteropathy were discussed in Chapter 31; cystic fibrosis is discussed in this chapter.

Cystic Fibrosis This congenital disorder of unknown etiology involves a generalized dysfunction of exocrine glands. The incidence is 1 per 2,000 live births. About 10 million persons in the United States are carriers of the gene. The median age of survival in the United States is 21 for males and 17 years for females.[1]

Clinical Features. Pulmonary disease is a prominent feature. An abnormally thick mucus, produced in excessive amounts, obstructs the airways, leading to stasis and infection. Clinical manifestations include chronic cough with mucus production, shortness of breath upon exertion, clubbing of the fingers, failure to gain weight and cyanosis. Some 80 to 90 percent of children have gastrointestinal involvement. Obstruction of pancreatic ducts by thick mucus interferes with release of enzymes needed in digestion of proteins and fats. Malabsorption of fats is characterized by frequent, foul-smelling, loose stools. As much as 50 percent of the protein and fat may be present in the feces. In some instances obstruction of hepatic biliary ducts leads to portal hypertension and cirrhosis. Elevated levels of sodium and chloride—up to 2½ times normal—are found in sweat. Massive salt loss in hot weather may cause heat stroke.

Symptoms. During the neonatal period, cystic fibrosis may present as meconium ileus, or there may be insidious onset of malnutrition in infants with good appetite but who nevertheless fail to grow and gain weight. Passage of foul-smelling, bulky, soft stools, haggard appearance, marked enlargement of the abdomen, and tissue wasting, especially about the buttocks, occur. Appetite is often decreased because of bloating, cramping, and diarrhea.

Treatment. General treatment consists of controlling pulmonary complications by daily postural drainage to loosen mucus plugs for airways, and use of antibiotics to reduce the likelihood of infection; maintaining good nutrition; the use of pancreatic extract; and prevention of abnormal salt loss.

Dietary Modification. A number of studies have indicated that growth and weight gain are inadequate in most children with cystic fibrosis.[2,3] Weight gain

appears to be better in children with mild disease. Poor appetite is common when there is extensive pulmonary involvement. Cystic children vary widely in their tolerance to foods and no single diet is appropriate for all patients. The levels of protein, fat, and carbohydrate must be adjusted individually for each child. Generally speaking, a diet high in calories, 120 to 150 kcal per kg, and protein, 3 to 4 g per kg, is needed to permit satisfactory weight gain and to replace protein lost in the stools. Protein hydrolysates such as Pregestimil for infants, or Portagen for older children, may be indicated. These formulas contain MCT, which is useful if dietary fat is not well tolerated. (See Chapter 31.) Pancreatic extract is taken with each meal. Additional B-complex vitamins, ascorbic acid, and aqueous preparations of fat-soluble vitamins are commonly prescribed. Iron supplementation may also be needed. Additional salt is needed in hot weather. Additions of food are made much more gradually than for healthy infants and children. Distribution of food into six small feedings is often advisable, especially in younger children. Some older children develop diabetes secondary to cystic fibrosis. The diabetes is usually mild and is easily controlled with insulin. Ketoacidosis is uncommon.

Inflammatory Bowel Disease The characteristics, symptoms, and clinical findings in regional enteritis (Crohn's disease) and ulcerative colitis were discussed in Chapter 30. The incidence of these diseases in children appears to be increasing.[4] Although treatment goals are similar in adults and children, satisfactory growth is an additional concern in children. Growth failure may be due to steroid therapy or insufficient energy and nutrient intake. Malnutrition occurs as a result of inadequate oral intake, increased fecal losses of nutrients, increased nutrient requirements, and malabsorption.

Most patients experience weight loss and increased intestinal protein losses. Nutritional deficiencies include anemia due to malabsorption of folate, iron, or vitamin B-12; deficiencies of calcium, magnesium, and potassium secondary to diarrhea; deficiencies of fat-soluble vitamins, and zinc. Lactose intolerance is often a feature.

Dietary Management. With the exception of lactose, restricted diets are not usually indicated in children with Crohn's disease. Some children tolerate lactose-hydrolyzed milk better than regular milk. The diet should be adequate in all nutrients, and oral supplements are indicated if an adequate nutrient intake cannot otherwise be assured. A diet high in protein and low in fiber with vitamin supplements is usually recommended. In some cases enteral feeding or parenteral nutrition methods produce a temporary remission of symptoms.[5]

Nutritional Effects of Drug Therapy. Sulfasalazine, often used in treatment of ulcerative colitis, interferes with absorption of folate. Requirements for ascorbic acid, folate, vitamin B-6, and vitamin D are increased when prednisone is used.[6]

Milk-Induced Colitis This is a manifestation of allergy to cow's milk protein which occurs in 1 to 3 percent of children, most often between the ages of 1 and 4 months. The response to the ingestion of milk is almost immediate in some and may lead to colic, spitting up of the feeding, irritability, diarrhea, and respiratory disorders. A delayed reaction may occur hours to days following the ingestion of milk, and thus it becomes difficult to determine the exact cause. The incidence of hypochromic anemia in some infants has been attributed to sensitivity to milk. Following the ingestion of milk by these sensitive infants, some blood is lost from the gastrointestinal tract. This may average several milliliters per day and may go unnoticed until the anemia becomes apparent months later. It occurs less commonly in infants who were breast fed for the first few months of life than in those who were formula fed. Often the family history is positive for respiratory, cutaneous, or food allergies. Biopsy specimens of the rectal mucosa give the appearance of ulcerative colitis. (See Chapter 30.)

The diagnosis is based chiefly on the response to the withdrawal of milk, and often beef, from the diet. Improvement when milk is eliminated, and relapse upon re-introduction of milk, suggest the diagnosis. Some clinicians require two or three positive challenges to confirm the diagnosis.[4] Intolerance to chicken, fish, and rice has also been reported in infants intolerant to cow's milk protein.[7]

Dietary Management. The treatment consists of elimination of cow's milk, and often beef, from the diet. Improvement in appearance of the colon is noted within a few days. Goat's milk and soy formulas* are tolerated by some infants but are also strong antigens. Infants who become sensitized to soy protein may develop rectal bleeding similar to that seen in allergy to cow's milk protein. Nutramigen,† a casein hydroly-

*Prosobee (Soy Protein Isolate) (Mead Johnson & Company, Evansville, Ind.).

† Nutramigen (Mead Johnson & Company, Evansville, Ind.).

sate, is used. Most children tolerate cow's milk protein by the age of 3 years; however, a significant proportion develop other types of allergies.

Diabetes

The first patient treated with insulin prepared by Banting and Best in 1922 was a 14-year-old diabetic boy. Approximately 1 in every 2,500 children under 16 years is diabetic.

Insulin-Dependent Diabetes The etiology, metabolic aberrations, diagnostic tests, and clinical characteristics of insulin-dependent (type I) diabetes have been described in Chapter 36. The disease in children differs in a number of important respects from that in adults. The onset of symptoms is usually more abrupt and the disease usually increases in severity during the period of growth. A seasonal incidence has been noted, with an increase in new cases during the autumn and winter months. Some evidence suggests that viruses such as mumps or measles may precipitate the disease or may trigger an autoimmune response in some genetically predisposed children.[5] In contrast with the adult, obesity is uncommon; in fact, when first seen the diabetic child is likely to be underweight and not growing because he or she has not been metabolizing food adequately.

All diabetic children need insulin, since there appears to be few if any functioning cells of the islets of Langerhans. The maintenance of control between acidosis on the one hand and hypoglycemia on the other is often difficult because of the greater frequency of infections and the erratic physical activity and emotional control.

Psychologic Considerations Too often the child and parents feel that the child is different from other children and that there is a certain stigma attached to the diabetic state. If the child experiences insulin reactions, he or she will be afraid to participate in the activities of other children and may become more dependent on parents. The diabetic adolescent is likely to be especially difficult to control. Like other adolescents, he or she may rebel against authority, and may show independence by failure to keep the disease in good control.

The guidance of the child in all aspects of development, not only in the treatment of the diabetes, requires great patience, forbearance, and understanding on the part of the parent and physician. The child and the parent must recognize the interrelationship of diet, insulin, and activity and the importance of regulation. It is equally important that the child learn—and parents understand—that the child can take his or her place in the family and society just as the nondiabetic child.

Modification of the Diet   The principles of dietary modification for the diabetic child are similar to those for the adult. (See Chapter 36.) The nutritive requirements are the same as those for the normal child of the same age, size, and activity. (See Chapter 21.) Briefly, these needs are as follows:

Calories.   An intake of 48 to 100 kcal per kg (22 to 45 kcal per pound) is required according to age and activity.

Protein.   The recommended daily allowance is, for younger children, 1.5 g per kg (0.68 g per pound), and for older children, 1.0 g per kg (0.45 g per pound). The American Diabetes Association recommends that 12 to 20 percent of total calories be provided as protein.[8]

Carbohydrate.   From 50 to 60 percent of calories are from carbohydrate. About 70 percent of the carbohydrate is starch, with the remainder from lactose, fructose, or sucrose.

Fat.   The remaining calories are from fat, with an emphasis on polyunsaturated fats and restriction of saturated fats and cholesterol.

Other.   The additional calcium requirements are easily met when 3 to 4 cups of milk are included daily. Other minerals and vitamins are provided in satisfactory amounts when the exchange lists are used as the basis of meal planning. Children should receive vitamin D either in milk or as a supplement.

The diet prescription should be adjusted periodically to make allowances for satisfactory growth. Emphasis should be on day-to-day consistency in distribution of calories and carbohydrate for meals and snacks in accordance with the type and action of insulin and physical activity. Most children receive NPH insulin; thus, an appropriate division of calories and carbohydrate might be 2/10, 2/10, 3/10 for the three main meals and 1/10 at each of three snacks taken in the midmorning, midafternoon, and evening. Some clinicians favor regularity of calorie intake using a fixed dose of insulin, whereas others prefer adjustment of insulin dosage without changing the basic meal pattern. Children should receive a snack prior to exercise and should have available rapidly utilized carbohydrate such as juice, carbonated drinks, or candy to forestall the possibility of an insulin reaction during and after exercise.

Dietary Control   Although the life span of diabetic children has improved greatly, the incidence of degenerative diseases is unusually high after 10 to 20 years. The possibilities of diminished vision and even blindness, of coronary artery disease, and of kidney disease during the prime of life are serious, and as yet unsolved, problems. Retinopathy is present in most persons who have had diabetes for many years. Diabetic neuropathy is common in patients in whom the disease is long standing and poorly controlled. Renal disease accounts for half the deaths in insulin-dependent diabetics of many years.[9]

Measurement of hemoglobin A_{1C} (HbA_{1C}) is one means of assessing long-term control of hyperglycemia. The level of HbA_{1C} is normally less than 5 percent, but in persistent hyperglycemia may be 6 to 10 percent. Many investigators believe that the degenerative changes are related to persistent hyperglycemia and that the changes can be delayed many years if the diabetes is well controlled. Under such control the blood sugar is kept as nearly normal as possible and glycosuria is avoided for the most part.

Some pediatricians use a so-called *free diet*, allowing the child to eat all family foods but usually including snacks and restricting concentrated sweets and high-carbohydrate desserts. Enough insulin is given to metabolize food for normal growth and to avoid ketosis, but mild hyperglycemia and glycosuria are disregarded. At the other extreme are those pediatricians who maintain rigid chemical control and require weighed or carefully measured diets.

Insulin   In early stages of juvenile diabetes the pancreas sometimes produces small amounts of insulin, but this rapidly diminishes. As growth accelerates the insulin requirement increases greatly and control becomes much more difficult.

Some clinicians recommend at least two doses of intermediate-acting insulin for the desirable three-meal-plus-snacks pattern. The morning dose is a mixture of regular and NPH insulin. A second dose of intermediate-acting insulin is given late in the afternoon (about 5:00 P.M.). With this program the blood sugar is maintained as nearly normal as possible throughout the 24-hour day. This regimen is intended to avoid glycosuria or insulin reactions.

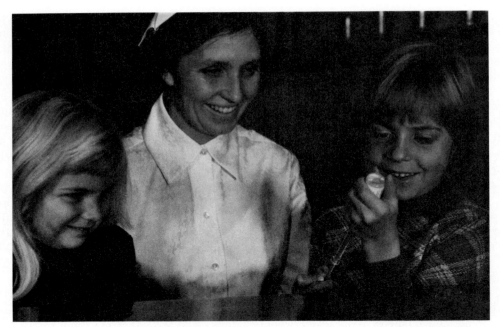

Figure 43-2. Success! Learning to measure his own insulin is an important first step toward independence for the young diabetic. (Courtesy, International Diabetes Center, Minneapolis.)

DIETARY COUNSELING

Whenever possible, initial hospitalization is desirable not only to stabilize the diabetes in the child but especially to set up an adequate program of education. The child and parents must face the issue of diabetes squarely, but also recognize that the child can live a happy, useful life. Regardless of the opinions about chemical or clinical control, pediatricians agree that close adherence to the diet at the beginning provides security and guidance for the child and parent during the period of adjustment to the disease. The initial diet could be one that provides few substitutions until the patient is thoroughly accustomed to it; then gradually the diet is liberalized with respect to the food choices until the meal exchange lists are used with ease. On festive occasions, such as birthdays and holidays, allowance for special treats should be made.

Children, like adults, need to be taught the nature of the disease, how to administer insulin, how to select the daily diet from the plan set up, how to test the urine, and how to keep records. (See Figure 43-2.) The importance of cleanliness and personal hygiene must be emphasized. The recognition of the signs of insulin reactions or of acidosis and what to do when these signs appear must be learned. See also pages 512 to 514 for further details on dietary counseling.

Diabetic camps provide an unusual educational opportunity for children to learn more about the care of themselves and also to learn the important social adjustments with other children. Such camps are well staffed with recreational leaders, nurses, dietitians, physicians, and laboratory technicians.

Renal Diseases

The causes of renal disease in children are similar to those in adults. The etiology, clinical manifestations, biochemical abnormalities, and principles of dietary modification are discussed in Chapter 40. These considerations hold for children as well, although quantitative differences must be taken into account. In this section nephrotic syndrome and chronic renal insufficiency in children are considered.

Nephrotic Syndrome

Symptoms and Clinical Findings The term NE-PHROTIC SYNDROME is used to describe a group of signs and symptoms that are characteristically seen in renal and systemic diseases. The syndrome is manifested by heavy proteinuria (more than 4 g in 24 hours), hypoalbuminemia, marked edema, and hypercholesterolemia. Albumin is lost in the largest amounts, but losses of other proteins such as ceruloplasmin, transferrin, gamma globulin, and thyroxine-binding protein increase susceptibility to infection. As the serum albumin level falls, the colloid osmotic pressure is no longer maintained and fluid moves into interstitial spaces, resulting in edema. Serum lipids, especially cholesterol, are markedly elevated, but the reasons are not clear.

The aims of therapy include control of infections and edema and establishment of good nutrition. Diuretics and sometimes sodium restriction are employed. Corticosteroids are used for some patients.

Modification of the Diet Patients with nephrosis have a particularly poor appetite, and the high-calorie high-protein diets that are often ordered are not necessarily consumed. Much attention must be given to the selection of foods that are acceptable to the child. With the loss of edema fluid the appetite usually improves. (See Figure 43-3.)

Diuretics are prescribed in the presence of edema. Some limit intake of salty foods, while others permit less than 2 g sodium per day and may limit sodium to 500 mg per day until edema is corrected. (See Chapter 39.)

The caloric intake should be based on the desirable weight for the child's height and body build. Unless the caloric intake is adequate, effective tissue regeneration cannot take place. The protein intake is generally a little higher than normal; about 3 to 4 g per kg is suitable for the preschool child and 2 to 3 g per kg for school-age children.

High protein supplements that are low in sodium are sometimes useful in boosting calorie intake. In some areas, low sodium fluid milk is available and can be used to increase the protein intake. Measures to reduce elevated lipids by altering the type and amount of dietary fat were discussed in Chapter 38.

Nutritional Effects of Drug Therapy. Diuretics such as thiazides and furosemide increase potassium losses in urine and may lead to hypokalemia unless preventive measures are taken. Potassium supplements or emphasis on foods that are rich in potassium are needed in these cases. (See Chapter 40.) Patients taking prednisone have increased need for pyridoxine, ascorbic acid, and vitamin D.[6]

Chronic Renal Insufficiency

A major problem in most children on long-term dialysis for chronic renal disease is growth failure. The etiology is complex and inadequate caloric intake is just one of the several factors involved. Poor appetite and multiple dietary restrictions make food less appealing.

Figure 43-3. The dietitian talks with a young child to determine what foods she likes. This is the first step in planning a diet that will meet the child's needs and that will be well accepted. (Courtesy, Hennepin County Medical Center, Minneapolis.)

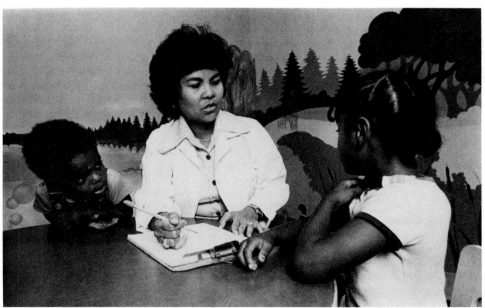

Dietary Considerations A major difficulty with the diet is providing adequate calories without exceeding the protein, mineral, and fluid allowances. The calorie intake needed for optimal growth is not known. Some recommend 70 kcal per kg in order to maintain nitrogen balance.[10] The protein allowance initially is limited to 0.5 g per kg per 24 hours and is provided chiefly in the form of high biologic value protein. As symptoms and biochemical values improve, and for children on dialysis, 1 to 2 g protein per kg is permitted daily. Foods containing relatively large amounts of incomplete proteins, such as peas and beans, are limited in the diet. Milk intake may also need to be limited due to its high sodium, potassium, and phosphorus content. Sodium is restricted if there is hypertension, edema, or excessive weight gain between dialyses. Hyperkalemia occurs and usually necessitates moderate potassium restriction, 1 mEq per kg per day.[10] Diuretics are also used to increase potassium excretion.

Children with chronic renal failure commonly experience hypocalcemia, hyperphosphatemia, and bone disease. The hypocalcemia and renal osteodystrophy are attributed primarily to impaired ability of the kidney to convert 25-hydroxycholecalciferol to 1,25-dihydroxycholecalciferol. Dietary phosphorus intake is restricted, and aluminum hydroxide is given to bind dietary phosphate. Calcium and vitamin D supplements are needed. A number of suitable commercial products and recipes low in protein, sodium, and potassium are available, but monotony and lack of palatability limit their acceptance by many patients. Supplements of the B-complex vitamins, folic acid, ascorbic acid, and trace minerals are needed, especially for patients on dialysis. Ferrous sulfate is recommended for patients who have iron-deficiency anemia.

Because of the many nutritional problems in this disease, parents of these children require much guidance in meal planning in order that they can provide appropriate foods that are acceptable to the child.

Epilepsy

The Nature of Epilepsy Epilepsy is a disease of the central nervous system characterized by loss of consciousness, which may last for only a few seconds, as in petit mal attacks, or which may be accompanied by convulsions, as in grand mal attacks. It occurs more frequently in children than in adults. The disease in no way affects the individual's mental ability, but unthinking relatives and friends sometimes attach an entirely unwarranted stigma to the disease and thus may increase the tension states in the individual.

Treatment Various drugs such as phenobarbital or phenytoin sodium or others have been employed with considerable success in the treatment of epilepsy and have largely replaced the ketogenic diet once so widely used. As a rule, a normal diet for the individual's age and activity is prescribed when drug therapy is used. Low biotin levels in plasma, folate deficiency, anemia, and osteomalacia have been attributed to use of these drugs. Phenytoin may interfere with the metabolism of vitamin K or of vitamin D.[11] Gastric distress associated with valproic acid therapy can be minimized by giving the drug with meals.

Some individuals with minor motor seizures and petit mal epilepsy who do not respond to drug therapy have been successfully managed with a ketogenic diet. The purpose of the diet is to produce ketosis by limiting very severely the amount of available glucose and increasing markedly the intake of fat so that complete combustion of fats cannot take place. Plasma ketones (acetone, acetoacetic acid, and beta-hydroxybutyric acid) gradually rise as glycogen stores become depleted. The accumulation of ketone bodies has a favorable effect on the irritability and restlessness of the child and does not dull the mental function as some drugs do. Preschool-age children seem to benefit most, presumably because higher plasma ketone levels can be achieved with the diet in this age group than in older children. A rapid reversal of the anticonvulsant effect occurs when even small amounts of carbohydrate are ingested, and leads to seizures as the plasma ketones fall.

Some of the difficult features of the diet are that it permits selection from only a very limited list of foods, is severely restricted in carbohydrate, is unpalatable, lacks bulk, deviates sharply from customary food patterns, and requires great care in planning and preparation. A careful evaluation of the probable success of the diet for each patient and the ability of the parents to understand and adhere to the regulations is essential.

Modification of the Diet Sufficient calories for normal weight and for the maintenance of normal growth are necessary. The allowances recommended by Mike[12] are

Age (years)	kcal per kg
2–3	100 to 80
3–5	80 to 60
5–10	79 to 55

Protein. An allowance of 1 g protein per kg of body weight is sufficient, but may be increased to 1.5 g per kg for the older child.

Carbohydrate and Fat. The nonprotein calories are so divided that a ketogenic to antiketogenic ratio of approximately 3:1 or 4:1 is maintained. Ketogenic factors (fatty acids) in the diet include 90 percent of the fat, and about 50 percent of the protein. The antiketogenic factors in the diet (available glucose) are derived fom 100 percent of the carbohydrate, plus approximately 50 percent of the protein and 10 percent of the fat. Obviously, to achieve a 3:1 or 4:1 ratio, the carbohydrate must be sharply restricted and the fat intake greatly increased. The level of carbohydrate usually needs to be less than 30 g if ketosis is to be produced, but should never be less than 10 g daily.

The diet for a 5-year-old child weighing 25 kg illustrates the calculation of a diet prescription

1. Kcal: $25 \times 70 = 1750$
2. Protein: $25 \times 1 = 25$ gm
3. Kcal from protein: $25 \times 4 = 100$
4. Kcal from carbohydrate and fat:
   $1750 - 100 = 1650$

If we allow 25 g carbohydrate, the fat intake would need to be 172 g as noted in the following calculations:

5. Kcal from carbohydrate: $25 \times 4 = 100$
6. Kcal from fat: $1,650 - 100 = 1,550$
7. Grams of fat: $1,550 \div 9 = 172$

The fatty acid-to-glucose ratio of this diet is as follows:

$$\frac{FA}{AG} = \frac{0.50(25) + 0.9(172)}{0.50(25) + 0.1(172) + 1.0(25)} = \frac{167}{55} = \frac{3}{1}$$

The maintenance of a constant acidosis requires that the protein, fat, and carbohydrate for the day be divided in three equal meals. The urine shows a positive test for acetoacetic acid when acidosis is being maintained.

Minerals and Vitamins. Calcium carbonate, gluconate, or lactate is prescribed to furnish calcium. An iron supplement providing 7 to 10 mg elemental iron is also given. The vitamin needs are met by giving an aqueous multivitamin preparation.

Management of the Diet For the first 24 to 72 hours the child is given nothing but water, usually restricted to 500 to 1,000 ml. Hunger disappears as ketosis increases. When ketosis is marked the diet is initiated, but is not forced until the transition has been accomplished. During this period nausea and vomiting may occur.

The diet may be calculated by using the values for individual foods as in Table A-1, or by using food groupings such as those developed by Mike[12] or Lasser.[13] The meal exchange lists are not satisfactory for the calculation. The predominant foods in the diet are carefully restricted amounts of meat, cheese, and eggs; cream, butter, bacon, mayonnaise; and restricted amounts of low-carbohydrate vegetables and fruits. Other foods are avoided: sugar-containing beverages; breads and cereals; desserts such as cake, cookies, ice cream, pastries, pie, puddings; milk; all sweets including sugar, jellies, candy, preserves; vegetables and fruits high in carbohydrate.

The diet must be weighed on a gram scale, and all food must be consumed at each meal. Foods may not be saved for later consumption. If no improvement occurs within 6 weeks, there is nothing to be gained by further continuance of the diet. If improvement does occur, the diet must be continued for a year or longer. Gradually the diet is liberalized with very small increases in the carbohydrate and corresponding caloric decreases in the fat. Table 43-1 illustrates a sample calculation for the ketogenic diet.

Signore[14] has described a ketogenic diet using medium-chain triglycerides. Inasmuch as medium-chain triglycerides are more ketogenic than conventional food fats, more carbohydrate is permitted on this diet. Foods need not be weighed.

Feeding Handicapped Children

Cerebral Palsy This is a disorder in which motor control is disturbed due to brain damage. It affects some 300,000 children in the United States. A significant proportion weigh less than 2,500 g at birth. Cerebral anoxia may be an etiologic factor in these infants. Feeding problems are common in children with cerebral palsy.

Reverse Swallowing Wave. When the motor system of the tongue and throat is affected, food is not pushed back to the throat; instead, the tongue motion pushes the food forward. Initially such children must be tube fed, but in time they learn to put food at the back of the tongue and, by tilting the head backward, learn to swallow. These children often become severely undernourished because feeding is such a prolonged process. Concentrated foods with maximum

Table 43-1. **Sample Calculation for Ketogenic Diet***

Food	No. of Units	Household Measure	Weight (g)	Protein (g)	Fat (g)	Carbohydrate (g)
Breakfast						
Orange juice	4	⅙ cup	40	—	—	4.0
Canadian bacon	6	¾ slice	21	6.0	3.0	—
Whipping cream	2½	½ cup	115	2.5	42.5	3.8
Cellu wafers						
Butter	2	2¼ teaspoons	12	—	10.9	—
Apricot spread (Cellu)	½	1 teaspoon	5	—	—	0.5
				8.5	56.4	8.3
Luncheon or Supper						
Beef, lean	6	⅔ ounce	21	6.0	3.0	—
Tomato, raw	1	¼ small	25	0.2	—	1.0
Whipping cream	2½	½ cup	115	2.5	42.5	3.8
Peach, raw	3	⅓ small	30	—	—	3.0
Butter	2	2¼ teaspoons	12	—	10.9	—
Cellu wafers						
Blackberry jelly (Cellu)	½	1 teaspoon	5	—	—	0.5
				8.7	56.4	8.3
Dinner						
Cheddar cheese	5	⅔ ounce	20	5.0	5.0	—
Strawberries	4	4 large	40	—	—	4.0
Whipping cream	2½	½ cup	115	2.5	42.5	3.8
Butter	2	2¼ teaspoons	12	—	10.9	—
Cellu wafers						
Apricot spread (Cellu)	½	1 teaspoon	5	—	—	0.5
				7.5	58.4	8.3
Total for the day (Prescribed order)				24.7 (25.0)	171.2 (172.0)	24.9 (25.0)

$$\frac{\text{Ketogenic factors}}{\text{Antiketogenic factors}} = \frac{166.4}{54.4} = 3.1$$

* Based on plan described by Lasser, J. L., and Brush, M. K.: "An Improved Ketogenic Diet for Treatment of Epilepsy," *J. Am. Diet. Assoc.*, **62**:281–85, 1973.

protein and calorie value should be emphasized to keep the volume to a minimum. Vitamin and mineral supplements are usually required.

Athetoids are those who are constantly in motion and who thus burn up a great deal of energy. Although they require a high-calorie high-protein diet, the ingestion of the necessary amounts of food is difficult because of the constant motion. Feeding is quite time consuming and emphasis should be placed on concentrated foods of high caloric value. Children should be encouraged to feed themselves by giving them foods that they can pick up with their fingers such as pieces of fruit and sandwiches. Many devices have been developed as aids in feeding. (See page 398.)

Spastics are very limited in their activity and they may also be indulged in eating by their parents or caregivers. Consequently they gain excessive amounts of weight, and the obesity in turn further restricts their ability to get around. These individuals require marked restriction of caloric intake without jeopardizing the intake of protein, minerals, and vitamins.

Cleft Palate The incidence of cleft palate is 1 in 2,500 births, and that of cleft lip 1 per 1,000 births. Surgery for cleft palate is often not completed for several years. In addition to the needs for normal development, the infant and child must build up reserves for surgery, the promotion of healing, and the development of normal healthy gums and teeth. Several considerations should be borne in mind in feeding these children.

1. Infants may have difficulty in sucking, but most learn to use chewing movements to get the milk out of the nipple. An enlarged nipple opening is helpful. A Beniflex feeder with crosscut nipple is used in some cases. Some babies may be fed with a medicine dropper. Feeding in an upright position is helpful.
2. To counteract the tendency to choke, liquids should be taken in small amounts and swallowed slowly.
3. More frequent "burpings" are necessary because of the large amount of air that may be swallowed.
4. Spicy and acid foods often irritate the mouth and nose and should be avoided. If orange juice is not well taken, ascorbic acid supplements should be prescribed.
5. Among the foods that may get into the opening of the palate are peanut butter, peelings of raw fruit, nuts, leafy vegetables, and creamed dishes. Some children have no difficulty with any foods.
6. Puréed foods may be diluted with milk, fruit juice, or broth and given from a bottle with a large nipple opening. Some babies accept purées well if they are thickened with vanilla wafer or graham cracker crumbs.
7. The time required for feeding may be long and requires much patience on the part of parent and nurse. For the older child, five or six small meals may be better than three.

When surgery has been performed, a liquid or puréed diet is offered until healing is complete.

Mental Retardation   Some 3 percent of persons in the United States are estimated to be mentally retarded. It is often difficult to distinguish the truly retarded child from one who functions at a retarded level because of environmental factors. From 85 to 90 percent of the retarded are designated as mildly retarded (educable) and have an IQ between 50 and 75.

This type tends to be associated with disadvantaged socioeconomic groups such as children of migrant farm workers who are deprived of opportunities for intellectual, cultural, or social development. Approximately 10 percent of the mentally retarded are moderately retarded; that is, they have an IQ between 35 and 50 (trainable). The profoundly retarded individual with an IQ below 35 is believed to account for 5 percent of the mentally retarded and presents the problems in feeding; however, even the profoundly retarded can be trained to eat properly and to use good table manners.

The nutritional requirements of the mentally retarded child and adult are like those of the individual of normal mental development. The nurse can help parents to understand the problems of feeding by giving encouragement and support.

The mentally retarded child may be kept on the bottle too long, thus increasing the difficulties of introducing other foods. The child may eat very slowly, and feeding may be messy. Hand sucking and vomiting are not uncommon. To obtain adequate food intake for growth may require frequent, small feedings, and certainly an abundance of patience and ingenuity. One must strike a balance between overprotectiveness and lack of caring.

Retarded individuals, like normal persons, have an active emotional life. They feel the shunning of others and failure to achieve, but will respond to loving attention. They resist new foods, have definite likes and dislikes, and find it difficult to manage eating. They respond to the color of foods and like all children are fond of sweets.

When individuals are able to feed themselves, they should be permitted to do so even though feeding may be messy. Food must be presented in a form that can be easily managed. Foods may be eaten with the fingers for a long time until simple utensils can be managed. Children unable to support themselves should be held in a sitting position while they are being fed.

CASE STUDY 28

Ten-year-old Boy with Diabetes Mellitus (Puerto Rican)

Mr. and Mrs. G and their three children migrated from Puerto Rico to New York City 2 years ago when Mr. G found work in the garment industry. The family lives in a four-room flat in Spanish Harlem. Only Spanish is spoken in the home. Mr. and Mrs. G have a limited understanding of En-

glish, but they are unable to read English. Their 10-year-old son, José, speaks English fairly fluently and often serves as the interpreter for the family.

Since he was diagnosed with type I insulin-dependent diabetes mellitus 6 months ago, José has had several insulin reactions during school hours. He is very active and enjoys contact sports. However, he has difficulty matching his food intake with exercise so that he does not develop hypoglycemia. He has gym 2 days a week before lunch, and he has developed insulin reactions after playing strenuous games such as kickball and volleyball. His classmates tease him about acting strangely and eating candy bars during gym class. José has told his friends nothing about his diabetes because he is afraid they will tease him all the more and not play with him.

José has been taking a fixed dose of 16 units NPH and 8 units of regular U-100 insulin before breakfast each morning. He usually gives his own insulin in either his upper arms or thighs. He does not test his urine at school, although he has written "0/0" in his diabetic record book in the noon-hour slot. He thinks that his record should show as many negatives as possible.

The dietitian at the outpatient clinic has been working with José and his mother to develop a realistic meal plan that will fit within their meager income, account for food preferences, and provide needed nutrients for José's growth. José weighs 28 kg (61½ lb) and is 140 cm (55 in.) tall. Mrs. G has difficulty understanding and planning José's 2,300 kcal diabetic diet. The main source of protein in the G family's diet consists of legumes. They rarely have meat and they eat few green or leafy vegetables. Lard and olive oil are used in cooking. Favorite foods include viandas, legumes, chicken, and bacalao.

During a recent clinic visit, a public health referral was made to help José and his family adapt the treatment plan to the school and home environment. The public health nurse met with José's homeroom teacher, the school food service manager, and the school nurse. José's gym class was changed to after lunch, and the rationale for extra food intake before strenuous exercise was explained to the teachers. The public health nurse made plans for follow-up visits with José and his mother to educate them further regarding the day-to-day management of José's diabetes.

Pathophysiologic Correlations

1. What metabolic changes explain each of the symptoms typically seen in uncontrolled type I diabetes mellitus: polydipsia; weight loss; loss of consciousness; Kussmaul's respirations?

2. How can you explain the frequent insulin reactions that José was having during school hours?

3. How would you describe the symptomatic differences between ketoacidosis and hypoglycemia to Mrs. G?

4. List some factors believed to play a role in the etiology of insulin-dependent diabetes mellitus.

Nutritional Assessment

5. What is the normal weight range for José?

6. List the foods that are eaten most often by Puerto Rican people.

7. What foods are used sparingly by most Puerto Rican people?

8. Why is consideration of the supplementary value of proteins important in planning diets for Puerto Ricans?

Planning the Diet

9. List the objectives that you would set up for planning José's diet.

10. Why is it important to regulate the intake of protein and fat as well as that of carbohydrate?

11. The physician ordered the following diet for José: carbohydrate, 310 g; protein, 85 g; fat, 80 g. How many calories does this diet contain? Calculate the percentage of calories that are derived from fat.

12. The dietitian calculated the diet prescribed for José and arranged the exchanges for three meals and three snacks as follows:
    a. Using Table A-4, calculate the carbohydrate, protein, and fat provided for the day by the following pattern.
    b. Write a menu for 1 day according to the above distribution.

13. What level of protein is recommended for José from the table of Recommended Dietary Allowances? Examine the calculations for José's diet and state the problem that would be encountered if protein were restricted to the recommended level.

	Breakfast	Mid-morning	Lunch	Mid-afternoon	Dinner	Bedtime
Milk	½	1	1	1		½
Vegetables			1		2	
Fruit	1			1	2	1
Bread	3	1	3	1	4	1
Meat			1		2	
Fat	2	1	2		4	1

14. Why is José given both regular and NPH insulin? What is the duration of effect of each type of insulin? What adjustments in meal planning are required when these insulins are used?
15. Check the foods that would be most suitable to quickly correct signs of insulin shock: milk, sugar, butter, peanut butter sandwich, ginger ale, jelly beans, cheese, pineapple juice, diet cola.

Dietary Counseling
16. Which aspects of the diet should be emphasized in counseling the G family?
17. Suggest some practical ways by which the nurse could assist José in learning about the requirements of his diet.

18. José's mother has many questions and comments when the public health nurse makes her visit to the home. How would you respond to each of the following if you were the nurse?
   a. "What should we do when José's urine shows 2 percent sugar?"
   b. "José hasn't gained any weight for 2 months now."
   c. "José sneaks cookies and cake when I am not around."
   d. "My neighbor has diabetes but doesn't take insulin. When José grows up can he stop taking insulin?"
   e. "Will my other children get diabetes, too?"

References for the Case Study

Faro, B.:"Maintaining Good Control in Children with Diabetes," *Pediatr. Nurs.*, 9:368–73, 1983.
Hopper, S. V.: "Meeting the Needs of the Economically Deprived Diabetic," *Nurs. Clin. North Am*, 18:813–25, Dec. 1983.
Krause, K. L., and Madden, P.: "The Child with Diabetes Mellitus," *Nurs. Clin. North Am.*, 18:749–62, Dec. 1983.
Lindsey, N. M.: "Coping with Diabetes," *Nursing '83*, 13: 48–9, March 1983.
Skyler, J. S.: "Dietary Planning in Insulin-Dependent Diabetes Mellitus," *Pediatr. Ann.*, 12:652–7, 1983.
Yohai, F.: "Dietary Patterns of Spanish-Speaking People Living in the Boston Area," *J. Am. Diet. Assoc.*, 71:273–5, 1977.

Problems and Review

1. What dietary problems may be anticipated in children who must be hospitalized? How can these problems be overcome?
2. How can a schoolchild be helped to adjust to a prolonged therapeutic diet?
3. *Problem*. Plan a day's meals for a 3-year-old child with celiac disease for whom a gluten-restricted diet has been ordered. He is 34 inches tall and weighs 11 kg; he appears to be somewhat undernourished.
4. What are the similarities between celiac disease and cystic fibrosis? What differences are there?
5. List several ways in which milk intolerance may be manifested. What substances in milk have been shown to produce such sensitivity? List three products that may be used satisfactorily in place of a milk formula.
6. *Problem*. For a 2-year-old child with nephrosis plan a suitable diet containing 25 g protein and 1,200 kcal. How would you modify the diet for 500 mg sodium?
7. List some of the considerations to be kept in mind when planning the diet for a child undergoing chronic hemodialysis.

References

1. Gurwitz, D., et al.: "Perspectives in Cystic Fibrosis," *Pediatr. Clin. North Am.*, 26:603–15, 1979.
2. Hodges, P., et al.: "Nutrient Intake of Patients with Cystic Fibrosis," *J. Am. Diet. Assoc.*, 84:664–9, 1984.
3. Hubbard, V. S., and Mangruen, P. J.: "Energy Intake and Nutrition Counseling in Cystic Fibrosis," *J. Am. Diet. Assoc.*, 80:127–31, 1982.
4. Gryboski, J.: "Inflammatory Bowel Disease in Children," *Med. Clin. North Am.*, 64:1185–1202, 1980.
5. Ste. Marie, M.: "Symposium on the Treatment of Inflammatory Bowel Disease in Children and Adolescents," *Can. J. Surg.*, 25:495–8, 1982.
6. Moore, A. O., and Powers, D. E.: *Food–Medication Interactions*, 3rd ed. F-MI Publishing, Tempe, Arizona 1981.
7. Review: "Allergy to Other Dietary Proteins in Infants with Intolerance to Cow's Milk Protein," *Nutr. Rev.*, 40:333–5, 1982.
8. American Diabetes Association: "Principles of Nutrition and Dietary Recommendations for Individuals with Diabetes Mellitus, 1979," *Diabetes*, 28:1027–30, 1979.
9. Marshall, R. N.: "Juvenile Diabetes Mellitus," *Am. Fam. Physician*, 25: 193–8, January 1982.
10. Shane, R.: "Chronic Renal Failure," in *Pediatric Therapy*, 6th ed. C. V. Mosby Company, St. Louis, 1980.
11. Delgado-Eseveta, A.V., et al.: "The Treatable Epilepsies," *N. Engl. J. Med.*, 308:1576–84, 1983.
12. Mike, E. M.: "Practical Guide and Dietary Management of Children with Seizures Using the Ketogenic Diet, *Am. J. Clin. Nutr.*, 77:399–405, 1965.
13. Lasser, J. L., and Brush, M. K.: "An Improved Ketogenic Diet for Treatment of Epilepsy," *J. Am. Diet. Assoc.*, 62:281–85, 1973.
14. Signore, J. M.: "Ketogenic Diet Using Medium-Chain Triglycerides," *J. Am. Diet. Assoc*, 62:285–90, 1973.

44

Computer Applications in Clinical Nutrition*

Computer-age technology is influencing all facets of clinical nutrition practice. Microcomputers are being used in both the clinical and educational components of dietetics. Thus it behooves students of nutrition, dietetics, nursing, and other health care professions to seek education about computer terminology and technology[1] in order to capitalize on this trend and to use computers effectively to enhance their professional performance and competitiveness in today's high-tech environment.

The use of computers as an adjunct to the administrative aspects of health care is widely accepted. Historically computers were first applied to food service management, production, inventory, forecasting, recipe development, and other related areas. Those applications are reviewed in detail elsewhere.[2] The value of computers in direct clinical support roles and in the training and education of nutrition students continues to elicit controversy. This chapter will review computer applications in clinical nutrition, primarily as it relates to their use in nutritional assessment and in nutrition education.

Microcomputer applications will be emphasized, since it is possible to run, on microcomputers, large programs that were previously restricted to mainframes. With the recent dramatic reduction in price and size, and the increase in processing capability, reliability and availability, microcomputers are feasible for both professional and home use.

An in-depth review of computer hardware and software is beyond the scope of this chapter. Selected references are listed at the end of this chapter for those interested in initiating market investigation. However, new computer applications are proliferating at such a rate that it is difficult to stay current.

* Written by Darla E. Danford, M.P.H., D.Sc., R.D.; National Academy of Sciences, Washington, D.C.

Microcomputers

Software Any decision regarding a microcomputer purchase should begin with a thorough evaluation of software needs. There are many guides to assist in software evaluation.[1-7] Software trends are taking advantage of new hardware capabilities and are using interactive English languages that are understandable by uninitiated users. Many of the popular integrated packages that combine spread sheets, word processing and graphic generation are being adapted for use in nutrition settings.

Hardware Current and anticipated software application requirements determine the need for a micro-, mini-, or mainframe computer or timesharing services.[8] Software and hardware choices should be flexible enough to allow one to capitalize on new innovations, as they become available.

Hardware choices primarily consist of (1) *input devices*: traditional QWERTY keyboard, ergonomic keyboard, voice-recognition devices, touch screens, soft keys, bar code readers, light pen, mouse, joy stick, digitizer; (2) *monitors*: color, monotone, high resolution, liquid crystal; (3) *operating system*: CPM, DOS, UNIX; (4) *hardware family compatibility:* IBM PC, Apple II; (5) *storage devices*: floppy disc, hard disk, laser compact disk or videodisk, bubble memory, optical disk, laser-encoded holographic storage; and (6) *peripherals*: dot-matrix or letter-quality printers, laser printers, plotters, modems, voice synthesizers, local area network, and work-station connections. Descriptive information on these and other hardware options is available.[1,3]

Data Bases Most software used in nutrition application programs is oriented around a nutrient data base. Table 44-1 outlines the nutrient data bases commonly used.[19,20] The quality of a nutrient data base is

Table 44-1. Selected Computerized Nutrient Data Bases

Data Base Source	Reference Number*
Home & Garden Bulletin No. 72	9
Handbook No. 8	10
Handbook No. 456	11
National Nutrient Data Bank	12
NHLBI	13
Pennington & Church	14
NSMP	15
INFOODS	16
Mini List	17
Ohio State	18

*References listed at the end of this chapter.

crucial to the quality of nutritional care it supports. Issues the professional user should be concerned with include missing values that are either treated as zero or imputed; nonstandard conversion factors or number-rounding functions; inability to address biologic availability, storage losses, genetic differences, cooking losses, climatic factors, or the effect of food processing on nutrient composition; inflexible data bases that do not permit updates or changes in nutrient composition data; adequacy of the analyzed nutrient data, which differ by food and by nutrient[21]; ability to enter foods by English food name, thereby avoiding transcription errors associated with numerical coding; and the inclusion of "smart" entry programs to minimize errors.[18-22] The effect of these problems is illustrated by recent comparative studies showing that the identical diet analyzed by different diet analysis data bases can generate different nutrient values.[21-24]

Computer Use in Nutritional Assessment

Microcomputers can enhance the quality of nutritional assessment in a variety of clinical settings. Computer applications will be reviewed as they relate to the traditional components of nutritional assessment discussed in Chapter 23.

Anthropometric and Body Composition Measurements Many of the measurement tools used in anthropometrics, such as weight scales, underwater weighing apparatus, whole-body counters, and skinfold calipers, are available interfaced directly to microcomputers through the use of built-in microprocessors (computer on a chip) and communication cables.

Direct interfacing of measurement device and of computer eliminates errors in the tedious process of first recording data by hand and then entering these data into the computer. Computer-interfaced systems are more expensive and are probably only cost effective in situations requiring large-scale use. Whether data are entered automatically or by hand, the microcomputer greatly enhances the speed of calculations, automatically does specified conversions and/or comparisons with standards, provides information storage for trend and research analysis, and provides instant retrieval capability and printout options. Standard value, range of values, formulas, and nomograms such as illustrated in the Appendix can be incorporated into nutrition software. (See Table 44-2.)

Examples of microcomputer-enhanced anthropometric measurements include circumference and skinfold measurements,[30-33] bone diameters,[33] height and weight,[30-33] resting energy expenditure,[30,31] basal metabolic rate,[30,32] respiratory quotients,[32] and hydrostatic weighing.[33] Computer printouts of these data are primarily used in clinical settings for patients on total parenteral nutrition.[30-32] Others have applied these measurements to generate computer prescriptions for nutrition and exercise regimes in healthy, free-living subjects.[33]

Clinical Assessment Chapter 23 contains an extensive list of the clinical signs and symptoms that should alert the health professional to the risk of nutritional deficiencies. Few computer applications have been developed to contribute effectively to this assessment area. Computer-enhanced simulations of symptoms in conjunction with an effective interactive questionnaire could be useful in patient information gathering as well as in student education. They could be especially helpful in teaching students to recognize rare nutrient-deficiency symptoms that are rarely encountered in hospitalized settings or that are unavailable at the time of teaching.

Table 44-2. Selected Computerized Data Base Standards

Nutritional Assessment	Reference Number*
Recommended Dietary Allowances	25
USRDA	26
Nutritive Quality Index	27
Height, weight	28
Resting energy expenditure	26, 29
Skinfolds	26, 27

*References listed at the end of this chapter.

Biochemical Assessment An advantage of computer use in biochemical assessment is direct data collection from the clinical laboratory, automatic storage, and data comparison with preset parameters. Computer programs frequently collect the analyzed laboratory value and compare it with a normal range for parameters as blood and urine vitamin, mineral, trace element, and macronutrient levels; skin tests; total white cell count; visceral protein values; and electrolytes.[30-34]

Diet Assessment An integral part of the nutritional assessment technique includes comparing the subject's nutrient intake over an established time period with a predetermined desirable intake range. (See Chapter 23.) There is a variety of software written for diet assessment and analysis:

Socratic dialogue to obtain diet history, including weight reduction, smoking habits, food preferences, and self-medication with nutritional supplements[35,36]

History taking combined with food models[36]

3-day[37] to 7-day[38] food records[4,22] with or without flagging of high-risk foods/nutrients, or printouts of nutrient density profiles[27]

Measurement of iron bioavailability of diet[39]

24-hour diet recalls[4,11,22]

Food-frequency records[40]

Epidemiologic surveys[13]

Microcomputers are excellent computational aids for calculating nutrient intakes, comparing actual with expected intakes, and statistically comparing individual with group intakes of populations at nutritional risk. Such application avoids the necessity of labor- and time-intensive, error-prone hand-calculation methods. Health care professionals can spend more time doing those tasks that are more difficult to computerize, namely, to interpret data for the subject and to make appropriate therapeutic recommendations.

There are extensive reviews of commercially available diet analysis software. The types and uses of computer diet analysis systems are limited only by imagination. Some notable software programs include uses in diet or meal planning for weight reduction, diet and exercise programs, fast-food-oriented diet plans, nutrient-balanced meal planners that utilize food preferences, meal planners that generate grocery shopping lists, and programs that list the best food sources of specified nutrients.[4,24,27,41] Examples of dietary guidelines (see Chapter 3) and standards for meal or diet comparison that are often incorporated into software are listed in Table 44-2.

Computer Use in Diet Counseling

The nutritional and dietary assessment applications discussed above are an integral part of inpatient, outpatient, and community diet counseling.

Interview Techniques Interviewing is not only essential to taking a nutritional history but it is a first step in any patient encounter. The initial interview most commonly includes the collection of demographic information and nutritional and relevant medical history data, as well as obtaining current information about food habits, drug history, diet intake, exercise, and lifestyle habits. The microcomputer has been used successfully with patients to ascertain this type of history.

Microcomputer use has several advantages. If the software is well written, the computer can carry on a friendly, informative dialogue with the patient, unlike the tedious written questionnaire that traditionally does not provide feedback. Utilization of branch functions in the program design can ensure that no pertinent questions are unanswered in the interview and that the interviewee will not be bothered by the asking of irrelevant questions. More importantly, computerized interviewing has been shown to save professional time and to obtain patient responses that are not biased by the interviewer. Studies have shown that patients are more honest about answering embarrassing questions asked by a computer than by a human interviewer.[42] The interview can easily be written in any foreign language. Studies reveal favorable reactions by interviewees to machine interviews.[42,43]

Sophisticated interview programs can collect information directly from patients when they first arrive in the clinic or hospital room, summarize the relevant nutritional data, and provide a printed summary before the patient is seen.[22,43] Interviewing can also be oriented to specific medical problems. Examples in the literature include applications in working with diabetes,[36,44] renal disease,[22] phenylketonuria,[45] heart disease,[13] and obesity.[4,35,46] History taken by computer has been shown to agree closely with one taken by health care professionals.[42] The same holds true for the interview used as part of a diet assessment, clinical examination, research study, patient monitoring or follow-up, diet instruction, and patient education.

Artificial Intelligence Artificial intelligence (AI) is no longer reserved for research computer scientists. Computers can now be programmed to make decisions as humans do, within a strictly limited domain. This application has potential in assisting nurses and dietitians in diagnosing nutritional problems, interpreting diagnostic tests, analyzing metabolic aberrations, detecting new genetic inborn errors, isolating drug–nutrient–metabolic problems, and planning appropriate diet therapies. AI in medicine has primarily been used to help design treatment protocols (by relying on accepted treatment patterns), to make diagnoses or analyses of the future risk of events (by using statistical probability matching from large patient data bases), and to create interactive advice systems (by utilizing facts in a process similar to human thinking). Proper use of AI techniques still involves human judgement for interpretation and application of the results.

Nutrition Care Plan Once the interview is conducted and the nutritional assessment data analyzed, a care plan must be devised. Computers can be a valuable adjunct to this process through their ability to quickly analyze diet information and plan diets that meet the patient's specific nutrient requirements. Generation of computerized care-plans may involve sophisticated kinetic or metabolic modeling[45] or specialized needs such as planning high-carbohydrate, high-fiber diets.[47] Preadmission computerized interviews can flag high-risk patients so that specialized care plans and early nutrition intervention can be initiated.

Patient instruction is time consuming, and very often professional time constraints prevent the patient from obtaining adequate diet instruction and being tested for accurate comprehension. Microcomputers can remedy this problem. The computer can teach patients about the background of their medical disorder, reinforce information about their therapeutic diet, help them apply diet requirements to their lifestyle, and show them how to make necessary diet changes. In addition, the patient can be computer tested as to their understanding of the above.[48] This allows the health professional to intervene and prevent problems associated with patient misunderstanding.

Bedside Monitoring Computers are increasingly being used in critical care and specialty areas of hospitals. The most comprehensive systems tie a bedside, nursing station, or desk computer into the existing computerized hospital information system (HIS). Computer-use possibilities include collecting patient data (ECG analysis, urine output measurements, drug doses) at the bedside, manipulating those data to assist the health professional with bedside care (drug-dose calculations, nutrient requirement needs, fluid and electrolyte requirements), automated control of correct infusion rate changes, and provision of instant data printouts when needed (graphs of weight, calorie, and protein intake changes over time.)[49,50]

Inpatients, especially those who are bedridden, and outpatients in waiting rooms or on dialysis usually have time to spare. The use of microcomputers to give self-instruction during this time not only makes their wait seem shorter but enhances their perceived and real quality of nutritional care. One example utilizes a portable microcomputer combined with an audio-video tutorial program that uses cartoons and pictorial self-tests.[51]

Charting and Follow-up Utilizing HIS, microcomputers can monitor all patient events, notify the proper department of needed tests and schedules, and provide instant access to medical records. Such microcomputer stations could be used by nurses and dietitians to enter their chart notes, to collate and retrieve demographic and laboratory data, to schedule tests and order changes, and to facilitate the writing and printing of discharge notes.[49,52]

As previously mentioned, computer technology permits data collection when the patient enters the clinic waiting room, and quick analysis for professional use and patient feedback is provided by the time the patient is seen. Despite the obvious advantages of such use, the professional must be critical of the limitations of computer-generated prescriptions. The computer cannot substitute for human clarification and interpretation of the results on a computerized printout. When these printouts are handed to patients without interpretation, or with computer-generated explanations, the patient very often misapplies the information and may make harmful behavioral or unnecessary modifications.

Computerized diet-counseling systems can facilitate follow-up and patient surveillance programs. One such system allows the dietitian to measure dietary compliance of the patient, to survey population subsets, and to compare the effectiveness of different dietary treatments for a particular diagnosis.[53]

Other Computer Applications

Research Computers have traditionally been used in clinical research centers to plan and measure selective or constant diets that satisfy nutrient constraints for balance studies[54]; to incorporate personal food preferences into research diet plans[55]; to facilitate protocol design, scheduling, and monitoring; and to do statistical analysis, and graphic and written printouts for research publication.

Nutrition surveys and epidemiologic studies often have the problem of huge data volumes to enter and analyze. The computer can permit quick data entry through the use of scanners or readers. Mainframe statistical packages required for sophisticated analysis of large data banks are now available for microcomputers. Electronic spread-sheet programs for microcomputers do basic statistics and generate quick graphic representations for smaller data sets.

Home Health Care Intelligent computer-controlled devices permit the use of sophisticated medical equipment in the home for chronic health care. Real-time computer-monitoring equipment can automatically change pump infusion rates or control infused drug dosages. Phones with microprocessor units in the professional's office can collect data and patient information automatically or at the patient's initiative. Computer applications in preventative medicine are popular for the consumer, such as the use of heart-rate monitors built into exercise bicycles.

Computer-Assisted Instruction

Computer-assisted instruction (CAI) was developed during the late 1950s. CAI may use computer terminals alone or may be enhanced with peripherals such as printers, graphics terminal, graphics tablet or with interfaces to tape recorders, videoplayers, slide projectors, or videodisks.

Software has evolved from the first IBM-authored CAI software (Coursewriter I), to a large-scale mainframe-oriented system (PLATO), to the utilization of medical oriented CAI languages (MUMPS), and to the current microcomputer CAI programs (PILOT).[6] Complicated educational programs with large data bases to be accessed by multiple simultaneous users generally require mainframes with "dumb" or "smart" (with built-in microcomputers) terminals.

CAI has been classified into four types of educational software:

Instructional[6]: Includes tutorials,[6,48,56] drill and practice,[6,56] dialogue formats,[6] and programmed instruction.[6] Usually boring, repetitive presentation of material, but most effective for subject matter requiring rote memorization.

Revelatory[6]: Includes inquiry-type dialogues and simulations,[6] Socratic-interview and self-assessment,[6,48] games and simulations,[6,48,56] and diagnostic simulations.[48] Tends to lead students through conceptual and discovery learning processes.

Conjectural[6]: Includes modeling formats,[6,48] problem solving,[6,56] and decision-support systems.[6] Generally use the computer to test ideas and theories.

Emancipatory[6]: Includes (1) computer-managed instruction,[6] which uses the computer to test, score, and develop instructional material based on the student's performance; (2) computational, statistics, administration,[6] information management, and retrieval,[56] which uses data-base management, spread-sheet, statistical, and financial software; and (3) word processing,[6] which handles text and document generation.

Elementary to College Education The literature outlines many CAI programs that have been tested in classroom settings. CAI can be successfully used by all age groups. Examples include

Nutrition games for grades 4 to 6[4,57]
Anatomy and nutrition for college students[58]
Protein chemical score concepts[59]
Digestion, food groups, and other basic nutrition concepts[4]
Upper-level computerized nutrition course[60]
Nutritional concepts for vegetarians[61]

Guidelines are available for those who wish to write their own CAI courses[61]; however, to do so is usually very expensive and requires the services of a programmer. It is more cost effective to purchase existing software.

Libraries of computerized nutrition examination questions are being developed and should soon be commercially available. One such software package contains tests on 197 topic headings with 41 subcategories (including foundations of nutrition, safety and adequacy of food supply, nutrition during growth and stress, nutrition prevention and treatment of disease, drug–nutrient interactions).[62] Test results from such examinations can be stored on the computer, providing the instructor with statistical treatments of the students' progress.

The problems inherent in the development of good CAI software for nutrition education are discussed elsewhere.[63] The obvious advantages of CAI are that they (1) provide immediate feedback to the student, which facilitates learning; (2) present standardized material that is free of facial or voice bias; (3) can simplify abstract information by the use of visual analogies; and (4) can simulate difficult real-life situations more easily and often less expensively.[6] The disadvantages are often associated with hardware (mechanical problems) and software (poor programming being used). The educational effectiveness of CAI in nutrition programs has yet to be effectively evaluated,[6] but it appears promising despite skepticism regarding its use or abuse.

Dietetic Internships   With the increasing number of microcomputers in hospitals, CAI for classroom and clinical experience education is becoming more feasible. Not only does this free instructor time for clinical responsibilities, but the computer can help the instructor and student use their one-on-one educational encounters more effectively. CAI enables users to progress at their own learning rate, provides immediate feedback, and avoids user embarrassment when repetition is required. Major advantages of computer simulation of clinical cases are the elimination of risk due to student error, the presentation of rare nutritional cases, and the ability to condense months of patient history into a short time period, giving the student the benefit of patient follow-up experience.

CAI programs have been developed to teach dietetic students about diet therapy,[64,65] about the emotional responses and behavioral characteristics of patients,[66] and about clinical encounters requiring problem solving[67] (exposure to the nurse care Kardex, medical records, interview with a hypothetical patient, a formulary, and nutrient catalog).

Consumer Education   Computerized education modules successfully used by consumers include nutrition for athletes, nutrition and exercise regimens, choosing nutritious snacks, vitamin supplementation facts and fallacies, sugar in the diet, salt and hypertension, weight control, diet and health, evaluating food shopping habits, and selecting good food sources of specified nutrients.[4,62] These types of interactive computer programs have been used successfully at health fairs and in conjunction with public health screening programs. It has been suggested that these types of programs be used in public places like cafeterias, grocery stores, and laundromats.[68]

Computer Interfaces

The educational and clinical applications of computers in nutrition have been enhanced by peripherals such as videodisks, cable TV, music, voice synthesizers, and slide shows. Microcomputers utilizing these peripherals have been shown to teach more effectively than the use of more traditional audiovisual aids such as films, videotapes, or slide presentations that tend to transfer information passively.[69,70] Computers, videotapes, and optical videodisk systems help students develop counseling, interviewing, and diagnostic skills that can be used in conjunction with role playing.[49,71] Handicapped students can learn and/or communicate utilizing voice-activated computers.[49]

One educational program that creatively utilizes such peripherals in two courses is described elsewhere.[72] The basic nutrition and food science course uses taped modules along with films, slides, videotapes, compressed-speed audio tapes, discussion groups, and CAI with workbooks—all evaluated by on-line computer testing. The nutrition course for dietetic, nutrition, nursing, and premedicine students uses a lecture method supplemented by film, slides, overhead transparencies, television commercials, telelectures, videotapes, computer simulations, and computer games. Each student seat in the classroom amphitheater has a response panel tied to a timeshare computer so that individual responses can be recorded and analyzed.

Telecommunications   Microcomputers have become so commonplace and affordable that professionals and students often have one in their home. This allows for remote communication using a modem and phone with the hospital laboratory, HIS, patient bedside, or nursing station computer.

From any microcomputer/modem one can access a number of professionally useful data banks. Information on such on-line bibliographic and information services as MEDLINE, BRS/Saunders (which includes 20 medical texts and journals as well as MEDLINE), MED/MAIL of the AMA/NET, and the American Association for Medical Sciences and Informatics are available in most medical libraries. Consumers can find useful drug- and medical-related information on commonly available on-line services for personal computer owners as CompuServe and The Source.

An important professional use of telecommunication trends is in continuing education. Televised satellite conferences can be enhanced by microcomputer access for direct question and communication with the headquartered site as well as remote examination testing for credits. Networking with other colleagues via computer and transmission and exchange of useful patient or research data will become widespread.

Other Computer Applications   A home- or work-based microcomputer can enhance professional productivity in a number of ways: word processing for text generation; data base management for data collection, storage, and research; spread sheets for financial planning, file and library inventory, and management; and slide production by photography from the monitor screen or the printout. Many journals now accept tables, text, and graphics for figures that have been computer generated. Book publishers often accept text sent on disks that are machine readable in ASCII.

Future

Decreasing costs and other technologic advances will continue to make microcomputers more practical for personal purchase. More sophisticated programming languages and further miniaturization of data storage on chips and other media will enhance CAI development, allowing large mainframe programs to be adapted to microcomputers in the hospital setting. Medical records and patient care will become even more automated. Patients will be able to carry their medical records, past diet histories, laboratory values, and so forth on a machine-readable credit card size disk. The portability of computers will become less of an issue as they become smaller. Eventually health professionals will be using hand-held calculator-size computers at the bedside and in clinical areas. Licensing and other types of examinations may be administered at home or at work on one's own microcomputer. Software compatibility will become more common as hardware configurations allow different brands of computers to communicate. In other words, if one can imagine it, the future probably will bring it. One's computer knowledge and application development can help shape the future utilization of computers in the health care profession.

Misuse Computers save us time, but they do not relieve us from our responsibility to ensure that the data are accurate and that they are applied appropriately. Likewise, computers do not replace the need for health care professionals; rather they exist to facilitate the work of the professional.

In light of exciting advances and applications, one must not forget that the use of a computer does not mean that the data it generates are more valid. If bad data are entered, poor data bases used, or invalid or inappropriate standards used, the printout will reflect these limitations. In addition, sources of error tend to become less visable as procedures are automated by computer.

The computer revolution promises to transform many facets of health care, giving us new tools for nutritional diagnosis and treatment while continuing to free us from number crunching and administrative paper work. Computer-assisted diet analysis programs will continue to dominate the consumer market. The potential abuses[73] and printout limitations illustrate the continued need for us as professionals to monitor and evaluate computer software generated for professional and consumer use. Guidelines will also have to be developed for CAI design and evaluation.

The computer mystique will continue to cause computer-generated output to be considered more valid than the same data generated by less automated methods. It remains our professional challenge to ensure that wide-scale misapplication is prevented while we continue to encourage and take advantage of the good things that computers have to offer.

References

1. Bates, W.: *The Computer Cookbook.* Quantum Press/ Doubleday, New York, 1984.
2. Youngwirth, J.: "The Evolution of Computers in Dietetics: A Review," *J. Am. Diet. Assoc.*, **82**:62–7, 1983.
3. Brand, S. ed.: *Whole Earth Software Catalog.* Quantum Press/Doubleday, New York, 1984.
4. Byrd-Bredbenner, C. and Pelican, S., eds.: "Perspectives on Computer Use in Nutrition Education," *J. Nutr. Educ.*, **16**:80–117, 1984.
5. Murphy, S. P., et al.: "Choosing a Diet Analysis System for Classroom Use," *J. Nutr. Educ.*, **16**:73–5, 1984.
6. McMurray, P., and Hoover, L. W.: "The Education Uses of Computers: Hardware, Software, and Strategies," *J. Nutr. Educ.*, **16**:39–43, 1984.
7. Byrd-Bredbenner, C., and Pelican, S.: "Software: How Do You Choose?," *J. Nutr. Educ.*, **16**:77–9, 1984.
8. Shapin, P. G.: "Guidelines for Deciding Between Micros, Minis, Mainframes, and Timesharing," in *Proceedings Computer Applications in Medical Care.* IEEE, N.J., 1982.
9. U.S. Department of Agriculture: *Nutritive Value of Foods. Home and Garden Bulletin No. 72*, Government Printing Office, Washington, D.C., 1981.
10. U.S. Department of Agriculture: *Composition of Foods—Raw, Processed, Prepared.* Agriculture Handbook No. 8., Government Printing Office, Washington, D.C., 1976–1983.
11. U.S. Department of Agriculture: *Nutritive Value of American Foods in Common Units.* Agriculture Handbook No. 456, Government Printing Office, Washington, D.C., 1975.
12. Hepburn, F. N.: "The USDA National Nutrient Data Bank," *Am. J. Clin. Nutr.*, **35**:1297–1301, 1982.
13. Dennis, B., et al.: "The NHLBI Nutrition Data System," *J. Am. Diet. Assoc.*, **77**:641–47, 1980.
14. Pennington, A. T., and Church, H. N.: *Food Values of Portions Commonly Used.* 13th ed. Harper & Row Publishers, New York, 1980.

15. Bacha, M. J.: "Nutrient Standard Menu Planning," *J. Nutr. Educ.*, **16**:64, 1984.

16. Rand, W. M., and Young, V. R.: "Report of a Planning Conference Concerning an International Network of Food Data Systems (INFOODS)," *Am. J. Clin. Nutr.*, **39**:144–51, 1984.

17. Pennington, J. A. T.: *Dietary Nutrient Guide.* Avi Publishing Co., Westport, Conn., 1976.

18. Schuam, K. D., et al.: "Patient-Oriented Dietetic Information System. II. Compiling a Computerized Nutrient Data Bank," *J. Am. Diet. Assoc.*, **63**:39–41, 1973.

19. Hoover, L. W., and Pelican, S.: "Nutrient Data Bases—Considerations for Educators," *J. Nutr. Educ.*, **16**:58–62, 1984.

20. Hoover, L. W., and Perloff, P. P.: "Computerized Nutrient Data Bases: II. Development of Model for Appraisal of Nutrient Data Base System Capabilities," *J. Am. Diet. Assoc.*, **82**:506–8, 1983.

21. Comptroller General: *Report to the Congress: What Foods Should Americans Eat? Better Information Needed on Nutritional Quality of Foods.* CED-80-68, 1980.

22. Danford, D. E.: "Computer Applications to Medical Nutrition Problems," *JPEN*, **5**:441–6, 1981.

23. Frank, G. C., et al.: "Comparison of Dietary Intake by Two Computerized Analysis Systems," *J. Am. Diet. Assoc.*, **84**:818–20, 1984.

24. Dwyer, J., and Suitor, C. W.: "Caveat Emptor: Assessing Needs, Evaluating Computer Options," *J. Am. Diet. Assoc.*, **84**:302–12, 1984.

25. Food and Nutrition Board: *Recommended Dietary Allowances*, 9th ed. National Academy of Sciences, Washington, D.C., 1980.

26. *U.S. RDA Comparison Charts.* National Dairy Council, Chicago, 1974.

27. Sorenson, A. W., et al.: "An Index of Nutritional Quality for a Balanced Diet," *J. Am. Diet. Assoc.*, **68**:236–42, 1976.

28. Weisell, R. C., and François, P. J.: "Reference Weight for Height Standards: An Easier Approach for Computerization," *Food Nutr.*, **8**:12–18, 1982.

29. Rainey-MacDonald, C. G., et al.: "Nomograms for Predicting Resting Energy Expenditure of Hospitalized Patients," *JPEN*, **6**:59–60, 1982.

30. Collins, C. D.: "Microcomputers and Nutritional Assessment," *Nutr. Supp. Serv.*, **3**:48–52, 1983.

31. Fisher, M., and Munro, I.: "A Computer Programme for Nutritional Surveillance," *Aust. N.Z. J. Surg.*, **50**:512–16, 1980.

32. Agarwal, N. R., et al.: "The Automated Metabolic Profile," *Crit. Care Med.*, **11**:546–50, 1983.

33. Katch, F. I., and Katch, V. L.: "Computer Technology to Evaluate Body Composition, Nutrition, and Exercise," *Prev. Med.*, **12**:619–31, 1983.

34. Gale, R., et al.: "An Interactive Microcomputer Program for Calculation of Combined Parenteral and Enteral Nutrition for Neonates." *J. Pediatr. Gastroenterol. Nutr.*, **2**:653–8, 1983.

35. Witschi, J., et al.: "A Computer-Based Dietary Counseling System," *J. Am. Diet. Assoc.*, **69**:385–90, 1976.

36. Evans, S. N., and Gormican, A.: "The Computer in Retrieving Dietary History Data," *J. Am. Diet. Assoc.*, **63**:397–402, 1973.

37. Smith, A. E., and Lloyd-Still, J. D.: "Value of Computerized Dietary Analysis in Pediatric Nutrition: An Analysis of 147 Patients," *J. Pediatr.*, **103**:820–4, 1983.

38. Johnson, R. L., et al.: "Nutrient Analysis System—A Computerized Seven-Day Food Record System," *J. Am. Diet. Assoc.*, **83**:667–71, 1983.

39. Monsen, E. R., and Balintfy, J. L.: "Calculating Dietary Iron Bio-Availability: Refinement and Computerization," *J. Am. Diet. Assoc.*, **80**:307–11, 1982.

40. Baghurst, K. I., et al.: "A Computerized Dietary Analysis System For Use With Diet Diaries or Food Frequency Questionnaires," *Commun. Health Studies*, **8**:11–18, 1984.

41. Wheeler, L. A., and Wheeler, M. L.: "Review of Microcomputer Nutrient Analysis and Menu Planning Programs," *MD Computing*, **1**:42–51, 1984.

42. Lucas, R. W., et al.: "Computer Interrogation of Patients," *Br. Med. J.*, **2**:623–5, 1976.

43. Slack, W., et al.: "Dietary Interviewing by Computer," *J. Am. Diet. Assoc.*, **69**:514–17, 1976.

44. Bryant, D., et al.: "Computerized Surveillance of Diabetic Patient/Health Care Delivery System Interfaces," *Diabetes Care*, **1**:141–5, 1978.

45. Hjelm, M., et al.: "Computer Model of the Metabolism of Phenylalanine in Normal Subjects and in Patients with Phenylketonuria," *Comp. Prog. Biomed.*, **18**:21–32, 1984.

46. Miller, L. G.: "Computerized Interviewing System for the Obese," *J. Nutr. Educ.*, **8**:169–171, 1976.

47. Suitor, C. W., et al.: "Planning High-Carbohydrate, High-Fiber Diets With a Microcomputer," *J. Am. Diet. Assoc.*, **82**:279–82, 1983.

48. Williams, C. S., and Burnet, L. W.: "Future Applications of the Microcomputer in Dietetics," *Hum. Nutr: Appl. Nutr.*, **38A**:99–109, 1984.

49. Milholland, D. K., and Cardona, V. D.: "Computers at the Bedside," *Am. J. Nurs.*, **83**:1304–7, 1983.

50. McLaurin, N. K., et al.: "Computer-Generated Graphic Evaluation of Nutritional Status in Critically Injured Patients," *J. Am. Diet. Assoc.*, **82**:49–52, 1983.

51. Lawson, V. K., et al.: "An Audio-Tutorial Aid for Dietary Instruction in Renal Dialysis," *J. Am. Diet. Assoc.*, **69**:390–6, 1976.

52. Talbert, J. L., et al.: "Case History of a Hospital Information System," *J. Am. Diet. Assoc.*, **68**:45–6, 1976.

53. Bryant, O., et al.: "Computerized Surveillance of Diabetic Patient/Health Care Delivery System Interfaces," *Diabetes Care*, **1**:144–49, 1980.

54. Wheeler, M. L., and Wheeler, L. A.: "Nutrient Menu Planning for Clinical Nutrition Research Centers," *J. Am. Diet. Assoc.*, **67**:346–50, 1975.

55. Oexmann, M. J.: "Automated Diet Construction for Clinical Research," *J. Am. Diet. Assoc.*, **82**:75, 1983.

56. Schroeder, L. A., and Driscoll, D. L.: "Computerized Learning for Clinical and Nonclinical Students," *J. Am. Diet. Assoc.*, **83**:163–66, 1983

57. Hills, A. M.: "A Computer-Assisted Nutrition Education Unit for Grades 4–6," *J. Nutr. Educ.*, **15**:19, 1983.

58. Molleson, A.: "DIETAN—A Computer-Assisted Pro-

gram on Anatomy and Nutrition," *J. Am. Diet. Assoc.*, **68**:46–7, 1976.

59. Dubin, S., et al.: "A Computer Graphic Method for Teaching Protein Chemical Score Concepts," *J. Nutr. Educ.*, **14**:18–20, 1982.

60. Caster, W. O.: " Computer Use for Nutrition Majors," *J. Nutr. Educ.*, **16**:76G, 1984.

61. Ries, C. P., et al.: "Authoring a CAI Lesson in Nutrition Education," *J. Nutr. Educ.*, **16**:51–2, 1984.

62. Boker, J. R., et al.: "Nutrition Test-Item Bank," *J. Nutr. Educ.*, **16**:56, 1984.

63. Nijus, H. P., et al.: "Some Problem-Solving Techniques Applied to Nutrition Education Software," *J. Nutr. Educ.*, **16**:53–6, 1984.

64. Schroeder, L., and Thiele, V. F.: "Renal Diet Therapy—A Computer-Assisted Instruction Model," *J. Nutr. Educ.* **13**:(1) 111–14, 1981.

65. Argo, J. K., et al.: "A Computer-Managed Instruction System Applied to Dietetic Education," *J. Am. Diet. Assoc.*, **79**:450–2, 1981.

66. Hummel, T. J., et al.: "CLIENT 1: A Computer Pro-gram Which Stimulates Client Behavior in an Initial Interview," *J. Couns. Psychol.*, **22**:164–9, 1975.

67. Breese, M. S., et al.: "Computer-Simulated Clinical Encounters," *J. Am. Diet. Assoc.*, **70**:382–4, 1977.

68. Sorenson, A. W., et al.: "Personal Computers for Health," *Prof. Nutr.*, **15**:1–3,6, 1983.

69. Hon, D. C.: "Space Invaders, Videodiscs, and the Bench Connection," *Training Devel. J.*, **35**:10–16, 1981.

70. Maruyama, F. T., and Forester, J. D.: "Programs with Color, Sound, and Graphics," *J. Nutr. Educ.*, **16**:57, 1984.

71. Dow, R. M.: "Simulations Teach Management and Nutrition Counseling Skills," *J. Am. Diet. Assoc.*, **79**:453–5, 1981.

72. Short, S. H.: "Media in Teaching College Level Nutrition," *J. Am. Diet. Assoc.*, **66**:581–7, 1975.

73. Rogan, A., and Yu, S.: "Some Problems with Nutritional Analysis Software," *J. Nutr. Educ.*, **16**:65–6, 1984.

APPENDIXES

TABULAR MATERIALS

TABLE A-1 EXPLANATION

Table A-1 shows the food values in 730 commonly used foods. Foods are listed alphabetically under the following main headings: dairy products; eggs; fats and oils; fish, shellfish, meat, and poultry; fruits and fruit products; grain products; legumes (dry), nuts, and seeds; sugars and sweets; vegetables and vegetable products; and miscellaneous items. Part of the explanation offered in the bulletin is reproduced here*:

Most of the foods listed are in ready-to-eat form. Some are basic products widely used in food preparation, such as flour, fat, and cornmeal....

The approximate measure shown for each food is in cups, ounces, pounds, some other well-known unit, or a piece of certain size. The cup measure refers to the standard measuring cup of 8 fluid ounces or one half pint of liquid. The ounce refers to one-sixteenth of a pound avoirdupois, unless fluid ounce is indicated. The weight of a fluid ounce varies according to the food measured....

The values for food energy (calories) and nutrients shown in Table A-1 are the amounts present in the edible part of the item, that is, in only that portion customarily eaten—corn without cob, meat without bone, potatoes without skin, European-type grapes without seeds. If additional parts are eaten—the potato skin, for example—

amounts of some nutrients obtained will be somewhat greater than shown....

New fatty acid values are given for dairy products, eggs, meats, some grain products, nuts, and soups. The values are based on recent comprehensive research by USDA to update and extend tables for fatty acid content of foods.

Niacin values are for preformed niacin occurring naturally in foods. The values do not include additional niacin that the body may form from tryptophan, an essential amino acid in the protein of most foods. Among the better sources of tryptophan are milk, meat, eggs, legumes, and nuts.

Values have been calculated from the ingredients in typical recipes for many of the prepared items such as biscuits, corn muffins, macaroni and cheese, custard, and many dessert-type items.

Values for toast and cooked vegetables are without fat added, either during preparation or at the table. Some destruction of vitamins, especially ascorbic acid, may occur when vegetables are cut and shredded. Since such losses are variable, no deduction has been made.

For meat, values are for meat cooked and drained of the drippings. For many cuts, two sets of values are shown: meat including fat and meat from which the fat has been removed either in the kitchen or on the plate.

A variety of manufactured items—some of the milk products, ready-to-eat breakfast cereals, imitation cream products, fruit drinks, and various mixes—are included in Table A-1. Frequently these foods are fortified with one or more nutrients. If nutrients are added, this information is on the label. Values shown here for these foods are usually based on products by several manufacturers and may differ somewhat from the values provided by any one source.

*Adams, C. F., and Richardson, M.: *Nutritive Value of Foods.* Home and Garden Bulletin 72, Agricultural Research Service, U.S. Department of Agriculture, Washington, D.C., revised 1977.

Table A-1. Nutritive Values of the Edible Parts of Foods*

(Dashes (—) denote lack of reliable data for a constituent believed to be present in measurable amount)

Nutrients in Indicated Quantity

Foods, Approximate Measures, Units and Weight (edible part unless footnotes indicate otherwise)		Weight Grams	Water Percent	Food Energy Calories	Protein (g)	Fat (g)	Fatty Acids Saturated (total) (g)	Unsaturated Oleic (g)	Unsaturated Linoleic (g)	Carbohydrate (g)	Calcium (mg)	Phosphorus (mg)	Iron (mg)	Potassium (mg)	Vitamin A Value I.U.	Thiamin (mg)	Riboflavin (mg)	Niacin (mg)	Ascorbic Acid (mg)
DAIRY PRODUCTS (CHEESE, CREAM, IMITATION CREAM, MILK; RELATED PRODUCTS)																			
Butter. See Fats, oils; related products																			
Cheese																			
Natural																			
Blue	1 oz	28	42	100	6	8	5.3	1.9	0.2	1	150	110	0.1	73	200	0.01	0.11	0.3	0
Camembert (3 wedges per 4-oz container)	1 wedge	38	52	115	8	9	5.8	2.2	.2	Trace	147	132	.1	71	350	.01	.19	.2	0
Cheddar																			
Cut pieces	1 oz	28	37	115	7	9	6.1	2.1	.2	Trace	204	145	.2	28	300	.01	.11	Trace	0
	1 cu in	17.2	37	70	4	6	3.7	1.3	.1	Trace	124	88	.1	17	180	Trace	.06	Trace	0
Shredded	1 cup	113	37	455	28	37	24.2	8.5	.7	1	815	579	.8	111	1,200	.03	.42	.1	0
Cottage (curd not pressed down)																			
Creamed (cottage cheese, 4% fat):																			
Large curd	1 cup	225	79	235	28	10	6.4	2.4	.2	6	135	297	.3	190	370	.05	.37	.3	Trace
Small curd	1 cup	210	79	220	26	9	6.0	2.2	.2	6	126	277	.3	177	340	.04	.34	.3	Trace
Low fat (2%)	1 cup	226	79	205	31	4	2.8	1.0	.1	8	155	340	.4	217	160	.05	.42	.3	Trace
Low fat (1%)	1 cup	226	82	165	28	2	1.5	.5	.1	6	138	302	.3	193	80	.05	.37	.3	Trace
Uncreamed (cottage cheese dry curd, less than ½% fat)	1 cup	145	80	125	25	1	.4	.1	Trace	3	46	151	.3	47	40	.04	.21	.2	0
Cream	1 oz	28	54	100	2	10	6.2	2.4	.2	1	23	30	.3	34	400	Trace	.06	Trace	0
Mozzarella, made with																			
Whole milk	1 oz	28	48	90	6	7	4.4	1.7	.2	1	163	117	.1	21	260	Trace	.08	Trace	0
Part skim milk	1 oz	28	49	80	8	5	3.1	1.2	.1	1	207	149	.1	27	180	.01	.10	Trace	0
Parmesan, grated																			
Cup, not pressed down	1 cup	100	18	455	42	30	19.1	7.7	.3	4	1,376	807	1.0	107	700	.05	.39	.3	0
Tablespoon	1 tbsp	5	18	25	2	2	1.0	.4	Trace	Trace	69	40	Trace	5	40	Trace	.02	Trace	0
Ounce	1 oz	28	18	130	12	9	5.4	2.2	.1	1	390	229	.3	30	200	.01	.11	.1	0
Provolone	1 oz	28	41	100	7	8	4.8	1.7	.1	1	214	141	.1	39	230	.01	.09	Trace	0
Ricotta, made with																			
Whole milk	1 cup	246	72	1,790	28	32	20.4	7.1	.7	7	509	389	.9	257	1,210	.03	.48	.3	0
Part skim milk	1 cup	246	74	340	28	19	12.1	4.7	.5	13	669	449	1.1	308	1,060	.05	.46	.2	0
Romano	1 oz	28	31	110	9	8	—	—	—	1	302	215	—	—	160	—	.11	Trace	0
Swiss	1 oz	28	37	105	8	8	5.0	1.7	.2	1	272	171	Trace	31	240	.01	.10	Trace	0
Pasteurized process cheese																			
American	1 oz	28	39	105	6	9	5.6	2.1	.2	Trace	174	211	.1	46	340	.01	.10	Trace	0
Swiss	1 oz	28	42	95	7	7	4.5	1.7	.1	1	219	216	.2	61	230	Trace	.08	Trace	0
Pasteurized process cheese food, American	1 oz	28	43	95	6	7	4.4	1.7	.1	2	163	130	.2	79	260	.01	.13	Trace	0
Pasteurized process cheese spread, American	1 oz	28	48	82	5	6	3.8	1.5	.1	2	159	202	.1	69	220	.01	.12	Trace	0
Cream, sweet																			
Half-and-half (cream and milk)	1 cup	242	81	315	7	28	17.3	7.0	.6	10	254	230	.2	314	260	.08	.36	.2	2
	1 tbsp	15	81	20	Trace	2	1.1	.4	Trace	1	16	14	Trace	19	20	.01	.02	Trace	Trace
Light, coffee, or table	1 cup	240	74	470	6	46	28.8	11.7	1.0	9	231	192	.1	292	1,730	.08	.36	.1	2
	1 tbsp	15	74	30	Trace	3	1.8	.7	.1	1	14	12	Trace	18	110	Trace	.02	Trace	Trace

Food	Measure																		
Whipping, unwhipped (volume about double when whipped)																			
Light	1 cup	239	64	700	5	74	46.2	18.3	1.5	7	166	146	0.1	231	2,690	0.06	0.30	0.1	1
Light	1 tbsp	15	64	45	Trace	5	2.9	1.1	.1	Trace	10	9	Trace	15	170	Trace	.02	Trace	Trace
Heavy	1 cup	238	58	820	5	88	54.8	22.2	2.0	7	154	149	Trace	179	3,500	.05	.26	Trace	1
Heavy	1 tbsp	15	58	80	Trace	6	3.5	1.4	.1	Trace	10	9	Trace	11	270	Trace	.02	Trace	Trace
Whipped topping (pressurized)	1 cup	60	61	155	2	13	8.3	3.4	.3	7	61	54	Trace	88	550	.02	.04	Trace	0
Whipped topping (pressurized)	1 tbsp	3	61	10	Trace	1	.4	.2	Trace	Trace	3	4	Trace	4	30	Trace	Trace	Trace	0
Cream, sour	1 cup	230	71	495	7	48	30.0	12.1	1.1	10	268	195	.1	331	1,820	.08	.34	.2	2
Cream, sour	1 tbsp	12	71	25	Trace	3	1.6	.6	.1	1	14	10	Trace	17	90	Trace	.02	Trace	Trace
Cream products, imitation (made with vegetable fat)																			
Sweet																			
Creamers																				
Liquid (frozen)	1 cup	245	77	335	2	24	22.8	.3	Trace	28	23	157	.1	467	1,220†	0	0	0	0
Liquid (frozen)	1 tbsp	15	77	20	Trace	1	1.4	Trace	0	2	1	10	Trace	29	110	0	0	0	0
Powdered	1 cup	94	2	515	5	33	30.6	.9	Trace	52	21	397	Trace	763	190[1]	0	.16	0	0
Powdered	1 tsp	2	2	10	Trace	1	.7	Trace	0	1	Trace	8	Trace	16	Trace[1]	0	Trace	0	0
Whipped topping																				
Frozen	1 cup	75	50	240	1	19	16.3	1.0	.2	17	5	6	.1	14	1,650	0	0	0	0
Frozen	1 tbsp	4	50	15	Trace	1	.9	.1	Trace	1	Trace	Trace	Trace	1	130	0	0	0	0
Powdered, made with whole milk	1 cup	80	67	150	3	10	8.5	.6	.1	13	72	69	Trace	121	290[1]	.02	.09	Trace	1
Powdered, made with whole milk	1 tbsp	4	67	10	Trace	Trace	.4	Trace	Trace	1	4	3	Trace	6	10	Trace	Trace	Trace	Trace
Pressurized	1 cup	70	60	185	1	16	13.2	1.4	.2	11	4	13	Trace	13	330	0	0	0	0
Pressurized	1 tbsp	4	60	10	Trace	1	.8	.1	Trace	1	Trace	1	Trace	1	20	0	0	0	0
Sour dressing (imitation sour cream) made with nonfat dry milk	1 cup	235	75	415	8	39	31.2	4.4	1.1	11	266	205	.1	380	120[2]	.09	.38	.2	2
Sour dressing (imitation sour cream) made with nonfat dry milk	1 tbsp	12	75	20	Trace	2	1.6	.2	.1	1	14	10	Trace	19	Trace	.01	.02	Trace	Trace
Ice cream. See Milk desserts, frozen																			
Ice milk. See Milk desserts, frozen																			
Milk																			
Fluid																				
Whole (3.3% fat)	1 cup	244	88	150	8	8	5.1	2.1	.2	11	291	228	.1	370	310[2]	.09	.40	.2	2
Lowfat (2%) No milk solids added	1 cup	244	89	120	8	5	2.9	1.2	.1	12	297	232	.1	377	500	.10	.40	.2	2
Milk solids added Label claim less than 10 g of protein per cup	1 cup	245	89	125	9	5	2.9	1.2	.1	12	313	245	.1	397	500	.10	.42	.2	2
Label claim 10 or more grams of protein per cup (protein fortified)	1 cup	246	88	135	10	5	3.0	1.2	.1	14	352	276	.1	447	500	.11	.48	.2	2
Lowfat (1%) No milk solids added	1 cup	244	90	100	8	3	1.6	.7	.1	12	300	235	.1	381	500	.10	.41	.2	2
Milk solids added Label claim less than 10 g of protein per cup	1 cup	245	90	105	9	2	1.5	.6	.1	12	313	245	.1	397	500	.10	.42	.2	2
Label claim 10 or more grams of protein per cup (protein fortified)	1 cup	246	89	120	10	3	1.8	.7	.1	14	349	273	.1	444	500	.11	.47	.2	2
Nonfat (skim) No milk solids added	1 cup	245	91	85	8	Trace	.3	.1	Trace	12	302	247	.1	406	500	.09	.37	.2	2
Milk solids added Label claim less than 10 g of protein per cup	1 cup	245	90	90	9	1	.4	.1	Trace	12	316	255	.1	416	500	.10	.43	.2	2
Label claim 10 or more grams of protein per cup (protein fortified)	1 cup	246	89	100	10	1	.4	.1	Trace	14	352	275	.1	446	500	.11	.48	.2	3
Buttermilk	1 cup	245	90	100	8	2	1.3	.5	Trace	12	285	219	.1	371	80[3]	.08	.38	.1	2
Canned																				
Evaporated, unsweetened Whole milk	1 cup	252	74	340	17	19	11.6	5.3	.4	25	657	510	.5	764	610[3]	.12	.80	.5	5
Skim milk	1 cup	255	79	200	19	1	.3	.1	Trace	29	738	497	.7	845	1,000[4]	.11	.79	.4	3
Sweetened, condensed	1 cup	306	27	980	24	27	16.8	6.7	.7	166	868	775	.6	1,136	1,000[3]	.28	1.27	.6	8

†Numbered footnotes appear at the end of this table, pages 640 to 648.

*Adams, C. F., and Richardson, M.: Nutritive Value of Foods. Home and Garden Bulletin 72. Agricultural Research Service, U.S. Department of Agriculture, Washington, D.C., revised 1977.

Table A-1. (Continued)

Foods, Approximate Measures, Units and Weight (edible part unless footnotes indicate otherwise)		Weight (Grams)	Water (Percent)	Food Energy (Calories)	Protein (g)	Fat (g)	Fatty Acids Saturated (total) (g)	Unsaturated Oleic (g)	Unsaturated Linoleic (g)	Carbohydrate (g)	Calcium (mg)	Phosphorus (mg)	Iron (mg)	Potassium (mg)	Vitamin A Value (I.U.)	Thiamin (mg)	Riboflavin (mg)	Niacin (mg)	Ascorbic Acid (mg)
Milk (continued)																			
Dried																			
Buttermilk	1 cup	120	3	465	41	7	4.3	1.7	.2	59	1,421	1,119	.4	1,910	3260	.47	1.90	1.1	7
Nonfat instant																			
Envelope, net wt, 3.2 oz[5]	1 envelope	91	4	325	32	1	.4	.1	Trace	47	1,120	896	.3	1,552	62,160	.38	1.59	.8	5
Cup[7]	1 cup	68	4	245	24	Trace	.3	.1	Trace	35	837	670	.2	1,160	61,610	.28	1.19	.6	4
Milk beverages																			
Chocolate milk (commercial)																			
Regular	1 cup	250	82	210	8	8	5.3	2.2	.2	26	280	251	.6	417	300	.09	.41	.3	2
Lowfat (2%)	1 cup	250	84	180	8	5	3.1	1.3	.1	26	284	254	.6	422	500	.10	.42	.3	2
Lowfat (1%)	1 cup	250	85	160	8	3	1.5	.7	.1	26	287	257	.6	426	500	.10	.40	.2	2
Eggnog (commercial)	1 cup	254	74	340	10	19	11.3	5.0	.6	34	330	278	.5	420	890	.09	.48	.3	4
Malted milk, home-prepared with 1 cup of whole milk and 2 to 3 heaping tsp of malted milk powder (about ¾ oz)																			
Chocolate, milk	1 cup	265	81	235	9	9	5.5	—	—	29	304	265	.5	500	330	.14	.43	.7	2
Powder	¾ oz																		
Natural, milk	1 cup	265	81	235	11	10	6.0	—	—	27	347	307	.3	529	380	.20	.54	1.3	2
Powder	¾ oz																		
Shakes, thick[8]																			
Chocolate, container, net wt, 10.6 oz.	1	300	72	355	9	8	5.0	2.0	.2	63	396	378	.9	672	260	.14	.67	.4	0
Vanilla, container, net wt., 11 oz.	1	313	74	350	12	9	5.9	2.4	.2	56	457	361	.3	572	360	.09	.61	.5	0
Milk desserts, frozen																			
Ice cream																			
Regular (about 11% fat)																			
Hardened	½ gal	1,064	61	2,155	38	115	71.3	28.8	2.6	254	1,406	1,075	1.0	2,052	4,340	.42	2.63	1.1	6
	1 cup	133	61	270	5	14	8.9	3.6	.3	32	176	134	.1	257	540	.05	.33	.1	1
Container	3-fl oz	50	61	100	2	5	3.4	1.4	.1	12	66	51	Trace	96	200	.02	.12	.1	Trace
Soft serve (frozen custard)	1 cup	173	60	375	7	23	13.5	5.9	.6	38	236	199	.4	338	790	.08	.45	.2	1
Rich (about 16% fat), hardened	½ gal	1,188	59	2,805	33	190	118.3	47.8	4.3	256	1,213	927	.8	1,771	7,200	.36	2.27	.9	5
	1 cup	148	59	350	4	24	14.7	6.0	.5	32	151	115	.1	221	900	.04	.28	.1	1
Ice milk																			
Hardened (about 4.3% fat)	½ gal	1,048	69	1,470	41	45	28.1	11.3	1.0	232	1,409	1,035	1.5	2,117	1,710	.61	2.78	.9	6
	1 cup	131	69	185	5	6	3.5	1.4	.1	29	176	129	.1	265	210	.08	.35	.1	1
Soft serve (about 2.6% fat)	1 cup	175	70	225	8	5	2.9	1.2	.1	38	274	202	.3	412	180	.12	.54	.2	1
Sherbert (about 2% fat)	½ gal	1,542	66	2,160	17	31	19.0	7.7	.7	469	827	594	2.5	1,585	1,480	.26	.71	1.0	31
	1 cup	193	66	270	2	4	2.4	1.0	.1	59	103	74	.3	198	190	.03	.09	.1	4
Milk desserts, other																			
Custard, baked	1 cup	265	77	305	14	15	6.8	5.4	.7	29	297	310	1.1	387	930	.11	.50	.3	1
Puddings																			
From home recipe																			
Starch base																			
Chocolate	1 cup	260	66	385	8	12	7.6	3.3	.3	67	250	255	1.3	445	390	.05	.36	.3	1
Vanilla (blancmange)	1 cup	255	76	285	9	10	6.2	2.5	.2	41	298	232	Trace	352	410	.08	.41	.3	2
Tapioca cream	1 cup	165	72	220	8	8	4.1	2.5	.5	28	173	180	.7	223	480	.07	.30	.2	2
From mix (chocolate) and milk																			
Regular (cooked)	1 cup	260	70	320	9	8	4.3	2.6	.2	59	265	247	.8	354	340	.05	.39	.3	2
Instant	1 cup	260	69	325	8	7	3.6	2.2	.3	63	374	237	1.3	335	340	.08	.39	.3	2

Food	Measure	Grams	Water (%)	Food energy (cal)	Protein (g)	Fat (g)	Saturated (g)	Monounsat. (g)	Polyunsat. (g)	Carbohydrate (g)	Calcium (mg)	Phosphorus (mg)	Iron (mg)	Potassium (mg)	Vitamin A (IU)	Thiamin (mg)	Riboflavin (mg)	Niacin (mg)	Ascorbic acid (mg)
Yogurt																			
With added milk solids																			
Made with lowfat milk																			
Fruit-flavored[9] container	8 oz	227	75	230	10	3	1.8	.6	.1	42	343	269	.2	439	120[10]	.08	.40	.2	1
Plain container	8 oz	227	85	145	12	4	2.3	.8	.1	16	415	326	.2	531	150[10]	.10	.49	.3	2
Made with nonfat milk container	8 oz	227	85	125	13	Trace	.3	.1	Trace	17	452	355	.2	579	20[10]	.11	.53	.3	2
Without added milk solids																			
Made with whole milk container	8 oz	227	88	140	8	7	4.8	1.7	.1	11	274	215	.1	351	280	.07	.32	.2	1
EGGS																			
Eggs, large (24 oz per dozen)																			
Raw																			
Whole, without shell	1 egg	50	75	80	6	6	1.7	2.0	.6	1	28	90	1.0	65	260	.04	.15	Trace	0
White	1 white	33	88	15	3	Trace	0	0	0	Trace	4	4	Trace	45	0	Trace	.09	Trace	0
Yolk	1 yolk	17	49	65	3	6	1.7	2.1	.6	Trace	26	86	.9	15	310	.04	.07	Trace	0
Cooked																			
Fried in butter	1 egg	46	72	85	5	6	2.4	2.2	.6	1	26	80	.9	58	290	.03	.13	Trace	0
Hard-cooked, shell removed	1 egg	50	75	80	6	6	1.7	2.0	.6	1	28	90	1.0	65	260	.04	.14	Trace	0
Poached	1 egg	50	74	80	6	6	1.7	2.0	.6	1	28	90	1.0	65	260	.04	.13	Trace	0
Scrambled (milk added) in butter; also omelet	1 egg	64	76	95	6	7	2.8	2.3	.6	1	47	97	.9	85	310	.04	.16	Trace	0
FATS, OILS; RELATED PRODUCTS																			
Butter																			
Regular (1 brick or 4 sticks per lb)																			
Stick (½ cup)	1 stick	113	16	815	1	92	57.3	23.1	2.1	Trace	27	27	.2	29	3,470[11]	.01	.04	Trace	0
Tablespoon (about ⅛ stick)	1 tbsp	14	16	100	Trace	12	7.2	2.9	.3	Trace	3	3	Trace	4	430[11]	Trace	Trace	Trace	0
Pat (1 square, ⅓ in high, 90 per lb)	1 pat	5	16	35	Trace	4	2.5	1.0	.1	Trace	1	1	Trace	1	150[11]	Trace	Trace	Trace	0
Whipped (6 sticks or two 8-oz containers per lb)																			
Stick (½ cup)	1 stick	76	16	540	1	61	38.2	15.4	1.4	Trace	18	17	.1	20	2,310[11]	Trace	.03	Trace	0
Tablespoon (about ⅛ stick)	1 tbsp	9	16	65	Trace	8	4.7	1.9	.2	Trace	2	2	Trace	2	290[11]	Trace	Trace	Trace	0
Pat (1¼ in square, ⅓ in high; 120 per lb)	1 pat	4	16	25	Trace	3	1.9	.8	.1	Trace	1	1	Trace	1	120[11]	0	0	0	0
Fats, cooking (vegetable shortenings)	1 cup	200	0	1,770	0	200	48.8	88.2	48.4	0	0	0	0	0	—	0	0	0	0
	1 tbsp	13	0	110	0	13	3.2	5.7	3.1	0	0	0	0	0	—	0	0	0	0
Lard	1 cup	205	0	1,805	0	205	81.0	83.8	20.5	0	0	0	0	0	0	0	0	0	0
	1 tbsp	13	0	115	0	13	5.1	5.3	1.3	0	0	0	0	0	0	0	0	0	0
Margarine																			
Regular (1 brick or 4 sticks per lb)																			
Stick (½ cup)	1 stick	113	16	815	1	92	16.7	42.9	24.9	Trace	27	26	.2	29	3,750[12]	.01	.04	Trace	0
Tablespoon (about ⅛ stick)	1 tbsp	14	16	100	Trace	12	2.1	5.3	3.1	Trace	3	3	Trace	4	470[12]	Trace	Trace	Trace	0
Pat (1 in square, ⅓ in high; 90 per lb)	1 pat	5	16	35	Trace	4	.7	1.9	1.1	Trace	1	1	Trace	1	170[12]	Trace	Trace	Trace	0
Soft, two 8-oz containers per lb	1 cont.	227	16	1,635	1	184	32.5	71.5	65.4	Trace	53	52	.4	59	7,500[12]	.01	.08	.1	0
Whipped (6 sticks per lb)																			
Stick (½ cup)	1 stick	76	16	545	1	61	11.2	28.7	16.7	Trace	18	17	.1	20	2,500[12]	Trace	.03	Trace	0
Tablespoon (about ⅛ stick)	1 tbsp	9	16	70	Trace	8	1.4	3.6	2.1	Trace	2	2	Trace	2	310[12]	Trace	Trace	Trace	0
Oils, salad or cooking:																			
Corn	1 cup	218	0	1,925	0	218	27.7	53.6	125.1	0	0	0	0	0	—	0	0	0	0
	1 tbsp	14	0	120	0	14	3.3	3.3	7.8	0	0	0	0	0	—	0	0	0	0
Olive	1 cup	216	0	1,910	0	216	30.7	154.4	17.7	0	0	0	0	0	—	0	0	0	0
	1 tbsp	14	0	120	0	14	1.9	9.7	1.1	0	0	0	0	0	—	0	0	0	0
Peanut	1 cup	216	0	1,910	0	216	37.4	98.5	67.0	0	0	0	0	0	—	0	0	0	0
	1 tbsp	14	0	120	0	14	2.3	6.2	4.2	0	0	0	0	0	—	0	0	0	0
Safflower	1 cup	218	0	1,925	0	218	20.5	25.9	159.8	0	0	0	0	0	—	0	0	0	0
	1 tbsp	14	0	120	0	14	1.3	1.6	10.0	0	0	0	0	0	—	0	0	0	0
Soybean oil, hydrogenated (partially hardened)	1 cup	218	0	1,925	0	218	31.8	93.1	75.6	0	0	0	0	0	—	0	0	0	0
	1 tbsp	14	0	120	0	14	2.0	5.8	4.7	0	0	0	0	0	—	0	0	0	0
Soybean-cottonseed oil blend, hydrogenated	1 cup	218	0	1,925	0	218	38.2	63.0	99.6	0	0	0	0	0	—	0	0	0	0
	1 tbsp	14	0	120	0	14	2.4	3.9	6.2	0	0	0	0	0	—	0	0	0	0

Table A-1. (Continued)

								Nutrients in Indicated Quantity											
							Fatty Acids												
								Unsaturated											
Foods, Approximate Measures, Units and Weight (edible part unless footnotes indicate otherwise)	Weight Grams	Water Percent	Food Energy Calories	Protein (g)	Fat (g)	Saturated (total) (g)	Oleic (g)	Linoleic (g)	Carbohydrate (g)	Calcium (mg)	Phosphorus (mg)	Iron (mg)	Potassium (mg)	Vitamin A Value I.U.	Thiamin (mg)	Riboflavin (mg)	Niacin (mg)	Ascorbic Acid (mg)
Salad dressings																			
Commercial																			
Blue cheese																			
Regular	15	32	75	1	8	1.6	1.7	3.8	1	12	11	Trace	6	30	Trace	.02	Trace	Trace	1 tbsp
Low-calorie (5 Cal per tsp)	16	84	10	Trace	1	.5	.3	Trace	1	10	8	Trace	5	30	Trace	.01	Trace	Trace	1 tbsp
French																			
Regular	16	39	65	Trace	6	1.1	1.3	3.2	3	2	2	.1	13	—	—	—	—	—	1 tbsp
Low calorie (5 Cal per tsp)	16	77	15	Trace	1	.1	.1	.4	2	2	2	.1	13	—	—	—	—	—	1 tbsp
Italian																			
Regular	15	28	85	Trace	9	1.6	1.9	4.7	1	2	1	Trace	2	Trace	Trace	Trace	Trace	—	1 tbsp
Low calorie (2 Cal per tsp)	15	90	10	Trace	1	.1	.1	.4	Trace	Trace	1	Trace	2	Trace	Trace	Trace	Trace	—	1 tbsp
Mayonnaise	14	15	100	Trace	11	2.0	2.4	5.6	Trace	3	4	.1	5	40	Trace	.01	Trace	—	1 tbsp
Mayonnaise type																			
Regular	15	41	65	Trace	6	1.1	1.4	3.2	2	2	4	Trace	1	30	Trace	Trace	Trace	—	1 tbsp
Low calorie (8 Cal per tsp)	16	81	20	Trace	2	.4	.4	1.0	2	3	4	Trace	1	40	Trace	Trace	Trace	—	1 tbsp
Tartar sauce, regular	14	34	75	Trace	8	1.5	1.8	4.1	1	3	4	.1	11	30	Trace	Trace	Trace	Trace	1 tbsp
Thousand Island																			
Regular	16	32	80	Trace	8	1.4	1.7	4.0	2	2	3	.1	18	50	Trace	Trace	Trace	Trace	1 tbsp
Low calorie (10 Cal per tsp)	15	68	25	Trace	2	.4	.4	1.0	2	2	3	.1	17	50	Trace	Trace	Trace	Trace	1 tbsp
From home recipe																			
Cooked type[3]	16	68	25	1	2	.5	.6	.3	2	14	15	.1	19	80	.01	.03	Trace	Trace	1 tbsp
FISH, SHELLFISH, MEAT, POULTRY; RELATED PRODUCTS																			
Fish and shellfish																			
Bluefish, baked with butter or margarine	85	68	135	22	4	—	—	—	0	25	244	.6	—	40	.09	.08	1.6	—	3 oz
Clams																			
Raw, meat only	85	82	65	11	1	—	—	—	2	59	138	5.2	154	90	.08	.15	1.1	8	3 oz
Canned, solids and liquid	85	86	45	7	1	—	Trace	Trace	2	47	116	3.5	119	—	.01	.09	.9	—	3 oz
Crabmeat (white or king), canned, not pressed down	135	77	135	24	3	.6	.4	.1	1	61	246	1.1	149	—	.11	.11	2.6	—	1 cup
Fish sticks, breaded, cooked, frozen (stick, 4 by 1 by 1/2 in)	28	66	50	5	3	—	—	—	2	3	47	.1	—	0	.01	.02	.5	—	1 stick
Haddock, breaded, fried[14]	85	66	140	17	5	1.4	2.2	1.2	5	34	210	1.0	296	—	.03	.06	2.7	—	3 oz
Ocean perch, breaded, fried[14]	85	59	195	16	11	2.7	4.4	2.3	6	28	192	1.1	242	—	.10	.10	1.6	2	1 fillet
Oysters, raw, meat only (13-19 medium Selects)	240	85	160	20	4	1.3	.2	.1	8	226	343	13.2	290	740	.34	.43	6.0	—	1 cup
Salmon, pink, canned, solids and liquid	85	71	120	17	5	.9	.8	.1	0	167[15]	243	.7	307	60	.03	.16	6.8	—	3 oz
Sardines, Atlantic, canned in oil, drained solids	85	62	175	20	9	3.0	2.5	.5	0	372	424	2.5	502	190	.02	.17	4.6	—	3 oz
Scallops, frozen, breaded, fried, reheated	90	60	175	16	8	—	—	—	9	—	—	—	—	—	—	—	—	—	6
Shad, baked with butter or margarine, bacon	85	64	170	20	10	—	—	—	0	20	266	.5	320	30	.11	.22	7.3	—	3 oz
Shrimp																			
Canned meat	85	70	100	21	1	.1	.1	Trace	1	98	224	2.6	104	50	.01	.03	1.5	—	3 oz
French fried[16]	85	57	190	17	9	2.3	3.7	2.0	9	61	162	1.7	195	—	.03	.07	2.3	—	3 oz
Tuna, canned in oil, drained solids	85	61	170	24	7	1.7	1.7	.7	0	7	199	1.6	—	70	.04	.10	10.1	—	3 oz
Tuna salad[17]	205	70	350	30	22	4.3	6.3	6.7	7	41	291	2.7	—	590	.08	.23	10.3	2	1 cup
Meat and meat products																			
Bacon, (20 slices per lb, raw), broiled or fried, crisp	15	8	85	4	8	2.5	3.7	.7	Trace	2	34	.5	35	0	.08	.05	.8	—	2 slices

Food	Measure	Grams	Water (%)	Food energy (cal)	Protein (g)	Fat (g)	Saturated (g)	Oleic (g)	Linoleic (g)	Carbohydrate (g)	Calcium (mg)	Phosphorus (mg)	Iron (mg)	Potassium (mg)	Vitamin A (IU)	Thiamin (mg)	Riboflavin (mg)	Niacin (mg)	Ascorbic acid (mg)
Beef[18], cooked																			
Cuts braised, simmered or pot roasted																			
Lean and fat (piece, 2½ by 2½ by ¾ in)	3 oz	85	53	245	23	16	6.8	6.5	.4	0	10	114	2.9	184	30	.04	.18	3.6	—
Lean only	2.5 oz	72	62	140	22	5	2.1	1.8	.2	0	10	108	2.7	176	10	.04	.17	3.3	—
Ground beef, broiled																			
Lean, 10% fat, patty	3 oz	85	60	185	23	10	4.0	3.9	.3	0	10	196	3.0	261	20	.08	.20	5.1	—
Lean, 21% fat, patty	2.9 oz	82	54	235	20	17	7.0	6.7	.4	0	9	159	2.6	221	30	.07	.17	4.4	—
Roast, oven cooked, no liquid added																			
Relatively fat, such as rib																			
Lean and fat (2 pieces, 4⅛ by 2¼ by ¼ in)	3 oz	85	40	375	17	33	14.0	13.6	.8	0	8	158	2.2	189	70	.05	.13	3.1	—
Lean only	1.8 oz	51	57	125	14	7	3.0	2.5	.3	0	6	131	1.8	161	10	.04	.11	2.6	—
Relatively lean, such as heel of round																			
Lean and fat (2 pieces, 4⅛ by 2¼ by ¼ in)	3 oz	85	62	165	25	7	2.8	2.7	.2	0	11	208	3.2	279	10	.06	.19	4.5	—
Lean only	2.8 oz	78	65	125	24	3	1.2	1.0	.1	0	10	199	3.0	268	Trace	.06	.18	4.3	—
Steak																			
Relatively fat-sirloin, broiled																			
Lean and fat (piece, 2½ by 2½ by ¾ in)	3 oz	85	44	330	20	27	11.3	11.1	.6	0	9	162	2.5	220	50	.05	.15	4.0	—
Lean only	2.0 oz	56	59	115	18	4	1.8	1.6	.2	0	7	146	2.2	202	10	.05	.14	3.6	—
Relatively lean-round, braised																			
Lean and fat (piece, 4⅛ by 2¼ by ½ in)	3 oz	85	55	220	24	13	5.5	5.2	.4	0	10	213	3.0	272	20	.07	.19	4.8	—
Lean only	2.4 oz	68	61	130	21	4	1.7	1.5	.2	0	9	182	2.5	238	10	.05	.16	4.1	—
Beef, canned																			
Corned beef	3 oz	85	59	185	22	10	4.9	4.5	.2	0	17	90	3.7	—	—	.01	.20	2.9	—
Corned beef hash	1 cup	220	67	400	19	25	11.9	10.9	.5	24	29	147	4.4	440	—	.02	.20	4.6	—
Beef, dried, chipped	2½-oz	71	48	145	24	4	2.1	2.0	.1	0	14	287	3.6	142	—	.05	.23	2.7	0
Beef and vegetable stew	1 cup	245	82	220	16	11	4.9	4.5	.2	15	29	184	2.9	613	2,400	.15	.17	4.7	17
Beef potpie (home recipe), baked[19] (piece, ⅓ of 9-in-diam. pie)	1 piece	210	55	515	21	30	7.9	12.8	6.7	39	29	149	3.8	334	1,720	.30	.30	5.5	6
Chili con carne with beans, canned	1 cup	255	72	340	19	16	7.5	6.8	.3	31	82	321	4.3	594	150	.08	.18	3.3	—
Chop suey with beef and pork (home recipe)	1 cup	250	75	300	26	17	8.5	6.2	.7	13	60	248	4.8	425	600	.28	.38	5.0	33
Heart, beef, lean, braised	3 oz	85	61	160	27	5	1.5	1.1	.6	1	5	154	5.0	197	20	.21	1.04	6.5	1
Lamb, cooked																			
Chop, rib (3 per lb with bone), broiled																			
Lean and fat	3.1 oz	89	43	360	18	32	14.8	12.1	1.2	0	8	139	1.0	200	—	.11	.19	4.1	—
Lean only	2 oz	57	60	120	16	6	2.5	2.1	.2	0	6	121	1.1	174	—	.09	.15	3.4	—
Leg roasted																			
Lean and fat (2 pieces, 4⅛ by 2¼ by ¼ in)	3 oz	85	54	235	22	16	7.3	6.0	.6	0	9	177	1.4	241	—	.13	.23	4.7	—
Lean only	2.5 oz	71	62	130	20	5	2.1	1.8	.2	0	9	169	1.4	227	—	.12	.21	4.4	—
Shoulder, roasted																			
Lean and fat (3 pieces, 2½ by 2½ by ¼ in)	3 oz	85	50	285	18	23	10.8	8.8	.9	0	9	146	1.0	206	—	.11	.20	4.0	—
Lean only	2.3 oz	64	61	130	17	6	3.6	2.3	.2	0	8	140	1.0	193	—	.10	.18	3.7	—
Liver, beef, fried[20] (slice, 6½ by 2⅜ by ⅜ in)	3 oz	85	56	195	22	9	2.5	3.5	.9	5	9	405	7.5	323	45,390[2]	.22	3.56	14.0	23
Pork, cured, cooked																			
Ham, light cure, lean and fat, roasted (2 pieces, 4⅛ by 2¼ by ¼ in)[22]	3 oz	85	54	245	18	19	6.8	7.9	1.7	0	8	146	2.2	199	0	.40	.15	3.1	—
Luncheon meat																			
Boiled ham, slice (8 per 8-oz pkg.)	1 oz	28	59	65	5	5	1.7	2.0	.4	0	3	47	.8	—	0	.12	.04	.7	—
Canned, spiced or unspiced — Slice, approx. 3 by 2 by ½ in	1 slice	60	55	175	9	15	5.4	6.7	1.0	1	5	65	1.3	133	0	.19	.13	1.8	—
Pork, fresh[18], cooked																			
Chop, loin (cut 3 per lb with bone), broiled																			
Lean and fat	2.7 oz	78	42	305	19	25	8.9	10.4	2.2	0	9	209	2.7	216	0	.75	.22	4.5	—
Lean only	2 oz	56	53	150	17	9	3.1	3.6	.8	0	7	181	2.2	192	0	.63	.18	3.8	—
Roast, oven cooked, no liquid added																			
Lean and fat (piece, 2½ by 2½ by ¾ in)	3 oz	85	46	310	21	24	8.7	10.2	2.2	0	9	218	2.7	233	0	.78	.22	4.8	—
Lean only	2.4 oz	68	55	175	20	10	3.5	4.1	.8	0	9	211	2.6	224	0	.73	.21	4.4	—

Table A-1. (Continued)

Nutrients in Indicated Quantity

Foods, Approximate Measures, Units and Weight (edible part unless footnotes indicate otherwise)		Weight Grams	Water Percent	Food Energy Calories	Protein (g)	Fat (g)	Fatty Acids Saturated (total) (g)	Unsaturated Oleic (g)	Unsaturated Linoleic (g)	Carbohydrate (g)	Calcium (mg)	Phosphorus (mg)	Iron (mg)	Potassium (mg)	Vitamin A Value I.U.	Thiamin (mg)	Riboflavin (mg)	Niacin (mg)	Ascorbic Acid (mg)
Pork, fresh, cooked (continued)																			
Shoulder cut, simmered																			
Lean and fat (3 pieces, 2½ by 2½ by ¼ in)	3 oz	85	46	320	20	26	9.3	10.9	2.3	0	9	118	2.6	158	0	.46	.21	4.1	—
Lean only	2.2 oz	63	60	135	18	6	2.2	2.6	.6	0	8	111	2.3	146	0	.42	.19	3.7	—
Sausages (see also Luncheon meat)																			
Bologna, slice (8 per 8-oz pkg.)	1 slice	28	56	85	3	8	3.0	3.4	.5	Trace	2	36	.5	65	—	.05	.06	.7	—
Braunschweiger, slice (6 per 6-oz pkg.)	1 slice	28	53	90	4	8	2.6	3.4	.8	1	3	69	1.7	—	1,850	.05	.41	2.3	—
Brown and serve (10-11 per 8-oz pkg.), browned	1 link	17	40	70	3	6	2.3	2.8	.7	Trace	1	12	.3	—	—	.02	.01	.2	—
Deviled ham, canned	1 tbsp	13	51	45	2	4	1.5	1.8	.4	0	1	12	.3	—	0	.02	.01	.2	—
Frankfurter (8 per 1-lb pkg.), cooked (reheated)	1 frank.	56	57	170	7	15	5.6	6.5	1.2	1	3	57	.8	—	—	.08	.11	1.4	—
Meat, potted (beef, chicken, turkey), canned	1 tbsp	13	61	30	2	2	—	—	—	0	—	—	—	—	—	Trace	.03	.2	—
Pork link (16 per 1-lb pkg.), cooked	1 link	13	35	60	2	6	2.1	2.4	.5	Trace	1	21	.3	35	0	.10	.04	.5	—
Salami																			
Dry type, slice (12 per 4-oz pkg.)	1 slice	10	30	45	2	4	1.6	1.6	.1	Trace	1	28	.4	—	—	.04	.03	.5	—
Cooked type, slice (8 per 8-oz pkg.)	1 slice	28	51	90	5	7	3.1	3.0	.2	Trace	3	57	.7	—	—	.07	.07	1.2	—
Vienna sausage (7 per 4-oz can)	1	16	63	40	2	3	1.2	1.4	.2	Trace	1	24	.3	—	—	.01	.02	.4	—
Veal, medium fat, cooked, bone removed																			
Cutlet (4⅛ by 2¼ by ½ in), braised or broiled	3 oz	85	60	185	23	9	4.0	3.4	.4	0	9	196	2.7	258	—	.06	.21	4.6	—
Rib (2 pieces, 4⅛ by 2¼ by ¼ in), roasted	3 oz	85	55	230	23	14	6.1	5.1	.6	0	10	211	2.9	259	—	.11	.26	6.6	—
Poultry and poultry products																			
Chicken, cooked																			
Breast, fried[23], bones removed, ½ breast (3.3 oz with bones)	2.8 oz	79	58	160	26	5	1.4	1.8	1.1	1	9	218	1.3	—	70	.04	.17	11.6	—
Drumstick, fried[23], bones removed (2 oz with bones)	1.3 oz	38	55	90	12	4	1.1	1.3	.9	Trace	6	89	.9	—	50	.03	.15	2.7	—
Half broiler, broiled, bones removed (10.4 oz with bones)	6.2 oz	176	71	240	42	7	2.2	2.5	1.3	0	16	355	3.0	483	160	.09	.34	15.5	—
Chicken, canned, boneless	3 oz	85	65	170	18	10	3.2	3.8	2.0	0	18	210	1.3	117	200	.03	.11	3.7	3
Chicken à la king, cooked (home recipe)	1 cup	245	68	470	27	34	12.7	14.3	3.3	12	127	358	2.5	404	1,130	.10	.42	5.4	12
Chicken and noodles cooked (home recipe)	1 cup	240	71	365	22	18	5.9	7.1	3.5	26	26	247	2.2	149	430	.05	.17	4.3	Trace
Chicken chow mein																			
Canned	1 cup	250	89	95	7	Trace	—	—	—	18	45	85	1.3	418	150	.05	.10	1.0	13
From home recipe	1 cup	250	78	255	31	10	2.4	3.4	3.1	10	58	293	2.5	473	280	.08	.23	4.3	10
Chicken pot pie (home recipe), baked[19], (piece, ⅓ of 9-in diam. pie)	1	232	57	545	23	31	11.3	10.9	5.6	42	70	232	3.0	343	3,090	.34	.31	5.5	5
Turkey, roasted, flesh without skin																			
Dark meat, piece, 2½ by 1⅝ by ¼ in	4	85	61	175	26	7	2.1	1.5	1.5	0	—	—	2.0	338	—	.03	.20	3.6	—
Light meat, piece, 4 by 2 by ¼ in	2	85	62	150	28	3	.9	.6	.7	0	—	—	1.0	349	—	.04	.12	9.4	—
Light and dark meat																			
Chopped or diced	1 cup	140	61	265	44	9	2.5	1.7	1.8	0	11	351	2.5	514	—	.07	.25	10.8	—
Pieces (1 slice white meat, 4 by 2 by ¼ in with 2 slices dark meat, 2½ by 1⅝ by ¼ in)	3	85	61	160	27	5	1.5	1.0	1.1	0	7	213	1.5	312	—	.04	.15	6.5	—

FRUITS AND FRUIT PRODUCTS

Food	Measure	Grams	Water (%)	Food energy	Protein	Fat	Saturated	Oleic	Linoleic	Carbohydrate	Calcium	Phosphorus	Iron	Potassium	Vitamin A	Thiamin	Riboflavin	Niacin	Ascorbic acid
Apples, raw, unpeeled, without cores																			
2¾-in diam. (about 3 per lb with cores)	1 apple	138	84	80	Trace	1	—	—	—	20	10	14	.4	152	120	.04	.03	.1	6
3¼-in diam. (about 2 per lb with cores)	1 apple	212	84	125	Trace	1	—	—	—	31	15	21	.6	223	190	.06	.04	.2	8
Applejuice, bottled or canned[24]	1 cup	248	88	120	Trace	Trace	—	—	—	30	15	22	1.5	250	—	.02	.05	.2	2[25]
Applesauce, canned:																			
Sweetened	1 cup	255	76	230	1	Trace	—	—	—	61	10	13	1.3	166	100	.05	.03	.1	3[25]
Unsweetened	1 cup	244	89	100	Trace	Trace	—	—	—	26	10	12	1.2	190	100	.05	.02	.1	2[25]
Apricots:																			
Raw, without pits (about 12 per lb with pits)	3	107	85	55	1	Trace	—	—	—	14	18	25	.5	301	2,890	.03	.04	.6	11
Canned in heavy syrup (halves and syrup)	1 cup	258	77	220	2	Trace	—	—	—	57	28	39	.8	604	4,490	.05	.05	1.0	10
Dried:																			
Uncooked (28 large or 37 medium halves per cup)	1 cup	130	25	340	7	1	—	—	—	86	87	140	7.2	1,273	14,170	.01	.21	4.3	16
Cooked, unsweetened, fruit and liquid	1 cup	250	76	215	4	1	—	—	—	54	55	88	4.5	795	7,500	.01	.13	2.5	0
Apricot nectar, canned	1 cup	251	85	145	1	Trace	—	—	—	37	23	30	.5	379	2,380	.03	.03	.5	36[26]
Avocados, raw, whole, without skins and seeds																			
California, mid- and late-winter (with skin and seed, 3⅛-in diam.; wt., 10 oz)	1	216	74	370	5	37	5.5	22.0	3.7	13	22	91	1.3	1,303	630	.24	.43	3.5	30
Florida, late summer and fall (with skin and seed, 3⅝-in diam.; wt., 1 lb)	1	304	78	390	4	33	6.7	15.7	5.3	27	30	128	1.8	1,836	880	.33	.61	4.9	43
Bananas without peel (about 2.6 per lb with peel)	1	119	76	100	1	Trace	—	—	—	26	10	31	.8	440	230	.06	.07	.8	12
Banana flakes	1 tbsp	6	3	20	Trace	Trace	—	—	—	5	2	6	.2	92	50	.01	.01	.2	Trace
Blackberries, raw	1 cup	144	85	85	2	1	—	—	—	19	46	27	1.3	245	290	.04	.06	.6	30
Blueberries, raw	1 cup	145	83	90	1	1	—	—	—	22	22	19	1.5	117	150	.04	.09	.7	20
Cantaloupe. See Muskmelons																			
Cherries:																			
Sour (tart), red, pitted, canned, water pack	1 cup	244	88	105	2	Trace	—	—	—	26	37	32	.7	317	1,660	.07	.05	.5	12
Sweet, raw, without pits and stems	10	68	80	45	1	Trace	—	—	—	12	15	13	.3	129	70	.03	.04	.3	7
Cranberry juice cocktail, bottled, sweetened	1 cup	253	83	165	Trace	Trace	—	—	—	42	13	8	.8	25	Trace	.03	.03	.1	81[27]
Cranberry sauce, sweetened, canned, strained	1 cup	277	62	405	Trace	1	—	—	—	104	17	11	.6	83	60	.03	.03	.1	6
Dates:																			
Whole, without pits	10	80	23	220	2	Trace	—	—	—	58	47	50	2.4	518	40	.07	.08	1.8	0
Chopped	1 cup	178	23	490	4	1	—	—	—	130	105	112	5.3	1,153	90	.16	.18	3.9	0
Fruit cocktail, canned, in heavy syrup	1 cup	255	80	195	1	Trace	—	—	—	50	23	31	1.0	411	360	.05	.03	1.0	5
Grapefruit																			
Raw, medium, 3¾-in diam. (about 1 lb 1 oz)																			
Pink or red with peel[28]	½	241	89	50	1	Trace	—	—	—	13	20	20	.5	166	540	.05	.02	.2	44
White with peel[28]	½	241	89	45	1	Trace	—	—	—	12	19	19	.5	159	10	.05	.02	.2	44
Canned, sections with syrup	1 cup	254	81	180	2	Trace	—	—	—	45	33	36	.8	343	30	.08	.05	.5	76
Grapefruit juice:																			
Raw, pink, red, or white	1 cup	246	90	95	1	Trace	—	—	—	23	22	37	.5	399	(29)	.10	.05	.5	93
Canned, white:																			
Unsweetened	1 cup	247	89	100	1	Trace	—	—	—	24	20	35	1.0	400	20	.07	.05	.5	84
Sweetened	1 cup	250	86	135	1	Trace	—	—	—	32	20	35	1.0	405	30	.08	.05	.5	78
Frozen, concentrate, unsweetened:																			
Undiluted, 6-fl oz can	1 can	207	62	300	4	1	—	—	—	72	70	124	.8	1,250	60	.29	.12	1.4	286
Diluted with 3 parts water by volume	1 cup	247	89	100	1	Trace	—	—	—	24	25	42	.2	420	20	.10	.04	.5	96
Dehydrated crystals, prepared with water (1 lb yields about 1 gal)	1 cup	247	90	100	1	Trace	—	—	—	24	22	40	.2	412	20	.10	.05	.5	91
Grapes, European type (adherent skin), raw																			
Thompson seedless	10	50	81	35	Trace	Trace	—	—	—	9	6	10	.2	87	50	.03	.02	.2	2
Tokay and Emperor, seeded types	10[30]	60	81	40	Trace	Trace	—	—	—	10	7	11	.2	99	60	.03	.02	.2	2
Grape juice																			
Canned or bottled	1 cup	253	83	165	1	Trace	—	—	—	42	28	30	.8	293	—	.10	.05	.5	Trace[25]
Frozen concentrate, sweetened:																			
Undiluted, 6-fl oz can	1 can	216	53	395	1	Trace	—	—	—	100	22	32	.9	255	40	.13	.22	1.5	32[31]
Diluted with 3 parts water by volume	1 cup	250	86	135	1	Trace	—	—	—	33	8	10	.3	85	10	.05	.08	.5	10[31]

Table A-1. (Continued)

Nutrients in Indicated Quantity

Foods, Approximate Measures, Units and Weight (edible part unless footnotes indicate otherwise)	Weight (Grams)	Water (Percent)	Food Energy (Calories)	Protein (g)	Fat (g)	Saturated (total) (g)	Unsaturated Oleic (g)	Linoleic (g)	Carbohydrate (g)	Calcium (mg)	Phosphorus (mg)	Iron (mg)	Potassium (mg)	Vitamin A Value (I.U.)	Thiamin (mg)	Riboflavin (mg)	Niacin (mg)	Ascorbic Acid (mg)
Grape drink, canned	1 cup	250	86	135	Trace	Trace	—	—	—	35	8	10	.3	88	—	32.03	32.03	.3	(32)
Lemon, raw, size 165, without peel and seeds (about 4 per lb with peels and seeds)	1	74	90	20	1	Trace	—	—	—	6	19	12	.4	102	10	.03	.01	.1	39
Lemon juice																			
Raw	1 cup	244	91	60	1	Trace	—	—	—	20	17	24	.5	344	50	.07	.02	.2	112
Canned, or bottled, unsweetened	1 cup	244	92	55	1	Trace	—	—	—	19	17	24	.5	344	50	.07	.02	.2	102
Frozen, single strength, unsweetened, 6-fl oz can	1 can	183	92	40	1	Trace	—	—	—	13	13	16	.5	258	40	.05	.02	.2	81
Lemonade concentrate, frozen																			
Undiluted, 6-fl oz can	1 can	219	49	425	Trace	Trace	—	—	—	112	9	13	.4	153	40	.05	.06	.7	66
Diluted with 4⅓ parts water by volume	1 cup	248	89	105	Trace	Trace	—	—	—	28	2	3	.1	40	10	.01	.02	.2	17
Limeade concentrate, frozen																			
Undiluted, 6-fl oz can	1 can	218	50	410	Trace	Trace	—	—	—	108	11	13	.2	129	Trace	.02	.02	.2	26
Diluted with 4⅓ parts water by volume	1 cup	247	89	100	Trace	Trace	—	—	—	27	3	3	Trace	32	Trace	Trace	Trace	Trace	6
Lime juice																			
Raw	1 cup	246	90	65	1	Trace	—	—	—	22	22	27	.5	256	20	.05	.02	.2	79
Canned, unsweetened	1 cup	246	90	65	1	Trace	—	—	—	22	22	27	.5	256	20	.05	.02	.2	52
Muskmelons, raw, with rind, without seed cavity																			
Cantaloupe orange-fleshed (with rind and seed cavity, 5-in diam., 2⅓ lb)	½33	477	91	80	2	Trace	—	—	—	20	38	44	1.1	682	9,240	.11	.08	1.6	90
Honey dew (with rind and seed cavity, 6½-in diam., 5¼ lb)	1/1033	226	91	50	1	Trace	—	—	—	11	21	24	.6	374	60	.06	.04	.9	34
Oranges, all commercial varieties, raw																			
Whole, 2⅝-in diam., without peel and seeds (about 2½ per lb with peel and seeds)	1	131	86	65	1	Trace	—	—	—	16	54	26	.5	263	260	.13	.05	.5	66
Sections without membranes	1 cup	180	86	90	2	Trace	—	—	—	22	74	36	.7	360	360	.18	.07	.7	90
Orange juice																			
Raw, all varieties	1 cup	248	88	110	2	Trace	—	—	—	26	27	42	.5	496	500	.22	.07	1.0	124
Canned, unsweetened	1 cup	249	87	120	2	Trace	—	—	—	28	25	45	1.0	496	500	.17	.05	.7	100
Frozen concentrate																			
Undiluted, 6-fl oz can	1 can	213	55	360	5	Trace	—	—	—	87	75	126	.9	1,500	1,620	.68	.11	2.8	360
Diluted with 3 parts water by volume	1 cup	249	87	120	2	Trace	—	—	—	29	25	42	.2	503	540	.23	.03	.9	120
Dehydrated crystals, prepared with water (1 lb yields about 1 gal)	1 cup	248	88	115	1	Trace	—	—	—	27	25	40	.5	518	500	.20	.07	1.0	109
Orange and grapefruit juice																			
Frozen concentrate																			
Undiluted, 6-fl oz can	1 can	210	59	330	4	1	—	—	—	78	61	99	.8	1,308	800	.48	.06	2.3	302
Diluted with 3 parts water by volume	1 cup	248	88	110	1	Trace	—	—	—	26	20	32	.2	439	270	.15	.02	.7	102
Papayas, raw, ½-in cubes	1 cup	140	89	55	1	Trace	—	—	—	14	28	22	.4	328	2,450	.06	.06	.4	78
Peaches																			
Raw																			
Whole, 2½-in diam., peeled, pitted (about 4 per lb with peels and pits)	1	100	89	40	1	Trace	—	—	—	10	9	19	.5	202	341,330	.02	.05	1.0	7
Sliced	1 cup	170	89	65	1	Trace	—	—	—	16	15	32	.9	343	342,260	.03	.09	1.7	12
Canned, yellow-fleshed, solids and liquid (halves or slices)																			
Syrup pack	1 cup	256	79	200	1	Trace	—	—	—	51	10	31	.8	333	1,100	.03	.05	1.5	8
Water pack	1 cup	244	91	75	1	Trace	—	—	—	20	10	32	.7	334	1,100	.02	.07	1.5	7

Food	Measure	Grams	Water (%)	Food energy (cal)	Protein (g)	Fat (g)				Carbohydrate (g)	Calcium (mg)	Phosphorus (mg)	Iron (mg)	Potassium (mg)	Vitamin A (IU)	Thiamin (mg)	Riboflavin (mg)	Niacin (mg)	Ascorbic acid (mg)
Dried																			
Uncooked	1 cup	160	25	420	5	1	—	—	—	109	77	187	9.6	1,520	6,240	.02	.30	8.5	29
Cooked, unsweetened, halves and juice	1 cup	250	77	205	3	1	—	—	—	54	38	93	4.8	743	3,050	.01	.15	3.8	5
Frozen, sliced, sweetened																			
10-oz container	1	284	77	250	1	Trace	—	—	—	64	11	37	1.4	352	1,850	.03	.11	2.0	[35]116
Cup	1 cup	250	77	220	1	Trace	—	—	—	57	10	33	1.3	310	1,630	.03	.10	1.8	[35]103
Pears																			
Raw, with skin, cored																			
Bartlett, 2½-in diam. (about 2½ per lb with cores and stems)	1	164	83	100	1	1	—	—	—	25	13	18	.5	213	30	.03	.07	.2	7
Bosc, 2½-in diam. (about 3 per lb with cores and stems)	1	141	83	85	1	1	—	—	—	22	11	16	.4	83	30	.03	.06	.1	6
Anjou, 3-in diam. (about 2 per lb with cores and stems)	1	200	83	120	1	1	—	—	—	31	16	22	.6	260	40	.04	.08	.2	8
Canned, solids and liquid, syrup pack, heavy (halves or slices)	1 cup	255	80	195	1	1	—	—	—	50	13	18	.5	214	10	.03	.05	.3	3
Pineapple																			
Raw, diced	1 cup	155	85	80	1	Trace	—	—	—	21	26	12	.8	226	110	.14	.05	.3	26
Canned, heavy syrup pack, solids and liquid																			
Crushed, chunks, tidbits	1 cup	255	80	190	1	Trace	—	—	—	49	28	13	.8	245	130	.20	.05	.5	18
Slices and liquid																			
Large, slice; In liquid	1; 2¼ tbsp	105	80	80	Trace	Trace	—	—	—	20	12	5	.3	101	50	.08	.02	.2	7
Medium, slice; In liquid	1; 1¼ tbsp	58	80	45	Trace	Trace	—	—	—	11	6	3	.2	56	30	.05	.01	.1	4
Pineapple juice, unsweetened, canned	1 cup	250	86	140	1	Trace	—	—	—	34	38	23	.8	373	130	.13	.05	.5	[27]80
Plums																			
Raw, without pits																			
Japanese and hybrid (2⅛-in diam., about 6½ per lb with pits)	1	66	87	30	Trace	Trace	—	—	—	8	8	12	.3	112	160	.02	.02	.3	4
Prune-type (1½-in diam., about 15 per lb with pits)	1	28	79	20	Trace	Trace	—	—	—	6	3	5	.1	48	80	.01	.01	.1	1
Canned, heavy syrup pack (Italian prunes), with pits and liquid																			
Cup	1 cup[16]	272	77	215	1	Trace	—	—	—	56	23	26	2.3	367	3,130	.05	.05	1.0	5
Portion[16]	3; 2¾ tbsp	140	77	110	1	Trace	—	—	—	29	12	13	1.2	189	1,610	.03	.03	.5	3
Prunes, dried, "softenized," with pits																			
Uncooked, extra large or large	4; 5[16]	49	28	110	1	Trace	—	—	—	29	22	34	1.7	298	690	.04	.07	.7	1
Cooked, unsweetened, all sizes, fruit and liquid	1 cup[16]	250	66	255	2	1	—	—	—	67	51	79	3.8	695	1,590	.07	.15	1.5	2
Prune juice, canned or bottled	1 cup	256	80	195	1	Trace	—	—	—	49	36	51	1.8	602	—	.03	.03	1.0	5
Raisins, seedless																			
Cup, not pressed down	1 cup	145	18	420	4	Trace	—	—	—	112	90	146	5.1	1,106	30	.16	.12	.7	1
Packet, ½ oz (1½ tbsp)	1	14	18	40	Trace	Trace	—	—	—	11	9	14	.5	107	Trace	.02	.01	.1	Trace
Raspberries, red																			
Raw, capped, whole	1 cup	123	84	70	1	1	—	—	—	17	27	27	1.1	207	160	.04	.11	1.1	31
Frozen, sweetened, 10-oz container	1 cont.	284	74	280	2	1	—	—	—	70	37	48	1.7	284	200	.06	.17	1.7	60
Rhubarb, cooked, added sugar																			
From raw	1 cup	270	63	380	1	Trace	—	—	—	97	211	41	1.6	548	220	.05	.14	.8	16
From frozen, sweetened	1 cup	270	63	385	1	1	—	—	—	98	211	32	1.9	475	190	.05	.11	.5	16
Strawberries																			
Raw, whole berries, capped	1 cup	149	90	55	1	1	—	—	—	13	31	31	1.5	244	90	.04	.10	.9	88
Frozen, sweetened																			
Sliced, 10-oz container	1 cont.	284	71	310	1	1	—	—	—	79	40	48	2.0	318	90	.06	.17	1.4	151
Whole, 1-lb container (about 1¾ cups)	1 cont.	454	76	415	2	1	—	—	—	107	59	73	2.7	472	140	.09	.27	2.3	249
Tangerine, raw, 2⅜-in. diam., size 176, without peel (about 4 per lb with peels and seeds)	1	86	87	40	1	Trace	—	—	—	10	34	15	.3	108	360	.05	.02	.1	27
Tangerine juice, canned, sweetened	1 cup	249	87	125	1	Trace	—	—	—	30	44	35	.5	440	1,040	.15	.05	.2	54
Watermelon, raw, 4 by 8 in. wedge with rind and seeds (1/16 of 32⅔-lb melon, 10 by 16 in)[37]	1	926	93	110	2	1	—	—	—	27	30	43	2.1	426	2,510	.13	.13	.9	30

Table A-1. (Continued)

Foods, Approximate Measures, Units and Weight (edible part unless footnotes indicate otherwise)		Weight Grams	Water Percent	Food Energy Calories	Protein (g)	Fat (g)	Fatty Acids: Saturated (total) (g)	Fatty Acids: Unsaturated: Oleic (g)	Fatty Acids: Unsaturated: Linoleic (g)	Carbohydrate (g)	Calcium (mg)	Phosphorus (mg)	Iron (mg)	Potassium (mg)	Vitamin A Value I.U.	Thiamin (mg)	Riboflavin (mg)	Niacin (mg)	Ascorbic Acid (mg)
GRAIN PRODUCTS																			
Bagel, 3-in diam.																			
Egg	1	55	32	165	6	2	.5	.9	.8	28	9	43	1.2	41	30	.14	.10	1.2	0
Water	1	55	29	165	6	1	.2	.4	.6	30	8	41	1.2	42	0	.15	.11	1.4	0
Barley pearled, light uncooked	1 cup	200	11	700	16	2	.3	.2	.8	158	32	378	4.0	320	0	.24	.10	6.2	0
Biscuits, baking powder, 2-in diam. (enriched flour, vegetable shortening)																			
From home recipe	1	28	27	105	2	5	1.2	2.0	1.2	13	34	49	.4	33	Trace	.08	.08	.7	Trace
From mix	1	28	29	90	2	3	.6	1.1	.7	15	19	65	.6	32	Trace	.09	.08	.8	Trace
Breadcrumbs (enriched)[38]																			
Dry, grated	1 cup	100	7	390	13	5	1.0	1.6	1.4	73	122	141	3.6	152	Trace	.35	.35	4.8	Trace
Soft, see White bread																			
Breads																			
Boston brown bread, canned, slice, 3¼ by ½ in[38]	1 slice	45	45	95	2	1	.1	.2	.2	21	41	72	.9	131	390	.06	.04	.7	0
Cracked-wheat bread (¼ enriched wheat flour, ¾ cracked wheat)[38]																			
Loaf, 1 lb	1 loaf	454	35	1,195	39	10	2.2	3.0	3.9	236	399	581	9.5	608	Trace	1.52	1.13	14.4	Trace
Slice (18 per loaf)	1 slice	25	35	65	2	1	.1	.2	.2	13	22	32	.5	34	Trace	.08	.06	.8	Trace
French or vienna bread, enriched[38]																			
Loaf, 1 lb	1 loaf	454	31	1,315	41	14	3.2	4.7	4.6	251	195	386	10.0	408	Trace	1.80	1.10	15.0	Trace
Slice																			
French (5 by 2½ by 1 in)	1 slice	35	31	100	3	1	.2	.4	.4	19	15	30	.8	32	Trace	.14	.08	1.2	Trace
Vienna (4¾ by 4 by ½ in)	1 slice	25	31	75	2	1	.2	.3	.3	14	11	21	.6	23	Trace	.10	.06	.8	Trace
Italian bread, enriched																			
Loaf, 1 lb	1 loaf	454	32	1,250	41	4	.6	.3	1.5	256	77	349	10.0	336	0	1.80	1.10	15.0	0
Slice, 4½ by 3¼ by ¾ in	1 slice	30	32	85	3	Trace	Trace	Trace	.1	17	5	23	.7	22	0	.12	.07	1.0	0
Raisin bread, enriched[38]																			
Loaf, 1 lb	1 loaf	454	35	1,190	30	13	3.0	4.7	3.9	243	322	395	10.0	1,057	Trace	1.70	1.07	10.7	Trace
Slice (18 per loaf)	1 slice	25	35	65	2	1	.2	.3	.2	13	18	22	.6	58	Trace	.09	.06	.6	Trace
Rye Bread																			
American light (⅔ enriched wheat flour, ⅓ rye flour)																			
Loaf, 1 lb	1 loaf	454	36	1,100	41	5	0.7	0.5	2.2	236	340	667	9.1	658	0	1.35	0.98	12.9	0
Slice (4¾ by 3¾ by 7/16 in)	1 slice	25	36	60	2	Trace	Trace	Trace	.1	13	19	37	.5	36	0	.07	.05	.7	0
Pumpernickel (⅔ rye flour, ⅓ enriched wheat flour)																			
Loaf, 1 lb	1 loaf	454	34	1,115	41	5	.7	.5	2.4	241	381	1,039	11.8	2,059	0	1.30	.93	8.5	0
Slice (5 by 4 by ⅜ in)	1 slice	32	34	80	3	Trace	.1	Trace	.2	17	27	73	.8	145	0	.09	.07	.6	0
White bread, enriched[38]																			
Soft-crumb type																			
Loaf, 1 lb	1 loaf	454	36	1,225	39	15	3.4	5.3	4.6	229	381	440	11.3	476	Trace	1.80	1.10	15.0	Trace
Slice, (18 per loaf)	1 slice	25	36	70	2	1	.2	.3	.3	13	21	24	.6	26	Trace	.10	.06	.8	Trace
Slice, toasted	1 slice	22	25	70	2	1	.2	.3	.3	13	21	24	.6	26	Trace	.08	.06	.8	Trace
Slice (22 per loaf)	1 slice	20	36	55	2	1	.2	.2	.2	10	17	19	.5	21	Trace	.08	.05	.7	Trace
Slice, toasted	1 slice	17	25	55	2	1	.2	.2	.2	10	17	19	.5	21	Trace	.06	.05	.7	Trace
Loaf, 1½ lb	1 loaf	680	36	1,835	59	22	5.2	7.9	6.9	343	571	660	17.0	714	Trace	2.70	1.65	22.5	Trace
Slice (24 per loaf)	1 slice	28	36	75	2	1	.2	.3	.3	14	24	27	.7	29	Trace	.11	.07	.9	Trace
Slice, toasted	1 slice	24	25	75	2	1	.2	.3	.3	14	24	27	.7	29	Trace	.09	.07	.9	Trace
Slice (28 per loaf)	1 slice	24	36	65	2	1	.2	.3	.2	12	20	23	.6	25	Trace	.10	.06	.8	Trace
Slice, toasted	1 slice	21	25	65	2	1	.2	.3	.2	12	20	23	.6	25	Trace	.08	.06	.8	Trace

Food	Measure																		
Cubes	1 cup	30	36	80	3	1	.2	.3	.3	15	25	29	.8	32	Trace	.12	.07	1.0	Trace
Crumbs	1 cup	45	36	120	4	1	.3	.5	.5	23	38	44	1.1	47	Trace	.18	.11	1.5	Trace
Firm-crumb type																			
Loaf, 1 lb	1 loaf	454	35	1,245	41	17	3.9	5.9	5.2	228	435	463	11.3	549	Trace	1.80	1.10	15.0	Trace
Slice (20 per loaf)	1 slice	23	35	65	2	1	.2	.3	.3	12	22	23	.6	28	Trace	.09	.06	.8	Trace
Slice, toasted	1 slice	20	24	65	2	1	.2	.3	.3	12	22	23	.6	28	Trace	.07	.06	.8	Trace
Loaf, 2 lb	1 loaf	907	35	2,495	82	34	7.7	11.8	10.4	455	871	925	22.7	1,097	Trace	3.60	2.20	30.0	Trace
Slice (34 per loaf)	1 slice	27	35	75	2	1	.2	.3	.3	14	26	28	.7	33	Trace	.11	.06	.9	Trace
Slice, toasted	1 slice	23	24	75	2	1	.2	.3	.3	14	26	28	.7	33	Trace	.09	.06	.9	Trace
Whole wheat bread																			
Soft-crumb type[18]																			
Loaf, 1 lb	1 loaf	454	36	1,095	41	12	2.2	2.9	4.2	224	381	1,152	13.6	1,161	Trace	1.37	.45	12.7	Trace
Slice (16 per loaf)	1 slice	28	36	65	3	1	.1	.2	.2	14	24	71	.8	72	Trace	.09	.03	.8	Trace
Slice, toasted	1 slice	24	24	65	3	1	.1	.2	.2	14	24	71	.8	72	Trace	.07	.03	.8	Trace
Firm-crumb type[18]																			
Loaf, 1 lb	1 loaf	454	36	1,100	48	14	2.5	3.3	4.9	216	449	1,034	13.6	1,238	Trace	1.17	.54	12.7	Trace
Slice (18 per loaf)	1 slice	25	36	60	3	1	.1	.2	.2	12	25	57	.8	68	Trace	.06	.03	.7	Trace
Slice, toasted	1 slice	21	24	60	3	1	.1	.2	.2	12	25	57	.8	68	Trace	.05	.03	.7	Trace
Breakfast, cereals																			
Hot type, cooked																			
Corn (hominy) grits degermed																			
Enriched	1 cup	245	87	125	3	Trace	Trace	Trace	.1	27	2	25	.7	27	[40]Trace	.10	.07	1.0	0
Unenriched	1 cup	245	87	125	3	Trace	Trace	Trace	.1	27	2	25	.2	27	[40]Trace	.05	.02	.5	0
Farina, quick cooking enriched	1 cup	245	89	105	3	Trace	Trace	Trace	.1	22	147	[41]113	[42]	25	0	.12	.07	1.0	0
Oatmeal or rolled oats	1 cup	240	87	130	5	2	.4	.8	.9	23	22	137	1.4	146	0	.19	.05	.2	0
Wheat, rolled	1 cup	240	80	180	5	1	—	—	—	41	19	182	1.7	202	0	.17	.07	2.2	0
Wheat, whole-meal	1 cup	245	88	110	4	1	—	—	—	23	17	127	1.2	118	0	.15	.05	1.5	0
Ready-to-eat																			
Bran flakes (40% bran), added sugar, salt, iron, vitamins	1 cup	35	3	105	4	1	—	—	—	28	19	125	12.4	137	1,650	.41	.49	4.1	12
Bran flakes with raisins, added sugar, salt, iron, vitamins	1 cup	50	7	145	4	1	—	—	—	40	28	146	17.7	154	2,350	.58	.71	5.8	18
Corn flakes																			
Plain, added sugar, salt, iron, vitamins	1 cup	25	4	95	2	Trace	—	—	—	21	[41]	9	.6	30	1,180	.29	.35	2.9	9
Sugar-coated, added salt, iron, vitamins	1 cup	40	2	155	2	Trace	—	—	—	37	1	10	1.0	27	1,880	.46	.56	4.6	14
Corn, puffed, plain, added sugar, salt, iron, vitamins	1 cup	20	4	80	2	1	—	—	—	16	4	18	2.3	—	940	.23	.28	2.3	7
Corn, shredded, added sugar, salt, iron, thiamin, niacin	1 cup	25	3	95	2	Trace	—	—	—	22	1	10	.6	—	0	.11	.05	.5	0
Oats, puffed, added sugar, salt, minerals, vitamins	1 cup	25	3	100	3	1	—	—	—	19	44	102	2.9	—	1,180	.29	.35	2.9	9
Rice, puffed																			
Plain, added iron, thiamin, niacin	1 cup	15	4	60	1	Trace	—	—	—	13	3	14	.3	15	0	.07	.01	.7	0
Presweetened, added salt, iron, vitamins	1 cup	28	3	115	1	0	—	—	—	26	3	14	[44]1.1	43	1,250	.38	.43	5.0	[45]15
Wheat flakes, added sugar, salt, iron, vitamins	1 cup	30	4	105	3	Trace	—	—	—	24	12	83	[41]	81	1,410	.35	.42	3.5	11
Wheat, puffed: Plain, added iron, thiamin, niacin	1 cup	15	3	55	2	Trace	—	—	—	12	4	48	.6	51	0	.08	.03	1.2	0
Presweetened, added salt, iron, vitamins	1 cup	38	3	140	3	Trace	—	—	—	33	7	52	[44]1.6	63	1,680	.50	.57	6.7	[45]20
Wheat, shredded, plain																			
oblong biscuit	1	25	7	90	2	1	—	—	—	20	11	97	.9	87	0	.06	.03	1.1	0
Spoon-size	½ cup																		
Wheat germ, without salt and sugar, toasted	1 tbsp	6	4	25	2	1	—	—	—	3	3	70	.5	57	10	.11	.05	.3	1
Buckwheat flour light, sifted	1 cup	98	12	340	6	1	.2	.4	.4	78	11	86	1.0	314	0	.08	.04	.4	0
Bulgur, canned, seasoned	1 cup	135	56	245	8	4	—	—	—	44	27	263	1.9	151	0	.08	.05	4.1	0
Cake icings. See Sugars and Sweets																			

Table A-1. (Continued)

Nutrients in Indicated Quantity

Foods, Approximate Measures, Units and Weight (edible part unless footnotes indicate otherwise)		Weight Grams	Water Percent	Food Energy Calories	Protein (g)	Fat (g)	Fatty Acids Saturated (total) (g)	Unsaturated Oleic (g)	Linoleic (g)	Carbohydrate (g)	Calcium (mg)	Phosphorus (mg)	Iron (mg)	Potassium (mg)	Vitamin A Value I.U.	Thiamin (mg)	Riboflavin (mg)	Niacin (mg)	Ascorbic Acid (mg)
Cakes made from cake mixes with enriched flour[46]																			
Angelfood																			
Whole cake (9¾-in diam. tube cake)	1 cake	635	34	1,645	36	36	—	—	—	377	603	756	2.5	381	0	.37	.95	3.6	0
Piece, 1/12 of cake	1 piece	53	34	135	3	Trace	—	—	—	32	50	63	.2	32	0	.03	.08	.3	0
Coffeecake																			
Whole cake (7¾ by 5⅝ by 1¼ in.)	1 cake	430	30	1,385	27	41	11.7	16.3	8.8	225	262	748	6.9	469	690	.82	.91	7.7	1
Piece, 1/6 of cake	1 piece	72	30	230	5	7	2.0	2.7	1.5	38	44	125	1.2	78	120	.14	.15	1.3	Trace
Cupcakes, made with egg, milk, 2½-in diam.																			
Without icing	1	25	26	90	1	3	.8	1.2	.7	14	40	59	.3	21	40	.05	.05	.4	Trace
With chocolate icing	1	36	22	130	2	5	2.0	1.6	.6	21	47	71	.4	42	60	.05	.06	.4	Trace
Devil's food with chocolate icing																			
Whole, 2 layer cake (8- or 9-in diam.)	1 cake	1,107	24	3,755	49	136	50.0	44.9	17.0	645	653	1,162	16.6	1,439	1,660	1.06	1.65	10.1	1
Piece, 1/16 of cake	1 piece	69	24	235	3	8	3.1	2.8	1.1	40	41	72	1.0	90	100	.07	.10	.6	Trace
Cupcake, 2½-in diam	1	35	24	120	2	4	1.6	1.4	.5	20	21	37	.5	46	50	.03	.05	.3	Trace
Gingerbread																			
Whole cake (8-in square)	1 cake	570	37	1,575	18	39	9.7	16.6	10.0	291	513	570	8.6	1,562	Trace	0.84	1.00	7.4	Trace
Piece, 1/9 of cake	1	63	37	175	2	4	1.1	1.8	1.1	32	57	63	.9	173	Trace	.09	.11	.8	Trace
White, 2 layer with chocolate icing:																			
Whole cake (8- or 9-in diam)	1 cake	1,140	21	4,000	44	122	48.2	46.4	20.0	716	1,129	2,041	11.4	1,322	680	1.50	1.77	12.5	2
Piece, 1/16 of cake	1	71	21	250	3	8	3.0	2.9	1.2	45	70	127	.7	82	40	.09	.11	.8	Trace
Yellow, 2 layer with chocolate icing																			
Whole cake (8- or 9-in diam.)	1	1,108	26	3,735	45	125	47.8	47.8	20.3	638	1,008	2,017	12.2	1,208	1,550	1.24	1.67	10.6	2
Piece, 1/16 of cake	1	69	26	235	3	8	3.0	3.0	1.3	40	63	126	.8	75	100	.08	.10	.7	Trace
Cakes made from home recipes using enriched flour[47]																			
Boston cream pie with custard filling																			
Whole cake (8-in diam.)	1	825	35	2,490	41	78	23.0	30.1	15.2	412	553	833	8.2	[48]734	1,730	1.04	1.27	9.6	2
Piece, 1/12 of cake	1	69	35	210	3	6	1.9	2.5	1.3	34	46	70	.7	[48]61	140	.09	.11	.8	2
Fruitcake, dark																			
Loaf, 1-lb (7½ by 2 by 1½ in)	1	454	18	1,720	22	69	14.4	33.5	14.8	271	327	513	11.8	2,250	540	.72	.73	4.9	2
Slice, 1/30 of loaf	1	15	18	55	1	2	.5	1.1	.5	9	11	17	.4	74	20	.02	.02	.2	Trace
Plain sheet cake																			
Without icing																			
Whole cake (9-in square)	1	777	25	2,830	35	108	29.5	44.4	23.9	434	497	793	8.5	[48]614	1,320	1.21	1.40	10.2	2
Piece, 1/9 of cake	1	86	25	315	4	12	3.3	4.9	2.6	48	55	88	.9	[48]68	150	.13	.15	1.1	Trace
With uncooked white icing;																			
Whole cake (9-in square)	1	1,096	21	4,020	37	129	42.2	49.5	24.4	694	548	822	8.2	[48]669	2,190	1.22	1.47	10.2	2
Piece, 1/9 of cake	1	121	21	445	4	14	4.7	5.5	2.7	77	61	91	.8	[48]74	240	.14	.16	1.1	Trace
Pound[49]																			
Loaf, 8½ by 3½ by 3¼ in	1	565	16	2,725	31	170	42.9	73.1	39.6	273	107	418	7.9	345	1,410	.90	.99	7.3	0
Slice, 1/17 of loaf	1	33	16	160	2	10	2.5	4.3	2.3	16	6	24	.5	20	80	.05	.06	.4	0
Spongecake																			
Whole cake (9¾-in diam. tube cake).	1	790	32	2,345	60	45	13.1	15.8	5.7	427	237	885	13.4	687	3,560	1.10	1.64	7.4	Trace
Piece, 1/12 of cake	1	66	32	195	5	4	1.1	1.3	.5	36	20	74	1.1	57	300	.09	.14	.6	Trace
Cookies made with enriched flour[50,51]																			
Brownies with nuts																			
Home-prepared, 1¾ by 1¾ by ⅞ in																			
From home recipe	1	20	10	95	1	6	1.5	3.0	1.2	10	8	30	.4	38	40	.04	.03	.2	Trace
From commercial recipe	1	20	11	85	1	4	.9	1.4	1.3	13	9	27	.4	34	20	.03	.02	.2	Trace
Frozen, with chocolate icing,[52] 1½ by 1¾ by ⅞ in	1	25	13	105	1	5	2.0	2.2	.7	15	10	31	.4	44	50	.03	.03	.2	Trace

Food	Measure	Weight (g)	Water (%)	Food energy (cal)	Protein (g)	Fat (g)	Fatty acids — Saturated (g)	Oleic (g)	Linoleic (g)	Carbohydrate (g)	Calcium (mg)	Phosphorus (mg)	Iron (mg)	Potassium (mg)	Vitamin A (IU)	Thiamin (mg)	Riboflavin (mg)	Niacin (mg)	Ascorbic acid (mg)
Chocolate chip — Commercial, 2¼-in diam., ⅜ in thick	4	42	3	200	2	9	2.8	2.9	2.2	29	16	48	1.0	56	50	.10	.17	.9	Trace
From home recipe, 2⅓-in diam.	4	40	3	205	2	12	3.5	4.5	2.9	24	14	40	.8	47	40	.06	.06	.5	Trace
Fig bars, square (1⅝ by 1⅝ by ⅜ in) or rectangular (1½ by 1¾ by ½ in)	4	56	14	200	2	3	.8	1.2	.7	42	44	34	1.0	111	60	.04	.14	.9	Trace
Gingersnaps, 2-in diam., ¼ in thick	4	28	3	90	2	2	.7	1.0	.6	22	20	13	.7	129	20	.08	.06	.7	0
Macaroons, 2¾-in diam., ¼ in thick	2	38	4	180	2	9	—	—	—	25	10	32	.3	176	0	.02	.06	.2	0
Oatmeal with raisins, 2⅝ in diam., ¼ in thick	4	52	3	235	3	8	2.0	3.3	2.0	38	11	53	1.4	192	30	.15	.10	1.0	Trace
Plain, prepared from commercial chilled dough, 2½-in diam., ¼ in thick	4	48	5	240	2	12	3.0	5.2	2.9	31	17	35	.6	23	30	.10	.08	.9	0
Sandwich type (chocolate or vanilla), 1¾-in diam., ⅜ in thick	4	40	2	200	2	9	2.2	3.9	2.2	28	10	96	.7	15	0	.06	.10	.7	0
Vanilla wafers, 1¾-in diam., ¼ in thick	10	40	3	185	2	6	—	—	—	30	16	25	.6	29	50	.10	.09	.8	0
Cornmeal — Whole-ground, unbolted, dry form	1 cup	122	12	435	11	5	.5	1.0	2.5	90	24	312	2.9	346	620[53]	.46	.13	2.4	0
Bolted (nearly whole-grain), dry form	1 cup	122	12	440	11	4	.5	.9	2.1	91	21	272	2.2	303	590[53]	.37	.10	2.3	0
Degermed, enriched — Dry form	1 cup	138	12	500	11	2	.2	.4	.9	108	8	137	4.0	166	610[53]	.61	.36	4.8	0
Cooked	1 cup	240	88	120	3	Trace	Trace	.1	.2	26	2	34	1.0	38	140[53]	.14	.10	1.2	0
Degermed, unenriched — Dry form	1 cup	138	12	500	11	2	.2	.4	.9	108	8	137	1.5	166	610[53]	.19	.07	1.4	0
Cooked	1 cup	240	88	120	3	Trace	Trace	.1	.2	26	2	34	.5	38	140[53]	.05	.02	.2	0
Crackers[38] — Graham, plain, 2½-in square	2	14	6	55	1	1	.3	.5	.3	10	6	21	.5	55	0	.02	.08	.5	0
Rye, wafers, whole-grain 1⅞ by 3½ in	2	13	6	45	2	Trace	—	—	—	10	7	50	.5	78	0	.04	.03	.2	0
Saltines, made with enriched flour	4	11	4	50	1	1	.3	.5	.4	8	2	10	.5	13	0	.05	.05	.4	0
Danish pastry (enriched flour), plain without fruit or nuts[54] — Packaged ring, 12 oz	1	340	22	1,435	25	80	24.3	31.7	16.5	155	170	371	6.1	381	1,050	.97	1.01	8.6	Trace
Round piece, about 4¼-in diam. by 1 in	1	65	22	275	5	15	4.7	6.1	3.2	30	33	71	1.2	73	200	.18	.19	1.7	Trace
Ounce	1 oz	28	22	120	2	7	2.0	2.7	1.4	13	14	31	.5	32	90	.08	.08	.7	Trace
Doughnuts, made with enriched flour[38] — Cake type, plain, 2½-in diam., 1 in high	1	25	24	100	1	5	1.2	2.0	1.1	13	10	48	.4	23	20	.05	.05	.4	Trace
Yeast-leavened, glazed, 3¾-in diam., 1¼ in high	1	50	26	205	3	11	3.3	5.8	3.3	22	16	33	.6	34	25	.10	.10	.8	0
Macaroni, enriched, cooked (cut lengths, elbows, shells) — Firm stage (hot)	1 cup	130	64	190	7	1	—	—	—	39	14	85	1.4	103	0	.23	.13	1.8	0
Tender stage — Cold macaroni	1 cup	105	73	115	4	Trace	—	—	—	24	8	53	.9	64	0	.15	.08	1.2	0
Hot macaroni	1 cup	140	73	155	5	1	—	—	—	32	11	70	1.3	85	0	.20	.11	1.5	0
Macaroni (enriched) and cheese: Canned[55]	1 cup	240	80	230	9	10	4.2	3.1	1.4	26	199	182	1.0	139	260	.12	.24	1.0	Trace
From home recipe (served hot)[56]	1 cup	200	58	430	17	22	8.9	8.8	2.9	40	362	322	1.8	240	860	.20	.40	1.8	Trace
Muffins made with enriched flour[38] — From home recipe — Blueberry, 2⅜-in diam., 1½ in high	1	40	39	110	3	4	1.1	1.4	.7	17	34	53	.6	46	90	.09	.10	.7	Trace
Bran	1	40	35	105	3	4	1.2	1.4	.8	17	57	162	1.5	172	90	.07	.10	1.7	Trace
Corn (enriched degermed cornmeal and flour), 2⅜-in diam., 1½ in high	1	40	33	†125	3	4	1.2	1.6	.9	19	42	68	.7	54	120[57]	.10	.10	.7	Trace
From mix, egg, milk — Plain, 3-in diam., 1½ in high	1	40	38	120	3	4	1.0	1.7	1.0	17	42	60	.6	50	40	.09	.12	.9	Trace
Corn, 2⅜-in diam., 1½ in high[58]	1	40	30	130	3	4	1.2	1.7	.9	20	96	152	.6	44	100[57]	.08	.09	.7	Trace
Noodles (egg noodles), enriched, cooked	1 cup	160	71	200	7	2	—	—	—	37	16	94	1.4	70	110	.22	.13	1.9	0
Noodles, chow mein, canned	1 cup	45	1	220	6	11	—	—	—	26	—	—	—	—	—	—	—	—	—

Table A-1.   (Continued)

Nutrients in Indicated Quantity

Foods, Approximate Measures, Units and Weight (edible part unless footnotes indicate otherwise)		Weight Grams	Water Percent	Food Energy Calories	Pro-tein (g)	Fat (g)	Fatty Acids Satu-rated (total) (g)	Unsaturated Oleic (g)	Lino-leic (g)	Carbo-hydrate (g)	Calcium (mg)	Phos-phorus (mg)	Iron (mg)	Potas-sium (mg)	Vitamin A Value I.U.	Thiamin (mg)	Ribo-flavin (mg)	Niacin (mg)	Ascorbic Acid (mg)
Pancakes, (4-in diam.)[38]																			
Buckwheat, made from mix (with buckwheat and enriched flours) egg and milk added	1 cake	27	58	55	2	2	.8	.9	.4	6	59	91	.4	66	60	.04	.05	.2	Trace
Plain																			
Made from home recipe using enriched flour	1 cake	27	50	60	2	2	.5	.8	.5	9	27	38	.4	33	30	.06	.07	.5	Trace
Made from mix with enriched flour, egg and milk added	1 cake	27	51	60	2	2	.7	.7	.3	9	58	70	.3	42	70	.04	.06	.2	Trace
Pies, piecrust made with enriched flour, vegetable shortening (9-in diam.)																			
Apple																			
Whole pie	1	945	48	2,420	21	105	27.0	44.5	25.2	360	76	208	6.6	756	280	1.06	.79	9.3	9
Sector, 1/7 of pie	1	135	48	345	3	15	3.9	6.4	3.6	51	11	30	.9	108	40	.15	.11	1.3	2
Banana cream																			
Whole pie	1	910	54	2,010	41	85	26.7	33.2	16.2	279	601	746	7.3	1,847	2,280	.77	1.51	7.0	9
Sector, 1/7 of pie	1	130	54	285	6	12	3.8	4.7	2.3	40	86	107	1.0	264	330	.11	.22	1.0	1
Blueberry																			
Whole pie	1	945	51	2,285	23	102	24.8	43.7	25.1	330	104	217	9.5	614	280	1.03	.80	10.0	28
Sector, 1/7 of pie	1	135	51	325	3	15	3.5	6.2	3.6	47	15	31	1.4	88	40	.15	.11	1.4	4
Cherry																			
Whole pie	1	945	47	2,465	25	107	28.2	45.0	25.3	363	132	236	6.6	992	4,160	1.09	.84	9.8	Trace
Sector, 1/7 of pie	1	135	47	350	4	15	4.0	6.4	3.6	52	19	24	.9	142	590	.16	.12	1.4	Trace
Custard																			
Whole pie	1	910	58	1,985	56	101	33.9	38.5	17.5	213	874	1,028	8.2	1,247	2,090	.79	1.92	5.6	0
Sector, 1/7 of pie	1	130	58	285	8	14	4.8	5.5	2.5	30	125	147	1.2	178	300	.11	.27	.8	0
Lemon meringue																			
Whole pie	1	840	47	2,140	31	86	26.1	33.8	16.4	317	118	412	6.7	420	1,430	.61	.84	5.2	25
Sector, 1/7 of pie	1	120	47	305	4	12	3.7	4.8	2.3	45	17	59	1.0	60	200	.09	.12	.7	4
Mince																			
Whole pie	1	945	43	2,560	24	109	28.0	45.9	25.2	389	265	359	13.3	1,682	20	.96	.86	9.8	9
Sector, 1/7 of pie	1	135	43	365	3	16	4.0	6.6	3.6	56	38	51	1.9	240	Trace	.14	.12	1.4	1
Peach																			
Whole pie	1	945	48	2,410	24	101	24.8	43.7	25.1	361	95	274	8.5	1,408	6,900	1.04	.97	14.0	28
Sector, 1/7 of pie	1	135	48	345	3	14	3.5	6.2	3.6	52	14	39	1.2	201	990	.15	.14	2.0	4
Pecan																			
Whole pie	1	825	20	3,450	42	189	27.8	101.0	44.2	423	388	850	25.6	1,015	1,320	1.80	.95	6.9	Trace
Sector, 1/7 of pie	1	118	20	495	6	27	4.0	14.4	6.3	61	55	122	3.7	145	190	.26	.14	1.0	Trace
Pumpkin																			
Whole pie	1	910	59	1,920	36	102	37.4	37.5	16.6	223	464	628	7.3	1,456	22,480	.78	1.27	7.0	Trace
Sector, 1/7 of pie	1	130	59	275	5	15	5.4	5.4	2.4	32	66	90	1.0	208	3,210	.11	.18	1.0	Trace
Piecrust (home recipe) made with enriched flour and vegetable shortening, baked 9-in. diam.	1	180	15	900	11	60	14.8	26.1	14.9	79	25	90	3.1	89	0	.47	.40	5.0	0
Piecrust mix with enriched flour and vegetable shortening, 10-oz pkg prepared and baked	2 crusts	320	19	1,485	20	93	22.7	39.7	23.4	141	131	272	6.1	179	0	1.07	.79	9.9	0
Pizza (cheese) baked, 4¾-in. sector; ⅛ of 12-in diam. pie.[19]	1	60	45	145	6	4	1.7	1.5	0.6	22	86	89	1.1	67	230	.16	.18	1.6	4
Popcorn, popped																			
Plain, large kernel	1 cup	6	4	25	1	Trace	Trace	.1	.2	5	1	17	.2	—	—	—	.01	.1	0
With oil (coconut) and salt added, large kernel	1 cup	9	3	40	1	2	1.5	.2	.2	5	1	19	.2	—	—	—	.01	.2	0
Sugar coated	1 cup	35	4	135	2	1	.5	.2	.4	30	2	47	.5	—	—	—	.02	.4	0

Food	Measure	Grams	Water (%)	Food energy (cal)	Protein (g)	Fat (g)	Saturated (g)	Oleic (g)	Linoleic (g)	Carbohydrate (g)	Calcium (mg)	Phosphorus (mg)	Iron (mg)	Potassium (mg)	Vitamin A (IU)	Thiamin (mg)	Riboflavin (mg)	Niacin (mg)	Ascorbic acid (mg)
Pretzels, made with enriched flour																			
Dutch, twisted, 2¾ by 2⅝ in	1	16	5	60	2	1	—	—	—	12	4	21	.2	21	0	.05	.04	.7	0
Thin, twisted, 3¼ by 2¼ by ¼ in	10	60	5	235	6	3	—	—	—	46	13	79	.9	78	0	.20	.15	2.5	0
Stick, 2¼ in long	10	3	5	10	Trace	Trace	—	—	—	2	1	4	Trace	4	0	.01	.01	.1	0
Rice, white, enriched																			
Instant, ready-to-serve, hot	1 cup	165	73	180	4	Trace	Trace	Trace	Trace	40	5	31	1.3	—	0	.21	(59)	1.7	0
Long grain																			
Raw	1 cup	185	12	670	12	1	.2	.2	.2	149	44	174	5.4	170	0	.81	.06	6.5	0
Cooked, served hot	1 cup	205	73	225	4	Trace	.1	.1	.1	50	21	57	1.8	57	0	.23	.02	2.1	0
Parboiled																			
Raw	1 cup	185	10	685	14	1	.2	.1	.2	150	111	370	5.4	278	0	.81	.07	6.5	0
Cooked, served hot	1 cup	175	73	185	4	Trace	.1	.1	.1	41	33	100	1.4	75	0	.19	.02	2.1	0
Rolls, enriched[38]																			
Commercial																			
Brown-and-serve (12 per 12-oz pkg.), browned	1 roll	26	27	85	2	2	.4	.7	.5	14	20	23	.5	25	Trace	.10	.06	.9	Trace
Cloverleaf or pan, 2½-in diam., 2 in high	1 roll	28	31	85	2	2	.4	.6	.4	15	21	24	.5	27	Trace	.11	.07	.9	Trace
Frankfurter and hamburger (8 per 11½-oz pkg.)	1 roll	40	31	120	3	2	.5	.8	.6	21	30	34	.8	38	Trace	.16	.10	1.3	Trace
Hard, 3¾-in diam., 2 in high	1 roll	50	25	155	5	2	.4	.6	.5	30	24	46	1.2	49	Trace	.20	.12	1.7	Trace
Hoagie, or submarine, 11½ by 3 by 2½-in	1 roll	135	31	390	12	4	.9	1.4	1.4	75	58	115	3.0	122	Trace	.54	.32	4.5	Trace
From home recipe																			
Cloverleaf, 2½-in diam., 2 in high	1 roll	35	26	120	3	3	.8	1.1	.7	20	16	36	.7	41	30	.12	.12	1.2	Trace
Spaghetti, enriched, cooked:																			
Firm stage, "al dente," served hot	1 cup	130	64	190	7	1	—	—	—	39	14	85	1.4	103	0	.23	.13	1.8	0
Tender stage, served hot	1 cup	140	73	155	5	1	—	—	—	32	11	70	1.3	85	0	.20	.11	1.5	0
Spaghetti (enriched) in tomato sauce with cheese																			
From home recipe	1 cup	250	77	260	9	9	2.0	5.4	.7	37	80	135	2.3	408	1,080	.25	.18	2.3	13
Canned	1 cup	250	80	190	6	2	.5	.3	.4	39	40	88	2.8	303	930	.35	.28	4.5	10
Spaghetti (enriched) with meatballs and tomato sauce																			
From home recipe	1 cup	248	70	330	19	12	3.3	6.3	1.0	39	124	236	3.7	665	1,590	.25	.30	4.0	22
Canned	1 cup	250	78	260	12	10	2.2	3.3	3.9	29	53	113	3.3	245	1,000	.15	.18	2.3	5
Toaster pastries	1	50	12	200	3	6	—	—	—	36	54	[60]67	1.9	[60]74	500	.16	.17	2.1	(60)
Waffles, made with enriched flour, 7-in diam.[38]																			
From home recipe	1	75	41	210	7	7	2.3	2.8	1.4	28	85	130	1.3	109	250	.17	.23	1.4	Trace
From mix, egg and milk added	1	75	41	205	7	8	2.8	2.9	1.2	27	179	257	1.0	146	170	.14	.22	.9	Trace
Wheat flours																			
All-purpose or family flour, enriched																			
Sifted, spooned	1 cup	115	12	420	12	1	.2	.1	.5	88	18	100	3.3	109	0	.74	.46	6.1	0
Unsifted, spooned	1 cup	125	12	455	13	1	.2	.1	.5	95	20	109	3.6	119	0	.80	.50	6.6	0
Cake or pastry flour, enriched, sifted, spooned	1 cup	96	12	350	7	1	.1	.1	.3	76	16	70	2.8	91	0	.61	.38	5.1	0
Self-rising, enriched, unsifted, spooned	1 cup	125	12	440	12	1	.2	.2	.5	93	331	583	3.6	—	0	.80	.50	6.6	0
Whole wheat, from hard wheats, stirred	1 cup	120	12	400	16	2	.4	.2	1.0	85	49	446	4.0	444	0	.66	.14	5.2	0
LEGUMES (DRY), NUTS, SEEDS; RELATED PRODUCTS																			
Almonds, shelled																			
Chopped (about 130 almonds)	1 cup	130	5	775	24	70	5.6	47.7	12.8	25	304	655	6.1	1,005	0	.31	1.20	4.6	Trace
Slivered, not pressed down (about 115 almonds)	1 cup	115	5	690	21	62	5.0	42.2	11.3	22	269	580	5.4	889	0	.28	1.06	4.0	Trace
Beans, dry																			
Common varieties as Great Northern, navy, and others																			
Cooked, drained																			
Great Northern	1 cup	180	69	210	14	1	—	—	—	38	90	266	4.9	749	0	.25	.13	1.3	0
Pea (navy)	1 cup	190	69	225	15	1	—	—	—	40	95	281	5.1	790	0	.27	.13	1.3	0
Canned, solids and liquid																			
White with																			
Frankfurters (sliced)	1 cup	255	71	365	19	18	—	—	—	32	94	303	4.8	668	330	.18	.15	3.3	Trace
Pork and tomato sauce	1 cup	255	71	310	16	7	2.4	2.8	.6	48	138	235	4.6	536	330	.20	.08	1.5	5
Pork and sweet sauce	1 cup	255	66	385	16	12	4.3	5.0	1.1	54	161	291	5.9	536	330	.15	.10	1.3	—
Red kidney	1 cup	255	76	230	15	1	—	—	—	42	74	278	4.6	673	10	.13	.10	1.5	—
Lima, cooked, drained	1 cup	190	64	260	16	1	—	—	—	49	55	293	5.9	1,163	—	.25	.11	1.3	—

Nutrients in Indicated Quantity

Foods, Approximate Measures, Units and Weight (edible part unless footnotes indicate otherwise)		Weight Grams	Water Percent	Food Energy Calories	Protein (g)	Fat (g)	Fatty Acids Saturated (total) (g)	Unsaturated Oleic (g)	Unsaturated Linoleic (g)	Carbohydrate (g)	Calcium (mg)	Phosphorus (mg)	Iron (mg)	Potassium (mg)	Vitamin A Value I.U.	Thiamin (mg)	Riboflavin (mg)	Niacin (mg)	Ascorbic Acid (mg)
Blackeye peas, dry, cooked (with residual cooking liquid)	1 cup	250	80	190	13	1	—	—	—	35	43	238	3.3	573	30	.40	.10	1.0	—
Brazil nuts, shelled (6–8 large kernels)	1 oz	28	5	185	4	19	4.8	6.2	7.1	3	53	196	1.0	203	Trace	.27	.03	.5	—
Cashew nuts, roasted in oil	1 cup	140	5	785	24	64	12.9	36.8	10.2	41	53	522	5.3	650	140	.60	.35	2.5	—
Coconut meat, fresh																			
Piece, about 2 by 2 by ½ in	1 piece	45	51	155	2	16	14.0	.9	.3	4	6	43	.8	115	0	.02	.01	.2	1
Shredded or grated, not pressed down	1 cup	80	51	275	3	28	24.8	1.6	.5	8	10	76	1.4	205	0	.04	.02	.4	2
Filberts (hazelnuts), chopped (about 80 kernels)	1 cup	115	6	730	14	72	5.1	55.2	7.3	19	240	388	3.9	810	—	.53	—	1.0	Trace
Lentils, whole, cooked	1 cup	200	72	210	16	Trace	—	—	—	39	50	238	4.2	498	40	.14	.12	1.2	0
Peanuts, roasted in oil, salted (whole, halves, chopped)	1 cup	144	2	840	37	72	13.7	33.0	20.7	27	107	577	3.0	971	—	.46	.19	24.8	0
Peanut butter	1 tbsp	16	2	95	4	8	1.5	3.7	2.3	3	9	61	.3	100	—	.02	.02	2.4	0
Peas, split, dry, cooked	1 cup	200	70	230	16	1	—	—	—	42	22	178	3.4	592	80	.30	.18	1.8	—
Pecans, chopped or pieces (about 120 large halves)	1 cup	118	3	810	11	84	7.2	50.5	20.0	17	86	341	2.8	712	150	1.01	.15	1.1	2
Pumpkin and squash kernels, dry, hulled	1 cup	140	4	775	41	65	11.8	23.5	27.5	21	71	1,602	15.7	1,386	100	.34	.27	3.4	—
Sunflower seeds, dry, hulled	1 cup	145	5	810	35	69	8.2	13.7	43.2	29	174	1,214	10.3	1,334	70	2.84	.33	7.8	—
Walnuts																			
Black																			
Chopped or broken kernels	1 cup	125	3	785	26	74	6.3	13.3	45.7	19	Trace	713	7.5	575	380	.28	.14	.9	—
Ground (finely)	1 cup	80	3	500	16	47	4.0	8.5	29.2	12	Trace	456	4.8	368	240	.18	.09	.6	—
Persian or English, chopped (about 60 halves)	1 cup	120	4	780	18	77	8.4	11.8	42.2	19	119	456	3.7	540	40	.40	.16	1.1	2
SUGARS AND SWEETS																			
Cake icings																			
Boiled, white																			
Plain	1 cup	94	18	295	1	0	0	0	0	75	2	2	Trace	17	0	Trace	0.03	Trace	0
With coconut	1 cup	166	15	605	3	13	11.0	.9	Trace	124	10	50	0.8	277	0	0.02	0.07	0.3	0
Uncooked																			
Chocolate made with milk and butter	1 cup	275	14	1,035	9	38	23.4	11.7	1.0	185	165	305	3.3	536	580	.06	.28	.6	1
Creamy fudge from mix and water	1 cup	245	15	830	7	16	5.1	6.7	3.1	183	96	218	2.7	238	Trace	.05	.20	.7	Trace
White	1 cup	319	11	1,200	2	21	12.7	5.1	.5	260	48	38	Trace	57	860	Trace	.06	Trace	Trace
Candy																			
Caramels, plain or chocolate	1 oz	28	8	115	1	3	1.6	1.1	.1	22	42	35	.4	54	Trace	.01	.05	.1	Trace
Chocolate																			
Milk, plain	1 oz	28	1	145	2	9	5.5	3.0	.3	16	65	65	.3	109	80	.02	.10	.1	Trace
Semisweet, small pieces (60 per oz)	1 cup	170	1	860	7	61	36.2	19.8	1.7	97	51	255	4.4	553	30	.02	.14	.9	0
Chocolate-covered peanuts	1 oz	28	1	160	5	12	4.0	4.7	2.1	11	33	84	.4	143	Trace	.10	.05	2.1	Trace
Fondant, uncoated (mints, candy corn, other)	1 oz	28	8	105	Trace	1	.1	.3	.1	25	4	2	.3	42	0	Trace	Trace	Trace	0
Fudge, chocolate, plain	1 oz	28	8	115	1	3	1.3	1.4	.6	21	22	24	.3	42	Trace	.01	.03	.1	Trace
Gum drops	1 oz	28	12	100	Trace	Trace	—	—	—	25	2	Trace	.1	1	0	0	Trace	Trace	0
Hard	1 oz	28	1	110	0	Trace	—	—	—	28	6	2	.5	1	0	0	0	0	0
Marshmallows	1 oz	28	17	90	1	Trace	—	—	—	23	5	2	.5	2	0	0	Trace	Trace	0
Chocolate-flavored beverage powders (about 4 heaping tsp per oz)																			
With nonfat dry milk	1 oz	28	2	100	5	1	.5	.3	Trace	20	167	155	.5	227	10	.04	.21	.2	1
Without milk	1 oz	28	1	100	1	1	.4	.2	Trace	25	9	48	.6	142	—	.01	.03	.1	0
Honey, strained or extracted	1 tbsp	21	17	65	Trace	0	0	0	0	17	1	1	.1	11	0	Trace	.01	.1	Trace

Food	Measure	Grams	Water (%)	Food energy (cal)	Protein (g)	Fat (g)	Saturated	Oleic	Linoleic	Carbohydrate (g)	Calcium (mg)	Phosphorus (mg)	Iron (mg)	Potassium (mg)	Vit. A (IU)	Thiamin (mg)	Riboflavin (mg)	Niacin (mg)	Ascorbic acid (mg)
Jams and preserves	1 tbsp	20	29	55	Trace	Trace	—	—	—	14	4	2	.2	18	Trace	Trace	Trace	Trace	Trace
Packet	1	14	29	40	Trace	Trace	—	—	—	10	3	1	.1	12	Trace	Trace	Trace	Trace	Trace
Jellies	1 tbsp	18	29	50	Trace	Trace	—	—	—	13	4	1	.3	14	Trace	Trace	Trace	Trace	1
Packet	1	14	29	40	Trace	Trace	—	—	—	10	3	1	.2	11	Trace	Trace	Trace	Trace	1
Syrups																			
Chocolate-flavored syrup or topping																			
Thin type	2 tbsp	38	32	90	1	1	.5	.3	Trace	24	6	35	.6	106	Trace	.01	.03	.2	0
Fudge type	2 tbsp	38	25	125	2	5	3.1	1.6	.1	20	48	60	.5	107	60	.02	.08	.2	Trace
Molasses, cane																			
Light (first extraction)	1 tbsp	20	24	50	—	—	—	—	—	13	33	9	.9	183	—	.01	.01	Trace	—
Blackstrap (third extraction)	1 tbsp	20	24	45	—	—	—	—	—	11	137	17	3.2	585	—	.02	.04	.4	—
Sorghum	1 tbsp	21	23	55	—	—	—	—	—	14	35	5	2.6	—	—	—	.02	Trace	—
Table blends, chiefly corn, light and dark	1 tbsp	21	24	60	0	0	0	0	0	15	9	3	.8	1	0	0	0	0	0
Sugars																			
Brown, pressed down	1 cup	220	2	820	0	0	0	0	0	212	187	42	7.5	757	0	.02	.07	.4	0
White																			
Granulated	1 cup	200	1	770	0	0	0	0	0	199	0	0	.2	6	0	0	0	0	0
	1 tbsp	12	1	45	0	0	0	0	0	12	0	0	Trace	Trace	0	0	0	0	0
Packet	1	6	1	23	0	0	0	0	0	6	0	0	Trace	Trace	0	0	0	0	0
Powdered, sifted, spooned into cup	1 cup	100	1	385	0	0	0	0	0	100	0	0	.1	3	0	0	0	0	0
VEGETABLE AND VEGETABLE PRODUCTS																			
Asparagus, green																			
Cooked, drained																			
Cuts and tips, 1½- to 2-in lengths																			
From raw	1 cup	145	94	30	3	Trace	—	—	—	5	30	73	.9	265	1,310	.23	.26	2.0	38
From frozen	1 cup	180	93	40	6	Trace	—	—	—	6	40	115	2.2	396	1,530	.25	.23	1.8	41
Spears, ½-in diam. at base:																			
From raw, spears	4	60	94	10	1	Trace	—	—	—	2	13	30	.4	110	540	.10	.11	.8	16
From frozen, spears	4	60	92	15	2	Trace	—	—	—	2	13	40	.7	143	470	.10	.08	.7	16
Canned, ½-in diam. at base, spears	4	80	93	15	2	Trace	—	—	—	3	15	42	1.5	133	640	.05	.08	.6	12
Beans																			
Lima, immature seeds, frozen, cooked, drained																			
Thick-seeded types (Fordhooks)	1 cup	170	74	170	10	Trace	—	—	—	32	34	153	2.9	724	390	.12	.09	1.7	29
Thin-seeded types (baby limas)	1 cup	180	69	210	13	Trace	—	—	—	40	63	227	4.7	709	400	.16	.09	2.2	22
Snap																			
Green																			
Cooked, drained																			
From raw (cuts and French style)	1 cup	125	92	30	2	Trace	—	—	—	7	63	46	.8	189	680	.09	.11	.6	15
From frozen																			
Cuts	1 cup	135	92	35	2	Trace	—	—	—	8	54	43	.9	205	780	.09	.12	.5	7
French style	1 cup	130	92	35	2	Trace	—	—	—	8	49	39	1.2	177	690	.08	.10	.4	9
Canned, drained solids (cuts)	1 cup	135	92	30	2	Trace	—	—	—	7	61	34	2.0	128	630	.04	.07	.4	5
Yellow or wax																			
Cooked, drained																			
From raw (cuts and French style)	1 cup	125	93	30	2	Trace	—	—	—	6	63	46	.8	189	290	.09	.11	.6	16
From frozen (cuts)	1 cup	135	92	35	2	Trace	—	—	—	8	47	42	.9	221	140	.09	.11	.5	8
Canned, drained solids (cuts)	1 cup	135	92	30	2	Trace	—	—	—	7	61	34	2.0	128	140	.04	.07	.4	7
Beans, mature. See Beans, dry and Blackeye peas, dry																			
Beans sprouts (mung)																			
Raw	1 cup	105	89	35	4	Trace	—	—	—	7	20	67	1.4	234	20	.14	.14	.8	20
Cooked, drained	1 cup	125	91	35	4	Trace	—	—	—	7	21	60	1.1	195	30	.11	.13	.9	8
Beets																			
Cooked, drained, peeled																			
Whole beets, 2-in diam.	2 beets	100	91	30	1	Trace	—	—	—	7	14	23	.5	208	20	.03	.04	.3	6
Diced or sliced	1 cup	170	91	55	2	Trace	—	—	—	12	24	39	.9	354	30	.05	.07	.5	10
Canned, drained solids																			
Whole beets, small	1 cup	160	89	60	2	Trace	—	—	—	14	30	29	1.1	267	30	.02	.05	.2	5
Diced or sliced	1 cup	170	89	65	2	Trace	—	—	—	15	32	31	1.2	284	30	.02	.05	.2	5
Beet greens, leaves and stems, cooked drained	1 cup	145	94	25	2	Trace	—	—	—	5	144	36	2.8	481	7,400	.10	.22	.4	22
Blackeye peas, immature seeds, cooked and drained																			
From raw	1 cup	165	72	180	13	1	—	—	—	30	40	241	3.5	625	580	.50	.18	2.3	28
From frozen	1 cup	170	66	220	15	1	—	—	—	40	43	286	4.8	573	290	.68	.19	2.4	15

Table A-1. (Continued)

Foods, Approximate Measures, Units and Weight (edible part unless footnotes indicate otherwise)		Weight Grams	Water Percent	Food Energy Calories	Protein (g)	Fat (g)	Fatty Acids Saturated (total) (g)	Unsaturated Oleic (g)	Linoleic (g)	Carbohydrate (g)	Calcium (mg)	Phosphorus (mg)	Iron (mg)	Potassium (mg)	Vitamin A Value I.U.	Thiamin (mg)	Riboflavin (mg)	Niacin (mg)	Ascorbic Acid (mg)
Broccoli, cooked, drained																			
From raw																			
Stalk, medium size	1 stalk	180	91	45	6	1	—	—	—	8	158	112	1.4	481	4,500	.16	.36	1.4	162
Stalks, cut into ½-in pieces	1 cup	155	91	40	5	Trace	—	—	—	7	136	96	1.2	414	3,880	.14	.31	1.2	140
From frozen																			
Stalk, 4½ to 5 in long	1 stalk	30	91	10	1	Trace	—	—	—	1	12	17	.2	66	570	.02	.03	.2	22
Chopped	1 cup	185	92	50	5	1	—	—	—	9	100	104	1.3	392	4,810	.11	.22	.9	105
Brussels sprouts, cooked, drained																			
From raw, 7–8 sprouts (1¼ to 1½-in diam.)	1 cup	155	88	55	7	1	—	—	—	10	50	112	1.7	423	810	.12	.22	1.2	135
From frozen	1 cup	155	89	50	5	Trace	—	—	—	10	33	95	1.2	457	880	.12	.16	.9	126
Cabbage																			
Common varieties																			
Raw																			
Coarsely shredded or sliced	1 cup	70	92	15	1	Trace	—	—	—	4	34	20	0.3	163	90	.04	.04	.2	33
Finely shredded or chopped	1 cup	90	92	20	1	Trace	—	—	—	5	44	26	.4	210	120	.05	.05	.3	42
Cooked, drained	1 cup	145	94	30	2	Trace	—	—	—	6	64	29	.4	236	190	.06	.04	.4	48
Red, raw, coarsely shredded	1 cup	70	90	20	1	Trace	—	—	—	5	29	25	.6	188	30	.06	.04	.3	43
Savoy, raw, coarsely shredded or sliced	1 cup	70	92	15	2	Trace	—	—	—	3	47	38	.6	188	140	.04	.06	.2	39
Cabbage, celery (also called pe-tsai or wongbok), raw, 1-in pieces	1 cup	75	95	10	1	Trace	—	—	—	2	32	30	.5	190	110	.04	.03	.5	19
Cabbage, white mustard (also called bokchoy or pakchoy), cooked, drained	1 cup	170	95	25	2	Trace	—	—	—	4	252	56	1.0	364	5,270	.07	.14	1.2	26
Carrots																			
Raw, without crowns and tips, scraped																			
Whole, 7½ by 1⅛ in, or strips, 2½ to 3 in long, 18 strips	1	72	88	30	1	Trace	—	—	—	7	27	26	.5	246	7,930	.04	.04	.4	6
Grated	1 cup	110	88	45	1	Trace	—	—	—	11	41	40	.8	375	12,100	.07	.06	.7	9
Cooked (crosswise cuts) drained	1 cup	155	91	50	1	Trace	—	—	—	11	51	48	.9	344	16,280	.08	.08	.8	9
Canned																			
Sliced, drained solids	1 cup	155	91	45	1	Trace	—	—	—	10	47	34	1.1	186	23,250	.03	.05	.6	3
Strained or junior (baby food)	2 tbsp	28	92	10	Trace	Trace	—	—	—	2	7	6	.1	51	3,690	.01	.01	.1	1
Cauliflower																			
Raw, chopped	1 cup	115	91	31	3	Trace	—	—	—	6	29	64	1.3	339	70	.13	.12	.8	90
Cooked, drained																			
From raw (flower buds)	1 cup	125	93	30	3	Trace	—	—	—	5	26	53	.9	258	80	.11	.10	.8	69
From frozen (flowerets)	1 cup	180	94	30	3	Trace	—	—	—	6	31	68	.9	373	50	.07	.09	.7	74
Celery, Pascal type, raw																			
Stalk, large outer, 8 by 1½ in, at root end	1 stalk	40	94	5	Trace	Trace	—	—	—	2	16	11	.1	136	110	.01	.01	.1	4
Pieces, diced	1 cup	120	94	20	1	Trace	—	—	—	5	47	34	.4	409	320	.04	.04	.4	11
Collards, cooked, drained																			
From raw (leaves without stems)	1 cup	190	90	65	7	1	—	—	—	10	357	99	1.5	498	14,820	.21	.38	2.3	144
From frozen (chopped)	1 cup	170	90	50	5	1	—	—	—	10	299	87	1.7	401	11,560	.10	.24	1.0	56
Corn, sweet																			
Cooked, drained																			
From raw, ear 5 by 1¾ in	1 ear[61]	140	74	70	2	1	—	—	—	16	2	69	.5	151	[62]310	.09	.08	1.1	7
From frozen																			
Ear, 5 in long	1 ear[61]	229	73	120	4	1	—	—	—	27	4	121	1.0	291	[62]440	.18	.10	2.1	9
Kernels	1 cup	165	77	130	5	1	—	—	—	31	5	120	1.3	304	[62]580	.15	.10	2.5	8
Canned																			
Cream style	1 cup	256	76	210	5	2	—	—	—	51	8	143	1.5	248	[62]840	.08	.13	2.6	13
Whole kernel																			
Vacuum pack	1 cup	210	76	175	5	1	—	—	—	43	6	153	1.1	204	[62]740	.06	.13	2.3	11
Wet pack, drained solids	1 cup	165	76	140	4	1	—	—	—	33	8	81	.8	160	[62]580	.05	.08	1.5	7

Cowpeas. See Blackeye peas

Food	Measure	Grams	Water (%)	Food energy (cal)	Protein (g)	Fat (g)	Saturated	Oleic	Linoleic	Carbohydrate (g)	Calcium (mg)	Phosphorus (mg)	Iron (mg)	Potassium (mg)	Vitamin A (IU)	Thiamin (mg)	Riboflavin (mg)	Niacin (mg)	Ascorbic acid (mg)
Cucumber slices, ⅛-in thick, with peel (large, 2⅛-in diam.; slices small, 1¾-in diam. slices) — large	6	28	95	5	Trace	Trace	—	—	—	1	7	8	.3	45	70	.01	.01	.1	3
With peel, small slices	8	28	95	5	Trace	Trace	—	—	—	1	7	8	.3	45	70	.01	.01	.1	3
Without peel, large slices	6½	28	96	5	Trace	Trace	—	—	—	1	5	5	.1	45	Trace	.01	.01	.1	3
Without peel, small slices	9	28	96	5	Trace	Trace	—	—	—	1	5	5	.1	45	Trace	.01	.01	.1	3
Dandelion greens, cooked, drained	1 cup	105	90	35	2	1	—	—	—	7	147	44	1.9	244	12,290	.14	.17	—	19
Endive, curly (including escarole), raw, small pieces	1 cup	50	93	10	1	Trace	—	—	—	2	41	27	.9	147	1,650	.04	.07	.3	5
Kale, cooked, drained, from raw (leaves without stems and midribs)	1 cup	110	88	45	5	1	—	—	—	7	206	64	1.8	243	9,130	.11	.20	1.8	102
Kale, from frozen (leaf style)	1 cup	130	91	40	4	1	—	—	—	7	157	62	1.3	251	10,660	.08	.20	.9	49
Lettuce, raw — Butterhead, as Boston types, head, 5-in diam	1[63]	220	95	25	2	Trace	—	—	—	4	57	42	3.3	430	1,580	.10	.10	.5	13
Butterhead, leaves, outer	1	15	95	Trace	Trace	Trace	—	—	—	Trace	5	4	.3	40	150	.01	.01	Trace	1
Butterhead, leaves, inner	2	15	95	Trace	Trace	Trace	—	—	—	Trace	5	4	.3	40	150	.01	.01	Trace	1
Crisphead, as Iceberg, head, 6-in diam	1[64]	567	96	70	5	1	—	—	—	16	108	118	2.7	943	1,780	.32	.32	1.6	32
Crisphead, wedge, ¼ of head	1	135	96	20	1	Trace	—	—	—	4	27	30	.7	236	450	.08	.08	.4	8
Crisphead, pieces, chopped or shredded	1 cup	55	96	5	Trace	Trace	—	—	—	2	11	12	.3	96	180	.03	.03	.2	3
Looseleaf (bunching varieties including romaine or cos), chopped or shredded pieces	1 cup	55	94	10	1	Trace	—	—	—	2	37	14	.8	145	1,050	.03	.04	.2	10
Mushrooms, raw, sliced or chopped	1 cup	70	90	20	2	Trace	—	—	—	3	4	81	.6	290	Trace	.07	.32	2.9	2
Mustard greens, without stems and midribs, cooked, drained	1 cup	140	93	30	3	1	—	—	—	6	193	45	2.5	308	8,120	.11	.20	.8	67
Okra pods, 3 by ⅝ in, cooked	10	106	91	30	2	Trace	—	—	—	6	98	43	.5	184	520	.14	.19	1.0	21
Onions, mature, raw, chopped	1 cup	170	89	65	3	Trace	—	—	—	15	46	61	.9	267	[65]Trace	.05	.07	.3	17
Onions, mature, raw, sliced	1 cup	115	89	45	2	Trace	—	—	—	10	31	41	.6	181	[65]Trace	.03	.05	.2	12
Onions, mature, cooked (whole or sliced), drained	1 cup	210	92	60	3	Trace	—	—	—	14	50	61	.8	231	[65]Trace	.06	.06	.4	15
Young green onions, bulb (⅜-in diam.) and white portion of top	6	30	88	15	Trace	Trace	—	—	—	3	12	12	.2	69	Trace	.02	.01	.1	8
Parsley, raw, chopped	1 tbsp	4	85	Trace	Trace	Trace	—	—	—	Trace	7	2	.2	25	300	Trace	.01	Trace	6
Parsnips, cooked (diced or 2-in lengths)	1 cup	155	82	100	2	1	—	—	—	23	70	96	.9	587	50	.11	.12	.2	16
Peas, green, canned, whole, drained solids	1 cup	170	77	150	8	1	—	—	—	29	44	129	3.2	163	1,170	.15	.10	1.4	14
Peas, green, canned, strained (baby food)	2 tbsp	28	86	15	1	Trace	—	—	—	3	3	18	.3	28	140	.02	.03	.3	3
Peas, green, frozen, cooked, drained	1 cup	160	82	110	8	Trace	—	—	—	19	30	138	3.0	216	960	.43	.14	2.7	21
Peppers, hot, red, without seeds, dried (ground chili powder, added seasonings)	1 tsp	2	9	5	Trace	Trace	—	—	—	1	5	4	.3	20	1,300	.02	.02	.2	Trace
Peppers, sweet (about 5 per lb, whole, stems and seeds removed), raw	1 pod	74	93	15	1	Trace	—	—	—	4	7	16	.5	157	310	.06	.06	.4	94
Peppers, sweet, cooked, boiled, drained	1 pod	73	95	15	1	Trace	—	—	—	3	7	12	.4	109	310	.05	.05	.4	70
Potatoes, cooked, baked, peeled after baking (about 2 per lb, raw)	1	156	75	145	4	Trace	—	—	—	33	14	101	1.1	782	Trace	.15	.07	2.7	31
Boiled (about 3 per lb, raw), peeled after boiling	1	137	80	105	3	Trace	—	—	—	23	10	72	.8	556	Trace	.12	.05	2.0	22
Boiled, peeled before boiling	1	135	83	90	3	Trace	—	—	—	20	8	57	.7	385	Trace	.12	.05	1.6	22
French-fried, strip, 2 to 3½ in long, prepared from raw	10	50	45	135	2	7	1.7	1.2	3.3	18	8	56	.7	427	Trace	.07	.04	1.6	11
French-fried, frozen, oven heated	10	50	53	110	2	4	1.1	.8	2.1	17	5	43	.9	326	Trace	.07	.01	1.3	11
Hashed brown, prepared from frozen	1 cup	155	56	345	3	18	4.6	3.2	9.0	45	28	78	1.9	439	Trace	.11	.03	1.6	12
Mashed, prepared from raw, milk added	1 cup	210	83	135	4	2	—	—	—	27	50	103	.8	548	40	.17	.11	2.1	21
Mashed, milk and butter added	1 cup	210	80	195	4	9	5.6	2.3	.2	26	50	101	.8	525	360	.17	.11	2.1	19
Mashed, prepared from dehydrated flakes (without milk), water, milk, butter, and salt added	1 cup	210	79	195	4	7	3.6	2.1	.2	30	65	99	.6	601	270	.08	.08	1.9	11

643

Table A-1. (Continued)

Foods, Approximate Measures, Units and Weight (edible part unless footnotes indicate otherwise)	Weight Grams	Water Percent	Food Energy Calories	Protein (g)	Fat (g)	Fatty Acids Saturated (total) (g)	Unsaturated Oleic (g)	Unsaturated Linoleic (g)	Carbohydrate (g)	Calcium (mg)	Phosphorus (mg)	Iron (mg)	Potassium (mg)	Vitamin A Value I.U.	Thiamin (mg)	Riboflavin (mg)	Niacin (mg)	Ascorbic Acid (mg)
Potato chips, 1¾ by 2½ in oval cross section	10	2	115	1	8	2.1	1.4	4.0	10	8	28	.4	226	Trace	.04	.01	1.0	3
Potato salad, made with cooked salad dressing	1 cup	76	250	7	7	2.0	2.7	1.3	41	80	160	1.5	798	350	.20	.18	2.8	28
Pumpkin, canned	1 cup 245	90	80	2	1	—	—	—	19	61	64	1.0	588	15,680	.07	.12	1.5	12
Radishes, raw (prepackaged) stem ends, rootlets cut off	4 18	95	5	Trace	Trace	—	—	—	1	5	6	.2	58	Trace	.01	.01	.1	5
Sauerkraut, canned, solids and liquid	1 cup 235	93	40	2	Trace	—	—	—	9	85	42	1.2	329	120	.07	.09	.5	33
Southern peas. See Blackeye peas																		
Spinach																		
Raw, chopped	1 cup 55	91	15	2	Trace	—	—	—	2	51	28	1.7	259	4,460	.06	.11	.3	28
Cooked, drained From raw	1 cup 180	92	40	5	1	—	—	—	6	167	68	4.0	583	14,580	.13	.25	.9	50
From frozen Chopped	1 cup 205	92	45	6	1	—	—	—	8	232	90	4.3	683	16,200	.14	.31	.8	39
Leaf	1 cup 190	92	45	6	1	—	—	—	7	200	84	4.8	688	15,390	.15	.27	1.0	53
Canned, drained solids	1 cup 205	91	50	6	1	—	—	—	7	242	53	5.3	513	16,400	.04	.25	.6	29
Squash, cooked Summer (all varieties), diced, drained	1 cup 210	96	30	2	Trace	—	—	—	7	53	53	.8	296	820	.11	.17	1.7	21
Winter (all varieties), baked, mashed	1 cup 205	81	130	4	1	—	—	—	32	57	98	1.6	945	8,610	.10	.27	1.4	27
Sweetpotatoes Cooked (raw, 5 by 2 in; about 2½ per lb) Baked in skin, peeled	1 114	64	160	2	1	—	—	—	37	46	66	1.0	342	9,230	.10	.08	.8	25
Boiled in skin, peeled	1 151	71	170	3	1	—	—	—	40	48	71	1.1	367	11,940	.14	.09	.9	26
Candied, 2½- by 2-in piece	1 105	60	175	1	3	2.0	.8	.1	36	39	45	.9	200	6,620	.06	.04	.4	11
Canned Solid pack (mashed)	1 cup 255	72	275	5	1	—	—	—	63	64	105	2.0	510	19,890	.13	.10	1.5	36
Vacuum pack, piece 2¾ by 1 in	1 40	72	45	1	Trace	—	—	—	10	10	16	.3	80	3,120	.02	.02	.2	6
Tomatoes Raw, 2⅗-in diam. (3 per 12 oz pkg.)	1[66] 135	94	25	1	Trace	—	—	—	6	16	33	.6	300	1,110	.07	.05	.9	6[7][28]
Canned, solids and liquid	1 cup 241	94	50	2	Trace	—	—	—	10	6[8]14	46	1.2	523	2,170	.12	.07	1.7	41
Tomato catsup	1 cup 273	69	290	5	1	—	—	—	69	60	137	2.2	991	3,820	.25	.19	4.4	41
	1 tbsp 15	69	15	Trace	Trace	—	—	—	4	3	8	.1	54	210	.01	.01	.2	2
Tomato juice, canned Cup	1 cup 243	94	45	2	Trace	—	—	—	10	17	44	2.2	552	1,940	.12	.07	1.9	39
Glass (6 fl oz)	1 182	94	35	2	Trace	—	—	—	8	13	33	1.6	413	1,460	.09	.05	1.5	29
Turnips, cooked, diced	1 cup 155	94	35	1	Trace	—	—	—	8	54	37	.6	291	Trace	.06	.08	.5	34
Turnip greens, cooked, drained From raw (leaves and stems)	1 cup 145	94	30	3	Trace	—	—	—	5	252	49	1.5	—	8,270	.15	.33	.7	68
From frozen (chopped)	1 cup 165	93	40	4	Trace	—	—	—	6	195	64	2.6	246	11,390	.08	.15	.7	31
Vegetables, mixed, frozen, cooked	1 cup 182	83	115	6	1	—	—	—	24	46	115	2.4	348	9,010	.22	.13	2.0	15
MISCELLANEOUS ITEMS Baking powders for home use Sodium aluminum sulfate With monocalcium phosphate monohydrate	1 tsp 3.0	2	5	Trace	Trace	0	0	0	1	58	87	—	5	0	0	0	0	0
With monocalcium phosphate monohydrate, calcium sulfate	1 tsp 2.9	1	5	Trace	Trace	0	0	0	1	183	45	—	—	0	0	0	0	0
Straight phosphate	1 tsp 3.8	2	5	Trace	Trace	0	0	0	1	239	359	—	6	0	0	0	0	0
Low sodium	1 tsp 4.3	2	5	Trace	Trace	0	0	0	2	207	314	—	471	0	0	0	0	0

Nutrients in Indicated Quantity

Food	Measure	Grams	Water (%)	Food energy (cal)	Protein (g)	Fat (g)	Fat, Saturated (g)	Fat, Oleic (g)	Fat, Linoleic (g)	Carbohydrate (g)	Calcium (mg)	Phosphorus (mg)	Iron (mg)	Potassium (mg)	Vitamin A (IU)	Thiamin (mg)	Riboflavin (mg)	Niacin (mg)	Ascorbic acid (mg)
Barbecue sauce	1 cup	250	81	230	4	17	2.2	4.3	10.0	20	53	50	2.0	435	900	.03	.03	.8	13
Beverages, alcoholic																			
Beer	12 fl oz	360	92	150	1	0	0	0	0	14	18	108	Trace	90	—	.01	.11	2.2	—
Gin, rum, vodka, whisky:																			
80-proof, jigger	1½ fl oz	42	67	95	—	0	0	0	0	Trace	—	—	—	1	—	—	—	—	—
86-proof, jigger	1½ fl oz	42	64	105	—	0	0	0	0	Trace	—	—	—	1	—	—	—	—	—
90-proof, jigger	1½ fl oz	42	62	110	—	0	0	0	0	Trace	—	—	—	1	—	—	—	—	—
Wines																			
Dessert	3½ fl oz	103	77	140	Trace	0	0	0	0	8	8	—	—	77	—	.01	.02	.2	—
Table	3½ fl oz	102	86	85	Trace	0	0	0	0	4	9	10	.4	94	—	Trace	.01	.1	—
Beverages, carbonated, sweetened, nonalcoholic																			
Carbonated water	12 fl oz	366	92	115	0	0	0	0	0	29	—	—	—	—	0	0	0	0	0
Cola type	12 fl oz	369	90	145	0	0	0	0	0	37	—	—	—	—	0	0	0	0	0
Fruit-flavored sodas and Tom Collins mixer	12 fl oz	372	88	170	0	0	0	0	0	45	—	—	0	—	0	0	0	0	0
Ginger ale	12 fl oz	366	92	115	0	0	0	0	0	29	—	—	0	—	0	0	0	0	0
Root beer	12 fl oz	370	90	150	0	0	0	0	0	39	—	—	0	0	0	0	0	0	0
Chili powder. See Peppers, hot, red																			
Chocolate:																			
Bitter or baking	1 oz	28	2	145	3	15	8.9	4.9	.4	8	22	109	1.9	235	20	.01	.07	.4	0
Semisweet, see Candy, chocolate																			
Gelatin, dry, envelope	1	7	13	25	6	Trace	0	0	0	0	—	—	—	—	—	—	—	—	—
Gelatin, dessert prepared with gelatin dessert powder and water	1 cup	240	84	140	4	0	0	0	0	34	0	—	—	—	—	—	—	—	—
Mustard, prepared yellow	1 tsp	5	80	5	Trace	Trace	—	—	—	Trace	4	4	.1	7	—	—	Trace	—	—
Olives, pickled, canned:[69]																			
Green (giant 2, extra large 3, medium 4)		16	78	15	Trace	2	.2	1.2	.1	Trace	8	2	.2	7	40	Trace	Trace	—	—
Ripe, Mission (large 2, medium 3, small 2)		10	73	15	Trace	2	.2	1.2	.1	Trace	9	1	.1	2	10	Trace	Trace	—	—
Pickles, cucumber																			
Dill, medium, whole, 3¾ in long, 1¼-in diam	1	65	93	5	1	Trace	—	—	—	1	17	14	.7	130	70	Trace	.01	—	4
Fresh-pack, slices 1½-in diam., ¼ in thick	2	15	79	10	Trace	Trace	—	—	—	3	5	4	.3	—	20	Trace	Trace	—	1
Sweet, gherkin, small whole about 2½ in long, ¾-in diam.	1	15	61	20	Trace	Trace	—	—	—	5	2	2	.2	—	10	Trace	Trace	—	1
Relish, finely chopped, sweet	1 tbsp	15	63	20	Trace	Trace	—	—	—	5	3	2	.1	—	—	—	—	—	—
Popcorn. See under Grain Products																			
Popsicle, 3-fl oz size	1	95	80	70	0	0	0	0	0	18	0	—	Trace	—	0	0	0	0	0
Soups																			
Canned, condensed																			
Prepared with equal volume of milk																			
Cream of chicken	1 cup	245	85	180	7	10	4.2	3.6	1.3	15	172	152	.5	260	610	.05	.27	.7	2
Cream of mushroom	1 cup	245	83	215	7	14	5.4	2.9	4.6	16	191	169	.5	279	250	.05	.34	.7	1
Tomato	1 cup	250	84	175	7	7	3.4	1.7	1.0	23	168	155	.8	418	1,200	.10	.25	1.3	15
Prepared with equal volume of water																			
Bean with pork	1 cup	250	84	170	8	6	1.2	1.8	2.4	22	63	128	2.3	395	650	.13	.08	1.0	3
Beef broth, bouillon, consomme	1 cup	240	96	30	5	0	0	0	0	3	Trace	31	.5	130	Trace	Trace	.02	1.2	—
Beef noodle	1 cup	240	93	65	4	3	.6	.7	.8	7	7	48	1.0	77	50	.05	.07	1.0	Trace
Clam chowder, Manhattan type (with tomatoes, without milk)	1 cup	245	92	80	2	3	.5	.4	1.3	12	34	47	1.0	184	880	.02	.02	1.0	0
Cream of chicken	1 cup	240	92	95	3	6	1.6	2.3	1.1	8	24	34	.5	79	410	.02	.05	.5	Trace
Cream of mushroom	1 cup	240	90	135	2	10	2.6	1.7	4.5	10	41	50	.5	98	70	.02	.12	.7	Trace
Minestrone	1 cup	245	90	105	5	3	.7	.9	1.3	14	37	59	1.0	314	2,350	.07	.05	1.0	—
Split pea	1 cup	245	85	145	9	3	1.1	1.2	.4	21	29	149	1.5	270	440	.25	.15	1.5	1
Tomato	1 cup	245	91	90	2	2	.5	.5	1.0	16	15	34	.7	230	1,000	.05	.05	1.2	12
Vegetable beef	1 cup	245	92	80	5	2	—	—	—	10	12	49	.7	162	2,700	.05	.05	1.0	—
Vegetarian	1 cup	245	92	80	4	2	—	—	—	13	20	39	1.0	172	2,940	.05	.05	1.0	—

Table A-1. (Continued)

| | | | | | | Fatty Acids | | | | | | | | | | | | |
| | | | | | | | Unsaturated | | | | | | | | | | | |
Foods, Approximate Measures, Units and Weight (edible part unless footnotes indicate otherwise)	Weight Grams	Water Percent	Food Energy Calories	Protein (g)	Fat (g)	Saturated (total) (g)	Oleic (g)	Linoleic (g)	Carbohydrate (g)	Calcium (mg)	Phosphorus (mg)	Iron (mg)	Potassium (mg)	Vitamin A Value I.U.	Thiamin (mg)	Riboflavin (mg)	Niacin (mg)	Ascorbic Acid (mg)
Soups (continued)																		
Dehydrated																		
Bouillon, cube ½ in	1 cube	4	4	5	1	Trace	—	—	—	Trace	—	—	—	—	4	—	—	—	—	—
Mixes																		
Unprepared																		
Onion	1½-oz	43	3	150	6	5	1.1	2.3	1.0	23	42	49	.6	238	30	.05	.03	.3	6
Prepared with water																		
Chicken noodle	1 cup	240	95	55	2	1	—	—	—	8	7	19	.2	19	50	.07	.05	.5	Trace
Onion	1 cup	240	96	35	1	1	—	—	—	6	10	12	.2	58	Trace	Trace	Trace	Trace	2
Tomato vegetable with noodles	1 cup	240	93	65	2	1	—	—	—	12	7	19	.2	29	480	.05	.02	.5	5
Vinegar, cider	1 tbsp	15	94	Trace	Trace	0	0	0	0	1	1	1	.1	15	—	—	—	—	—
White sauce, medium, with enriched flour	1 cup	250	73	405	10	31	19.3	7.8	.8	22	288	233	.5	348	1,150	.12	.43	.7	2
Yeast																		
Baker's, dry, active	1 pkg	7	5	20	3	Trace	—	—	—	3	3	90	1.1	140	Trace	.16	.38	2.6	Trace
Brewer's, dry	1 tbsp	8	5	25	3	Trace	—	—	—	3	[7]17	140	1.4	152	Trace	1.25	.34	3.0	Trace

[1]Vitamin A value is largely from beta-carotene used for coloring. Riboflavin value for powdered creamer apply to product with added riboflavin.

[2]Applies to product without added vitamin A. With added vitamin A, value is 500 international units (IU).

[3]Applies to product without vitamin A added.

[4]Applies to product with added vitamin A. Without added vitamin A, value is 20 IU.

[5]Yields 1 qt of fluid milk when reconstituted according to package directions.

[6]Applies to product with added vitamin A.

[7]Weight applies to product with label claim of 1⅓ cups equal 3.2 oz.

[8]Applies to products made from thick shake mixes and that do not contain added ice cream. Products made from milk shake mixes are higher in fat and usually contain added ice cream.

[9]Content of fat, vitamin A, and carbohydrate varies. Consult the label when precise values are needed for special diets.

[10]Applies to product made with milk containing no added vitamin A.

[11]Based on year-round average.

[12]Based on average vitamin A content of fortified margarine. Federal specifications for fortified margarine require a minimum of 15,000 IU of vitamin A per pound.

[13]Fatty acid values apply to product made with regular-type margarine.

[14]Dipped in egg, milk or water, and breadcrumbs; fried in vegetable shortening.

[15]If bones are discarded, value for calcium will be greatly reduced.

[16]Dipped in egg, breadcrumbs, and flour or batter.

[17]Prepared with tuna, celery, salad dressing (mayonnaise type), pickle, onion, and egg.

[18]Outer layer of fat on the cut was removed to within approximately ½ inch of the lean. Deposits of fat within the cut were not removed.

[19]Crust made with vegetable shortening and enriched flour.

[20]Regular-type margarine used.

[21]Value varies widely.

[22]About one fourth of the outer layer of fat on the cut was removed. Deposits of fat within the cut were not removed.

[23]Vegetable shortening used.

[24]Also applies to pasteurized apple cider.

[25]Applies to product without added ascorbic acid. For value of product with added ascorbic acid, refer to label.

[26]Based on product with label claim of 45 percent of U.S. RDA in 6 fl oz.

[27]Based on product with label claim of 100 percent of U.S. RDA in 6 fl oz.

[28]Weight includes peel and membranes between sections. Without these parts, the weight of the edible portion is 123 g for pink grapefruit and 118 g for white grapefruit.

[29]For white-fleshed varieties, value is about 20 IU per cup; for red-fleshed varieties, 1,080 IU.

[30]Weight includes seeds. Without seeds, weight of the edible portion is 57 g.

[31]Applies to product without added ascorbic acid. With added ascorbic acid, based on claim that 6 fl oz of reconstituted juice contain 45 percent or 50 percent of the U.S. RDA, value in milligrams is 108 or 120 for a 6-fl oz can, 36 or 40 for 1 cup of diluted juice.

[32]For products with added thiamin and riboflavin but without added ascorbic acid, values in milligrams would be 0.60 for thiamin, 0.80 for riboflavin, and trace for ascorbic acid. For products with only ascorbic acid added, value varies with the brand. Consult the label.

[33]Weight includes rind. Without rind, the weight of the edible portion is 272 g for cantaloupe and 149 g for honey dew.

[34]Represents yellow-fleshed varieties. For white-fleshed varieties, value is 50 IU for 1 peach, 90 IU for 1 cup of slices.

[35]Value represents products with added ascorbic acid. For products without added ascorbic acid, value in milligrams is 116 for a 10-oz container, 103 for 1 cup.

[36]Weight includes pits. After removal of the pits, the weight of the edible portion is 258 g for canned plums, 133 g for plums, 43 g for uncooked prunes, and 213 g for cooked prunes.

[37]Weight includes rind and seeds. Without rind and seeds, weight of the edible portion is 426 g.

[38]Made with vegetable shortening.

[39]Applies to product made with white cornmeal. With yellow cornmeal, value is 30 IU.

[40]Applies to white varieties. For yellow varieties, value is 150 IU.

[41]Applies to products that do not contain di-sodium phosphate. If disodium phosphate is an ingredient, value is 162 mg.

[42]Value may range from less than 1 mg to about 8 mg, depending on the brand. Consult the label.

[43]Value varies with the brand. Consult the label.

[44]Value varies with the brand. Consult the label.

[45]Applies to product with added ascorbic acid. Without added ascorbic acid, value is trace.

[46]Excepting angelfood cake, cakes were made from mixes containing vegetable shortening; icings, with butter.

[47]Excepting spongecake, vegetable shortening used for cake portion; butter, for icing. If butter or margarine used for cake portion, vitamin A values would be higher.

[48]Applies to product made with a sodium aluminum-sulfate type baking powder. With a low-sodium-type baking powder containing potassium, value would be about twice the amount shown.

[49]Equal weights of flour, sugar, eggs, and vegetable shortening.

[50]Products are commercial unless otherwise specified.

[51]Made with enriched flour and vegetable shortening except for macaroons which do not contain flour or shortening.

[52]Icing made with butter.

[53]Applies to yellow varieties; white varieties contain only a trace.

[54]Contains vegetable shortening and butter.

[55]Made with corn oil.

[56]Made with regular margarine.

[57]Applies to product made with yellow cornmeal.

[58]Made with enriched degermed cornmeal and enriched flour.

[59]Product may or may not be enriched with riboflavin. Consult the label.

[60]Value varies with the brand. Consult the label.

[61]Weight includes cob. Without cob, weight is 77 g for raw corn, 126 g for frozen corn.

[62] Based on yellow varieties. For white varieties, value is trace.

[63]Weight includes refuse of outer leaves and core. Without these parts, weight is 163 g.

[64]Weight includes core. Without core, weight is 539 g.

[65]Value based on white-fleshed varieties. For yellow-fleshed varieties, value in international units is 70 for chopped onions, 50 for sliced onions, and 80 for cooked onions.

[66]Weight includes cores and stem ends. Without these parts, weight is 123 g.

[67]Based on year-round average. For tomatoes marketed from November through May, value is about 12 mg; from June through October, 32 mg.

[68]Applies to product without calcium salts added. Value for products with calcium salts added may be as much as 63 mg for whole tomatoes, 241 mg for cut forms.

[69]Weight includes pits. Without pits, weight is 13 g for green olives, 9 g for ripe olives.

[70]Value may vary from 6 to 60 mg.

TABLE A-2. MINERAL AND VITAMIN CONTENT OF FOODS

Explanatory Notes. The data in this table are intended to provide assistance in the planning of diets for sodium content and for some minerals and vitamins for which recommended allowances have been set. The data were derived from many sources listed below.

These values for minerals and vitamins must be regarded as tentative inasmuch as analyses in many instances have included only a small number of food samples. Wide variations for a nutrient in a given kind of food may occur depending upon the variety of breed, the growing conditions, the processing techniques, the storage conditions, the preparation within the home, and the methods used for analyses.

Sodium. The sodium values for commercially canned vegetables assume 0.6 percent salt concentration in the regular pack. Salt is ordinarily added to canned meats, fish, poultry, soups; cured meats; cheeses; baked products including breads, quick breads, rolls, cakes, cookies, pies; ready-to-eat and cooked breakfast cereals; salad dressings; butter and margarine.

The amount of salt added to some foods is so highly variable that the values listed in the table pertain to the unsalted product. Included are cooked fresh and frozen vegetables; cooked fresh meats, fish, and poultry; cooked legumes; cooked macaroni, spaghetti, and noodles.

Vitamin E. The table lists the values for alpha-tocopherol. Vitamin E activity is shown by eight tocopherols. Of these alpha-tocopherol is the most active. Assuming the alpha-tocopherol activity to be 1.0, the corresponding activity of other tocopherols is as follows: beta-tocopherol, 0.4; gamma-tocopherol, 0.1; delta-tocopherol, 0.01; alpha-tocotrienol, 0.3; beta-tocotrienol, 0.05; and gamma-tocotrienol, 0.01.

The alpha-tocopherol content of a food slightly underestimates the total vitamin E activity. However, for some foods other tocopherols predominate, and hence the total tocopherol value would considerably overestimate the vitamin E activity.

In values for copper, zinc, and vitamin E, two decimal places are used when the value is less than 0.1. This does not imply greater accuracy, but indicates the presence of some of the nutrients in these food.

Sources of Data for Table A-2

DONG, M. H. et al.: "Thiamin, Riboflavin, and Vitamin B_6 Contents of Selected Foods, as Served," *J. Am. Diet. Assoc.*, **76**:156–60, 1980.

FREELAND, J. H. and COUSINS, R. J.: "Zinc Content of Selected Foods," *J. Am. Diet. Assoc.*, **68**:526–9, 1976.

GODDARD, M. S., et al.: *Provisional Table on the Nutrient Content of Frozen Vegetables.* U.S. Department of Agriculture, Hyattsville, Md., 1979.

GREGOR, J. L., et al.: "Magnesium Content of Selected Foods," *J. Food Sci.*, **43**:1610, 1978.

HAEFLEIN, K. A., and RASMUSSEN, A. I.: "Zinc Content of Selected Foods," *J. Am. Diet. Assoc.*, **70**:610–16, 1977.

McLAUGHLIN, P. J., and WEIHRAUCK, J. L.: "Vitamin E Content of Foods," *J. Am. Diet. Assoc.*, **75**:647–65, 1979.

MEYER, B. H. et al.: "Pantothenic Acid and Vitamin B_6 in Beef," *J. Am. Diet. Assoc.*, **54**:122–5, 1969.

MURPHY, E. W., et al.: "Provisional Tables on the Zinc Content of Foods," *J. Am. Diet. Assoc.*, **66**:345–55, 1975.

ORR, M. L.: *Pantothenic Acid, Vitamin B_6 and Vitamin B_{12} in Foods.* Home Economics Research Report No. 36, Agricultural Research Service, U.S. Department of Agriculture, Washington, D.C., 1969.

PENNINGTON, J. A.: *Dietary Nutrient Guide.* AVI Publishing Co., Inc., Westport, Conn., 1976.

PENNINGTON, J. T., and CALLOWAY, D. H.: "Copper Content of Foods," *J. Am. Diet Assoc.*, **63**:143–53, 1973.

PERLOFF, B. P., and BUTRUM, R. R.: "Folacin in Selected Foods," *J. Am. Diet. Assoc.*, **70**:161–72, 1977.

POLANSKY, M. M.: "Vitamin B_6 Components in Fresh and Dried Vegetables," *J. Am. Diet. Assoc.*, **54**:118–21, 1969.

POSATI, L. P., and ORR, M. L.: *Composition of Foods: Dairy and Egg Products*, Ag. Handbook 8–1, U.S. Department of Agriculture, Washington, D.C., 1976.

WATT, B. K., and MERRILL, A. L.: *Composition of Foods— Raw, Processed, Prepared*, Ag. Handbook No. 8, U.S. Department of Agriculture, Washington, D.C., 1963.

Table A-2. Mineral and Vitamin Content of Foods: Sodium, Magnesium, Copper, and Zinc; Folacin, Pantothenic Acid, Vitamin B-6, Vitamin B-12, and Vitamin E
(Values for 100 gm food, edible portion)

Item No.	Food	Sodium (mg)	Magnesium (mg)	Copper (mg)	Zinc (mg)	Folacin (µg)	Pantothenic Acid (µg)	Vitamin B-6 (µg)	Vitamin B-12 (µg)	Vitamin E (mg)
1	Almonds, fried	4	270	0.8 [1]	—[2]	96	470	100	0	24.0 R[3]
2	roasted, salted	198		—	2.6	—	250	95	0	—
3	Apple, raw, not peeled	1	8	.09	.05	8	105	30	0	.6
4	Apple juice, bottled	1	4	.2	.03	tr	—	30	0	.01
5	Applesauce, sweetened	2	5	.4	.1	1	85	30	0	.05
6	Apricots, raw	1	12	.1	.04	3	240	70	0	
7	canned	1	7	.05	.04	1	92	54	0	
8	dried, uncooked	26	62	.4	.1	14	753[1]	169[1]	0	.9
9	cooked	7	20		—	—	—	—	0	
10	Apricot nectar	tr	6		—	—	100	40	0	
11	Asparagus, green, cooked	1	20 R	.1	1.0	60	600	200	0	2.0
12	canned, regular pack	236	—	.2	—	27	195	55	0	.4
13	low sodium	3								
14	frozen, spears, cooked	1	14	.1	.6	109	410	155	0	1.4 R
15	Avocado	4	45	.4	.4	51	1,070	420	0	1.6
16	Bacon, cooked, drained	1,021	25	.5	4.8	—	330 R	125 R	0.7	.5 R
17	Canadian, cooked	2,555	24							
	Baking powder, home use									
18	sodium aluminum phosphate	10,953								
19	straight phosphate	8,220								
20	tartrate	7,300								
21	low sodium, commercial	6								
22	Banana	1	33	.2	0.2	28	260	510	0	.3
23	Barley, pearled, light	3	37	.2	—	—	503	224	0	.02
	Beans, immature									
24	Lima, cooked	1	67	.4	—	34	130	—	0	—
25	canned, regular pack	236	—	—	—	13		90	0	—
26	low sodium	4								
27	frozen, Fordhook, cooked	101	48 R	.06	.05	31 R	240	150	0	—
28	snap, green, cooked	4	32 R	.1	.3	40	190 R	80 R	0	.02 R
29	canned, regular pack	236	14	.04	.3	12	75	40	0	.03
30	low sodium	2								
31	frozen, cooked	1	21 R	0.5	.2	28	135	70	0	.1
32	snap, yellow, cooked	3	—	—	—	32	250 R	—	0	—
33	canned, regular pack	236						42	0	
34	low sodium	2							0	—

No.	Food									
	Beans, mature									
35	Lima, dry	4	180	.7	2.8	113	975	580	0	7.7
36	cooked	2	—	.2	.9	43	—	—	0	—
37	red, dry	10	163	.8	—	133	500	441	0	2.1
38	cooked	3	—	.4	—	37	—	—	0	—
39	soy, dry	—	—	.3	.7	171	—	670	0	.9
40	cooked	2	170	—	—	129	—	—	0	—
41	white, common, dry	19	—	.3	2.8	—	725	560	0	.3
42	cooked	7	—	.9	1.0	—	—	—	0	—
43	canned, pork with tomato sauce	463	37	—	—	129	—	—	—	—
44	Bean sprouts, Mung, cooked	4	—	.2	1.0	24	92	—	0	.06 R
	Beef									
45	all cuts, lean, broiled, roasted, average	60	29	.2	—	10	—	—	0	.4 R
46	simmered, average	60	18	—	5.8	4	620 R	160	1.8 R	—
47	corned, cooked	1,740	25	—	6.2	—	—	—	—	—
48	hash, canned	540	20	—	1.9	2	560	148	1.8	—
49	dried	4,300	—	—	2.0	—	—	242	.8	.03
50	hamburger	47	21	.06 R	—	4	—	—	1.8	—
51	pot pie, commercial	366	—	—	4.4	—	320	48	1.68	.4
52	stew, with vegetables, canned	411	—	.02	1.4	3	—	—	—	—
53	home recipe	37	17	—	—	—	—	120	.65	.2
54	Beets, cooked	43	25	.2	.05	78	150 R	55 R	.65	.2
55	canned, regular pack	236	15	.1	—	3	100	50	0	.03
56	low-sodium pack	46	—	—	—	—	—	—	0	.03
57	Beet greens, cooked	76	106	.1	.5	60	250	100	0	—
	Beverages, alcoholic									
58	beer	7	10	.07	.03	—	80	60	0	1.5 R
59	gin	1	10	.01	.1	—	—	—	0	—
60	wine, table	5	—	—	—	—	30	40	0	—
	Beverages, nonalcoholic									
61	cola	2	2	.04	.02	—	—	—		—
62	fruit drinks	3	3	—	.02	—	—	—		—
63	Biscuits, baking powder, enriched	626	—	.3	1.0	7	330	—	0	—
64	self-rising flour[4]	630	—	—	—	—	—	—		—
65	Biscuits, dough, commercial, in can	868	—	—	—	—	—	—		—
66	Blackberries, raw	1	30	.2	.05	14	240	50	0	.6
67	Blueberries, raw	1	6	.2	.05	6	156	67	0	—
68	frozen, sweet	1	4	—	—	8	121	54	0	—
69	Bluefish, baked or broiled	104	—	—	—	—	—	—		—
70	Bouillon cubes	24,000	—	—	—	—	—	—		—
	Bran. See Cereals									
71	Brazil nuts	1	225	1.5	5.1	4	231	170	0	6.5

Table A-2. (Continued)

Item No.	Food	Sodium (mg)	Magnesium (mg)	Copper (mg)	Zinc (mg)	Folacin (µg)	Pantothenic Acid (µg)	Vitamin B-6 (µg)	Vitamin B-12 (µg)	Vitamin E (mg)
	Breads									
72	Boston brown	251	—	.3	—	—	—	—	—	—
73	corn, southern style, degermed meal	591	33	—	—	—	607	81		
74	cracked wheat	529	35	.2	1.2	25	378	92	0	
75	French, Italian, Vienna	580	22	.4	.9	9	400	53	0	
76	raisin	365	24	.2	1.2	12	450	40	0	
77	rye, American	557	42	.2	1.6	23	500	100	0	
78	pumpernickel	569	71	—	1.1	—	430	160	0	.1
79	white, 3–4% milk solids	507	22	.2	.6	39	760	40	tr	.1
80	whole wheat, 2% nonfat solids	527	78	.2	1.8	58	448	180	tr	.5 R
81	Broccoli spears, cooked	10	24 R	.1	.2	56	525	112	0	
82	frozen, cooked	12	21	.04	.3	54	420	170	0	
83	Brussels sprouts, cooked	10	29 R	.08	.4	36	(frozen)	175 (frozen)	0	.9
84	Butter, salted	826	2	.03	.05	3	—	3	tr	1.6
85	unsalted	under 10								
86	Cabbage, raw	20	14	.08	.4	66	205	160	0	1.7
87	cooked, small amount water	14	6	.09	.4	18	112	100	0	
88	Cabbage, celery or Chinese	23	14	—	—	83	—	—	0	.1
	Cakes, home recipe									
89	angel food	283	25	.05	.3	3	200	tr	tr	
90	chocolate with icing	235	42	.3	1.0	6	200		.1	
91	fruit cake, dark	158	—	.1						
92	gingerbread	237								
93	plain with icing	229								
94	plain, without icing	300			.2		300	40[5]		2.6
95	pound	110	—	.09	—	7		22		1.1
96	sponge	167	8			7				
	Candy									
97	caramels	226	—	.04	—	7	100	tr	0	.2
98	chocolate, milk, plain	94	58	.5	.5			tr		1.1
99	fudge, plain	190								
100	hard	32	tr	.09		0	0	0	0	0
101	marshmallow	39	4	.2	.03				0	
102	mint, chocolate coated	52								
103	peanut brittle	31	—			—		—		
104	Cantaloupe	12	16	.05	.02	30	250	86	0	.1
105	Carrots, raw	47	23	.1	.4	32	280	150	0	.4
106	cooked	33	13	.08	.3	24	280	28	0	.4
107	canned, regular pack	236	—	—	.3	3	130	30	0	
108	low sodium	39								

No.	Food									
109	Cashew nuts, not salted	15	267	.7	4.4	68	1,300	—	0	.2
110	Cauliflower, raw	13	24	.07	.3	55	1,000	210	0	.03
111	cooked	9	—	.06	—	34	835	170	0	
112	frozen, cooked	10	13 R	.02	.2	—	540	190	0	
113	Celery, raw	126	22	.07	.1	12	429	60	0	.4
114	cooked	88	—	.1	—	—	—	—	0	
	Cereals, breakfast									
115	bran, wheat, crude	9	490	1.5	9.8	258	335	—	0	
116	bran flakes (40% bran)	925	—	.6	3.6	—	875	384	0	1.5
117	bran flakes with raisins	800								
118	corn, puffed	1,060					288		0	.09
119	corn, shredded	988							0	.08
120	cornflakes	1,005	16	.1	.3	12	185	65	0	.1
121	cornflakes, sugar coated	775								
122	corn grits, dry, white, degermed	1	20	—	.4	24	—	147	0	.1
123	cooked	—	3	.05	.1	2	165	34	0	.04
124	cornmeal, degermed, dry	1	47	.1	.8	7			0	
125	cooked		7		.1	9				
126	cornmeal, whole ground, dry	1	106	—	1.8	24	580	250	0	.2
127	farina, regular, dry	2	25	.2	.5	24	515	67	0	
128	cooked, salted	144	3	.03	.06	4	85	15	0	
129	instant cooking, cooked	188	4							
130	oatmeal, dry	2	144	.6	3.4	52	1,500	140	0	1.5
131	cooked, salted	218	21	.03	.5				0	
132	rice flakes	987	25	.3	1.4	8	340	125	0	.04
133	rice, puffed, no salt	2	—	.4	1.4	23	378	75	0	.06
134	wheat and barley, malted, dry	1	168	.6	3.6	33			0	1.1
135	cooked	72	31		.5	49				
136	wheat, rolled, cooked	tr								
137	wheat flakes	1,032	102	.4	1.4	47	469	292	0	.4
138	wheat, puffed, no salt	4	—	.4	2.6		—	170	0	.7
139	wheat, shredded, plain	3	133	—	2.8	50	706	244	0	.4
140	Chard, Swiss, cooked	86	65 R		—	42	172 R	—	0	
	Cheese									
141	Camembert	842	20	—	2.4	62	1,364	227	1.3	
142	cheddar or American	620	28	.1	3.1	18	413	74	1.0	.6
143	cheddar, process	1,189[6]	31	.06	3.6	11	558	80	1.1	
144	cottage, creamed	405	5	.02	.4	12	213	67	.6	
145	uncreamed	406	6	—	.4	13	242	76	.7	
146	cream	296	6	.04	.5	13	271	47	.4	
147	Gouda	819	29	—	3.9	21	340	80	—	
148	Mozzarella	373	19	—	2.2	7	64	56	.7	
149	Parmesan	1,862	51	.4	3.2	8	527	105	—	
150	Swiss	260	36	.1	3.9	6	429	83	1.7	
151	Cherries, raw, sweet	2	14	.1	.1	8	261	32	0	
152	canned, syrup	1	9	.06	—	3	—	30	0	.1

Table A-2. (Continued)

Item No.	Food	Sodium (mg)	Magnesium (mg)	Copper (mg)	Zinc (mg)	Folacin (µg)	Pantothenic Acid (µg)	Vitamin B-6 (µg)	Vitamin B-12 (µg)	Vitamin E (mg)
153	Chicken broiled, dark without skin	86	—	.2 R	2.8	7	1,000	325	.4	.4
154	light without skin	64	19	.1 R	.9	4	800	683	.5	.3
155	Chicken, canned, boneless	—	12	.1	2.0	2	850	300	.8	.3
156	Chicken potpie, frozen, commercial	411	11	—	—	—	—	86	—	—
157	Chickpeas (garbanzos) dry	8	—	—	2.7	199	320	160	0	—
158	boiled, drained	—	—	—	1.4	102		45	0	
159	Chicory	7	13	—	—	52	140	103	—	
160	Chili concarne, canned with beans	531	—	—	—	—				
161	Chili powder with seasoning	1,574	169	—	2.3	14	190	35		
162	Chocolate, bitter	4	292	2.7	.9				0	
163	Chocolate syrup, thin	52	63	.4				80		
164	Clams, raw, soft, meat only	36	—	—	1.5	—	300			
165	hard, round, meat only	205	—	—	1.5	—				
166	canned	—	115	—	1.2	2	300	83		.2
167	Cocoa, breakfast, dry	6	420	3.6	5.6				0	.2
168	processed with alkali	717								.7
169	Coconut, fresh, shredded	23	46	.5	—	24	200	44	0	
170	dried, sweetened	—	77	.6	—	—	200	33	0	
171	Coffee, instant, dry	72	456	1.0	.6	—	400	32	0	
172	beverage	1	4	.02	.03		4	tr	0	
173	Collards, cooked	25	57	.3	.7	102 R	450 (frozen)	195 (frozen)	0	
174	Cookies, fig bars	252	—	.2	1.2	4	400	100		
175	oatmeal	170	2	.1	1.3	4	—	—	0	
176	plain, assorted	365	15	.07	.3	9	300	60	0	2.6
177	Corn, sweet, cooked	tr	48 R	.07 R	.4	33 R	540 R	161 R	0	1.2
178	canned, whole kernel, regular pack	236	19	.06	.2	8	220	200	0	.01
179	low-sodium pack	2								
180	Cowpeas, dry, cooked	8	230	.2	1.2	133 R	1,050	562	0	
181	Crabmeat, canned	1,000	34	1.5	4.3	20	600	300	10	1.2
182	Crackers, graham	670	51	.2	1.1	25	540	65	0	
183	saltines, soda	1,100	29	.04	.6	20	500	68	0	
184	Cranberry juice	1						22		
185	Cranberry sauce	1	2							
186	Cream, half and half	41	10	.1	.5	2	289	39	.3	2.6
187	light, coffee	40	9	.1	.3	2	276	32	.2	1.2
188	whipping, light	34	7	.1	.3	4	59	28	.2	.4
189	Cucumber, not peeled	6	11	.06	.2	15	250	42	0	
190	Dandelion greens, cooked	44	36 R	—	—		—	—	0	.2
191	Dates, domestic	1	58	.2	—	21	780	153	0	2.5 R

No.	Food									
192	Doughnuts, cake type	501	23	.1	.5	8	387⁵	—		.7
193	Duck, flesh, raw	74	—	.4	—	16	220 R	81 R	2.8	
194	Eggplant, cooked	1	16 R	.1 R	—	65		120	0	.03
195	Egg, whole, raw	138	12	.1	1.4	16	1,727	3	1.5	.7
196	white, raw	152	9	.05	.02		241	310	.07	
197	yolk, raw	49	15	.3	3.0	152	4,429	20	3.8	2.1
198	Endive, curly	14	10	—	—	49	90	20	0	
	Fats. See Oils, Shortening									
199	Figs, raw	2	20	.1	—	14	300	113	0	
200	canned	2	—	—	—		69	—	0	
201	dried, uncooked	34	71	.3	—	9	435	175	0	
202	Filberts (hazelnuts)	78	—	1.3	3.1	72				23.8
203	Flounder, raw	78	—	.2	.7	21	850	170	1.2	.4
204	Flour, all purpose	2	25	.2	.7	5	465	60	0	.03
205	cake	2	—	—	.3	78	320	45	0	.04
206	rye, light	1	73	.4	—	38	720	90	0	.4
207	whole wheat	3	113	.5	2.4		1,100	340	0	.8
208	Fruit cocktail	5	7	.03	.02		—	33	0	
209	Gelatin, dry	—	33	1.1	—	0	0	0	0	
210	sweetened, ready-to-eat	51	3	.02	—				0	
211	Grapefruit, fresh	1	12	.04	.05	11	283	34	0	.3
212	canned	1	11	.04	—		120	20	0	
213	Grapefruit juice, canned	1	—	.01	.03	21	130	11	0	.1
214	frozen, diluted	1	9	—	—		162	14	0	
215	Grapes, American	3	13	.09	.3	7	126	80⁵	0	
216	Grape juice, bottled	2	12	.01	—	2	40	18	0	
217	Haddock, raw	61	24	.2	.7	10	130	180	1.3	.4
218	fried, (dipped in egg, milk, bread crumbs)	177	24	.2	—				1.3	
219	Heart, beef, lean, raw	86	18	.3	1.0	5	100	180	11.0	.6
220	Herring, raw, Pacific	74	—	.2	—		2,500	250	2.0	1.1
221	smoked, hard	6,231	—	—	—			—	7.0	
222	Honey, strained	5	3	.04	.08	3	500	200	0	
223	Honeydew melon	12	—	.06	.07	5	200	20	0	
224	Ice cream, chocolate	—	23	.1	—		207	56		
225	vanilla, 10 percent fat	87	14	.02	1.1	2	492		.5	
226	Ice milk, vanilla, hardened	80	14	—	.4	2	505	46	.7	
227	Jams and preserves	12	5	.3	.04		—	65	0	.09
228	Jellies	17	4	.1	—			25		.09
229	Kale, cooked, leaves with stems	43	37	.05	.2	60 R	376 R	185 R	0	
230	Lamb, lean cut, dry heat	70	21	.06 R	4.3	3	550 R	275 R	2.2 R	.2
231	Lard	0	0	.03	.2		—	20	0	1.2
232	Lasagna	490	25	—	.8	22	—	20	—	
233	Lemon juice, fresh	1	8	.08	.01	12	103	—	0	
234	Lemonade, frozen, diluted	tr	1	.01	.01	5	11	46	0	
235	Lentils, dry, boiled	9	11	.09	3.1	36	—	5	—	.06
236	Lettuce, crisp head	9	—	.09	.4	37	200	55⁵	0	.4
237	loose leaf, romaine	9	—	.09	.4	44	200	60	0	
238	Lime juice, fresh or canned	1	—	—	—	4	314		0	

Table A-2. (Continued)

Item No.	Food	Sodium (mg)	Magnesium (mg)	Copper (mg)	Zinc (mg)	Folacin (µg)	Pantothenic Acid (µg)	Vitamin B-6 (µg)	Vitamin B-12 (µg)	Vitamin E (mg)
	Liver, cooked, fried									
239	beef	184	18	2.80 R	5.1	145	7,700 R	840 R	80 R	.6
240	calf	118	26	7.9 R	6.1	—	8,000 R	670 R	60 R	.3
241	chicken, simmered	60	—	.3 R	3.4	—	—	—	25	
242	pork	111	24	1.1 R	2.2	145	6,400 R	650 R	32 R	
243	Lobster, cooked or canned	210	22	1.7 R	1.5	17	1,500 R	—	.5 R	1.5 R
244	Macaroni, dry	2	48	.1	.5	12	—	64	0	.02
245	cooked, firm	1	20	.02	.7	4	150	25	0	
246	Macaroni and cheese	543	20	.04		5	200	23	.4	
247	Margarine, corn oil, stick, salted	987		.04	.2	2				12.9
248	safflower, soybean, stick									17.8
249	soybean, stick									3.1
250	Milk, fresh, whole	49	13	.04	.4	5	314	42	.36	.06
251	fresh, skim	52	11	.02	.4	5	329	40	.38	tr
252	buttermilk	130	14	.03		11	307	36	.22	
253	evaporated, undiluted	106	24	.1	.8	8	638	50	.16	
254	nonfat dry	549	117	.5	4.5	50	3,235	345	4.0	
255	Milk, goat	50	14	.05	.3	1	310	46	.07	
256	Milk, human	17	3	.05	.2	5	223	11	.05	.9
257	Milk beverages chocolate flavored with skim milk	64	18		.4	6	261	49	.35	
258	malted with whole milk	81	16		.4	8	289	68	.39	
259	Molasses, light	15	46	1.4		10[5]	350[5]	200[5]	0	.4
260	black strap	96	258	1.4						
261	Muffins, plain	441	23	.2	1.2	7	500	19	.2	
262	Mushrooms, raw	15	—	1.0	1.3	24	2,200	125	0	.08
263	canned	400	8	.4		4	1,000	60	0	
264	Mustard, prepared, yellow	1,252	48	.09	.2	60	164 R	133 R	0	
265	Mustard greens, cooked	18	27	.08		5	—	17	0	1.8
266	Nectarine	6	13	.2			—	88	tr	2.0
267	Noodles, enriched, dry	5	126		.6	2	200	7	tr	
268	cooked	2	—			0	0	0	0	
269	Oil, corn	0	0	0	0	0	0	0	0	14.3[7]
270	Okra, raw	2	41	.1		24	215	45	0	
271	Olives, green	2,400	22	.3	.08		18	14	0	
272	ripe	813	—	.4	.3	1	15		0	
273	Onions, green, raw	5	21	.04	.3	36	144	—	0	
274	mature, raw	10	12	.1	.3	25	130	130	0	.1
275	cooked	7	—	.07	—	10	100	100	0	
276	Orange, peeled	1	11	.06	.2	46	250	60	0	.2

No.	Food								
277	Orange juice, fresh,	1	11	.08	.02	55	190	40	0	.04
278	canned	1			.02	55	150	35	0	
279	frozen, diluted	1	10	.01	.02	55	164	28	0	
280	Oysters, Eastern, raw	73	32	17.1	74.7	11	250	50	18	.9
281	Pancakes, wheat, home recipe	425	—	.05	.8	9 (canned)	720	20	tr	
282	Papayas, raw	3	—	.01			218	—	0	
283	Parsley	45	41	.5		116	300	164	0	1.7
284	Parsnips, cooked	8	32 R			67	600[1]	90[1]	0	1.0 R
285	Peaches, raw	1	10	.09	.2	8	170	24	0	
286	canned	2	6	.05	.1	1	50	19	0	
287	dried	16	48	—	—	5		100[1]	0	
288	cooked with sugar	4	15							
289	frozen	2	6							
290	Peanuts, roasted	5	5		3.0	4	132	18	0	7.8
291	salted	418	175	1.0	2.9	106	2,100	400	0	8.3
292	Peanut butter	607	175	.6	2.9	79	—	330	0	7.0
293	Pears, raw	2	173	.2		14	70	17	0	.5
294	canned	1	7	.04	.3		22	14	0	
295	Peas, green, cooked	1	5	.2	.7	25	—	109	0	.1 R
296	canned, regular pack	236	18	.2	.8	10	150	50	0	
297	low sodium pack	3	20							
298	frozen, not thawed	129	24	.1	.8	53	315	130	0	.1
299	Peas, dried, split	40	180		3.2	51	2,000	130	0	.09
300	cooked	13	—	.3	1.1	20	220	20	0	
301	Pecans	tr	142	1.4	—	24	1,707	183	0	1.2
302	Peppers, sweet, green, raw	13	18	.1	.06	19	230	260	0	.7
303	Perch, Atlantic, raw	79	12		—	9				1.2
304	Pickles, dill	1,428	—	.2	.3	4	225	75[5]	0	
305	relish, sweet	712	—	.5	.06					
306	Pie, home recipe apple	301	5	.06	.09	4	110	—	0	1.6
307	cherry	304	—	.04	.04				0	
308	custard	287	—				946		—	
309	lemon meringue	282	—	—					—	
310	mince	448	—	.09	.05				—	
311	pumpkin	214	—		.4		519	57	—	
312	Piecrust, baked	611	—	.1	.5					
313	Pike, walleye, raw	51	—	.2						
314	Pineapple, raw	1	13	.06	.2	11	160	88	0	.5
315	canned	1	8	.1	.2	1	100	74	0	
316	Pineapple juice, canned	1	12	.05	.2	1	100	96	0	.1
317	Pizza, cheese	702	—	.3	1.2	37				
318	Plums, raw	2	9	.1		6	186	52	0	
319	canned, purple	1	5			1	72	27	0	
320	Popcorn, salted, with oil	1,940	—	.4	3.0			204		
321	Pork, fresh, lean, roast	65	29	.06	3.1	5	790 R	259	.7 R	
322	picnic ham, simmered	65	18		4.0					.08 R

Table A-2. (Continued)

Item No.	Food	Sodium (mg)	Magne-sium (mg)	Copper (mg)	Zinc (mg)	Folacin (µg)	Panto-thenic Acid (µg)	Vitamin B-6 (µg)	Vitamin B-12 (µg)	Vitamin E (mg)
323	Pork, cured, ham, light cure	930	20	.03	4.0	11	675 R	400 R	.6 R	.3
324	canned, spiced or unspiced	1,100	—	.09			—	360		.3
325	Potatoes, baked, no skin	4	18	.2	.5	10	400	138	0	.06 R
326	boiled, unsalted	2	—	.1	.3	7	400	174	0	.04
327	french fried	6	17	.3	.3	22	540 (frozen)	180 (frozen)	0	.2
328	mashed, with milk, table fat, salted	331 (variable to)	14	.1	.4	10	200	100	0	
329	Potato chips	1,000	55	.3	.8	10	500	180	0	4.3
330	Pretzels	1,680 (variable)	24	.2	1.1		540	19	0	.2
331	Prunes, dried, uncooked	4	40	.3		4	460	240		
332	cooked	2	20	.2	.3					
333	Prune juice, canned	2	10	.02	.01					
	Pudding									
334	bread with raisin	201	—	.08						
335	chocolate	56	19							
336	cornstarch (blanc mange)	65	8	.04					—	
337	custard, baked	79			.1	4			—	
338	rennin, using mix	46	—	.03					—	
339	rice with raisin	71	—	.04	.3				—	
340	tapioca cream	156	—						—	
341	Pumpkin, canned, unsalted	2	12 R	.1		19	400	56	0	1.0
342	Radishes	18	15	.09	.3	24	184	75	0	
343	Raisins, dried	27	35	.3	.2	4	45	240	0	.7
344	Raspberries, red, raw	1	20			5	240	60	0	.3
345	frozen	1				5	270	38	0	
346	Rhubarb, cooked	2	13	.1	.1	7 R	70	25	0	.03 R
347	Rice, white, dry	5	24	.2	1.3	—	550	170	0	.1
348	cooked, salted	374	8	.02	.4	16	225	35	0	
349	Rolls, commercial, plain	506	21	.2	1.0		310	35	—	.04
350	sweet	389	20							
351	whole wheat	564								
352	Rutabagas, cooked	4	15 R			21	160[1]	100[1]	0	
353	Rye wafers	882	—	.3						
354	Salad dressings									
355	blue cheese	1,094			.3					
356	commercial, mayonnaise type	586			.1					
357	French	1,370	10		.08					
358	home cooked	728								
359	mayonnaise	597	2	.2	.2					
360	Thousand Island	700	6	.2	.1	3				

658

No.	Food									
361	Salmon, fresh, broiled	64	40	.2	.8	4	220	670	3.9	1.4
362	canned	387	30	.07	.9	20	550	300	6.9	
363	Sardines, Pacific, canned in tomato sauce	400	24	.04	2.6	16	700	160	10.0	
364	Sauerkraut	747	—	.1	.9		93	130	0	
	Sausage									
365	bologna	1,300	14	.02	1.8	5	—	100	—	.06
366	frankfurters	1,100	13	.08	2.0	4	430	140	1.3	
367	liverwurst			3.0	7.3	30	2,660	200	14.0	.4
368	pork links	958	16			14 R	682	165	.5	.2
369	salami		11							.1
370	Scallops	265	18	.1 R	1.3	16 R	132 R		1.2 R	.6
371	Sesame seed			1.6		96	608		0	
372	Shad, raw	54								
373	baked with table fat	79								
374	Sherbet, orange	46	8		.7	7	32	13	.08	
375	Shrimp, raw	140	42	.6 R	1.5	15	220	100	.9	.4
	canned, dry pack		51	.2	2.1		210	60	—	
376	Soup, canned, diluted with equal part water									
377	bean with pork	403	—	—	—					
378	beef bouillon	326	—	.01	—					
379	beef noodle	382	—	.04	1.4					
380	chicken noodle	408	10	—						
381	clam chowder, Manhattan	383	—		.6	7				
382	cream (mushroom) prepared with milk	424	5	—	.5	3		54	.2	
383	minestrone	406	—							
384	pea, green	367	—	.1	.8		80	40		
385	tomato	396	9	.04	.1					
386	vegetable with beef broth	345	11	.2	1.6	6	140			
387	Spaghetti, dry	2	—		—	12	—			
388	cooked, tender	1	—							
389	Spaghetti, with meatballs, canned	488	—	.2						
390	Spinach, raw	71	88	.1	.8	193	300	280	0	1.9
391	cooked	50	—	.1	.7	91	75	130 (frozen)	0	
392	canned, regular pack	236	63	—	.8	49	65 (frozen)	70 (frozen)	0	.02
393	low-sodium pack	32								
394	Squash, summer, cooked	1	16	.08	.2	10	173	63	0	
395	winter, cooked	1	17			12	280 (frozen)	91 (frozen)	0	.1
396	Strawberries, raw	1	12	—	.08	16	340	55	0	.1
397	frozen	1	9	—	.07	9	135	43	0	.2
398	Sugar, brown	30	—	.4					0	
399	granulated	1	tr	.02	.06				0	
400	Sunflower seeds	30	38	1.8		38	1.420	1.130	0	49.5

Table A-2. (Continued)

Item No.	Food	Sodium (mg)	Magnesium (mg)	Copper (mg)	Zinc (mg)	Folacin (µg)	Pantothenic Acid (µg)	Vitamin B-6 (µg)	Vitamin B-12 (µg)	Vitamin E (mg)
401	Sweetpotatoes, baked	12	31	.1	.08 R	12	820 R	218 R	0	4.6 R
402	boiled	10	—	.2		18	700	200	0	
403	Syrup, table blend	68		.4			200			
404	Tangerine, raw	2	—	.07		21		67	0	
405	juice, canned	1					—	32	0	
406	Tapioca, dry	3	4	.06					0	
407	Tea, instant, powder		395		.02	8				
408	beverage		22							
409	Tomato, raw	3	14	.5	.2	39	330	100	0	.3
410	canned, regular pack	130	12	.1	.2	4	230	90	0	
411	low-sodium pack	3		.2						
412	Tomato catsup, regular	1,042	21	.6	.3	5	—	107	0	
413	Tomato juice, canned, regular pack	200	10	.07	.04	7	250	192	0	.2
414	low-sodium pack	3							0	
415	Tongue, beef, braised	61	16 R	.07 R			2,000	100	2.2	
416	Tuna, in oil	800	—	.1	1.0	15	320	425		
417	Turkey, dark, roasted	99	—	.1	4.4	7	1,128	—	—	.6
418	light, roasted	82	28	.1	2.1	5	591	—	—	
419	Turnips, cooked	34	7	.04	.09	20 R	200 R	90 R	0	.03
420	Turnip greens, canned, regular pack	236	58 R			95 R	68		0	2.2
421	frozen, not thawed	23	27	.06	.2	—	54	140	0	
422	Veal, lean, roasted	80	19	.1 R	4.1	17	900	345	1.9	.05
423	stewed	80	—	—	4.2	3	1,060 R	400 R	1.8 R	.05
424	Vinegar, cider	1	1	.09	.1			1		
425	Waffles, home recipe	475	28				650	38	0	
426	Walnuts, black	3	190	1.4	2.3	77			0	
427	English	2	131	.07		66	900	730	0	.9
428	Watermelon	1	8			8	300	68	0	
429	Wheat germ	827	336	2.4	14.3	328	1,200	1,150	0	14.1
430	Yeast, compressed	16	59				3,500	600	0	
431	dry, active	52	—	5.0		4,090	11,000	2,000	0	.08
432	dry, brewer's	121	231			3,909	12,000	2,500	0	.08
433	Yogurt, from partially skimmed milk	46	12		.5	11	389	32	.4	

[1] Source of data does not indicate whether value is for raw or cooked food; it is assumed that it represents the raw food.

[2] Dashes denote lack of reliable data for a constituent believed to be present in a measurable amount.

[3] The letter "R" following value indicates that the only available data were on a raw sample of that food.

[4] Based on use of self-rising flour containing anhydrous monocalcium phosphate.

[5] Nature of sample not clearly defined.

[6] Value based on use of 1.5 percent anhydrous disodium phosphate as the emulsifying agent; if the emulsifying agent does not contain sodium the value is 650 mg.

[7] Vitamin E content, as alpha-tocopherol in other oils; coconut, 0.4; cottonseed, 35.3; olive, 11.9; peanut, 11.6; safflower, 34.1; sesame, 1.4; soybean, 11.0; sunflower, 59.5; wheat germ, 149.4.

Table A-3. Dietary Fiber in Selected Plant Foods*†

	Measure	Weight (g)	Total Dietary Fiber (g)	Noncellulosic Poly-saccharides (g)	Cellulose (g)	Lignin (g)
Apple, flesh	1 medium	138	1.96	1.29	0.66	0.01
Apple peel only		100	3.71	2.21	1.01	.49
Banana	1 small	119	2.08	1.33	.44	.31
Beans, baked, canned	1 cup	255	18.53	14.45	3.59	.48
Beans, runner, boiled	1 cup	125	4.19	2.31	1.61	.26
Beverages, concentrated						
Cocoa		100	43.27	11.25	4.13	27.9
Chocolate		100	8.20	2.61	1.16	4.43
Coffee and chicory essence		100	.79	.73	.02	.04
Instant coffee		100	16.41	15.55	.53	.33
Brazil nuts	1 ounce	30	2.32	1.08	.65	.59
Bread, white	1 slice	25	.68	.50	.18	tr
whole-meal	1 slice	25	2.13	1.49	.33	.31
Broccoli, tops, cooked	1 cup	155	6.36	4.53	1.78	.05
Brussels sprouts, cooked	1 cup	155	4.43	3.08	1.24	.11
Cabbage, cooked	1 cup	145	4.10	2.55	1.00	.55
Carrots, young, cooked	1 cup	155	5.74	3.44	2.29	tr
Cauliflower, cooked	1 cup	125	2.25	.84	1.41	tr
Cereals						
All-Bran	1 ounce	30	8.01	5.35	1.80	.86
Corn flakes	1 cup	25	2.75	1.82	.61	.33
Grapenuts	¼ cup	30	2.10	1.54	.38	.17
Puffed Wheat	1 cup	15	2.31	1.55	.39	.37
Rice Krispies	1 cup	30	1.34	1.04	.23	.07
Shredded Wheat	1 biscuit	25	3.07	2.20	.66	.21
Special K	1 cup	30	1.64	1.10	.22	.32
Sugar Puffs	1 cup	30	1.82	1.20	.30	.33
Cherries, flesh and skin	10 cherries	68	.84	.63	.17	.05
Cookies						
Ginger	4 snaps	28	.56	.41	.08	.07
Oatmeal	4 cookies	52	2.08	1.64	.21	.22
Short, sweet	4 cookies	48	.80	.68	.05	.06
Corn, sweet,						
cooked	1 cup	165	7.82	7.11	.51	.20
canned	1 cup	165	9.39	8.20	1.06	.13
Flour						
bran		100	44.0	32.7	8.05	3.23
white	1 cup	115	3.62	2.90	.69	.03
whole-meal	1 cup	120	11.41	7.50	2.95	.96
Grapefruit, canned,						
fruit and syrup	½ cup	100	.44	.34	.04	.06
Guavas, canned,						
fruit and syrup	½ cup	100	3.64	1.67	1.17	.80
Jam, strawberry	1 tablespoon	20	.22	.17	.02	.03
Lettuce, raw	⅙ head	100	1.53	.47	1.06	tr
Mangoes, canned,						
fruit and syrup	½ cup	100	1.00	.65	.32	.03
Marmalade, orange	1 tablespoon	20	.14	.13	.01	tr
Onions, raw	1 cup sliced	100	2.10	1.55	.55	tr
Oranges, mandarin	1 cup	200	.58	.44	.08	.06
Parsnips, raw	1 cup diced	100	4.90	3.77	1.13	tr
Peanuts	1 ounce	30	2.79	1.92	.51	.36
Peanut butter	1 tablespoon	16	1.21	.90	.31	tr
Peaches, flesh and skin	1 peach	100	2.28	1.46	.20	.62
Pears, flesh only	1 pear	164	4.00	2.16	1.10	.74
peel only		100	8.59	3.72	2.18	2.67
Peas, frozen, raw		100	7.75	5.48	2.09	.18
canned, drained	1 cup	170	13.35	8.84	3.91	.60

	Measure	Weight (g)	Total Dietary Fiber (g)	Noncellulosic Polysaccharides (g)	Cellulose (g)	Lignin (g)
Peppers, cooked	1 pod	73	.68	.43	.25	tr
Pickles	1 ounce	30	.46	.27	.15	.04
Plums	1 plum	66	1.00	.65	.15	.20
Potatoes, raw	1 medium	135	4.73	3.36	1.38	tr
canned, drained		100	2.51	2.23	.28	tr
Potato chips	10 chips	20	.64	.41	.22	tr
Raisins, Sultana	1 ounce	30	1.32	.72	.25	.35
Rhubarb, raw		100	1.78	.93	.70	.75
Strawberries, raw	1 cup	149	2.65	1.39	1.04	.22
canned, fruit and syrup	½ cup	100	1.00	.48	.20	.33
Tomatoes, raw	1 medium	135	1.89	.88	.61	.41
canned, drained	1 cup	240	2.04	1.08	.89	.07
Turnips, raw		100	2.20	1.50	.70	tr

* Adapted from: Southgate, D. A. T. et al: "A Guide to Calculating Intakes of Dietary Fibre," *J. Human Nutr.*, **30:**303–13, 1976.

† Household measures and approximate equivalent weights from Adams, C. F., and Richardson, M.: *Nutritive Value of Foods*, HG 72. U.S. Department of Agriculture, Washington, D.C., 1977. (See Table A-1.)

Table A-4. Exchange Lists for Meal Planning*

Exchange List	Carbohydrate (g)	Protein (g)	Fat (g)	Calories
Starch/Bread	15	3	trace	80
Meat				
Lean	—	7	3	55
Medium-Fat	—	7	5	75
High-Fat	—	7	8	100
Vegetable	5	2	—	25
Fruit	15	—	—	60
Milk				
Skim	12	8	trace	90
Low-fat	12	8	5	120
Whole	12	8	8	150
Fat	—	—	5	45

"The Exchange Lists are the basis of a meal planning system designed by a committee of the American Diabetes Association and The American Dietetic Association. While designed primarily for people with Diabetes and others who must follow special diets, the Exchange Lists are based on principles of good nutrition that apply to everyone. © 1986 American Diabetes Association, Inc., American Dietetic Association."

List 1. Starch/Bread List. 15 g carbohydrate, 3 g protein, a trace of fat, and 80 kcal per item.

Cereals/Grains/Pasta		Dried Beans/Peas/Lentils	
Bran cereals, concentrated*	⅓ cup	Beans and peas (cooked)* (such as kidney, white, split, blackeye)	⅓ cup
Bran cereals, flaked* (such as Bran Buds,® All Bran®)	½ cup	Lentils (cooked)*	⅓ cup
Bulgur (cooked)	½ cup	Baked beans*	¼ cup
Cooked cereals	½ cup		
Cornmeal (dry)	2 ½ tbsp.		
Grapenuts	3 tbsp.	Starchy Vegetables	
Grits (cooked)	½ cup	Corn*	½ cup
Other ready-to-eat		Corn on cob, 6 in. long*	1
unsweetened cereals	¾ cup	Lima beans*	½ cup
Pasta (cooked)	½ cup	Peas, green (canned or frozen)*	½ cup
Puffed cereal	1 ½ cup	Plantain	½ cup
Rice, white or brown		Potato, baked	1 small (3 oz.)
cooked	⅓ cup	Potato, mashed	½ cup
Shredded wheat	½ cup	Squash, winter (acorn, butternut)	¾ cup
Wheat germ	3 tbsp.	Yam, sweet potato, plain	⅓ cup

Bread		Saltine-type crackers	6
Bagel	½ (1 oz.)	Whole wheat crackers,	2–4 slices (¾ oz.)
Bread sticks, crisp, 4 in. long × ½ in.	2 (⅔ oz.)	no fat added (crisp	
Croutons, low fat	1 cup	breads, such as Finn®,	
English muffin	½	Kavli®, Wasa®)	
Frankfurter or hamburger bun	½ (1 oz.)		
Pita, 6 in. across	½	**Starch Foods Prepared with Fat**	
Plain roll, small	1 (1 oz.)	*(Count as 1 starch/bread serving, plus 1*	
Raisin, unfrosted	1 slice (1 oz.)	*fat serving.)*	
Rye, pumpernickel	1 slice (1 oz.)	Biscuit, 2½ in. across	1
Tortilla, 6 in. across	1	Chow mein noodles	½ cup
White (including French, Italian)	1 slice (1 oz.)	Corn bread, 2 in. cube	1 (2 oz.)
Whole wheat	1 slice (1 oz.)	Cracker, round butter type	6
		French fried potatoes,	
Crackers/Snacks		2 in. to 3½ in. long	10 (1½ oz.)
Animal crackers	8	Muffin, plain, small	1
Graham crackers, 2½ in. square	3	Pancake, 4 in. across	2
Matzoth	¾ oz.	Stuffing, bread (prepared)	¼ cup
Melba toast	5 slices	Taco shell, 6 in. across	2
Oyster crackers	24	Waffle, 4½ in. square	1
Popcorn (popped, no fat added)	3 cups	Whole wheat crackers, fat	
Pretzels	¾ oz.	added (such as Triscuits®)	4–6 (1 oz.)
Rye crisp, 2 in. × 3½ in.	4		

* 3 g or more of fiber per serving.

List 2. **Meat. Lean Meat and Substitutes:** 0 g carbohydrate, 7 g protein, 3 g fat, and 55 kcal per item

Beef	USDA Good or Choice grades of lean beef, such as round, sirloin, and flank steak; tenderloin; and chipped beef*	1 oz.		Oysters	6 medium
				Tuna (canned in water)*	¼ cup
				Herring (uncreamed or smoked)	1 oz.
				Sardines (canned)	2 medium
Pork	Lean pork, such as fresh ham; canned, cured or boiled ham*; Canadian bacon*, tenderloin.	1 oz.	**Wild Game**	Venison, rabbit, squirrel	1 oz.
				Pheasant, duck, goose (without skin)	1 oz.
			Cheese	Any cottage cheese	¼ cup
Veal	All cuts are lean except for veal cutlets (ground or cubed). Examples of lean veal are chops and roasts.	1 oz.		Grated parmesan	2 tbsp.
				Diet cheeses (with less than 55 calories per ounce)*	1 oz.
			Other	95% fat-free luncheon meat	1 oz.
Poultry	Chicken, turkey, Cornish hen (without skin)	1 oz.		Egg whites	3 whites
				Egg substitutes with less than 55 calories per ¼ cup	¼ cup
Fish	All fresh and frozen fish	1 oz.			
	Crab, lobster, scallops, shrimp, clams (fresh or canned in water)*	2 oz.			

* 400 mg or more of sodium per exchange

Medium-Fat Meat and Substitutes: 0 g carbohydrate, 7 g protein, 5 g fat, and 75 kcal per item

Beef	Most beef products fall into this category. Examples are: all ground beef, roast (rib, chuck, rump), steak (cubed, Porterhouse, T-bone), and meatloaf.	1 oz.	**Cheese**	Skim or part-skim milk cheeses, such as:	
				Ricotta	¼ cup
				Mozzarella	1 oz.
				Diet cheeses (with 56–80 calories per ounce)*	1 oz.
Pork	Most port products fall into this category. Examples are: chops, loin roast, Boston butt, cutlets.	1 oz.	**Other**	86% fat-free luncheon meat*	1 oz.
				Egg (high in cholesterol, limit to 3 per week)	1
Lamb	Most lamb products fall into this category. Examples are: chops, leg, and roast.	1 oz.		Egg substitutes with 56–80 calories per ¼ cup	¼ cup
Veal	Cutlet (ground or cubed, unbreaded)	1 oz.		Tofu (2½ in. × 2¾ in. × 1 in.)	4 oz.
Poultry	Chicken (with skin), domestic duck or goose (well-drained of fat), ground turkey	1 oz.		Liver, heart, kidney, sweetbreads (high in cholesterol)	1 oz.
Fish	Tuna (canned in oil and drained)*	¼ cup			
	Salmon (canned)*	¼ cup			

* 400 mg or more of sodium per exchange

High-Fat Meat and Substitutes: 0 g carbohydrate, 7 g protein, 8 g fat, and 100 kcal; High in saturated fat, cholesterol, and calories. Use no more than three times a week.

Beef	Most USDA prime cuts of beef, such as ribs, corned beef*	1 oz.	Sausage, such as Polish, Italian*	1 oz.	
			Knockwurst, smoked	1 oz.	
Pork	Spareribs, ground pork, pork sausage (patty or link)*	1 oz.	Bratwurst	1 oz.	
			Frankfurter (turkey or chicken)*	1 frank (10/lb.)	
Lamb	Patties (ground lamb)	1 oz.			
Fish	Any fried fish product	1 oz.	Peanut butter (contains unsaturated fat)	1 tbsp.	
Cheese	All regular cheeses, such as American, Blue, Cheddar, Monterey, Swiss*	1 oz.	**Count as one high-fat meat plus one fat exchange:**		
Other	Luncheon meat, such as bologna, salami, pimento loaf*	1 oz.	Frankfurter (beef, pork, or combination)*	1 frank (10/lb.)	

* 400 mg or more of sodium per exchange

List 3. Vegetable. 5 g carbohydrate, 2 g protein, and 25 kcal per cup raw vegetables or ½ cup cooked

Artichoke (1/2 medium)	Cabbage, cooked	Mushrooms, cooked	Spinach, cooked
Asparagus	Carrots	Okra	Summer squash (crookneck)
Beans (green, wax, Italian)	Cauliflower	Onions	Tomato (one large)
Bean sprouts	Eggplant	Pea pods	Tomato/vegetable juice*
Beets	Greens (collard, mustard, turnip)	Peppers (green)	Turnips
Broccoli	Kohlrabi	Rutabaga	Water chestnuts
Brussels sprouts	Leeks	Sauerkraut*	Zucchini, cooked

Starchy vegetables such as corn, peas, and potatoes are found on the Starch/Bread List.

For free vegetables, see Free Food List on page 000.

* 400 mg or more of sodium per exchange

List 4. Fruit. 15 g carbohydrate and 60 kcal per item

Fresh, Frozen, and Unsweetened Canned Fruit

Apple (raw, 2 in. across)	1 apple	Mango (small)	½ mango
Applesauce (unsweetened)	½ cup	Nectarine (1½ in. across)*	1 nectarine
Apricots (medium, raw) or	4 apricots	Orange (2½ in. across)	1 orange
Apricots (canned)	½ cup, or 4 halves	Papaya	1 cup
		Peach (2¾ in. across)	1 peach, or ¾ cup
Banana (9 in. long)	½ banana		
Blackberries (raw)*	¾ cup	Peaches (canned)	½ cup, or 2 halves
Blueberries (raw)*	¾ cup		
Cantaloupe (5 in. across)	⅓ melon	Pear	½ large, or 1 small
(cubes)	1 cup		
Cherries (large, raw)	12 cherries	Pears (canned)	½ cup or 2 halves
Cherries (canned)	½ cup		
Figs (raw, 2 in. across)	2 figs	Persimmon (medium, native)	2 persimmons
Fruit cocktail (canned)	½ cup	Pineapple (raw)	¾ cup
Grapefruit (medium)	½ grapefruit	Pineapple (canned)	⅓ cup
Grapefruit (segments)	¾ cup	Plum (raw, 2 in. across)	2 plums
Grapes (small)	15 grapes	Pomegranate*	½ pomegranate
Honeydew melon (medium)	⅛ melon	Raspberries (raw)*	1 cup
(cubes)	1 cup	Strawberries (raw, whole)*	1¼ cup
Kiwi (large)	1 kiwi	Tangerine (2½ in. across)	2 tangerines
Mandarin oranges	¾ cup	Watermelon (cubes)	1¼ cup

Dried Fruit		Fruit Juice	
Apples*	4 rings	Apple juice/cider	½ cup
Apricots*	7 halves	Cranberry juice cocktail	⅓ cup
Dates	2½ medium	Grapefruit juice	½ cup
Figs*	1½	Grape juice	⅓ cup
Prunes*	3 medium	Orange juice	½ cup
Raisins	2 tbsp.	Pineapple juice	½ cup
		Prune juice	⅓ cup

* 3 or more g of fiber per serving

List 5. Milk.
Skim/very low fat, 12 g carbohydrate, 8 g protein, trace fat, and 90 kcal per item; low fat, 12 g carbohydrate, 8 g protein, 5 g fat, and 120 kcal per item; whole, 12 g carbohydrate, 8 g protein, 8 g fat, and 150 kcal per item.

Skim and Very Lowfat Milk		Whole Milk	
skim milk	1 cup	The whole milk group has much more fat per serving than the skim and lowfat groups. Whole milk has more than 3¼ % butterfat. Try to limit your choices from the whole milk group as much as possible.	
½% milk	1 cup		
1% milk	1 cup		
lowfat buttermilk	1 cup	whole milk	1 cup
evaporated skim milk	½ cup	evaporated whole milk	½ cup
dry nonfat milk	⅓ cup	whole plain yogurt	8 oz.
plain nonfat yogurt	8 oz.		

Lowfat Milk	
2% milk	1 cup fluid
plain lowfat yogurt (with added nonfat milk solids)	8 oz.

List 6. Fat.
5 g fat, and 45 kcal per item.

Unsaturated Fats			
		Salad dressing, mayonnaise-type	2 tsp.
Avocado	⅛ medium		
Margarine	1 tsp.	Salad dressing, mayonnaise-type, reduced-calorie	1 tbsp.
†Margarine, diet	1 tbsp.		
Mayonnaise	1 tsp.		
†Mayonnaise, reduced-calorie	1 tbsp.	†Salad dressing (all varieties)	1 tbsp.
		Salad dressing, reduced-calorie	2 tbsp.
Nuts and Seeds:		*(Two tablespoons of low-calorie salad dressing is a free food.)*	
Almonds, dry roasted	6 whole		
Cashews, dry roasted	1 tbsp.	Saturated Fats	
Pecans	2 whole	Butter	1 tsp.
Peanuts	20 small or 10 large	Bacon	1 slice
		Chitterlings	½ ounce
Walnuts	2 whole	Coconut, shredded	2 tbsp.
Other nuts	1 tbsp.	Coffee whitener, liquid	2 tbsp.
Seeds, pine nuts, sunflower (without shells)	1 tbsp.	Coffee whitener, powder	4 tsp.
Pumpkin seeds	2 tsp.	Cream (light, coffee, table)	2 tbsp.
Oil (corn, cottonseed, safflower, soybean, sunflower, olive, peanut)	1 tsp.	Cream, sour	2 tbsp.
		Cream (heavy, whipping)	1 tbsp.
†Olives	10 small or 5 large	Cream cheese	1 tbsp.
		†Salt pork	¼ ounce

* 400 mg or more of sodium per serving.

† If more than one or two servings are eaten', these foods have 400 mg or more of sodium.

Free Foods. Each item contains less than 20 kcal per serving. Use up to three servings a day of a food with a specified serving size. Use as desired those foods without a specified serving size.

Drinks	Fruit	Salad greens	Sugar substitutes
Bouillon or broth	Cranberries,	Endive	(saccharin,
without fat†	unsweetened	Escarole	aspartame)
Bouillon, low-sodium	(½ cup)	Lettuce	Whipped topping
Carbonated drinks,	Rhubarb, unsweetened	Romaine	(2 tbsp.)
sugar-free	(½ cup)	Spinach	
Carbonated water			Condiments
Club soda	Vegetables	Sweet Substitutes	Catsup (1 tbsp.)
Cocoa powder,	*(raw, 1 cup)*	Candy, hard, sugar-free	Horseradish
unsweetened	Cabbage	Gelatin, sugar-free	Mustard
(1 tbsp.)	Celery	Gum, sugar-free	Pickles, dill
Coffee/Tea	Chinese cabbage*	Jam/Jelly, sugar-free	unsweetened†
Drink mixes, sugar-free	Cucumber	(2 tsp.)	Salad dressing,
Tonic water, sugar-free	Green onion	Pancake syrup,	low-calorie (2 tbsp.)
	Hot peppers	sugar-free (1–2 tbsp.)	Taco sauce (1 tbsp.)
Nonstick pan spray	Mushrooms		Vinegar
	Radishes		
	Zucchini*		

* 3 grams or more of fiber per serving.

† 400 mg or more of sodium per serving.

Table A-5. **Cholesterol Content of the Edible Portion of Food***

Food	Household Measure	Weight (g)	Cholesterol (mg)
Beef, lean, trimmed of separable fat, cooked	3 ounces	85	(77)†
Beef-vegetable stew			
Home recipe	1 cup	245	63
Canned	1 cup	245	36
Beef potpie			
Home prepared, baked	⅓ 9-in. pie	210	44
Commercial, frozen, unheated	1 pie	216	38
Brains, raw		100	>2,000
Butter	1 tablespoon	14	35
Buttermilk, from nonfat milk	1 cup	245	5
Cakes, home recipes			
Chocolate, chocolate frosting	1/16 9-in. diam.	75	32
Fruitcake, dark	1/30 8-in. loaf	15	7
Sponge	1/12 10-in. diam.	66	162
Yellow, chocolate frosting	1/16 9-in. diam.	75	33
Baked from mixes			
Angel food	1/12 10-in. diam.	53	0
Chocolate, with eggs, chocolate frosting	1/16 9-in. diam.	69	33
	cupcake, small	36	17
Gingerbread	1/9 8-in. square	63	trace
White, 2 layer, chocolate frosting	1/16 9-in. diam.	71	1
Yellow, 2 layer, with eggs, chocolate frosting	1/16 9-in. diam.	75	36
Caviar, sturgeon, granular	1 tablespoon	16	>48
Cheeses, natural			
Blue	1 ounce	28	(24)
Camembert	triangular wedge	38	(35)
Cheddar, milk or sharp	1 ounce	28	28
Cottage, creamed, 1 percent fat	1 cup	267	23
4 percent fat	1 cup	245	48
Uncreamed	1 cup	200	13

Food	Household Measure	Weight (g)	Cholesterol (mg)
Cheeses, natural (continued)			
Cream cheese	1 tablespoon	14	16
Edam	1 ounce	28	(29)
Mozzarella, part skim	1 ounce	28	18
Muenster	1 ounce	28	(25)
Parmesan, grated	1 cup	100	(113)
Provolone	1 ounce	28	(28)
Ricotta, part skim	1 ounce	28	(14)
Swiss	slice, rectangular	35	35
Pasteurized process, American	1 ounce	28	(25)
Swiss	1 ounce	28	(26)
Pasteurized process spread	1 tablespoon	14	(9)
Cheese soufflé, home recipe	¼ of 7-in. diam.	110	184
Chicken, breast, cooked meat and skin	½ breast	92	74
meat only	½ breast	80	63
Drumstick, meat and skin	1 drumstick	52	47
meat only	1 drumstick	43	39
Chicken à la king, home recipe	1 cup	245	185
Chicken fricassee, home recipe	1 cup	240	96
Chicken potpie, home recipe	⅓ 9-in. diam.	232	71
Commercial, frozen, unheated	1 pie	227	29
Chop suey with meat, home recipe	1 cup	250	64
Canned	3 ounces	85	10
Chow mien, without noodles, home recipe	1 cup	250	77
Clams,‡ raw, meat only	1 cup (19 large or soft or 7 round chowders)	227	114
Cod, raw, flesh only	3½ ounces	100	50
Cookies			
Brownies with nuts, home recipe	1 brownie 1¾ in. square	20	17
Ladyfingers	4 ladyfingers	44	157
Corn pudding	1 cup	245	102
Corn bread, home recipe	piece, 2½ in. square	83	58
Baked from mix	piece	55	38
	muffin	40	28
Crab, steamed, meat only	1 cup	125	100
Canned, meat only	1 cup	160	(161)
Cream, half and half	1 tablespoon	15	6
Light, coffee	1 tablespoon	15	10
Sour	1 tablespoon	12	8
Whipped topping (pressurized)	1 cup	60	51
Heavy whipping (unwhipped)	1 tablespoon	15	20
Cream puff, custard filling	1 cream puff	130	188
Custard, baked	½ cup	133	139
Egg, whole	1 large	50	252
White	one	33	0
Yolk	one	17	252
Flounder, raw, flesh only	3½ ounces	100	50
Frog legs, raw (refuse: 35 percent)	3½ ounces	100	50
Gizzard, chicken, cooked	3 ounces	85	(166)
Turkey, cooked	3 ounces	85	196
Haddock, raw, flesh only	3½ ounces	100	60
Halibut, cooked, flesh only	piece, 6½ × 2½ × ⅝ in.	125	(60)
Heart, beef, cooked	1 cup chopped	145	(398)
Herring, raw, flesh only	3½ ounces	100	85
Ice cream, 10 percent fat	1 cup	133	53
Frozen custard or French	1 cup	133	97
Ice milk, hardened	1 cup	131	26
Soft-serve	1 cup	175	36
Kidneys, all kinds, cooked	1 cup sliced	140	(1,125)

667

Food	Household Measure	Weight (g)	Cholesterol (mg)
Lamb, lean, trimmed, cooked	3 ounces	85	(85)
Lard	1 cup	205	195
Liver, including beef, calf, hog, lamb, cooked	3 ounces	85	(372)
Chicken, cooked	1 liver	25	(187)
Turkey, cooked	1 cup chopped	140	839
Lobster, cooked, meat only	1 cup cubed	145	123
Lobster Newburg, with butter, egg yolks, sherry, cream	1 cup	250	456
Macaroni and cheese, home recipe	1 cup	200	42
Mackerel, broiled	piece 8½ × 2½ × ½ in.	105	(106)
Margarine			
All vegetable fat	1 tablespoon	14	0
⅔ animal fat, ½ vegetable fat	1 tablespoon	14	7
Milk, whole	1 cup	244	34
Low fat, 1 percent with 1 to 2 percent nonfat milk solids	1 cup	246	14
2 percent fat with 1 to 2 percent nonfat milk solids	1 cup	246	22
Nonfat, skim	1 cup	245	5
Canned, undiluted evaporated	1 cup	252	79
Condensed sweetened	1 cup	306	105
Dry, to make 1 quart diluted	1⅓ cups	91	20
Chocolate beverage, commercial flavored milk drink with 2 percent added butterfat	1 cup	250	20
Flavored milk	1 cup	250	32
Cocoa, homemade	1 cup	250	35
Muffins, plain, home recipe	1 muffin	40	21
Noodles, whole egg, dry	8-ounce package	227	213
Cooked	1 cup	160	50
Chow mein, canned	1 cup	45	5
Oysters,§ meat only, raw	1 cup, 13–19 medium; 19–31 small; 4–6 Pacific medium	240	120
Canned, solids and liquid	3 ounces	85	(38)
Oyster stew, home prepared, 1 part oysters, 2 parts milk	1 cup	240	63
Pancakes, mix, with eggs, milk	cake 6-in. diam.	73	54
Pepper, stuffed with beef and crumbs	pepper with 1⅛ cup stuffing	185	56
Pies, baked			
Apple			0
Custard	⅛ of 9-in. diam.	114	120
Lemon chiffon	⅛ of 9 in. diam.	81	137
Lemon meringue	⅛ of 9-in. diam.	105	98
Peach			0
Pumpkin	⅛ of 9-in. diam.	114	70
Popovers, home recipe	1 popover (from ¼ cup batter)	40	59
Pork, lean, trimmed, cooked	3 ounces	85	(75)
Potatoes, au gratin, milk, cheese	1 cup	245	36
Scalloped, milk	1 cup	245	14
Salad, mayonnaise, hard-cooked egg	1 cup	250	162
Pudding, chocolate, mix	1 cup	260	30
Vanilla, home recipe (blanc mange)	1 cup	255	35
Rabbit, domesticated, cooked	1 cup diced	140	(127)
Rice pudding with raisins	1 cup	265	29
Roe, salmon, raw	1 ounce	28	101
Salad dressing			
Mayonnaise, commercial	1 tablespoon	14	10
Salad dressing, home recipe	1 tablespoon	16	12
Mayonnaise-type, commercial	1 tablespoon	15	8
Salmon, red, broiled steak (refuse: 12 percent)	6¾ × 2½ × 1 in.	145	(59)
Canned, solids and liquid	3 ounces	85	30
Sardines, drained solids	can—3¼ ounces	92	129

Food	Household Measure	Weight (g)	Cholesterol (mg)
Sausage, frankfurter, all meat	1 frank	56	(34)
Scallops,‖ muscle only, steamed	3 ounces	85	(45)
Shrimp, raw, flesh only	3½ ounces	100	150
Canned, drained solids	1 cup–22 large or 76 small	128	192
Spaghetti with meatballs in tomato sauce			
Home recipe	1 cup	248	75
Canned	1 cup	250	39
Sweetbreads (thymus), cooked	3 ounces	85	(396)
Tapioca cream pudding	1 cup	165	159
Tartar sauce, regular	1 tablespoon	14	7
Trout, raw, flesh only	3½ ounces	100	55
Tuna, canned in oil, drained	can (No. ½); 5½ ounces	157	102
Canned in water, solids, and liquid	can (No. ½); 6½ ounces	184	(116)
Turkey, cooked, light meat, without skin	3 ounces	85	65
Dark meat, without skin	3 ounces	85	86
Turkey potpie, home prepared	⅓ 9-in. diam.	232	71
Commercial, frozen	1 pie	227	20
Veal, lean, cooked	3 ounces	85	(84)
Waffles, mix, egg, milk	1 waffle 9 × 9 in.	200	119
Welsh rarebit	1 cup	232	71
White sauce, thin	1 cup	250	36
Medium	1 cup	250	33
Thick	1 cup	250	30
Yogurt, nonfat, plain or vanilla	carton; 8 ounces	227	17
Fruit flavored	carton; 8 ounces	227	15

* Adapted from Feeley, R. M. et al.: "Cholesterol Content of Foods," *J. Am. Diet. Assoc.*, **61:**134–49, 1972.

  † Numbers in parentheses indicate imputed values.

  ‡Cholesterol accounts for about 40 percent of the total sterol content of clams.

  § Cholesterol accounts for about 40 percent of the total sterol of oysters.

  ‖ Cholesterol accounts for about 30 percent of total sterol of scallops.

Table A-6. Nutritive Values of Selected Fast Foods*

Food Item	Weight (g)	Energy (kcal)	Protein (g)	Fat (g)	Cholesterol (mg)	Carbohydrate (g)	Calcium (mg)	Sodium (mg)	Iron (mg)	A IU	Thiamin (mg)	Riboflavin (mg)	Niacin (mg)	Ascorbic Acid (mg)
ARBY'S®†														
Regular Roast Beef	142	350	22	15	45	32	80	880	3.6	**	0.30	0.34	5.0	**
Super Roast Beef	277	620	30	28	85	61	100	1,420	5.4	**	.53	.43	7.0	**
Beef'N Cheddar	170	484	29	21	70	46	250	1,745	1.8	200	.68	.43	4.0	**
Chicken Breast Sand.	206	584	27	28	56	55	100	1,323	3.6	**	.23	.25	10.0	**
Arby's Butter Croissant	59	220	5	10	50	28	40	225	1.1	300	.15	.14	0.8	**
Bacon & Egg Croissant	128	420	16	25	440	32	60	550	1.8	750	.30	.51	2.0	**
Potato Cakes (2)	99	190	2	9	—	24	**	476	0.4	**	**	**	0.8	18
Horsey Sauce®	28	120	tr	6	—	25	**	—	**	**	**	**	**	**
Cherry Turnover	85	320	2	20	—	32	20	254	0.7	**	tr	tr	0.4	1
BURGER KING®!														
Whopper® Sandwich	261	630	26	36		50	40	995	2.7	**	.06	.26	4.0	**
Whopper® with Cheese	289	740	32	45		52	150	1,435	2.7	**	.12	.34	3.0	**
Double Beef Whopper®	337	850	44	52		52	20	1,080	4.5	**	.09	.43	6.0	**
Double Beef Whopper® with Cheese	365	950	50	60		54	150	1,535	3.6	**	.09	.43	6.0	**
Hamburger	110	290	15	13		29	40	525	2.7	**	.15	.17	6.0	**
Cheeseburger	124	350	18	17		30	40	730	2.7	**	.12	.17	6.0	**
Double Cheeseburger	179	530	30	31		32	80	990	2.7	**	.15	.26	12.0	**
Onion Rings	76	270	3	16		29	80	450	0.4	**	.06	**	**	**
Chocolate Shake	282	340	8	10		57	250	280	—	**	.12	.26	**	**
HARDEE'S FOOD SYSTEMS, INC.														
Hamburger	110	305	17	13		29	23	682	3.6	57	0.55	0.58	6.4	2
Cheeseburger	116	335	17	17		29	48	789	2.7	749	.51	.32	5.5	2
Big Deluxe	248	546	29	26	77	48	98	1,083	6.7	398	.50	.73	10.6	42
Roast Beef Sandwich	143	377	20	17	57	36	56	1,030	6.3	542	.93	.19	3.7	3
Hot Ham and Cheese	148	376	23	15	59	37	207	1,067	3.8	178	.37	.74	2.5	
Fisherman's Fillet	196	469	25	20	80	47	139	1,013	2.2	319	.18	.29	3.4	0
Chef Salad	329	277	23	16	179	10	212	517	2.4	632	.42	.39	5.9	10
Chicken Fillet	192	510	27	26	57	42	83	360	4.8	1,098	.52	.63	9.5	13
Biscuit	82	275	5	13	3	35	149	650	2.4	44	.34	.24	.7	0
Steak Biscuit w/Egg	162	527	20	31	298	41	151	973	5.8	772	.39	.58	3.4	0
Sausage Biscuit	112	413	10	26	29	34	139	864	2.8	45	.36	.22	2.8	0
JACK IN THE BOX®														
Hamburger	98	276	13	12	29	30	69	521	2.6	49	0.35	0.24	3.3	1
Cheeseburger	113	323	15	15	42	32	157	749	2.7	305	.35	.27	3.3	1
Jumbo Jack	205	485	26	26	64	38	97	905	6.9	348	.51	.21	7.0	5
Regular Taco	81	191	8	11	21	16	97	406	1.1	397	.07	.18	1.1	**

Chicken Supreme	228	601	31	36	60	39	235	1,582	3.0	456	.52	.37	10.5	4
Moby Jack (fish, cheese)	137	444	16	25	47	39	159	820	2.2	274	.40	.25	2.9	**
Sausage Croissant (egg, cheese)	156	584	22	43	187	28	169	1,012	2.9	530	.59	.51	4.7	**
Breakfast Jack (egg, ham, cheese)	126	307	19	13	203	30	168	871	3.0	441	.47	.41	3.0	12
Chicken Strips Dinner	321	689	40	30	100	65	114	1,213	4.0	417	.45	.30	18.6	8
Sirloin Steak Dinner	334	699	38	27	75	75	216	969	9.6	167	.67	.50	12.4	4
Pita Pocket Supreme	165	284	22	8	43	30	84	953	2.4	247	.78	.33	7.8	3
Cheese Nachos	170	571	15	35	37	49	367	1,154	1.5	511	.10	.19	1.0	9
Supreme Nachos	298	718	23	40	55	66	414	1,782	3.2	1,013	.15	.25	3.3	3
French Fries	68	221	2	12	8	27	10	164	.5	0	.08	.03	1.2	
Stawberry Shake	328	320	10	7	25	55		240	.5		.08	.03	1.2	3
KENTUCKY FRIED CHICKEN														
Wing	42	136	10	9	55	4	22	302	0.7	<9	0.03	0.04	2.3	<1
Extra Crispy™	53	201	11	14	59	9	15	312	.7	<11	.06	.09	2.9	<1
Drumstick	47	117	12	7	63	3	12	207	.8	<10	.04	.09	2.4	<1
Extra Crispy™	58	155	13	9	66	5	11	263	1.0	<12	.07	.11	3.1	<1
Side Breast	69	199	16	12	70	7	50	558	1.0	<14	.06	.08	5.7	<1
Extra Crispy™	85	286	17	18	65	14	57	564	1.1	<17	.12	.13	5.4	<2
Thigh	88	257	18	18	109	7	34	566	1.5	<18	.08	.16	4.0	<2
Extra Crispy™	107	343	20	23	109	13	49	549	1.5	<22	.12	.19	5.4	<2
2-Piece Colonel's Special Dinner, Extra Crispy™ (Wing, Thigh)	371	902	36	48	176	58	135	1,529	6.4	255	.31	.35	10.3	37
Cole Slaw	91	121	1	8	7	13	32	255	0.5	55	.03	<.02	.02	32
LONG JOHN SILVER'S®														
Fish w/Batter (2 pc.)	136	366	22	22			21							
Chicken Planks® (4 pc.)	166	457	27	23			35							
Ocean Scallops (6 pc.)	120	283	11	13			30							
Shrimp w Batter (6)	88	268	8	13			30							
Breaded Oysters (6)	156	441	13	19			53							
Hushpuppies (3 pc.)	45	153	3	7			20							
Cole Slaw	113	138	1	8			16							
McDONALD'S® RESTAURANTS														
Hamburger	102	255	12	10	25	30	51	520	2.3	82	0.25	0.18	4.0	2
Cheeseburger	115	307	15	14	37	30	132	767	2.4	345	.25	.23	3.8	2
Quarter Pounder®	166	424	24	22	67	33	63	735	4.1	133	.32	.28	6.5	2
Quarter Pounder® with Cheese	194	524	30	31	96	32	219	1,236	4.3	660	.31	.37	7.4	3
Big Mac®	204	563	26	33	86	41	157	1,010	4.0	530	.39	.37	6.5	2
Filet-O-Fish®	139	432	14	25	47	37	93	781	1.7	180	.26	.20	2.6	1
Egg McMuffin®	138	327	19	15	229	31	226	885	2.9	591	.47	.44	3.8	1
Hot Cakes w/butter, syrup	214	500	8	10	47	94	103	1,070	2.2	257	.26	.36	2.2	5
Hash Brown Potatoes	55	125	2	7	7		5	325	0.4	14	.06	.01	0.8	4
Regular Fries	58	220	3	12	9	26	9	109	.6	17	.12	.02	2.3	13
Vanilla Shake	291	352	9	8	31	60	329	201	.6	349	.12	.70	0.3	3
Hot Fudge Sundae	164	310	7	11	18	46	215	175	.6	230	.07	.31	1.1	2
Apple Pie	85	253	2	14	12	29	14	398	.6	34	.02	.02	.2	1

Table A-6. (Continued)

Food Item	Weight (g)	Energy (kcal)	Protein (g)	Fat (g)	Cholesterol (mg)	Carbohydrate (g)	Minerals Calcium (mg)	Sodium (mg)	Iron (mg)	A IU	Vitamins Thiamin (mg)	Riboflavin (mg)	Niacin (mg)	Ascorbic Acid (mg)
TACO BELL														
Bean Burrito	166	343	11	12		48	98	272	2.8	1,657	0.37	0.22		15
Beef Burrito	184	466	30	21		37	83	327	4.6	1,675	.30	.39		15
Beefy Tostada	192	331	18	18		23	208	138	3.4	3,450	.16	.27		13
Bell Beefer®	123	221	15	7		23	40	231	2.6	2,961	.15	.20		10
Bell Beefer® w/Cheese	137	278	19	12		23	147	330	2.7	3,146	.16	.27		10
Burrito Supreme®	225	457	21	22		43	121	367	3.8	3,462	.33	.35		16
Combination Burrito	175	404	21	16		43	91	300	3.7	1,666	.34	.31		15
Enchirito®	207	454	25	21		42	259	1,175	3.8	1,178	.31	.37		10
Taco	78	192	12	11		11	120	79	2.5	120	.09	.16		
Tostada	156	259	10	11		18	191	101	2.3	3,152	.18	.15		10

* Sources of Data (Additional information available from these firms):

Arby's, Inc. One Piedmont Center, 3495 Piedmont Road N.E. Atlanta, GA 30305. Nutritional Analysis by Technological Resources, Camden, NJ.

Burger King Corporation, Consumer Information, P.O. Box 520783, General Mail Facility, Miami, FL 33152. Analysis by WARF Institute, Madison, WI and Campbell Labs, Camden, NJ.

Hardee's Food Systems, Inc., 1233 N. Church St., Rocky Mount, NC 27801.

Jack In the Box, Foodmaker, Inc., 9330 Balboa Ave., San Diego, CA 92123. Analyses by Raltech Scientific Services, Madison, WI.

Kentucky Fried Chicken, Public Affairs Dept., P.O. Box 32070, Louisville, KY 40232. Analyses by Raltech Scientific Services, Madison, WI.

Long John Silver's, Jerrico, 101 Jerrico Drive, P.O. Box 11988, Lexington, KY 40579. Analyses by Food and Nutrition Service, U. Kentucky.

McDonald's Corporation, Consumer and Community Affairs, One McDonald's Plaza, Oak Brook, Il 60521. Analyses by Raltech Scientific Services Madison, WI.

Taco Bell, 16808 Armstrong Avenue, Irvine, CA 92714. Nutritional values calculated from ''Nutritive Values in Common Foods,'' Hdbk 456, U.S. Deparment of Agriculture, Washington, DC.

† Values for calcium, iron, vitamin A, thiamin, riboflavin, and niacin calculated from percentages of USRDA reported (Arby's and Burger King).

** Product provided less than 2 per cent of the USRDA for this nutrient.

Table A-7. Physical Growth NCHS Percentiles
Girls: Birth to 36 Months (Length/Age and Weight/Age)*

NAME _____ RECORD # _____

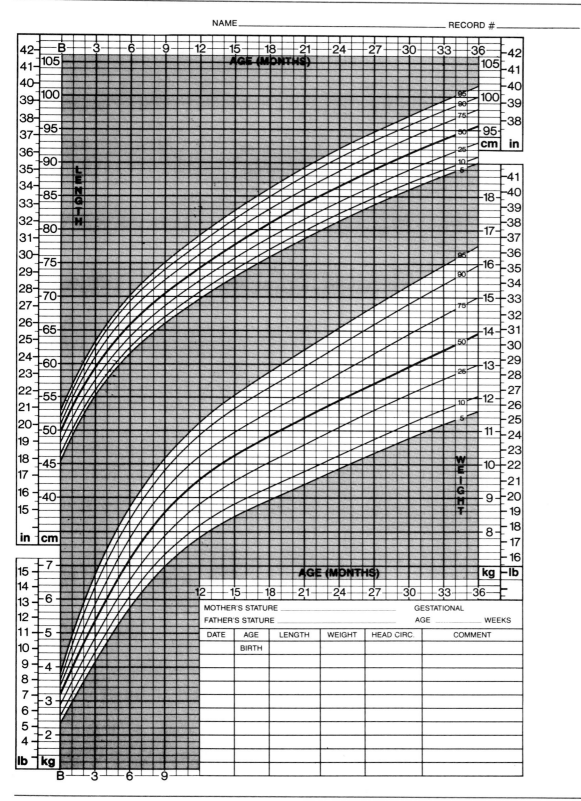

MOTHER'S STATURE _____ GESTATIONAL

FATHER'S STATURE _____ AGE _____ WEEKS

DATE	AGE	LENGTH	WEIGHT	HEAD CIRC.	COMMENT
	BIRTH				

* Courtesy, Ross Laboratories, Columbus, Ohio. Adapted from Hamill, P. V. V., et al.: "Physical Growth: National Center for Health Statistics," *Am. J. Clin. Nutr.*, **32:**607–29, 1979. Data from National Center for Health Statistics (NCHS) Hyattsville, Maryland.

Table A-8. Physical Growth NCHS Percentiles
Girls: Birth to 36 Months (Head Circumference/Age and Length/Weight)*

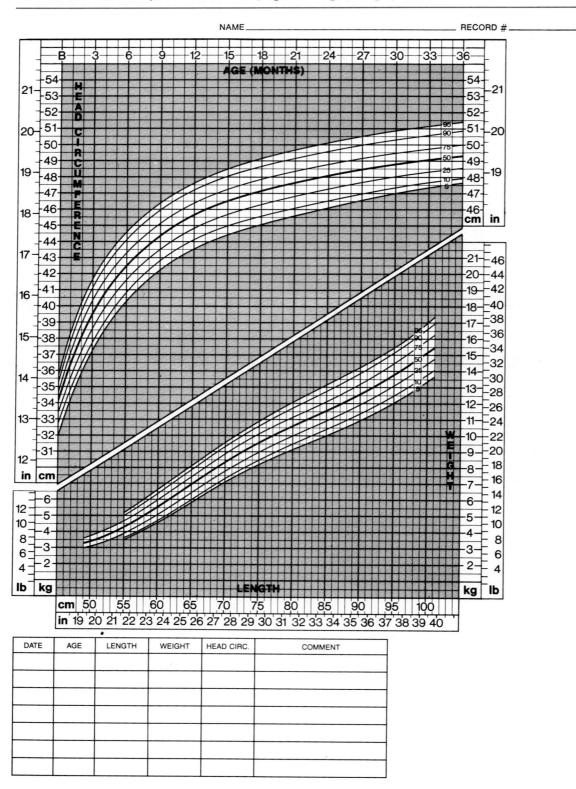

DATE	AGE	LENGTH	WEIGHT	HEAD CIRC.	COMMENT

* Courtesy, Ross Laboratories, Columbus, Ohio. Adapted from Hamill, P. V. V., et al.: "Physical Growth: National Center for Health Statistics," *Am. J. Clin. Nutr.*, **32**:607–29, 1979. Data from National Center for Health Statistics (NCHS) Hyattsville, Maryland.

674

Table A-9. Physical Growth NCHS Percentiles
Girls: 2 to 18 Years (Stature/Age and Weight/Age)*

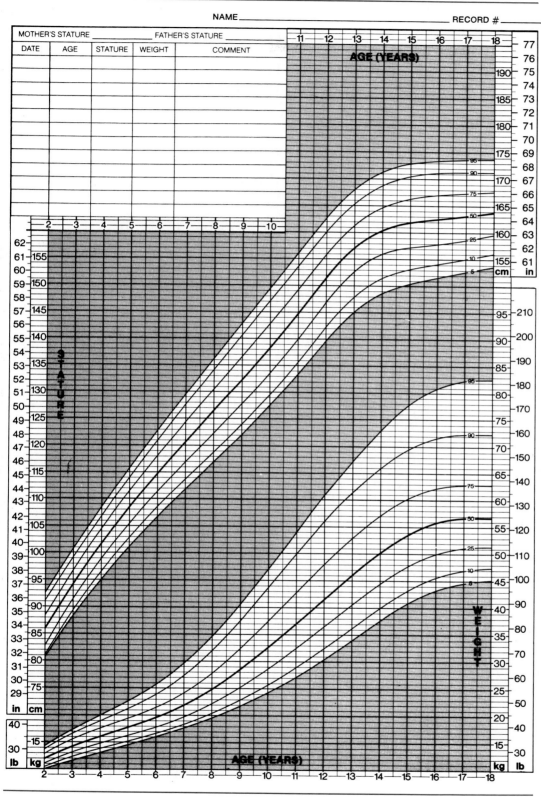

* Courtesy, Ross Laboratories, Columbus, Ohio. Adapted from Hamill, P. V. V., et al.: "Physical Growth: National Center for Health Statistics," *Am. J. Clin. Nutr.*, **32:**607–29, 1979. Data from National Center for Health Statistics (NCHS) Hyattsville, Maryland.

Table A-10. Physical Growth NCHS Percentiles
Girls: Prepubescent (Stature/Weight)*

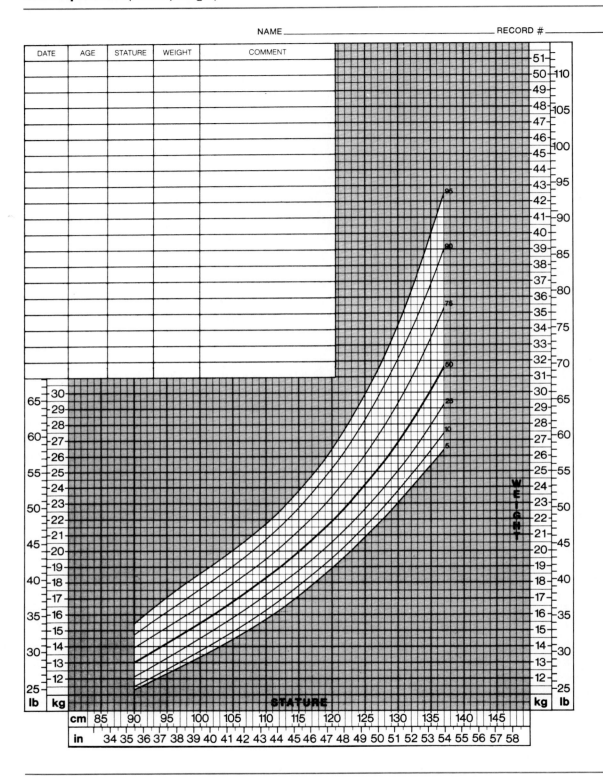

* Courtesy, Ross Laboratories, Columbus, Ohio. Adapted from Hamill, P. V. V., et al.: "Physical Growth: National Center for Health Statistics," *Am. J. Clin. Nutr.*, **32:**607–29, 1979. Data from National Center for Health Statistics (NCHS) Hyattsville, Maryland.

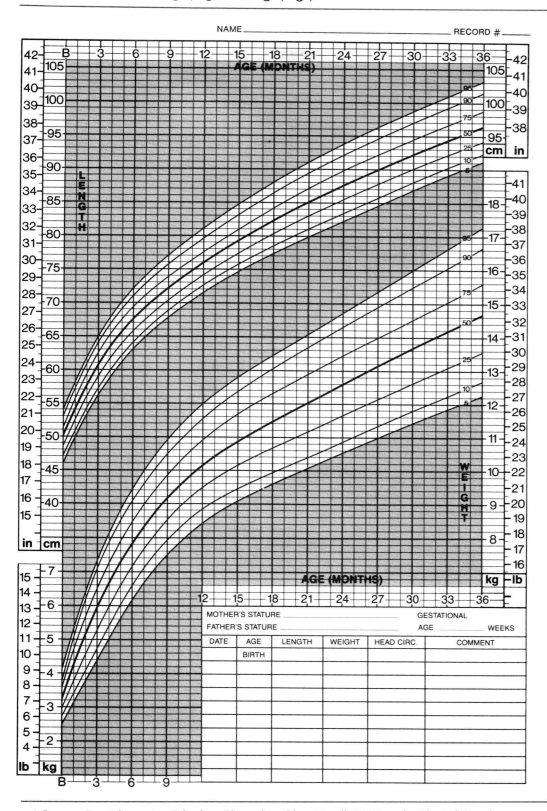

NAME _____ RECORD # _____

* Courtesy, Ross Laboratories, Columbus, Ohio. Adapted from Hamill, P. V. V., et al.: "Physical Growth:
National Center for Health Statistics," *Am. J. Clin. Nutr.*, **32:**607–29, 1979. Data from National Center for
Health Statistics (NCHS) Hyattsville, Maryland.

NAME_____ RECORD #_____

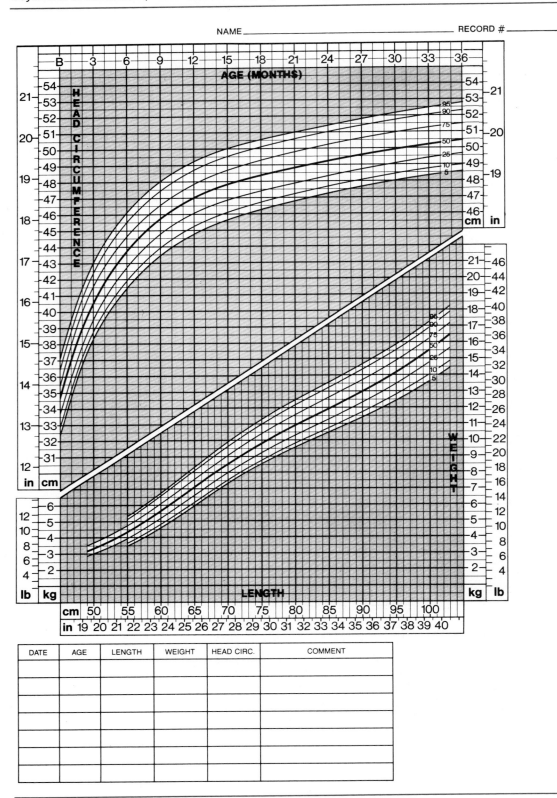

DATE	AGE	LENGTH	WEIGHT	HEAD CIRC.	COMMENT

* Courtesy, Ross Laboratories, Columbus, Ohio. Adapted from Hamill, P. V. V., et al.: "Physical Growth: National Center for Health Statistics," *Am. J. Clin. Nutr.*, **32**:607–29, 1979. Data from National Center for Health Statistics (NCHS) Hyattsville, Maryland.

678

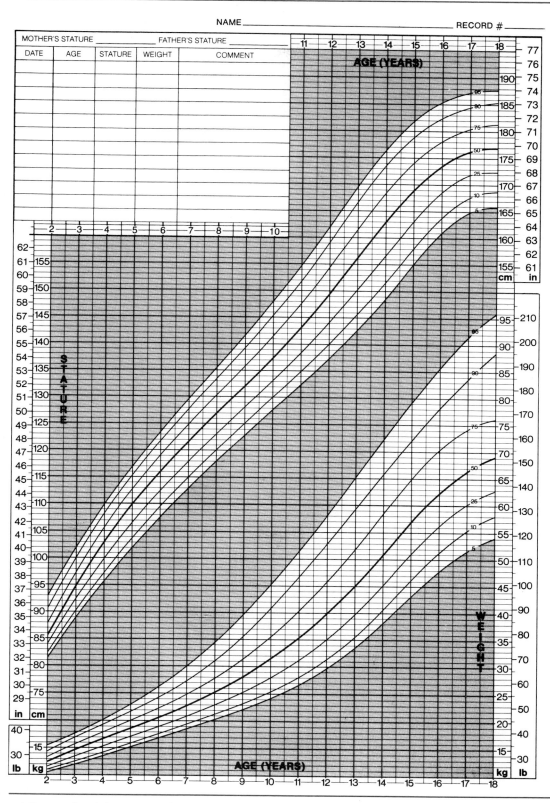

* Courtesy, Ross Laboratories, Columbus, Ohio. Adapted from Hamill, P. V. V., et al.: "Physical Growth: National Center for Health Statistics," *Am. J. Clin. Nutr.*, **32**:607–29, 1979. Data from National Center for Health Statistics (NCHS) Hyattsville, Maryland.

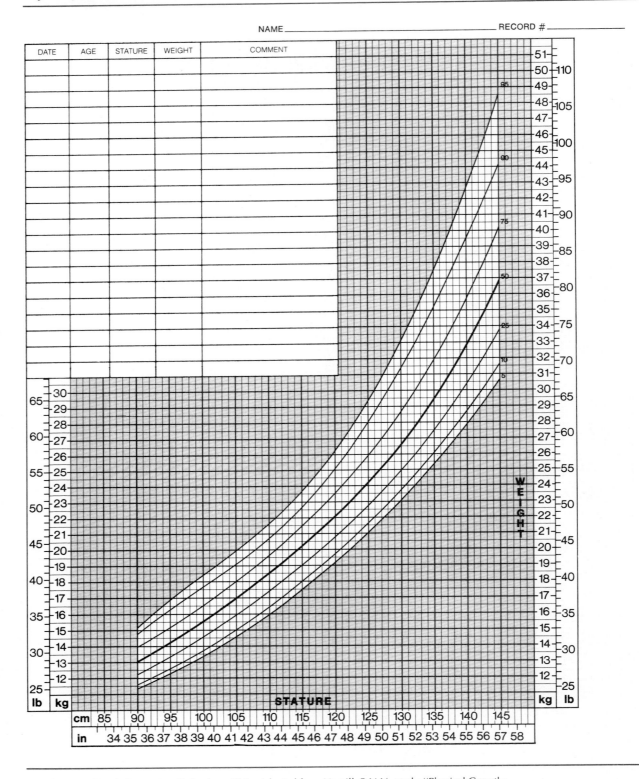

* Courtesy, Ross Laboratories, Columbus, Ohio. Adapted from Hamill, P. V. V., et al.: "Physical Growth: National Center for Health Statistics," *Am. J. Clin. Nutr.,* **32:**607–29, 1979. Data from National Center for Health Statistics (NCHS) Hyattsville, Maryland.

Table A-15. Determination of Body Frame
Determination of Body Frame According to Wrist Measurement*

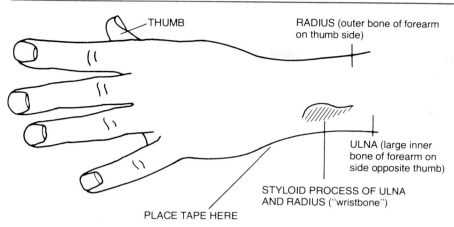

The wrist is measured distal to styloid process of radius and ulna at smallest circumference. Use height without shoes and inches for wrist size to determine frame type from this chart. *

BODY FRAME TYPE

Small Frame   Medium Frame   Large Frame

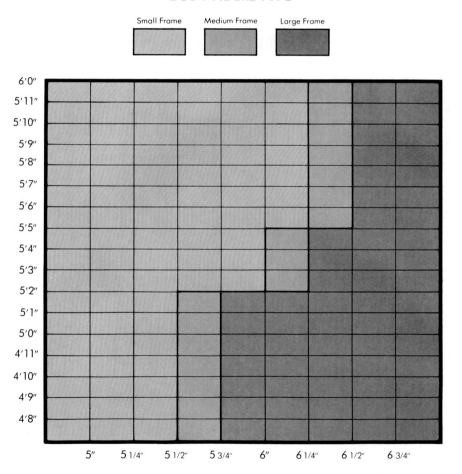

Table A-15. **(Continued)**

Body Frame According to Height : Wrist Circumference ("r")

$$r = \frac{\text{height, cm}}{\text{wrist circumference}}$$

	Small	Medium	Large
Males, "r" values	10.4	10-4-9.6	9.6
Females, "r" values	10.9	10.9-9.9	9.9

Body Frame According to Elbow Breadth

1. Extend arm, and bend forearm upward at 90° angle with fingers kept straight. Inside of wrist is toward the body.
2. Apply calipers to either side of the two prominent bones of the elbow. Read measurement in centimeters.
3. Determine frame size from the following table.

Frame size by elbow breadth (cm) of the US male and female adults derived from the combined NHANES and II data sets*

Age yr	Frame Size		
	Small	Medium	Large
Males			
18–24	≤6.6	>6.6 and <7.7	≥7.7
25–34	≤6.7	>6.7 and <7.9	≥7.9
35–44	≤6.7	>6.7 and <8.0	≥8.0
45–54	≤6.7	>6.7 and <8.1	≥8.1
55–64	≤6.7	>6.7 and <8.1	≥8.1
65–74	≤6.7	>6.7 and <8.1	≥8.1
Females			
18–24	≤5.6	>5.6 and <6.5	≥6.5
25–34	≤5.7	>5.7 and <6.8	≥6.8
35–44	≤5.7	>5.7 and <7.1	≥7.1
45–54	≤5.7	>5.7 and <7.2	≥7.2
55–64	≤5.8	>5.8 and <7.2	≥7.2
65–74	≤5.8	>5.8 and <7.2	≥7.2

* Used by permission. Frisancho, A. R.: "New Standards of Weight and Body Composition by Frame Size and Height for Assessment of Nutritional Status of Adults and the Elderly," *Am. J. Clin. Nutr.*, **40**:808–19, 1984.

Table A-16. Heights and Weights for Men and Women*†

Men				**Women**			
	Small Frame	Medium Frame	Large Frame		Small Frame	Medium Frame	Large Frame
Height	(pounds)**			Height	(pounds)#		
5 ft. 2 in.	128–134	131–141	138–150	4 ft. 10 in.	102–111	109–121	118–131
5 ft. 3 in.	130–136	133–143	140–153	4 ft. 11 in.	103–113	111–123	120–134
5 ft. 4 in.	132–138	135–145	142–156	5 ft. 0 in.	104–115	113–126	122–137
5 ft. 5 in.	134–140	137–148	144–160	5 ft. 1 in.	106–118	115–129	125–140
5 ft. 6 in.	136–142	139–151	146–164	5 ft. 2 in.	108–121	118–132	128–143
5 ft. 7 in.	138–145	142–154	149–168	5 ft. 3 in.	111–124	121–135	131–147
5 ft. 8 in.	140–148	145–157	152–172	5 ft. 4 in.	114–127	124–138	134–151
5 ft. 9 in.	142–151	148–160	155–176	5 ft. 5 in.	117–130	127–141	137–155
5 ft. 10 in.	144–154	151–163	158–180	5 ft. 6 in.	120–133	130–144	140–159
5 ft. 11 in.	146–157	154–166	161–184	5 ft. 7 in.	123–136	133–147	143–163
6 ft. 0 in.	149–160	157–170	164–188	5 ft. 8 in.	126–139	136–150	146–167
6 ft. 1 in.	152–164	160–174	168–192	5 ft. 9 in.	129–142	139–153	149–170
6 ft. 2 in.	155–168	164–178	172–197	5 ft. 10 in.	132–145	142–156	152–173
6 ft. 3 in.	158–172	167–182	176–202	5 ft. 11 in.	135–148	145–159	155–176
6 ft. 4 in.	162–176	171–187	181–207	6 ft. 0 in.	138–151	148–162	158–179

* Metropolitan Life Insurance Company, New York, 1983. Data from 1979 Build Study. Society of Actuaries and Associates of Life Insurance Medical Directors of America, 1980.
† Weight at ages 25 to 59 based on lowest mortality.
** Weight in indoor clothing weighing 5 pounds, shoes with 1-inch heel.
# Weight in indoor clothing weighing 3 pounds, shoes with 1-inch heel.

Table A-17.   Weight of Men Aged 18 to 74 Years by Age and Height: Selected Percentiles, United States, 1971-74*†

Left panel — Weight in pounds

Age and Height	5th	10th	25th	50th	75th	90th	95th
18–24 years							
62 in.							
63 in.							
64 in.	118	120	133	145	151	186	187
65 in.	111	112	121	134	145	164	193
66 in.	116	125	146	155	165	172	179
67 in.	121	131	140	153	173	187	203
68 in.	124	132	142	153	168	180	195
69 in.	133	139	147	161	182	208	224
70 in.	129	137	146	162	179	195	213
71 in.	141	146	157	170	187	202	228
72 in.	140	147	155	168	185	214	228
73 in.	132	157	164	180	201	229	247
74 in.	134	148	159	197	218	228	234
75 in.							
76 in.							
25–34 years							
62 in.							
63 in.	109	110	130	155	159	196	197
64 in.	111	126	133	148	161	195	206
65 in.	123	128	136	150	162	194	201
66 in.	129	134	145	157	176	191	194
67 in.	134	136	152	167	182	199	207
68 in.	129	140	149	164	181	196	201
69 in.	140	148	154	167	194	225	233
70 in.	141	148	159	180	197	215	253
71 in.	128	142	154	175	193	212	224
72 in.	154	157	168	185	210	224	244
73 in.	156	165	176	192	211	224	241
74 in.	157	158	167	182	217	226	244
75 in.							
76 in.							
35–44 years							
62 in.							
63 in.							
64 in.	125	139	151	160	173	183	184
65 in.	121	125	137	159	169	190	192
66 in.	124	132	144	164	181	192	203
67 in.	134	147	159	172	185	206	211
68 in.	140	150	162	177	194	204	209
69 in.	140	147	153	169	189	199	208
70 in.	143	147	166	185	198	207	218
71 in.	155	159	169	186	199	223	232
72 in.	138	140	169	197	222	237	243
73 in.	159	172	186	204	225	258	277
74 in.							
75 in.							
76 in.							

Right panel — Weight in pounds

Age and Height	5th	10th	25th	50th	75th	90th	95th
45–54 years							
62 in.							
63 in.	107	136	143	154	161	168	169
64 in.	101	126	140	159	193	224	236
65 in.	116	131	143	161	177	189	211
66 in.	136	137	151	165	179	194	200
67 in.	129	143	158	168	185	202	215
68 in.	126	130	154	173	185	210	223
69 in.	136	142	162	176	190	215	220
70 in.	143	147	164	184	199	211	234
71 in.	134	153	169	190	199	220	236
72 in.	156	164	176	193	213	225	240
73 in.	144	156	173	192	217	222	234
74 in.							
75 in.							
76 in.							
55–64 years							
62 in.							
63 in.							
64 in.	104	124	140	154	165	182	201
65 in.	112	128	146	162	177	196	209
66 in.	123	131	152	165	176	186	193
67 in.	128	135	145	167	182	204	229
68 in.	130	146	154	171	182	201	214
69 in.	139	146	154	172	188	209	238
70 in.	139	149	165	177	198	224	236
71 in.	153	154	167	187	203	214	232
72 in.	131	132	157	182	213	215	239
73 in.	158	160	171	194	202	212	233
74 in.							
75 in.							
76 in.							
65–74 years							
62 in.	120	124	138	148	155	172	179
63 in.	112	121	132	144	156	177	182
64 in.	110	121	132	148	161	175	182
65 in.	118	124	141	156	170	181	288
66 in.	117	129	147	159	175	189	199
67 in.	127	135	153	167	180	197	212
68 in.	126	137	152	167	182	204	214
69 in.	139	143	152	168	187	209	214
70 in.	139	149	161	177	193	214	236
71 in.	146	153	178	190	204	218	230
72 in.	143	149	161	185	202	211	233
73 in.							
74 in.							
75 in.							
76 in.							

* National Center for Health Statistics: *Weight by Height and Age for Adults 18–74 Years: United States, 1971–74.* Vital and Health Statistics, Series 11, No 208 (DHEW Pub. No PHS 79–1656).

† Examined persons were measured without shoes; clothing weight ranged from 0.20 to 0.62 pound, which was not deducted from weights shown.

Table A-18. Weight of Women Aged 18-74 Years by Age and Height: Selected Percentiles, United States, 1971-74*†

Age and Height	Percentile							Age and Height	Percentile						
	5th	10th	25th	50th	75th	90th	95th		5th	10th	25th	50th	75th	90th	95th
18–24 years	Weight in pounds							*45–54 years*	Weight in pounds						
57 in.								57 in.							
58 in.	87	90	106	112	131	155	157	58 in.							
59 in.	95	98	107	112	132	145	162	59 in.	94	100	105	148	165	169	174
60 in.	93	96	107	115	132	154	179	60 in.	110	112	118	135	170	214	216
61 in.	97	101	109	118	132	150	182	61 in.	100	108	120	140	154	181	196
62 in.	97	99	109	119	133	150	166	62 in.	108	111	120	134	153	172	195
63 in.	101	106	114	129	142	162	188	63 in.	110	112	125	143	163	187	215
64 in.	104	108	116	130	142	165	179	64 in.	119	123	130	147	167	191	209
65 in.	104	110	119	130	143	162	190	65 in.	116	126	134	150	166	194	217
66 in.	112	114	121	131	154	174	190	66 in.	127	129	139	151	165	186	201
67 in.	112	115	129	138	151	164	187	67 in.	123	124	141	152	183	194	217
68 in.	117	119	127	140	150	161	168	68 in.	132	138	146	186	191	197	212
69 in.	104	119	130	134	142	152	170	69 in.							
70 in.								70 in.							
25–34 years								*55–64 years*							
57 in.								57 in.							
58 in.	95	97	102	115	141	147	157	58 in.	70	86	101	119	126	181	200
59 in.	91	97	115	126	131	151	186	59 in.	110	112	127	141	161	167	179
60 in.	95	97	106	120	134	171	185	60 in.	103	105	122	145	161	177	188
61 in.	100	103	110	121	138	172	187	61 in.	100	110	128	148	166	183	190
62 in.	103	107	116	127	146	172	190	62 in.	106	116	128	139	164	187	199
63 in.	104	109	118	131	147	178	201	63 in.	109	118	132	147	176	203	223
64 in.	107	110	120	131	150	188	207	64 in.	109	117	129	147	169	191	208
65 in.	109	115	122	134	153	187	210	65 in.	110	119	141	151	171	200	225
66 in.	109	118	124	137	160	190	217	66 in.	90	100	127	151	175	209	223
67 in.	120	123	131	144	173	191	221	67 in.							
68 in.	125	129	137	152	172	217	237	68 in.							
69 in.	120	124	136	143	155	177	292	69 in.							
70 in.								70 in.							
35–44 years								*65–74 years*							
57 in.								57 in.	87	105	113	133	147	167	171
58 in.	94	95	107	118	141	182	216	58 in.	94	105	111	130	150	180	188
59 in.	97	102	117	132	147	171	209	59 in.	94	104	115	131	153	179	190
60 in.	104	109	116	124	149	173	193	60 in.	99	107	116	136	158	178	191
61 in.	101	106	113	128	147	164	180	61 in.	100	112	126	140	160	177	195
62 in.	108	111	121	134	150	181	199	62 in.	106	115	126	142	165	183	200
63 in.	109	114	124	136	164	195	206	63 in.	113	120	131	144	160	183	192
64 in.	111	114	125	138	166	195	210	64 in.	111	121	135	150	167	183	195
65 in.	118	123	131	147	174	201	219	65 in.	119	122	132	150	169	189	199
66 in.	118	121	130	145	167	214	239	66 in.	135	140	146	147	175	208	215
67 in.	123	124	130	146	162	205	235	67 in.	127	145	149	168	190	220	251
68 in.	123	125	145	160	179	240	268	68 in.	132	138	156	171	194	190	223
69 in.	139	143	152	167	184	230	300	69 in.							
70 in.								70 in.							

* National Center for Health Statistics: *Weight by Height and Age for Adults 18–74 Years, United States, 1971–74.* Vital and Health Statistics, Series 11, No 208 (DHEW Pub. No. PHS 79–1656).

† Examined persons were measured without shoes; clothing weight ranged from 0.20 to 0.62 pound, which was not deducted from weights shown.

Table A-19. Percentiles for Triceps Skinfold for Whites of the United States Health and Nutrition Examination Survey I of 1971 to 74*

Age group	N†	5	10	25	50	75	90	95	N†	5	10	25	50	75	90	95
				Males								Females				
1–1.9	228	6	7	8	10	12	14	16	204	6	7	8	10	12	14	16
2–2.9	223	6	7	8	10	12	14	15	208	6	8	9	10	12	15	16
3–3.9	220	6	7	8	10	11	14	15	208	7	8	9	11	12	14	15
4–4.9	230	6	6	8	9	11	12	14	208	7	8	8	10	12	14	16
5–5.9	214	6	6	8	9	11	14	15	219	6	7	8	10	12	15	18
6–6.9	117	5	6	7	8	10	13	16	118	6	6	8	10	12	14	16
7–7.9	122	5	6	7	9	12	15	17	126	6	7	9	11	13	16	18
8–8.9	117	5	6	7	8	10	13	16	118	6	8	9	12	15	18	24
9–9.9	121	6	6	7	10	13	17	18	125	8	8	10	13	16	20	22
10–10.9	146	6	6	8	10	14	18	21	152	7	8	10	12	17	23	27
11–11.9	122	6	6	8	11	16	20	24	117	7	8	10	13	18	24	28
12–12.9	153	6	6	8	11	14	22	28	129	8	9	11	14	18	23	27
13–13.9	134	5	5	7	10	14	22	26	151	8	8	12	15	21	26	30
14–14.9	131	4	5	7	9	14	21	24	141	9	10	13	16	21	26	28
15–15.9	128	4	5	6	8	11	18	24	117	8	10	12	17	21	25	32
16–16.9	131	4	5	6	8	12	16	22	142	10	12	15	18	22	26	31
17–17.9	133	5	5	6	8	12	16	19	114	10	12	13	19	24	30	37
18–18.9	91	4	5	6	9	13	20	24	109	10	12	15	18	22	26	30
19–24.9	531	4	5	7	10	15	20	22	1060	10	11	14	18	24	30	34
25–34.9	971	5	6	8	12	16	20	24	1987	10	12	16	21	27	34	37
35–44.9	806	5	6	8	12	16	20	23	1614	12	14	18	23	29	35	38
45–54.9	898	6	6	8	12	15	20	25	1047	12	16	20	25	30	36	40
55–64.9	734	5	6	8	11	14	19	22	809	12	16	20	25	31	36	38
65–74.9	1503	4	6	8	11	15	19	22	1670	12	14	18	24	29	34	36

Triceps skinfold percentiles (mm²)

* By permission from Dr. A. Roberto Frisancho, and *Am. J. Clin. Nutr.*, **34**:2541, 1981.

† N = number of persons on which data are based.

Table A-20. Age- and Sex-Specific Reference Values for Subscapular Skinfold (SSS) of U.S. Adults*

Age Group	Percentile[†]						
	5th	10th	25th	50th	75th	90th	95th
Men							
18–74	6.0[‡]	7.0	10.0	14.5	20.0	26.0	30.5
18–24	6.0	6.5	8.0	11.0	16.0	24.0	29.0
25–34	6.5	7.0	10.0	14.0	20.0	26.0	30.5
35–44	7.0	8.0	11.5	16.0	21.0	26.0	30.5
45–54	7.0	8.0	12.0	16.5	22.0	29.0	32.0
55–64	6.0	7.0	11.0	15.5	21.0	27.0	30.0
65–74	6.0	7.5	10.5	15.0	20.0	25.0	30.0
Women							
18–74	6.5	7.5	10.5	16.0	25.2	33.2	38.0
18–24	6.0	7.0	9.0	13.0	19.0	27.0	31.5
25–34	6.0	7.0	10.0	14.5	22.5	32.0	38.0
35–44	6.5	8.0	11.0	17.0	26.5	34.0	39.0
45–54	7.0	8.5	12.0	20.0	28.0	35.0	40.0
55–64	7.0	8.0	12.5	20.0	28.0	34.5	38.0
65–74	7.0	8.0	12.0	18.0	25.0	32.5	37.0

* Bishop, C. W.: "Reference Values for Arm Muscle Area, Arm Fat Area, Subscapular Skinfold Thickness, and Sum of Skinfold Thicknesses for American Adults," *JPEN*, **8**:515–22, 1984.

† These reference values were developed from data collected during the NHANES I, 1971 to 1974, and are representative of the adult noninstitutionalized civilian population of the United States as of November 1, 1972.

‡ Values are in units of mm.

Table A-21. Age- and Sex-Specific Reference Values for the Sum of Triceps and Subscapular Skinfold Thicknesses (SOS) for U.S. Adults*

Age Group	Percentile[†]						
	5th	10th	25th	50th	75th	90th	95th
Men							
18–74	11.5[‡]	13.5	19.0	26.0	34.5	44.0	51.0
18–24	10.0	12.0	15.0	21.0	30.0	41.0	51.0
25–34	11.5	13.5	19.0	26.0	35.5	45.0	54.0
35–44	12.0	15.0	21.0	28.0	36.0	44.0	48.5
45–54	13.0	15.0	21.0	28.0	37.0	46.0	53.0
55–64	12.0	14.0	20.0	26.0	34.0	44.0	48.0
65–74	11.5	14.0	19.5	26.0	34.0	42.5	49.0
Women							
18–74	18.5	22.0	28.5	39.0	53.0	65.0	73.0
18–24	17.0	19.0	24.0	31.0	41.5	54.5	64.0
25–34	18.5	20.5	26.5	35.0	48.0	64.0	73.0
35–44	20.0	23.0	30.0	40.5	55.0	68.0	75.0
45–54	22.0	25.0	33.5	45.0	58.0	69.5	78.5
55–64	19.0	25.0	33.0	46.0	58.0	68.0	73.0
65–74	20.0	25.0	32.0	41.0	52.5	63.0	70.0

* Bishop, C. W.: "Reference Values for Arm Muscle Area, Arm Fat Area, Subscapular Skinfold Thickness, and Sum of Skinfold Thicknesses for American Adults," *JPEN*, **8**:515–22, 1984.

† These reference values were developed from data collected during the NHANES I, 1971 to 1974, and are representative of the adult noninstitutionalized civilian population of the United States as of November 1, 1972.

‡ Values are in units of mm.

Table A-22. Percentiles of Upper Arm Circumference (mm) and Estimated Upper Arm Muscle Circumference (mm) for Whites of the United States Health and Nutrition Examination Survey I of 1971 to 1974*

Age Group	Arm circumference (mm)							Arm muscle circumference (mm)						
	5	10	25	50	75	90	95	5	10	25	50	75	90	95
	Males							Males						
1–1.9	142	146	150	159	170	176	183	110	113	119	127	135	144	147
2–2.9	141	145	153	162	170	178	185	111	114	122	130	140	146	150
3–3.9	150	153	160	167	175	184	190	117	123	131	137	143	148	153
4–4.9	149	154	162	171	180	186	192	123	126	133	141	148	156	159
5–5.9	153	160	167	175	185	195	204	128	133	140	147	154	162	169
6–6.9	155	159	167	179	188	209	228	131	135	142	151	161	170	177
7–7.9	162	167	177	187	201	223	230	137	139	151	160	168	177	190
8–8.9	162	170	177	190	202	220	245	140	145	154	162	170	182	187
9–9.9	175	178	187	200	217	249	257	151	154	161	170	183	196	202
10–10.9	181	184	196	210	231	262	274	156	160	166	180	191	209	221
11–11.9	186	190	202	223	244	261	280	159	165	173	183	195	205	230
12–12.9	193	200	214	232	254	282	303	167	171	182	195	210	223	241
13–13.9	194	211	228	247	263	286	301	172	179	196	211	226	238	245
14–14.9	220	226	237	253	283	303	322	189	199	212	223	240	260	264
15–15.9	222	229	244	264	284	311	320	199	204	218	237	254	266	272
16–16.9	244	248	262	278	303	324	343	213	225	234	249	269	287	296
17–17.9	246	253	267	285	308	336	347	224	231	245	258	273	294	312
18–18.9	245	260	276	297	321	353	379	226	237	252	264	283	298	324
19–24.9	262	272	288	308	331	355	372	238	245	257	273	289	309	321
25–34.9	271	282	300	319	342	362	375	243	250	264	279	298	314	326
35–44.9	278	287	305	326	345	363	374	247	255	269	286	302	318	327
45–54.9	267	281	301	322	342	362	376	239	249	265	281	300	315	326
55–64.9	258	273	296	317	336	355	369	236	245	260	278	295	310	320
65–74.9	248	263	285	307	325	344	355	223	235	251	268	284	298	306

Table A-22. (Continued)

	Arm circumference (mm)							Arm muscle circumference (mm)						
				Females							Females			
Age Group	5	10	25	50	75	90	95	5	10	25	50	75	90	95
1–1.9	138	142	148	156	164	172	177	105	111	117	124	132	139	143
2–2.9	142	145	152	160	167	176	184	111	114	119	126	133	142	147
3–3.9	143	150	158	167	175	183	189	113	119	124	132	140	146	152
4–4.9	149	154	160	169	177	184	191	115	121	128	136	144	152	157
5–5.9	153	157	165	175	185	203	211	125	128	134	142	151	159	165
6–6.9	156	162	170	176	187	204	211	130	133	138	145	154	166	171
7–7.9	164	167	174	183	199	216	231	129	135	142	151	160	171	176
8–8.9	168	172	183	195	214	247	261	138	140	151	160	171	183	194
9–9.9	178	182	194	211	224	251	260	147	150	158	167	180	194	198
10–10.9	174	182	193	210	228	251	265	148	150	159	170	180	190	197
11–11.9	185	194	208	224	248	276	303	150	158	171	181	196	217	223
12–12.9	194	203	216	237	256	282	294	162	166	180	191	201	214	220
13–13.9	202	211	223	243	271	301	338	169	175	183	198	211	226	240
14–14.9	214	223	237	252	272	304	322	174	179	190	201	216	232	247
15–15.9	208	221	239	254	279	300	322	175	178	189	202	215	228	244
16–16.9	218	224	241	258	283	318	334	170	180	190	202	216	234	249
17–17.9	220	227	241	264	295	324	350	175	183	194	205	221	239	257
18–18.9	222	227	241	258	281	312	325	174	179	191	202	215	237	245
19–24.9	221	230	247	265	290	319	345	179	185	195	207	221	236	249
25–34.9	233	240	256	277	304	342	368	183	188	199	212	228	246	264
35–44.9	241	251	267	290	317	356	378	186	192	205	218	236	257	272
45–54.9	242	256	274	299	328	362	384	187	193	206	220	238	260	274
55–64.9	243	257	280	303	335	367	385	187	196	209	225	244	266	280
65–74.9	240	252	274	299	326	356	373	185	195	208	225	244	264	279

* By permission from Dr. A. Roberto Frisancho, and *Am.J. Clin. Nutr.*, **34**:2542, 1981.

Table A-23. Age- and Sex-Specific Reference Values for Midupper Arm Muscle Area (AMA) of U.S. Adults*

Age Group	Percentile†						
	5th	10th	25th	50th	75th	90th	95th
Men							
18–74	45.0‡	49.0	54.9	61.9	69.9	78.5	84.3
18–24	44.1	47.3	53.0	58.8	66.4	75.3	83.0
25–34	46.8	50.8	55.9	62.6	71.9	79.9	86.2
35–44	49.9	52.2	58.4	65.4	73.1	82.0	86.9
45–54	46.0	49.5	55.9	62.7	70.9	79.0	84.6
55–64	41.3	47.3	54.8	61.9	69.8	76.7	80.7
65–74	40.1	44.7	50.9	57.5	64.6	71.3	75.2
Women							
18–74	27.0	28.8	32.5	37.7	44.3	53.2	59.6
18–24	25.0	27.1	30.1	33.8	38.7	44.4	49.5
25–34	26.7	28.3	32.0	36.3	41.6	49.4	56.3
35–44	27.4	29.4	33.8	38.5	45.9	54.4	59.9
45–54	28.1	30.1	34.0	39.4	46.8	56.5	61.7
55–64	27.4	30.1	34.4	40.6	47.5	54.9	62.7
65–74	27.4	30.3	34.5	40.4	47.6	55.7	62.7

 * Bishop, C. W.: "Reference Values for Arm Muscle Area, Arm Fat Area, Subscapular Skinfold Thickness, and Sum of Skinfold Thicknesses for American Adults," *JPEN*, **8**:515–22, 1984.
 † These reference values were developed from data collected during the NHANES I, 1971 to 1974, and are representative of the adult noninstitutionalized civilian population of the United States as of November 1, 1972.
 ‡ Values are in units of cm².

Table A-24. Age- and Sex-Specific References Values for Midupper Arm Fat Area (AFA) for U.S. Adults*

Age Group	Percentile†						
	5th	10th	25th	50th	75th	90th	95th
Men							
18–74	6.1‡	7.8	11.2	16.6	23.0	31.1	36.8
18–24	5.3	7.0	9.5	13.7	21.2	30.6	36.6
25–34	6.2	7.9	11.5	17.8	24.7	33.0	39.1
35–44	6.7	8.4	13.2	17.8	24.4	31.5	36.3
45–54	7.0	8.6	12.3	16.8	22.6	31.5	39.5
55–64	6.3	8.1	11.4	16.3	21.5	29.8	34.4
65–74	5.7	7.5	11.0	15.9	21.8	27.8	33.3
Women							
18–74	12.0	14.5	20.1	27.9	38.2	49.2	57.2
18–24	10.3	12.0	15.8	21.2	29.1	39.0	47.4
25–34	11.8	14.0	18.3	25.4	34.8	46.9	54.8
35–44	13.4	16.5	21.7	29.1	39.9	52.1	60.4
45–54	14.7	18.1	24.7	32.9	42.5	55.2	63.0
55–64	12.7	16.2	24.4	32.3	42.2	52.0	58.8
65–74	13.4	16.8	22.8	30.1	38.8	48.1	54.1

 * Bishop, C. W.: "Reference Values for Arm Muscle Area, Arm Fat Area, Subscapular Skinfold Thickness, and Sum of Skinfold Thicknesses for American Adults," *JPEN*, **8**:515–22, 1984.
 † These reference values were developed from data collected during the NHANES I, 1971 to 1974, and are representative of the adult noninstitutionalized civilian population of the United States as of November 1, 1972.
 ‡ Values are in units of cm².

Table A-25.   Arm Anthropometry Nomogram for Adults*

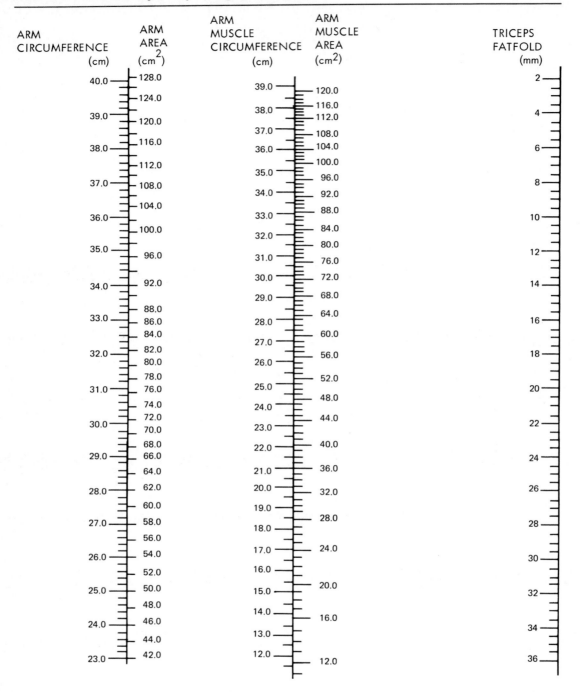

TO OBTAIN MUSCLE CIRCUMFERENCE:
1. LAY RULER BETWEEN VALUE OF ARM CIRCUMFERENCE AND FATFOLD
2. READ OFF MUSCLE CIRCUMFERENCE ON MIDDLE LINE

TO OBTAIN TISSUE AREAS:
1. THE ARM AREA AND MUSCLE AREA ARE ALONGSIDE THEIR RESPECTIVE CIRCUMFERENCES
2. FAT AREA = ARM AREA–MUSCLE AREA

* Source: Gurney, J. M., and Jelliffe, D. B.: "Arm Anthropometry in Nutritional Assessment: Nomogram for Rapid Calculation of Muscle Circumferences and Cross-Sectional Muscle and Fat Areas," *Am. J. Clin. Nutr.*, **26:**912–15, 1973.

Table A-26. Arm Anthropometry Nomogram for Children*

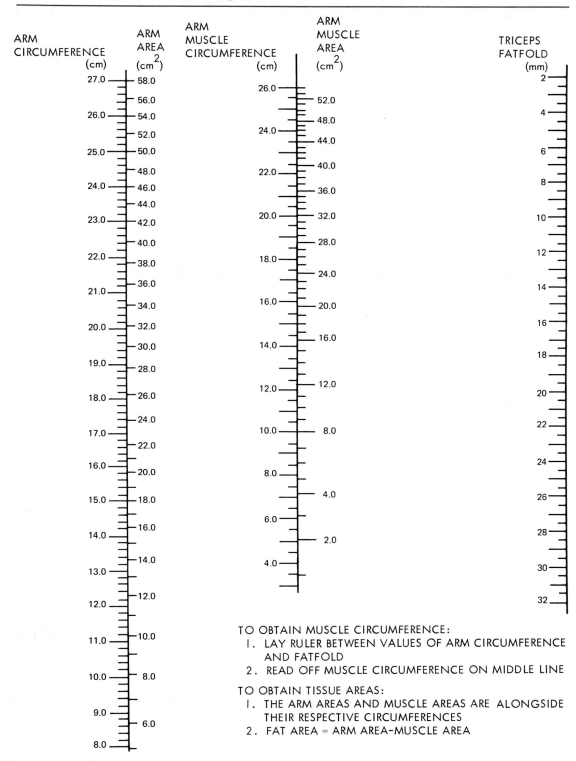

ARM CIRCUMFERENCE (cm)

ARM AREA (cm²)

ARM MUSCLE CIRCUMFERENCE (cm)

ARM MUSCLE AREA (cm²)

TRICEPS FATFOLD (mm)

TO OBTAIN MUSCLE CIRCUMFERENCE:
1. LAY RULER BETWEEN VALUES OF ARM CIRCUMFERENCE AND FATFOLD
2. READ OFF MUSCLE CIRCUMFERENCE ON MIDDLE LINE

TO OBTAIN TISSUE AREAS:
1. THE ARM AREAS AND MUSCLE AREAS ARE ALONGSIDE THEIR RESPECTIVE CIRCUMFERENCES
2. FAT AREA = ARM AREA—MUSCLE AREA

* Source: Gurney, J. M., and Jelliffe, D. B.: "Arm Anthropometry in Nutritional Assessment: Nomogram for Rapid Calculation of Muscle Circumference and Cross-Sectional Muscle and Fat Areas," *Am. J. Clin. Nutr.*, **26**:912–15, 1973.

Table A-27. Normal Constituents of Human Blood*†
(B = whole blood; P = plasma; S = serum)

Constituent	Normal Range		Examples of Deviations
PHYSICAL MEASUREMENTS			
Specific gravity (S)	1.025–1.029		
Bleeding time, capillary	1–3	min	
Prothrombin time (Quick, P)	10–20	sec	
Sedimentation rate (Wintrobe)			
Men	0–9	mm/hr	
Women	0–20	mm/hr	
Viscosity (water as unity) (B)	4.5–5.5		
ACID–BASE CONSTITUENTS			
Base, total fixed cations (Na + K + Ca + Mg) (S)	143–150	mEq/liter	Low in alkali deficit; diabetic acidosis
Sodium (S)	320–335	mg/dl	Low in alkali deficit; diabetic acidosis, excessive fluid administration
	139–146	mEq/liter	
Potassium (S)	16–22	mg/dl	High in acute infections, pneumonia, Addison's disease; low in diarrhea, vomiting, correction of diabetic acidosis
	4.1–5.6	mEq/liter	
Calcium (S)	9–11	mg/dl	High with excessive vitamin D, hyperparathyroidism; low in infantile tetany, steatorrhea, severe nephritis, defective vitamin D absorption
	4.5–5.5	mEq/Liter	
Calcium, ionized (S)	50–60	percent	
Magnesium (S)	2–3	mg/dl	High in chronic nephritis, liver disease; low in uremia, tetany, severe diarrhea
	1.65–2.5	mEq/Liter	
Chloride (S)	340–372	mg/dl	High in congestive heart failure, eclampsia, nephritis
	96–105	mEq/liter	
As NaCl (S)	560–614	mg/dl	
	96–105	mEq/liter	
Phosphorus, inorganic as P (S)			
Child	4.0–6.5	mg/dl	High in chronic nephritis, hypoparathyroidism; low during treatment of diabetic coma, hyperparathyroidism
Adult	2.5–4.5	mg/dl	
Sulfates as SO_4^{2-} (S)	2.5–5.0	mg/dl	
	0.5–1.0	mEq/liter	
Bicarbonate cation-binding power (S)	19–30	mEq/liter	
Serum protein cation-binding power (S)	15.5–18.0	mEq/liter	
Lactic acid (S)	10–20	mg/dl	
	1.1–2.2	mEq/liter	
pH at 38°C (B, P, or S)	7.30–7.45		High in uncompensated alkalosis; low in uncompensated acidosis
BLOOD GASES			
CO_2 content (venous S)	45–70	vol %	Low in primary alkali deficit, diarrhea; high in hypoventilation
	20.3–31.5	mM/liter	
CO_2 content (venous B)	40–60	vol %	
	18–27	mM/liter	
CO_2 tension (P_{CO_2}) arterial blood	35–45	mm Hg	P_{CO_2} in venous blood is about 6 mm higher than arterial or capillary blood
Oxygen content (arterial B)	15–22	vol %	High in polycythemia; low in emphysema
Oxygen content (venous B)	11–16	vol %	
Oxygen capacity (B)	16–24	vol %	
Oxygen tension (P_{O_2})	85–100	mm Hg	
CARBOHYDRATES			
Glucose			
Reducing substances (B)	90–120	mg/dl	High in diabetes mellitus; low in hyperinsulinism
"True"	60–85	mg/dl	
Glucose tolerance			
Fasting sugar	90–120	mg/dl	
Highest value	130–140	mg/dl	
Highest value reached in	45–60	minutes	
Return to fasting in	1.5–2.5	hr	

Constituent	Normal Range		Examples of Deviations
CARBOHYDRATES (continued)			
Lactose tolerance			
Fasting blood glucose (B)	90–120	mg/dl	In lactase deficiency the rise in blood glucose after
Increase in blood glucose after test dose lactose	20	mg/dl	test dose of lactose is less than 20 mg in 1 hour
Citric acid (B)	1.3–2.3	mg/dl	
(P)	1.6–2.7	mg/dl	
Lactic acid (see acid–base constituents)			
Pyruvic acid, fasting (B)	0.7–1.2	mg/dl	
ENYZMES			
Amylase (Somogyi) (S)	60–180	units/dl	High in acute pancreatitis, acute appendicitis
Lactic dehydrogenase (S)	25–100	units/ml	High in myocardial infarction
Lipase (S)	0.2–1.5	units/ml	High in pancreatitis
Leucine-aminopeptidase (S)	1–3.5	units/ml	High in hemolytic anemias
Phosphatase, alkaline			
(Bodansky) (S) Child	5–14	units/dl	High in rickets, bone cancer, Paget's disease,
Adult	1–4	units/dl	hyperparathyroidism, vitamin D inadequacy;
			indicates rapid bone growth in young
Transaminases			
Glutamic-oxalacetic (SGOT) (Karmen) (S)	10–40	units/ml	Increased within 24 hours in myocardial infarction;
			normal after 6 to 7 days
Glutamic-pyruvic (SGPT) (Karmen) (S)	5–35	units/ml	High in hepatic disease, and trauma after surgery
HEMATOLOGIC STUDIES			
Hematocrit			High in polycythemia; low in anemia, prolonged
Up to 2 years	31+	percent	iron deficiency
2 to 5 years	34+	percent	
6–12 years	36+	percent	
13–16 years—male	40+	percent	
13–16 years—female	36+	percent	
16+ years—males	44+	percent	
16+ years—females	33+	percent	
Pregnant	33+	percent	
Red blood cells	4.25–5.25	million per cu mm	High in polycythemia, dehydration; low in anemia, hemorrhage
White blood cells	5,000–9,000	per cu mm	Increased in acute infections, leukemias
Lymphocytes	1,500–3,000	per cu mm	Decreased in protein malnutrition
	25–30	percent	
Neutrophils	60–65	percent	
Monocytes	4–8	percent	
Eosinophils	0.5–4	percent	
Basophils	0–1.5	percent	
Platelets	125,000–300,000	per cu mm	
Hemoglobin (B)			High in polycythemia, dehydration; low in dietary
6–23 months	10+	g/dl	deficiency of iron, anemia
2–5 years	11+	g/dl	
6–12 years	11.5+	g/dl	
13–16 years—males	13.0+	g/dl	
13–16 years—females	11.5+	g/dl	
16+ years—males	14.0+	g/dl	
16+ years—females	12.0+	g/dl	
Pregnant (after 6 months)	11.0+	g/dl	
Iron (S)			High in hemochromatosis, liver disease, transfusion
Up to 2 years	30+	μg/dl	hemosiderosis; low in iron-deficiency anemia
2 to 5 years	40+	μg/dl	
6–12 years	50+	μg/dl	
12+ years—males	60+	μg/dl	
12+ years—females	40+	μg/dl	
Transferrin saturation			
Up to 2 years	15+	percent	
2 to 12 years	20+	percent	
12+ years—males	20+	percent	
12+ years—females	15+	percent	

Constituent	Normal Range		Examples of Deviations
HEMATOLOGIC STUDIES (continued)			
Iron-binding capacity (S)			High in anemia
Men	250–430	µg/dl	
Women	220–415	µg/dl	
Serum ferritin			
16+ years—males	77+	ng/ml	
16+ years—females	36+	ng/ml	
LIPIDS			
Acetone (S)	0.3–2.0	mg/dl	High in uncontrolled diabetes and starvation
Cholesterol, total (S)	125–225	mg/dl	High in uncontrolled diabetes mellitus, nephrosis,
esters	50–67	percent	hypothyroidism, hyperlipidemias
free	33–50	percent	
Fatty acids, unesterified (P)	8–31	mg/dl	
17-Hydroxycorticosteroids (P)	10–13.5	µg/dl	
Lipids, total (P)	570–820	mg/dl	
Phospholipid (S)	150–300	mg/dl	
Triglycerides (S)	30–140	mg/dl	Increased in hyperlipidemias
NITROGENOUS CONSTITUENTS			
Alpha-amino acid nitrogen (S)	3.5–5.5	mg/dl	High in severe liver disease; low in nephrosis
Ammonia (B)	40–70	µg/dl	High in liver disease
Creatinine (S)	0.5–1.2	mg/dl	Increased in renal insufficiency
Creatinine clearance endogenous (B)	120 ± 20	ml	Blood cleared per min by kidney; measure of glomerular filtration
Nonprotein N (NPN) (B)	25–35	mg/dl	High in acute glomerulonephritis, dehydration, metallic poisoning, intestinal obstruction, renal failure
Phenylalanine (S)	0.7–4	mg/dl	Increased in phenylketonuria
Urea nitrogen (BUN) (B)	8–18	mg/dl	High in renal failure, acute glomerulonephritis, mercury poisoning, dehydration; low in hepatic failure
Urea clearance (B)	75	ml/min C_m	C_m = maximal clearance
	54	ml/min C_s	C_s = standard clearance
Uric acid (S)	2–6	mg/dl	High in gout, nephritis, arthritis
PROTEINS			
Total protein (S)	6.5–7.5	g/dl	High in dehydration; low in liver disease, nephrosis
Albumin (S)	3.9–4.5	g/dl	Low in protein malnutrition, cirrhosis, proteinuria
Globulin (S)	2.3–3.5	g/dl	High in infections, liver disease, multiple myeloma
Albumin : globulin ratio	1.2–1.9		Low in liver disease, nephrosis
Fibrinogen (P)	0.2–0.5	g/dl	High in infections; low in severe liver disease
Ceruloplasmin (S)	16–33	mg/dl	
Gamma globulin (S)	0.7–1.2	gm/dl	
Hemoglobin (See Hematologic Studies)			
VITAMINS			
Ascorbic acid (S)	0.3–1.4	mg/dl	
Folic acid (*L. casei*) (S)	6–10	µµg/ml	
(*L. casei*) (B)	100–220	µµg/ml	
Niacin (S)	30–150	µg/dl	
Riboflavin (S)	2.3–3.7	µg/dl	
Thiamin (B)	5.5–9.5	µg/dl	
Tocopherol (S)	0.6–2.0	mg/dl	
Vitamin A (S)	25–90	µg/dl	
Carotene (S)	40–125	µg/dl	
Vitamin B-6 (B)	1–18	µg/dl	
Vitamin B-12 (S)	10–90	µg/dl	

Table A-27. **(Continued)**

Constituent	Normal Range		Examples of Deviations
MISCELLANEOUS			
Bilirubin (S)	0–1.5	mg/dl	High in red cell destruction, liver disease
Icterus index	4–6	units	High in jaundice
Copper (S)	80–240	μg/dl	Low in anemia, Wilson's disease
Lead (S)	1–3	μg/dl	
Manganese (S)	2–5	μg/dl	
Protein-bound iodine (PBI) (S)	3–8	μg/dl	High in hyperthyroidism; low in hypothyroidism
Zinc (S)	100–140	μg/dl	

* Units:
  ml = milliliters
  dl = deciliter (100 ml)
  mg = milligrams
  μg = micrograms
  μμg = micro-micrograms
  mEq = milliequivalents
  g = grams
  cu mm = cubic millimeters

$$\text{mEq per liter} = \frac{\text{mg per liter}}{\text{equivalent weight}}$$

$$\text{mM (millimoles) per liter} = \frac{\text{mg per liter}}{\text{molecular weight}}$$

$$\text{equivalent weight} = \frac{\text{atomic weight}}{\text{valence of element}}$$

volumes percent = mM per liter × 2.24

† Sources of data:
  Oser, B. L., ed.: *Hawk's Physiological Chemistry*, 14th ed. McGraw-Hill Book Company, New York, 1965, pp. 977–79.
  Robinson, H. W.: "Biochemistry," in *Rypins' Medical Licensure Examinations*, 11th ed. A. W. Wright, ed. J. B. Lippincott Company, Philadelphia, 1970, pp. 202–5.
  Ten-State Nutrition Survey in the United States, 1968–70. I. Historical Development. II. Demographic Data. U.S. Department of Health, Welfare and Education (HSM) 72–8130.
  Christakis, G.: "Nutritional Assessment in Health Programs," *Am. J. Publ. Health, Suppl.*, **63:**1–82, November 1973.

Table A-28. Normal Constituents of Urine

	Adult Values
Specific gravity	1.010–1.025
Reaction, pH	5.5–8.0
Volume, ml per 24 hr	800–1,600

	g per 24 hr
Total solids	55–70
Nitrogenous constituents	
Total nitrogen	10–17
Ammonia	0.5–1.0
Amino acid N	0.4–1
Creatine	None
Creatinine	1–1.5
Men, mg per kg per 24 hr	(mg) 23
Women, mg per kg per 24 hr	(mg) 18
Protein	None
Purine bases	0.016–0.060
Urea	20–35
Uric acid	0.5–0.7
Acetone bodies	0.003–0.015
Bile	None
Calcium	0.2–0.4
Chloride (as NaCl)	10–15
Glucose	None
Indican	0–0.030
Iron	0.001–0.005
Magnesium (as MgO)	0.15–0.30
Phosphate, total (as phosphoric acid)	2.5–3.5
Potassium (as K_2O)	2.0–3.0
Sodium (as Na_2O)	4.0–5.0
Sulfates, total (as sulfuric acid)	1.5–3.0

	Acceptable Levels (All Ages)
Vitamin Studies*	
Pyridoxine, μg per g creatinine	
1–3 years	90+
4–6 years	80+
7–9 years	60+
10–12 years	40+
13–15 years	30+
16+ years	20+
N-Methyl nicotinamide, mg per g creatinine	
All ages	6.0+
Pregnancy	2.5+
Riboflavin, μg per g creatinine	
1–3 years	500+
4–6 years	300+
7–9 years	270+
10–18 years	200+
16+ years	80+
Pregnancy	90+
Thiamin, μg per g creatinine	
1–3 years	175+
4–5 years	120+
6–9 years	180+
10–15 years	150+
16+ years	65+
Pregnancy	50+
Tryptophan load test (dose = 100 mg per kg)	
Xanthurenic acid excretion, mg	
Adults, 6 hours	up to 25
Adults, 24 hours	up to 75

* Adapted from *Ten State Nutrition Survey in the United States, 1968–70. I. Historical Development. II. Demographic Data.* U.S. Department of Health, Welfare and Education (HSM) 72–8130.

Table A-29. Conversions to and from Metric Measures*

If Measure Is In	Multiply By	To Find
Length		
inches	25.4	millimeters
inches	2.54	centimeters
feet	30.48	centimeters
feet	0.305	meters
centimeters	0.394	inches
meters	3.281	feet
Weight		
grains	64.799	milligrams
ounces (Av.)	28.35	grams
pounds (Av.)	454	grams
pounds	0.454	kilograms
grams	15.432	grains
grams	0.035	ounces (Av.)
grams	0.0022	pounds (Av.)
kilograms	2.205	pounds
Capacity		
teaspoons	4.7	milliliters
tablespoons	14.1	milliliters
fluid ounces	29.573	milliliters
cups (8 ounces)	238	milliliters
pints	0.473	liters
quarts	0.946	liters
milliliters	0.034	fluid ounces
liters	1.057	quarts
Energy units		
kilocalories	4.184	kilojoules
kilojoules	0.239	kilocalories
Temperature		
Fahrenheit	subtract 32; then multiply by 5/9	Celsius (Centigrade)
Celsius	multiply by 9/5; then add 32	Fahrenheit

* Metric equivalents
  1 kilogram (kg) = 1,000 grams
  1 gram (g) = 1,000 milligrams
  1 milligram (mg) = 1,000 micrograms
  1 microgram (mcg, μg, γ) = 1,000 nanograms
  1 nanogram (ng) = 1,000 picograms (pg)

Multiples
  deca- 10
  hecto- 10^2 (1000)
  kilo- 10^3 (1,000)
  mega- 10^6 (1,000,000)

Submultiples
  deci- = one tenth 10^{-1} (0.1)
  centi- = one hundredth 10^{-2} (0.01)
  milli- = one thousandth 10^{-3} (0.001)
  micro- = one millionth 10^{-6} (0.000,001)
  nano- = one billionth 10^{-9} (0.000,000,001)
  pico- = one trillionth 10^{-12} (0.000,000,000,001)

Table A-30. Summary Examples of Recommended Nutrient Intakes for Canandians[*][a][b]

Age	Sex	Weight (kg)	Pro-tein (g/day)[c]	Fat-Soluble Vitamins			Water-Soluble Vitamins			Minerals				
				Vitamin A (RE/day)[d]	Vitamin D (μg/day)[e]	Vitamin E (mg/day)[f]	Vitamin C (mg/day)	Folacin (μg/day)[g]	Vitamin B$_{12}$ (μg/day)	Calcium (mg/day)	Magnesium (mg/day)	Iron (mg/day)	Iodine (μg/day)	Zinc (mg/day)
Months														
0–2	Both	4.5	11[h]	400	10	3	20	50	0.3	350	30	0.4[i]	25	2[j]
3–5	Both	7.0	14[h]	400	10	3	20	50	0.3	350	40	5	35	3
6–8	Both	8.5	16[h]	400	10	3	20	50	0.3	400	45	7	40	3
9–11	Both	9.5	18	400	10	3	20	55	0.3	400	50	7	45	3
Years														
1	Both	11	18	400	10	3	20	65	0.3	500	55	6	55	4
2–3	Both	14	20	400	5	4	20	80	0.4	500	65	6	65	4
4–6	Both	18	25	500	5	5	25	90	0.5	600	90	6	85	5
7–9	M	25	31	700	2.5	7	35	125	0.8	700	110	7	110	6
	F	25	29	700	2.5	6	30	125	0.8	700	110	7	95	6
10–12	M	34	38	800	2.5	8	40	170	1.0	900	150	10	125	7
	F	36	39	800	2.5	7	40	170	1.0	1000	160	10	110	7
13–15	M	50	49	900	2.5	9	50	160	1.5	1100	220	12	160	9
	F	48	43	800	2.5	7	45	160	1.5	800	190	13	160	8
16–18	M	62	54	1000	2.5	10	55	190	1.9	900	240	10	160	9
	F	53	47	800	2.5	7	45	160	1.9	700	220	14	160	8
19-24	M	71	57	1000	2.5	10	60	210	2.0	800	240	8	160	9
	F	58	41	800	2.5	7	45	165	2.0	700	190	14	160	8
25–49	M	74	57	1000	2.5	9	60	210	2.0	800	240	8	160	9
	F	59	41	800	2.5	6	45	165	2.0	700	190	14[k]	160	8
50–74	M	73	57	1000	2.5	7	60	210	2.0	800	240	8	160	9
	F	63	41	800	2.5	6	45	165	2.0	800	190	7	160	8
75+	M	69	57	1000	2.5	6	60	210	2.0	800	240	8	160	9
	F	64	41	800	2.5	5	45	165	2.0	800	190	7	160	8
Pregnancy (additional)														
1st Trimester			15	100	2.5	2	0	305	1.0	500	15	6	25	0
2nd Trimester			20	100	2.5	2	20	305	1.0	500	20	6	25	1
3rd Trimester			25	100	2.5	2	20	305	1.0	500	25	6	25	2
Lactation (additional)			20	400	2.5	3	30	120	0.5	500	80	0	50	6

[*] Used by permission: Department of National Health and Welfare: *Recommended Nutrient Intakes for Canadians*, Canadian Government Publishing Centre, Ottawa, Canada, 1983.

[a] Recommended intakes of energy and of certain nutrients are not listed in this table because of the nature of the variables upon which they are based. The figures for energy are estimates of average requirements for expected patterns of activity. For nutrients not shown, the following amounts are recommended: thiamin 0.4 mg/1000 kcal (0.48 mg/5,000 kJ); riboflavin, 0.5 mg/1,000 kcal (0.6 mg/5,000 kJ); niacin, 7.2 NE/1000 kcal (8.6 NE/5,000 kJ); vitamin B$_6$, 15 μg, as pyridoxine, per gram of protein; phosphorus, same as calcium.

[b] Recommended intakes during periods of growth are taken as appropriate for individuals representative of the mid-point in each age group. All recommended intakes are designed to cover individual variations in essentially all of a healthy population subsisting on a variety of common foods available in Canada.

[c] The primary units are grams per kilogram of body weight. The figures shown here are only examples.

[d] One retinol equivalent (RE) corresponds to the biological activity of 1 μg of retinol, 6 μg of beta-carotene, or 12 μg of other carotenes.

[e] Expressed as cholecalciferol or ergocalciferol.

[f] Expressed as d-alpha-tocopherol equivalents, relative to which beta- and gamma-tocopherol and alpha-tocotrienol have activities of 0.5, 0.1, and 0.3, respectively.

[g] Expressed as total folate.

[h] Assumption that the protein is from breast milk or is of the same biological value as that of breast milk and that between 3 and 9 months adjustment for the quality of the protein is made.

[i] It is assumed that breast milk is the source of iron up to 2 months of age.

[j] Based on the assumption that breast milk is the source of zinc for the first 2 months.

[k] After the menopause the recommended intake is 7 mg day.

APPENDIX B. EXPLANATION

Appendix B lists some commonly used prescription drugs and some of the potential nutritional effects associated with use of these drugs. The listing of drugs is not all-inclusive and is intended to show representative examples within the various classes of drugs that may have adverse effects on nutrition. The reader is encouraged to consult the cited references at the end of Chapter 27 for more information on drug-nutrient interactions.

Table B-1. Food, Nutrient, and Drug Interactions

Class of Drug	Trade Name	Gastrointestinal Side Effects	Other Nutritional Effects	Proposed Mechanism	Dietary Precautions
ANTIINFECTIVES					
Antibiotics					
Tetracyclines	Cyclopar	Anorexia, nausea, vomiting, glossitis, dysphagia	Interferes with intestinal synthesis of vitamin K; ↓ absorption: calcium, iron, magnesium, zinc, xylose, amino acids, fat; ↑ urinary: ascorbic acid, riboflavin, nitrogen, amino acids, folate, niacin	Inhibits protein synthesis in susceptible microorganisms	Take on empty stomach with 8 oz. water; do not take milk or other dairy products or iron-containing foods within 3 hours of taking the drug
Chloramphenicols	Chloromycetin	Altered taste, nausea, vomiting, glossitis, stomatitis, diarrhea	Possible ↑ need: riboflavin, pyridoxine, vitamin B-12; ↑ urinary glucose	Interferes with or inhibits protein synthesis in intact cells and in cell-free systems	
Aminoglycosides					
Neomycin		Nausea, vomiting, diarrhea	↓ Absorption: fat, nitrogen, carotene, MCT, amino acids, glucose, lactose, sucrose, sodium, potassium, calcium, iron, vitamin B-12, fat-soluble vitamins	Interferes with bile acid metabolism	
Antifungal Agents					
Griseofluvin	Grisactin	Altered taste acuity, dry mouth, possible nausea, vomiting, epigastric distress, diarrhea		Appetite suppression	Take with meals, especially fat; no alcohol
Sulfonamides					
Sulfasalazine	Azulfidine	Anorexia, nausea, vomiting, stomatitis, gastric distress, diarrhea, pancreatitis, hepatitis	↓ Absorption: iron, folate; ↓ intestinal synthesis of vitamin K; ↑ urinary: protein, ascorbic acid		Take with food or water or after meals; encourage adequate fluid intake; recommend good food sources of folate

Class of Drug	Trade Name	Gastrointestinal Side Effects	Other Nutritional Effects	Proposed Mechanism	Dietary Precautions
ANTINEOPLASTICS					
Alkylating Agents					
Chlorambucil	Leukeran	Occasionally, gastrointestinal discomfort	Bone marrow depression, anemia, hyperuricemia	Transfer of alkyl group of drug to biochemically important cell constituents induces chromosomal changes in proliferating cells	Take 1 hour before breakfast or 2 hours after evening meal; encourage fluids
Cytosine arabinoside	Cytosar-U	Anorexia, nausea, vomiting, dysphagia, diarrhea, oral ulceration	Bone marrow suppression; anemia	Interferes with DNA synthesis; antagonist of deoxycytidine triphosphate; competitively inhibits DNA polymerase	
Miscellaneous Agents					
Cisplatin	Platinol	Taste alterations, nausea, vomiting	Bone marrow depression; ↓ blood levels: magnesium, calcium, potassium, phosphate, zinc; ↑ BUN; uric acid	Interferes with DNA synthesis	
Antimetabolites					
5-Fluoro-uracil	Fluorouracil	Taste alterations, nausea, vomiting, stomatitis, diarrhea, decreased appetite, GI bleeding	↑ need thiamin; anemia; hyperuricemia	Blocks the methylation reaction of deoxyuridylic acid to thymidylate, interfering with DNA synthesis and RNA formation	Take with water; not with acidic juices or meals
Methotrexate	Mexate	Altered taste acuity, anorexia, nausea, vomiting, ulcerative stomatitis, diarrhea, steatorrhea	↓ Absorption: B-12, carotene, folacin, fat, cholesterol, lactose, calcium; megaloblastic anemia; hyperuricemia; weight loss	Mucosal damage; inhibits DNA synthesis; it binds to dihydrofolate reductase and prevents reduction of folic acid to methylene tetrahydrofolate, an important methyl donor in DNA synthesis	Avoid alcohol; encourage fluid intake (2,000 ml); avoid vitamin supplements containing folic acid
CARDIOVASCULAR DRUGS					
Cardiac glycosides					
Digoxin	Lanoxin	Anorexia, nausea, vomiting, epigastric distress, abdominal pain, diarrhea	↑ Urinary: calcium, magnesium, potassium, zinc; hypokalemia		Avoid high sodium foods; ensure adequate potassium intake; avoid bran

Class of Drug	Trade Name	Gastrointestinal Side Effects	Other Nutritional Effects	Proposed Mechanism	Dietary Precautions
CARDIOVASCULAR DRUGS (continued)					
Antihypertensives					
Reserpine	Serpasil	Anorexia, nausea, vomiting, dry mouth, increased gastric secretion, diarrhea	↑ Sodium and water retention; ↑ weight	Depletes nerve terminals of norepinephrine and serotonin, with less neurotransmitter available to interact with receptors, results in relaxation of smooth muscle of blood vessels	
Guanethidine	Ismelin	Taste disturbances, nausea, vomiting, dryness of mouth, diarrhea	Fluid retention; possible anemia	Depletes norepinephrine reserves; inhibits its release	Avoid alcohol; may need to restrict sodium, calories
Hydralazine	Apresoline	Anorexia, nausea, vomiting, diarrhea	↑ Urinary: manganese, pyridoxine; sodium and water retention (long-term use)	Direct vasodilating action on vascular smooth muscle	Take with food; diet restricted in calories, sodium, and alcohol may be indicated
Methyldopa	Aldomet	Nausea, vomiting, dryness of mouth, glossitis, colitis, constipation, diarrhea, pancreatitis	↑ need for folacin, B-12; edema; weight gain	Stimulates central inhibitory alpha-adrenergic receptors, false neurotransmission, and/or reduction of plasma renin	Take with food; avoid alcohol; sodium and calorie restriction may be indicated
Antiarrhythmic Agents					
Propranolol hydrochloride	Inderal	Nausea, vomiting, dry mouth, constipation, diarrhea	↓ Carbohydrate tolerance; ↑ BUN	Beta-Adrenergic receptor blockade; direct effect on cardiac cell membrane; decreases rate and force of contraction of heart and cardiac output	Take with food for better absorption
Hypocholesterolemic Agents					
Cholestyramine	Questran	Anorexia, nausea, constipation, steatorrhea	Impaired uptake of iron into protoporphyrin; ↓ absorption of vitamins A, D, E, K, B-12, folacin, MCT, fat, glucose, carotene, iron; ↑ blood: triglycerides; ↓ blood/serum: calcium, B-12; ↑ urinary: calcium; edema; bloating; weight change	Binds bile salts in the intestine	Take with 4–6 oz water or non-carbonated beverages; low-cholesterol diet indicated; increase dietary fiber and fluids

Class of Drug	Trade Name	Gastrointestinal Side Effects	Other Nutritional Effects	Proposed Mechanism	Dietary Precautions
Hypocholes-terolemic Agents (continued)					
Clofibrate	Atromid-S	↓ Taste acuity, unpleasant after-taste, nausea, stomatitis, gastritis, diarrhea, dyspepsia	↓ Absorption of carotene, glucose, iron, MCT, B-12, electrolytes; ↓ carrier protein for vitamin E; ↑ urinary: protein; weight gain	Uncertain; may increase catabolism of VLDL to LDL and decrease synthesis of VLDL by liver	Take with food or after meals; low-choles-terol, low-triglycer-ide diet indicated
Nicotinic acid	Nitro-Bid	Nausea, vomiting, cramps, diarrhea, activation of peptic ulcer, dyspepsia	↓ Glucose tolerance; hyperglycemia; glycosuria	Stimulates lipoprotein lipase in adipose cells; increases lipolysis	Take with meals; avoid alcohol
Colestipol	Colestid	Constipation, GI irritation	Interferes with absorption of vitamins A, D, E, K; ↓ serum: cholesterol	Binds and removes bile acids	Mix with water or other fluids
DIURETICS					
Chlorothiazide	Diuril	Anorexia, nausea, vomiting, dry mouth, GI irritation, constipation or diarrhea, pancreatitis	↑ Blood/serum: uric acid, calcium, glucose; ↓ blood/serum: sodium, potassium, chloride, phosphate, mag-nesium; ↑ urinary: sodium, potassium, zinc, riboflavin, chloride, magnesium, uric acid, glucose	Enhances excretion of sodium and potassium	Take with food; use alcohol with caution; ensure adequate intake of potassium and magnesium; diet may need to be restricted in sodium, calories; avoid licorice, MSG
Ethacrynic acid	Edecrin	Anorexia, nausea, vomiting, dysphagia, abdominal discomfort, diarrhea	Possible ↓ carbohydrate tolerance; ↑ urinary: calcium, magnesium, potassium, zinc, uric acid	Increases sodium and potassium excretion	Take after meals; avoid alcohol; ensure adequate intake of potassium and magnesium
Furosemide	Lasix	Anorexia, nausea, vomiting, cramping, dry mouth, thirst, constipation, diarrhea, pancreatitis	↑ blood/serum: glucose, BUN, uric acid, zinc; ↓ blood/serum: sodium, potassium, chloride, calcium, magnesium; ↑ urinary: glucose, potassium, sodium, calcium, chloride, magnesium, zinc; anemia.	Increases sodium and potassium excretion	Diet may also need to be restricted in calories and sodium
Spironolactone	Aldactone	Nausea, cramping, dry mouth, diarrhea	↑ Blood/serum: potassium, BUN; ↓ blood/serum: sodium, chloride; ↑ urinary: sodium, chloride; ↓ urinary: potassium		
Triamterene	Dyazide	Nausea, vomiting, dry mouth, constipation, diarrhea	↓ Serum: B-12, folate, sodium, chloride; ↑ blood/serum: uric acid, potassium; ↑urinary: calcium, sodium, chloride, uric acid; ↓ urinary: potassium	Promotes sodium excretion	Take with food or milk; avoid excessive potassium intake

Table B-1. (Continued)

Class of Drug	Trade Name	Gastrointestinal Side Effects	Other Nutritional Effects	Proposed Mechanism	Dietary Precautions
DRUGS AFFECTING THE CENTRAL NERVOUS SYSTEM					
Barbiturates Phenobarbital		Anorexia, nausea, vomiting, diarrhea	↓ Vitamins D and K in children; ↑ urinary: ascorbic acid; ↓ absorption: thiamin; ↑ blood/serum: folacin, B-12, pyridoxine, calcium, magnesium, vitamin D; osteomalacia		Take with meals; avoid alcohol; ensure adequate intake of vitamin D containing foods
Sedatives Chloral hydrate	Noctec	Nausea, vomiting, unpleasant taste in mouth, gastritis, diarrhea			Take with liquid; avoid alcohol
Antianxiety Agents Diazepam	Valium	Nausea, vomiting, constipation	Can stimulate appetite, increasing food intake; possible anemia		Take with food or water; avoid alcohol
Anticonvulsants Phenytoin	Dilantin	Nausea, vomiting, gastric distress, constipation	Increased blood glucose, glycosuria; ↑ need for ascorbic acid; interferes with folic acid absorption; ↓ blood: folacin, B-12, pyridoxine, vitamin D, calcium; osteomalacia, rickets	May interfere with enzyme that converts folic acid to monoglutamate form; may interfere with hepatic metabolism of folic acid	Take with food or milk; avoid alcohol
Antidepressants Monoamine oxidase inhibitors (MAO)	Eutonyl	Anorexia, nausea, vomiting, dry mouth, constipation, appetite stimulation	Weight gain, severe headache, hypertension, intracranial hemorrhage when taken with tyramine-containing foods	Uncertain; believed to prevent MAO from metabolizing epinephrine, serotonin; these amines then accumulate and increase the concentration of neurotransmitters released upon nerve stimulation	Avoid alcohol and tyramine-containing foods; use caffeine containing beverages in moderation
Tricyclic antidepressants	Elavil	Altered taste sensation, anorexia, nausea, vomiting, stomatitis, constipation, diarrhea, dry mouth	↑ or ↓ blood glucose; weight gain	Prevents reuptake of norepinephrine and/or serotonin into storage granule of presynaptic nerve, resulting in increased concentrations of the neurotransmitters in the synapse	Take with food or milk; avoid alcohol
Anorexiants Dextro-amphetamine	Dexedrine	Anorexia, nausea, cramps, metallic taste, constipation, diarrhea	Weight loss; ↓ tissue ascorbic acid levels	Stimulation of the satiety center in limbic and hypothalamus areas of brain	When used for adjunctive treatment of exogenous obesity, low-calorie diet is recommended

Table B-1.   (Continued)

Class of Drug	Trade Name	Gastrointestinal Side Effects	Other Nutritional Effects	Proposed Mechanism	Dietary Precautions
DRUGS AFFECTING THE CENTRAL NERVOUS SYSTEM (continued)					
Analgesics and Antipyretics					
Acetylsalicylic acid	Aspirin	Nausea, dyspepsia, GI irritation	Antagonizes vitamin K; ↓ serum folate, iron; electrolyte imbalance; ↑ urinary: ascorbic acid, thiamin, potassium, amino acids, glucose	Damages lining of stomach and intestine, leading to chronic blood loss	Take on empty stomach for more rapid absorption; limit alcohol
Antiinflamma-tory Agents					
Ibuprofen	Motrin	Anorexia, nausea, vomiting, indiges-tion, stomatitis, ↓ appetite, flatulence, diarrhea, GI bleeding, peptic ulceration	Edema; weight gain; anemia	Inhibition of prostaglandin synthesis	Take with food or milk; avoid alcohol
Indomethacin	Indocin	Anorexia, nausea, vomiting, abdom-inal distress, constipation, diarrhea	↑ Blood/serum: glucose, BUN, ascorbic acid; ↑ urinary glucose, amino acids; iron deficiency; weight gain		Take with food or milk; avoid alcohol
Phenyl-butazone	Butazolidin	Anorexia, nausea, vomiting, stoma-titis, GI distur-bances, peptic ulceration with hemorrhages, hepatitis	↓ Folate; ↑ urinary: protein, uric acid; ↑ blood/serum: sodium, chloride; anemia Fluid and sodium retention		Take with food or milk; low-sodium diet may be indicated; avoid alcohol
Antigout Agents					
Allopurinol	Zyloprim	Metallic taste, anorexia, vomiting, abdominal pain, diarrhea	Anemia	Inhibitor of xanthine oxidase, resulting in decreased levels of uric acid	Avoid alcohol; take after meals with fluids; encourage high fluid intake (2 liters per day)
Colchicine	Colchicine	Anorexia, nausea, vomiting, abdominal cramping, diarrhea	Bone marrow depression; may decrease absorption of B-12, carotene, fat, calcium, iron, sodium, folacin, potassium, nitrogen, lactose; ↓ blood/serum: cholesterol	Intestinal mucosal damage	Take with water and with food to decrease gastric irritation; encourage fluids (2,000 ml); avoid alcohol; gradual weight reduction recommended
Probenecid	Benemid	Anorexia, nausea, vomiting, abdominal discomfort, constipation, diarrhea	↓ Intestinal absorption of riboflavin, amino acids; ↑ urinary: riboflavin, calcium, magnesium, sodium, potassium, phosphate, chloride; anemia	Inhibits tubular reabsorption of uric acid	Take with food or milk; encourage fluids; avoid alcohol

Class of Drug	Trade Name	Gastrointestinal Side Effects	Other Nutritional Effects	Proposed Mechanism	Dietary Precautions
DRUGS AFFECTING THE CENTRAL NERVOUS SYSTEM (continued)					
Antiparkinson Agents					
Levodopa	Larodopa	Anorexia, nausea, vomiting, dry mouth, bitter taste, dysphagia, abdominal distress, GI bleeding, duodenal ulcer, constipation, diarrhea	↑ Need for ascorbic acid, B-6; ↓ absorption of tryptophan, phenylalanine, tyrosine; ↑ urinary: sodium, potassium; ↓ hemoglobin, hematocrit; hypertension; weight change	Inhibits normal metabolism of vitamin B-6 by forming drug–vitamin complexes and by inhibiting the pyridoxyl kinase enzyme	Take with foods; limit foods high in amino acids and those high in pyridoxine; avoid coffee; avoid vitamin supplements containing pyridoxine hydrochloride
Antituberculars					
Isoniazid	INH	Anorexia, nausea, vomiting, dry mouth, epigastric distress	↑ Urinary pyridoxine; ↓B-12 absorption, iron absorption; ↑ need for folic acid; ↓ absorption of vitamin E; possible pellagra symptoms; tyramine-type reactions with some food; hyperglycemia	Interferes with formation of pyridoxal phosphate; the latter combines with a hydrazine derivative and is excreted in urine as a complex	Take on empty stomach with water; avoid alcohol; prophylactic vitamin B-6 therapy; may need to avoid foods high in pressor amines
GASTROINTESTINAL AGENTS					
Antacids					
Nonsystemic aluminum hydroxide gel	Amphojel	Constipation	↓Absorption: vitamin A, D; inactivates: thiamin; phosphate depletion	Combines with food phosphates to form insoluble aluminum phosphate; retards phosphate absorption	Take with or immediately after meals; ensure adequate dietary phosphate intake (except in chronic renal disease)
Miscellaneous					
Cimetidine	Tagamet	Bitter taste, constipation, transient diarrhea, possible malabsorption		Binds to histamine receptors in the gastric mucosa, thereby inhibiting release of gastric acid	Take with food
Cathartics					
Mineral oil		Possible anorexia, flatulence, indigestion	Interferes with absorption of fat-soluble vitamins, carotene, calcium, phosphorus, potassium, and glucose; weight loss	Solubilizes nutrients; physical barrier to absorption	Take between meals or at bedtime without food
Bisacodyl	Dulcolax	Nausea, abdominal cramps, diarrhea, fluid and electrolyte losses	↓ Serum: potassium (prolonged use)	Acts directly on colonic mucosa to produce normal peristalsis throughout colon	Take on empty stomach with 8 oz water
Antidiarrheal Agents					
Systemic agents					
diphenoxylate hydrochloride with atropine	Lomotil	Anorexia, nausea, vomiting, abdominal cramps, dryness of mouth		Inhibits GI motility	Take with food; avoid alcohol

Class of Drug	Trade Name	Gastrointestinal Side Effects	Other Nutritional Effects	Proposed Mechanism	Dietary Precautions
HORMONES AND HORMONE ANTAGONISTS					
Adrenocortico-steroids					
Glucocorti-coids					
Cortisol			↑ Urinary excretion: ascorbic acid, calcium, potassium, zinc, nitrogen; inhibits protein synthesis; ↓ absorption: calcium, phosphate; ↑ need for ascorbic acid, B-6, folacin, vitamin D; ↓ serum: zinc; ↑ blood: glucose, triglycerides, cholesterol		Take with food; low-sodium, high-potassium diet; increase protein; caution against alcohol
Oral contra-ceptives		Nausea, vomiting, abdominal pain, constipation, diarrhea	↑ Need for B-6, ascorbic acid; ↓ serum: ascorbic acid, B-12, riboflavin, folate, pyridoxine, magnesium, zinc; edema; weight gain	May interfere with enzyme activity involved in conversion of folic acid to monoglu-tamate (absorb-able) form	Avoid foods high in sodium
MISCELLANEOUS					
Penicillamine	Cuprimine	Anorexia, nausea, vomiting, decreased taste acuity, diarrhea	↑ Requirement for pyridoxine; ↑ excretion: zinc, iron, copper, pyridoxine; possible iron-defi-ciency, anemia	Chelating agent	Increase fluid intake; Take 1 hour before or 3 hours after meals. Wilson's disease: avoid high copper foods; prophylactic vitamin B-6 therapy. Cystinuria: encourage high fluid intake especially at bedtime and during the night

APPENDIX C. SAMPLE FORM FOR A DIETARY HISTORY AND NUTRITIONAL ASSESSMENT

(NOTE: Health professionals should always extract as much of the needed data as possible from the medical record before interviewing the client.)

Personal Data

Name _____ Identification Number _____

Address _____ Telephone _____

_____ Sex _____ Age _____ Marital: S M W D

Ethnic Origin _____ Religion _____ Education (no. yrs) _____

Occupation _____ Hours of work _____ Travel time to work _____

Family: lives alone _____ lives with _____

Housing: Room _____ Apartment _____ Single House _____

Income: employment _____ public assistance _____ Food Stamps _____ S.S. _____ Other _____

Diagnosis

Anthropometric Data (see inside back cover for calculations and Appendix Tables A-7 to A-20 for standards)

Height: in _____ cm _____

   NCHS percentile (child) _____

Weight: lb _____ kg _____

   NCHS percentile (child) _____

Usual weight: lb _____ kg _____

Recent weight change: _____

   planned? _____

Body frame: S M L

Weight range for frame: _____

Triceps skinfold: mm _____ % std. _____

Arm circumference: mm _____ % std. _____

Arm muscle circumference: mm _____ % std. _____

Status: satisfactory _____

    over 20 percent underwt. _____

    over 20 percent overwt. _____

    over 10 percent unplanned change _____

Nutrition-Related Problems

Poor vision _____

Poor hearing _____

Change in appetite _____

Change in taste/smell _____

Chewing difficulty _____

Dysphagia _____

Nausea/vomiting _____

Heartburn _____

Diarrhea/constipation _____

Food allergy _____

Lactose intolerance _____

Food Profile

Meals at home/wk (no.) _____

Meals away/wk (no.) _____

   Which? _____

   Type facility? _____

Meals skipped: which? _____

   How often? _____

Snacks: how often? _____

Eating binges? _____

Modified diet? _____

   How long? _____

Supplements: Vitamin _____

   Mineral _____

   Other _____

Food preparation:

   Facilities: adequate _____ none _____

    hot plate _____ toaster/oven _____

    refrigerator _____

   Transportation to market? _____

   Who shops for food? _____

   Who prepares food? _____

Clinical Signs *(see Table 23–1, page 337)*

Hair _____

Skin _____

Eyes _____

Ears _____

Lips _____

Gums _____

Teeth _____

Nails _____

Posture _____

Muscles _____

Extremities _____

Other _____

Laboratory Data *(See Table A-27 for standards)*

Hemoglobin _____ g/dl

Hematocrit _____ percent

TIBC _____ μg/dl

Serum transferrin _____ mg/dl

Total lymphocytes _____ cu mm

Glucose _____ mg/dl

Total protein _____ g/dl

Serum albumin _____ g/dl

Blood urea nitrogen _____ mg/dl

Cholesterol _____ mg/dl

Triglycerides _____ mg/dl

Sodium _____ mg/dl

Potassium _____ mg/dl

Calcium _____ mg/dl

Phosphorus _____ mg/dl

Other _____

Lifestyle

Sleep: hours _____

Hobbies: _____

Exercise: kind _____

How often? _____

Activity level: bed _____ sedentary _____

moderately active _____ active _____

Smoking: _____ how much? _____

Drug/alcohol use _____

_____

Medications: prescribed _____

_____

over the counter _____

Summary

Twenty-Four-Hour Dietary Recall

Time: Where:	Time: Where:	Time: Where:
Snacks:	Snacks:	Snacks:

Food-Frequency List	Usual Serving Size	Number Times			Usual Serving Size	Number Times	
		Daily	Weekly			Daily	Weekly
Fruit: citrus or				Peanut butter			
vitamin-C rich				Dry beans, peas			
other				Nuts			
Vegetable: yellow				Fats: butter			
green leafy				reg. margarine			
potato				soft margarine			
other				salad dressings			
				cream			
Bread: enriched/				fried food			
whole grain				Sweets: sugar			
biscuits/muffins				jam, jelly, honey			
pastry/donuts				candy			
Breakfast cereal				cake, cookies			
cooked				pie, pastry			
dry, plain				Snacks: chips			
dry, sweetened				crackers			
Rice, pasta				pretzels			
				other			
Milk: Skim, 1%,				Beverages: water			
2%, whole				coffee/tea			
Ice cream				decaf.			
Cheese				soda, reg./diet			
Eggs				hard liquor			
Beef, pork, lamb				wine/beer			
Bacon, sausage							
Cold cuts, franks							
Fish							
Poultry							

Suggested Student Activities

1. Compare 24-hour recall with Daily Food Guide (page 30).
   Which food groups are supplied in adequate amounts?
   Which food groups are provided in inadequate amounts?
   What nutrients are likely to be in deficient supply?
2. Calculate the food values for the total number of exchanges in each category. For foods that do not appear in the Exchange Lists, look up the caloric, protein, fat, and carbohydrate values in Table A-1.

Exchange List	Number of Exchanges	C (g)	P (g)	F (g)	Energy (kcal)
Milk: whole					
nonfat					
Vegetables					
Fruit					
Bread					
Meat: low-fat					
medium-fat					
high-fat					
Fat					
Other foods (e.g., snacks, chips, alcohol)					
Total day's intake					

3. Calculate the Resting Metabolic Expenditure (see inside back cover). Compare with actual energy intake. See Problem 2.
4. Develop a problem list and plans to correct the problems identified.

Problem List	Goals	Plans to Achieve Goals

Common Abbreviations

AcCoA: acetyl coenzyme A
ACTH: adrenocorticotropic hormone
ADH: antidiuretic hormone
ADP: adenosine 5'-diphosphate
AFA: arm fat area
AMA: arm muscle area
AMP: adenosine 5'-phosphate
ATP: adenosine 5'-triphosphate
ATPase: adenosine triphosphatase

BEE: basal energy expenditure
BHA: butylated hydroxyanisole
BHT: butylated hydroxytoluene
bid: twice daily
BMR: basal metabolic rate
BUN: blood urea nitrogen
BV: biologic value

C: Celsius, centigrade
CAD: coronary artery disease
cc: cubic centimeter
CF: crude fiber
CHD: coronary heart disease
CHI: creatinine height index
cm: centimeter
CVA: cerebrovascular accident
CVD: cardiovascular disease

DES: diethylstilbesterol
DF: dietary fiber
dl: deciliter
DNA: deoxyribonucleic acid
DOPA: dioxy- or dihyroxyphenylalanine

EAA: essential amino acid
EFA: essential fatty acid
EPA: Environmental Protection Agency

F: fahrenheit
FAD: flavin adenine dinucleotide, oxidized form
FADH: flavin adenine dinucleotide, reduced form
FAO: Food and Agriculture Organization
FDA: Food and Drug Administration
FFA: free fatty acid
FMN: flavin mononucleotide
FSH: follicle-stimulating hormone
FTC: Federal Trade Commission

GFR: glomerular filtration rate
GI: gastrointestinal

g: gram(s)
GOT: glutamate oxalacetate transaminase
GRAS: generally recognized as safe
GTF: glucose tolerance factor

HANES: Health and Nutrition Examination Survey
Hb: hemoglobin
HbO_2: oxyhemoglobin
Hct: hematocrit
HDL: high-density lipoprotein
HHS: Health and Human Services, Department of
HMS: hexose monophosphate shunt
hs: at bedtime

IDDM: insulin-dependent diabetes mellitus
IF: intrinsic factor
IGT: impaired glucose tolerance
IHD: ischemic heart disease
INQ: index of nutritional quality
IU: international unit

J: joule

kcal: kilocalorie
kg: kilogram
kJ: kilojoule

lb: pound
LBW: low birth weight
LCT: long-chain triglyceride
LDL: low-density lipoprotein
LH: luteinizing hormone
LTT: lactose tolerance test

μg: microgram
MAC: midarm circumference
MAMC: midarm muscle circumference
MAO: monoamine oxidase
MCT: medium-chain triglyceride
mEq: milliequivalent
mg: milligram(s)
ml: milliliter(s)
mm: millimeter(s)
MRFIT: Multiple Risk Factor Intervention Trial
mRNA: messenger ribonucleic acid
MSG: monosodium glutamate
MSUD: maple syrup urine disease

NAD: nicotinamide adenine dinucleotide
NADP: nicotinamide adenine dinucleotide phosphate

NAS: National Academy of Science
NE: niacin equivalent
NEFA: nonesterified fatty acid
NFCS: National Food Consumption Survey
ng: nanogram(s)
NIDDM: noninsulin-dependent diabetes mellitus
NPN: nonprotein nitrogen
npo: nothing by mouth
NPU: net protein utilization
NRC: National Research Council

OGTT: oral glucose tolerance test
oz: ounce

PABA: para-amino benzoic acid
PBI: protein-bound iodine
pc: after meals
PCBs: polychlorinated biphenyls
PEM: protein-energy malnutrition
PER: protein efficiency ratio
pg: picogram(s)
pH: hydrogen ion concentration
PKU: phenylketonuria
POMR: problem-oriented medical record
ppm: parts per million
P : S: polyunsaturated to saturated fatty acid ratio
PTH: parathyroid hormone
PUFA: polyunsaturated fatty acid

qid: four times daily

RDA: Recommended Dietary Allowances
RE: retinol equivalent
RNA: ribonucleic acid

RNase: ribonuclease
RQ: respiratory quotient

SDA: specific dynamic action
SGA: small for gestational age
SGOT: serum glutamate oxalacetate transaminase
SGPT: serum glutamate pyruvate transaminase
SOAP: subjective, objective, assessment, plan
SSS: subscapular skinfold

tbsp: tablespoon
TCA: tricarboxylic acid cycle
alpha-TE: alpha-tocopherol equivalent
TIBC: total iron-binding capacity
tid: three times daily
TPN: total parenteral nutrition
TPP: thiamin pyrophosphate
tRNA: transfer ribonucleic acid
TSF: triceps skinfold
TSH: thyroid-stimulating hormone
tsp: teaspoon

UNESCO: United Nations Educational, Scientific and Cultural Organization
UNICEF: United Nations Children's Fund
USDA: United States Department of Agriculture
USHHS: United States Department of Health and Human Services
USP: United States Pharmacopoeia
USRDA: United States Recommended Dietary Allowances

VLDL: very-low-density lipoproteins

WHO: World Health Organization
WIC: Women, Infants and Children Nutrition Program

Glossary

acetoacetic acid (as'et-o-as-e'tik): a 4-carbon keto acid; one of the acetone bodies in diabetic urine

acetone (as'et-ōn): dimethyl ketone; accumulates in the blood and excretions when fats are incompletely oxidized as in diabetes mellitus; gives fruity odor to the breath

acetylcholine (as'et-il-kō'lēn): an acetic acid ester of choline; involved in nerve transmission, and other important physiologic functions

acetyl coenzyme A (as'et-il co-en'zīm): condensation product of acetic acid and coenzyme A; form by which 2-carbon fragment enters the tricarboxylic acid cycle

achlorhydria (a-klor-hi'drī-ah): absence of hydrochloric acid in gastric juice

acid: a substance that gives off or donates protons (H^+ ions)

acidosis (as-īd-o'sis): condition caused by accumulation of an excess of acids (anions) in the body, or by excessive loss of base (mineral cations) from the body

active transport: the movement of substances across cell membranes by pumping against a concentration gradient; requires source of energy

adenine (ad'en-in): one of the purines (bases) that are constituents of nucleic acid

adenosine triphosphate (ad-en'o-sin tri-fos'fāt): a compound consisting of 1 molecule each of adenine and ribose and 3 molecules of phosphoric acid; two of the phosphate groups are held by high-energy bonds; ATP

adipose (ad'ip-ōs): fat; fatty

aerobic (a-er-o'-bik): living in presence of air

albumin(al-bu'min): a protein in tissues and body fluids soluble in water and coagulated by heat; principal protein in blood regulating osmotic pressure; lactalbumin of milk

aldehyde (al'de-hīd): any of a large group of compounds containing the grouping -CHO

aldosterone (al-dos'ter-ōn): a steroid hormone produced by the adrenal cortex; increases sodium retention and potassium loss

alkalosis (al-kah-lo'sis): increased alkali reserve (blood bicarbonate) of the blood and other body fluids; caused by excessive ingestion of sodium bicarbonate, persistent vomiting, or hyperventilation; pH of blood is usually increased

allergen (al'ler-jen): substance (usually protein) capable of producing altered response of cell, resulting in manifestation of allergy

amino acid (am-īn'-o as'id): an organic acid containing an amino (NH_2) group; the building blocks of protein molecules

amylase (am'ilās): salivary or pancreatic enzyme that hydrolyzes starch; ptyalin, amylopsin

amylopectin (am'il-o-pek'tin): polysaccharide found in starch consisting of branched chains of glucose

amylose (am'il-ōs): polysaccharide of starch consisting of unbranched chains of glucose

anabolism (an-ab'oh-lizm): processes for building complex substances from simple substances

anaerobic (an-aer-oh'bik): living in the absence of oxygen

androgen (an'dro-jen): a substance such as testosterone that produces male sex characteristics

anemia (an-e'me-ah): deficiency in the circulating hemoglobin, red blood cells, or packed cell volume

anion (an'i-on): an ion that contains a negative charge of electricity and therefore goes to a positively charged anode

anorexia (an-o-rek'se-ah): loss of appetite

anthropometry (an-thro-pom'et-re): branch of anthropology dealing with comparative measurements of the parts of the human body

anti-: a prefix meaning against or opposing; e.g., antiscorbutic means preventing scurvy

antibiotic (an'ti-bi-ot'ik): a substance that inhibits the growth of bacteria

antibody (an'te-bod-e): a protein substance produced in an organism as a response to the presence of an antigen

antigen (an'ti-jen): any substance such as bacteria or foreign protein that, as a result of contact with tissues of the animal body, produces an immune response; an increased reaction such as hypersensitivity may result

antiketogenesis (an-ti-ke-tō-jen'es-is): the prevention of ketosis by stimulating the tricarboxylic acid cycle and thus bringing about oxidation of the ketone bodies

antimetabolite (an-ti-met-ab'-o-līt): a substance that interferes with the activity of a metabolite

antioxidant (an-te-ok'sid-ant): a substance that prevents deterioration by hindering oxidation, e.g., tocopherols prevent oxidation and rancidity of fats

antivitamin (an-ti-vi'tah-min): a substance similar in structure to a vitamin that interferes with the activity of that vitamin

anuria (au-u're-ah): lack of urinary secretion

apathy (ap'ath-e): indifference; lack of interest or concern

apatite (ap'ah-tīt): complex calcium phosphate salt giving strength to bones

apoenzyme (ap-o-en'zīm): the protein part of an enzyme

arabinose (ar-ab'in-ose): a 5-carbon sugar found in fruits and root vegetables

arachidonic acid (ar-ak-id-on'ik): a 20-carbon fatty acid with four double bonds; the physiologically functioning essential fatty acid

arginase (ar'jin-ās): enzyme that splits arginine to urea and ornithine

arginine (ar'jin-in): a diamino acid; required for growth but not required by adults

arteriosclerosis (ar-te-re-o-skle-ro'sis): thickening and hardening of the inner walls of the arteries

ascites (a-si'tēz): accumulation of fluid in the abdominal cavity

ascorbic acid (a-skor'bik): water soluble vitamin required for collagenous intercellular substance; prevents scurvy; also known as vitamin C

-ase: suffix that is used in naming an enzyme; for example, peptidase

aspartame (a'spar-tām): a dipeptide of phenylalanine and aspartic acid; used as artificial sweetener

asymptomatic (a-sim-tō-mat'ik): without symptoms

ataxia (a-tak'se-ah): loss of ability of muscular coordination

atherosclerosis (ath-er-o-skle-ro'sis): thickening of the walls of blood vessels by deposits of fatty materials, including cholesterol

atony (at'o-ne): a lack of normal tone or strength

atrophy (at'ro-fe): a wasting away of cell, tissue, or organ

autosome (aw'tō-sōm): any chromosome other than a sex chromosome

avidin (av'id-in): protein substance in raw egg white which binds biotin and prevents its absorption from the digestive tract

azotemia (a-zo-te'me-ah): elevated levels of nitrogenous constituents in the blood; uremia

basal metabolism (ba'zal me-tab'o-lizm): energy expenditure of the body at rest in the postabsorptive state

base (bās): substance that combines with an acid to form a salt; any molecule or ion that will add on a hydrogen ion

beikost (bī-koost): foods given to the infant at weaning

benign (bi-nīn'): mild nature of an illness; with reference to a neoplasm, not malignant

beriberi (ber'ē-ber'ē): a deficiency disease caused by lack of thiamin and characterized by extreme weakness, polyneuritis, emaciation, edema, and cardiac failure

beta-hydroxybutyric acid (ba-tah-hi-drox'e-bu-tir'-ik): a 4-carbon intermediate in oxidation of fatty acids; one of the acetone bodies excreted in the urine in uncontrolled diabetes

bio- (bi-o-): prefix denoting life

bioassay (bi'-o-as-say): testing of activity or potency, as of a vitamin or hormone, on an animal or microorganism

biologic value: a measure of the effectiveness of a nutrient, such as protein, in the living organism

biopsy (bi'op-sē): examination of a piece of tissue removed from a living subject

biotin (bi'o-tin): a vitamin of the B complex; participates in fixation of carbon dioxide in fatty acid synthesis

Bitot's spots (be'tōz): gray, shiny spots on the conjunctiva resulting from malnutrition, especially vitamin A deficiency

botulism (bot'u-lizm): frequently fatal poisoning caused by toxin produced in inadequately sterilized canned food by the *Clostridium botulinum*

buffer (buf'er): a mixture of an acid and its conjugate base that is capable of neutralizing either an acid or a base without appreciably changing the original acidity or alkalinity, e.g., H_2CO_3/HCO_3-

cachexia (kah-kek'si-ah): general lack of nutrition and wasting

calciferol (kal-sif'er-ol): vitamin D_2, fat-soluble vitamin of plant origin formed by irradiation of ergosterol; prevents rickets

calcification (kal-sif-ik-a'shun): hardening of tissue by a deposit of calcium and also magnesium salts

calcitonin (kal-sit-oh'-nin): hormone secreted by the thyroid gland; hypocalcemic effect; opposes action of parathormone

calculus (kal'ku-lus): an abnormal concretion occurring in any part of the body; usually consists of mineral salts around an organic nucleus

calorie (kal'o-rē): a unit of heat measurement; in nutrition, the kilocalorie is the amount of heat required to raise the temperature of 1 kg water 1°C

calorimetry (kal-or-im'et-rē): measurement of heat produced by the body, or from a food; *direct*: measure of heat produced by a subject in a closed chamber; *indirect*: measurement of heat by determining consumption of oxygen and sometimes carbon dioxide and calculating the amount of heat produced

carbonic acid (kar-bon'ik): the acid formed when carbon dioxide is dissolved in water; H_2CO_3

carboxylase (kar-bok'sil-ās): a thiamin-containing enzyme that catalyzes the removal of the carboxyl group of alpha keto acids, e.g., decarboxylation of pyruvic acid

carboxypeptidase (kar-box-e-pep'tid-ās): an intestinal enzyme that catalyzes the splitting of peptides

carcinogen (kar-sin'-o-gen): a substance that causes cancer

carotene (kar'o-tēn): precursor of vitamin A; yellow plant pigments occurring abundantly in dark green leafy and deep yellow vegetables

casein (ka'se-in): principal protein in milk; a phosphoprotein

catabolism (kat-ab'o-lizm): process for breaking down complex substances to simpler substances; usually yields energy

catalyst (kat'ah-list): a substance that in minute amounts initiates or modifies the speed of a chemical or physical change without itself being changed

catecholamine (kat'e-kol'-am-in): any of a group of compounds that are functionally related, such as epinephrine, norepinephrine, and dopamine

cation (kat'i-on): an ion that carries a positive charge and migrates to the negatively charged pole

cell-mediated immunity: thymus-dependent lymphocytes (T cells) comprise a major defense against mycobacteria, viruses, and fungi

cellulose (sel'u-lōs): the structural fibers of plants; an indigestible polysaccharide

cephalin (sef'al-in): a phospholipid in brain and nervous tissue

ceruloplasmin (ser-ul'o-plaz-min): copper-containing protein in blood plasma

cheilosis (ki-lo'sis): lesions of the lips and the angles of the mouth; characteristic of riboflavin deficiency

chelation (ke-la′shun): formation of a bond between a metal ion and two or more polar groupings of a single molecule

cholecalciferol (ko-le-kal-sif′er-ol): vitamin D_3 formed from 7-dehydrocholesterol

cholecystitis (ko-le-sis-ti′tis): inflammation of the gallbladder

cholecystokinin (ko-le-sis-tō-kin′in): hormone produced in duodenum in presence of fat; stimulates contraction of gallbladder and release of bile

cholelithiasis (ko-le-lith-i′a-sis): gallstones in the gallbladder

cholesterol (ko-les′ter-ol): a sterol found in animal foods and made within the body; a constituent of gallstones and of atheroma

choline (ko′lēn): a nitrogenous base that donates methyl groups; a component of lecithin and acetylcholine

chondroitin sulfate (kon-droi′tin): a mucopolysaccharide widely distributed in skin and cartilage

chylomicrons (ki′lo-mi′krons): large molecules of fat occurring in lymph and plasma after a fat-rich meal; consist of triglycerides attached to a small amount of protein

citric acid (sit′rik): an organic acid containing three carboxyl groups; one of compounds in the Krebs or citric acid cycle; a constituent of citrus fruits

Clostridium (klos-trid′i-um): a genus of bacteria, chiefly anaerobic, found in soils and in the intestinal tract, e.g., *botulinum*, *perfringens*

coagulation (ko-ag-u-la′shun): process of clot formation, as in heating of an egg, curdling of milk

cobalamine (ko-bal′ah-min): compound containing cobalt grouping found in vitamin B-12

cocarboxylase (ko-kar-box′il-ās): thiamin-containing coenzyme of carboxylase

coenzyme (ko-en′zīm): prosthetic group of an enzyme; for example, a vitamin, that conjugates with a protein molecule to form an active enzyme

coenzyme A: a complex nucleotide containing pantothenic acid; combines with acetyl groups to yield active acetate that can enter the Krebs cycle; involved in fatty acid oxidation and synthesis and cholesterol synthesis

colitis (ko-li′tis): inflammation of the colon

collagen (kol′aj-in): protein matrix of bone, cartilage, and connective tissue

colloid (kol′oid): matter dispersed through another medium; particles are larger than crystalline molecules but not large enough to settle out; do not pass through an animal membrane

colostrum (ko-los′trum): milk secreted during the first few days after the birth of a baby

coma (ko′mah): state of unconsciousness

complement system: a system of protein fractions that interact and are involved in several defenses against viruses, inactivation of endotoxins, bacteriolysis, and lysis of virus-infected cells

complementarity: the ability of one substance to supply a missing substance in another; e.g., one food supplies amino acids lacking in another, thus providing a "complete" amino acid mixture

congenital (kon-jen′it-al): existing at or before birth with reference to certain physical or mental traits

coronary (kor′o-na-re): like a crown; related to blood vessels supplied to the heart muscle

cortex (kor′tex): outer layers of an organ, e.g., adrenal cortex

cortisone (kor′ti-sōn): hormone of the adrenal cortex; influences carbohydrate metabolism

creatine (kre′at-in): a nitrogenous constituent essential for muscle contraction

creatinine (kre-at′in-in): a nitrogen-containing substance derived from catabolism of creatine and present in the urine

cretinism (kre′tin-izm): severe thyroid deficiency resulting in mental retardation; usually congenital

crude fiber: plant fiber that remains after sample has been treated with sulfuric acid and sodium hydroxide; chiefly cellulose and lignin

cryptoxanthine (kript-o-zan′thin): a yellow pigment present in some foods; precursor of vitamin A

-cyte: suffix meaning cell; for example, adipocyte

cytochrome (si′tō-krom): a respiratory enzyme; consists of a number of hemochromogens; undergoes alternate reduction and oxidation

cytoplasm (si′to-plazm): substance within the cell exclusive of the nucleus

cytosine (si′to-sin): one of the nitrogenous bases in nucleic acid

deamination (de-am-in-a′shun): removal of the amino (NH_2) group from an amino acid

dehydrocholesterol, 7- (de-hi-dro-ko-les′ter-ol): cholesterol derivative in the skin that is converted to vitamin D

dehydrogenases (de-hi-dro′jen-ās-es): enzymes that catalyze oxidation by transferring hydrogen to a hydrogen acceptor

denaturation (de-na-tur-a′shun): the alteration of the natural properties of a substance by physical or chemical means; e.g., heat coagulation of protein

deoxyribonucleic acid (DNA) (de-ok′se-ri-bo-nu-kla′ik): giant molecule in cell nucleus that determines hereditary traits; consists of four bases attached to ribose and phosphate

dermatitis (der-mat-i′tis): inflammation of the surface of the skin

dextrin (dex′trin): intermediate product in breakdown of starches; a polysaccharide

dicoumarin (di-koo′mah-rin): antiprothrombin; anticlotting factor first isolated from sweet clover

dietary fiber: plant fibers that include cellulose, hemicelluloses, lignin, mucilages and gums, and pectin

diffuse (dif-us′): not localized

diffusion: the movement of particles from an area of higher concentration to one of lower concentration

diglyceride (di-glis′er-id): a fat containing 2 fatty acid molecules

disaccharidase (di-sak′ar-id-ās): enzyme which hydrolyzes disaccharides

disaccharide (di-sak′ar-id): a carbohydrate that yields two simple sugars upon hydrolysis; sucrose, maltose, lactose

distal (dis′tal): part of structure farthest from the point of attachment

diuresis (di-u-re′sis): increased secretion of urine

diverticulum (di-ver-tik′u-lum): a pouch opening from a tubular organ such as the colon

duodenum (du-o-de′num): first portion of the small intestine, extending from the pylorus to the jejunum

dynamic equilibrium: tendency to maintain equilibrium of normal body states

dys-: prefix meaning bad, painful, or difficult

dysgeusia (dis-goo'se-ah): perverted sense of taste; "bad" taste

dysosmia (dis-ahs'-me-ah): impaired sense of smell; obnoxious odor

dyspepsia (dis-pep'se-ah): indigestion or upset stomach

dysphagia (dis-fa'je-ah): difficulty in swallowing

dyspnea (disp'ne-ah): difficulty or distress in breathing

eclampsia (ĕ-klamp'se-ah): convulsions occurring during pregnancy and associated with edema, hypertension, and proteinuria

edema (ĕ-de'mah): presence of abnormal amounts of fluid in intercellular spaces

elastin (ĕ-las'tin): insoluble yellow elastic protein in connective tissue

electrolyte (el-ek'tro-lit): any substance which dissociates into ions when dissolved and thus conducts an electric current

emaciation (e-ma-se-a'shun): wasting of the body; excessive leanness

-emia: suffix that denotes a condition of the blood; for example, hypoglycemia

emulsion (e-mul'shun): a system of two immiscible liquids in which one is finely divided and held in suspension by another

endemic (en-dem'-ik): prevalence of a disease in a given region

endo-: prefix meaning inner or within

endocrine (en'do-krin): pertaining to glands that secrete substances into the blood for control of metabolic processes

endogenous (en-doj'en-us): originating in the cells or tissues of the body

endoplasmic reticulum (en'do-plaz-mik ret-ic'u-lum): the system of membranes within the cell that permits communication between cellular, nuclear, and extracellular environment

endosperm (en'do-sperm): reserve food material of the plant; the starch center of the cereal grain

enrichment: the addition of thiamin, riboflavin, niacin, and iron to refined cereal products

enter-: combining term denoting intestine

enteritis (en-ter-i'tis): inflammation of the intestine

enterocrinin (en-ter-o-kri'nin): hormone of small intestine that stimulates secretion of intestinal juice

enterogastrone (en-ter-o-as'trōn): hormone secreted by duodenal mucosa upon stimulation by fat; inhibits secretion of gastric juice and reduces motility

enterohepatic cycle (en-ter-o-hep-at'ik): the circulation of bile from the liver to the gallbladder to the intestine and back to the liver

enterokinase (en-ter-o-kīn'ās): enzyme of intestinal juice that converts trypsinogen to trypsin

enteropathy (en-ter-op'ath-e): any disease of the intestine

enzyme (en'zīm): an organic compound of protein nature produced by living tissue to accelerate metabolic reactions; hydrolases, oxidases, transferases, dehydrogenases, peptidases, and others

epidemiology (ep-i-dem'-e-ol-o-ji): the science of epidemic diseases; factors that influence frequency and distribution of disease

epinephrine (ep-in-ef'rin): secretion of the medulla of the adrenal gland that stimulates energy metabolism; adrenaline

epithelium (ep-ith-e'le-um): the covering layer of the skin and mucous membranes

ergogenic (er'go-jen'ik): tendency to increase work; often referred to foods that are mistakenly believed to have special energy-producing effects

ergosterol (er-gos'ter-ol): a sterol found chiefly in plants; when exposed to ultraviolet light becomes vitamin D

erythrocyte (er-ith'ro-sīt): mature red blood cell

erythropoiesis (er-ith-ro-po-e'sis): formation of red blood cells

essential amino acid: an amino acid that must be supplied in the diet

essential fatty acid: a fatty acid that must be present in the diet; linoleic acid, arachidonic acid

estrogen (es'tro-jen): hormone secreted by the ovary

etiology (e-te-ol'o-je): cause of a disease

exacerbation (ex-as-er-ba'shun): increase in severity of symptoms

exocrine (eks'o-krin): pertaining to a gland that secretes outwardly; opposed to endocrine

exogenous (ex-oj'en-us): originating or produced from the outside

extracellular (extra-sel'u-lar): situated or occurring outside the cells

exudate (ex'u-dāt): a fluid discharged into the tissues or any cavity

familial (fam-il'e-al): common to a family

fatty acids (fat'e): open-chain monocarboxylic acids containing only carbon, hydrogen, and oxygen

favism (fa'vism): condition caused by eating certain species of beans, e.g., *Vicia fava*

febrile (feb'ril): feverish; having a fever

ferritin (fer'it-in): water-soluble storage form of iron in the body; composed of protein (apoferritin) and colloidal ferric iron

fibrosis (fi-bro'sis): formation of fibrous tissue in repair processes

fistula (fis'tu-lah): a tubelike ulcer leading from an abscess cavity or organ to the surface, or from one abscess cavity to another

flatulence (flat'u-lens): distention of stomach or intestines with gases

flavin adenine dinucleotide, FAD (fla'vin ad'en-in di-nu'kle-o-tīd): a coenzyme consisting of riboflavin and adenosine diphosphate required for the action of various dehydrogenases

flavin mononucleotide, FMN (fla'vin mon-o-nu'kle-o-tīd): a riboflavin-containing coenzyme involved in the action of dehydrogenases

flavoprotein (fla-vo-pro'te-in): a conjugated protein that contains a flavin and is involved in tissue respiration

fluoridation (floo-or-id-a'shun): the addition of fluoride to water to reduce tooth decay

fluorosis (floo-o-ro'sis): mottling of teeth because of excess ingestion of fluoride

folacin (fo'lah-sin): folic acid, a vitamin of the B complex

folic acid (fo'lik): a vitamin of the B complex necessary for the maturation of red blood cells and synthesis of nucleo-proteins; also known as folacin and pteroylglutamic acid

follicle (fol'ikl): small excretory sac or gland, e.g., hair follicle, ovarian follicle

fortification (for-ti-fik-a'shun): the addition of one or more nutrients to a food to make it richer than the unprocessed food, e.g., vitamin D milk

fructose (fruk'tōs): a 6-carbon sugar found in fruits and honey; also obtained from the hydrolysis of sucrose; fruit sugar; levulose

galactose (gal-ak'tos): a single sugar resulting from the hydrolysis of lactose

galactosemia (gal-ak'tō-se'me-ah): accumulation of galactose in the blood owing to a hereditary lack of an enzyme to convert galactose to glucose; accompanied by severe mental retardation

gastrectomy (gas-trek'tō-me): surgical removal of part or all of the stomach

gastrin (gas'trin): hormone secreted by pyloric mucosa that stimulates secretion of hydrochloric acid by parietal cells

gene (jēn): the functional unit of heredity carried by a chromosome

genetic (jen-et'ik): congenital or inherited

-genic: suffix meaning to produce or give rise to; for example, ketogenic

geriatric (je-rĭ-at'rik): pertaining to the science of old age

gingivitis (jin-jĭ-vi'tis): inflammation of the gums

gliadin (gli'ad-in): a protein fraction of wheat gluten

globulin (glob'u-lin): a class of proteins insoluble in water and alcohol; serum globulin, lactoglobulin, myosin

glomerulus (glom-er'u-lus): the tuft of capillaries at the beginning of each tubule in the kidney

glossitis (glos-i'tis): inflammation of the tongue

glucagon (gloo'kag-on): hormone produced by the alpha cells of the islets of Langerhans; raises blood sugar by increasing glycogen breakdown

glucocorticoid (glu-ko-kor'-tĭ-koid): hormone produced by the adrenal cortex that influences glucose metabolism

glucogenic (glu-ko-jen'ik): glucose forming

gluconeogenesis (glu'ko-ne-o-jen'e-sis): formation of glucose from noncarbohydrate sources, namely, certain amino acids and glycerol

glucose (glu'kōs): a single sugar occurring in fruits and honey; also obtained by the hydrolysis of starch, sucrose, maltose, and lactose; the sugar found in the blood; dextrose; grape sugar

glutathione (glu-ta-thi'ōn): a tripeptide of glycine, glutamic acid, and cystine; can act as hydrogen acceptor and hydrogen donor

gluten (glu'ten): protein in wheat and other cereals that gives elastic quality to a dough

glyceride (glis'er-id): organic ester of glycerol; fats are esters of fatty acids and glycerol

glycerol (glis'er-ol): a 3-carbon alcohol derived from the hydrolysis of fats

glycogen (gli'ko-jen): polysaccharide produced from glucose by the liver or the muscle; "animal" starch

glycogen loading: a dietary-exercise regimen to increase muscle storage of glycogen; low-carbohydrate intake plus heavy exercise for several days followed by a high-carbohydrate diet and minimal exercise.

glycogenesis (gli'ko-jen-ĭ-sis): formation of glycogen from glucose by the liver or muscle

glycogenolysis (gli-ko-jen-ol'ĭ-sis): enzymatic breakdown of glycogen to glucose

glycolysis (gli-kol'ĭ-sis): the anaerobic conversion of glucose to pyruvic and lactic acids, an energy-yielding process

glycosuria (gli-ko-su're-ah): presence of sugar in the urine

goiter (goi'ter): enlargement of the thyroid gland

goitrogen (goi'tro-jen): a substance that leads to goiter

guanine (gwan'in): one of the nitrogenous bases in nucleic acids

hem-, hema-, hemo-: prefixes referring to blood

hematocrit (he-mat'o-krit): separation of red cells from the plasma

hematuria (he-mat-u're-ah): condition in which urine contains blood

heme (hēm): deep red pigment consisting of ferrous iron linked to protoporphyrin

heme iron: form of iron in hemoglobin and in myoglobin that is absorbed intact

hemicellulose (hem-i-sel'u-los): indigestible polysaccharides that form the cell wall of plants

hemochromatosis (hem-o-kro-ma-to'sis): a condition in which excessive iron absorption leads to skin pigmentation and deposits of hemosiderin in the liver and other organs

hemoglobin (he-mo-glo'bin): the iron–protein pigment in the red blood cells; carries oxygen to the tissues

hemolytic (he-mo-lit'ik): causing separation of hemoglobin from the red blood cells

hemopoietic, hematopoietic (he-mo-poi-et'ik): concerned with the formation of blood

hemorrhage (hem'or-ej): loss of blood from the vessels; bleeding

hemosiderin (he'mo-sid'er-in): water-insoluble storage form of iron in the body

heparin (hep'ar-in): a mucopolysaccharide that prevents clotting of blood

hepatic (hep-at'ik): pertaining to the liver

hepatomegaly (hep-at-o-meg'ah-le): enlargement of the liver

heterozygous (het-er-o-zi'gus): possessing dissimilar pairs of genes for any hereditary trait

hexose (heks'ōs): a 6-carbon sugar; glucose, fructose, galactose

histidine (his'tid-in): an essential amino acid

homeostasis (ho-me-o-sta'sis): tendency to maintain equilibrium in normal body states

homozygous (ho-mo-zi'gus): having identical pairs of genes for any given pair of hereditary traits

hormone (hor'mōn): substance produced by an organ to produce a specific effect in another organ

hospice (hos'pis): a home for the sick; a program of integrated services for the terminally ill

humoral immunity (hu'mor-al im-mu'nit-e): thymus-independent lymphocytes (B cells) that produce immunoglobulins: IgG, IgM, IgA, IgD, and IgE

hydrogenation (hi'dro-jen-a'shun): the addition of hydrogen to a compound, such as an unsaturated fatty acid to produce a solid fat

hydrolysate (hi-drol'is-āt): the product of hydrolysis; e.g., protein hydrolysate is a mixture of the constituent amino acids when the protein molecule is split by acids, alkalies, or enzymes

hydrolysis (hi-drol′is-is): the splitting up of a product by the addition of water

hydroxyapatite (hī-drok′sē-ap′a tīt): a naturally occurring mineral crystal containing calcium, phosphorus, hydrogen, and oxygen

hyper-: a prefix meaning above, beyond, or excessive

hypercalcemia (hi-per-kal-se′me-ah): abnormally high calcium level in the blood

hypercalciuria (hi-per-kal-se-u′re-ah): abnormal calcium excretion in the urine

hyperchlorhydria (hi-per-klor-hi′dre-ah): increased hydrochloric acid secretion by stomach cells

hyperchromic (hi-per-krōm′ik): abnormally high color

hyperemia (hy-per-e′me-ah): excess of blood in any part of the body

hyperesthesia (hi-per-es-the′zī-ah): increased sensitivity to touch or pain

hyperglycemia (hi-per-glī-se′me-ah): an excess of sugar in the blood

hyperkalemia (hi-per-kah-le′me-ah): an increased level of potassium in the blood

hyperkinesis (hi-per-kin-e′sis): one of a group of terms used to describe disruptive, inattentive, and other behavioral problems in children

hyperlipoproteinemia (hi-per-li-po-pro-te-ne′me-ah): increased concentration of lipoproteins in the blood

hypernatremia (hi-per-na-tre′me-ah): increased level of sodium in the blood

hyperphagia (hi-per-fay′je-ah): increased appetite; overeating

hyperplasia (hi-per-pla′se-ah): abnormal multiplication of normal cells

hypertension (hi-per-ten′shun): elevated blood pressure

hypertriglyceridemia (hi-per-tri-glis-er-id-e′me-ah): increased blood levels of triglycerides

hypertrophic (hi-per-tro′fik): pertaining to enlargement of an organ due to increase in size of its constituent cells

hyperuricemia (hi-per-u-ris-e′me-ah): excess of uric acid in the blood as in gout

hypervitaminosis (hi-per-vi-tah-min-o′sis): condition produced by excessive ingestion of vitamins, especially vitamins A and D

hypo-: prefix meaning lack or deficiency

hypoalbuminemia (hi-po-al-bu-min-e′me-ah): low albumin level of the blood

hypocalcemia (hi-po-kal-se′me-ah): blood calcium level below normal

hypochlorhydria (hi-po-klor-hid′re-ah): decreased secretion of hydrochloric acid by the cells of the stomach

hypochromic (hi-po-krom′ik): below normal color; e.g., pale red blood cells lacking hemoglobin

hypogeusia: diminished sense of taste

hypoglycemia (hi-po-gli-se′me-ah): a lower than normal level of glucose in the blood

hypokalemia (hi-po-kal-e′me-ah): decreased potassium level in the blood

hyposmia (hi-pos′mi-ah): diminished sense of smell

hypothalamus (hi-po-thal′am-us): a group of nuclei at the base of the brain; includes centers of appetite control, cells that produce antidiuretic hormone

iatrogenic (i-at′ro-jen′ik): relating to an abnormal condition in a patient resulting from inadvertent or erroneous treatment by a physician

idiopathic (id-e-o-path′ik): pertaining to a disease of unknown origin

idiosyncrasy (id-e-o-sin′kra-se): a susceptibility to action of food or drugs that is characteristic or peculiar to an individual person

ileum (il′e-um): lower portion of the small intestine extending from the jejunum to the cecum

ileus (il′e-us): obstruction of the bowel

infarction (in-fark′shun): the formation of an area of dead tissue resulting from obstruction of blood vessels supplying the part

inositol (in-os′it-ol): a 6-carbon alcohol found especially in cereal grains; combines with phosphate to form phytic acid

insulin (in′su-lin): hormone secreted by beta cells of the islets of Langerhans; promotes utilization of glucose and lowers blood sugar

interstitial (in-ter-stish′-al): situated in spaces between tissues

intra-: prefix meaning within

intracellular (in-trah-sel′u-lar): within the cell

intravenous (in-trah-ve′nus): into or from within a vein

intrinsic factor (in-trin′sik): mucoprotein in gastric juice that facilitates absorption of vitamin B-12

iodopsin (i-o-dop′sin): pigment found in cones of the retina; visual violet

ion (i′on): an atom or group of atoms carrying a charge of electricity; e.g., cations, anions

ionize (i′on-īz): to separate molecules into electrically charged atoms or group of atoms; the number of negative charges exactly equals the number of positive charges

ischemia (is-ke′me-ah): a local deficiency of blood, chiefly from narrowing of the arteries

isocaloric (i-sō-kal-or′ik): containing an equal number of calories

isoleucine (i-sō-lu′sin): an essential amino acid

isotypes (i′so-tōps): atoms of the same element having the same atomic numbers and chemical properties but differing in the nuclear masses

-itis: suffix denoting inflammation; for example, colitis

jaundice (jon′dis): condition characterized by elevated bilirubin level of the blood and deposit of bile pigments in skin and mucous membranes

jejunum (je-joo′num): middle portion of small intestine; extends from duodenum to ileum

joule (jool): the unit of energy in the metric system; 1 calorie equals 4.184 joules (J)

keratin (ker′at-in): an insoluble sulfur-containing protein found in the skin, nails, hair

keratomalacia (ker′at-o-mal-a′shah): dryness and ulceration of the cornea resulting from vitamin A deficiency

keto-: a prefix denoting the presence of the carbonyl (CO) group

ketogenesis (ke-to-jen′es-is): formation of ketones from fatty acids and some amino acids

alpha-ketoglutaric acid (ke-tō-gloo-tar′ik): one of the intermediates in the tricarboxylic acid cycle; also the product of oxidative deamination of glutamic acid

ketone (ke'tōn): any compound containing a ketone (CO) grouping

ketosis (ke-tō'sis): condition resulting from incomplete oxidation of fatty acids, and the consequent accumulation of ketones, acetone, beta-hydroxybutyric acid, and acetoacetic acid

kilocalorie (kil'o-ka'lo-re): the unit of heat used in nutrition; the amount of heat required to raise 1,000 g water 1°C (from 15.5 to 16.5°C); also known as the large calorie

Krebs cycle: the cycle through which acetyl coenzyme A is oxidized to produce ATP; also known as tricarboxylic acid cycle and citric acid cycle

kwashiorkor (kwash-e-or'kor): deficiency disease related principally to protein lack and seen in severely malnourished children

labile (la'bil): chemically unstable

lactalbumin (lak-tal-bu'min): a protein in milk

lactic acid (lak'tik): 3-carbon acid produced in milk by bacterial fermentation of lactose; also produced during muscle contraction by anaerobic glycolysis

lactose (lak'tōs): a disaccharide composed of glucose and galactose; milk sugar

lamina propria (lam'in-ah pro'pre-ah): connective-tissue structure that supports the epithelial cells of the intestinal mucosa

lecithin (les'ith-in): a phospholipid occurring in nervous and organ tissues, and in egg yolk

leucine (lu'sin): an essential amino acid

lignin (lig'nin): woody part of plants; a noncarbohydrate component of dietary fiber

limiting amino acid: that amino acid that is in shortest supply in relationship to synthetic needs and therefore limits synthesis

linoleic acid (lin-o-le'ic): an 18-carbon essential fatty acid with two double bonds

linolenic acid (lin-o-len'ik): an 18-carbon fatty acid with three double bonds; not essential

lipase (lip'ās): an enzyme that hydrolyzes fat

lipid (lip'id): a term for fats including neutral fats, oils, fatty acids, phospholipids, cholesterol

lipogenesis (lip-o-jen'es-is): formation of fat

lipolysis (lip-ol'is-is): the splitting of fat

lipoprotein (li-po-pro'te-in): a conjugated protein that incorporates lipids to facilitate transportation of the lipids in an aqueous medium

lipotropic (lip-o-trop'ik): pertaining to substances that prevent accumulation of fat in the liver

lithiasis (li-thi'a-sis): the formation of calculi of any kind

low-density lipoproteins: complexes of triglycerides, cholesterol, and phospholipids with proteins in the blood

lutein (lu'te-in): an orange pigment; internal secretion of the ovary which, with ovulin and folliculin, constitutes the hormone oophorin

lymphocytes (lim'fo-sites): white blood cells—B cells and T cells

lysine (li'sēn): a diamino essential amino acid

lysosomes (li'so-sōms): structures of cell cytoplasm that contain digestive enzymes

macrocyte (mak'ro-sīt): an abnormally large red blood cell

malaise (mal-āz'): discomfort, distress, or uneasiness

malignant (mal-ig'nant): occurring in severe form, frequently fatal; in tumors refers to uncontrollable growth as in cancer

maltose (mawl'tōs): a disaccharide resulting from starch hydrolysis; yields 2 molecules glucose on further hydrolysis

marasmus (mar-az'mus): extreme protein-calorie malnutrition marked by emaciation, especially severe in young children

matrix (ma'trix): the groundwork in which something is cast; for example, protein is the bone matrix into which mineral salts are deposited

megaloblast (meg'al-o-blast): primitive red blood cell of large size with large nucleus

menadione (men-a-di'on): synthetic compound with vitamin K activity

metabolic pool (met-ah-bol'ik): the assortment of nutrients available at any given moment of time for the metabolic activities of the body, e.g., amino acid pool, calcium pool

metabolism (me-tab'o-lism): physical and chemical changes occurring within the organism; includes synthesis of biologic materials and breakdown of substances to yield energy

metabolite (me-tab'oh-līt): any substance that results from physical and chemical changes within the organism

metastasis (met-ass'tah-sis): shifting of disease from one part of the body to another; in cancer, the location of tumors away from the primary tumor

methionine (meth-i'o-nin): an essential sulfur-containing amino acid

micelle (mis-el'): a microscopic particle of lipids and bile salts

microcyte (mi'kro-sīt): small red blood cell

microvilli (mi'kro-vil'li): minute structures visible by electron microscope, present on surface of mucosal epithelium; the "brush border"

milliequivalent, mEq (mil'li-e-kwiv'ah-lent): concentration of a substance per liter of solution; obtained by dividing the milligrams per liter by the equivalent weight

mitochondria (mit-o-kon'dre-ah): rod-shaped or round structures in cell that trap energy-rich ATP

monosaccharide (mon-o-sak'ar-id): a single sugar not affected by hydrolysis; includes glucose, fructose, galactose

monounsaturated (mon-o-un-sat'u-ra-ted): having a single double bond as in a fatty acid, e.g., oleic acid

morbidity (mor-bid'it-e): the proportion of disease to health in a community

motility (mo-til'it-e): ability to move spontaneously

mucin (mu'sin): a substance containing mucopolysaccharides secreted by goblet cells of the intestine and other glandular cells; has a protective and lubricating action

mucopolysaccharide (mu'ko-pol-e-sak'er-id): any of a group of polysaccharides combined with other groups such as protein

mucoprotein (mu'ko-pro'te-in): a conjugated protein containing a carbohydrate group such as chondroitin sulfate

mucosa (mu-ko'sah): membrane lining the gastrointestinal, respiratory, and genitourinary tracts

mycotoxin (my-ko-tok'sin): toxins produced by molds that grow on grains and nuts

myelin (my'el-in): lipid–protein complex surrounding nerve fibers

myo-: prefix meaning muscle

myocardium (mi-o-kar'de-um): the heart muscle

myoglobin (mi-o-glo'bin): an iron-protein complex in muscle that transports oxygen; somewhat similar to hemoglobin

myosin (mi'o-sin): a soluble protein in muscle; combines with actin to form actomyosin, an enzyme that catalyzes the dephosphorylation of ATP during muscle contraction

necrosis (ne-kro'sis): death of a cell or cells or of a portion of tissue

neonatal (ne-o-na'tal): pertaining to the newborn

neoplasm (ne'o-plasm): new or abnormal, uncontrolled growth, such as a tumor

nephron (nef'fron): the functional unit of the kidney consisting of the tuft of capillaries known as the glomerulus attached to the renal tubule

neuropathy (nu-rop'ath-e): disease of the nervous system

neurotransmitter (nu'ro-trans-mit-er): a chemical substance that relays nerve impulses, thus enabling cells to communicate; dopamine, norepinephrine, serotonin

niacin (ni'ah-sin): a water-soluble B-complex vitamin required for cell respiration; antipellagra factor

niacin equivalent: the total niacin available from the diet including preformed niacin plus that derived from the metabolism of tryptophan; 60 mg tryptophan = 1 mg niacin

nicotinic acid: niacin

nitrosamine (ni-tros'am-in): a compound formed in the stomach when nitrate combines with an amine; a carcinogen

nocturia (nok-tu're-ah): excessive urination at night

nonheme iron: the form of iron not associated with hemoglobin or myoglobin; iron in plant foods, eggs, dairy products; also some of iron in meat products

norepinephrine (nor-ep-in-ef'rin): a neurotramsmitter derived from tyrosine; also a vasoconstrictor

nucleic acid (nu-kle'ik): complex organic acid containing four bases—adenine, guanine, cytosine, and thymine—attached to ribose and phosphate

nucleoprotein (nu-kle-o-pro'te-in): conjugated protein found in the nuclei of cells; yields a protein fraction and nucleic acid

nucleotide (nu'kle-o-tid): a hydrolytic product of nucleic acid; contains one purine or pyrimidine base and a sugar phosphate

nutrient (nu'tre-ent): chemical substance in foods which nourishes, e.g., amino acid, fat, calcium

nutrient density: the ratio of the nutritive value of a food or diet to its caloric contribution

nyctalopia (nik-tal-o'pe-ah): night blindness

oleic acid (o-le'ik): an 18-carbon fatty acid containing one double bond

oliguria (ol-ig-u're-ah): scanty secretion of urine

-ology: suffix meaning science of, study of

ophthalmia (of-thal'me-ah): inflammation of the eye

opsin (op'sin): the protein portion of the light sensitive pigment (rhodopsin) of the eye

osmolality (os-mo-lal'it-e): the number of molecules and ionic particles per kg of solution

osmosis (oz-mo'sis): the passage of a solvent from the lesser to the greater concentration when two solutions are separated by a membrane

ossification (os-if-ik-a'shun): formation of bone

osteo-: prefix meaning bone

osteoblast (os'te-o-blast): bone-forming cell

osteoclast: large cell formed in bone marrow that is involved in absorption and removal of osseous tissue

osteomalacia (os-te-o-mal-a'se-ah): softening of the bone, chiefly in adults

osteoporosis (os-te-o-po-ro'sis:) reduction of the quantity of bone, occurring principally in women after middle age

-otomy: suffix meaning to cut into, e.g., lobotomy, phlebotomy

oxalic acid (oks-al'ik): a dicarboxylic acid present in foods such as spinach, chard, rhubarb; forms insoluble salts with calcium

oxaloacetic acid (oks-al-o-as-e'tik): a 3-carbon ketodicarboxylic acid; an intermediate in the tricarboxylic acid cycle

oxidation (oks-id-a'shun): increase in positive charges on an atom or loss of negative charges

oxytocin (oks'e-to-sin): hormone of posterior pituitary that promotes uterine contraction and milk-releasing action

palmitic acid (pal-mit'ik): a 16-carbon fatty acid widespread in foods

pancreozymin (pan'kre-o-zi'min): hormone produced in duodenal mucosa that stimulates secretion of pancreatic enzymes

pantothenic acid (pan-to-then'ik): one of the B-complex vitamins

parathormone (par-at-hor-mōn): secretion of parathyroid gland that regulates calcium and phosphorus metabolism

parenchyma (par-en'ki-mah): functional tissue of an organ or gland as distinct from its supporting framework

parenteral (par-en'ter-al): by means other than through the gastrointestinal tract; nutrients by vein or into subcutaneous tissues

paresthesia (par-es-the'zi-ah): abnormal sensation such as numbness, burning, prickling

parturition (par-tu-rish'un): giving birth to a child

path-, patho-, pathy: combining forms meaning disease, e.g., *patho*genic, nephro*pathy*

pathology (path-ol'o-je): science dealing with disease; structural and functional changes caused by disease

pectin pek'tin): a polysaccharide found in many fruits and having gelling properties

pellagra (pel-lah'gra): a deficiency disease of the skin, gastrointestinal tract, and nervous system caused by lack of niacin

pentose (pen'tōs): a simple sugar containing 5 carbon atoms; ribose, arabinose, xylose

peptide linkage (pep'tid): the CO-NH linkage of two amino acids by condensation of the amino group of one amino acid with the carboxyl group of another amino acid

peptone (pep'ton): an intermediate product of protein digestion

perinatal (per-ī-na'tal): pertaining to before, during, or after the time of birth

periodontal (pe-re-o-don'tal): around a tooth

peristalsis (per-is-tal'sis): the rhythmic, wavelike movement produced by muscles of the small intestine to move food forward

phagocyte (fag'o-sīt): a cell capable of ingesting bacteria for other foreign material

phenylalanine (fen-il-al'ah-nin): an essential amino acid

phenylketonuria (fe-nil-ke-to-nu're-ah): excretion of phenylpyruvic acid and other phenyl compounds in urine because of congenital lack of an enzyme required for conversion of phenylalanine to tyrosine

phospholipid (fos'fo-lip'id): a fatlike compound that contains a phosphate and another group such as a nitrogen base in addition to glycerol and fatty acids, e.g., lecithin, cephalin

phosphoprotein (fos-fo-pro'te-in): a conjugated protein that contains phosphorus, e.g., nucleoprotein, casein

phosphorylate (fos-fo'ril-ate): to introduce a phosphate grouping into an organic compound, e.g., glucose monophosphate produced by action of enzyme *phosphorylase*

photosynthesis (fo-to-sin'the-sis): the process whereby the chlorophyll in green plants utilizes the energy from the sun to synthesize carbohydrate from carbon dioxide and water

phytic acid (fi'tik): a phosphoric acid ester of inositol found in seeds; interferes with absorption of calcium, magnesium, iron, zinc

pica (pi'kah): a hunger for substances not fit for food

pinocytosis (pin-o-si-to'sis): the taking up of droplets (e.g., fat) by a cell by surrounding the liquid with part of the membrane

plaque (plak): any patch or flat area; atherosclerotic plaque is a deposit of lipid material in the blood vessel

plasma (plaz'mah): fluid portion of the blood before clotting has taken place

poly-: prefix meaning much or many

polyneuritis (pol-e-nu-ri'tis): inflammation of a number of nerves

polypeptide (pol-e-pep'tid): a compound consisting of more than three amino acids; an intermediate stage in protein digestion

polyphagia (pol-e-fa'je-ah): excessive eating

polysaccharide (pol-e-sak'ar-id): a class of carbohydrates containing many single sugars; includes starch, glycogen, dextrins, pectins, cellulose, and others.

polyunsaturated fatty acid: fatty acids containing two or more double bonds; linoleic, linolenic, and arachidonic acids

porphyrin (por'fir-in): a pigmented compound containing four pyrrole nuclei joined in a ring structure; combines with iron in hemoglobin

postprandial (post-pran'de-al): after a meal

prealbumin (pre-al-bu'min): a thyroxine linking plasma protein with a high tryptophan content

precursor: anything that precedes another or from which another is derived; for example, carotene is a precursor to vitamin A

preeclampsia (pre'eh-klamp'se-ah): toxemia of late pregnancy; albuminuria, edema, and hypertension

prenatal (pre-na'tal): preceding birth

progesterone (pro-jes'ter-on): hormone of corpus luteum that prepares endometrium for reception and development of the fertilized ovum

prognosis (prog-no'sis): forecast of probable results from attack of disease

prolactin (pro-lak'tin): hormone of the anterior lobe of the hypophysis that stimulates milk secretion

prophylaxis (pro-fil-ak'sis): prevention of disease

prostaglandins (pros-tah-glan'dins): a group of hormones derived from polyunsaturated fatty acids and produced by a number of organs; alter transmission of nerve cells; modify response to other hormones

prosthetic group (pros-thet'ik): chemical group attached to a molecule such as protein; non-protein part of an enzyme

protease (pro'te-as): an enzyme that digests protein

protein efficiency ratio: a measure of the quality of a protein by calculating the weight gain of an experimental animal per gram of protein fed

proteinuria (pro'te-in-u'ri-ah): excretion of protein in the urine

proteolytic (pro'te-o-lit'ik): effecting the hydrolysis of protein

prothrombin (pro-throm'bin): factor in blood plasma for blood clotting; precursor of thrombin

protoplasm (pro'to-plazm): form of living matter in all cells

provitamin (pro-vi'tah-min): precursor of a vitamin

proximal (prok'sim-al): nearest to the head or point of attachment

pteroylglutamic acid (ter'o-il-glu-tam'ik): folic acid

puerperium (pur-pe'ri-um): the period after labor until involution of the uterus

purine (pur'in): organic compounds containing heterocyclic nitrogen structures that are catabolized to uric acid; supplied especially by flesh foods and synthesized in the body

pyridoxal phosphate (pir-i-dok'sal fos'fate): a coenzyme that contains vitamin B-6

pyridoxine (pi-ri-dox'in): one of the forms of vitamin B-6

pyruvic acid (pi-ru'vik): a 3-carbon ketoacid; an intermediate in glucose metabolism

regurgitation (re-gur-jit-a'shun): the backward flow of food; casting up of undigested food

relapsing (re-laps'ing): return of symptoms

remission (re-mish'un): a lessening of the severity or temporary abatement of symptoms

renal (re'nal): pertaining to the kidney

renal threshold: the level of concentration of a substance in the blood beyond which it is excreted in the urine

renin: enzyme produced by the kidney; pressor substance

rennin (ren'in): enzyme in gastric juice that coagulates milk protein

repletion (rep-le'shun): to fill up; to restore

resection (re-sek'shun): removal of part of an organ

residue (rez'i-du): remainder; the contents remaining in the intestinal tract after digestion of food; includes fiber and other unabsorbed products

resorption (re-sorp'shun): a loss of substance, e.g., loss of mineral salts from bone

reticulocyte (re-tik'u-lo-sit): a young red blood cell occurring during active blood regeneration

reticuloendothelium (re-tik'u-lo-en-do-the'le-um): a system of macrophages concerned with phagocytosis; present in spleen, liver, bone marrow, connective tissues, and lymph nodes

retinal, retinene (ret'in-al): vitamin A aldehyde

retinol (ret'in-ol): vitamin A alcohol

retinol equivalent: a measure of the total vitamin A activity; includes vitamin A and the activity available from the carotenes

retinopathy (ret-in-op'ath-e): degenerative disease of the retina

rhodopsin (ro-dop′sin): visual purple; pigment of the rods of the retina bleached by light; vitamin A required for regeneration

riboflavin (ri′bo-fla′vin): heat-stable B-complex vitamin and a constituent of flavin enzymes; vitamin B-2

ribonucleic acid, RNA (ri-bo-nu-kle′ik): molecules in cytoplasm which serve for transfer of amino acid code from nucleus and the synthesis of protein

ribose (ri′bōs): 5-carbon sugar; a constituent of nucleic acid

ribosomes (ri′bo-sōms): dense particles in cell cytoplasm that are the site of protein synthesis

rickets (rik′ets): a deficiency disease of the skeletal system caused by a lack of vitamin D or calcium or both, and often resulting in bone deformities

risk factor: a factor related to a disease but not necessarily a cause

saccharin (sak′ah-rin): a noncaloric sweetener that is 300 to 500 times as sweet as sugar

Salmonella (sal-mon-nel′ah): group of bacteria causing intestinal infection; frequently contaminates foods

saponification (sap-on′if-ik-a′shun): the action of alkali on a fat to form a soap

satiety (sat-i′et-e): feeling of satisfaction following meals

saturated (sat′u-ra-ted): a state in which a substance holds the most of another substance that it can

scurvy (skur′vē): a deficiency disease caused by lack of ascorbic acid and leading to swollen bleeding gums, hemorrhages of the skin and mucous membranes, and anemia

secretin (se′-kre-tin): a hormone secreted by the epithelium of the duodenum upon stimulation by the acid chyme; stimulates secretion of pancreatic juice and bile

sepsis (sep′sis): disease producing organisms or toxins in the blood or tissues

serotonin (ser-o-to′nin): a neurotransmitter with a structure similar to tryptophan

serum (se′rum): the fluid portion of the blood that separates from the blood cells after clotting

siderophilin (sid′er-o-fil′in): an iron-transferring protein; transferrin

somatic (so′mat′ik): refers to the frame or trunk of the body

somatostatin (so-mat′o-stat′in): a hormone that inhibits the release of glucagon from the pancreas

sorbitol (sor′bit-ol): a 6-carbon sugar alcohol with a sweet taste; used commercially to maintain moisture and inhibit crystal formation

sphincter (sfink′ter): a muscle surrounding and closing an orifice

sphingomyelin (sfing-go-mi′el-in): a phospholipid found in the brain, spinal cord, and kidney

stachyose (stack′e-ose): a polysaccharide found in some tubers and plant foods

staphylococcus (staf′il-o-kok′es): group of bacteria that produce heat-resistant toxins, a common cause of food poisoning

stasis (sta′sis): retardation or cessation of flow of blood in the vessels; congestion

steapsin (ste-ap′sin): a hormone in pancreatic juice that hydrolyzes fat; lipase

stearic acid (ste′rik): a saturated fatty acid containing 18 carbon atoms

steatorrhea (ste-at-o-re′ah): excessive amount of fat in the feces

stenosis (sten-o′sis): narrowing of a passage

steroid (ster′oid): a group of compounds similar in structure to cholesterol; includes bile acids, sterols, sex hormones

sterol (ste′rol): an alcohol of high molecular weight; cholesterol, ergosterol

stomatitis (sto-ma-ti′tis): inflammation of the mucous membranes of the mouth

sub-: prefix denoting beneath, or less than normal

substrate (sub′strat): substance upon which an enzyme acts

succinic acid (suk-sen′ik): a 3-carbon dicarboxylic acid that is an intermediate in the tricarboxylic acid cycle

sucrose (su′krōs): cane or beet sugar; a disaccharide that yields glucose and fructose when hydrolyzed

syn-: prefix meaning with, together

syndrome (sin′drōm): a set of symptoms occurring together

synergism (sin′er-jizm): the joint action of agents which when taken together increases each other's effectiveness

synthesis (sin′thes-is): process of building up a compound

systemic (sis-tem′ik): pertaining to the body as a whole

tachycardia (tak-e-kar′de-ah): rapid beating of the heart

testosterone (tes-tos′ter-ōn): testicular hormone responsible for male secondary sex characteristics

tetany (tet′an-e): a condition marked by intermittent muscular contraction accompanied by fibrillar tremors and muscular pains; seen in hypocalcemia, alkalosis

thiamin (thi′am-in): a B-complex vitamin; with phosphate forms coenzymes of decarboxylases; essential for carbohydrate metabolism

thio-: prefix meaning sulfur-containing

threonine (thre′o-nin): an essential amino acid

thrombus (throm′bus): a clot in a blood vessel formed by coagulation of blood

thymine (thi′min): one of the four nitrogenous bases in nucleic acid

thyroxine (thī-rok′sin): iodine-containing hormone produced by the thyroid gland; regulates the rate of energy metabolism

tocopherol (tok-of′er-ōl): vitamin E; antioxidant alcohol occurring in vegetable germ oils; alpha-, beta-, gamma-, delta-tocopherol

tox-: prefix meaning poison

toxemia of pregnancy (tok-se′me-ah): a disorder of pregnancy characterized by hypertension, edema, albuminuria

transamination (trans′am-in-a′shun): transfer of an amino group to another molecule, e.g., transfer to a keto acid, thus forming another amino acid

transferase (trans′fer-ās): an enzyme that transfers a chemical grouping from one compound to another, for example, transaminase, transphosphorylase

transferrin (trans-fer′in): iron-binding protein for transport of iron in blood; siderophilin

trauma (traw-mah): wound or injury usually inflicted suddenly

trichinosis (trik-in-o′sis): illness caused by eating raw pork that is infested by *Trichinella spiralis*, a worm

triglyceride (tri-glis′er-id): an ester of glycerol and three fatty acids

trypsin (trip′sin): a protein-digesting enzyme secreted by the pancreas and released into the small intestine

tryptophan (trip′tōfan): an essential amino acid that contains the indole ring

tyramine (tir'am-en): a pressor amine that has an action similar to epinephrine; reproduced by decarboxylation of tyrosine; found especially in cheeses and some wines

tyrosine (ti'ro-sin): semiessential amino acid; spares phenylalanine; the amino acid in thyroxine

urea (u-re'ah): chief nitrogenous constituent of the urine; formed by the liver when amino acids are deaminated

uremia (u-re'me-ah): presence of urinary constituents in the blood resulting from deficient secretion of urine

uric acid (u-rik): a nitrogenous constituent formed in the metabolism of purines; excreted in the urine; blood levels increased in gout

valine (va'lin): an essential amino acid

vegan (ve-gan): one who excludes all animal foods from his or her diet

vegetarian: one who excludes one or more classes of animal foods from his or her diet; thus, vegans, lactovegetarian, lacto-ovo-vegetarian

villus (vil'us): fingerlike projection of the intestinal mucosa

viosterol (vi-os'ter-ol): vitamin D formed by irradiation of ergosterol

visceral (vis'er-al): relating to the organs

visual purple: photosensitive pigment found in the rods of the retina; rhodopsin

vitamin (vi'tah-min): organic compound occurring in minute amounts in foods and essential for numerous metabolic reactions; fat-soluble A, D, E, and K; water-soluble ascorbic acid and B complex including thiamin, riboflavin, niacin, pantothenic acid, biotin, vitamin B-6, vitamin B-12, folacin, and others

xanthine (zan'thin): an intermediate in the metabolism of purines; related to uric acid

xanthomatosis (zan-thō-mat-o'sis): accumulation of lipids in the form of tumors in various parts of the body

xerophthalmia (zer-of-thal'me-ah): dry infected eye condition caused by lack of vitamin A

xerosis (ze-ro'sis): abnormal dryness of skin and eye

xylose (zi'los): a 5-carbon aldehyde sugar that is not metabolized by the body

zein (za'in): a protein of low biologic value present in corn

zymogen (zi'mo-jen): the inactive form of an enzyme

Index

Tables are indicated by the letter "t." Illustrations are indicated in **bold face** type. Footnotes are indicated by the letter "n."

Criteria for Nutritional Assessment

Anthropometric Measurements

Body Frame—see Table A–15, page 681
Weight for body frame and height—see Table A–16, page 682
Weight for height, percentiles—see Table A–17, A–18

$$\text{Body Mass Index (BMI)} = \frac{\text{Weight, kg}}{\text{Height}^2,\ \text{m}}$$

Desirable BMI: males, 20–25; females, 19–24
Triceps skinfold (TSF)—see Table A–19, page 685
Subscapular skinfold (SSS)—see Table A–20, page 686
Sum of TSF and SSS—see Table A–21, page 686
Arm circumference and arm muscle circumference—see Table A–22, page 687
Arm muscle area—see Table A–23, page 689
Arm fat area—see Table A–24, page 689

$$\text{Creatinine Height Index (CHI)} = \frac{\text{Measured Urinary Creatinine}}{\text{Ideal Urinary Creatinine}} \times 100$$

Ideal Urinary Creatinine Values

Men*		Women†	
Height (cm)	Ideal Creatinine (mg)	Height (cm)	Ideal Creatinine (mg)
157.5	1288	147.3	830
160.0	1325	149.9	851
162.6	1359	152.4	875
165.1	1386	154.9	900
167.6	1426	157.5	925
170.2	1467	160.6	949
172.7	1513	162.6	977
175.3	1555	165.1	1006
177.8	1596	167.6	1044
180.3	1642	170.2	1076
182.9	1691	172.7	1109
185.4	1739	175.3	1141
188.0	1785	177.8	1174
190.5	1831	180.3	1206
193.0	1891	182.9	1240

* Creatinine coefficient (men) = 23 mg/kg of ideal body weight.

† Creatinine coefficient (women) = 18 mg/kg of ideal body weight.

$$\text{Nitrogen Balance} = \frac{\text{Protein Intake}}{6.25} - (\text{Urinary Urea Nitrogen} + 4)$$

Immune Status

$$\text{Total Lymphocyte Count (TLC)} = \frac{\%\ \text{Lymphocytes} \times \text{W.B.C.}}{100}$$